SURGERY

Official Publication

SOCIETY OF UNIVERSITY SURGEONS

SOCIETY FOR VASCULAR SURGERY

Volume 76

July—December, 1974

THE C. V. MOSBY COMPANY
St. Louis

VOLUME 76

Printed in the United States of America

Volume 76 *Number* 1

SURGERY

CONTENTS, JULY, 1974

SOCIETY OF UNIVERSITY SURGEONS

page 1 **Myonecrosis in chronic experimental vasospasm.** John F. Alksne, M.D., *San Diego, Calif.*

8 **Contraction of experimental wounds. I. Inhibiting wound contraction by using a topical smooth muscle antagonist.** John W. Madden, M.D., Duncan Morton, Jr., M.D., *and* Erle E. Peacock, Jr., M.D., *Tucson, Ariz.*

16 **Radioimmunoassay for mouse mammary tumor virus–associated antigen.** P. Lo Gerfo, M.D., G. Silverstein, *New York, N. Y., and* J. Charney, *Camden, N. J.*

23 **Immune cytolysis of human tumor cells mediated by xenogeneic "immune" RNA: Implications for immunotherapy.** Yosef H. Pilch, M.D., Larry L. Veltman, M.D., *and* David H. Kern, Ph.D., *Los Angeles, Calif.*

continued on page 7

Vol. 76, No. 1, July, 1974, SURGERY is published monthly by The C. V. Mosby Company, 11830 Westline Industrial Drive, St. Louis, Mo. 63141.

Annual subscription rates.

	U. S.	*Canada, Mexico*	*Other countries*
Institutional*	$29.00	$32.00	$32.75
Personal†	$21.00	$24.00	$24.75
Student, intern, resident†	$14.70	$17.70	$18.45

Single copies are $3.50 postpaid. Remittances should be made by check, draft, post office or express money order, payable to this Journal.

*Institutional (multiple-reader) subscriptions are available to public and private libraries, schools, hospitals, and clinics; city, county, state, provincial, and national government bureaus and departments; and all commercial and private institutions and organizations.
†Personal subscriptions and all student-rate subscriptions must be in the names of, billed to, and paid by individuals. All student-rate requests must indicate training status and name of institution.

Subscriptions may begin at any time.

Second class postage paid at St. Louis, Mo. Printed in the U. S. A.

CONTENTS *continued*

page 35 **An immunosuppressive peptide fraction in the serum of cancer patients.** A. H. Glasgow, M.D., J. O. Menzoian, M.D., R. B. Nimberg, D.M.D., S. R. Cooperband, M.D., K. Schmid, Ph.D., *and* J. A. Mannick, M.D., *Boston, Mass.*

43 **Distinction of allogeneic immunity from tumor-specific immunity in man.** Leon C. Parks, M.D., William J. Smith, *and* G. Melville Williams, M.D., *Baltimore, Md.*

50 **Immune surveillance and tumor dissemination: In vitro comparison of the B_{16} melanoma in primary and metastatic form.** Leonard I. Goldman, M.D., B. A. Flaxman, M.D., *Philadelphia, Pa.,* G. Wernick, B.S., *and* J. B. Zabriskie, M.D., *New York, N. Y.*

57 **Pulmonary vascular impedance in chronic pulmonary hypertension.** Ronald C. Elkins, M.D., Marvin D. Peyton, M.D., *and* Lazar J. Greenfield, M.D., *Oklahoma City, Okla.*

65 **Airway resistance regulation of dynamic compliance.** John F. Neville, Jr., M.D., Jeffrey Askanazi, Peter B. Kane, M.D., *and* Watts R. Webb, M.D., *Syracuse, N. Y.*

72 **Mechanisms of oxygen inhibition of pulmonary surfactant synthesis.** Helena Gilder, M.D., *and* Charles K. McSherry, M.D., *New York, N. Y.*

80 **Effect of immunosuppression and lung transplantation upon surfactant.** John A. Drews, M.D., Donald F. Tierney, M.D., *and* John R. Benfield, M.D., *Los Angeles, Calif.*

88 **Immunologic injury induced by ex vivo perfusion of canine renal autografts.** R. S. Filo, Commander (MC) USNR, L. G. Dickson, Captain (MC) USN, E. A. Suba, *and* K. W. Sell, Captain (MC) USN, *Bethesda, Md.*

101 **The kidney cell crossmatch in retransplantation.** James C. Pierce, M.D., Ph.D., *and* Hyung M. Lee, M.D., *Richmond, Va.*

112 **Passive enhancement of canine renal allografts with polyspecific $F(ab')_2$ fragments.** Simon F. G. Wren, M.D., Antonio C. P. Martins, M.D., Ulrich Von Haefen, M.D., George J. Busch, M.D., Gordon E. Katske, M.D., Thomas L. Koppenheffer, Ph.D., Thongdee Shaipanich, M.D., *and* Richard E. Wilson, M.D., *Boston, Mass.*

continued on page 9

CONTENTS *continued*

page 121 **Renal allograft prolongation using phytomitogens to mask graft antigens.** Luis A. Toledo-Pereyra, M.D., Prasanta K. Ray, Ph.D., Clive O. Callender, M.D., John S. Najarian, M.D., *and* Richard L. Simmons, M.D., *Minneapolis, Minn.*

129 **Functional characterization of blocking antibody after human renal transplantation.** Joshua Miller, M.D., Judith Lifton, Faye Rood, George Kyriakides, M.D., Kazimiera Y. Gajl-Peczalska, M.D., Edmond J. Yunis, M.D., *and* Brack G. Hattler, Jr., M.D., *Minneapolis, Minn., and Tucson, Ariz.*

142 **Tolerance to myocardial tissue allografts by pretreatment with cross-reactive streptococcal membrane antigen.** Robert J. Ellis, M.D., John B. Zabriskie, M.D., *and* Paul A. Ebert, M.D., *New York, N. Y.*

150 **Prolongation of rat cardiac allograft survival by a new immunosuppressant: Chicken anti–rat lymphocyte globulin.** R. E. Morris, B.A., S. G. Souther, M.D., E. Dong, Jr., M.D., L. M. Vistnes, M.D., *and* N. E. Shumway, M.D., *Stanford, Calif.*

160 **Effects of pulmonary embolism on regional myocardial blood flow.** H. Newland Oldham, Jr., M.D., Jimmy L. Cox, M.D., Harvey I. Pass, B.A., Andrew S. Wechsler, M.D., *and* David C. Sabiston, Jr., M.D., *Durham, N. C.*

170 **The training of surgeons: How many, in what, and by whom? Panel discussion.** Leonard D. Miller, M.D., *Philadelphia, Pa.,* William B. Saxbe, Jr., M.D., M.P.H., *Boston, Mass.,* Edward F. X. Hughes, M.D., M.P.H., *New York, N. Y.,* Richard M. Bergland, M.D., *Hershey, Pa.,* James A. O'Neill, Jr., M.D., *Nashville, Tenn.,* Mark M. Ravitch, M.D., *Pittsburgh, Pa.,* Bruce Barton, M.S., *Pittsburgh, Pa.,* Frank C. Spencer, M.D., *New York, N. Y., and* Francis D. Moore, M.D., *Boston, Mass.*

Volume 76 *Number* 2

SURGERY

CONTENTS, AUGUST, 1974

EDITORIALS

page 199 **Too many surgeons?** Claude E. Welch, M.D., *Boston, Mass.*

202 **A computer logic program in the operating room.** Mark M. Ravitch, M.D., *Pittsburgh, Pa.*

ORIGINAL COMMUNICATIONS

204 **Boris Petrov, great Russian surgeon, and the Sklifosovsky Institute of Emergency Surgery.** Owen H. Wangensteen, M.D., *Minneapolis, Minn.*

209 **The current status of vena caval replacement.** J. P. Scherck, M.D., M. D. Kerstein, M.D., *and* H. C. Stansel, Jr., M.D., *New Haven, Conn.*

234 **Long-term results of hepatic portoenterostomy for biliary atresia: Special reference to postoperative portal hypertension.** Masahiko Miyata, M.D., Minoru Satani, M.D., Takashi Ueda, M.D., *and* Eizo Okamoto, M.D., *Osaka, Japan*

continued on page 7

Vol. 76, No. 2, August, 1974, SURGERY is published monthly by The C. V. Mosby Company, 11830 Westline Industrial Drive, St. Louis, Mo. 63141.

Annual subscription rates.

	U. S.	*Canada, Mexico*	*Other countries*
Institutional*	$29.00	$32.00	$32.75
Personal†	$21.00	$24.00	$24.75
Student, intern, resident†	$14.70	$17.70	$18.45

Single copies are $3.50 postpaid. Remittances should be made by check, draft, post office or express money order, payable to this Journal.

*Institutional (multiple-reader) subscriptions are available to public and private libraries, schools, hospitals, and clinics; city, county, state, provincial, and national government bureaus and departments; and all commercial and private institutions and organizations.
†Personal subscriptions and all student-rate subscriptions must be in the names of, billed to, and paid by individuals. All student-rate requests must indicate training status and name of institution.

Subscriptions may begin at any time.

Second class postage paid at St. Louis, Mo. Printed in the U. S. A.

CONTENTS *continued*

page 238 **Attitudes of British graduates on surgical research fellowships in the United States.** Michael J. Knight, F.R.C.S., *London, England, and* Ceri M. Griffiths, F.R.C.S.(C), *Galveston, Texas*

243 **Changes and trends in graduate medical education and credentialling.** J. W. Humphreys, Jr., M.D., *Philadelphia, Pa.*

252 **The fate of kidney transplants from donors with minor renal abnormalities.** Panayiotis K. Spanos, M.D., Richard L. Simmons, M.D., Luca C. Rattazzi, M.D., Marvin E. Goldberg, M.D., *and* John S. Najarian, M.D., *Minneapolis, Minn.*

259 **Adjuncts to the abdominal wall reconstruction following extensive cancer surgery.** Tomoo Tajima, M.D., *and* John C. McDonald, M.D., *New Orleans, La.*

263 **Proteolysis of preformed protein in wound nutrition.** H. Paul Ehrlich, Ph.D., Harold Tarver, Ph.D., *and* Thomas K. Hunt, M.D., *San Francisco, Calif.*

267 **Rabbit anti–rat lymphocyte serum-induced lymphopenia in thoracic duct lymph and peripheral blood.** Roland Girardet, Eli A. Friedman, *and* Karl E. Karlson, *Brooklyn, N. Y.*

272 **Effect of single dose irradiation on isolated perfused canine kidney.** G. H. Malek, M.D., M. J. S. Richards, M.D., P. M. Burkholder, M.D., *and* W. L. Caldwell, M.D., *Madison, Wis.*

278 **Effect of complete parenteral nutrition including fat emulsion on plasma lipid.** Yoshiko Koga, M.D., Keiichi Ikeda, M.D., *and* Kiyoshi Inokuchi, M.D., D.Sc., *Fukuoka, Japan*

286 **Thrombosis in the superior mesenteric and portal veins: Report of a case treated with thrombectomy.** Sven-Erik Bergentz, M.D., Björn Ericsson, M.D., Ulla Hedner, M.D., Lennart Leandoer, M.D., *and* Inga Marie Nilsson, M.D., *Malmö, Sweden*

291 **Control of capillary bleeding by topical application of microcrystalline collagen.** Lars M. Vistnes, M.D., David A. Goodwin, M.D., *Palo Alto, Calif.,* John H. Tenery, M.D., *Fort Worth, Texas,* George A. Ksander, M.S., *and* Ronald P. Gruber, M.D., *Palo Alto, Calif.*

295 **Effect of aspirin on microaggregate formation in banked blood.** Paul J. Arrington, M.S., *and* J. Judson McNamara, M.D., *Honolulu, Hawaii*

continued on page 9

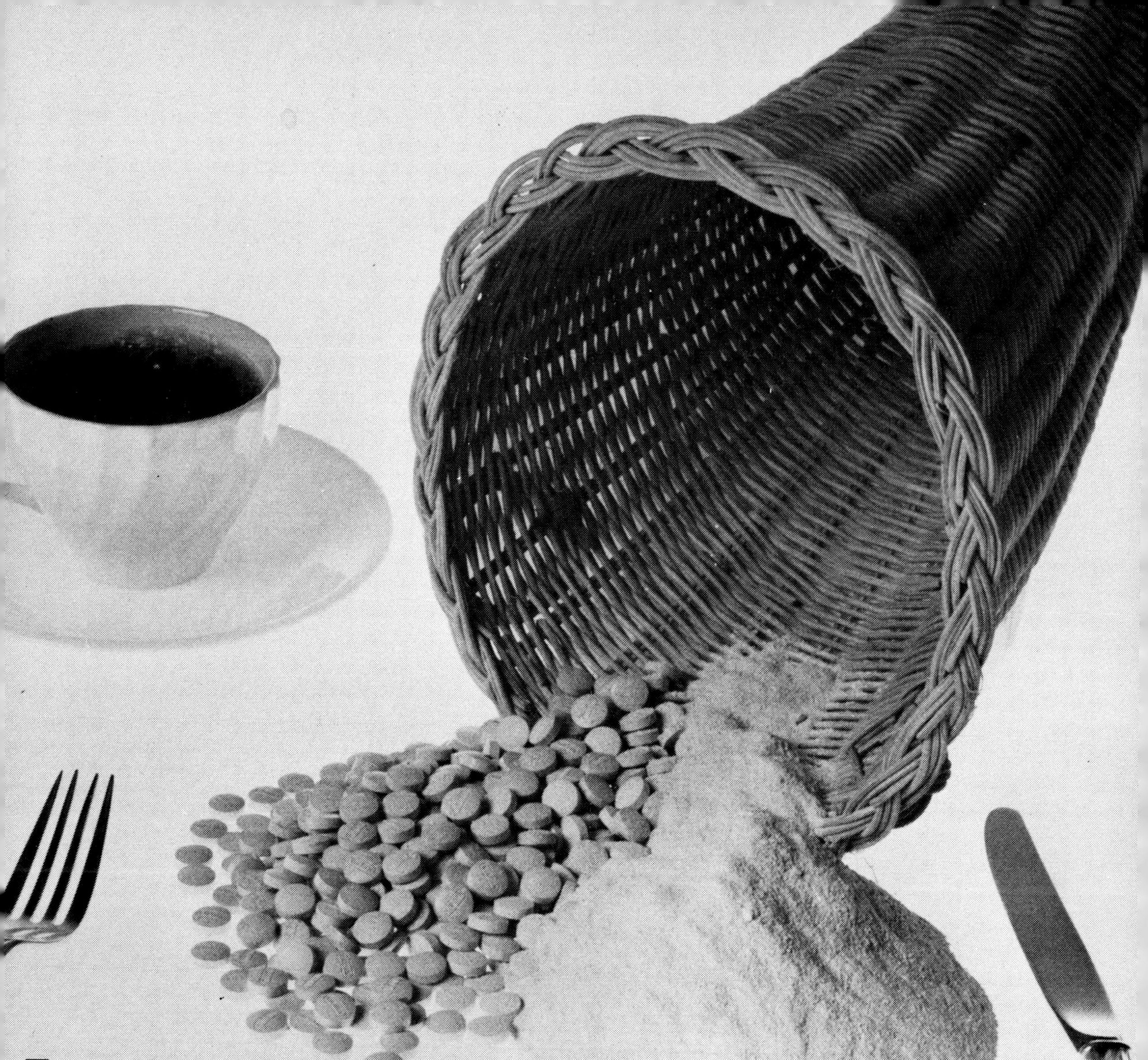

CONTENTS *continued*

page 298 **Preliminary results of a computer logic program for the operative management of colon cancer.** Carl O. Knutson, M.D., *Louisville, Ky., and* Francis R. Watson, Ph.D., *Columbia, Mo.*

309 **Teratomas in infancy and childhood: Experience with 81 cases.** G. Hossein Mahour, M.D., M.Sc.(Surgery), Morton M. Woolley, M.D., Sulochana N. Trivedi, M.D., *and* Benjamin H. Landing, M.D., *Los Angeles, Calif.*

319 **Choledochoduodenostomy: An 18 year study of 175 consecutive cases.** George A. Degenshein, M.D., *Brooklyn, N. Y.*

325 **Trace elements in normal and malignant human breast tissue.** Arthur E. Schwartz, M.D., *New York, N. Y.,* George W. Leddicotte, Sc.D., Richard W. Fink, Ph.D., *Atlanta, Ga., and* Eugene W. Friedman, M.D., *New York, N. Y.*

BRIEF CLINICAL REPORTS

330 **Duodenal duplication cysts: Diagnosis and operative management.** Norman B. Ackerman, M.D., Ph.D., *Kansas City, Mo.*

334 **Hepatic and splenic lymphangiomatosis with skeletal involvement: Report of a case and review of the literature.** Morris J. Asch, M.D., Arthur H. Cohen, M.D., *and* Thomas C. Moore, M.D., *Torrance, Calif.*

340 **Ischemic colitis following rectal prolapse.** Y. Kawarada, M.D., S. Satinsky, M.D., *and* T. Matsumoto, M.D., Ph.D., F.A.C.S., *Philadelphia, Pa.*

LETTERS TO THE EDITORS

344 **Is the author the writer? Who cares?** John H. Lavin, *Oradell, N. J.*

344 **Reply: Authorship in scholarly journals.** Lois DeBakey, Ph.D., *Houston, Texas*

345 **A splendid statement on a taboo subject.** R. Gordon Holcombe, Jr., M.D., *Lake Charles, La.*

346 **Myocardial glycogen.** George L. Blackburn, M.D., Ph.D., *Cambridge, Mass.*

346 **Reply.** Robert L. Hewitt, M.D., *and* Theodore Drapanas, M.D., *New Orleans, La.*

347 **Debridement.** David Patey, *Hythe, Kent, England*

continued on page 11

CONTENTS *continued*

page 347 **The role of débridement—Reply to Mr. Patey's Interrogatory.** Owen H. Wangensteen, M.D., *Minneapolis, Minn.*

350 **Anatomic approach to vagotomy.** Charles A. Griffith, M.D., *Bellevue, Wash.*

352 **Reply: The vagaries of the vagus.** John E. Skandalakis, M.D., Ph.D., F.A.C.S., *Atlanta, Ga.*

352 **Phagocytosis.** H. Gans, M.D., Ph.D., *New York, N. Y.*

353 **Reply.** Nicholas R. Di Luzio, Ph.D., Isik Olcay, M.D., *and* Theodore Drapanas, M.D., *New Orleans, La.*

355 **Subclavian steal syndrome.** David J. Mozersky, Lt. Col., USAF, MC, *Lackland Air Force Base, Texas*

355 **Reply.** Harry H. LeVeen, M.D., *Brooklyn, N. Y.*

356 **Painless removal of sutures.** Leon Bialostozky, M.D., *Mexico*

357 **Value of intraoperative tests in vagotomy.** Miles J. Gullickson, M.D., *Rockford, Ill.*

357 **Central venous catheter maintenance.** Dong K. Kim *and* Joseph G. Fortner, *New York, N. Y.*

358 **Bifurcation of canine abdominal aorta.** R. Adar, M.D., *Boston, Mass.*

Volume 76 *Number* 3

SURGERY

CONTENTS, SEPTEMBER, 1974

EDITORIALS

page 359 **The Carrel-Guthrie letters revisited.** L. G. Walker, Jr., M.D., *Charlotte, N. C.*

363 **Ischemia and the gastric mucosal barrier: A note of caution.** W. P. Ritchie, Jr., M.D., Ph.D., *Charlottesville, Va.*

367 **The academic surgical body count.** B. Eiseman, M.D., *Denver, Colo.*

372 **Physician supply, residency programs, and the foreign medical graduate.** Lucian L. Leape, M.D., *Boston, Mass.*

ORIGINAL COMMUNICATIONS

376 **Adrenalectomy with chemotherapy in the treatment of advanced breast cancer: Objective and subjective response rates; duration and quality of life.** Francis D. Moore, M.D., Susan Bland VanDevanter, M.D., Caryl Magnus Boyden, M.S., Jacob Lokich, M.D., *and* Richard E. Wilson, M.D., *Boston, Mass.*

continued on page 7

Vol. 76, No. 3, September, 1974, SURGERY is published monthly by The C. V. Mosby Company, 11830 Westline Industrial Drive, St. Louis, Mo. 63141.

Annual subscription rates.

	U. S.	*Canada, Mexico*	*Other countries*
Institutional*	$29.00	$32.00	$32.75
Personal†	$21.00	$24.00	$24.75
Student, intern, resident†	$14.70	$17.70	$18.45

Single copies are $3.50 postpaid. Remittances should be made by check, draft, post office or express money order, payable to this Journal.

*Institutional (multiple-reader) subscriptions are available to public and private libraries, schools, hospitals, and clinics; city, county, state, provincial, and national government bureaus and departments; and all commercial and private institutions and organizations.
†Personal subscriptions and all student-rate subscriptions must be in the names of, billed to, and paid by individuals. All student-rate requests must indicate training status and name of institution.

Subscriptions may begin at any time.

Second class postage paid at St. Louis, Mo. Printed in the U. S. A.

CONTENTS *continued*

page 391 **Safe limits of hemodilution in cardiopulmonary bypass.** Yasunaru Kawashima, M.D., Zengo Yamamoto, M.D., *and* Hisao Manabe, M.D., *Osaka, Japan*

398 **Positive-contrast peritoneography for accurate delineation of diaphragmatic abnormalities.** John J. White, M.D., C.M., Kook Sang Oh, M.D., *and* J. Alex Haller, Jr., M.D., *Baltimore, Md.*

405 **Effect of ethanol, acetylsalicylic acid, acetaminophen, and ferrous sulfate on gastric mucosal permeability in man.** Michael J. Gordon, M.D., John J. Skillman, M.D., Bruce G. Edwards, B.S., *and* William Silen, M.D., *Boston, Mass.*

413 **Axillo-axillary bypass with cephalic vein for correction of subclavian steal syndrome.** Herbert Dardik, M.D., *and* Irving Dardik, M.D., *Englewood, N. J., and Bronx, N. Y.*

419 **Gastrin concentrations in upper gastrointestinal mucosa in dogs.** Larry C. Watson, M.D., David D. Reeder, M.D., Horst D. Becker, M.D., Lavenia LaGrone, *and* James C. Thompson, M.D., *Galveston, Texas*

423 **Effect of ischemia on hepatic parenchymal and reticuloendothelial function in the baboon.** Klaus Holper, M.D., Isik Olcay, M.D., Akio Kitahama, M.D., Robert H. Miller, M.D., Lawrence Brettschneider, M.D., Theodore Drapanas, M.D., Rafael A. Trejo, M.D., Ph.D., *and* Nicholas R. Di Luzio, Ph.D., *New Orleans, La.*

433 **British surgery today: Perspective of a James IV surgical traveler.** Keith A. Kelly, M.D., *Rochester, Minn.*

439 **Body responses and recovery after 2½ hour hypothermic circulatory arrest.** Yoshio Kondo, M.D., M. Don Turner, Ph.D., Jose Bebin, M.D., *and* James D. Hardy, M.D., *Jackson, Miss.*

447 **Ischemic tolerance of the canine autotransplanted lung.** Yoshio Kondo, M.D., M. Don Turner, Ph.D., John V. Cockrell, M.D., *and* James D. Hardy, M.D., *Jackson, Miss.*

454 **A model for cardiogenic shock by coronary artery microembolization in calves.** Richard M. Satava, Jr., M.D., *and* Dwight C. McGoon, M.D., *Rochester, Minn.*

461 **Results of renal transplantation in 100 children.** Claude V. DeShazo, M.D., Richard L. Simmons, M.D., Dorothy M. Bernstein, M.D., Maureen M. DeShazo, Justine Willmert, R.N., *and* John S. Najarian, M.D., *Minneapolis, Minn.*

continued on page 9

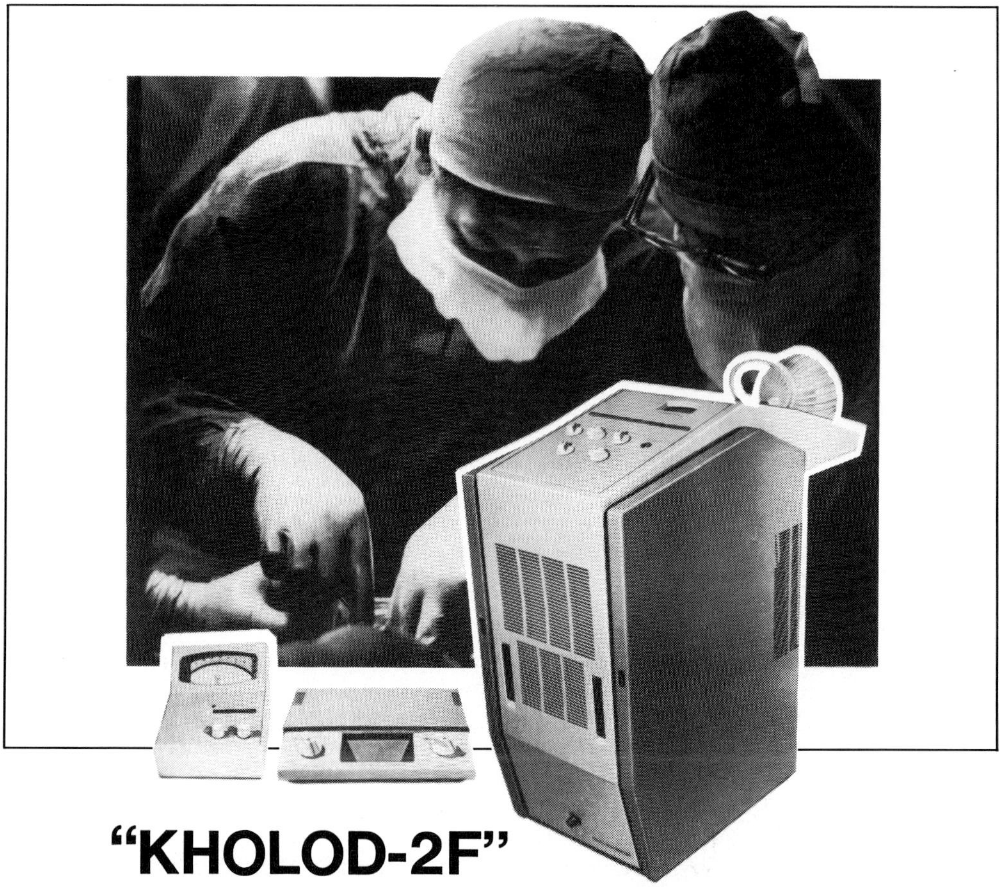

CONTENTS *continued*

page 469 **In vitro demonstration of altered antigenicity of metastases from a primary methylcholanthrene-induced sarcoma.** Robert P. Faraci, M.D., *Bethesda, Md.*

474 **Role of endotoxin and bacteria in long-term survival of preserved small-bowel allografts.** Luis H. Toledo-Pereyra, M.D., Leopoldo Raij, M.D., Richard L. Simmons, M.D., *and* John S. Najarian, M.D., *Minneapolis, Minn.*

482 **Coronary blood flow and myocardial reactive hyperemia in the ischemic dog heart.** William E. Elzinga, Ph.D., David B. Skinner, M.D., F.A.C.S., Mary F. Dutka, B.S., R.N., *and* Vincent L. Gott, M.D., F.A.C.S., *Baltimore, Md., and Chicago, Ill.*

490 **A chickenpox epidemic in a pediatric burn unit.** W. H. Weintraub, M.D., J. R. Lilly, *and* J. G. Randolph, *Washington, D. C.*

495 **Intestinal absorption of intake antigenic protein.** Andrew L. Warshaw, M.D., *and* W. Allan Walker, M.D., *Boston, Mass.*

500 **Dissolution of gallstones with bile salts, lecithin, and heparin.** Laurence Y. Cheung, M.D., Edwin Englert, Jr., M.D., Frank G. Moody, M.D., *and* Eugene E. Wales, *Salt Lake City, Utah*

BRIEF CLINICAL REPORTS

504 **A technique for in situ repair of bipolar transvenous pacemaker electrode.** Michael L. Gelfand, M.D., *and* Robert M. Blumenberg, M.D., Schenectady, N. Y.

506 **Subclavian artery aneurysm; sequela of thoracic outlet syndrome.** Stephen J. Mathes, M.D., *and* Atef A. Salam, M.D., *Atlanta, Ga.*

511 **Cystic adventitial degeneration of the common femoral artery.** Daniel K. Lowe, M.D., Frederick G. Winegarner, M.D., *and* John E. Jesseph, M.D., *Indianapolis, Ind.*

CLINICAL REVIEW

515 **Pathogenesis of peptic ulcer: A selective review.** John J. Skillman, M.D., *Boston, Mass.*

LETTERS TO THE EDITORS

524 **Lower abdominal tenderness following traumatic rupture of the spleen.** John L. Butsch, M.D., *and* Winfield L. Butsch, M.D., *Buffalo, N. Y.*

525 **An inverted Dacron patch graft.** Frank W. LoGerfo, M.D., *Baltimore, Md.*

Space Age Microbicidal Power

Prep with BETADINE®

Surgical Scrub/Solution/Aerosol Spray

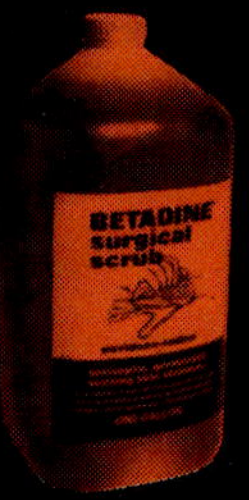

For optimal preoperative skin degerming—BETADINE Surgical Scrub. Chosen by NASA for Apollo 11/12/14 splashdowns, BETADINE Surgical Scrub provides a golden microbicidal lather for prepping the operative site... kills both gram-positive and gram-negative bacteria (including antibiotic-resistant strains), fungi, viruses, protozoa and yeasts... promptly achieves full microbicidal effect with each usage. (In the rare instance of local irritation or sensitivity, discontinue use in the individual.)

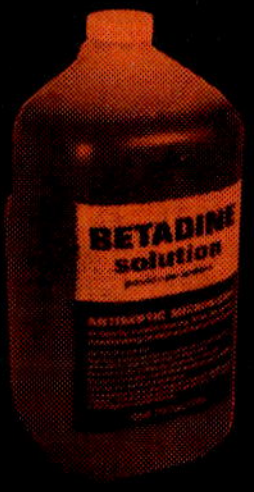

To enhance antisepsis—BETADINE Solution or BETADINE Aerosol Spray. After initial prepping with BETADINE Surgical Scrub, paint the operative area with BETADINE Solution (chosen by NASA for the Skylab mission), or spray with BETADINE Aerosol Spray...both are fully microbicidal and film-forming... maintain microbicidal activity in the presence of blood, pus and serum...treated area may be bandaged, taped or covered by a cast.

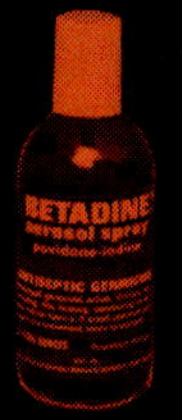

To help maintain postoperative antisepsis—Reapply BETADINE Solution or BETADINE Aerosol Spray after suturing and during redressing. BETADINE microbicides are virtually nonirritating and do not stain skin and natural fabrics.

PHOTOGRAPH: SKYLAB IN ORBIT, COURTESY OF THE NATIONAL AERONAUTICS AND SPACE ADMINISTRATION.

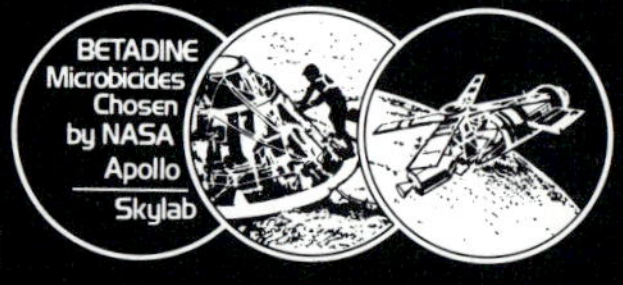

Purdue Frederick

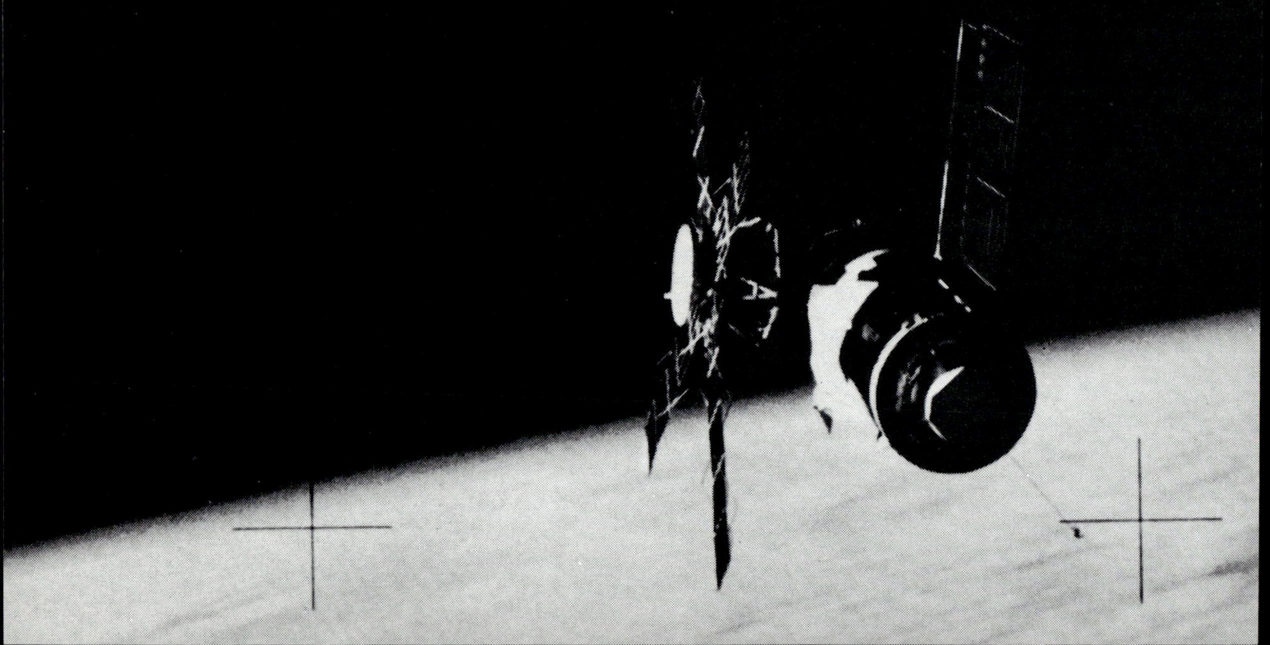

Volume 76 *Number* 4

SURGERY

CONTENTS, OCTOBER, 1974

ORIGINAL COMMUNICATIONS

page 527 **Evaluation of pulmonary function in the ischemic, nonventilated canine lung.** Eric W. Fonkalsrud, M.D., Isao Higashijima, M.D., Abdel K. Sarwat, M.D., Eitoku Arima, M.D., *and* Manuel Sanchez, *Los Angeles, Calif.*

533 **Impaired gluconeogenesis in dogs with *E. coli* bacteremia.** A. C. Groves, M.D., F.R.C.S.(C), L. I. Woolf, Ph.D., P. J. O'Regan, M.B., C. Beach, B.Sc.(Oxon.), C. Hasinoff, B.Sc., *and* W. H. Sutherland, M.D., F.R.C.S.(C), *Vancouver, B. C., Canada*

542 **Accumulation of lymphotoxin-secreting lymphoid cells in rat heart allografts.** Gale A. Granger, Ph.D., *Irvine, Calif., and* Thomas C. Moore, M.D., *Los Angeles, Calif.*

546 **Experience with autotransfusion in the surgical management of trauma.** George J. Reul, Jr., M.D., R. Thomas Solis, M.D., S. Donald Greenberg, M.D., Kenneth L. Mattox, M.D., *and* Hartwell H. Whisennand, M.D., *Houston, Texas*

556 **Thymectomy in the young pig: Effects on the level of circulating thymic hormone.** M. Lacombe, M.D., F. Perner, M.D., M. Dardenne, M.D., *and* J. F. Bach, M.D., *Paris, France*

continued on page 7

Vol. 76, No. 4, October, 1974, SURGERY is published monthly by The C. V. Mosby Company, 11830 Westline Industrial Drive, St. Louis, Mo. 63141.

Annual subscription rates.

	U. S.	*PUAS, Mexico*	*Canada, other countries*
Institutional*	$30.00	$34.75	$35.50
Personal†	$21.00	$25.75	$26.50
Student, intern, resident†	$14.70	$19.45	$20.20

Single copies are $3.50 postpaid. Remittances should be made by check, draft, post office or express money order, payable to this Journal.

*Institutional (multiple-reader) subscriptions are available to public and private libraries, schools, hospitals, and clinics; city, county, state, provincial, and national government bureaus and departments; and all commercial and private institutions and organizations.

†Personal subscriptions and all student-rate subscriptions must be in the names of, billed to, and paid by individuals. All student-rate requests must indicate training status and name of institution.

Subscriptions may begin at any time.

CONTENTS *continued*

page 560 **Cardiopulmonary effects of volume loading of primates in endotoxin shock.** Lazar J. Greenfield, M.D., Richard H. Jackson, Ronald C. Elkins, M.D., Jacqueline J. Coalson, Ph.D., *and* Lerner B. Hinshaw, Ph.D., *Oklahoma City, Okla.*

573 **Anti–HL-A antibodies: Failure to correlate with renal allograft rejection.** Clive O. Callender, M.D., Richard L. Simmons, M.D., Edmund J. Yunis, M.D., Luis H. Toledo-Pereyra, M.D., Maureen T. M. DeShazo, B.S., *and* John S. Najarian, M.D., *Minneapolis, Minn.*

581 **Follow-up study of the endorectal pull-through operation for the treatment of Hirschsprung's disease, with special reference to intestinal anastomosis.** Kisaku Satomura, M.D., Zheng Hang-Long, M.D., Satoshi Ohnishi, M.D., Kaoru Kumada, M.D., Yoshihiko Kisaka, M.D., Hidehiro Yamazaki, M.D., Katsuhiko Komaki, M.D., Nobuhiko Tanigawa, M.D., *Kyoto, Japan,* Keibun Hara, M.D., *Shiga, Japan,* Sumio Tominaga, M.D., *Kobe, Japan, and* Kenichi Kinoshita, M.D., *Ehime, Japan*

587 **Combined use of ^{131}I hippurate blood clearance and bladder/kidney ratio data in the early detection, classification, and management of accelerated rejection of human renal transplants.** Thomas C. Moore, M.D., *and* Michael Hayes, M.D., *Torrance, Calif.*

601 **Transhepatic metabolism after end-to-side portacaval shunt in the young pig.** Rosemary Hickman, M.D., Ch.M., James H. Crosier, M.B., Ch.B., Stuart J. Saunders, M.D., F.R.C.P., *and* John Terblanche, Ch.M., F.C.S.(SA), *Cape Town, South Africa*

608 **Removal of 5-hydroxytryptamine and norepinephrine from the pulmonary vascular space of man: Influence of cardiopulmonary bypass and pulmonary arterial pressure on these processes.** C. N. Gillis, Ph.D., L. H. Cronau, M.D., Ph.D., N. M. Greene, M.D., *and* G. L. Hammond, M.D., *New Haven, Conn.*

617 **Another look at rejection in pig liver homografts.** C. Battersby, M.S., F.R.C.S., W. S. Egerton, M.D., F.R.A.C.S., Glenda Balderson, B.Sc., J. F. Kerr, Ph.D., F.R.C.P.A., *and* W. Burnett, Ch.M., F.R.C.S., *Brisbane, Australia*

624 **Alveolar morphometrics: Effects of positive end-expiratory pressure.** Benedict D. T. Daly, M.D., David A. Hughes, M.D., *and* John C. Norman, M.D., *Houston, Texas*

630 **Allograft tolerance in the absence of circulating antibodies.** R. Nowygrod, M.D., D. E. R. Sutherland, M.D., R. J. Howard, M.D., *and* J. S. Najarian, M.D., *Minneapolis, Minn.*

continued on page 9

CONTENTS *continued*

page 637 **Pulmonary hypertension in acute hemorrhagic pancreatitis.** Denis F. J. Halmagyi, M.D., D.Sc., J. H. Karis, M.D., *New York, N. Y.*, F. G. Stenning, M.B., B.S., *Melbourne, Australia, and* D. Varga, B.Sc., *Sydney, Australia*

643 **Reticuloendothelial function: Determinant for survival following hepatic ischemia in the baboon.** Isik Olcay, M.D., Klaus Holper, M.D., Akio Kitahama, M.D., Robert H. Miller, M.D., Theodore Drapanas, M.D., Rafael A. Trejo, M.D., Ph.D., *and* Nicholas R. Di Luzio, Ph.D., *New Orleans, La.*

CLINICAL REVIEW

654 **The use of lymphangiography in melanoma.** Irving M. Ariel, M.D., F.A.C.S., F.A.C.N.M., *New York, N. Y.*

BRIEF CLINICAL REPORTS

666 **Post-traumatic renovascular hypertension.** M. N. Sechas, M.D., S. N. Plessas, M.D., *and* G. D. Skalkeas, M.D., *Athens, Greece*

671 **Staged palliative resection of recurrent carcinoma of the neck using an extra anatomic carotid bypass.** Clyde O. Hagood, Jr., M.D., F.A.C.S., Colonel, USAF(MC), David J. Mozersky, M.D., Major, USAF(MC), *and* Fulton W. Fite, M.D., F.A.C.S., Colonel, USAF(MC), *Lackland Air Force Base, Texas*

674 **Spontaneous (pathologic) rupture of spleen in malignancies.** G. P. Karakousis, M.D., *and* E. G. Elias, M.D., *Buffalo, N. Y.*

678 **Salmonella endocarditis treated with prosthetic valve replacement: A case report.** Noriaki Yamamoto, M.D., Oscar Magidson, M.D., Christian Posner, M.D., A. Michael Mendez, M.D., Pablo Zubiate, M.D., *and* Jerome Harold Kay, M.D., *Los Angeles, Calif.*

LETTERS TO THE EDITORS

682 **Disseminated intravascular coagulation.** Robert M. Hardaway, III, M.D., Brigadier General, MC, *El Paso, Texas*

684 **Reply.** Seymour I. Schwartz, M.D.

Volume 76 Number 5

SURGERY

CONTENTS, NOVEMBER, 1974

ORIGINAL COMMUNICATIONS

page 685 **The choice of treatment for operable carcinoma of the breast.** C. D. Haagensen, M.D., *New York, N. Y.*

715 **Penetrating vascular injuries of the thoracic outlet.** Robert L. Hewitt, M.D., Arnett D. Smith, M.D., Mathis L. Becker, M.D., Edward S. Lindsey, M.D., James B. Dowling, M.D., *and* Theodore Drapanas, M.D., *New Orleans, La.*

723 **Directional Doppler studies of supraorbital artery flow in internal carotid stenosis and occlusion.** Frank W. LoGerfo, M.D., *and* G. Robert Mason, M.D., *Baltimore, Md.*

729 **A comparison of gastric emptying before and after vagotomy with antrectomy and vagotomy with pyloroplasty.** I. A. Donovan, F.R.C.S., I. F. Gunn, F.R.A.C.S., Anne Brown, J. Alexander-Williams, M.D., Ch.M., F.R.C.S., *Birmingham, England, and* R. J. Clarke, M. D., F.R.C.S., *Somerset, England*

continued on page 7

Vol. 76, No. 5, November, 1974, SURGERY is published monthly by The C. V. Mosby Company, 11830 Westline Industrial Drive, St. Louis, Mo. 63141.

Annual subscription rates.

	U. S.	*PUAS, Mexico*	*Canada, other countries*
Institutional*	$30.00	$34.75	$35.50
Personal†	$21.00	$25.75	$26.50
Student, intern, resident†	$14.70	$19.45	$20.20

Single copies are $3.50 postpaid. Remittances should be made by check, draft, post office or express money order, payable to this Journal.

*Institutional (multiple-reader) subscriptions are available to public and private libraries, schools, hospitals, and clinics; city, county, state, provincial, and national government bureaus and departments; and all commercial and private institutions and organizations.
†Personal subscriptions and all student-rate subscriptions must be in the names of, billed to, and paid by individuals. All student-rate requests must indicate training status and name of institution.

Subscriptions may begin at any time.

Second class postage paid at St. Louis, Mo. Printed in the U. S. A.

CONTENTS *continued*

page 733 **Effect of aging, organ allografting, and surgical stress on rat thymus histidine decarboxylase activity.** Thomas C. Moore, M.D., Michael C. Sinclair, M.D., Columbus D. McAlpin, M.D., Griffith A. Weber, A.B., *and* Carlos A. E. Lemmi, M.A., *Torrance, Calif.*

741 **Complications of related kidney donation.** Panyiotis K. Spanos, M.D., Richard L. Simmons, M.D., Ernest Lampe, M.D., Luca C. Rattazzi, M.D., Carl M. Kjellstrand, M.D., Frederick C. Goetz, M.D., *and* John S. Najarian, M.D., *Minneapolis, Minn.*

748 **New method of reconstruction of the alimentary canal after total gastrectomy.** Józef Kalemba, M.D., *and* Bogdan Lazarkiewicz, M.D., *Wroclaw, Poland*

754 **The need for pediatric surgeons as determined by the volume of work and the mode of delivery of surgical care.** Mark M. Ravitch, M.D., *and* Bruce A. Barton, M.S., *Pittsburgh, Pa.*

764 **The effect of sepsis on acute gastric ulcerations in the rat.** R. Rasche, M.D., *and* W. C. Butterfield, M.D., *Waterbury, Conn.*

771 **Uveitis and vitiligo associated with BCG treatment for malignant melanoma.** Robert C. Donaldson, M.D., Samuel A. Canaan, Jr., M.D., Robert B. McLean, M.D., *and* Lauren V. Ackerman, M.D., *St. Louis, Mo.*

779 **Effect of sera obtained from normal and partially hepatectomized rats and patients on the growth of cells in tissue culture.** Achilles A. Demetriou, M.D., Eli Seifter, Ph.D., *and* Stanley M. Levenson, M.D., *Bronx, N. Y.*

786 **The hemodynamic response to positive end-expiratory ventilation in hypovolemic patients.** Alden H. Harken, M.D., Murray F. Brennan, M.D., Beverly Smith, R.N., *and* Ernest M. Barsamian, M.D., *Roxbury and Boston, Mass.*

794 **Lymphocyte output by the isolated perfused rabbit thymus.** O. Ekwueme, M.D., F.R.C.S., *and* A. P. M. Forrest, B.Sc., M.D., Ch.M., F.R.C.S., *Cardiff, Wales*

804 **The influence of glucose on gastrin and insulin release in the enteroinsular axis.** Stanley R. Friesen, M.D., Robert E. Bolinger, M.D., *and* Joseph L. Kyner, M.D., *Kansas City, Kan.*

continued on page 9

CONTENTS *continued*

CLINICAL REVIEW

page 811 **The elective surgical treatment of chronic duodenal ulcer: A critical review.** Leslie Wise, M.D., *and* Walter F. Ballinger, M.D., *St. Louis, Mo.*

BRIEF CLINICAL REPORTS

827 **Aberrant pancreas causing pyloric obstruction.** Yoichi Matsumoto, M.D., Yoshio Kawai, M.D., *and* Ken Kimura, M.D., *Kobe, Japan*

830 **Solitary rectal ulcer: A cause of life-threatening hemorrhage.** Herman Delancy, M.D., *and* William Stroud Hitch, M.D., *Savannah, Ga.*

833 **Occlusion of popliteal artery caused by popliteal cysts.** James D. Schlenker, M.D., Kent Johnston, M.D., *and* Jerry S. Wolkoff, M.D., *Cleveland, Ohio*

837 **Successful balloon membranotomy for obstruction of the hepatic portion of the inferior vena cava.** Shoji Euguchi, M.D., Yoshimi Takeuchi, M.D., *and* Ken-ichi Asano, M.D., *Niigata, Japan*

841 **Femorofemoral bypass.** L. M. Gazzola, M.D., S. A. Hirsch, M.D., *and* G. I. Kaufer, M.D., *Pittsburgh, Penn.*

845 **Coronary artery aneurysms in a 9-year-old child.** John E. Liddicoat, M.D., Szabolcs M. Bekassy, M.D., Manus J. O'Donnell, M.D., *and* Michael E. De Bakey, M.D., *Houston, Texas*

LETTERS TO THE EDITORS

848 **Buerger's disease—the need for diagnostic criteria.** Raphael Adar, M.D., F.A.C.S., *Tel Aviv, Israel*

848 **Reply.** Shigehiko Shionoya, M.D., *Nagoya, Japan*

Space Age Microbicidal Power

Prep with BETADINE®
Surgical Scrub/Solution/Aerosol Spray

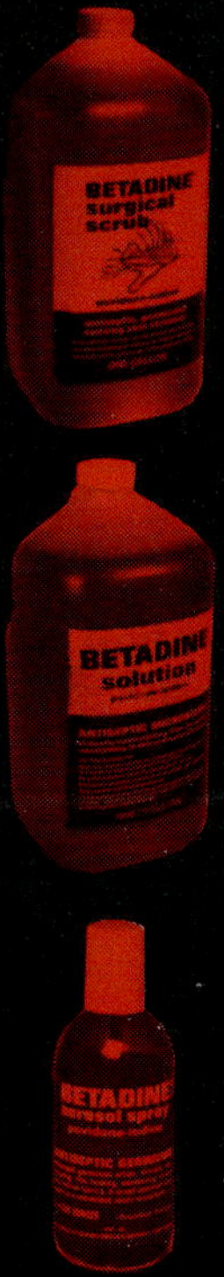

For optimal preoperative skin degerming—BETADINE Surgical Scrub. Chosen by NASA for Apollo 11/12/14 splashdowns, BETADINE Surgical Scrub provides a golden microbicidal lather for prepping the operative site... kills both gram-positive and gram-negative bacteria (including antibiotic-resistant strains), fungi, viruses, protozoa and yeasts... promptly achieves full microbicidal effect with each usage. (In the rare instance of local irritation or sensitivity, discontinue use in the individual.)

To enhance antisepsis—BETADINE Solution or BETADINE Aerosol Spray. After initial prepping with BETADINE Surgical Scrub, paint the operative area with BETADINE Solution (chosen by NASA for the Skylab mission), or spray with BETADINE Aerosol Spray...both are fully microbicidal and film-forming... maintain microbicidal activity in the presence of blood, pus and serum...treated area may be bandaged, taped or covered by a cast.

To help maintain postoperative antisepsis—Reapply BETADINE Solution or BETADINE Aerosol Spray after suturing and during redressing. BETADINE microbicides are virtually nonirritating and do not stain skin and natural fabrics.

PHOTOGRAPH: SKYLAB IN ORBIT, COURTESY OF THE NATIONAL AERONAUTICS AND SPACE ADMINISTRATION.

BETADINE Microbicides Chosen by NASA Apollo Skylab

Purdue Frederick

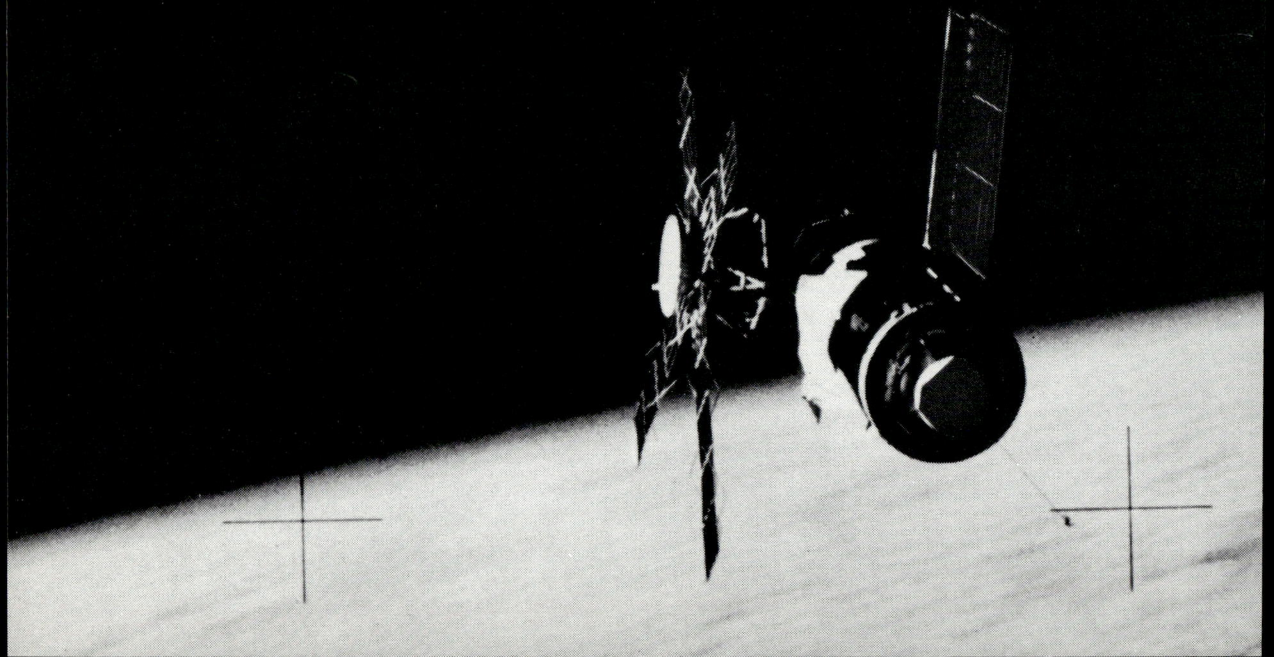

Volume 76 *Number* 6

SURGERY

CONTENTS, DECEMBER, 1974

SOCIETY FOR VASCULAR SURGERY

page 849 **The beginnings of Vascular Surgery.** W. Andrew Dale, *Nashville, Tenn.*

867 **Long-term evaluation of the celiac band syndrome.** William E. Evans, M.D., *Columbus, Ohio*

872 **Deceptive patterns of renal artery stenosis.** Richard H. Dean, M.D., Henry Burko, M.D., James P. Wilson, M.D., Joseph H. Mulherin, M.D., *and* John H. Foster, M.D., *Nashville, Tenn.*

882 **Carotid cavernous fistula: Direct repair with preservation of carotid.** Dwight Parkinson, M.D., Allan R. Downs, M.D., Lawrence L. Whytehead, M.D., *and* Walter B. Syslak, M.D., *Winnipeg, Manitoba, Canada*

890 **Juxtarenal aortic occlusion.** Richard W. Starrett, M.D., *and* Ronald J. Stoney, M.D., *San Francisco, Calif.*

continued on page 5

Vol. 76, No. 6, December, 1974, SURGERY is published monthly by The C. V. Mosby Company, 11830 Westline Industrial Drive, St. Louis, Mo. 63141.

Annual subscription rates.

	U. S.	*PUAS* Mexico*	*Canada, other countries*
Institutional**	$30.00	$34.75	$35.50
Personal†	$21.00	$25.75	$26.50
Student, intern, resident†	$14.70	$19.45	$20.20

*(*Postal Union of the Americas and Spain)*

Single copies are $3.50 postpaid. Remittances should be made by check, draft, post office or express money order, payable to this Journal.

**Institutional (multiple-reader) subscriptions are available to public and private libraries, schools, hospitals, and clinics; city, county, state, provincial, and national government bureaus and departments; and all commercial and private institutions and organizations.

†Personal subscriptions and all student-rate subscriptions must be in the names of, billed to, and paid by individuals. All student-rate requests must indicate training status and name of institution.

Subscriptions may begin at any time.

Second class postage paid at St. Louis, Mo. Printed in the U. S. A.

Fifth of The Life Series/Medical Incorporated

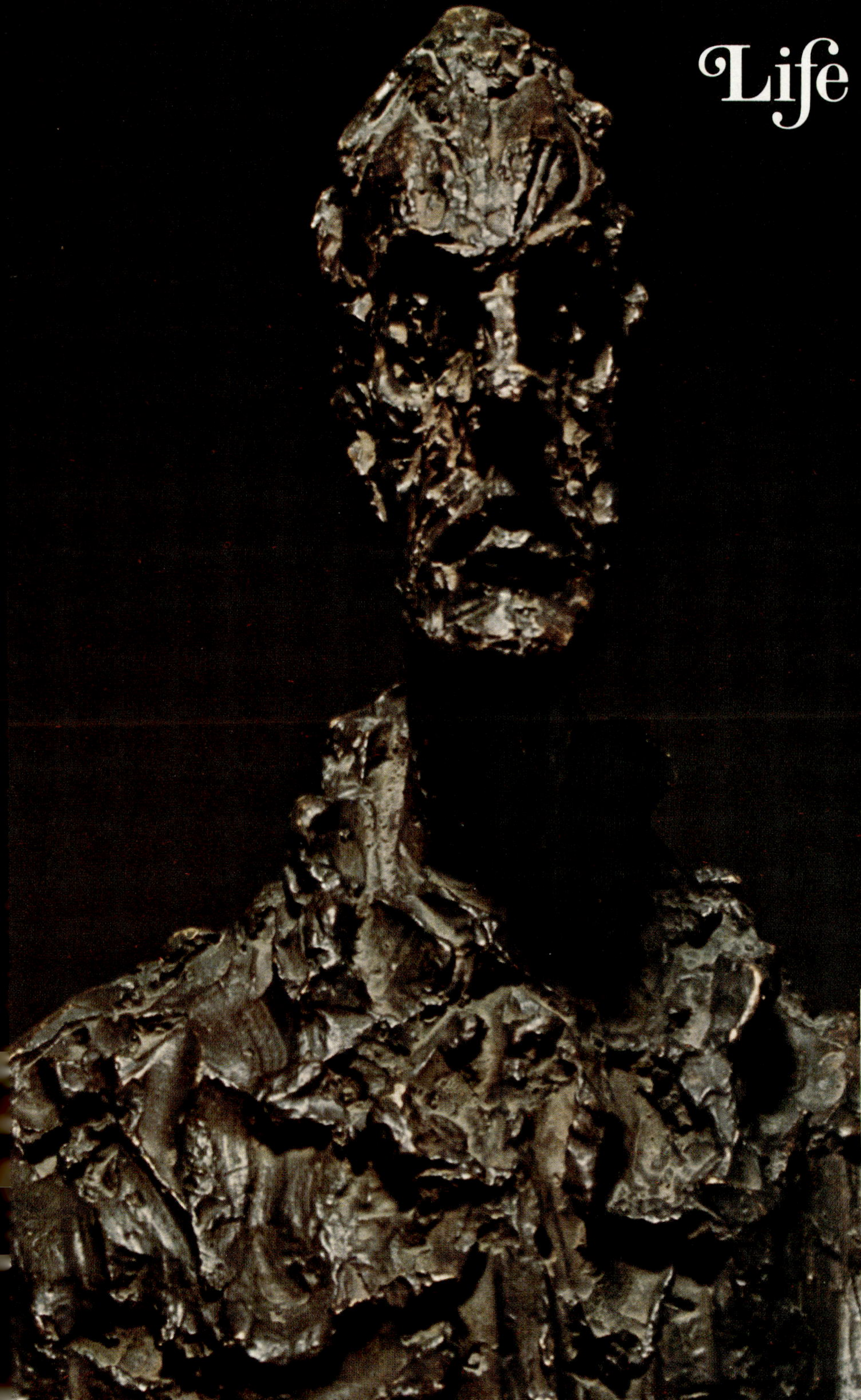

Alberto Giacometti, "HEAD OF DIEGO" from the Collection of Walker Art Center, Minneapolis.

Life

. . . one crowded hour . . .
worth an age without a n
Sir Walter

The Lillehei-Kaster™ Piv
Disc Prosthetic Heart Val
designed to meet the rec
ments of hemodynamic
ciency with minimal grad
and regurgitant flows at p
iologic outputs. Over four y
of clinical experience has
stantiated the benefits anc
ability of this design. 1-4

The Pivoting Disc Prost
presents these outstan
features:

Increased Effective Flow
- largest effective orifice
- highest cardiac output
- lower pressure gradients
- minimal regurgitation
- controlled marginal back

Minimal Flow Obstruction
- low incidence of hemolys
- optimized central lamina
- negligible flow stasis
- spontaneous disc respor

Blood Compatible Materia
- free-floating Pyrolite® di
- low profile titanium hous

Our technical specialists
be pleased to demonstra
Pivoting Disc Prosthesis
discuss clinical and labo
findings.

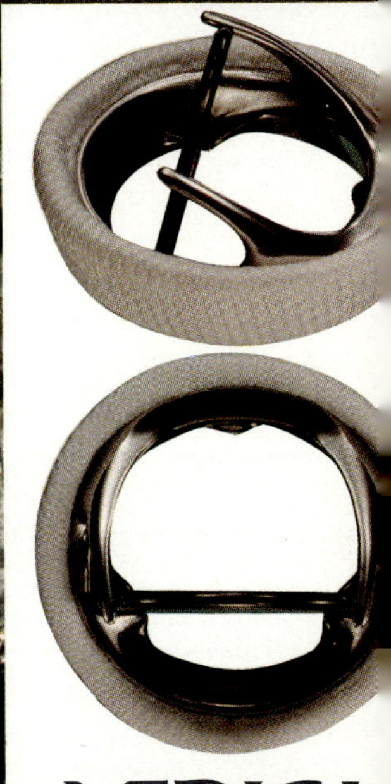

MEDICA
incorporate

1974
EDICAL INCORPORATED • 9605 WEST JEFFERSON TRAIL • INVER GROVE HEIGHTS, MN 55075 • 612/452-3000

Borst HG, et al: Aortic Valve Replacement with the Lillehei-Kaster Prosthesis; two years experience in 125 patients without using anticoagulants for isolated valve replacement. Presented to the European Society of Cardiovascular Surgery, 23rd Congress, July 3, 1974. In Press.

Gibson TC, et al: Echocardiographic and Phonocardiographic characteristics of the Lillehei-Kaster Mitral Valve Prosthesis. Circulation 49:434, 1974.

Lillehei CW, et al: Heart Valve Replacement with the Lillehei-Kaster Pivoting Disc Prosthesis. Presented at the Southern African Cardiac Society 8th Biennial Cardiac Congress, 1972.

Lillehei CW, et al: A New Central Flow Pivoting Disc Aortic and Mitral Prosthesis: Initial Clinical Experience, Am J Cardiol 26:688, 1970.

Pyrolite is the registered trademark of the General Atomic Company.

CONTENTS *continued*

page 898 **Pathogenesis and clinical significance of splenic artery aneurysms.** James C. Stanley, M.D., *and* William J. Fry, M.D., *Ann Arbor, Mich.*

910 **Surgical therapy for venous stasis.** Ralph G. De Palma, M.D., *Cleveland, Ohio*

918 **Sinusoidal shunt fraction by radioextraction ratio.** E. L. Bradley, III, M.D., D. L. Quinton, B.S., L. G. Martin, M.D., Evangelos Kourias, M.D., *and* James Larose, M.D., *Atlanta, Ga.*

925 **Objective assessment of late results of aortocoronary bypass operation.** Hooshang Bolooki, M.D., F.R.C.S.(C), Richard J. Thurer, M.D., Ali Ghahramani, M.D., Abelardo Vargas, M.D., Willis Williams, M.D., *and* Gerard Kaiser, M.D., *Miami, Fla.*

935 **Total cardiopulmonary bypass with a new microporous Teflon membrane oxygenator.** K. E. Karlson, M.D., Ph.D., W. R. Murphy, M.D., M. Kakvan, M.D., P. Anthony, B.A., G. N. Cooper, Jr., M.D., P. D. Richardson, Ph.D., *and* P. M. Galletti, M.D., Ph.D., *Providence, R. I.*

946 **Complications following the contoured Dacron baffle in correction of transposition of the great arteries.** George J. Reul, Jr., M.D., Denton A. Cooley, M.D., Frank M. Sandiford, M.D., *and* Grady L. Hallman, M.D., *Houston, Texas*

955 **Management of carotid artery injuries.** Erwin R. Thal, M.D., William H. Snyder, III, M.D., *Dallas, Texas,* Robert J. Hays, M.D., *Amarillo, Texas, and* M. O. Perry, M.D., *Dallas, Texas*

963 **The modified bovine arterial graft: A clinical study.** Bruce S. Cutler, M.D., Jesse E. Thompson, M.D., R. Don Patman, M.D., Alfred V. Persson, M.D., *and* Philip D. Manfredi, M.D., *Dallas, Texas*

974 **Experience with open mitral commissurotomy in 100 consecutive patients.** Michael J. Mullin, M.D., Richard M. Engelman, M.D., O. Wayne Isom, M.D., Arthur D. Boyd, M.D., Ephraim Glassman, M.D., *and* Frank C. Spencer, M.D., *New York, N. Y.*

983 **Clinical and hemodynamic comparisons of Kay-Shiley, Starr-Edwards No. 6520, and Reis-Hancock porcine xenograft mitral valves.** John W. Brown, M.D., P. David Myerowitz, M.D., Michael S. Cann, M.D., Stephen B. Colvin, M.D., Charles L. McIntosh, M.D., *and* Andrew G. Morrow, M.D., *Bethesda, Md.*

continued on page 7

CONTENTS *continued*

page 992 **The deleterious effect of immediate postoperative prosthesis in below-knee amputation for ischemic disease.** Steven I. Cohen, M.D., Leon D. Goldman, M.D., Edwin W. Salzman, M.D., *and* Donald J. Glotzer, M.D., *Boston, Mass.*

1002 **The acutely ischemic upper extremity: Selective management.** Charles R. Sachatello, M.D., Calvin B. Ernst, M.D., *and* Ward O. Griffen, Jr., M.D., *Lexington, Ky.*

1010 **Reoperation for residual defects after repair of tetralogy of Fallot.** Aldo R. Castaneda, M.D., Robert M. Sade, M.D., John Lamberti, M.D., *Boston, Mass., and* Demetre M. Nicoloff, M.D., *Minneapolis, Minn.*

1018 **A 6 year clinical experience with arteriovenous fistulas and bypasses for hemodialysis.** Victor R. Zerbino, M.D., David A. Tice, M.D., Lois A. Katz, M.D., *and* Bernard D. Nidus, M.D., *New York, N. Y.*

1024 **Caution regarding autotransfusion.** S. Edwin Duncan, M.D., William H. Edwards, M.D., *and* W. Andrew Dale, M.D., *Nashville, Tenn.*

1031 **Structural changes during preparation of autogenous venous grafts.** William M. Abbott, M.D., Steven Wieland, B.S., *and* W. Gerald Austen, M.D., *Boston, Mass.*

INDEX

1043 **Index**

Volume 76 Number 1

SURGERY

JULY, 1974

Society of University Surgeons

Myonecrosis in chronic experimental vasospasm

John F. Alksne, M.D., *San Diego, Calif.*

The word "vasospasm" may be a misnomer: vasonecrosis is revealed by electronmicroscopy. Preventive measures based on this hypothesis may be more effective in controllong vasospasm than therapeutic measures applied after the damage has occurred.

From the Division of Neurological Surgery, University of California, San Diego, Calif.

CLINICALLY, cerebral arterial spasm persists as one of the major factors responsible for the morbidity and deaths associated with intracranial hemorrhage. Attempts to treat vasospasm in patients have been unsuccessful and its etiology and mechanism remain unclear. Intensive investigations in animals during the past 10 years have demonstrated that experimental cerebral vasospasm is biphasic,[2] that it can be produced experimentally by arterial injury,[14] subarachnoid blood injection,[15] or application of vasoactive chemicals.[6, 11, 12] It is associated with depletion of catecholamines from arterial adrenergic nerve endings,[10] and with reduction in cerebral blood flow.[5] Recent experiments demonstrate a predominant first phase of spasm when vessel injury is produced without hemorrhage and a predominant second phase of spasm where hemorrhage is added.[3]

Most investigators studying spasm have focused primarily on the large vessels at the base of the brain. The observation by Bloor[1] that some patients with severe spasm of the circle of Willis have very little alteration of cerebral blood flow, whereas some patients with minimal spasm of the circle of Willis have a marked reduction in cerebral blood flow, suggests, however, that the critical vessels causing a reduction in flow may be the small, penetrating arteries and arterioles. These vessels have been extensively examined by both light and electronmicroscopy in their normal state. A perivascular space contain-

Presented at the Thirty-fifth Annual Meeting of the Society of University Surgeons, St. Louis, Mo., Feb. 14-16, 1974.

Reprint requests: John F. Alksne, M.D., Division of Neurological Surgery, University of California, San Diego, Calif. 92110.

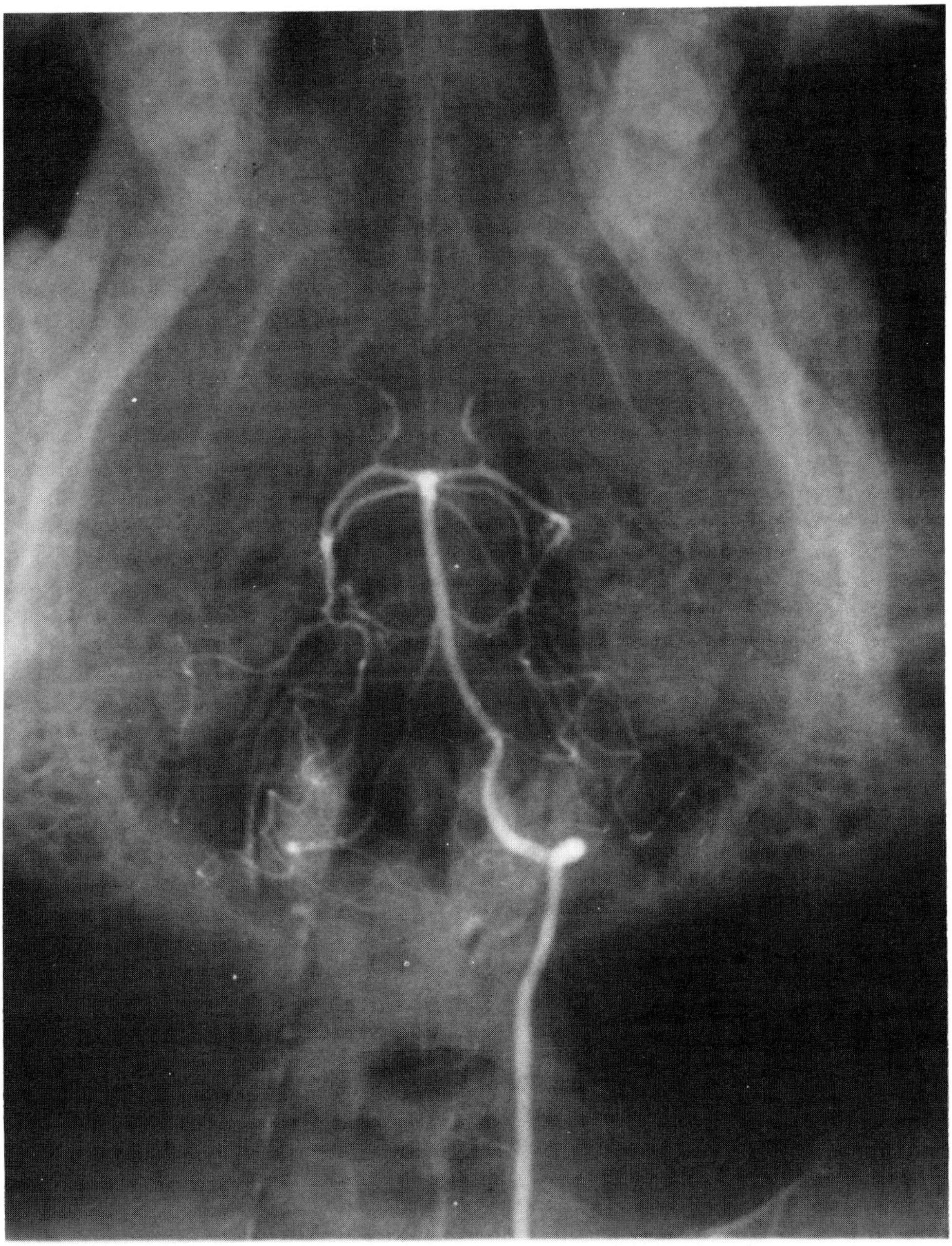

Fig. 1. Subtraction vertebral angiogram showing normal monkey vertebral-basilar artery circulation. Note normal caliber of vessels.

ing elements of pia arachnoid accompanies all arteries as they leave the subarachnoid space to enter brain substance, and separates the basement membrane of the vessel from the glial basement membrane.[4, 7] Arteries greater than 50 μ in diameter have been shown by fluorescence microscopy to have abundant adrenergic nerve endings.[10] Electronmicroscopy has confirmed the presence of nerve endings on large arteries,[9] and demonstrated that the small penetrating arteries and arterioles which are devoid of nerve terminals are still invested with smooth muscle cells.[13] These small muscular vessels are surrounded by a perivascular space which is in direct communication with the subarachnoid space. The perivascular space disappears along with the smooth muscle cells when the basement membrane of the arteriole fuses with the glial-basement membrane of the brain. This occurs at the capillary level and up to this point, at least, a potential perivascular space exists.[8]

The resistance of clinical spasm to any type of pharmacologic relaxation suggests that persistent spasm may be secondary to a pathologic change in the vascular wall. Light microscope examination of arteries from human patients dying from vasospasm, and examination of arteries from animals with experimental spasm, have revealed no lesions.[16] The animal studies included only the large arteries from the base of the brain, and the specimens were not taken at a time when the vessels were known to be in spasm.

The presence of sympathetic nerve endings on cerebral vessels and the depletion of their catecholamine after subarachnoid hemorrhage suggest that the sympathetic nervous system could play a role in intracranial arterial spasm. The report that the administration of alpha adrenergic blocking agents prior to the subarachnoid hemorrhage will prevent cerebral arterial spasm supports this hypothesis but the failure of blocking agents to relieve the spasm once it is present indicates that some alteration in the contractile process has occurred. Our studies indicate that excessive sympathetic stimulation will profoundly affect the structure of the smooth muscle cells.

METHODS

All experiments have been performed on monkeys under surital anesthesia. Utilizing sterile technique, a C_2 laminectomy was performed and the dura and arachnoid were opened under magnification. A silicone rubber catheter was inserted immediately beneath the C_2 root and then directed cephalad, ventral to the spinal cord, into the prepontine cistern. The catheter was brought out between the paraspinous muscle, occluded, and left beneath the skin for subsequent injections.

Following the satisfactory placement of a prepontine catheter, each animal underwent vertebral angiography by the transfemoral, catheter approach. The catheter was positioned in the left subclavian artery at the origin of the left vertebral artery.

After satisfactory control angiograms had been obtained, the test material was injected into the prepontine cistern through the silicone catheter. Experimental animals received either norepinephrine or nonheparinized whole blood. The norepinephrine was administered as a standard dose of 2 mg. of the amine, an alpha-adrenergic stimulator, either as supplied in its commercial base* or in powdered form* dissolved in the animal's own spinal fluid. The nonheparinized whole blood was withdrawn from the animal's own arterial system and 8 c.c. were injected with simultaneous monitoring of intracranial pressure. Control animals received either injection base alone, without norepinephrine, isoproterenol, a beta-adrenergic stimulator, or saline.

Immediately after injection of the test material, repeat vertebral arteriograms were performed, and again repeated at one hour, two days, four days, eight days, and 10 days following injection. The presence or absence of vasospasm was noted and graded as mild, moderate, or severe.

At the termination of each experiment, the monkey was killed by transcardiac perfusion with glutaraldehyde-paraformaldehyde fixative. The intra-arterial pressure was continually monitored during the perfusion to insure that it did not go above the animal's normal systolic pressure. The brain was immediately removed and the basilar artery excised, postfixed in phosphate-buffered osmium tetroxide, imbedded in epon, and sectioned for electronmicroscopy. Similar arterial samples were imbedded in paraffin for light microscopy.

RESULTS

All animals receiving subarachnoid norepinephrine injections showed biphasic vasospasm, although the degree of spasm varied from animal to animal. The first phase of spasm began immediately and lasted for 10

*Levophed, Winthrop Laboratories, New York.

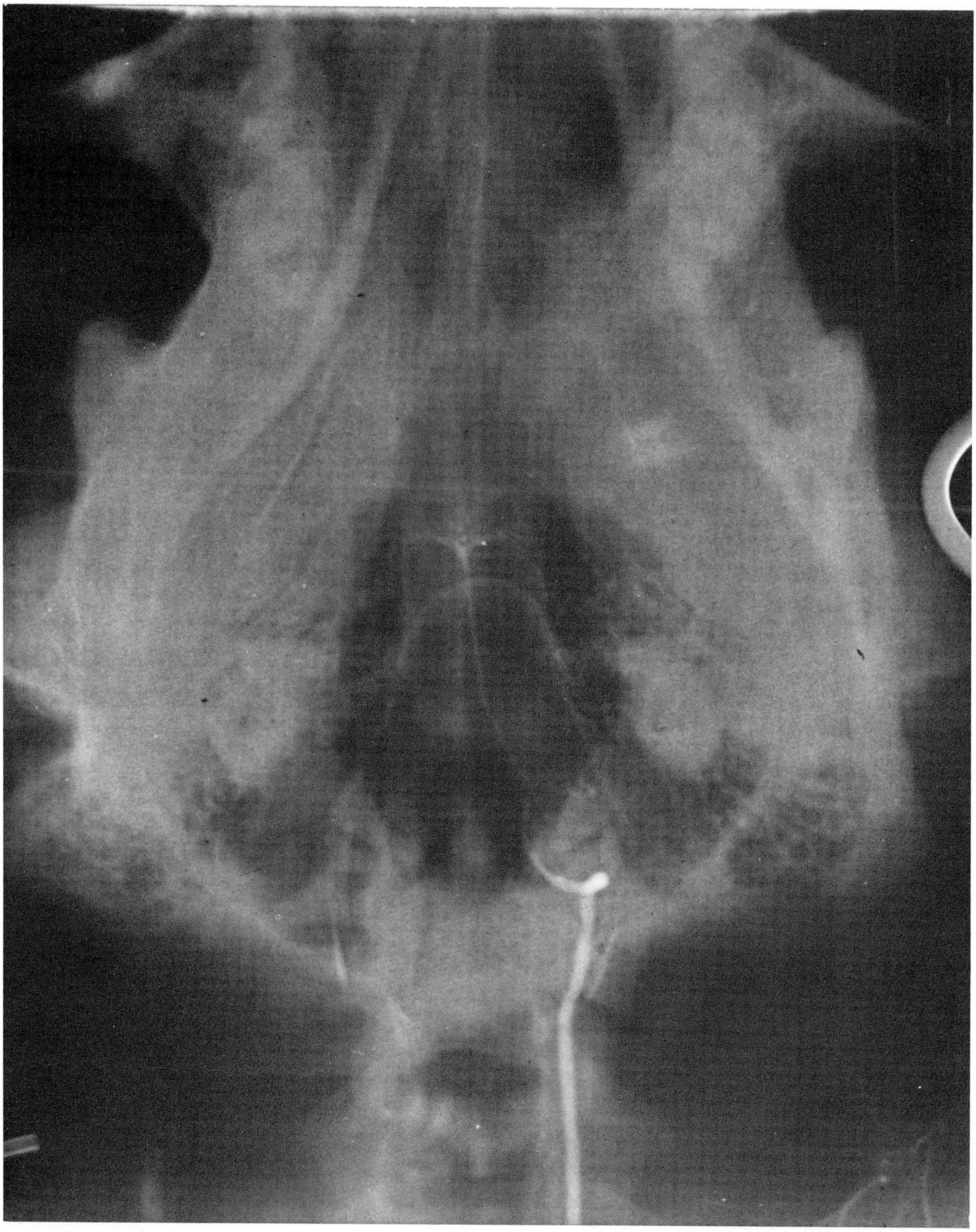

Fig. 2. Subtraction vertebral angiogram on same monkey as Fig. 1, four days after intracisternal injection of 8 c.c. of blood. Note marked reduction in caliber of vertebral and basilar arteries beginning at point where vertebral artery enters the cranial cavity. This picture is similar to what is interpreted as "vasospasm" on human angiograms.

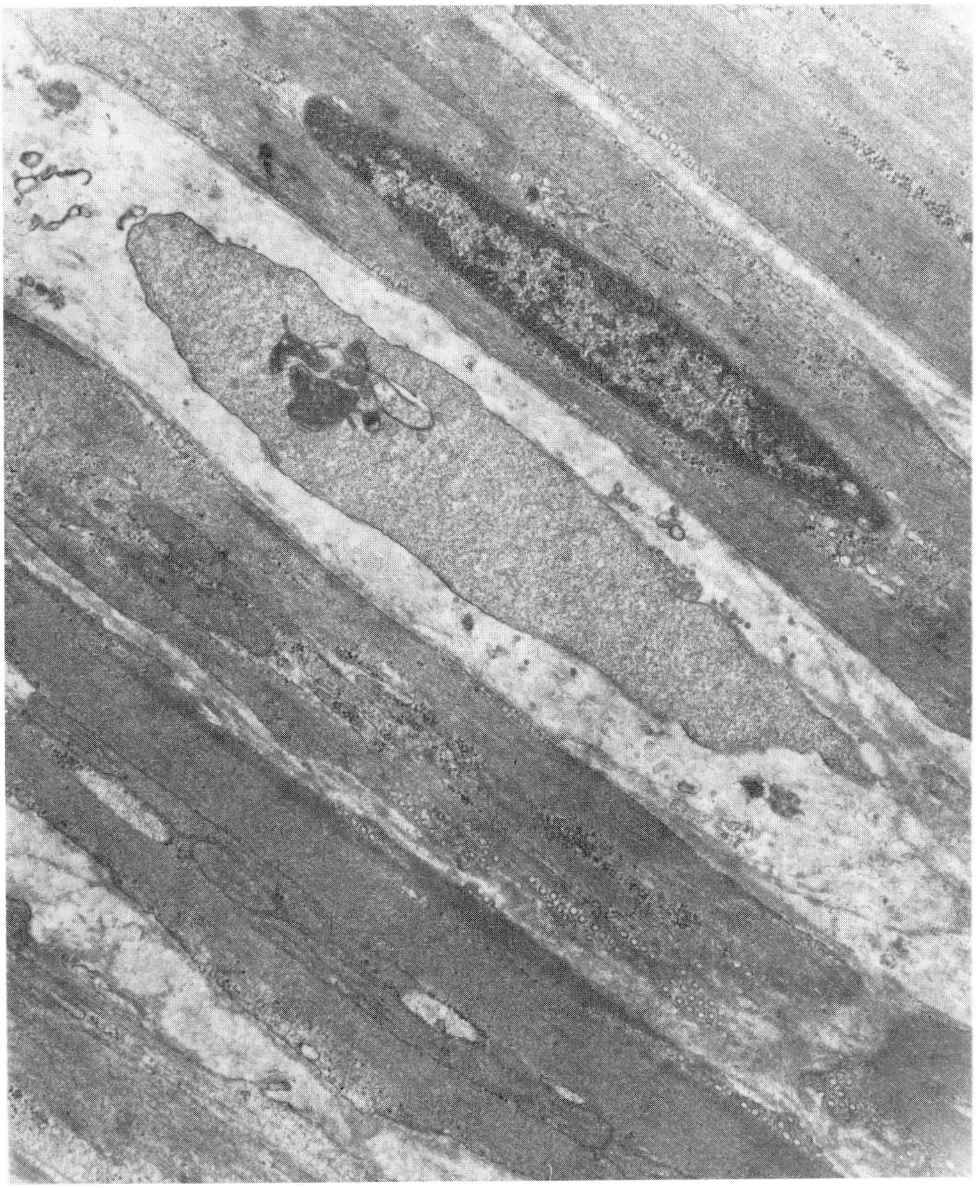

Fig. 3. Electronmicrograph of smooth muscle cells in wall of basilar artery showing a necrotic muscle fiber between other normal fibers. Note the complete absence of myofilaments in the damaged muscle cell. The arterial wall was removed from an animal with demonstrated vasospasm on angiography. (Original magnification ×28,000; reduced 30 percent.)

to 15 minutes. The second phase began between four to 24 hours postinjection and lasted eight to 10 days. The monkeys showed no untoward clinical effect during this interval.

The vasospasm, as measured angiographically, was less consistent following the subarachnoid injection of blood. When visualized acutely, it was also visualized chronically, however, and appeared to be more severe than that produced by norepinephrine. Of the seven animals injected with blood, only three demonstrated unquestionable spasm (Figs. 1 and 2).

Electronmicroscopy of the basilar arteries of all animals killed during the chronic phase of angiographically demonstrated vasospasm showed significant pathological changes in

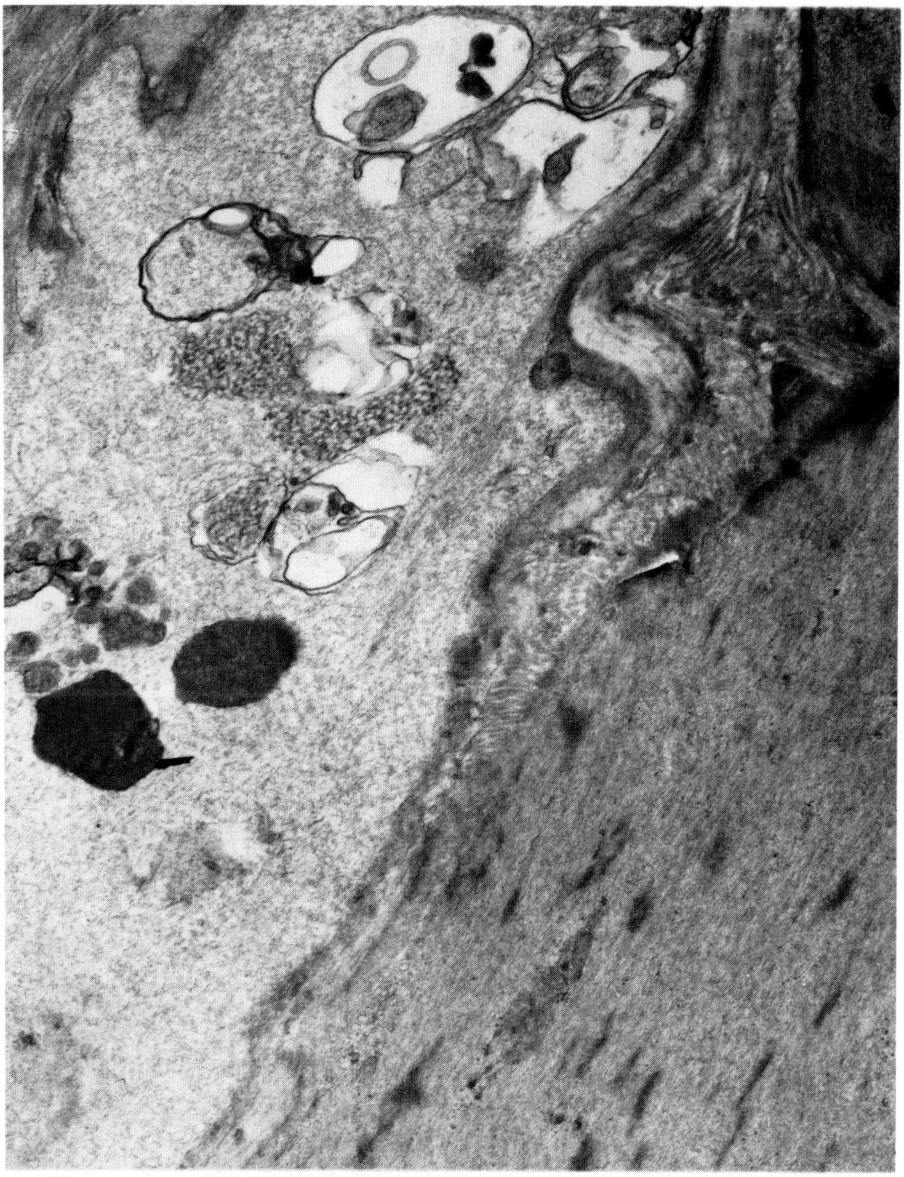

Fig. 4. Electronmicrograph of necrotic smooth muscle cell showing loss of myofilaments and presence of intracytoplasmic inclusions (×40,000). (Original magnification ×40,000; reduced 30 percent.)

the smooth muscle cells of the media. These changes consisted of fragmentation of myofilaments, disruption of the sarcolemma, and lipid inclusions within abnormal smooth muscle cells (Figs. 3 and 4). The abnormal cells were scattered randomly throughout the vessel wall with markedly distorted cells frequently lying adjacent to normal-appearing cells. The damaged cells were more frequently found close to the internal elastic lamina than to the adventitia. In both intact and fragmented muscle fibers, the mitochondria appeared normal. The pathologic changes were similar in both norepinephrine-induced and blood-induced chronic vasospasm.

DISCUSSION

The detection of damaged or necrotic smooth muscle cells in association with chronic intracranial arterial vasospasm suggests that actual arterial injury may be important in the etiology of such spasm. If the vasonecrosis were seen only after subarachnoid blood injection, it would be possible to explain it as secondary to some toxic chemical liberated from the clotted blood. Since it also occurs after a single injection of norepinephrine, however, it would appear more likely to be secondary to the initial insult.

The observation that the blood and norepinephrine produce chronic vasospasm with a similar time course and vasonecrosis with similar lesions suggests that both agents may alter the vessel wall by the same mechanisms. Since it has already been demonstrated that subarachnoid blood injection causes liberation of naturally occurring catecholamines, it seems reasonable to postulate that excessive vasoactive amine stimulation produces the vasonecrosis which leads to chronic vasospasm.

Similar electronmicroscopic observations have been made during the study of vessel walls of animals with experimental hypertension. This suggests that the phenomena described may not be applicable only to cerebral arteries but may represent a universal response to excessive sympathetic stimulation. Further study is necessary to elucidate the mechanism and significance of the reaction.

REFERENCES

1. Bloor, B.: Personal communication, 1970.
2. Brawley, B. W., et al.: The biphasic response of cerebral vasospasm in experimental subarachnoid hemorrhage, J. Neurosurg. **28:** 1, 1968.
3. Echlin, F.: Experimental vasospasm, acute and chronic, due to blood in the subarachnoid space, J. Neurosurg. **35:** 646, 1971.
4. Jones, E. G.: On the mode of entry of blood vessels into the cerebral cortex, J. Anat. **106:** 507, 1970.
5. Kagstrom, E., et al.: Changes in cerebral blood flow after subarachnoid hemorrhage, Proc. Third Int. Congress of Neurol. Surg. of World Fed. Neurol. Soc., Amsterdam, 1965, Excerpta Med. Fdn., p. 629.
6. Karlsberg, P., et al.: Effect of various pharmacological agents on cerebral arteries, Neurology **13:** 772, 1963.
7. Maynard, E. A., Shultz, R. L., and Pease, D. C.: Electronmicroscopy of the vascular bed of rat cerebral cortex, Am. J. Anat. **100:** 409, 1957.
8. Nelson, E., Blinzinger, K., and Hager, H.: Electronmicroscopic observations of subarachnoid and perivascular spaces of the Syrian hamster brain, Neurology **11:** 285, 1961.
9. Nelson, E., and Rennels, M.: Innervation of intracranial arteries, Brain **93:** 475, 1970.
10. Peerless, S. J., and Yasargil, M. G.: Adrenergic innervation of the cerebral blood vessels in the rabbit, J. Neurosurg. **35:** 148, 1971.
11. Raynor, R. B., McMurtry, J. G., and Pool, J. L.: Cerebrovascular effects of topically applied serotonin in the cat, J. Neurol. **11:** 190, 1961.
12. Rosenblum, W. I.: Cerebral arteriolar spasm inhibited by β-adrenergic blocking agents, Arch. Neurol. **21:** Sept. 1969.
13. Samarasinghe, D. D.: The innervation of the cerebral arteries in the rat: an electronmicroscope study, J. Anat. **99:** 815, 1965.
14. Simeone, F. A., et al.: Prolonged experimental cerebral vasospasm, J. Neurosurg. **29:** 357, 1968.
15. Stasikowski, J.: Further physiological observations during induced basilar artery spasm in cats and dogs, J. Surg. Res. **10:** 47, 1970.
16. Weir, B., et al.: Vasospasm in response to repeated subarachnoid hemorrhages in the monkey, J. Neurosurg. **33:** 395, 1970.

Contraction of experimental wounds. I. Inhibiting wound contraction by using a topical smooth muscle antagonist

John W. Madden, M.D., Duncan Morton, Jr., M.D., *and* **Erle E. Peacock, Jr., M.D.,** *Tucson, Ariz.*

Several investigators have described unique cells in contracting granulation tissue with structural features suggesting both smooth muscle and fibroblast functions. Additional biochemical and physiological data imply that myofibroblasts participate actively in wound contraction. Paired symmetrical full-thickness dorsal skin wounds were made in 60 rabbits. One wound was dressed with saline daily and served as control. The second was dressed with beta-diethylaminoethyldiphenylthio acetate (Trocinate), a powerful smooth muscle antagonist. Various concentrations of Trocinate were applied for ten days, then discontinued, and wounds observed an additional five days. Rates of collagen and noncollagenous protein synthesis and concentrations were measured using incorporation of H^3-proline. Saline-treated wounds contracted normally, but wounds treated with Trocinate did not contract during the treatment period. Wounds contracted rapidly over 48 hours after Trocinate removal, suggesting a specific inhibition of myofibroblast contractility. Decreasing concentrations of Trocinate produced decreasing inhibition of contraction. Light and electron microscopy showed no evidence of cytotoxicity. Wound contraction is inhibited significantly by local application of a smooth muscle antagonist. Rapid resumption of normal wound contraction following therapy, a dose-response effect, normal protein metabolism, and normal morphological findings suggest that the smooth muscle antagonist may be a specific inhibitor of myofibroblast contraction. These data plus those obtained from human biopsy specimens suggest that a variety of fibro-contractive diseases of man might be controlled by pharmacological inhibition of myofibroblast contraction.

From the Department of Surgery, University of Arizona College of Medicine, Tucson, Ariz.

WITH TIME, full-thickness defects in any mobile area of mammalian skin undergo dramatic changes in size and shape. After a two- to three-day latent period, wounds begin to contract and, by ten days, are less than 30 percent of their original area.[3] Experimental data support the concept that living cells rather than alterations in extracellular mesenchymal material, supply the force moving wound edges together.[19] Recently, Gabbiani and co-workers have identified a specific cell type in granulation tissue which may represent the contractile element.[5] This unique cell combines ultrastructural features of both the fibroblast and smooth muscle cell. Modified fibroblasts ("myofibroblasts") are found free in the connective tissue space without a plasmalemma and have a well-developed system of rough endoplasmic reticulum, both features characteristic of fibroblasts. In addition, myofibroblasts possess deeply indented nuclei, a highly developed system of cytoplasmic

Supported by United States Public Health Grant No. AM 14047, National Institute of Arthritis and Metabolic Diseases, Bethesda, Md.

Presented at the Thirty-fifth Annual Meeting of the Society of University Surgeons, St. Louis, Mo., Feb. 14-16, 1974.

microfilaments, dense bodies, and desmosomes, all features typical of smooth muscle cells.[6] Modified fibroblasts have been identified in contracting tissues from several animal species and in a variety of human fibrocontractive diseases.[5, 12, 13]

Although proving that atypical cells, which are identifiable on ultrastructural criteria alone, supply the motive force for wound contraction is difficult, other data supports this interpretation. In addition to observing myofibroblasts in situations where fibrous tissue undergoes active shortening, biochemical measurements demonstrate that granulation tissue with no skeletal muscle fibers present contains as much actomyosin as pregnant uterus.[6] Human anti-smooth muscle sera label the cytoplasm of myofibroblasts.[9] Granulation tissue containing significant numbers of atypical fibroblasts contracts actively in vitro, behaving as vascular smooth muscle tissue. Strips of tissue excised from ten-day-old granulating wounds contract actively upon addition of 5-hydroxytryptamine, bradykinin, angiotensin, vasopressin, and epinephrine; agents inhibiting contraction of smooth muscle also prevent contraction of granulation tissue in vitro.[14] In addition, avascular fibrous tissue containing large numbers of myofibroblasts contracts in vitro, suggesting that modified fibroblasts themselves rather than newly formed blood vessels are the contractile elements.[17]

If wound contraction is the result of myofibroblastic activity and if myofibroblasts respond to pharmacological agents as smooth muscle cells respond, smooth muscle antagonists should effect the kinetics of wound contraction significantly. The following experiments were performed to test the hypothesis that wound contraction can be inhibited specifically by a topically applied anti-smooth muscle agent.

MATERIALS AND METHODS

Model. California white rabbits of both sexes, weighing between 1.5 and 2.5 kilograms, were caged individually and maintained on standard rabbit chow, cabbage supplement, and water as needed. One day before wounding, dorsal and lateral thoracic skin was shaved closely with electric clippers. Under acepromazine (2 mg. per kilogram) and paraldehyde (0.3 ml. per kilogram) anesthesia, dorsal thoracic skin was prepared with alcohol and symmetrical 4 cm.^{2} areas, 3 cm. from the midline, were tattooed with the use of plexiglass template, 21 gauge needle, and India ink. The template marked the corners and two intermediate positions on each side of a 2 cm. square. Thus, the area for excision was identified with 12 permanent marks. Full-thickness skin was excised immediately within the boundaries of the tattooed dots; the panniculus muscle was preserved. Wounds were dressed individually with cotton balls and isolated from each other with polyethylene drapes cemented at the midline; both dressings were reinforced with gauze sponges and circumferential wraps of elastic bandage. Polyethylene catheters were incorporated into the dressings so that each wound could be treated separately with test solutions. Preliminary experiments demonstrated that this technique isolated each wound effectively; cross-contamination with test solutions did not occur.

At each daily dressing change, wound area was measured by tracing the tattooed marks onto transparent acetate, transferring the traced area onto paper of standard weight, and determining area by weighing the paper cutout.[1] Repeated measurements of the same wound by several observers demonstrated an error of less than two percent by using this technique. One of the paired wounds was selected randomly as the experimental and the second as a control; thus, each animal served as his own control.

Preliminary experiments demonstrated that the contraction of kinetics of a single wound made on the dorsum of the rabbit were not affected by a second wound. Therefore, comparing contraction rates in randomized paired wounds is valid. Unbuffered test solutions of Trocinate in saline had a pH of five. Electrolyte solutions buffered from pH 4.8 through 6.5 with osmolarities over the range created by adding the test

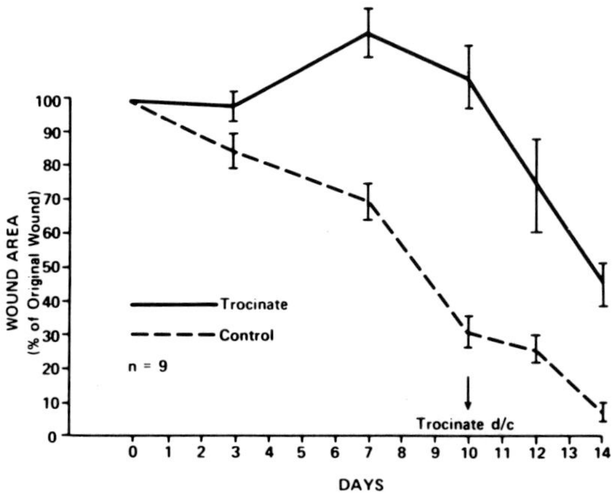

Fig. 1. Area of full-thickness skin wounds treated with saline or 0.02M Trocinate twice daily. When Trocinate was discontinued on the tenth day, wound contraction began immediately; rate of contraction was greater during next four days than control rate during any period.

concentrations of Trocinate to saline did not affect contraction kinetics. Therefore, using normal saline as a control is valid. Although the same template was used to mark all wounds, minor variations in initial wound size occurred. For adequate comparison, area is expressed as a percentage of the initial wound size. To obtain this figure, wound area at any given time was divided by the initial wound area for that specific wound and multiplied by 100.

Experiment 1. Ten rabbits had the experimental wound moistened with a 0.02M solution of beta-diethylaminoethyldiphenylthioacetate (Trocinate) dissolved in saline immediately after wounding and twice daily for ten days. The control wound was treated identically with saline solution. After the area measurements on the tenth day, Trocinate was discontinued and both wounds were moistened with saline and measured daily for an additional four days. In a second group of four animals, panniculus muscle was excised as well as skin and wounds treated as described.

Experiment 2. Two groups of ten rabbits were treated for ten days as in Experiment 1 with 0.015M and 0.01M solutions of Trocinate and saline.

Experiment 3. Five rabbits were treated with 0.02M Trocinate and saline for ten days. Biopsies of the central granulation tissue and the wound edge were obtained on the second, sixth, and tenth day after wounding. Tissue was fixed in Formalin, embedded and sectioned by using standard techniques, and stained with hematoxylin and eosin and Mallory's trichrome.

Experiment 4. Six rabbits were treated with 0.02M Trocinate and saline for ten days. On the tenth day, rabbits were killed, and the central granulation tissue was excised from each wound, leaving the panniculus carnosis intact. Twenty-four hours prior to killing, each animal was given 1 mCi. of H^3-proline (specific activity, 5 Ci. per micromole, New England Nuclear Corporation) intraperitoneally. Excised samples were pulverized under liquid nitrogen, dried to a constant weight, and weighed. Total protein and total hydroxyproline were measured in aliquots of each sample with the use of Lowry's[11] and Woessner's[20] methods. Specific activities of collagenous and non-collagenous proteins were determined by using the Juva-Prockop method.[10]

RESULTS

Experiment 1. During the first three days, control wounds decreased in area by approximately 15 percent. By ten days, the area of control wounds was only 30 percent of initial measurements; by fourteen days, control wounds measured less than ten percent of initial area (Table I). These measurements are comparable to published figures on the contraction of dressed, full-thickness wounds.[3] In contrast, wounds treated twice daily with an 0.02M solution of Trocinate in saline did not contract. By the tenth day, Trocinate-treated wounds were over 100 percent of their initial area (Table I). When Trocinate was discontinued, the experimental wounds contracted rapidly, losing over 30 percent of their area within the first two days (Fig. 1). Rapid contraction continued throughout the four-day observation period. Removing the panniculus had no effect on contraction kinetics or on the effectiveness of Trocinate treatment.

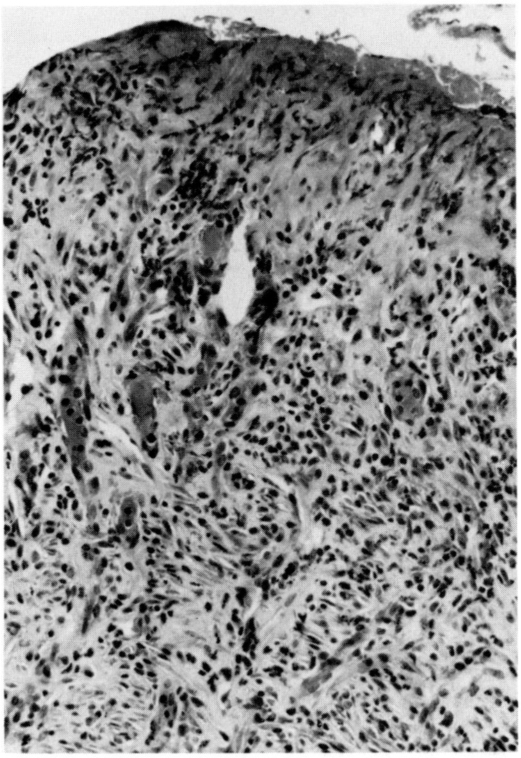

Fig. 2. Microphotograph of ten-day-old control wound. Surface composed of fibrin and inflammatory cells. Deeper areas contain fibroblasts, monocytes, and collagen fibers. (Mallory's trichrome. Original magnification ×250.)

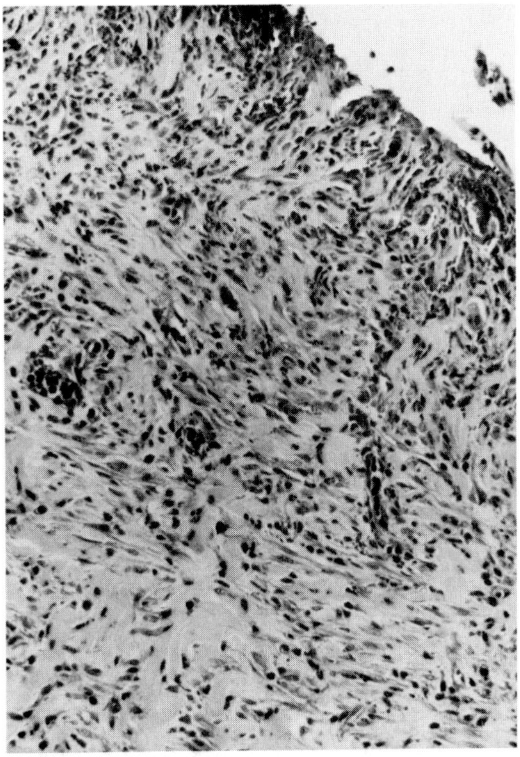

Fig. 3. Microphotograph of ten-day-old wound treated with 0.02M Trocinate. Surface area contains larger numbers of polymorphonuclear leukocytes than control wounds. Deeper areas appear less cellular than in the specimen shown in Fig. 2, but differences of even greater magnitude occurred within groups. (Mallory's trichrome. Original magnification ×250.)

Experiment 2. Intermediate concentrations of Trocinate produced intermediate inhibition of wound contraction (Table I). Mean area at three days was the same in all groups. From the third through the tenth day, however, treated wounds contracted at rates distributed between the control and 0.02M Trocinate values.

Experiment 3. By the second day, treated and control wounds showed a typical inflammatory exudate on the surface composed of fibrin, red blood cells, and polymorphonuclear leukocytes. By the sixth day, epithelial cells were present on the surface of the granulation tissue near the wound edges and appeared to be migrating normally. By the tenth day, both wounds demonstrated abundant granulation tissue composed of capillaries, acute and chronic inflammatory cells, fibroblasts, and large amounts of collagen (Figs. 2 and 3). Granulation tissue from Trocinate-treated wounds contained slightly greater numbers of polymorphonuclear leukocytes than the control wounds; there were no other histological differences between the two groups. The quantity of new vascular tissue, invasion pattern and number of fibroblasts, epithelial migration rates, and pattern of collagen fibers seemed identical in both groups. Although cellular debris was present on the surface, picnotic cells and cellular debris were not prominent in the depths of either control or experimental wounds.

Grossly, Trocinate-treated wounds had a fine, white, pliable surface coating. After removing Trocinate and starting saline irrigations, the surface characteristics of the

Table I. *Area of treated and control wounds (percent of initial wound area, mean ± S.E.)*

Experiment	No.	Days after wounding: 0	3	7	10*	12	13	14
Control	25	100	85 ± 1	67 ± 6	31 ± 4	26 ± 3	12 ± 3	7.8 ± 2
0.02M Trocinate	10	100	97 ± 5	119 ± 6†	106 ± 9†	74 ± 13†	51 ± 9†	41 ± 6†
0.015M Trocinate	10	100	89 ± 4	75 ± 6	60 ± 7			
0.01M Trocinate	6	100	101 ± 5	73 ± 4	48 ± 5			

*Trocinate discontinued at day 10; all wounds dressed with saline thereafter.

†Significantly different than controls, $p < 0.01$.

Table II. *Protein determinations in ten-day-old granulation tissue*

	No.	Total protein: µg protein/mg. dry weight ± SE	Total protein: dpm/µg protein ± SE	Collagen: µmoles hydroxyproline/mg. dry weight ± SE	Collagen: dpm hydroxyproline/µmoles hydroxyproline ± SE
Control	6	530.2 ± 46.2	1.34 ± 0.44	3,866 ± 198	1,634 ± 631
0.02M Trocinate	6	430.0 ± 14.7	1.56 ± 0.52	4,031 ± 175	1,621 ± 651

experimental wounds did not change. In spite of the whitish surface, experimental wounds contracted rapidly once Trocinate was discontinued.

Experiment 4. Total protein and total hydroxyproline measurements were identical in treated and control wounds (Table II). Because each animal served as his own control, specific activity of the proline pool was the same in both wounds. Therefore, specific activity of hydroxyproline and the total incorporation of H^3-proline into protein reflect rate of collagen and non-collagenous protein synthesis. There were no differences in synthetic rates between treated and control wounds (Table II).

DISCUSSION

We selected Trocinate as our test drug because Trocinate inhibits contraction by affecting smooth muscle cells directly, rather than influencing parasympathetic or sympathetic nerve function. Trocinate is as effective as papaverine in preventing $BaCl_2$ induced contractions of human uterus and more than twice as effective in inhibiting contraction of intestinal muscle.[15] In a separate series of in vitro experiments to be reported elsewhere, we demonstrated that Trocinate was as effective in reversing 5-hydroxytryptamine–induced contractions of ten-day-old rabbit granulation tissue as papaverine. Although complete bioavailability studies have not been performed, Trocinate, an ester of a thioacid, should be absorbed rapidly from mucosal and open surfaces. Trocinate has been used clinically as a smooth muscle relaxant for bladder and ureteral spasm.

Our data demonstrate that Trocinate, applied topically, inhibits wound contraction completely. Although this observation supports our hypothesis that wound contraction can be prevented by specific inhibition of myofibroblastic activity, similar effects can be obtained by non-specific cellular toxins. Reynolds and associates[16] injected dinitrophenol, an uncoupler of oxidative phosphorylation, into the granulation tissue of contracting wounds and stopped contraction immediately. Higton and James[8] incubated twelve-day-old splinted granulation tissue in a medium containing potassium cyanide and demonstrated a marked decrease in in vitro contraction. Grillo and Potsaid[7] irradiated contracting wounds and retarded contraction significantly. Billingham and Russell[3] and, later, Stephens and co-workers[18] administered systemic steroid hormones and observed a significant retardation in wound contraction. Any agent killing cells or affecting normal metabolic function seems to inhibit the contraction process. Although proving that the topical application of a smooth muscle antagonist inhibits wound contraction by specifically inhibiting myofibroblastic activity is impossible, immediate resumption of rapid contraction after discontinuing Trocinate, a dose-response effect, normal histological findings, and normal protein metabolism are consistent with a specific inhibition of cell function rather than a non-specific toxic effect.

When Trocinate was removed at ten days, wound contraction resumed immediately without a latent interval. Within 48 hours, wound size was reduced 32 percent. More important, rate of contraction was rapid. Within four days, experimental wounds were comparable in size to ten-day-old control wounds. These data suggest that Trocinate paralyzes rather than destroys the contraction mechanism. In many ways, Trocinate-treated wounds resemble splinted wounds. Ten-day-old open wounds prevented from contracting by mechanical splints contract rapidly when the constraint is removed.[2] Within 48 hours, liberated wounds lose over 40 percent of their area. Trocinate seems to be acting as a pharmacological splint.

Applying intermediate concentrations of Trocinate produced a dose-response curve. Although these data do not prove specificity, they suggest that specific receptor sites on the contraction mechanism are being affected by the drug.

Toxic compounds produce typical histological changes when applied to susceptible tissues. In addition to creating a violent inflammatory response, dead and fragmented cells are a prominent feature. Histological comparisons of Trocinate-treated and control wounds showed only minor morphological variations. Although there were increased numbers of polymorphonuclear leukocytes in some experimental wounds, individual variation was large, and this observation could not account for the marked differences in contraction rates. Dead or fragmented cells were not prominent in either group. These observations suggest that Trocinate produces reversible effects on living cells rather than cytotoxicity.

Regardless of their mode of action, most metabolic poisons produce significant effects on protein metabolism. Any agent altering energy pathways, membrane integrity, or redox reactions ultimately reduces protein synthesis significantly. Trocinate treatment has no effect on protein accumulation or rate of protein synthesis. More important, collagen production by fibroblasts was normal under Trocinate treatment. Neither collagen accumulation, rate of collagen synthesis, nor morphologic patterns of collagen fiber aggregation were affected by Trocinate applications. These data suggest that Trocinate alters cell function specifically and produces few significant toxic effects.

Our data suggest that the pharmacological control of wound contraction in clinical situations where contraction creates permanent deformity may be possible. As an example, if wound contraction could be prevented following massive burns of the neck and extremities until permanent skin grafts could be applied, significant contractures might be avoided. Recently, the differentiation and subsequent contraction of myofibroblasts has been implicated as a cause of several human fibrocontractive diseases. Myofibroblastic cells have been identified as the major cell type in the nodules of Dupuytren's contracture,[4] in transverse carpal ligament from idiopathic carpal tunnel syndrome, in digital theca and tendon nodules from triggering tenosynovitis[12] and in interosseous muscles from ischemic contracture.[13] If fibrocontractive diseases are produced by myofibroblastic cell activity, our data suggest that pharmacological treatment programs may be devised to prevent or reverse the disease process.

SUMMARY AND CONCLUSIONS

1. Topical application of Trocinate, an inhibitor of smooth muscle activity, prevents

contraction of full-thickness skin wounds in rabbits. Control wounds in the same animals contract normally.

2. Accelerated wound contraction begins immediately after removing the smooth muscle antagonist.

3. Inhibition of wound contraction correlates with concentration of the Trocinate solution applied.

4. Histological examination of treated and control wounds did not demonstrate significant morphological differences.

5. Total protein and total collagen accumulation are not altered by Trocinate treatment. Rate of collagen and non-collagenous protein synthesis are identical in treated and control wounds.

6. Our data suggest that Trocinate produces a specific inhibition of the contraction mechanism rather than a non-specific toxic effect.

The authors acknowledge gratefully the techical assistance of Mr. Kenneth K. Keown, Jr., Ms. Linda M. Tillema, and members of the Surgical Biology Laboratory Staff.

REFERENCES

1. Abercrombie, M., Flint, M. H., and James, D. W.: Collagen formation and wound contraction during repair of small excised wounds in the skin of rats, J. Embryol. Exp. Morph. 2: 264, 1954.
2. Abercrombie, M., James, D. W., and Newcombe, J. F.: Wound contraction in rabbit skin, studied by splinting the wound margins, J. Anat. **94:** 170, 1960.
3. Billingham, R. E., and Russell, P. S.: Studies on wound healing, with special reference to contracture in experimental wounds in rabbits' skin, Ann. Surg. **144:** 961, 1956.
4. Gabbiani, G., and Majno, G.: Dupuytren's contracture: Fibroblast contraction? An ultrastructural study, Am. J. Pathol. **66:** 131, 1972.
5. Gabbiani, G., Ryan, G. B., and Majno, G.: Presence of modified fibroblasts in granulation tissue and their possible role in wound contraction, Experimentia. **27:** 549, 1971.
6. Gabbiani, G., Hirschel, B. J., Ryan, G. B., Statkov, P. R., and Majno, G.: Granulation tissue as a contractile organ: A study of structure and function, J. Exp. Med. **135:** 719, 1972.
7. Grillo, H. C., and Potsaid, M. S.: Studies in wound healing. IV. Retardation of contraction by local x-irradiation and observations relating to the origin of fibroblast in repair, Ann. Surg. **154:** 741, 1961.
8. Higton, D. I. R., and James, D. W.: The effect of potassium cyanide on wound contraction, studied in vitro, Br. J. Surg. **51:** 698, 1964.
9. Hirschel, B. J., Gabbiani, G., Ryan, G. B., and Majno, G.: Fibroblasts of granulation tissue: Immunofluorescent staining with anti-smooth muscle serum, Proc. Soc. Exp. Biol. Med. **138:** 466, 1971.
10. Juva, K., and Prockop, D. J.: Modified procedure for the assay of H^3- or C^{14}-labeled hydroxyproline, Ann. Biochem. **15:** 77, 1966.
11. Lowry, O. H., Rosebrough, N. J., Farr, A. L., and Randall, R. J.: Protein measurement with the Folin phenol reagent, J. Biol. Chem. **193:** 265, 1951.
12. Madden, J. W.: On "the contractile fibroblast," Plast. Reconstr. Surg. **52:** 291, 1973.
13. Madden, J. W., Carlson, E. C., and Hines, J.: Presence of modified fibroblasts in ischemic contracture of intrinsic hand musculature: An ultrastructural study, J. Bone Joint Surg. In press.
14. Majno, G., Gabbiani, G., Hirschel, B. J., Ryan, G. B., and Statkov, P. R.: Contraction of granulation tissue in vitro: Similarity to smooth muscle, Science **173:** 548, 1971.
15. Ramsey, H., and Richardson, A. G.: Studies on the pharmacology of beta-diethylaminoethyldiphenylthioacetate, a synthetic antispasmodic, J. Pharmacol. Exp. Therap. **89:** 131, 1947.
16. Reynolds, B. L., Leveque, T. F., Codington, J. B., Mansberger, A. R., and Buxton, R. W.: Wound healing. II. Chemical influence of contraction and migration of regenerate, Am. Surg. **25:** 540, 1959.
17. Ryan, G. B., Cliff, W. J., Gabbiani, G., Irle, C., Statkov, P. R., and Majno, G.: Myofibroblasts in an avascular fibrous tissue, Lab. Invest. **29:** 197, 1973.
18. Stephens, F. O., Dunphy, J. E., and Hunt, T. K.: Effect of delayed administration of corticosteroids on wound contraction, Ann. Surg. **173:** 214, 1971.
19. Van Winkle, W., Jr.: Wound contraction, Surg. Gynecol. Obstet. **125:** 131, 1967.
20. Woessner, J. F., Jr.: The determination of hydroxyproline in tissue and protein samples containing small portions of this amino acid, Arch. Biochem. **93:** 440, 1961.

DISCUSSION

Dr. Thomas Knight Hunt (San Francisco, Calif.). This very interesting material about the fibroblast brings up some other questions about the very nature of the fibroblast itself. Many of you may recall the difficulty pathologists have had over the last several decades deciding whether the cell in atheromata is a fibroblast or a myoblast; now there is perfectly good information to suggest that it is both. Fibroblasts also undertake other forms. For instance, a number of cultures of epithelial cells and other types of muscle cells, and so forth, will produce collagen. It appears that it may be true that the fibroblast is a development of a large number of cells, and I think this is a fundamental questioning of an old concept that the fibroblast is a unique cell.

My request for clarification involves an old definition that many of us are careful to make: What is the difference between contracture and contraction? It is widely held that contraction is that which occurs, as best seen, in the back of the neck and involves the closure by intussusceptive growth of tissue; contracture is that thing which limits the motions of joints.

Personally, I think there is overlap. These data certainly suggest that we might be able to prevent such problems as stricture of the esophagus by the use of these pharmacological materials. Yet contracture does have other properties. For instance, it occurs in areas that have already been epithelialized, and it probably has something to do with cross-binding of collagen in the new form, reinjury, patient's avoidance of pain.

Dr. Marshall J. Orloff (San Diego, Calif.). I would just like to ask Dr. Madden if he has tried to stimulate, by pharmacologic means, the contraction of the myofibrils.

Dr. Paul Richard Schloerb (Kansas City, Kan.). What is the effect on epithelial growth?

Dr. John W. Madden (closing). I do not think we have any argument at all in terms of contraction versus contracture. Contraction is an active process which brings the wound edges together in any open wound present for a long time. Contracture is the end result of that process: the fixed shortening that is usually present when wounds are epithelialized. What I am talking about is influencing the active contraction, or the active movement of wound edges together.

The question of what are these cells and where do they come from is exciting. We have been able to find patients who have a peculiar disease called intrinsic contracture of the interosseous muscles, that have a number of these cells, but unlike some of Gabbiani's patients and our other patients who have these cells, it looks as if there is a continuum between smooth muscle cells and standard fibroblasts.

As you know, Russell Ross, in culturing smooth muscle cells, has been able to show without any question that they do produce collagen in culture and that they also produce glycose aminoglycans.

As far as attempting to make cells contract faster—it turns out that if you take out strips of granulation tissue from the center of a ten-day-old wound, put them in a waterbath, add 5-hydroxytryptamine, they do not contract. Nothing happens. It turns out that myofibroblasts within that tissue are in a state of maximum contraction. If you take the tissue, then, and stretch it, or add a resistance to it, then add 5-hydroxytryptamine to it, it contracts.

Now, in many other instances—for example the fibrous capsules that form around blood clots in the peritoneal cavity—they do not have any vessels in them, and they are not in this state of permanent contraction. They have a lot of myofibroblasts. If you put those in waterbaths and add 5-hydroxytryptamine, or other agents, they contract readily, without being stretched. However, in vitro you can do this quite nicely. You can take cyanide, or materials like this, and prevent in vitro contraction, but you can also speed up the contraction by adding ATP or a number of other energy substances which will make these tissues contract. In the granulating wound, they are normally under a state of maximum contraction, but you can alter them in vitro.

There is no effect whatsoever on the rate of epithelialization or the patterns of epithelialization in these wounds that were treated with Trocinate.

Radioimmunoassay for mouse mammary tumor virus–associated antigen

P. Lo Gerfo, M.D., G. Silverstein, *New York, N. Y., and* **J. Charney,** *Camden, N. J.*

Mouse mammary tumor virus (MTV) was labeled with I^{125} and rebanded in 1.18 Gm. per milliliter of sucrose. Rebanded labeled intact particles were used in this assay. An inhibition double-antibody assay was employed that allowed viral antigen detection in a 1:25,000 dilution of RIII mouse milk. The quantity of this viral-associated antigen (VAA) in Paris RIII and C-57 BL milk was determined. Milk from a tumor-free colony of C-57 BL mice contains detectable amounts of VAA. Although inhibition curves from milk of these animals was similar to those obtained with purified virus, this finding does not imply that these animals shed intact virus into their milk. The levels of VAA in C-57 BL animals who received MTV during the neonatal period correlated with the eventual development of mammary tumors, and it was easy to predict which animals were susceptible to tumor development. Inhibition curves with Tween-treated virus and intact virus suggest that envelop antigen was being detected by the assay.

From the Department of Surgery, College of Physicians and Surgeons of Columbia University, and the Institute for Cancer Research, New York, N. Y., and the Institute for Medical Research, Camden, N. J.

SEVERAL INVESTIGATORS have described methods of detecting antigens related to murine mammary tumor virus (MTV).[2, 4, 10] Detection of these soluble viral associated antigens (VAA's) in C-57 BL mouse milk by immunodiffusion (ID) techniques has been used to determine virus infectivity in these animals.[5, 6, 7] Fifty percent of C-57 BL mice injected with MTV during the neonatal period have detectable VAA in their milk at first lactation. This percentage increases markedly when third lactation specimens are tested. The correlation of tumor development with demonstrable VAA's is excellent.[6] The immunodiffusion techniques, however, lack the sensitivity for in depth studies of tissues and ID negative milk specimens. In addition, it is difficult to quantitate the amount of VAA's present. The current investigation was undertaken to develop a radioimmunoassay for MTV associated antigens which would increase our ability to detect these antigens and provide for antigen quantitation.

Supported by the Overlook Fund and Cancer Research Center Grant No. CA-13-696-01.

Presented at the Thirty-fifth Annual Meeting of the Society of University Surgeons, St. Louis, Mo., Feb. 14-16, 1974.

METHODS AND MATERIALS

MTV was isolated from Paris RIII/Haag milk (Columbia University) using a sucrose density gradient.[12] MTV was also prepared from mouse mammary tumors by tumor tissue disruption, sonification, and density gradient centrifugation. Most of the intact virus particles were found at a sucrose density of 1.18 Gm. per milliliter. The 260 nm./280 nm. ratio on this virus band was 1.10 to 1.17 depending on the MTV preparation tested.[15] Viral protein determinations were

Vol. 76, No. 1, pp. 16-22

done on Tween 80–treated virus (0.25 percent Tween at 56° C. for 30 minutes) using the method of Lowry and associates.[11]

Purified MTV prepared from milk was used to produce antisera in adult New Zealand rabbits.[7] Absorption of the MTV antisera was accomplished by using tissue and milk from a tumor-free strain of C-57 BL mice. Two milliliters of milk were added to 1 ml. of rabbit antiserum. To ensure complete absorption, liver, spleen, and mammary tissue (1 Gm. of each) was homogenized in 15 ml. of phosphate-buffered saline (PBS) (0.05 M phosphate, pH 7.4) and added to the latter. This mixture was incubated at 37° C. for one hour and then overnight at 4° C. The solution was then cleared by centrifugation at 12,000× gravity. The incubation, refrigeration, and centrifugation were repeated three times.

Radiolabeled MTV was prepared by the method of Hunter and Greenwood.[9] The final reaction mixture contained 5 mc: I^{125}, 50 μg of MTV, and 0.1 mg. of chloramine T in 0.3 ml. The reaction was allowed to proceed for 1.5 minutes and then stopped by the addition of 0.24 mg. of sodium metabisulfite. The mixture was drawn up in PBS (5 ml.) and dialyzed against 4 L. of saline at 4° C. The dialysate was changed eight times in an 18 hour period. The labeled virus was then rebanded on a discontinuous sucrose gradient at 35,000× gravity for 90 minutes. Most of the labeled material was found in the 1.18 Gm. per milliliter band and this was used for all assays. Electron microscopy was carried out on this labeled rebanded material.[15] The diluent used throughout this study consisted of a one percent solution of Plasmanate* in phosphate-buffered (0.01 M phosphate Ph 7.4) and 0.01 percent sodium azide.

A dilution curve was carried out in 1 ml. centrifuge tubes which contained 0.2 ml. of diluent and 50 μl of anti-MTV antiserum at the appropriate dilution. As a control, preimmunization rabbit serum was run at the same dilutions. After incubation at 37° C. for one hour, I^{125} MTV (20,000 c.p.m. per 0.1 ml.) was added, and the tubes were reincubated for one hour at 37° C. The appropriate dilution of sheep anti-rabbit globulin was added,[11] and a final incubation of one hour at 37° C. was performed. The tubes were placed in the cold (4° C.) overnight and diluent was added to fill each tube (0.7 ml.). The tubes were spun at 7,000× gravity for ten minutes to separate the antigen antibody complexes. The supernatant and precipitate were counted, and the percentage of I^{125} bound to the antigen antibody complexes was determined.

A standard inhibition curve was carried out by adding purified virus (0.1 ml.), diluent (0.1 ml.), and a constant amount of antisera (50 μl of a 1:1000 dilution). After incubation at 37° C. for one hour, I^{125} MTV (20,000 c.p.m. per 0.1 ml.) was added, and the tubes were reincubated for one hour at 37° C. The appropriate dilution of sheep anti-rabbit globulin was added,[11] and a final incubation of one hour at 37° C. was performed. The tubes were placed in the cold (4° C.) overnight and diluent was added to fill each tube (0.7 ml.). The tubes were spun at 7,000× gravity for ten minutes to separate the antigen antibody complexes. The supernatant and precipitate were counted and the percentage of I^{125} bound to the antigen antibody complexes was determined. Inhibition curves on C-57 BL and RIII milk were carried out in a similar manner, except that diluted milk was substituted for purified virus. Studies on mouse milk were carried out on Tween-treated specimens except where indicated. In order to have sample values fall in the sensitive area of the inhibition curve, most specimens had to be diluted 20:1, and those with high titers required dilutions as high as 100:1. Immunodiffusion studies on mouse milk were carried out as previously described.[5] Inhibition curves with Rauscher virus and Gross leukemia were done by substituting these viruses in place of purified MTV.*

*Cutler Laboratories, Berkeley, Calif.

*Rauscher leukemia virus from Balb C mice and Gross leukemia virus from C-57 BL mice were kindly supplied by Dr. Kuff, Columbia University, Institute for Cancer Research, New York, N. Y.

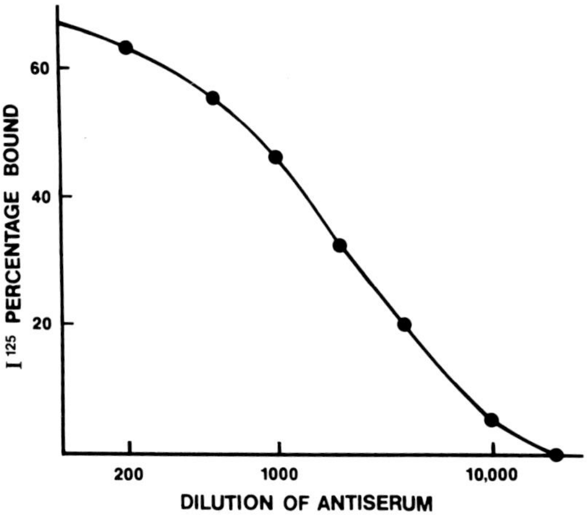

Fig. 1. Titration of rabbit anti-MTV serum using constant amount of MTV-I^{125} and increasing dilutions of antiserum. Percentage of the I^{125} bound to antigen-antibody complexes using a double-antibody precipitation technique is plotted on ordinate. This graph represents the dilution of the antiserum added. The final antiserum dilution would be 6.05 times greater.

Virus-free C-57 BL mice which normally do not develop tumors were inoculated with MTV during the neonatal period and milk was obtained from individual animals at the first and third lactation.[5] These milk specimens were then studied for the presence of viral antigens by using immunodiffusion and radioimmunoassay techniques. The mice were followed for a period of 18 months to determine which animals would develop tumors. The results of the immunodiffusion testing for VAA on the first and third lactations has been previously correlated with eventual tumorigenesis.[5] On the basis of these studies, the animals were divided into three groups. Animals belonging in Group I were those whose milk did not contain viral antigen(s) at first or third lactation. Group I animals never developed tumors. Animals belonging in Group II were those whose initial milk specimen was negative for viral antigen(s), but which eventually shed viral antigen(s) into their milk at the third lactation. Eighty-six percent of these Group II animals developed tumors. Group III contained those animals whose milk contained viral antigen(s) at both first and third lactation. Ninety percent of Group III animals developed tumors. Milk from these three groups was then analyzed for VAA by radioimmunoassay.

RESULTS

Electron microscopy studies on I^{125}-labeled virus show intact B type particles with little or no cellular debris. The dilution curve obtained with the use of this virus is shown in Fig. 1. The MTV antisera bound 70 to 74 percent of the labeled virus at a 1:200 antiserum dilution. This binding was completely blocked by prior absorption of the antisera with purified MTV prepared from milk, RIII tumor tissue, or milk from RIII mice which contained virus.

The standard inhibition curve obtained with purified virus is shown in Fig. 2. Fifteen nanograms of VAA can be detected with this assay. The inhibition curves with Tween-treated virus, iodinated virus, and virus prepared from tumor tissue extracts were identical (the latter not illustrated). This indicates that the antigenic site being detected on the virus is not altered by treatment with Tween or by our labeling process. No inhibition of binding was seen with purified Rauscher leukemia virus (RLV) or Gross leukemia virus (GLV) at any antiserum dilution. Addition of RLV to milk containing small quantities of VAA did not increase the amount of inhibition.

Analysis of third lactation Tween-treated RIII milk is shown in Table I. All specimens were positive by ID for viral antigen. These specimens contained 200 to 400 μg of VAA per milliliter. This represents a dry weight for the virus. Since the virus contains significant quantities of lipid (30 percent), the weight of hydrated virus would presumably be greater. Milk from a tumor-free colony of C-57 BL mice which never contains VAA by ID contained significant amounts of VAA when tested by RIA (Table I). The quantities of VAA as determined by RIA were 1/25 to 1/50 of that found in RIII specimens. Inhibition studies carried out with C-57 BL milk having the largest quantities of VAA were identical to those obtained with purified virus (Fig. 2). The density of this in-

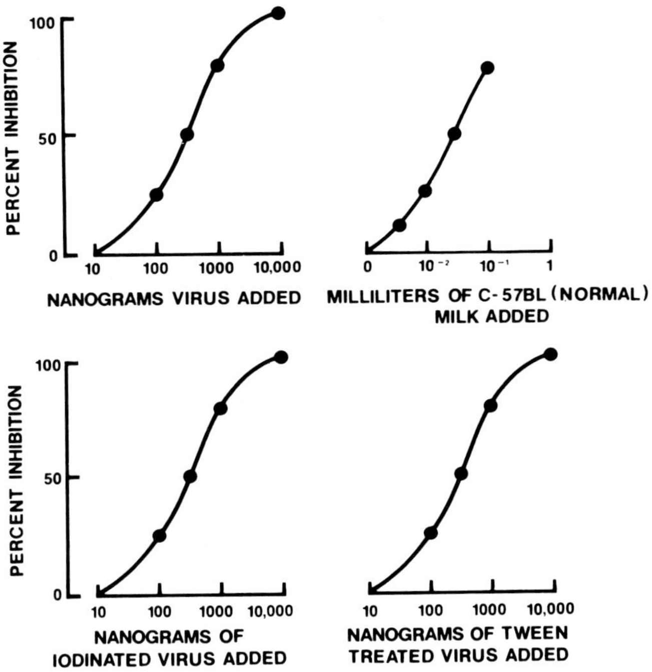

Fig. 2. Inhibition curves obtained by addition of purified MTV, C-57 BL milk, iodinated MTV, or Tween-treated MTV to a constant amount of MTV antisera and MTV-I^{125}. The final antisera dilution is 6,050. Percentage inhibition is plotted on the ordinate.

hibiting antigen in C-57 BL milk was less than that of purified MTV (1.12 Gm. per milliliter or less vs. 1.18 Gm. per milliliter). This suggests that the inhibiting substance in C-57 BL milk contains the same antigenic site as that found in MTV but that it is nonviral in nature. Complete blocking of the antisera could be obtained by prior absorption with large amounts of C-57 BL milk (100:1). It is possible, of course, that this material was adhering to the MTV in RIII milk and was not part of the virus itself. In order to test this, RLV was added to C-57 BL milk and the density of the inhibiting material was determined. Again, the density of the inhibiting substance was less than that of purified RLV, indicating that the material did not bind to RLV.

It is possible to induce mammary tumors in some C-57 BL mice by infecting them with virus in the neonatal period. There is a good correlation with the presence of viral antigens in milk at the third lactation by ID and eventual tumor development.[6, 7] It is therefore important to establish a similar correlation by using a RIA to detect viral antigens. After infection with MTV, each C-57 BL mouse had its milk examined at the first and third lactation by using ID and RIA. All milk specimens that were positive for viral antigens by ID contained greater than 40 μg per milliliter of VAA as determined by RIA. All specimens negative by ID con-

Table I. *Levels of viral-associated antigen determined by radioimmunoassay (µl/ml. of milk)*

*RIII**	*C-57†*
400	8.2
228	12.0
460	16.4
346	14.2
410	9.2
324	9.4
318	10.3
474	10.7
298	11.4
540	8.7

*Third lactation specimens. Ninety-six percent of these mice developed tumors. All specimens were positive by immunodiffusion.

†Random lactations (3 to 5). Tumor-free colony. All specimens were negative by immunodiffusion.

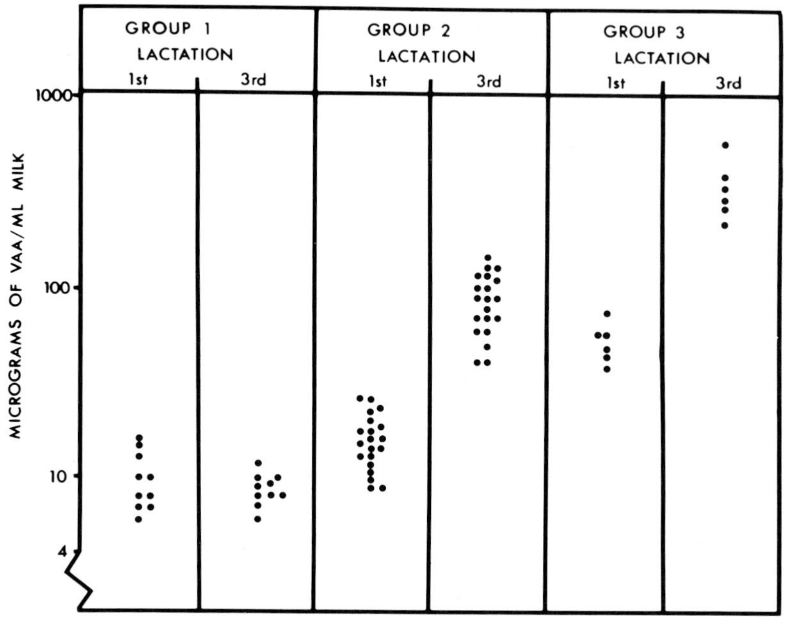

Fig. 3. C-57 BL mice infected with MTV. Group I were mice whose milk did not contain viral antigen(s) by ID at first or third lactation. These animals never developed tumors. Group II were mice whose milk was negative for viral antigen(s) at first lactation but had viral antigen(s) present by ID at third lactation. Eighty-six percent of Group II animals developed tumors. Group III were mice whose milk contained viral antigen(s) by ID at first and third lactation. Ninety-two percent of animals in Group III developed tumors. The level of VAA was determined by radioimmunoassay.

tained less than 16 μg per milliliter of VAA.

Milk from Group I animals which never developed tumors contained less than 16 μg per milliliter of VAA at both first and third lactations (Fig. 3). Group III animals which have a 92 percent tumor incidence and whose milk was positive by ID at first and third lactation all produced milk containing greater than 40 μg per milliliter regardless of lactation tested. Group II animals which have an 86 percent tumor incidence and negative first lactation milk specimens by ID had variable amounts of VAA by RIA (8 to 30 μg per milliliter) at the first lactation. The third lactation specimen in all instances contained greater than 40 μg per milliliter. In essence we can say that all animals which developed tumor shed at the least 40 μg per milliliter of VAA into their milk at third lactation.

DISCUSSION

A radioimmunoassay has been developed to detect antigens associated with mouse mammary tumor virus. There is no cross-reactivity with other common mouse oncogenic RNA viruses. Inhibition studies which use MTV prepared from tumor tissue and milk indicate that we are not studying a milk protein absorbed on the surface of the virus. Using this assay, we have been able to detect as little as 15 ng. of virus antigen and have been able to quantitate the amounts of this antigen in mouse milk. Paris RIII mice shed large amounts of viral antigen into their milk even at early lactations.

The antisera used in this study are multivalent[7] and may be detecting several viral antigens. Investigations are now underway to determine which antigen(s) is being detected. At the present time, it seems reasonable to postulate that viral surface antigen(s) may be involved since intact virus particles are employed as the radiolabeled antigen. In favor of this hypothesis is the fact that Tween treatment, which would be expected to expose internal viral antigen(s),[13, 14] does not increase the amount of inhibition or change the shape of the inhibition curve. The presence of small amounts of VAA in C-57 BL mouse milk from a virus-free colony suggests that envelop antigen(s) coded by the genetic material in the host is being detected.[1] At least three viral envelop antigens have been reported and Blair[2] provides some evidence that a common envelop antigen exists.

The finding of VAA in virus-free C-57 BL milk was unexpected, and it would be tempting to attribute this to an incompletely absorbed cross-reacting antigen. Inhibition curves using C-57 BL milk strongly support the view that the antigen is truly viral related. It has been suggested by other investigators that every mouse strain carries the genetic information for MTV and that this information may be only partially expressed.[12] VAA may in part represent this expression and does not necessarily imply that intact virus are present. In fact, our studies have shown that the antigen(s) present in C-57 BL milk does not have the density of intact MTV, and we believe it is the membrane antigen on host cells which would become viral envelop if virus replication took place. The presence of such an antigen may be interpreted to imply that these host cells are genetically susceptible to MTV infection.

In view of these results, absorption of our antiserum with C-57 BL milk might be open to criticism. However, since our antiserum is not virus-specific without absorption of antibodies against milk protein, some form of absorption with mouse milk is necessary. This absorption results in a slight decrease in our antiserum titer against virus but does not affect our assay. If extensive absorption with C-57 BL milk is carried out (100:1) complete blocking of the antiserum activity takes place. This problem of milk absorption is a difficult one since the antiserum might be detecting a milk protein which adheres to the virus surface. Our data suggests that this is not so because virus prepared directly from mammary tumor extracts produces the same inhibition curve as virus prepared from milk. In addition, when RLV is added to milk containing small quantities of VAA, no increase in inhibition occurs, as determined by radioimmunoassay. If milk protein were binding to the virus surface, it must therefore bind to MTV and not RLV.

The predictive value of RIA in identifying animals susceptible to tumor development was identical to that previously reported for ID.[7] The high levels of VAA in milk from mice susceptible to tumor development did not always occur until the third lactation, and the time required to carry out predictive studies was not shortened by use of RIA. The increase of VAA above background levels probably represents an increase in viral envelop antigen associated with active virus replication rather than just an increase in virus. This hypothesis will require testing in other mouse models. The correlation between the ID data and data obtained by RIA does not mean that both methods are detecting the same antigen(s). Preliminary information in our laboratory would suggest that the antigen detected by radioimmunoassay is intact membrane which does not diffuse in gel.

REFERENCES

1. Bentvelzen, P., Daams, J. H., Hageman, P., Calafat, J., and Timmermans, A.: Interaction between viral and genetic factors in the origin of mammary tumors in mice, J. Natl. Cancer Inst. **48:** 1089, 1972.
2. Blair, P. B.: Immunology of the mouse mammary tumor virus (MTV): A qualitative in vitro assay for MTV, Nature **208:** 165, 1965.
3. Blair, P. B.: Immunology of the mouse mammary tumor virus: Comparison of the antigenicity of mammary tumor virus obtained from several strains of mice, Cancer Res. **30:** 625, 1970.
4. Blair, P. B., and Weiss, D. W.: Immunology of the mouse mammary tumor virus: Comparison of mammary tumor virus with the agent found in C3Hf/Crgl mice, J. Natl. Cancer Inst. **36:** 423, 1966.
5. Charney, J., Pullinger, B. D., and Moore, D. H.: A rapid assay for Bittner virus by the immunologic detection of virus antigen in the milk of inoculated mice, Proc. Am. Assoc. Cancer Res. **9:** 13, 1968.
6. Charney, J., Pullinger, B. D., and Moore, D. H.: Conference on Immunology of Mouse Mammary Tumors, Institute for Medical Research, Camden, N. J., Nov., 1968, Science **163:** 1230, 1968.
7. Charney, J., Pullinger, B. D., and Moore, D. H.: Development of an infectivity assay

for mouse mammary tumor virus, J. Natl. Cancer Inst. **43:** 1289, 1969.
8. Hales, L. N., and Randall, R. J.: Immunoassay of insulin with insulin-antibody precipitate, J. Biochem. **88:** 137, 1963.
9. Hunter, W. M., and Greenwood, F. C.: Preparation of I^{131} labeled growth hormone, Nature **194:** 495, 1964.
10. Lezhneva, O. M.: A comparative study of the antigenic structure of the lactating mammary gland of high and low cancer strain mice, Probl. Oncol. (U.S.S.R.) (English trans.) **7:** 62, 1961.
11. Lowry, O. H., Rosebrough, N. J., Farr, A. L., and Randall, R. J.: Protein measurement with the Folin phenol reagent, J. Biol. Chem. **193:** 265, 1951.
12. Lyons, M. J., and Moore, D. H.: Isolation of the mouse mammary tumor virus: Chemical and morphological studies, J. Natl. Cancer Inst. **35:** 549, 1965.
13. Nowinski, R. C., Old, L. J., Geering, G., and Boyse, E. A.: A soluble antigen of the mammary tumor virus, Virology **31:** 1, 1967.
14. Nowinski, R. C., Sarkar, N. H., Old, L. J., et al.: Characteristics of the structural components of the mouse mammary tumor virus. II. Viral proteins and antigens, Virology **46:** 21, 1971.
15. Sarkar, N. H., Nowinski, R. C., and Moore, D. H.: Characteristics of the structural components of the mouse mammary tumor virus. I. Morphological and biochemical studies, Virology **46:** 1, 1971.

DISCUSSION

Dr. Yosef H. Pilch (Torrance, Calif.). Have you had a chance as yet to screen either human milk or human serum for these antigens and have you attempted to do these studies in patients with breast cancer, as opposed to normal patients?

Dr. Paul Lo Gerfo (closing). We really have not done any human studies. However, we would like to.

I would rather work with a human antiserum against a human particle. However, to label the human particles has been a very, very difficult thing, because it is very hard to free them from the other cellular debris. Spiegelman has developed a method of using cores of viruses, and maybe we can do it using that.

The only comment I would like to make is that we really do not know what the relationship of this virus is to human cancer, and I do not want anyone to go away with the idea that I really, strongly feel that it causes human cancer. The idea is that in humans you can find this virus distributed in almost any milk you would look at. If you take milk samples at random from populations, you can find it distributed all over. Whether it causes human breast cancer is really open to question.

The second thing is that probably, if it is related to human breast cancer, it would probably be more related to something like lobular carcinoma, which is more in line with the mouse model than the average carcinoma we see.

The one thing that is important about this study, though, is that we are not looking at a virus, really. We are looking at a genetic make-up of the cell. That is really the key. I think the goal would be to work with cell membranes and to look for genetic differences between people in the normal human population and people with breast cancer.

Immune cytolysis of human tumor cells mediated by xenogeneic "immune" RNA: Implications for immunotherapy

Yosef H. Pilch, M.D., Larry L. Veltman, M.D., *and* **David H. Kern, Ph.D.,** *Los Angeles, Calif.*

Using a quantitative assay for lymphocyte-mediated cytotoxicity, it showed that normal, nonimmune human lymphocytes were converted to effector cells specifically cytotoxic to human tumor cells in vitro by incubation with "immune" RNA extracted from the lymphoid organs of specifically immunized guinea pigs or sheep. Lymphocytes incubated without RNA or with control RNA preparations failed to show cytotoxic activity. These immune responses were abrogated when the "immune" RNA was treated with RNase prior to incubation with lymphocytes. Treatment with DNase or pronase did not alter the activity of the "immune" RNA. RNA concentrations as low as 100 μg per milliliter were active in this system.

From the Department of Surgery, Harbor General Hospital, Torrance, Calif., The Tumor Immunology Laboratory, Veterans Administration Hospital, Sepulveda, Calif., and the UCLA School of Medicine, Los Angeles, Calif.

INTEREST in the role of ribonucleic acids extracted from specifically sensitized lymphoid cells as mediators of immune responses was initiated in 1961 when Fishman and Adler[7, 8] demonstrated that RNA, extracted from normal rat macrophages exposed in vitro to T2 phage could transfer to normal, nonimmune rat lymph node cells the capacity to produce specific antibodies to T2 phage antigen. Mannick and Egdahl[10] and, subsequently, Sabbadini and Sehon[19] demonstrated that immunity to skin allografts could be transferred to previously untreated rabbits by the intravenous administration of autologous spleen cells which have been preincubated with RNA extracted from the lymphoid organs of specifically immunized donor rabbits. Alexander and associates[1] reported growth retardation and occasional temporary regression of benzpyrene-induced sarcomas in rats treated by footpad injections of RNA extracted from lymph cells of sheep immunized with the particular rat tumor being treated.

Ramming and Pilch,[12-15, 18] and Deckers and Pilch[4] then applied the above models to the mediation of anti-tumor immune responses and were able to show, in mouse and rat tumor-host systems, that tumor-specific transplantation immunity could be conferred upon previously untreated, syngeneic animals by the administration of syngeneic lymphoid cells preincubated with xenogeneic "immune" RNA extracted from the lymphoid organs of guinea pigs previously immunized with the tumor to be treated. Confirmation of the capacity of xenogeneic "immune" RNA to mediate cellular immune responses was provided by Paque and Dray.[11] They incubated xenogeneic "immune" RNA, ex-

Supported in part by United States Public Health Service Grant No. CA 14846, Grant No. ET-28 from the American Cancer Society, and by research funds from the Veterans Administration.

Presented at the Thirty-fifth Annual Meeting of the Society of University Surgeons, St. Louis, Mo., Feb. 14-16, 1974.

tracted from the lymphoid organs of monkeys immunized with complete Freund's adjuvant or with the H37RA strain of *M. tuberculosis,* with normal, nonimmune human leukocytes, and they demonstrated that these leukocytes would then mediate the inhibition of migration of guinea pig peritoneal exudate cells when tuberculin was added to the medium. This was the first report of the interspecies transfer of a cellular immune response from animal to man with "immune" RNA.

In the present paper, we report the transfer of cellular immune responses to human tumor cells in vitro mediated by xenogeneic "immune" RNA. In these studies, normal, nonimmune human lymphocytes were converted into "killer cells," which effected immune cytolysis of human tumor cells, by incubation with "immune" RNA extracted from the lymph nodes and spleens of sheep or guinea pigs which had previously been immunized with cells from the particular human tumor being studied.

MATERIALS AND METHODS

The tumors employed were: (1) a human gastric adenocarcinoma, RI-H, established in tissue culture in our laboratory by primary explant from a surgical specimen, and studied in its twelfth to fourteenth passage; (2) a human adenocarcinoma of the breast, BT-20, obtained from Dr. E. Lasfargues, and studied in its three hundredth to three hundred tenth passage; (3) a human malignant melanoma, ED-H, explanted from a surgical specimen in our laboratory and studied in its eighteenth to twenty-fifth passage; and (4) a human melanoma, RO-H, established from a primary explant, in its tenth to fifteenth passage. These cells were maintained in RPMI 1640 supplemented with 20 percent fetal calf serum, which contained 0.15 percent glutamine, 0.25 mg. per milliliter of amphotericin B, 100 I.U. per milliliter of penicillin, and 100 mg. per milliliter of streptomycin or with 20 percent human serum containing the same additives. When cells from the thirteenth passage of the RI-H line were injected into the cheek pouch of an immunosuppressed hamster, a tumor developed which was histologically similar to the original tumor. Between 10^7 and 10^8 viable tumor cells (determined by exclusion of 0.4 percent trypan blue) in 3 ml. RPMI 1640 were emulsified in an equal volume of complete Freund's adjuvant and injected, intradermally into all four extremities of sheep at weekly intervals for three consecutive weeks. In most instances, tumor cells for immunization were harvested from monolayer cultures with 0.2 percent trypsin; in one instance (a melanoma), tumor cells were obtained from a fresh surgical specimen. Ten days after the last injection, the animals were killed, and the spleen and mesenteric lymph nodes were harvested and immediately frozen in dry ice. Hartley guinea pigs were also immunized by the administration of 10^7 tumor cells in 0.5 ml. of medium emulsified in an equal volume of complete Freund's adjuvant and injected in 0.25 ml. aliquots into each foot pad. A simultaneous intraperitoneal injection of 10^7 tumor cells in 0.5 ml. medium without adjuvant was also given. These animals were killed ten days later, and the axillary and inguinal lymph nodes and the spleens were frozen in dry ice.

"Immune" RNA was extracted from the frozen lymphoid tissue by the hot phenol method of Ramming and Pilch.[18] Control RNA preparations were also extracted from the spleens and lymph nodes of other guinea pigs and other sheep were immunized with complete Freund's adjuvant only. The RNA content was determined by the Orcinol reaction, the DNA content was determined by the diphenylamine reaction of Dische,[6] and the protein concentration by the method of Lowry.[9] In some experiments, "immune" RNA was treated with ribonuclease, deoxyribonuclease, or pronase as previously described by Ramming and Pilch.[18] The RNA preparations were also analyzed with respect to their sedimentation characteristics by ultracentrifugation in five to twenty percent continuous sucrose gradients.[18]

In early experiments, heparinized blood (120 ml.) was drawn by venopuncture from

Table I. *Immune cytolysis of RI-H tumor cells mediated by "immune" RNA**

	Experiment 1 *RNA donor: Sheep*		*Experiment 2* *RNA donor: Sheep*		*Experiment 3* *RNA donor: Guinea pig*	
	Cytotoxicity index	*p*	*Cytotoxicity index*	*p*	*Cytotoxicity index*	*p*
Leukocytes incubated with:						
"Immune" RNA†	0.45 ± 0.08		0.30 ± 0.05		0.41 ± 0.13	
"Immune" RNA + ribonuclease‡	0.18 ± 0.14	< 0.05	0.38 ± 0.05	< 0.005	−0.37 ± 0.08	< 0.005
Freund's adjuvant RNA§	−0.10 ± 0.18	< 0.005	−0.30 ± 0.05	< 0.005	−0.20 ± 0.10	< 0.005
No RNA	0.0 ± 0.14	< 0.01	0.0 ± 0.15	< 0.01	0.0 ± 0.07	< 0.025

*Only leukocyte-to-target cell ratios of 500:1 are included in the table. Six replicate wells were used for each determination and mean cytotoxicity indices with their standard deviations are presented. The p values were calculated by Student's t test for unpaired data and represent differences between "immune" RNA and the various control groups.

†RNA from the lymphoid organs of animals immunized with RI-H tumor cells.

‡"Immune" RNA treated with ribonuclease prior to incubation with leukocytes.

§RNA from the lymphoid organs of animals immunized with Freund's adjuvant only.

normal human volunteers, and the red cells were allowed to sediment following the addition of ten percent Plasmagel* at 37° C. for one hour. The white cell–rich supernatant was then centrifuged at 1000 × g for ten minutes and treated with 0.85 percent ammonium chloride at room temperature for five minutes to lyse residual red blood cells. The remaining leukocytes were washed twice with RPMI 1640 and counted. In subsequent experiments, purified lymphocyte populations were prepared from heparinized blood specimens on Ficol-Isopaque gradients, suspended in RPMI 1640 with 40 percent agamma human serum and ten percent dimethylsulfoxide (DMSO), and frozen in liquid nitrogen at 1° C. per minute. Prior to use, the lymphocytes were thawed at 37° C. and washed twice with RPMI 1640 to remove DMSO. One ml. RPMI 1640 containing 1.5 × 10^7 lymphocytes (or leukocytes) was incubated with 1 ml. of the appropriate RNA preparation at a concentration of 2 mg. per milliliter for 20 minutes at 37° C. in a gyrotory shaking water bath. The cells were washed twice with RPMI 1640 supplemented with 20 percent fetal calf serum and diluted to the appropriate cell concentration for addition to the target cells (see below).

The assay for immune cytolysis employed was a modification of the ^{125}I-iododeoxyuridine (^{125}IDU) assay of Cohen and associates.[3] Tumor cells were harvested from monolayer cultures with 0.2 percent trypsin, washed once in medium, counted, and diluted so that 10^6 cells were contained in 4 ml. of medium. This cell suspension was then added to 30 ml. plastic tissue culture flasks. At this time, 1 ml. of medium containing 60 μc ^{125}IDU* and 10^{-6}M FUDR (fluorodeoxyuridine)† was added to the flask. After incubation at 37° C. for 24 hours, the cells were trypsinized, washed twice in medium, counted, and diluted to a concentration of 10^4 cells per milliliter. One thousand tumor cells in 0.1 ml. medium were added to each well of Falcon Microtest II plates.‡ The RNA-incubated lymphocytes (or control lymphocytes) were then added to each well, in 0.2 ml. of medium, in lymphocyte:target cell ratios of from 2000:1 to 100:1. The plates were incubated at 37° C. for 48 hours, and the wells were then washed four times with medium to remove debris and dead tumor cells which detached from the well bottoms during the incubation. After drying in air, the plates were sprayed with Aeroplast,§ and the individual wells were separated by cutting the plates with a band saw. The radioactivity in each well was

*Roger Bellon Laboratories, Neuilly, France.

*NEX-072, New England Nuclear, Boston, Mass.
†Hoffmann-LaRoche, Nutley, N. J.
‡Falcon Plastics, Oxnard, Calif.
§Parke-Davis, Detroit, Mich.

measured in an automatic gamma counting system.* The counts recorded were then a measure of the viable tumor cells which remained adherent to the well bottoms and not killed by the lymphocytes. Six replicate wells were prepared identically for each lymphocyte to target cell ratio for each lymphocyte preparation. The mean and standard error of the mean were calculated for each group of wells, and a cytotoxicity index (CI) was calculated by the following formula:

$$CI = \frac{\text{mean CPM with no RNA-mean CPM with experimental RNA}}{\text{mean CPM with no RNA}}$$

Statistical comparison of groups was by Student's t test for unpaired data.

RESULTS

Immune cytolysis of RI-H tumor cells. The results of three typical early experiments using buffy coat leukocytes as effector cells are given in Table I. In experiments 1 and 2, xenogeneic "immune" RNA extracted from the lymphoid organs of sheep immunized with RI-H tumor cells were incubated with normal human leukocytes, and in experiment 3, the "immune" RNA was extracted from the lymph nodes and spleens of immunized guinea pigs. The optimal leukocyte-to-tumor cell ratio was found to be 500:1. Higher ratios resulted in an unacceptable degree of nonspecific lysis, and lower ratios were usually less effective or ineffective. In experiment 1, the cytotoxicity index (CI) obtained with leukocytes incubated with RNA extracted from the lymphoid organs of immunized sheep ("immune" RNA) was 0.45 ± 0.08. The CI for leukocytes incubated with no RNA was 0 ± 0.14. The difference was significant at p value < 0.01. Leukocytes incubated with RNA extracted from the lymphoid organs of a sheep immunized with complete Freund's adjuvant only (Freund's adjuvant RNA) gave a CI for –0.10 ± 0.18, a value significantly different ($p < 0.005$) from "immune" RNA but not different from the leukocyte preparation incubated with no RNA. When the same "immune" RNA preparation was treated with ribonuclease prior to incubation with leukocytes, a CI of 0.18 ± 0.14 was obtained. This value was significantly different from the CI obtained with untreated "immune" RNA ($p < 0.05$) but not different from the other two control leukocyte preparations. In this particular experiment, the ribonuclease used did not completely degrade the "immune" RNA. This was evident from the profile obtained upon analysis of this RNA preparation on a sucrose density gradient. When a fresh preparation of ribonuclease was utilized in experiments 2 and 3, complete degradation of the "immune" RNA resulted, and all immunologic activity was abrogated. In experiment 2, also with the use of sheep "immune" RNA, results similar to those of experiment 1 were obtained. The leukocytes incubated with "immune" RNA gave a CI of 0.30 ± 0.05. This was a significantly greater cytotoxicity index than those obtained with leukocytes incubated without RNA (CI = 0 ± 0.15; $p < 0.01$), leukocytes incubated with Freund's adjuvant RNA (CI = 0.30 ± 0.05; $p < 0.005$). Again, the CI of the three control leukocyte preparations were not statistically different from each other. In experiment 3, guinea pig "immune" RNA was employed instead of sheep RNA but all other parameters were the same. The CI for leukocytes incubated with guinea pig "immune" RNA was 0.41 ± 0.13. This was a significantly higher cytotoxicity index than those obtained with leukocytes incubated without RNA (CI = 0 ± 0.07; $p < 0.025$), leukocytes incubated with Freund's adjuvant RNA (CI = –0.20 ± 0.1; $p < 0.005$), and leukocytes incubated with "immune" RNA treated with ribonuclease (CI = –0.37 ± 0.08; $p < 0.005$). The cytotoxicity indices for control leukocyte preparations were not statistically different from one another. Note that in all three experiments there was no significant difference between the cytotoxicity indices obtained with control RNA preparations.

When purified lymphocyte populations, prepared on Ficol-Isopaque gradients were incubated with the RNA instead of buffy

*Series 1185 Automatic Gamma Counting System, Nuclear Chicago, Chicago, Ill.

Table II. *Immune cytolysis of RI-H tumor cells mediated by "immune" RNA from the lymphoid organs of immunized sheep**

	Experiment 4 Lymphocyte-to-target cell ratio = 100:1		Experiment 5 Lymphocyte-to-target cell ratio = 200:1		Experiment 6 Lymphocyte-to-target cell ratio = 100:1		Experiment 7 Lymphocyte-to-target cell ratio = 100:1	
	Cytotoxicity index	p	Cytotoxicity index	p	Cytotoxicity index	p	Cytotoxicity index	p
Lymphocytes incubated with:								
"Immune" RNA†	0.60 ± 0.06		0.84 ± 0.02		0.69 ± 0.07		0.60 ± 0.06	
"Immune" RNA + ribonuclease‡	Not done		Not done		−0.08 ± 0.14	< 0.005	0.05 ±0.02	< 0.005
"Immune" RNA + deoxyribonuclease§	Not done		0.84 ± 0.03	N.S.	Not done		Not done	
"Immune" RNA + pronase‖	Not done		Not done		Not done		0.53 ± 0.06	N.S.
Freund's adjuvant RNA¶	0.22 ± 0.05	< 0.005	0.22 ± 0.13	< 0.005	0.12 ± 0.24	< 0.05	Not done	
No RNA	0.0 ± 0.10	< 0.005	0.0 ± 0.19	< 0.005	0.0 ± 0.14	< 0.005	0.0 ± 0.04	< 0.005

*Six replicate wells were used for each determination and mean cytotoxicity indices with their standard deviations are presented. The p values were calculated by Student's t test for unpaired data and represent differences between "immune" RNA and the various control groups. In these experiments, purified lymphocyte populations were employed rather than buffy coat leukocytes.

†RNA from the lymphoid organs of sheep immunized with RI-H tumor cells.

‡"Immune" RNA treated with ribonuclease prior to incubation with lymphocytes.

§"Immune" RNA treated with deoxyribonuclease prior to incubation with lymphocytes.

‖"Immune" RNA treated with pronase prior to incubation with lymphocytes.

¶RNA from the lymphoid organs of animals immunized with Freund's adjuvant only.

coat leukocytes, the magnitude of the cytotoxicity observed was increased and the lymphocyte-to-target cell ratio could be significantly reduced (from 500:1 to 100:1 or 200:1). These data are presented in Table II. From these results, it may be seen that, at a lymphocyte-to-target cell ratio of 100:1, CI's of from 0.60 to 0.69 were obtained in a very consistent fashion. Since lymphocytes account for 20 to 40 percent of the total peripheral white blood cells in man, this result is quite consistent with what would be expected assuming that one or more population of lymphocytes are the active effector cell population. By effecting approximately a fivefold increase in lymphocyte concentration, the leukocyte-to-target cell ratio could be reduced by a factor of 5 with no loss (or even an increase) in cytotoxicity.

When the active "immune" RNA preparations were pretreated with deoxyribonuclease (experiment 5) at an enzyme-to-substrate ratio of 1:50 (based on the actual amount of DNA in the sample) or with pronase (experiment 7) at an enzyme-to-substrate ratio of 1:20 (based on the actual amount of protein in the sample) and then incubated with leukocytes, the resultant cytotoxicity index was not significantly altered. The fact that deoxyribonuclease and pronase treatment of the "immune" RNA preparations did not affect the transfer of immunity and that ribonuclease treatment of the "immune" RNA abrogated the response offers

Table III. *Immune cytolysis of RI-H tumor cells mediated by "immune" RNA from the lymphoid organs of immunized sheep**

	Experiment 8 Lymphocyte-to-target cell ratio 100:1		Experiment 9 Lymphocyte-to-target cell ratio 100:1	
	Cytotoxicity index	p	Cytotoxicity index	p
Concentration of "immune" RNA†				
No RNA	0.0 ± 0.14		0.0 ± 0.06	
2.0 mg. RNA/ml.	0.69 ± 0.07	< 0.005	0.53 ± 0.06	< 0.005
1.0 mg. RNA/ml.	0.79 ± 0.02	< 0.005	0.36 ± 0.02	< 0.005
0.5 mg. RNA/ml.	0.62 ± 0.03	< 0.005	N.D.	
0.25 mg. RNA/ml.	N.D.‡		0.21 ± 0.05	< 0.05
0.10 mg. RNA/ml.	N.D.		0.17 ± 0.07	< 0.05

*Six replicate wells were used for each determination and mean cytotoxicity indices with their standard deviations are presented. The p values were calculated by Student's t test for unpaired data and represent differences between no RNA and the various other groups. In these experiments purified lymphocyte populations were employed rather than buffy coat leukocytes.

†RNA from the lymphoid organs of sheep immunized with RI-H tumor cells.

‡Not done.

Table IV. *Immune cytolysis of BT-20 tumor cells mediated by "immune" RNA from the lymphoid organs of immunized guinea pigs**

	Experiment 1 Lymphocyte-to-target cell ratio = 200:1		Experiment 2 Lymphocyte-to-target cell ratio = 200:1		Experiment 3 Lymphocyte-to-target cell ratio = 200:1		Experiment 4 Lymphocyte-to-target cell ratio = 200:1	
	Cytotoxicity index	p	Cytotoxicity index	p	Cytotoxicity index	p	Cytotoxicity index	p
Lymphocytes incubated with:								
"Immune" RNA†	0.57 ± 0.10		0.54 ± 0.05		0.73 ± 0.06		0.71 ± 0.08	
"Immune" RNA + ribonuclease‡	Not done		0.11 ± 0.09	< 0.005	−0.02 ± 0.06	< 0.005	−0.02 ± 0.06	< 0.005
"Immune" RNA + deoxyribonuclease§	Not done		Not done		Not done		0.48 ± 0.06	N.S.
"Immune" RNA + pronase‖	Not done		Not done		Not done		0.68 ± 0.03	N.S.
Freund's adjuvant RNA¶	0.21 ± 0.30	< 0.05	Not done		0.17 ± 0.04	< 0.005	Not done	
No RNA	0.0 ± 0.36	< 0.05	0.0 ± 0.05	< 0.005	0.0 ± 0.04	< 0.005	0.0 ± 0.05	< 0.005

*Six replicate wells were used for each determination and mean cytotoxicity indices with their standard deviations are presented. The p values were calculated by Student's t test for unpaired data and represent differences between "immune" RNA and the various control groups. In these experiments purified lymphocyte populations were employed as effector cells.

†RNA from the lymphoid organs of guinea pigs immunized with BT-20 tumor cells.

‡"Immune" RNA treated with ribonuclease prior to incubation with lymphocytes.

§"Immune" RNA treated with deoxyribonuclease prior to incubation with lymphocytes.

‖"Immune" RNA treated with pronase prior to incubation with lymphocytes.

¶RNA from the lymphoid organs of animals immunized with Freund's adjuvant only.

Table V. *Immune cytolysis of melanoma cells mediated by "immune" RNA**

	Experiment 1 Target cell line: RO-H RNA donor: Sheep		*Experiment 2 Target cell line: ED-H RNA donor: Sheep*		*Experiment 3 Target cell line: ED-H RNA donor: Guinea pig*	
	Cytotoxicity index	*p*	*Cytotoxicity index*	*p*	*Cytotoxicity index*	*p*
Lymphocytes incubated with:						
"Immune" RNA†	0.53 ± 0.12		0.37 ± 0.05		0.30 ± 0.02	
Freund's adjuvant RNA‡	−0.20 ± 0.08	< 0.005	−0.30 ± 0.10	< 0.005	0.07 ± 0.04	< 0.05
No RNA	0.0 ± 0.08	< 0.005	0.0 ± 0.08	< 0.005	0.0 ± 0.03	< 0.005

*Only lymphocyte-to-target cell ratios of 500:1 are included in the table. Six replicate wells were used for each determination and mean cytotoxicity indices with their standard deviations are presented. The p values were calculated by Student's t test for unpaired data and represent differences between "immune" RNA and the various control groups. Purified lymphocyte populations were employed as effector cells.

†RNA from the lymphoid organs of animals immunized with melanoma cells.

‡RNA from the lymphoid organs of animals immunized with Freund's adjuvant only.

strong evidence that one or more moieties of RNA were responsible for the immunological activity of these preparations.

Attempts were then made to determine the effect of varying the RNA concentration upon the magnitude of the immune response observed. The concentration of RNA in which the lymphocytes were incubated was progressively reduced so that a dose-response curve might be established and a threshold RNA concentration determined. The results of these experiments are depicted in Table III. From these data, it can be seen that reducing the RNA concentration from 2.0 to 1.0 mg. per milliliter or even to 0.5 mg. per milliliter had little effect on the response, but reducing the concentration still further to 0.25 mg. per milliliter resulted in approximately a 50 percent decrease in cytotoxicity. Further reducing the RNA concentration to 0.10 mg. per milliliter reduced cytotoxicity still further, but this result remained significantly different from that obtained with no RNA.

Immune cytolysis of BT-20 tumor cells. Experiments similar to those described above for the RI-H cell line were performed by utilizing the BT-20 cell line. In these experiments guinea pig RNA was used. The results are depicted in Table IV. Again, xenogeneic "immune" RNA induced normal, nonimmune human lymphocytes to become cytotoxic to BT-20 cells in a consistent and reproducible fashion. RNA from guinea pigs immunized with Freund's adjuvant only was inactive. The activity was abolished by treatment of the "immune" RNA preparations with RNAase but was not affected by treatment with DNAase or pronase.

Immune cytolysis of melanoma cells (ED-H and RO-H). In these experiments, two types of "immune" RNA preparations were studied: (1) RNA from the lymphoid organs of guinea pigs immunized with ED-H cells, and (2) RNA from the lymphoid organs of a sheep immunized with melanoma cells from a fresh surgical specimen obtained from a third melanoma patient H. O. The results of these experiments are tabulated in Table V. Of particular interest is the fact that RNA from the lymphoid organs of a sheep immunized with melanoma cells from one patient, H. O., was effective in mediating cytotoxic immune responses directed against melanoma cells from two other patients, R. O. and E. D.

A critical experiment was then performed in an autologous system with the use of autologous lymphocytes obtained from the same patient from whom the ED-H cell line originated. These lymphocytes were incubated with the sheep anti-melanoma "immune" RNA and reacted with cells from the patient's own tumor in vitro. The patient's lymphocytes which incubated without RNA served as a control. When incubated with no RNA, the patient's lymphocytes were very slightly cytotoxic to his tumor cells (CI = 0.22 ± 0.05) as might be expected. However, when this patient's lymphocytes were incubated with "immune" RNA, the cytotoxicity index of his lymphocytes more than doubled (CI = 0.45 ± 0.02). This increase was significant at $p < 0.005$. At the same time, lymphocytes from a normal volunteer were incubated with this RNA. The resulting CI was 0.49 ± 0.05. It can be seen that the effect of "immune" RNA upon autologous lymphocytes (autologous with respect to the tumor cells) was equal in magnitude to its effect on normal, nonimmune allogeneic lymphocytes. In this autologous system, it appears likely that immune responses directed specifically against melanoma-associated antigens were mediated by the "immune" RNA. Again, it is important to remember that the anti-melanoma "immune" RNA was extracted from the lymphoid organs of a sheep immunized with melanoma cells from a different melanoma patient.

DISCUSSION

This series of experiments demonstrates the mediation of immune cytolysis of human tumor cells in vitro by normal, nonimmune human lymphocytes preincubated with xenogeneic, anti-tumor "immune" RNA extracted from the lymphoid organs of animals immunized with the particular human tumor being studied. This may be the first reported demonstration of the transfer, in vitro, of an immune response to cell surface antigens from animal to man. Only "immune" RNA from animals immunized with tumor cells mediated the conversion of normal human leukocytes to "killer cells," and RNA preparations extracted from the lymphoid organs of animals immunized with Freund's adjuvant were ineffective in conferring cytotoxic activity upon normal human lymphocytes.

Wilson and Wecker,[20] Bondevik and Mannick,[2] and Ramming and Pilch[16] showed that normal nonimmune lymphoid cells, incubated with allogeneic "immune" RNA extracted from the lymphoid organs of rodents immunized against histocompatibility antigens, mediated specific immune cytolysis of allogeneic target cells in vitro. Ramming and Pilch[17] then demonstrated, in syngeneic system, that immune cytolysis of guinea pig tumor cells in vitro could be mediated by "immune" RNA extracted from the spleens of syngeneic guinea pigs that had previously been immunized to the particular tumor being studied. In these studies, the tumor cells, lymphoid cells, and RNA-donor animals were all from the same inbred strain and, therefore, it was apparent that the immune responses transferred by "immune" RNA were directed specifically at tumor-associated antigens. However, when xenogeneic sources of "immune" RNA are utilized, the determination of specificity becomes more difficult. In a murine tumor-host system employing xenogeneic "immune" RNA extracted from the lymphoid organs of immunized guinea pigs, Ramming and Pilch[17] provided convincing evidence that, when pig tumor cells in vitro could be mediated by "immune" RNA extracted from the spleens of syngeneic guinea pigs that had previously been immunized to the particular tumor being studied. In these studies, the tumor cells, lymphoid cells and RNA-donor animals were all from the same inbred strain and, therefore, it was apparent that the immune responses transferred by "immune" RNA were directed specifically at tumor-associated antigens. However, when xenogeneic sources of "immune" RNA are utilized, the determination of specificity becomes more difficult. In a murine tumor-host system employing xenogeneic "immune" RNA extracted from the lymphoid organs of immunized guinea pigs, Ramming and Pilch[18] provided convincing evidence that, when xenogeneic anti-tumor "immune" RNA is incubated with lymphoid cells that are syngeneic with the tumor cells, only immune responses directed against tumor-associated antigens are transferred.

Because the patients from whom the RI-H

and BT-20 tumor lines were established were dead, it was impossible for us to establish, within an autologous system (by utilizing lymphocytes from the primary autochthonous host), that the immune responses directed against those cells were specific for tumor-associated antigens, as distinct from immune responses directed against histocompatibility antigens. In these series of experiments, since the "immune" RNA was incubated with lymphocytes which were allogeneic with respect to the tumor cells, the immune responses observed were probably directed against histocompatibility antigens present on the tumor cells as well as to tumor-specific antigens. This problem of establishing specificity for tumor-specific antigens was overcome when lymphocytes that were autologous with the ED-H melanoma cell line were used in place of allogeneic lymphocytes. In that instance, histocompatibility differences between the lymphocytes and tumor cells were eliminated, and presumably the immune responses observed were directed solely against tumor-associated antigens.

A rational model for the immunotherapy of human cancer with xenogeneic "immune" RNA has been proposed by Deckers and Pilch.[5] In this model, xenogeneic "immune" RNA is extracted from the lymphoid organs of animals immunized with human tumor tissue removed at surgery. Autologous lymphocytes obtained from the patient by means of a mechanical blood cell separator would be incubated with xenogeneic "immune" RNA and returned to the patient by intravenous infusion. Alternately, the "immune" RNA might be given systemically by multiple intradermal or subcutaneous injections in a vehicle containing a ribonuclease inhibitor. Although it has not yet been administered to man, xenogeneic "immune" RNA offers several theoretical advantages over other methods for adoptive immunotherapy: (1) There is no need to give serum or plasma. Serum has been shown, in some situations, to contain factors which may block cell-mediated immune responses in vitro and which may facilitate tumor growth in vivo. (2) Intact leukocytes need not be given. This obviates the administration of allogeneic leukocytes which can sensitize the recipient to foreign histocompatibility antigens. Repeated transfusions of allogeneic leukocytes may then result in significant toxicity. Moreover, the immune elimination of allogeneic leukocytes may make subsequent transfusions of such cells ineffective for immunotherapy. "Immune" RNA contains no transplantation antigens. (3) There would be no danger of inducing a graft-vs.-host reaction in immunodeficient or immunosuppressed individuals. (4) "Immune" RNA itself is not a strong antigen, and, therefore, injections of RNA, even xenogeneic RNA, would not be expected to sensitize the recipient, to cause secondary syndromes, or to result in immune elimination of subsequent doses of RNA.

The immune cytolysis produced by lymphocytes preincubated with "immune" RNA may be due to completely cellular (cell to cell) mechanisms, e.g., T-cell killing. However, it is also possible that "immune" RNA induces the production of antibodies to cell surface antigens and that these antibodies play a significant role in mediating the cytotoxicity observed. Studies now in progress are aimed at detecting such antibodies and at elucidating the mechanism by which lymphocytes pre-incubated with "immune" RNA mediate cytotoxic reactions.

We thank Carol Drogemuller and Terri Matsumoto for expert technical assistance.

REFERENCES

1. Alexander, P., Delorme, E. J., Hamilton, G., and Hall, J. G.: Effect of nucleic acids from immune lymphocytes on rat sarcomata, Nature **213:** 569, 1967.
2. Bondevik, H., and Mannick, J. A.: RNA-mediated transfer of lymphocyte vs. target cell activity, Proc. Soc. Exp. Biol. Med. **129:** 264, 1968.
3. Cohen, A. M., Burdick, J. F., and Ketcham, A. S.: Cytotoxicity: An assay using ^{125}I-iododeoxyuridine labeled target cells, J. Immunol. **107:** 895, 1971.
4. Deckers, P. J., and Pilch, Y. H.: Transfer of immunity to tumor isografts by the systemic administration of xenogeneic "immune RNA, Nature **231:** 181, 1971.

5. Deckers, P. J., and Pilch, Y. H.: RNA-mediated transfer of tumor immunity—A new model for the immunotherapy of cancer, Cancer **28:** 1219, 1971.
6. Dische, Z.: *In* Chargaff, E., and Davidson, J. N., editors, The nucleic acids, New York, 1955, Academic Press, Inc., pp. 285-305.
7. Fishman, M. J.: Antibody formation in vitro, J. Exp. Med. **114:** 837, 1961.
8. Fishman, M. J., and Adler, F. L.: Antibody formation initiated in vitro. II. Antibody synthesis in X-irradiated recipients of diffusion chambers containing nucleic acid derived from macrophages incubated with antigen, J. Exp. Med. **117:** 595, 1963.
9. Lowry, O. H., Rosebrough, R. P., Farr, A. L., and Randall, R. J.: Protein measurement with the Folin phenol reagent, J. Biol. Chem. **193:** 265, 1951.
10. Mannick, J. A., and Egdahl, R. H.: Transfer of heightened immunity to skin homografts by lymphoid RNA, J. Clin. Invest. **43:** 2166, 1964.
11. Paque, R. E., and Dray, S.: Monkey to human transfer of delayed hypersensitivity in vitro with RNA extracts, Cell. Immunol. **5:** 30, 1972.
12. Pilch, Y. H., and Ramming, K. P.: Transfer of tumor immunity with ribonucleic acid, Cancer **26:** 630, 1970.
13. Pilch, Y. H., Ramming, K. P., and Deckers, P. J.: Transfer of immunity with RNA, Isr. J. Med. Sci. **7:** 246, 1971.
14. Pilch, Y. H., Ramming, K. P., and Deckers, P. J.: Induction of anti-cancer immunity with RNA, Ann. N. Y. Acad. Sci. **207:** 409, 1973.
15. Ramming, K. P., and Pilch, Y. H.: Mediation of immunity to tumor isografts in mice by heterologous ribonucleic acid, Science **168:** 492, 1970.
16. Ramming, K. P., and Pilch, Y. H.: RNA-mediated immune cytolysis to transplantation antigens in vitro, Surg. Forum **21:** 267, 1970.
17. Ramming, K. P., and Pilch, Y. H.: Transfer of tumor specific immunity with RNA: Demonstration by immune cytolysis of tumor cells in vitro, J. Natl. Cancer Inst. **45:** 543, 1970.
18. Ramming, K. P., and Pilch, Y. H.: Transfer of tumor-specific immunity with RNA: Inhibition of growth of murine tumor isografts, J. Natl. Cancer Inst. **46:** 735, 1971.
19. Sabbadini, E., and Sehon, A. H.: Acceleration of allograft rejection induced by RNA from sensitized donors, Int. Arch. Allergy Appl. Immunol. **32:** 55, 1967.
20. Wilson, D. B., and Wecker, E. E.: Conversion of "normal" lymphoid cells to an immunologically active status with RNA derived from isologous lymphoid tissues of specifically immunized rats, J. Immunol. **97:** 512, 1966.

DISCUSSION

Dr. Charles F. McKhann (Minneapolis, Minn.). The important question is: Is the immunity transferred by the RNA, or is it induced de novo? Is it transferred by informational RNA from the immunized lymphocytes to the unimmunized lymphocytes, or is it induced by the inclusion of small amounts of antigen that are in the RNA preparation and have been rendered superantigen by association with the RNA, as was found by Arthur Gottlieb in several other systems?

Is the RNA specific enough for the tumor to be safe in human studies? And we may have seen part of that already here. When one immunizes guinea pigs against guinea pig tumors, one has only the tumor-specific antigen—or if the strains are not the same, histocompatibility antigens—to worry about; but when one immunizes a guinea pig or a sheep against human tumor cells, one includes a much broader spectrum of antigens, which includes many strong normal antigens as well as the weak tumor antigens. And if the test system uses lymphocytes on tumor cells, they are found to be cytotoxic.

However, the real question is: What happens when the test system is used on cells that are not tumor cells—normal cells? The information that they get as RNA from xenogeneic sheep lymphocytes may be directed against many normal human cellular antigens.

What evidence do you have that you are not harming your lymphocytes with a sort of a sawed-off shotgun, capable of doing serious damage to normal cells in vivo, as well as to tumor cells themselves?

What is your criteria of a patient who has been cured of melanoma, when he is used as a donor for informational RNA, when we know that the possibility of this disease recurring five, ten, or fifteen years later is real?

Dr. Richard E. Wilson (Boston, Mass.). How soon after the cells are reacted can you find specificity of response, both in the animal and in the human studies?

Dr. John A. Mannick (Boston, Mass.). Dr. Wang, in our laboratory, has recently succeeded in showing that both in human tumors and in animal tumors that one can, with the use of xenogeneic RNA raised in guinea pigs, convert the cells of the tumor-bearing individual to reactivity in tissue culture specifically against the tumor cells used to immunize the guinea pigs that donated the RNA. In other words, this is, again, the kind of thing that you showed in one slide, Dr. Pilch; that sometimes the lymphocytes already react somewhat against the tumor, but the reaction is vastly increased after incubation with the xenogeneic RNA. We tend to believe that you are on a tumor-specific track.

I would like to ask a couple of technical questions also. Do you really have any evidence that RNA in incubation with lymphocytes causes them to transform into blast cells, as you showed in one of those slides?

I am interested to know whether those Ficol-Hypaque–purified cells were really all lymphocytes, or did they contain monocytes? It is rather important to settle whether or not the RNA actually comes from macrophage or macrophage precursors or whether it comes from lymphocytes.

Dr. Jay Collie Fish (Galveston, Texas). I would like to know if there is an estimate of the number of lymphocytes that would need to be exposed to RNA to produce a therapeutic effect and what number of lymphocytes are being obtained from the separator. Another source of great numbers of lymphocytes might be from thoracic duct cannulation, in which one might expect to get 10^{10} or 10^{11} of those cells per day.

Dr. Yosef H. Pilch (closing). There have been two types of immune RNA identified; one, the RNA antigen complex type of RNA, the so-called superantigen type of RNA, where antigen moieties, or antigenic determinants, can be identified in the RNA preparation and bound to the RNA. The second is what has been called "informative RNA," which is an RNA in which antigen cannot be detected by methods that so far have been employed and which is involved in allotypic transfers in model systems with the use of human immunity to sheep red blood cells. We have absolutely no knowledge, and no data, which would permit us to say which of these two types of immune RNA we are dealing with. Perhaps we are dealing with both.

In regard to whether we are transferring an immune response or inducing an immune response de novo, it is rather difficult for us to say. We assume that our donor guinea pig, or donor sheep, is now immune or is harboring an immune response to our tumor following the immunization we have used. We have not tested the immune responses of the RNA donor in this particular model. We have in other models used immune RNA from animals who have either had temporary tumor growth or who have had growing tumors. These animals can be demonstrated to resist a second tumor challenge, either following amputation of a growing tumor or by concomitant immunity, and we have used immune RNA from such animals, and found it to be active. I really do not know whether we are transferring an immune response or inducing one de novo. Presumably, if one believes in the clonal selection theory, all one has to do is just turn on a clone.

Regarding the specificity, certainly when one uses xenogeneic RNA, one has to infer specificity by a whole variety of contortions, controls, and these sorts of artifacts. We have, however, in studies which will appear in the January issue of the *Journal of the National Cancer Institute,* studied in detail immune RNA within a totally syngeneic rat model, where the RNA donor, the tumor cell, and the antilymphocyte are all from a single inbred strain of rat, by using RNA extracted either from the spleens of tumor-bearing rats or animals that have undergone surgical excision of a growing tumor. This system can be completely duplicated and confirmed with the same order of cytotoxic indices being obtained.

Regarding the question of using normal cells as target cells, we have not done this specifically. It is easier for us to use a normal tissue RNA—in other words, an RNA prepared following immunization to normal cells—rather than using the normal cells as target cells, since the growth rate of normal fibroblasts in tissue culture is so low that they do not take up the isotope well and are extremely difficult to use in our particular assay.

In the studies we reported a few years ago, we found that these immune RNA preparations were totally incapable of mediating graft-versus-host reactions in neonatal mice. I think there is a more serious question of: Would we ever produce facilitation of tumor growth through some inadvertent manipulation of the immune response?

Regarding what our criterion of "cure" is for melanoma patients submitted to leucophoresis on a continuous flow blood cell separator, we simply use the criterion that they are putatively cured by surgical excision, have a favorable prognosis, good in vitro evidence of possessing melanoma immunity, and have been free of disease for at least six months. We have almost completed a very extensive study on the hematologic and immunologic sequelae of a single cell separator run, and, of course, we cannot discuss it today, but we have reason to believe that one cell separator run does little, if anything, to either nonspecific or tumor-specific cellular immunity.

The RNA is incubated with the effector cells for twenty minutes at 37° C., then washed twice, and diluted to the appropriate dilution to give the appropriate lymphocyte-to-target cell ratio, and placed at once into the assay. Incubation in the assay is 48 hours. At the end of 48 hours, one gets the cytotoxicity index that I have showed you.

We have no direct evidence that the treatment of lymphoid cells with immune RNA transforms them into blast cells, and that was simply an impression based on a number of Professor Peter Alexander's theories regarding the immunoblast and its role in mediating antitumor immune responses.

In regard to the nature of the cell source of immune RNA, we do not know whether it is the macrophage or the lymphocyte. Our Ficol-Hypaque–prepared peripheral blood lymphocytes contain both monocytes and lymphocytes. We are dealing with about 85 percent lymphocytes; the rest are monocytes. We do not know which cell population we are turning on, nor do we know whether we are turning on T-cells or B-cells.

We also do not know whether we may, in fact, be dealing with a humoral antibody production which we are inducing, which then arms B-cells or activates macrophages. We do not know if we are mediating a T-cell killing effect.

The number of lymphocytes that we obtain from a single run on a continuous-flow blood cell separator is of the order of 7×10^9 to 1.4×10^{10} mononuclear cells; again, 85 to 90 percent are lymphocytes, the rest being monocytes. The number of tumor target cells in the assay is 2,000. Therefore, if you do the computation, the lymphocyte-to-target cell ratio being between 50 and 500, you can derive the number of lymphocytes we use.

The RNA is always incubated at that concentration indicated on the slide, in 5×10^7 lymphocytes. The RNA is extracted not from sheep blood, but from spleen and lymph node tissue of the sheep, and the same thing is true for the guinea pigs.

An immunosuppressive peptide fraction in the serum of cancer patients

A. H. Glasgow, M.D., J. O. Menzoian, M.D., R. B. Nimberg, D.M.D., S. R. Cooperband, M.D., K. Schmid, Ph.D., *and* **J. A. Mannick, M.D.,** *Boston, Mass.*

Serums from hospitalized cancer patients and noncancer patients as well as from normal volunteers were compared for immunosuppressive activity as measured by phytohemagglutinin stimulation of human peripheral lymphocytes in vitro. The serums were further fractionated to see if the immunosuppressive activity was present in a peptide fraction of the serum. The immunosuppressive activity of cancer serum was five to ten times greater than that of hospitalized noncancer patients or normal volunteers. Moreover, it was shown that a peptide subfraction of the serum contained the immunosuppressive activity.

From the Departments of Surgery and Biochemistry, Boston University, Boston, Mass.

In mammals, the cellular immune response has the capacity to destroy tumors or, at least, prevent the proliferation of tumor cells. Many patients with cancer manifest cellular immunity to their tumors.[3, 15, 16, 30, 31] However, in both human beings and other animals, despite the fact that the cells in many cancers are immunogens capable of eliciting a cellular immune response, those cells survive and grow.

Many patients with cancer manifest nonspecific suppression of cellular immunity and exhibit anergy.[8, 15, 22] Eilber and Morton[8] and Herberman[15] demonstrated that this general loss of cellular immunity to common bacterial antigens, to the hapten DNCB, or to tumor antigens correlates well with the extent and severity of the cancer. A number of reports have appeared in recent years that suggest circulating nonspecific cellular immunosuppressive factors in the serum of tumor-bearing humans and other animals.[2, 9, 11, 19, 22, 28, 29] Generally, immunosuppressive activity of these sera has been demonstrated by inhibition of lymphocyte activation induced by mitogens in vitro.

For several years this laboratory has been involved in studying an immunosuppressive factor, immunoregulatory alpha globulin (IRA), which we have found in the alpha globulins of normal human serum. Our isolation of IRA has progressed to the point where we have demonstrated that the factor(s) is contained in a 5,000 to 7,000 molecular weight polypeptide fraction, which electrophoretically migrates with, or is carried by, the serum alpha globulins.[26] Because of the suggestion that there might be some relationship between serum immunosuppressive factors and the phenomenon of anergy in cancer patients, we decided to investigate the immunosuppressive activity of serum from cancer patients and to determine if that

This study was supported by National Institutes of Health Grants No. CA-12209, AM-10824, GM-10374, and 5FO2DE44743.

Presented at the Thirty-fifth Annual Meeting of the Society of University Surgeons, St. Louis, Mo., Feb. 14-16, 1974.

immunosuppressive activity was contained in a fraction similar to IRA obtained from normal human serum.

METHODS AND MATERIALS

Population studied. Cancer patients were all hospitalized patients in whom the diagnosis of cancer was substantiated by tissue histology. They ranged in age from 42 to 87 years. They were eight men and five women. All had solid tumors, and none were receiving any chemotherapy or irradiation. Noncancer patients were, also, all hospitalized. None had known signs or symptoms of cancer. They ranged in age from 29 to 88 years and were equally divided by sex, five men and five women. "Normal" persons were medical school personnel in good health. They ranged in age from 23 to 37 years and consisted of three men and 12 women.

Serum collection. Peripheral venipuncture was used to obtain 30 to 200 ml. of blood. The blood was allowed to clot, and after clot retraction had developed, the serum was removed by centrifugation at 2,000 × g for 30 minutes.

Serum fractionation. Aliquots of serum were pooled, and 30 ml. of serum was then fractionated by DEAE ion exchange chromatography. The protein peaks from this separation were then desalted by gel filtration and concentrated by lyophilization. To obtain peptides, the first peak from DEAE, peak I, was acidified to pH 3.0 with the use of volatile buffers and separated by diafiltration with a PM-10 membrane* which retains species with molecular weights above 10,000. The ultrafiltrate, consisting of peptide, was desalted and concentrated by lyophilization.

Assay for immunosuppressive activity. To test for immunosuppressive activity, we measured inhibition of phytohemagglutinin (PHA)-induced proliferation of human peripheral lymphocytes, a method previously described by us.[5-7] Human peripheral lymphocytes were obtained by gravity sedimentation of heparinized blood. The serum layer after two hours of sedimentation at room temperature was then purified on sterile cotton wool columns. The cells were washed from the columns with minimal essential media (MEM).* After three washings and centrifugation, the cells were counted in a counting chamber. They invariably were 95 percent small lymphocytes that were 95 percent viable by trypan blue dye exclusion.

Tissue cultures were performed with 10^6 lymphocytes in 1 ml. of complete media and additives. All tubes contained ten percent fetal calf serum plus penicillin, streptomycin, and L-glutamine. The experimental tubes contained varying concentrations of protein or peptide samples from cancer patients, noncancer patients, or "normals." Control tubes contained a concentration of reference normal human serum equal to the greatest concentration of experimental protein or peptide being tested. The reference serum has been used in all our experiments, and, consistently, the counts in these tubes are equal to the counts of tubes which have no additional human serum added. The tubes were then maintained in stationary racks in a five percent CO_2–humidified environment at 37° C. for 48 hours. They were then pulsed by the addition of 4 μCi of tridiated thymidine. Sixteen to 18 hours later the cultures were sacrificed and stored in the frozen state. At the time that the cells were ready for counting, they were thawed and washed four times with saline, 2 ml. each time. Finally, 1 ml. of 0.01N sodium hydroxide was added to the cells. To this was added 5 ml. of "cocktail D," consisting of dioxane, napthalene, and 2.5-diphenyloxazole, and the liquid was then counted in a scintillation counter.

Calculation of immunosuppression in vitro.

Percent suppression =

$$1 - \frac{\text{(experimental tubes with PHA-control tubes)}}{\text{(control tubes with PHA-control tubes)}} \times 100$$

*Amicon, New Bedford, Mass.

*Gibco, New York, N. Y.

Calculation of immunosuppression units.

$$\text{Immunosuppression units} = \frac{\text{total weight of protein fraction}}{\text{smallest dose producing 100 percent suppression of PHA stimulation in vitro}}$$

RESULTS

The immunosuppressive activity of various sera. In order to have enough material for fractionation, the 13 cancer serums were divided into three pools, two with five samples and one with three samples. In a similar manner, the serums from noncancer hospitalized patients and from normal volunteers were also divided into two and three pools, respectively. For each of the four protein peaks, dose curves were determined so that it was possible to select the smallest dose of material producing 100 percent suppression of PHA-induced stimulation. Using this figure, we were able to calculate immunosuppression units so that we could determine the total amount of immunosuppressive activity in each of the peaks and in the total amount of serum. As can be seen in Table I, each of the three pools of cancer serum had immunosuppressive activity in peak I; however, in neither of the two noncancer pools or in the three normal pools was there any immunosuppressive activity in peak I. Immunosuppressive activity in peaks II and III was variable in cancer, noncancer, and normal patients but all serums tested had immunosuppressive activity in peak IV. The total immunosuppressive activity in the three pools of cancer serum range from 138 immunosuppressive units to 155 immunosuppression units. For noncancer hospitalized patients, the total immunosuppression units ranged from 23 to 30. For normal volunteers, the total amount of immunosuppression units ranged from 12 to 29. This indicates that all serum samples contain some immunosuppressive activity; however, the total amount of immunosuppressive activity in the serum of cancer patients was five to ten times greater than the immunosuppressive activity of noncancer hospitalized patients or normal volunteers. This difference in immunosuppressive activity could be related to the presence of a considerable amount of immunosuppressive activity in both peaks I and II of cancer serum. These peaks contained essentially no immunosuppressive activity in the serum of noncancer hospitalized patients or normal volunteers.

Table I. *Serum immunosuppressive activity*

Serum pool	*Diagnosis*	*Immunosuppression units**	
		Peak I	*Total*
1A	Cancer	77	140
1B	Cancer	103	155
1C	Cancer	68	138
2	Noncancer	0	30
2A	Noncancer	0	23
3A	Normals	0	24
3B	Normals	0	29
3C	Normals	0	12

*Calculation for immunosuppression units given in text.

Fractionation of immunosuppressive activity. Since we have previously demonstrated that the immunosuppressive activity of normal human serum could be found in a peptide fraction,[26] we followed similar fractionation procedures to obtain a peptide fraction from cancer serum. Because the amount of peptide that is obtained from the serum is a small fraction of the total serum protein, we began the peptide fractionation using peak I from the DEAE because this contained most of the immunosuppressive activity in all of the cancer serums. A portion of peak I from combined pools of 1A, 1B, and 1C was acidified and subjected to diafiltration on the PM-10 membrane. The ultrafiltrate was considered to be a peptide fraction since the filter retains molecular weight species greater than 10,000. Peak I after acidification, but before diafiltration, was then compared to the peptide fraction and to the retained proteins left in the filter after the removal of the peptide fraction. These fractions were compared by their ability to suppress PHA-induced proliferation of peripheral lymphocytes in vitro. As a control, peak I from the 3A, 3B, and 3C (normal) serum pools was combined and processed in a similar fashion. Table II demonstrates the dose-related per-

Table II. *Effect of peptide extraction on immunosuppressive activity*

Serum	Serum fraction	Dose-related percent suppression of PHA lymphocyte stimulation					
		7*	3.5	1.75	0.8	0.4	0.2
Pool 1 (1A + 1B+ 1C)	Protein peak I	100%	100%	70%	35%		
	Peptide fraction				100%	0	0
	Retained protein	100%	70%	0	0		

*Doses are given in milligrams per milliliter.

cent suppression of PHA-induced lymphocyte stimulation. The peak I protein from cancer serum was 100 percent suppressive at 7 and 3.5 mg., 70 percent suppressive at 1.75 mg. per milliliter, and 35 percent suppressive at 0.8 mg. per milliliter. The peptide fraction was 100 percent suppressive at 0.8 mg. per milliliter and was not suppressive at doses below this. The protein remaining behind in the ultrafilter was still 100 percent suppressive at 7 mg. per milliliter, but at 3.5 mg. per milliliter, it had become only 70 percent suppressive and it had no suppressive activity at 1.75 or 0.8 mg. per milliliter. In the control (normal human serum), there was no immunosuppressive activity even at 7 mg. per milliliter in peak I fraction. The peptide fraction also demonstrated no immunosuppressive activity when it was tested at 1.75 mg. per milliliter. It was not tested at higher doses because there was insufficient material. The retained protein was also not suppressive, even at 7 mg. per milliliter. This indicated that the immunosuppressive activity of cancer serum, as represented by the immunosuppressive activity of peak I, could be reduced by removing from it a peptide which contained immunosuppressive activity. This suggests that in cancer serum, as in normal serum, it is the peptide fraction which is responsible for the immunosuppression activity.

DISCUSSION

We have demonstrated that the serum of cancer patients has more immunosuppressive activity, as measured by suppression of PHA-induced proliferation of human peripheral lymphocytes in vitro, than the serum of non-cancer or hospitalized patients or normal volunteers. Moreover, we have demonstrated that the immunosuppressive activity of cancer serum is probably contained in a peptide fraction which is similar to an immunosuppressive peptide fraction isolated from normal human blood. This is of some significance, as we have postulated that the immunosuppressive peptide factor from normal human blood acts as a feedback regulator of cell-mediated immunity.[21] The data from this study are therefore suggestive that, in patients with cancer, the cancer may capitalize on an intrinsic immunoregulatory mechanism normally involved in the control of cellular immune responses.

The presence of naturally occurring nonspecific immunosuppressive factors in serum and/or lymphoid tissues has been thoroughly documented in man and laboratory animals. Beginning with the report by Kamrin[17] in 1959 that alpha globulins isolated from rat serum prolonged the survival of histoincompatible skin grafts, many investigators have been able to isolate humoral factors which suppress various T cell–mediated immune responses. Riggio and associates[27] have isolated immunosuppressive alpha globulins from pooled normal human serum and from the serum of patients undergoing rejection of a transplanted kidney. This material was assayed for immunosuppression by suppression of PHA-induced blastogenesis of human peripheral lymphocytes. Nelson[25] has isolated from mouse spleen cells a soluble factor which suppresses the response of spleen lymphocytes to PHA and allogeneic lymphocytes. Veit and Michael[33, 34] have found a naturally occurring mouse serum factor, an alpha globulin, which suppressed both primary and secondary plaque-forming cell responses to sheep red blood cells. The same factor did not inhibit the plaque-forming cell response to *E. coli* bacteria and lipopolysaccharide. Garcia-Giralt and associates[10] have isolated an immunosuppressive material from calf spleen and have shown that it is suppressive in vitro transformation induced by PHA or histoincompatible cells. Mowbray,[24] Carpenter and colleagues,[4] and Milton[23] have isolated an immunosuppressive alpha globulin fraction from mammalian serum as well as from bovine thymus, and they have shown that it suppresses a variety of T cell–dependent assay systems. Kiger and associates[18] have isolated a lymphocyte-specific inhibitory factor from calf thymus and have found that it acts on immune reactions in which T lymphocytes are involved.

We have demonstrated that IRA acts upon the lymphocyte to inhibit activation by both antigen and mitogen.[6] We have determined that this alpha globulin has its own receptor on the surface of lymphocytes which is different from that receptor necessary for mitogen activation.[6] The alpha globulin is ineffective once activation of lymphoid cells has begun and therefore, acts to antagonize the early events of antigen recognition.[13] We have also carried out in vivo studies with IRA isolated from human plasma and have observed in mice that this factor suppresses both the primary and secondary plaque-forming cell response to sheep red blood cells,[12] prolongs the survival of histoincompatible skin allografts,[20] and hinders immunosurveillance and suppresses cellular immunity to methylcholanthrene-induced tumors.[14] Recent investigations[21] demonstrate that this factor does not antagonize thymus-independent antigen reactions with B lymphocytes. We belive that this immunosuppressive factor(s) which is effective in suppressing T cell-mediated responses acts as a form of "feedback" control to regulate the cellular immune response.

There is evidence in support of the hypothesis that serum immunosuppressive humoral factors are produced or increased during immune stimulation. Veit and Michael[34] have demonstrated immunosuppressive activity in whole mouse serum and have shown that this activity increased considerably following antigenic stimulation of the mice with thymus-dependent antigens. Ambrose[1] has isolated an immunosuppressive factor in the serum-free medium of antigen-stimulated rabbit lymph node cultures. Riggio and co-workers[27] have found immunosuppressive alpha globulin in the plasma of patients undergoing the intense immune response which occurs during the acute rejection of a transplanted kidney. In a few patients followed sequentially, immunosuppressive activity was not detectable at a time prior to the rejection episode, nor was it detectable after the rejected kidney was removed. Thus, there is evidence that serum immunosuppressive factor(s) is produced as part of a T cell–mediated immune response. It is our hypothesis that tumors may either produce factors which mimic the "feedback" regulator or are able to manipulate the immune response so that the regulator is inappropriately produced.

REFERENCES

1. Ambrose, C. T.: Regulation of the secondary antibody response in vitro, J. Exp. Med. **137:** 1369, 1973.
2. Ashikawa, K., Inone, K., Shimizu, T., and Ishibashi, Y.: An increase of serum alpha-globulin in tumor bearing hosts and its immunological significance, Jap. J. Exp. Med. **41:** 339, 1971.
3. Black, M. M.: Human breast cancer: A model for cancer immunology, Isr. J. Med. Sci. **9:** 284, 1973.
4. Carpenter, C. B., Boylston, II, A. W., and Merrill, J. P.: Immunosuppressive alphaglobulin from bovine thymus, Cell. Immunol. **2:** 435, 1972.
5. Cooperband, S. R., Badger, A. M., Davis, R. C., Schmid, K., and Mannick, J. A.: Competitive blockade of lymphocyte stimulation by a serum immunoregulatory alphaglobulin (IRA), Transplant. Proc. **1:** 516, 1969.
6. Cooperband, S. R., Badger, A. M., Davis, R. C., Schmid, K., and Mannick, J. A.: The effect of immunoregulatory alphaglobulin (IRA) on lymphocyte stimulation in vitro, J. Immunol. **109:** 154, 1972.

7. Cooperband, S. R., Bondevik, H. E., Schmid, K., and Mannick, J. A.: Inhibition of the transformation of human lymphocytes by homologous globulin, Science **159:** 1243, 1969.
8. Eilber, F. T., and Morton, D. L.: Impaired immunologic reactivity and recurrence following cancer surgery, Cancer **25:** 362, 1970.
9. Field, E. J., and Caspary, E. A.: Lymphocyte sensitization in advanced malignant disease, Br. J. Cancer **26:** 164, 1972.
10. Garcia-Giralt, E., Morales, V. H., LaSalvia, E., and Mathé, G.: Suppression of graft vs. host reaction by a spleen extract, J. Immunol. **109:** 878, 1972.
11. Gatti, R. A.: Serum inhibitors of lymphocyte responses, Lancet **1:** 1351, 1971.
12. Glasgow, A. H., Cooperband, S. R., Occhino, J. C., Schmid, K., and Mannick, J. A.: Inhibition of secondary immune response in vivo by immunoregulatory alpha globulin (IRA), Proc. Soc. Exp. Biol. Med. **138:** 753, 1971.
13. Glasgow, A. H., Menzoian, J. O., Cooperband, S. R., Nimberg, R. B., Schmid, K., and Mannick, J. A.: Immunoregulatory alpha-globulin "failure" to inhibit antibody response when administered after antigen exposure, J. Immunol. **3:** 272, 1973.
14. Glasgow, A. H., Schmid, K., and Mannick, J. A.: Effect of immunoregulatory alpha globulins (IRA) on tumor immunity, Surg. Forum **23:** 120, 1972.
15. Herberman, R. B.: Cellular immunity to human tumor associated antigens, Isr. J. Med. Sci. **9:** 300, 1973.
16. Hellstrom, I., and Hellstrom, K. E., Pierce, G. E., and Yang, J. P. S.: Cellular and humoral immunity to different types of human neoplasms, Nature **220:** 1352, 1968.
17. Kamrin, B. B.: Successful skin homografts in mature non-litter mate rats treated with fractions containing alpha globulins, Proc. Soc. Exp. Biol. Med. **100:** 58, 1959.
18. Kiger, N., Florentin, I., and Mathé, G.: Some effects of a partially purified lymphocyte inhibiting factor from calf thymus, Transplantation **14:** 448, 1972.
19. McLaughlin, A. P., Kessler, W. O., Trimen, K., and Gittes, R. F.: Immune lymphocyte competence in urologic cancer, Surg. Forum **24:** 112, 1973.
20. Mannick, J. A., and Schmid, K.: Prolongation of allograft survival by a alpha globulin isolated from normal blood, Transplantation **5:** 1231, 1967.
21. Menzoian, J. O., Glasgow, A. H., Nimberg, R. B., Cooperband, S. R., Schmid, K., Saporoschetz, I., and Mannick, J. A.: Regulation of "T" lymphocyte function by immunoregulatory alpha globulin (IRA), J. Immunol. In press.
22. Menzoian, J. O., Scheinman, L., Glasgow, A. H., Saporoschetz, I., and Mannick, J. A.: Correlation between skin test reactivity and in vitro immunosuppressive activity of the serum of cancer patients, Surg. Forum **24:** 309, 1973.
23. Milton, J. D.: Effect of an immunosuppressive serum α-2 glycoprotein with ribonuclease activity on the proliferation of human lymphocytes in culture, Immunology **20:** 205, 1971.
24. Mowbray, J. F.: Effect of large doses of an α-2 glycoprotein fraction on the survival of rat skin homografts, Transplantation **1:** 15, 1963.
25. Nelson, D. S.: Mouse serum factor depressing lymphocyte transformation, Separatum Experientia **28:** 227, 1972.
26. Occhino, J. C., Glasgow, A. H., Cooperband, S. R., Mannick, J. A., and Schmid, K.: Isolation of an immunosuppressive peptide from human plasma, J. Immunol. **110:** 685, 1973.
27. Riggio, R. R., Schwartz, G. H., Bull, F. G., Stenzel, K. H., and Rubin, A. L.: α-2 globulins in renal graft rejection, Transplantation **8:** 689, 1969.
28. Sample, W. F., Gertner, H. R., and Chretien, P. B.: Inhibition of phytohemagglutinin-induced in vitro lymphocyte transformation by serum from patients with carcinoma, J. Natl. Cancer Inst. **46:** 1291, 1971.
29. Silk, M.: Effect of plasma from patients with carcinoma on in vitro lymphocyte transformation, Cancer **20:** 2087, 1967.
30. Southam, C. M.: Evidence of immunological reactions to autochthonous cancer in man, Eur. J. Cancer **1:** 173, 1965.
31. Stewart, T. H. M.: The presence of delayed hypersensitivity reactions in patients toward cellular extracts of their malignant tumors, Cancer **23:** 1380, 1969.
32. Suciu-Foca, N., Buda, J., McManus, J., Thiem, T., and Reemtsma, K.: Impaired responsiveness of lymphocytes and serum inhibiting factors in patients with cancer, Cancer Res. **33:** 2373, 1973.
33. Veit, B. C., and Michael, J. G.: Immune response suppression by an inhibitor in normal and immune mouse serum, Nature (New Biol.) **235:** 238, 1972.
34. Veit, B. C., and Michael, J. G.: Characterization of an immunosuppressive factor present in mouse serum, J. Immunol. **111:** 341, 1973.

DISCUSSION

Dr. Charles F. McKhann (Minneapolis, Minn.). We have been studying the immune capacity of animals' lymph node cells from mice to respond to exposure to tumor cells or tumor cell antigen extracts in culture when the lymph node cells come from the very same animals that are being exposed to the same antigens in culture afterwards. With the different times after removal of lymph node cells from the animals, one can see that there is a great peak in potentiation of the capacity of the lymph node cells to respond to exposure in vitro for as long as fourteen days, and after that there is a very abrupt falling off in response.

The background increases, indicating that probably these cells are being stimulated in vivo and reach a maximum capacity in vivo before they are removed to be further stimulated in vitro. At any rate, they cannot be further stimulated in vitro.

If the tumor is removed, the capacity to be stimulated or the capability of being stimulated in vitro again, comes back very promptly after the tumor is removed. The major difference found in these animals is that after about fourteen days free antigen is found in the circulation of these animals, indicating that the glass is essentially full and overflowing: that is, the immune response, the immune capacity of the animal, with respect to specific antigen has been completely saturated, and now we have free antigen left over in excess in the circulation which can be identified.

Is there any evidence that the material that you are finding is actually antigen from the tumor, because the antigen that we find is also of low molecular weight?

Dr. Nicholas A. Halasz (San Diego, Calif.). In order to achieve 100 percent inhibition of PHA-induced transformation, you are using somewhere between 40 and 700 mg. per 100 ml. of peptide, or of protein. Now, what sort of concentrations are present in these patients' plasma? How much do you have to concentrate in order to get this amount, granted that the transformation inhibition is not directly transferable to measurement in vivo of carcinostatic or carcinocytotoxic effect affecting these tumor cells.

I would be interested to know what the quantitative correlation is, how much serum contains—how does that correlate with the concentration you need to block blast transformation?

Dr. Yosef H. Pilch (Torrance, Calif.). I believe that Drs. Catalona and Creegan from the Surgery Branch of the National Cancer Institute reported a few years ago something similar when they looked at the intrinsic capacity of lymphocytes from cancer patients to be stimulated by PHA, and they found that certain cancer patients—and this correlated to a certain extent with the stage of the disease—whose lymphocytes would not transform. Very often they found that the reason they would not transform was not a defect in the lymphocytes per se but that there was an inhibitory factor in the serum. In fact, in some of these patients, one could take the serum and inhibit the PHA stimulation of quite normal lymphocytes from normal donors. Therefore, I believe that your observation has confirmation in their work.

My question is: I think all of us who do DNCB skin testing on cancer patients have noted instances in which patients with very large tumor masses who are DNCB-negative have their skin test reactivity restored following either resection of a large body burden of tumor by surgery or even under certain circumstances, following a good response to chemotherapy or radiation therapy.

I wondered if you had had the opportunity to sort out two things: In the patients with local disease—or with advanced disease, for that matter—does the amount of immunosuppressive effect in the serum in any way correlate with the body burden of tumor? Does the immunosuppressive activity of the serum ever disappear or decrease following surgical excision of tumor or a response to chemotherapy or radiation therapy?

Dr. Arthur H. Glasgow (closing). Let me again specify that the kind of suppression that we are talking about is nonspecific suppression of cellular immunity. This material that we have talked about today we assayed primarily in terms of its ability to suppress phytohemagglutinin-induced stimulation of human peripheral lymphocytes, but we have also looked at it in terms of suppressing other cellular immune responses; also, we always try to confirm the in vitro studies by using the material in vivo in the assay for sheep red cells in mice, since we have previously shown that this material does go across species barriers. Because we feel so strongly that this does work nonspecifically, we have not really looked to see if there is antigen in these animals. And we have not, because we are not looking for antigen specificity.

In terms of the quantitative aspects, all I can say is that in looking at cancer serums, we find that we can get suppression of PHA stimulation at 7 or 3.5 mg. per milliliter in tissue culture with material from peak 1 of DEAE ion exchange chromatography. Peak 1 is essentially 80 percent of the serum proteins. In normal patients, we never ever get suppression at 7 or 3.5 mg. In fact, we have to look out in the alpha globulins when we are talking about normal serum, and that is only about five percent of the peak 1 material. So I would say there is at least twenty times as much material in the cancer serums as there is in the normal serums, and one of the reasons that it took us so long to try to extract this material from cancer patients was our difficulty in the early days in reliably getting immunosuppressive activity from normal serum. To avoid that problem, we had gone to using Cohn fractions, because there already is concentration of the alpha globulins in some of the Cohn fractions.

In response to Dr. Pilch's question, we certainly do agree with the work of Cataloni. This gets us into the question of how the material is actually produced. I can briefly say that we have studied some patients after they have had resections of rather large tumor burdens, and we have found that in some of them, the amount of immunosuppressive activity has indeed gone down, in fact, we have converted some patients from negative to positive skin test responders.

In general, I think that we have postulated that the IRA functions as a feedback regulator of the immune response, and one would anticipate, in areas where there was a lot of antigenic stimulation, more of the IRA would be produced. If the source of antigenic stimulation is removed, then one would suspect that the amount of IRA would go down. The few times that we have looked at that, that has indeed been true.

Distinction of allogeneic immunity from tumor-specific immunity in man

Leon C. Parks, M.D., William J. Smith, *and* **G. Melville Williams, M.D.,** *Baltimore, Md.*

Tissue-cultured melanoma cells and their autogenous fibroblasts were used for microcytotoxicity testing for the prevalence and activity in normals and in melanoma patients of: (1) "killer" lymphocytes; (2) blocking effects of transplantation and progressor melanoma sera; and (3) anti-tumor IgG antibody. Three of nine (33 per cent) of the melanoma patients possessed specific lymphocytotoxicity against melanoma cells, and 12 of 34 (35 per cent) normal individuals possessed allogeneic lymphocytotoxicity against both melanoma and fibroblast cells. Sera from melanoma patients could block melanoma-specific systems but, unlike transplant sera, did not block allogeneic kill. Sera from all normals and eight of nine melanoma patients were unreactive to melanoma and fibroblast cells by mixed agglutination. Sera from one melanoma patient reacted to both cell lines. These findings suggest a reappraisal of the role of allogeneic immunity in testing for tumor immunity.

From the Division of Transplantation, the Department of Surgery, The Johns Hopkins University School of Medicine, Baltimore, Md.

THE EXISTENCE of cell-mediated immunity to human cancer as originally demonstrated by Hellstrom and associates[4, 5] has now been reported by many laboratories.[1, 7, 8] Tumor-specific immunity is said to exist when lymphocytes from a cancer patient possess cytotoxicity for tumor cells cultured from a malignancy histologically similar to that of the lymphocyte donor and do not react with other malignant or benign cells. Lymphocytes from normal individuals are said to react infrequently against tumor or normal cells with the possible exception that North American Negroes may possess natural antimelanoma activity.[6]

These findings and the uncertainty of successfully culturing any given tumor have encouraged the use of established tissue culture cell lines or one of the relatively few successful short-term cultures of malignant cells for studies of human tumor immunity. Such lines are infrequently accompanied by a parallel culture of autogenous benign cells which would provide controls for the detection of nontumor or allogeneic immunity.

However, the studies reported here demonstrate that the lymphocytes of nonsensitized individuals frequently possess marked cytotoxicity for tissue-cultured cells and that the reactivity is of similar degree for malignant and autogenous benign cells. If valid, such findings suggest that erroneous conclusions may be developed by studies of tumor immunity not invariably controlled for allogeneic immunity.

MATERIALS AND METHODS

Culture of target cells. Tumor cultures were inititated with the cell-laden super-

Supported by National Institutes of Health Grant No. HL-14132 and the Ortho Research Foundation.

Presented at the Thirty-fifth Annual Meeting of the Society for University Surgeons, St. Louis, Mo., Feb. 14-16, 1974.

natant obtained by mincing surgically removed tumor specimens in phosphate-buffered saline. This supernatant was placed into Falcon 3012 tissue culture flasks and incubated at 37° C. with 15 percent fetal calf serum* in McCoys 5A* medium containing penicillin 10 U. per milliliter. Promising colonies of malignant cells were separated and subcultured until a pure tumor cell population was obtained. Melanoma line H-81 is a heavily pigmented small cell obtained from subcutaneous metastasis in a blood group O male (E. G.) possessing HLA antigens 2, 3, 7. Melanoma line H-104 is a nonpigmented cuboidal cell obtained from a brain metastasis in a blood group A female (P. B.) possessing HLA antigens 1, 2, 12, W17.

The autogenous control fibroblasts H-82 (E. G.) and H-109 (P. B.) were obtained by explant of skin biopsies as was fibroblast line H-97 selected for its HLA antigens. Kidney lines HK-81 and HK-86 were obtained by explant of portions of rejected kidneys and were selected for study because of HLA antigenicity similar to the tumor lines. All lines studied were in their fifth to twelfth passage and had not been frozen. Routine cultures for microplasm using mycoplasm agar* were consistently negative.

Lymphocyte preparation. Fifty milliliters of whole blood was drawn into syringes containing 1,250 U. of heparin† and 7 ml. of Plasmagel,‡ mixed, and allowed to settle for 45 minutes. The lymphocyte-rich supernatant was ejected into Siliclad§ 40 ml. conical tubes underlayed by 15 ml. of Ficoll-Hypaque,|| (specific gravity, 1.077) at 18° C. and spun at 450 × g for 40 minutes. The interface was removed, layed onto 15 ml. of sera autogenous to the lymphocyte donor, and spun at 250 × g for ten minutes, effectively removing residual Ficoll-Hypaque. The pellet obtained was washed three times by suspending and centrifuging at 250 × g for ten minutes in serum-free McCoy's medium. Contaminating macrophages were removed by suspending the pellet in 5 ml. of media and placing this serially into three Falcon 3012 flasks for 15 minutes of incubation in each at 37° C. The nonabsorbed cells were again washed three times in serum-free media and diluted to the desired concentration for assay. This method provides a 99 percent pure lymphocyte preparation which appears free of Ficoll-Hypaque and macrophage-related cytotoxicity.

Cytotoxicity testing. Target cells were plated in Falcon microtiter trays at 75 to 150 cells per well and incubated for 24 hours before exposure to test lymphocytes and sera. Lymphocyte/target cell ratios of 10^3 to 1 were used except as noted. Test sera were heat inactivated at 56° C. for 45 minutes and used in a 1:5 dilution with McCoy's medium. The assay technique used was that described by Hellstrom and associates[5] with exposure of target cells to test sera for 45 minutes, removal of test sera, and exposure of target cells to lymphocytes in serum-free media for 45 minutes, and finally addition of fetal calf sera to a 15 percent concentration. The plates were then incubated in a humid five percent CO_2 atmosphere for 40 hours, stained, and optically counted. Cytotoxicity is expressed as the percent reduction of target cells in test wells compared with the count of control lymphocyte wells. Blocking activity is defined by the formula:

$$\%\ \text{Blocking} = 1 - \left(\frac{\dfrac{\text{control sera*}}{\text{control lymphs}} - \dfrac{\text{patient sera}}{\text{patient lymphs}}}{\dfrac{\text{control sera}}{\text{control lymphs}} - \dfrac{\text{control sera}}{\text{patient lymphs}}} \right)$$

*i.e., the number of cells in the wells containing control sera and control lymphs, etc.

Blocking activity of transplantation serum was studied with serum obtained from a patient with a perfectly functioning 3⅓-year-old cadaver kidney transplant. This patient had rejected his first transplant, but had not experienced any rejection crisis with his second.

Mixed agglutination. Target cells were pre-

*North American Biologics, Rockville, Md.

†Upjohn Beef Lung, Sodium Heparin, 1000 U. per milliliter.

‡Roger Bellon Laboratories, Neuilly, France.

§Siliclad, Clay Adams.

||Sigma-Winthrop.

Table I. *Cytotoxicity of reactive normal males on melanoma (H-81) and benign control cells (H-82) autogenous with the melanoma*

Lymphocyte donor	Target cell	Average No. target cells/well			% CMI
		Media control	Control lymphocytes	Test lymphocytes	
Normal blacks					
V. T.	H-81	83	90	24	73
	H-82	65	60	18	70
J. H.	H-81	43	41	1	98
	H-82	62	45	17	62
W. M.	H-81	83	90	19	79
	H-82	163	157	22	86
A. W.	H-81	43	41	6	85
	H-82	189	132	54	59
W. G.	H-81	141	97	6	94
	H-82	189	132	24	82
Normal whites					
M. P.	H-81	75	65	8	88
	H-82	190	150	21	86
R. C.	H-81	72	82	9	89
	H-82	71	76	29	62
D. E.	H-81	52	57	19	67
	H-82	66	64	18	72

pared from the H-81 melanoma and H-82 fibroblast lines. Target cells were prepared by placing 5×10^4 trypsinized cells into 100×10 mm. glass tubes and slant culturing them until a monolayer was obtained. Test sera was heat-inactivated at 56° C. for 45 minutes, diluted in phosphate-buffered saline, and reacted with the target cells for one hour at 37° C. The monolayer was then washed three times in PBS and exposed to indicator human D+ red cells, which had been sensitized with Ripley serum (an IgG anti-D), and reacted with an excess of goat anti-human IgG* for one hour at 37° C. Positive reactions were graded as 1 to 4+ on the basis of erythrocyte adherence to the tissue culture monolayer. A polyspecific serum from a hypersensitized transplant patient was used as a positive control.

RESULTS

Microcytotoxicity assay with lymphocytes from normal males. The lymphocytes from nine of 23 black males and from three of 11 white males produced cytotoxicity in excess of 50 percent on at least four assays against both H-81 (melanoma cells) and H-82 (fibroblast) cultured from the same melanoma patient. The degree of reactivity compared to lymphocytes from nonreactive individuals is illustrated in the eight examples shown in Table I. Nonreactor and control cells produced no significant cell kill while the cells from reactors regularly killed more than 50 percent of the target cells. Further, there were no large differences in the ability of reactive lymphocytes to kill fibroblasts and melanoma cells. While the lymphocytes from certain individuals appeared more reactive against melanoma cells, the lymphocytes from others were more active against the fibroblasts.

Cell-mediated immunity and blocking in patients with melanoma. The lymphocytes from three of nine patients with melanoma had in vitro cytotoxic activity against melanoma cells, unattended by cytotoxicity to the

*Hyland Laboratories.

Table II. *Melanoma-specific cell-mediated immunity and blocking activity in patients with rapidly progressing melanoma*

Patient	Date	Average No. of cells			% CMI	Average No. of cells with patient's lymphocytes and		Percent significant blocking
		Media control	Control's lympho-cytes	Patient's lympho-cytes		Control's serum	Patient's serum	
M. N.	8- 1-73	52	48	29	40	—	—	—
	8- 9-73	110	116	93	20	93	90	0
	8-16-73	87	84	64	24	—	—	—
A. L.	11- 7-73	174	212	140	34	140	156	22
	11-19-73	41	45	36	20	36	33	0
	1- 1-73	154	173	228	−32	228	224	0
T. G.	3-26-73	146	129	91	30	91	109	48
	4-24-73	179	179	131	27	131	157	54
	5- 2-73	26	27	19	27	19	23	50

Table III. *Failure of progressor melanoma sera to block black lymphocytotoxicity for melanoma*

Test lymphocyte donor	Test serum donor	Average No. of cells			% CMI	Average No. of cells with test lymphocytes and		Percent significant blocking
		Media control	Control lympho-cytes	Test lympho-cytes		Control serum	Test serum	
V. T.	V. T.	83	90	24	73	24	24	0
	T. G.	132	145	43	70	54	43	−12
	M. S.	107	102	24	76	28	24	0
S. S. (10^3:1)	S. S.	52	53	15	74	15	15	0
	T. G.	171	194	69	64	85	69	−15
	M. S.	207	180	70	61	71	70	0
	P. B.	207	180	56	69	71	56	−14
S. S. (10^2:1)	S. S.	128	148	114	23	114	114	0
	T. G.			107	28	114	107	−21
	M. S.			104	30	114	104	−29
	P. B.			108	27	114	108	−18

fibroblasts. In no instance was cytotoxicity in excess of 50 percent, and in most instances cytotoxicity was less than 30 percent. The lack of more dramatic CMI against melanoma may be attributed to our patient selection, because five of nine of our patients had systemic metastasis. Serial studies performed in the three patients presented in Table II illustrate an over-all suppression of CMI with the progression of malignancy.

Serum-blocking factors did not invariably accompany the progression of the disease. It is perhaps noteworthy that the combination of patient serum and cells augmented tumor growth (negative CMI) in one patient in the terminal stages of metastatic disease.

The effects of melanoma "blocking serum" upon normal lymphocytes demonstrating CMI to melanoma. The sera from three patients with progressive melanoma failed to reduce the cytotoxicity of normal lymphocytes for melanoma cells (Table III). It was possible that the allogeneic kill was so intensive that blocking activity was obscured. For this reason, the attacker lymphocyte–to–target cell ratio was reduced from 1,000:1 to 100:1. Even at this reduced attacker lymphocyte–to–target cell ratio, where CMI was only 23 percent, no significant blocking activity was present.

The blocking activity of transplantation sera. The sera from a patient with a well-tolerated cadaver transplant produced repeatable and significant blocking in reactions with two of five cell lines tested against the lymphocytes from one patient (Table IV). These data also demonstrate the specificity of the CMI present in this individual. Dramatic CMI was demonstrated in four of the five lines tested but was completely absent in the other.

The serum from the transplant recipient did not have a blocking activity in reactions between the lymphocytes from a second normal male and the same target lines. This may reflect quantitative differences for this individual displayed intense CMI to four of the five cell lines tested. However, the difference in blocking activity observed makes it unlikely that the depressed CMI is related to nonspecific factors and is consistent with interference of specific lymphocyte–antigen interaction.

Antibody reactions in patients with melanoma and normal individuals. Multiple-serum samples from nine patients with melanoma were tested against the H-81 and H-82 cell lines. Eight were nonreactive and one reacted weakly to both at titers of 1:30. The sera from nine normal blacks likewise proved to be nonreactive. The only sera that distinguished the melanoma from the fibroblast line was one obtained from a chimpanzee immunized to melanoma and kindly supplied by Dr. H. Siegler.[9] The chimpanzee sera produced strongly positive reactions to H-81 and dilutions of 1:270, and it was nonreactive against H-82.

DISCUSSION

The results reported must be interpreted in the context of the methodology applied. There appear to be only two reasonable alternative explanations for the identification of CMI in normal individuals by microcytotoxicity technique. Either the microcytotoxicity test system is too sensitive an indicator of CMI to be relevant and neither the tumor-specific nor the allogeneic immunity detected by this assay are significant, or both allogeneic immunity in normal individuals and tumor immunity in cancer patients exist and require controls for their separate identification. Of the two interpretations, we prefer the latter, for the presence of cell-mediated immunity and its attenuation by serum factors has been demonstrated to correspond to clinical events.[2, 3, 10, 11]

Thus, the most important observation derived from these studies is that the lymphocytes of both normal individuals and cancer patients frequently possess marked cytotoxicity against not only cultured tumor cells but also benign cells autogenous with the malignant cells. The finding that such reactivity is present against certain cell lines and not others and that some reactions are blocked by transplant sera while others are not suggests that the cytotoxicity is not related to extraneous factors such as the presence of Ficoll-Hypaque, macrophages, or infectious agents. Rather, the reactions by virtue of reproducibility and specificity are real biologic phenomena.

Table IV. *Blocking activity of transplantation serum (A.S.) on "allogeneic" cell-mediated immunity*

Target	*Lymph donor*	*Sera*	*% Cytotoxicity*	*% Blocking*
Fibroblast (1, 2, 12, W17)	V. T.	V. T.	45	
		A. S.	25	42
	W. M.	W.M.	94	
		A. S.	88	10
Fibroblast (2, 3, 7)	V. T.	V. T.	48	
		A. S.	29	40
	W. M.	W.M.	67	
		A. S.	67	0
Fibroblast (3, 7, 11)	V. T.	V. T.	0	
		A. S.	0	—
	W. M.	W.M.	0	
		A. S.	0	—
Kidney (2, 7, 8, 10)	V. T.	V. T.	50	
		A. S.	50	0
	W. M.	W.M.	28	
		A. S.	28	0
Kidney (2, 12)	V. T.	V. T.	41	N.D.
	W. M.	W.M.	100	N.D.

A possible explanation for the simultaneous malignant-benign cell reactivity observed is that cells thought to be melanoma were indeed fibroblastic. This possibility can be discounted because: (1) the H-81 line possesses distinctive morphology and is heavily pigmented; (2) lymphocytes from melanoma patients possess CMI to H-81 and not H-82; and (3) chimpanzee sera reportedly melanoma specific is strongly reactive against H-81 and not against H-82.

The availability of the paired cultured H-81 and H-82 cell lines allowed us to distinguish between tumor-related and allogeneic immunity. Three of nine (33 percent) of the melanoma patients studied possessed specific lymphocytotoxicity against melanoma as determined by: (1) lack of reactivity against control autogenous fibroblasts and (2) the demonstration of blocking of the activity by progressor sera. Twelve of 34 (35 percent) normal individuals possessed allogeneic lymphocytotoxicity against both H-81 and H-82 as determined by: (1) equivalent reactivity to both cell lines and (2) the demonstration of blocking of this activity by transplant sera and not by sera from progressor melanoma patients. The finding that normal blacks react as strongly against benign control cells as against autogenous melanoma cells is contrary to the view that blacks possess natural immunity to melanoma.

The mixed agglutination test was applied to determine whether patients with malignant melanoma possessed antibodies that cross-reacted with other melanoma cell lines and whether the IgG antibody detected by this technique correlated with the presence or absence of blocking activity determined by the microcytotoxicity assay. The results were unequivocably negative since none of the nine patients with melanoma whose sera were examined serially demonstrated any IgG antibody combining specifically with the melanoma cell line. Therefore, it is unlikely that blocking factors are simple IgG molecules combining with tumor antigens. Further, our hope of detecting blocking by a simple procedure was not realized.

The failure to detect any antibody accompaniment of the described lymphocyte reactivity has implications for transplantation. Neither standard cross-match techniques nor antigen-matching would have predicted the marked lymphocytotoxicity found in some of these nonsensitized individuals. Studies of the HLA antigen composition of attacker, target, and blocking subjects failed to identify a determinant related to CMI.

In summary, these findings support the recent report of Takasugi and associates,[12] which calls for a reappraisal of the role of allogeneic immunity in testing for tumor immunity. Clearly, the lymphocytes of normal individuals may react strongly against tissue-cultured malignant and benign tissues in a nontumor-specific fashion. Lymphocytes from cancer patients may possess similar nontumor-related cytotoxicity which will not be identified as such unless studies of cell-mediated immunity are routinely and simultaneously conducted against autogenous benign cells.

An even greater problem exists in the transfer of in vitro information to clinical practice. For example, the data presented in Table IV suggest that W. M. and V. T. are "primed" to four or five test cultures. Would in fact a transplant from the donor of the cell line not attacked in vitro fare better than the others? Precisely such experimental-clinical correlations must be carried out in sufficent numbers if meaning is to be given to the in vitro studies alleged to measure important immunological variables in man.

The authors wish to express their appreciation to Dr. Wilma Bias and her co-workers in The Johns Hopkins Tissue Typing Laboratory for their assistance in these studies.

REFERENCES

1. Bubenik, J., Perlmann, P., Helmstein, K., and Moberger, G.: Cellular and humoral immune responses to human urinary bladder carcinomas, Int. J. Cancer **5:** 310, 1970.
2. Byrne, M., Heppner, G., Stolbach, L., Cummings, F., McDonough, E., and Calabresi, P.: Correlation of tumor specific immunity with extent of disease in malignant melanoma, Proc. Am. Assoc. Cancer Res. **13:** 184, 1972.
3. Hellstrom, I., and Helstrom, K. E.: Some

recent studies on cellular immunity to human melanomas, Fed. Proc. **32:** 156, 1973.

4. Hellstrom, I., Hellstrom, K. E., Pierce, G. E., and Yang, J. P. S.: Cellular and humoral immunity to different types of human neoplasms, Nature **220:** 1352, 1968.
5. Hellstrom, I., Hellstrom, K. E., Sjogren, H. O., and Warner, G. A.: Demonstration of cell-mediated immunity to human neoplasms of various histologic types, Int. J. Cancer **7:** 1, 1971.
6. Hellstrom, I., Hellstrom, K. E., Sjogren, H. O., and Warner, G. A.: Destruction of cultivated melanoma cells by lymphocytes from healthy black (North American Negro) donors, Int. J. Cancer **11:** 116, 1973.
7. Jagarlamoody, S., Aust, J. C., Tew, R. H., and McKhann, C. F.: In vitro detection of cytotoxic cellular immunity against tumor-specific antigens using a radioisotopic technique, Proc. Natl. Acad. Sci. **68:** 1346, 1971.
8. Levy, N. L., Mahaley, M. S., and Day, E. D.: In vitro demonstration of cell-mediated immunity to human brain tumors, Cancer Res. **32:** 477, 1972.
9. Metzgar, R. S., Bergoc, R. M., Moreno, M. A., and Seigler, H. F.: Melanoma-specific antibodies produced in monkeys by immunization with human melanoma cell lines, J. Natl. Cancer Inst. **50:** 1065, 1973.
10. O'Toole, C., Perlmann, P., Unsgaard, B., Moberger, G., and Edsmyr, F.: Cellular immunity to human urinary bladder carcinoma: Correlation to clinical stage and radiotherapy, Int. J. Cancer **10:** 77, 1972.
11. O'Toole, C., Perlmann, P., Unsgaard, B., Moberger, G., and Edsmyr, F.: Cellular immunity to human urinary bladder carcinoma: Effect of surgery and preoperative irradiation, Int. J. Cancer **10:** 92, 1972.
12. Takasugi, M., Mickey, M. R., and Terasaki, P. I.: Reactivity of lymphocytes from normal persons on cultured tumor cells, Cancer Res. **33:** 2898, 1973.

DISCUSSION

Dr. Yosef H. Pilch (Torrance, Calif.). Different concentrations of lymphocytes will nonspecifically kill any target cell. In other words, if the lymphocyte number is raised high enough, one can nonspecifically kill virtually any target cell. How many different lymphocyte–target cell ratios were looked at in the data that you reported?

We routinely examine at least three lymphocyte-to–target cell ratios between 100 and 500 to 1. The susceptibility of different target cells to nonspecific killing by lymphocytes—in other words, the lymphocyte–target cell ratio at which this nonspecific killing will occur—varies from target cell to target cell. It is a very casual observation that normal fibroblasts may be more or less resistant to nonspecific kill than tumor cells from the same individual. Methodology is crucial to the whole message of the paper.

Dr. John C. McDonald (New Orleans, La.). Some of us have been interested for many years in the mixed lymphocyte reaction and have thought it quite peculiar that people who are presumably nonimmune to other people will give a nice blastogenic response in the mixed lymphocyte culture, when they will not do that to any other antigens that we know. It has raised a question as to whether or not all of us are not preimmune in one way or another, or presensitized to HL-A antigens, or some sort of self-identification antigens. And I wonder if what you are saying is that your studies would suggest that we are in fact carrying a certain amount of immunity to our other members of the species.

Dr. Leon C. Parks (closing). There are two issues. One is the issue of the lymphocyte concentrations, and we have titrated these individuals showing cytotoxicity extensively. We find that we can get kill from these very highly sensitized, or very reactive, individuals down at lymphocyte–tumor ratios of as low as 50 and 100 to 1. It is a profound degree of kill, and it is far stronger kill than we observe in a tumor system.

Drs. Bean from the Sloan-Kettering Institute and Pearlman from the Karolinska Institute have raised some concerns about the use of Ficoll-Hypaque in preparing lymphocytes, and we have been able to avoid that difficulty by washing our lymphocytes through autogenous sera. The lymphocytes are placed on top of autogenous sera when they come off the Ficoll-Hypaque, and after spinning, there is a clear layer of residual Ficoll left and a nice pellet of lymphocytes.

Following a suggestion by Dr. Lucas, we have also incorporated absorption of our lymphocyte preparations on plastic surfaces, after we get the lymphocytes, to remove all other macrophages. If one examines what he thinks is a pure lymphocyte preparation by this method, he finds that it contains a number of bands and polymorphonuclear leukocytes that will give nonspecific cytotoxicity if they are not removed. They have been removed from these studies.

And in answer to Dr. McDonald, I would simply like to agree with him.

Immune surveillance and tumor dissemination: In vitro comparison of the B_{16} melanoma in primary and metastatic form

Leonard I. Goldman, M.D., B. A. Flaxman, M.D., *Philadelphia, Pa.,* **G. Wernick, B.S.,** *and* **J. B. Zabriskie, M.D.,** *New York, N. Y.*

A comparison was made between the B_{16} melanoma in subcutaneous "primary" form and pulmonary metastases that spontaneously developed following amputation of the primary site. The primary tumors were always nonpigmented but the metastases were invariably black. Ultrastructural examination revealed that this difference was due to melanin deposition (presence of melanosomes) on premelanosomes in the metastases and an absence of pigment production in the premelanosomes of the primary cells. A mixed lymphocyte–tumor-cell reaction assayed immunologic difference between these cell types. Primary tumor cells induced a higher in vitro blastogenic response than did secondary cells. Immunization could be detected by pretreatment with live secondary cells employing the assay described above. Live primary cells produced an immunologically detectable response only when larger doses of mitomycin-pretreated cells were used as an immunogen, or when comparisons were made between experimental and control cultures performed simultaneously. These data suggest the existence of biological differences between primary and metastatic B_{16} melanoma.

From Temple University, Philadelphia, Pa., and Rockefeller University, New York, N. Y.

ANTIGENIC modulation between a primary lesion and its metastases might be one reason why tumors metastasize in spite of tumor-specific immunity. This highly theoretical and overly simplistic equation attempts to illustrate how immune selection might yield antigenic differences between primary tumors and their metastases.

Primary		Metastases
TSTA	immune	tsta
	⟶	
fetal	surveillance	FETAL

This investigation was supported in part by: Special Fellowship 1-FO3CA54348-01 and NIH Grant CA-11536 from the National Cancer Institute of the Department of Health, Education and Welfare.

Presented at the Thirty-fifth Annual Meeting of the Society of University Surgeons, St. Louis Mo., Feb. 14-16, 1974.

Reprint address: Leonard I. Goldman, M.D., c/o Lester M. Cramer, Department of Surgery, Temple University, Philadelphia, Pa. 19140.

The equation is based on the assumption that fetal and tumor-specific transplantation antigens (TSTA) exist on primary tumors and that the fetal antigens are less immunogenic since they may be recognized as "infantile self." The immune response directed against the more "foreign" antigens in the primary tumor would reduce the number that eventually metastasize; conversely, a lack of response to "self" antigens would allow relatively free replication in the metastases. The result would be a quantitative and/or qualitative antigenic difference between these two sites.

Previous workers employing transplantation and challenge techniques have reported the following differences. Kim[8] induced metastasizing adenocarcinomas in splenectomized and/or thymectomized syngeneic rats with methylcholanthrene. These tumors showed absent or lessened immunizing capacity when compared to nonmetastasizing tumors induced by the same carcinogen. Axelrad and Klein,[1] by employing hybrid hosts, demonstrated different H-gene requirements of metastatic tumors. Deichman and Kluchareva[4] and Sugarbaker and Cohen[11] have provided similar evidence in other tumor systems.

This study was undertaken to determine whether in vitro methods could detect antigenic differences between cells of primary and metastatic lesions in mice, preliminary to possible similar studies of human cancer.

METHODS

General. Young (six to eight weeks old) female $C_{57}Bl_6$ mice were used throughout. The B_{16} melanoma and animals were obtained from the Jackson Laboratory (Bar Harbor, Maine).

Tumors. Tumors were induced in the hind limbs of mice by the injection of 1×10^6 cells in 0.2 ml. of saline; palpable growth usually appeared by 10 days. Thirty-one days after injection the limbs were amputated under ether anesthesia and the tumor cells prepared as described below. If the limbs are not amputated animals invariably die from primary tumor bulk prior to the development of metastases. Pulmonary metastases were harvested when the animals were killed 20 days after amputation.

Tumor cell preparation. The primary and metastatic tumors were dissected from surrounding normal tissues and minced in Hank's balanced salt solution under aseptic conditions. The tumors were dissociated mechanically in 0.15 percent trypsin in Hank's solution at 37° C. for 30 minutes and the cells incubated in Earle's minimal essential medium (MEM) supplemented with 10 percent fetal calf serum for four to five days in a CO_2-air gas-phase incubator. Cell aliquots were freeze-stored at –70° C. in a mixture composed of glucose, minimal essential media, dimethylsulfoxide, and serum.[13] High levels of viability (90 percent), as measured by trypan blue exclusion, were seen when the cells were thawed and retrieved. In all cases live cells were harvested, stored to avoid antigenic change, and used when required. Comparison was always made between metastatic cells and the primary tumor from which they developed.

Measuring stimulation of DNA synthesis. Incorporation of ^{14}C thymidine* by splenic lymphocytes (R.C.) stimulated by the presence of mitomycin-treated tumor cells (S.C.) was measured by the method of Kanner and associates[7] with the semimicro modifications of Hartzman and associates.[5] Splenic cells, obtained from appropriate animals following inoculation, were dispersed by sieving through a wire screen (No. 60). Contaminating red cells were lysed with 0.83 percent ammonium chloride and the leukocytes were washed twice in saline. They were suspended in tissue culture medium (RPMI 1640, supplemented with glutamine, antibiotics, and 10 percent complement-inactivated fetal calf serum [No. 202169-NABI]) at concentrations of 2×10^5 cells per well on Microtest II plates (Falcon, Calif.). Mitomycin-C–treated tumor cells (50 μg per milliliter at 37° for 30 minutes) were added in varying concentrations and the cells then incubated at 37° in a CO_2-air gas-phase incubator. Viability was assessed by trypan blue exclusion counting in a standard hemocytometer. Phytohemagglutinin (PHA-Wellcome), a nonspecific lymphocyte mitogen, was added at the initiation of the culture to wells containing lymphocytes without tumor cells. On the third day of the culture ^{14}C-thymidine was added and 24 hours later the cells collected on glass wool filter paper. Aquasol† was added and the sample counted in a liquid scintillation counter. The results were expressed as radioactivity incorporated by stimulating cells and responding cells in combination divided by the sum of the radioactivities in both cell types cultured individually.

$$\text{Stimulation index} = \frac{\text{c.p.m. (S.C. + R.C.)}}{\text{c.p.m. S.C. + c.p.m. R.C.}}$$

*Nuclear Chicago, Chicago, Ill., or New England Nuclear, Boston, Mass.

†NEN, Chicago.

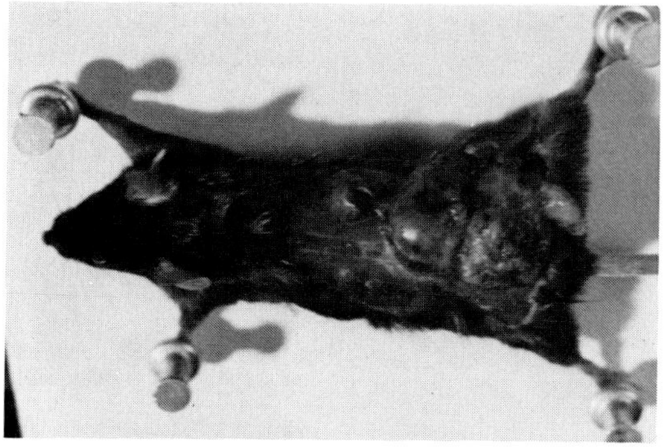

Fig. 1. B_{16} melanoma in "primary" subcutaneous form exhibiting absence of pigmentation.

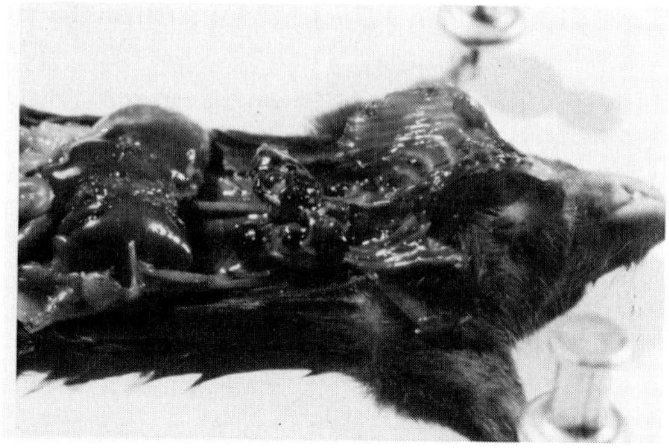

Fig. 2. Pulmonary metastases of B_{16} melanoma showing pigmentation.

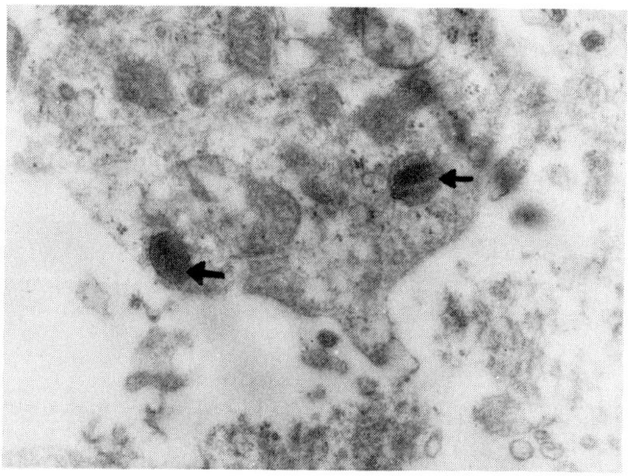

Fig. 3. Electron micrograph showing typical unmelanized premelanosomes (arrows) from a primary subcutaneous implant of B_{16} melanoma. (×30,000.)

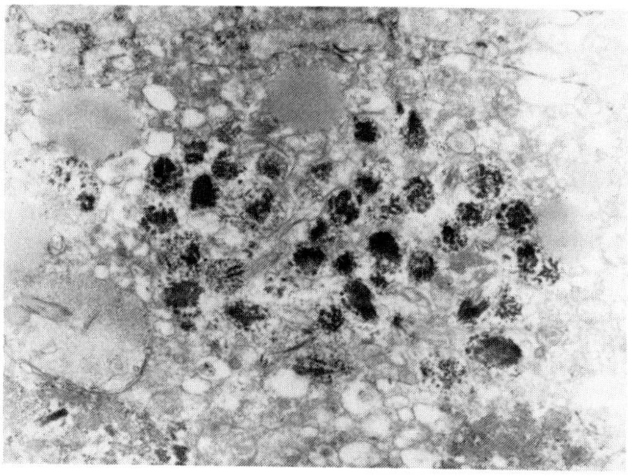

Fig. 4. Electron micrograph showing partially melanized premelanosomes in B_{16} melanoma from a metastatic lesion. (×30,000.)

All estimations were performed in triplicate.

Electron microscopy. For electron microscopy, small pieces of tissue were fixed in buffered 2.5 percent glutaraldehyde (pH 7.4), post-fixed in a 1:2 mixture of OsO_4 in collidine,[2] dehydrated through a graded series of alcohol to propylene oxide, and embedded in Araldite. Ultrathin sections were cut with a diamond knife. Sections were stained in lead citrate and uranyl acetate and examined in an AEI Corinth 175 electron microscope.

Study groups. The following groups of animals were compared to appropriate controls. Groups I and II were injected subcutaneously with 1×10^6 untreated primary or metastatic cells, respectively. In vitro stimulation by equal numbers of mitomycin-treated primary and metastatic cells was performed three to five days after injection.

Group III animals were injected intraperitoneally with 3×10^6 mitomycin-treated primary cells. Seven to 14 days later splenic lymphocytes from these animals and their controls were cultured in vitro with mitomycin-treated primary cells.

RESULTS

Gross and microscopic findings. B_{16} melanoma was slate gray, having lost its pigment through previous transplant generations. When implanted subcutaneously this color, as shown in Fig. 1, persisted.

The pulmonary metastases, seen in Fig. 2, were invariably deeply pigmented.

Ultrastructural examination of unpigmented primary tumors revealed the presence of cells with varying morphologic features. Most cells could not be readily classi-

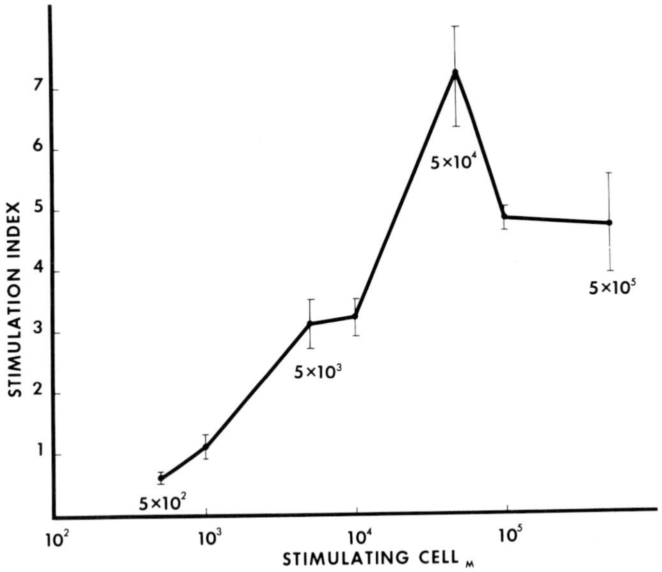

Fig. 5. Dose-response curve in 2×10^5 control splenic lymphocytes cultured in vitro with mitomycin-treated primary. Values expressed as mean stimulation index ± S.E.M.

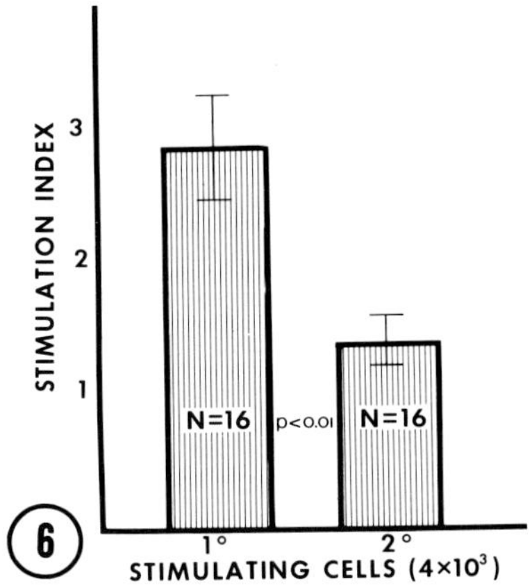

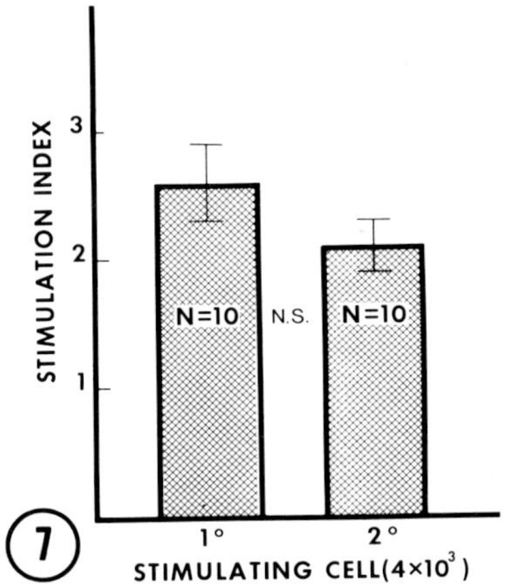

Fig. 6. Mean stimulation indices ± S.E.M. produced by primary and secondary cells in vitro on splenic lymphocytes from animals pretreated with live primary cells.

Fig. 7. Mean stimulation indices ± S.E.M. produced by primary and secondary cells in vitro on splenic lymphocytes from animals pretreated with live metastatic cells.

fied because of a lack of distinguishing characteristics. Some, however, had cytoplasmic organelles that resembled nonmelanized premelanosomes (Fig. 3). These organelles were oval, were demarcated by a distinct membrane, and possessed an internal structure of filaments having a repeating substructure. In the pigmented metastases, cells contained not only unpigmented and partially pigmented premelanosomes but also fully melanized melanosomes (Fig. 4). As was the case for primary tumors, many cells appeared to lack any specific cytoplasmic markers that would indicate their melanocytic origin.

Prior to assay of inoculated animals, an in vitro dose-response curve was performed. The mean stimulation indices and the standard errors which were developed in cultures of 2×10^5 control lymphocytes with varying concentrations of tumor cells are presented in Fig. 5. This curve, typical of blastogenic

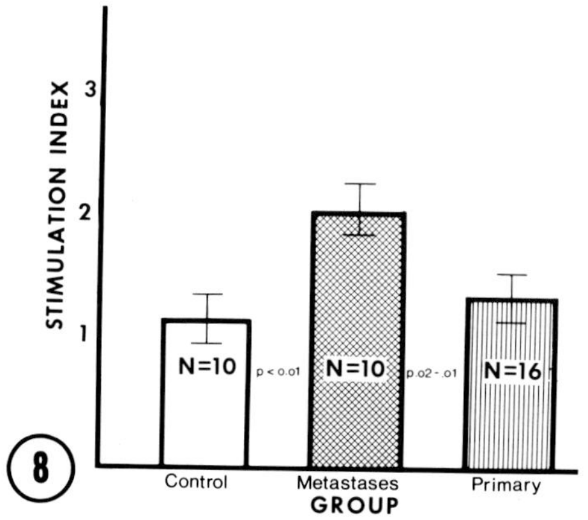

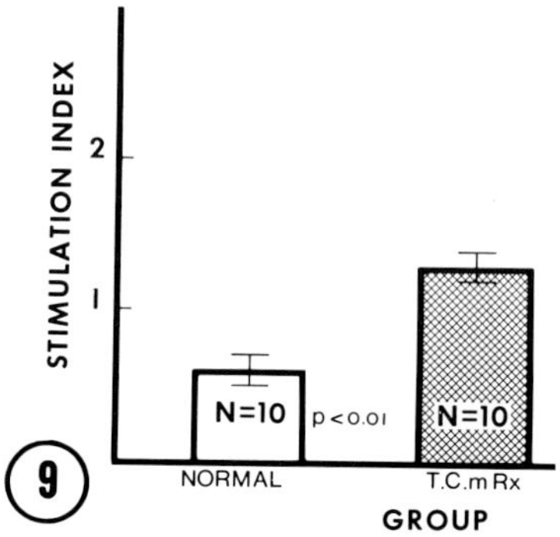

Fig. 8. Mean stimulation indices ± S.E.M. produced by secondary cells in vitro on splenic lymphocytes from controls and Groups I and II.

Fig. 9. Mean stimulation indices ± S.E.M. produced by primary cells in vitro on splenic lymphocytes from controls and animals immunized with 3×10^6 mitomycin-treated primary cells.

transformation with increasing antigen doses, reveals maximal stimulation at tumor cell concentrations of 5×10^4, a lymphocyte: tumor cell ratio of 4:1. At this concentration marked acidity was detected in the culture wells. For this reason we elected to use smaller tumor cell doses, in the ranges of 10^2 through 10^3 cells.

The stimulation indices produced by 4×10^3 primary and metastatic cells in Groups I and II are seen in Figs. 6 and 7. Group I animals, pretreated with 1×10^6 live primary cells, exhibited a stimulation index of 2.9 ± 0.4 (mean ± S.E.M.) with primary cells as antigen. Equal numbers of metastatic cells produce an index of 1.4 ± 0.2. This difference is significant at the 0.01 level (Fig. 6).

The injection of 1×10^6 metastatic cells three to five days prior to assay in Group II animals is shown in Fig. 7. Primary cells, in vitro, stimulated to the level of 2.6 ± 0.3. This is similar to Group I. The response to secondary cells, on the other hand, was increased to 2.1 ± 0.2. In this group there is no significant difference between the in vitro responses elicited by the two cell types. When a comparison is made between the effects of pretreatment regimen and the response to secondary cells alone, the following occurred (Fig. 8). Live metastatic cells injected subcutaneously enabled the splenic lymphocytes of these animals to increase their in vitro response to this antigen. This difference is significant when compared to both controls and those pretreated with live primary cells.

Controls show similar responses to Group I, with in vitro primary and secondary stimulation indices of 2.8 ± 0.4 and 1.2 ± 0.2, respectively. Since this indicated an apparent inability of live primary cells to show evidence of substantial antigenicity, we studied two alternatives for the detection of an immune response. The first employed higher concentrations of mitomycin-treated cells as an intraperitoneal immunogen (Fig. 9). The index of in vitro stimulation produced by 5×10^2 primary cells in controls is 0.6 ± 0.1. Pretreatment with 3×10^6 mitomycin-treated tumor cells, seven to 14 days prior to assay, increases the index to 1.3 ± 0.1. This difference is significant at the 99 percent confidence level.

The second alternative compared the lymphocyte primary tumor cell reactions between animals injected subcutaneously with 3×10^6 live primary cells and simultaneously cultured controls. These were done at intervals between three and 20 days following injection. Fig. 10 illustrates these findings. If the pooled data from three- and four-day animals is compared to controls, similarly pooled, no significant difference is seen because of high standard errors. On the other hand, changes can be seen by calculating the dif-

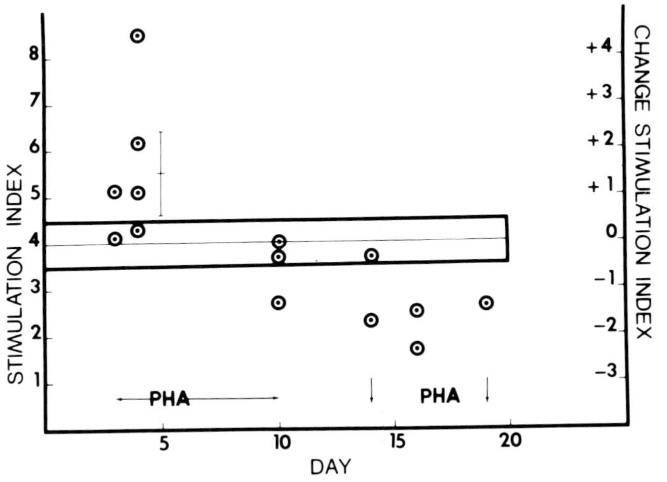

Fig. 10. Changes in the stimulation index of splenic lymphocytes from animals injected with 3×10^6 live primary cells compared to matched controls at varying periods following injection. Pooled data (mean stimulation index ± S.E.M.) shown for controls (horizontal bar) and combined three to four days (vertical bar) after injection.

ference between each animal and its matched control. At three and four days following immunization an increased stimulation index is seen. This disappears by the tenth day. Beyond this day the levels become depressed. PHA responses are unchanged during the early days, which suggests that the reaction to tumor cell antigen is immune specific. The depressed PHA response seen after the tenth day implies that generalized immunodepression has occurred and is probably related to the increasing tumor burden.

DISCUSSION

This study has identified certain differences between primary and metastatic B_{16} melanomas. The gross color changes noted were further studied by electron microscopy. Many cells from both primary and metastatic lesions could not be precisely identified as melanoma because they lacked premelanosomes (unpigmented or partially pigmented melanin granule) or melanosomes (fully pigmented melanin granule). In some cells of the unpigmented primary lesions, fully formed premelanosomes were present and identifiable by shape and internal structure. Melanin deposition was totally absent. In secondary lesions, however, the brown or black was due to the presence of cells containing both premelanosomes and melanosomes. These organelles were similar to those described for pigmented B_{16} melanomas in vivo and in vitro.[3, 6, 9, 10, 12] The morphologic difference between cells of primary and secondary origins is not the inability of either to form premelanosomes, but rather the latter's ability to produce melanin on the substructure of this organelle. The reason for this is unknown at present but may be due to some form of immune selection or environmental and/or organ-specific factors that allow pigment production to be expressed.

This intracellular difference could well be associated with plasma membrane changes and account for the immunologic findings we observed. In any case, at least two biologically distinct cell populations are noted. In every group studied, primary cells were capable of inducing a higher blastogenic response than were secondary cells. While this ability to transform lymphocytes cannot be directly equated to antigenicity, some relationship probably does exist. Further, the immunizing capability of these two cell types also differs. Metastatic cell pretreatment apparently sensitizes lymphocytes so that they show an increased in vitro responsiveness to identical cells. This was not seen in the pooled data from animals injected with live primary cells when they were compared to controls. It appears that the higher blastogenic responses produced by these cells in both sensitized and nonsensitized lymphocytes vary significantly between cultures. In any case, the use of mitomycin-pretreated cells as an immunogen—or use of concomitant, matched, control cultures—circumvents this problem. The immunologic assay described provides a means for further clarification of these observations.

The support, encouragement, and advice of Dr. Eugene Van Scott are gratefully appreciated. We thank Mrs. Dawn White for excellent technical assistance and Mrs. Shirley Peoples for administrative services.

REFERENCES

1. Axelrad, A., and Klein, G.: Differences in histocompatibility requirements between primary tumors and their metastases, Transplant. Bull. **3:** 100, 1956.
2. Bennett, H. S., and Luft, J. H.: S-collidine as a basis for buffering fixatives, J. Biophys. Biochem. Cytol. **6:** 113, 1959.
3. Demopoulos, H. B., Kasuga, T., Channing, A. A., and Bagdoyan, H.: Comparison of ultrastructure of B_{16} and S_{91} mouse melanomas, and correlation with group patterns, Lab. Invest. **14:** 108, 1965.
4. Deichman, G. I., and Kluchareva, T. E.: Loss of transplantation antigen in primary simian virus 40 induced tumors and their metastases, J. Natl. Cancer Inst. **36:** 647, 1966.
5. Hartzman, R. J., Segall, M., Bach, M. L., and Bach, F. H.: Histocompatibility matching. VI. Miniaturization of the mixed leucocyte culture test: A preliminary report, Transplantation **11:** 268, 1971.
6. Hu, F., Swedo, J. L., and Watson, J. H. L. Biological variations of B_{16} melanoma cells, *in* Montagna, W., and Hu, F., editors: Advances in biology of the skin, ed. 5, Oxford, 1967, Pergamon Press, vol. 8, pp. 549-579.
7. Kanner, S. P., Mardiney, M. R., Jr., and Mangi, R. J.: Experience with a mixed lymphocyte-tumor reaction as a method of detecting antigenic differences between normal and neoplastic cells, J. Immunol. **105:** 1052, 1970.
8. Kim, U.: Metastasizing mammary carcinoma in rats: Induction and study of their immunogenicity, Science **167:** 72, 1970.
9. Novikoff, A. B., Albala, A., and Biempica, L.: Ultrastructural and cytochemical observations on B_{16} Harding-Pussey mouse melanomas, J. Histochem. Cytochem. **16:** 299, 1968.
16: 299, 1968.
10. Seiji, M., Shimad, K., Birbeck, M. S. C., and Fitzpatrick, T. B.: Subcellular localization of melanin biosynthesis, Ann. N. Y. Acad. Sci. **100:** 497, 1963.
11. Sugarbaker, E. V., and Cohen, A. M.: Altered antigenicity in spontaneous pulmonary metastases from an antigenic murine sarcoma, SURGERY **72:** 155, 1972.
12. Wellings, S. R., and Siegel, B. V.: Electron microscopic studies on the subcellular origin and ultrastructure of melanin granules in mammalian melanomas, Ann. N. Y. Acad. Sci. **100:** 548, 1963.
13. Wood, N., et al.: A simple method of freezing and storing live lymphocytes, Tissue Antigens **2:** 27, 1972.

DISCUSSION

Dr. Richard E. Wilson (Boston, Mass.). This is a very interesting problem. In most tumor systems we have to be very careful about identifying antigenicity, particularly for tumor lines that have been carried for many generations, and this has been in part responsible for some of the differences in reports about whether or not metastases have the same antigenicity as the primary tumor or a different antigenicity from it.

We did some preliminary studies in our laboratory with methylcholanthrene-induced fibrosarcoma in the same mouse strain. Then, working only within the first 10 generations, we cloned four or five pulmonary metastases, and then back-challenged these, as well as the primaries. We found that they all had the same protective effect on the production of growth of a second challenge tumor.

You have to be very cautious about interpreting the potential concept of whether or not metastases are just specific cells or are representative of the total pattern, depending on the type of model you deal with.

Dr. Leonard I. Goldman (Closing). I agree with what you say, Dr. Wilson, and appreciate your comment. The only comment that I would like to make is that, with an in vitro approach such as this, this model does seem to have applicability to the human system.

Pulmonary vascular impedance in chronic pulmonary hypertension

Ronald C. Elkins, M.D., Marvin D. Peyton, M.D., *and* **Lazar J. Greenfield, M.D.,**
Oklahoma City, Okla.

Input impedance of a vascular bed gives a concise expression of pressure-flow relationships at the inlet of the bed and provides information about elasticity and other physical characteristics of the vessels. This study was designed to assess impedance changes in dogs with chronic pulmonary hypertension caused by repeated pulmonary embolization with acrylic beads. Mean pulmonary artery pressure of 34 to 52 mm. Hg and input resistance of 1,771 dyne sec. cm.$^{-5}$ (control dogs, 329 dyne sec. cm.$^{-5}$) were studied in five dogs. The impedance spectrum was significantly altered in the hypertensive dogs with an increase in the modulus and shift of the first minimum from 2.7 ± 0.1 c.p.s. in the control animals to 8.2 ± 0.5 c.p.s. The shift in the frequency of the first minimum is predominately due to either an apparent shift of the major reflecting sites or an increase in the phase velocity, whereas the alterations in characteristic impedance suggest an increase in the stiffness of the pulmonary arteries proximal to the reflecting sites. This increase in arterial stiffening as demonstrated by the impedance abnormality is associated with a significant increase in pulsatile power not normally recognized in calculations of steady flow.

From the Department of Surgery, University of Oklahoma Health Sciences Center, and the Veterans Administration Hospital, Oklahoma City, Okla.

PULMONARY vascular input impedance, the ratio of oscillatory pressure to oscillatory flow at the origin of the pulmonary artery, provides information about the dynamic properties of the pulmonary arterial system. In addition, estimates of the hydraulic energy required to move blood into the bed in a pulsatile fashion can be made. The pulmonary vascular input impedance has been studied in rabbits, dogs, and man[1-3, 6] and is highly frequency dependent so that the energy associated with pulmonary blood flow depends, in part, on the heart rate. Changes in the elasticity of the pulmonary arteries alter the pulmonary impedance spectrum significantly and affect the oscillatory power expenditure.

Pulmonary hypertension in man is associated with increased energy requirement for the movement of blood through the vascular bed, and this work has been recognized by potential power calculations based on mean flow and mean pressure. In the few instances in which pulmonary vascular impedance has been calculated in man, there is a corresponding increase in the pulsatile power dissipated in maintaining pulsatile flow. In some patients with normal or low pulmonary vascular resistance, the pulsatile power was significantly elevated, suggesting an alteration in the more proximal pulmonary arteries.[6]

Presented at the Thirty-fifth Annual Meeting of the Society of University Surgeons, St. Louis, Mo., Feb. 14-16, 1974.

Reprint requests: R. C. Elkins, M.D., Department of Surgery, University of Oklahoma Health Sciences Center, P.O. Box 26901, Oklahoma City, Okla. 73190.

In order to investigate further the alterations in pulmonary vascular impedance and hydraulic power caused by pulmonary hypertension, a group of dogs with repeated pulmonary embolization and chronic pulmonary hypertension was studied and forms the basis of this report.

METHODS

Adult mongrel dogs were screened for *Dirofilaria immitis,* and those selected for chronic study had base-line measurement of their pulmonary artery pressure. Under sterile technique, with the use of local anesthesia, the jugular veins were exposed and acrylic beads (3 by 4 mm.) were embolized to the pulmonary artery. This was repeated at one- to two-week intervals until the resting pulmonary artery pressure exceeded a mean pressure of 30 mm. Hg.

Five dogs were treated in this fashion and comprised the experimental group, and four dogs of similar size served as control subjects. All hemodynamic studies were done acutely and the following protocol was followed. The dogs were anesthetized with pentobarbital (20 mg. per kilogram of body weight) and ventilated with a volume-cycled respirator through an endotracheal tube. Under sterile conditions, a left thoracotomy was performed, and the proximal pulmonary artery was dissected from the surrounding tissue until an appropriately sized electromagnetic flow transducer could be placed around the main pulmonary artery. Flow transducers were selected so that they constricted the pulmonary artery ten to 15 percent. The pulmonary artery flow was measured with a Biotronix BL-610 flowmeter. Zero flow base line was taken as the integrated level during diastole. The flowmeter and transducers were calibrated in vivo by simultaneously recording the flowmeter signal and performing multiple thermal indicator dilution curves. Pulmonary artery and left atrial pressures were measured through short polyvinyl catheters (pvc) attached to P23db Statham pressure transducers. The pulmonary artery pressure was determined by inserting a short No. 23 gauge hypodermic needle which was attached to the pvc tubing into the pulmonary artery so that the bevel was facing the lateral wall of the artery. Left atrial pressure was measured by inserting the catheter into a segmental pulmonary vein and advancing it into the left atrium. The frequency response of the catheter system was determined by the pressure step method of McDonald.[4] The frequency response of the flowmeter was taken from data provided by the manufacturer. All computer calculations were made after appropriate corrections for these frequency responses.

All pressures and flow were recorded in analog form on magnetic tape (Honeywell Model 5600), and sections of the record obtained when the respirator was disconnected and the dog was apneic were selected for analysis. Analog-to-digital conversion was accomplished electronically (Hewlett-Packard 5610-A). Digital data were stored on magnetic discs and analyzed on a Hewlett-Packard 2100-A digital computer. The computation of impedance was based on harmonic analysis by computing the Discrete Fourier Transform on a specified data interval. From one to four beats comprised the data interval. The methods for calculation of impedance and hydraulic power with the use of harmonic analysis have previously been reported.[1, 5] In calculating hydraulic energy per unit time, or power, in the pulmonary artery, the total energy was separated into two components, potential (the product of pressure and volume) and kinetic (half the mass of the blood multiplied by the square of its velocity). These two components were further subdivided into a portion associated with mean pressure and flow (the energies that would exist if there were no oscillations around the means) and the part associated with pulsations. The methods for calculating these energy components have been described.[5]

In each experiment, the average input impedance modulus between 2 and 16 Hz. was calculated and designated the characteristic input impedance. This parameter is analogous to the characteristic impedance of a transmission line, which is defined as the

Table I. *Hemodynamics: Pulmonary hypertension**

Dog No.	Weight (Kg.)	Heart rate (beats/ min.)	PA flow (ml./sec.)	SV	Mean pressure (mm. Hg) PA	LA	PVR	z_0
Pulmonary hypertension								
4	21.0	150	27.4	11.0	34.3	2.5	1550	156
31	23.4	202	23.5	7.0	34.9	0.0	1983	106
45	28.0	138	55.3	24.1	50.0	3.0	1203	175
29	23.0	151	23.3	9.3	50.0	4.5	2605	230
2	27.0	157	43.3	16.5	52.1	3.0	1513	250
Control								
22	53.1	159	62.3	23.5	15.8	0.5	329	98
40	22.0	180	29.6	9.9	18.7	7.5	513	182
41	21.0	155	36.0	13.9	14.6	7.0	283	140
53	28.2	202	37.9	11.3	12.0	2.0	389	107

*SV = Stroke volume; PA = pulmonary artery; LA = left atrium; PVR = pulmonary vascular resistance; z_0 = characteristic impedance in dyne sec. cm.$^{-5}$.

impedance in the absence of reflected waves. In a vascular bed, it is determined by the dimensions and elastic properties of the blood vessels, predominately those of the large artery at the input.[4]

RESULTS

The experimental data are summarized in Table I for the five dogs with pulmonary hypertension and four control dogs. The cardiac output in the dogs with pulmonary hypertension average 2.1 L. per minute, which was significantly reduced from the control of 2.9 L. per minute. The mean pulmonary artery pressure averaged 44 mm. Hg (range: 34 to 52) with a mean left atrial pressure of 2.4 mm. Hg and an average pulmonary vascular resistance of 1,771 ± 543 dyne sec. cm.$^{-5}$ in the pulmonary hypertensive dogs. These compare to an average mean pulmonary artery pressure of 15.3 mm. Hg, a mean left atrial pressure of 4.2 mm. Hg, and an average pulmonary vascular resistance of 348 ± 118 dyne sec. cm.$^{-5}$ in the control dogs.

Impedance. The impedance spectra for the five pulmonary hypertensive dogs are displayed in Fig. 1. The impedance falls rapidly from a relatively high value at zero frequency to a first minimum between 7.8 and 12.6 c.p.s. (mean, 9.6 c.p.s.). Following the first minimum, the impedance appears to increase as frequency increases, but only in one dog is a distinct second maximum seen with a return of the impedance modulus toward zero. The impedance phase began as a negative value in all pulmonary hypertensive dogs and became progesively more positive with increasing frequency. The zero crossing of the impedance phase did not appear to correspond with the first minimum of the impedance modulus as seen in most previously reported studies but appeared to precede the first minimum by as much as 4 to 6 c.p.s.

The impedance spectra are displayed in the order of their increasing pulmonary artery pressure. Each curve represents the average value plotted from three or more separate determinations of the pulmonary vascular impedance from random portions of the analog record of each animal during a period when the respirator was off and the lungs were statically inflated to 3 cm. H_2O pressure.

The characteristic impedance is plotted for each dog and, in the pulmonary hypertensive dogs, averaged 183 dynes sec. cm.$^{-5}$ (4,488 dyne sec. cm.$^{-5}$ per kilogram when adjusted for body weight). This compared to a characteristic impedance of 132 dynes sec. cm.$^{-5}$ in the four control dogs. The average impedance spectra of the control dogs is displayed in Fig. 2. This impedance graph does not significantly differ from those previously reported in anesthetized open-chest dogs.[1, 5, 9]

Hydraulic power. The hydraulic power in

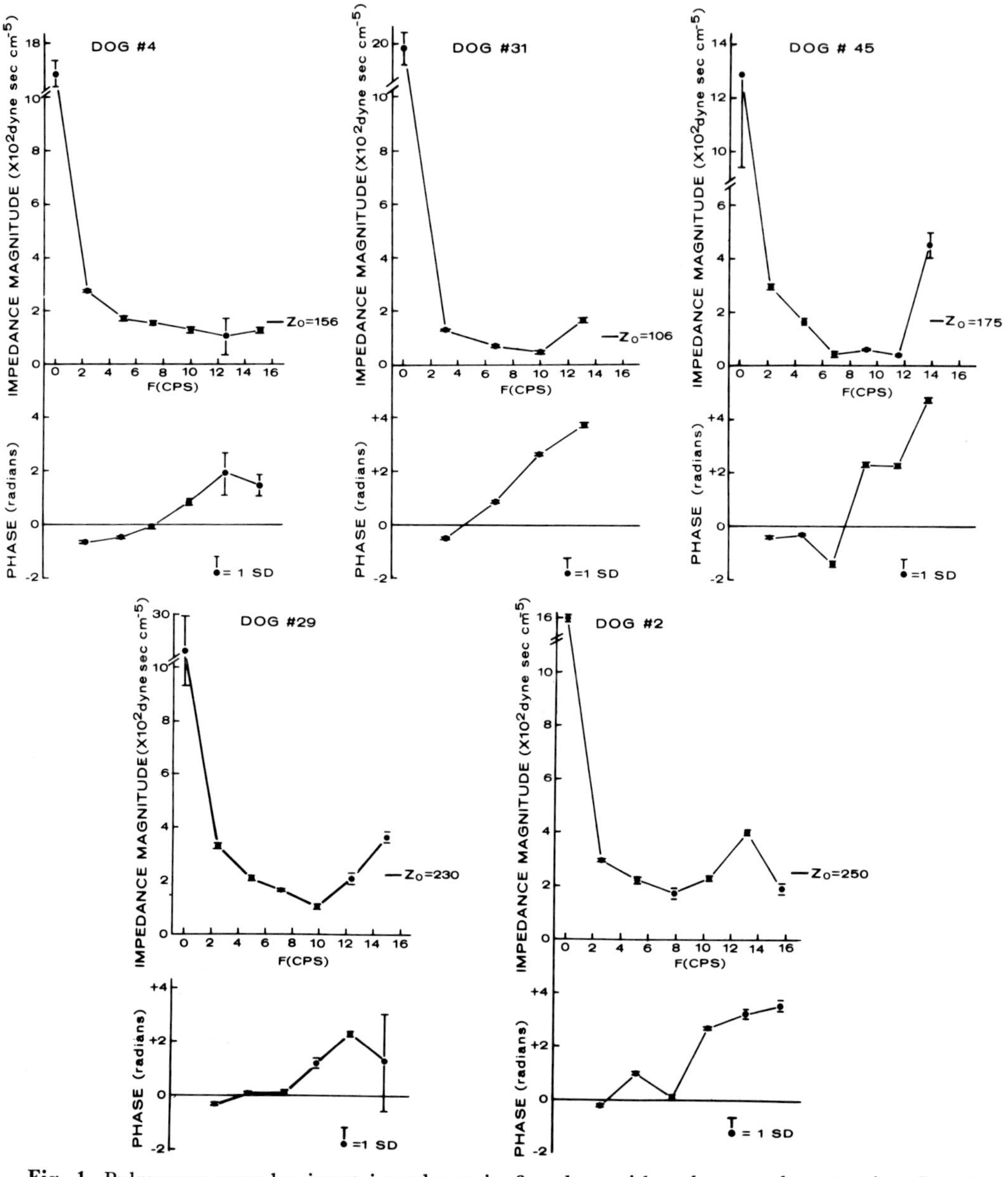

Fig. 1. Pulmonary vascular input impedance in five dogs with pulmonary hypertension. Input impedance modulus is in dyne sec. cm.$^{-5}$, and phase is in radians. Negative phase angles denotes that flow leads pressure. Pulmonary vascular input resistance is plotted at zero on the frequency scale. Impedance spectra are arranged in order of increasing pulmonary artery pressure ranging from 34.3 mm. Hg in Dog No. 4 to 52.1 mm. Hg in Dog No. 2.

each of the dogs is displayed in Table II. These values in the control dogs are very similar to those reported by Milnor and associates[5] in anesthetized open-chest dogs. The power associated with pulsations of flow in the pulmonary artery averaged 29 percent of the total input power, and the kinetic energy averaged nine percent of the total power in the control dogs. A comparison of the mean values for the control and experimental dogs are displayed in Fig. 3. The marked increase in hydraulic power associated with the increase in mean pulmonary artery pressure is seen as the mean term, and a similar increase is seen in the power associated with pulsatile flow. The ratio of the oscillatory power to the total power is 23 percent, which is similar to the values reported by Milnor and colleagues[6] in patients with pulmonary hypertension.

DISCUSSION

Impedance. The changes in input impedance spectra associated with pulmonary hypertension consist primarily of a rise in the characteristic impedance and a marked shift to the right of the first minimum of impedance. The shift to the right of the first minimum suggests a more proximal location of the major reflecting site in the pulmonary arteries or a significant rise in the phase velocity.[3, 4, 6] Our shift of the first minimum of impedance is greater than the shift reported by Reuben,[9] who noted a first minimum of 4.5 c.p.s. in patients with severe pulmonary hypertension (mean pulmonary artery pressure = 45 mm. Hg). The rise in characteristic impedance is suggestive of a decrease in compliance of the proximal pulmonary arteries. These changes in impedance are very similar to those reported by Bergel and Milnor[1] and Reuben[10] following the infusion of serotonin. However, the estimated characteristic impedance in the pulmonary hypertensive dogs, 183 dyne sec. cm.$^{-5}$, is slightly higher than that seen following the infusion of serotonin. In the two studies reported, the average increase in mean pulmonary artery pressure following the infusion of serotonin was 18.7 percent[1] and 74 percent,[10] and in the latter case a 17 percent increase in characteristic impedance was seen. The increase in characteristic impedance could be the result of passive decrease in pulmonary artery compliance resulting from the increased distending pressure or an actual histologic change in the wall of the pulmonary artery from the prolonged pulmonary hypertension. From data achieved by Patel and associates,[8] our observed increase in distending pressure (mean pulmonary artery pressure, 21 to 59 cm. H_2O) would produce a decrease in the volume distensibility of the pulmonary artery from 2.25 to 0.9 percent per centimeter of water. As the nominal wave velocity and the characteristic impedance of the artery are inversely proportional to the square root of the distensibility, this would result in a 58 percent increase in characteristic impedance, which is somewhat

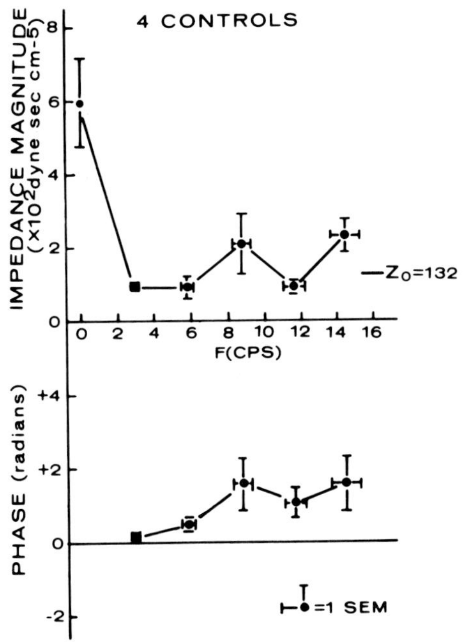

Fig. 2. The average input impedance for the four control dogs. The first minimum is at 4 c.p.s. and the first maximum is at 8.5 c.p.s.

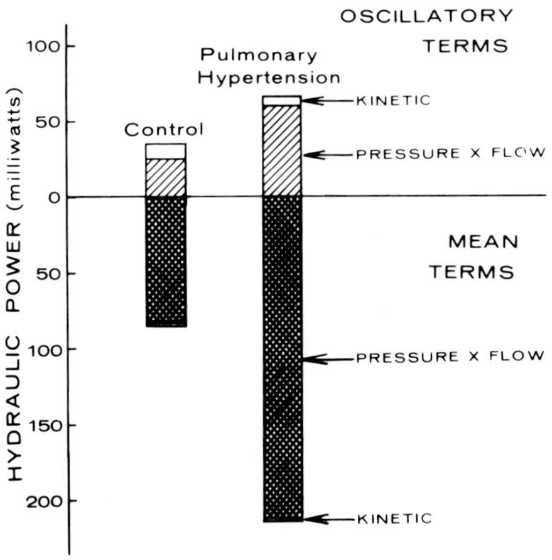

Fig. 3. Average hydraulic power associated with pulmonary arterial blood flow in control dogs and dogs with pulmonary hypertension.

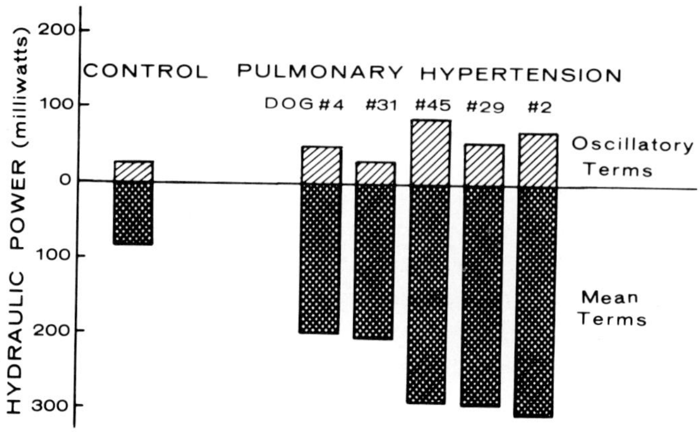

Fig. 4. The hydraulic power in the control dogs and in the five dogs with pulmonary hypertension with a normalized pulmonary blood flow. Kinetic power was omitted.

Table II. *Average hydraulic input power, chronic pulmonary hypertension, and controls (milliwatts)*

	Potential power			*Kinetic power*				
Dog No.	*Mean terms*	*Pulsatile*	*Combined*	*Mean terms*	*Pulsatile*	*Combined*	*Pulsatile/ total*	*Kinetic/ total*
Pulmonary hypertension								
4	125.0	29.1	145.2	0.41	3.80	4.21	0.21	0.03
31	109.4	21.3	130.7	0.11	2.80	2.97	0.18	0.02
45	369.6	124.1	493.7	0.69	6.23	6.92	0.27	0.01
29	155.7	48.0	203.7	0.11	2.60	2.70	0.25	0.01
2	300.4	84.5	384.8	1.61	12.86	14.47	0.24	0.04
Means	212.0	61.4	273.4	0.59	5.67	6.25	0.23	0.02
Control								
22	137.6	43.3	180.9	2.19	22.39	24.58	0.32	0.12
40	72.3	20.7	93.1	0.84	5.87	6.70	0.27	0.07
41	71.0	19.4	90.4	0.88	8.30	9.18	0.28	0.09
53	54.3	17.4	71.7	0.61	3.53	4.14	0.28	0.06
Means	83.8	25.2	109.0	1.13	10.02	11.15	0.29	0.09

higher than our observed increase in characteristic impedance of 39 percent but certainly within range of the expected value. The impedance changes associated with pulmonary hypertension are very similar to those reported by Milnor and co-workers[6] in man. However, the average characteristic impedance in man with pulmonary hypertension was significantly lower (46 dyne sec. cm.$^{-5}$), but this represented an increase of 100 percent over the normal in man as compared to our 39 percent increase. This difference between man and dog may be related to the type of pulmonary hypertension present, as the patients had involvement of the entire microcirculation whereas our experimental model only involved the more proximal pulmonary vascular system.

Hydraulic power. The calculations of hydraulic power in the experimental dogs demonstrate a significant increase in the mean terms as one would expect from the marked increase in pulmonary artery pressure. The ratio of oscillatory power to total power was reduced in the hypertensive dogs as compared to the control. In order to ensure that this reduction in the ratio of oscillatory power to total power was not the result of the reduced flow pulsations caused by a reduced cardiac output, calculations of hydraulic power based on a normalized input are displayed in Fig. 4. The normalized flow input consisted of the average cardiac output of the control dogs with the averaged harmonic content of their measured flow. This demonstrated a ratio of oscillatory power to total power (disregarding kinetic power) as displayed for each experimental dog ranging from 12 to 22 percent, with a mean of 17.6 percent. This is little difference from the actual observed values and does not correspond to the increased ratio of pulsatile power that was seen by Milnor and associates[6] in man. The increased ratio of pulsatile power demonstrated by Milnor and co-workers[6] is a reflection of the marked increase in the characteristic impedance with pulmonary hypertension in man, and our failure to demonstrate a similar increase in characteristic impedance may be related to experimental design as the animals had pulmonary hypertension for a relatively short period of time (four to six months) as compared to the prolonged pulmonary hypertension that would be seen in the patients reported. Also, the patients had involvement of their entire microvasculature, whereas the dogs had involvement of their more proximal pulmonary vascular bed. This also may be a species difference, as the main pulmonary arteries in dogs may not develop significant arterial stiffening as was suggested by the observed result in man.

Our results suggest that in pulmonary hypertension, there are significant changes in the pulmonary vascular input impedance and that these changes are compatible with a more proximal major reflecting site indicative of the obstruction of small pulmonary arteries by emboli or arteriolar narrowing. There is also evidence of increased stiffness of the proximal pulmonary artery, probably as the result of the increased distending pressure. This decrease in pulmonary artery compliance has significant consequences to the heart as a significant increase in hydraulic power is associated with pulsatile flow in pulmonary hypertension. These results do not confirm the relationship of decreased pulmonary artery compliance to a histologic alteration in the vessel wall, since the changes we have demonstrated can be explained by distension alone. The effects on the pulmonary vascularity of pulmonary hypertension secondary to chronic embolization may be quite different than the changes in the vascularity when the pulmonary hypertension is the result of pulmonary arteriolar narrowing caused by an elevated left atrial pressure. Further investigation into a model of pulmonary hypertension secondary to mitral valve obstruction is planned and hopefully will elucidate the differences between our studies and those reported in man.[6]

We acknowledge with gratitude the assistance of Mrs. Mary Lane in the performance of these studies and the assistance of Mr. Ed Malone in the development of the computer programs.

REFERENCES

1. Bergel, D. H., and Milnor, W. R.: Pulmonary vascular impedance in the dog, Circ. Res. **16:** 401, 1965.
2. Caro, C. G., and McDonald, D. A.: The relation of pulsatile pressure and flow in the pulmonary vascular bed, J. Physiol. **157:** 426, 1961.
3. Elkins, R. C., and Milnor, W. R.: Pulmonary vascular response to exercise in the dog, Circ. Res. **29:** 591, 1971.
4. McDonald, D. A.: Blood flow in arteries, London, 1960, Edward Arnold, Ltd.
5. Milnor, W. R., Bergel, D. H., and Bargainer, J. D.: Hydraulic power associated with pulmonary blood flow and its relation to heart rate, Circ. Res. **19:** 467, 1966.
6. Milnor, W. R., Conti, C. R., Lewis, K. B., and O'Rourke, M. F.: Pulmonary arterial pulse wave velocity and impedance in man, Circ. Res. **25:** 637, 1969.
7. Pace, J. B., Cox, R. H., and Alvarez-Vera, F., and Kaueman, G.: Influence of sympathetic nerve stimulation on pulmonary hydraulic input power, Am. J. Physiol. **222:** 196, 1972.
8. Patel, D. J., deFreitas, F. M., and Mallos, A. J.: Mechanical function of the main pulmonary artery, J. Appl. Physiol. **17:** 205, 1962.
9. Reuben, S. R.: Dynamics of the pulmonary circulation in health and disease, University of Oxford, Ph.D. Thesis, 1970.
10. Reuben, S. R., Swadling, J. P., Gersh, B. J., and Lee, G. de J.: Impedance and transmission properties of the pulmonary arterial system, Cardiovasc. Res. **5:** 1, 1971.

DISCUSSION

Dr. Benson Reid Wilcox (Chapel Hill, N. C.). In a three-segment transmission line model of the pulmonary circulation developed in our laboratory by Dr. Carroll Lucas, one can reproduce the results seen here in the modulus of impedance in pulmonary hypertensive dogs. However, in the phase angle, we tend to see a zero crossing or an inflexion point whenever we encounter a minimum or a maximum in the modulus of impedance. I notice you had a significant lag in yours, and I would be interested in your opinion as to why that is.

Second, in this model and in animal studies and in data we have collected from humans, whenever we encounter a phase angle of greater than 90 degrees, we also encounter a negative oscillatory power component. This is fairly straightforward in mathematical terms, but the physiological implications are a little less clear. For example, this may represent a power source within the pulmonary circulation, such as a venous pulse, or it may just be nonlinear interaction among the various harmonics. But I noticed that several of your phase angles were greater than 1.5 gradients, and I wondered if you did encounter this negative power component. If so, what do you think about it?

Dr. Ronald C. Elkins (closing). We have been very concerned about the phase angles that we have demonstrated in this group of animals, and we have spent a great deal of time looking at our computer calculations and in working carefully to be sure that we have corrected appropriately for the frequency response not only in our catheter system, but our amplification system. We have really come to the conclusion that this is what we are measuring.

The phase angle, theoretically, should never exceed $\pi/$ two radians, or 1.5. However, when it exceeds this, this probably represents some of the nonlinearities in the system that are very difficult to account for when a linear type approach is used, as we are using in this type of analysis.

The power components, when the phase angle clearly exceeds 2 π, is clearly negative. This may be associated with alterations in the compliance in the distal pulmonary vascular bed, but we are not sure. I think one of the problems that we are concerned about is that we have accepted zero as being the point where we talk about a phase angle change, but what we really, theoretically, should look for is the crossing point between the phase and the point that would be the terminal impedance. This may be either greater than zero or less than zero in terms of the phase angle of an individual vascular bed; I think it is going to require more work to sort this out.

Airway resistance regulation of dynamic compliance

John F. Neville, Jr., M.D., Jeffrey Askanazi, Peter B. Kane, M.D., *and* **Watts R. Webb, M.D.,**
Syracuse, N. Y.

Four methods of managing the lung during cardiopulmonary bypass were investigated: (1) continuous ventilation with no change in pre-bypass parameters, (2) continuous ventilation with addition of CO_2, (3) continuous ventilation with alternation of hypocapnia and normocapnia, and (4) static inflation.

From the Departments of Surgery and Anesthesiology, State University of New York, Upstate Medical Center.

During cardiopulmonary bypass, ventilation is no longer necessary to provide gas exchange. It is not clear how the lungs should be managed during this period nor has it been established whether it makes a difference in terms of subsequent lung function. We investigated the effect of four methods of managing the lung during bypass using pulmonary mechanics as an index of one aspect of lung function.

MATERIALS AND METHODS

Patients undergoing cardiopulmonary bypass through a midline sternotomy without entry into either pulmonary cavity were studied. Anesthesia consisted of morphine, N_2O, and O_2. Curare was used to provide muscle relaxation. A small amount of thiopental and succinylcholine were used to facilitate intubation. A modified Radford normogram was used to select the minute ventilation. If subsequent arterial P_{CO_2} measurement indicated that adjustments were necessary, this was done by altering the respiratory rate. A constant volume–constant flow generator (Fig. 1) was used with an open circuit. The average inspiratory flow rate was 0.7 L. per second. Once the proper ventilation had been established, a stable arterial P_{CO_2} was achieved for the pre-bypass period.

A pneumotachograph measured gas flow. This was electronically integrated to provide a volume signal. The flow transducer was calibrated volumetrically. Airway pressure was measured with a pressure transducer calibrated in cm. H_2O. An infra-red CO_2 analyzer was used to monitor end-expired CO_2. The electrical signals were recorded on a multichannel light beam galvanometer system. CO_2, pressure, flow, and volume were recorded at 15 minute intervals. Each recording consisted of three respiratory cycles, three sighs (3 × tidal volume), and three postsigh breaths.

The ventilator had an adjustable inspiratory hold. This was set at the minimum value which permitted easy identification of end-inspiratory pressure and volume. It was not long enough to alter airway pressure. With a

Presented at the Thirty-fifth Annual Meeting of the Society of University Surgeons, St. Louis, Mo., Feb. 14-16, 1974.

Reprint address: John F. Neville, Jr., M.D., Department of Surgery, State University of New York, Upstate Medical Center, Syracuse, N. Y. 13210.

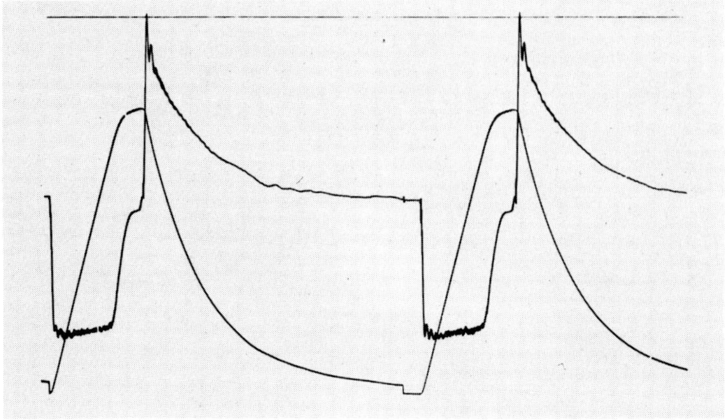

Fig. 1. Flow and volume pattern.

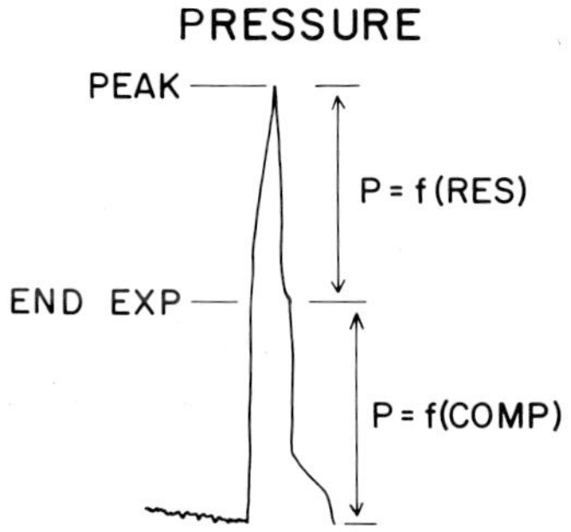

Fig. 2. Pressure corresponding to flow and volume in Fig. 1.

constant flow generator, the pressure at any point in time is equal to the sum of the pressures necessary to overcome resistance and elastic recoil. The latter is a function of volume. Inspection of Fig. 1 indicates that practically all of the inspired volume has been added at the point where flow suddenly drops to zero. Therefore, at this point the pressure consists of a flow-dependent factor and essentially all of the elastic recoil pressure. At the point of no flow, the pressure is due to elastic recoil alone. Fig. 2 shows the pressure corresponding to the flow and volume in Fig. 1. The difference between peak pressure and end-inspiratory pressure (PP-PEI) is a function of flow and resistance. The end-inspiratory pressure is a function of tidal volume and elastic recoil.

Resistance was calculated as (PP-PEI)/flow. Dynamic compliance was calculated as TV/PEI. Since flow was constant for any given patient, changes in resistance are immediately apparent from a corresponding change in the gradient between peak pressure and end-inspiratory pressure. With a constant tidal volume, changes in dynamic compliance will be manifest as reciprocal changes in end-inspiratory pressure. The inspiratory hold was too brief to permit intrapulmonary redistribution of gas; therefore, the end-inspiratory pressure is related to dynamic rather than static compliance. Esophageal pressure was not measured. Resistance and compliance include chest wall factors. The conditions of the study indicate that these should be constant; changes are attributed to the pulmonary component. Although measurements were made earlier, the baseline values for subsequent comparison were made with the sternal retractor in place, the pericardium open, but prior to caval cannulation. The post-bypass measurements were made under the same conditions. The bypass studies were made during total bypass with the pulmonary artery occluded and the left ventricle vented. Following bypass, it was necessary to increase the respiratory rate to restore normocapnia. This was done after the immediate post-bypass studies were obtained.

Patients were randomly assigned to one of four groups, consisting of seven patients each, which provided different methods of management of the lung during bypass: (1) continuous ventilation without changing the

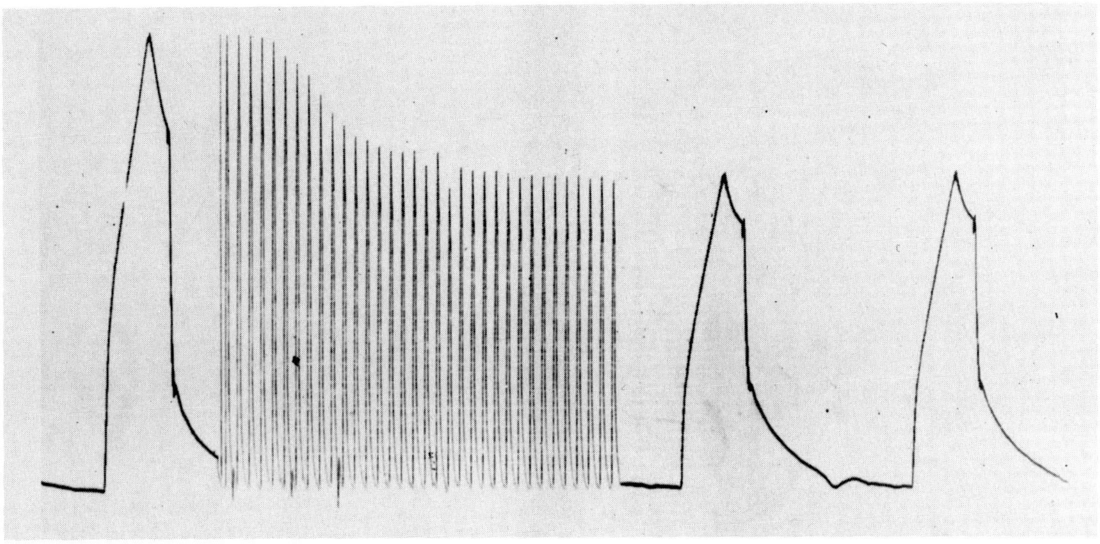

Fig. 3. CO_2 washin.

Table I. *Pulmonary mechanics: bypass/pre-bypass*

	High CO_2	Low CO_2	Alternating High	Alternating Low
Compliance	1.21	0.66	0.945	0.650
Resistance	0.97	2.48	1.40	2.90

pre-bypass parameters; this produced severe airway hypocapnia; (2) continuous ventilation with the addition of sufficient CO_2 to restore end-expiratory CO_2 to the pre-bypass levels; (3) continuous ventilation with alternating hypocapnia and normocapnia; (4) static inflation to 10 cm. H_2O for the duration of total bypass. No bypass measurements were obtained in the latter category. Arterial P_{CO_2} and P_{O_2} were maintained at normal levels by the oxygenator. The effect of CNS modification of mechanics were thereby minimized so that changes could be attributed to local effects within the lung.

RESULTS

All patients with airway hypocapnia responded with an increase in resistance and a decrease in compliance. This was found in both the continuous and the intermittent hypocapnia periods. It was also observed with the onset of total bypass. The changes became obvious at an end-expired CO_2 of one to two percent. Patients in whom hypocapnia was prevented showed an essentially constant level of resistance and compliance. In all patients subjected to alternating hypocapnia and normocapnia, correction of hypocapnia restored resistance and compliance to approximately pre-bypass levels. The effect of normocapnia and hypocapnia upon the ratio of bypass to pre-bypass compliance and resistance is shown in Table I. A typical pressure tracing is shown in Fig. 3 as CO_2 is washed back into a hypocapnic lung. The reduction in the resistive pressure gradient and end-inspiratory pressure is apparent.

Sighs were originally added to the protocol to eliminate any effects of monotonous ventilation upon the study. Unexpectedly this elicited another aspect of the effects of hypocapnia which can be best demonstrated by Fig. 4, which was obtained in a nonstudy patient to illustrate the point. When the lung was hypocapnic, the three sighs produce an immediate decrease in resistance with a

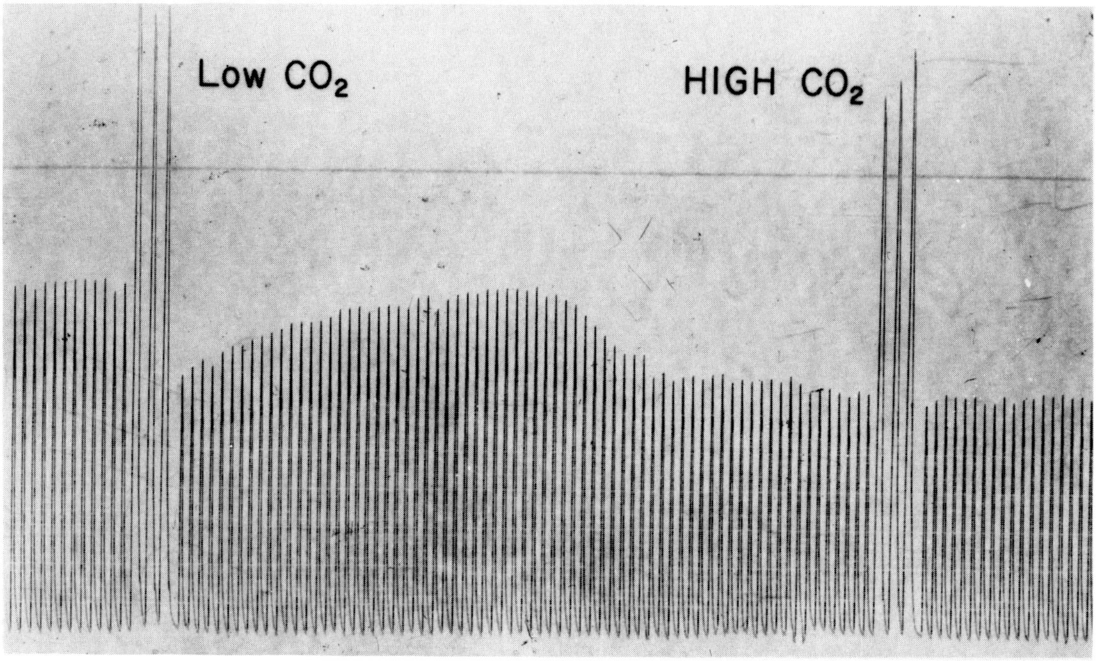

Fig. 4. CO_2 modification of sigh response.

Table II. *Percent change in pulmonary mechanics during bypass*

	Static inflation	*Vent, no* CO_2	*Vent, alt.* CO_2	*Vent,* CO_2
Resistance	+30	+30	+20	0
Compliance	0	−5	+13	+17

greater increase in compliance for the first post-sigh breath. With each subsequent breath, resistance and compliance revert toward the pre-sigh values. The values are changing on a breath-to-breath basis at a constant level of hypocapnia. In sharp contrast to this is the response to sighs with normocapnia. The post-sigh values either were the same as the pre-sigh values or occasionally showed an improved compliance. However, each post-sigh breath was the same as its predecessor.

There was some variation in the serial values of compliance and resistance but there was a 100 percent incidence of increased resistance and decreased compliance with either continuous or intermittent hypocapnia. There was a 100 percent incidence of the post-sigh pattern in the hypocapnic studies. This phenomenon was never seen in the normocapnic state. These responses represent an all-or-none response under the conditions of the study.

When the post-bypass values are compared to the pre-bypass values (Table II), there is a much greater spread in the responses than during bypass. The majority of patients who had either continuous or intermittent normocapnia showed an increase in compliance; those subjected to hypocapnia or static inflation did not. The difference between the CO_2 and non-CO_2 groups was significant at the five percent level. The data for resistance show a definite trend in that the increases in resistance—and especially the larger ones—were encountered primarily in the hypocapnic and static inflation categories. The variance was sufficiently great that these changes did not reach statistical significance. These post-bypass values were obtained at an arterial P_{CO_2} which was a variable amount above those obtained pre-bypass at the same ventilation. Patterson's[5] observations suggest that this may be the basis for the variability.

DISCUSSION

During inspiration, gas is not uniformly distributed throughout the lung. The distribution is regulated by the regional product of resistance and compliance (RC). The product of these is time in seconds. Areas of low resistance and high compliance get the maximum volume. Areas with low resistance and low compliance will be at the same alveolar pressure and therefore receive less volume. Areas with high resistance and high compliance will not be completely filled since the resistance limits the flow rate and therefore the volume delivered to the alveoli in the time available. The alveolar pressure will be less than airway pressure. Areas with high resistance and low compliance may or may not be completely filled, depending upon available time and the resistance. With the onset of expiration, gas flows from areas of high pressure into alveoli still capable of taking on volume. These areas then start emptying. This same phenomenon of internal redistribution occurs if the inspiratory volume is held. Now the airway pressure falls until it is uniform in all alveoli. This pressure and the tidal volume define the elastic recoil and dV/dP represents static compliance. This uneven gas distribution will be exacerbated by high gas flow rates with short inspiratory times. If resistance increases, the variation will also increase.

Compliance is defined as dV/dP. If it requires 10 cm. H_2O to increase the lung volume by 500 ml. the compliance will be 50 ml./cm. H_2O. If the tidal volume is divided equally between the lungs, the compliance of one lung is 25 ml./cm. H_2O and it would require 20 cm. H_2O to add 500 ml. to one lung. Obviously, compliance depends upon the lung volume to which the tidal volume is added. Specific compliance $[(dV/V) \times (1/dP)]$ obviates this problem but requires measurement of the end-expiratory lung volume. The latter is not a commonly available measurement. It must be remembered that changes in lung volume will produce corresponding changes in either dynamic or static compliance without a change in elastic properties.

We interpret our bypass data as follows: the primary effect of the low CO_2 is to increase the airway resistance. Since the time of inspiration was constant, the increased resistance and RC exacerbated the normal uneven distribution of inspired gas. Dynamic compliance is based upon the pressure at end inspiration before internal redistribution of the gas can occur. Since the same tidal volume is now added to a smaller effective lung volume, dynamic compliance must decrease. We have been able to prevent the effects of CO_2 upon compliance by decreasing the inspired flow rate and decreasing inspiratory time to achieve the same tidal volume. If the inspiratory time is long enough, all local RC time requirements are met and the tidal volume is more evenly distributed. During bypass this can be easily demonstrated. When the lungs are required to provide gas exchange, it is not feasible to increase inspiratory time sufficiently to utilize this therapeutically.

The difference in the response to sighs in the hypocapnic and normocapnic lung can be explained by airway closure in the hypocapnic group. In the normocapnic lung, either the sighs had no effect on the post-sigh parameters or there was some improvement in compliance. If the latter occurred, it persisted. In a separate pilot study, monotonous ventilation for one to two hours before administering sighs routinely produced an improvement in compliance in the post-sigh values whereas with 15 minute intervals between sighs there was a negligible change. This pattern suggests that the sighs open airways, increase effective lung volume, and thereby increase compliance. The improvement is maintained if the airways stay open. With hypocapnia, the sighs always decreased resistance somewhat but sharply increased compliance. The improvement was progressively lost on a breath-to-breath basis. The pattern strongly suggests that the sighs temporarily increased lung volume but in the presence of hypocapnia this improvement is rapidly lost, probably by reclosure of airways.

The present studies pertain to both lungs in parallel. Severinghaus[11] and Swenson[12] and their colleagues showed that the mechanisms apply to just one lung. If CO_2 is regulating the tone of bronchial smooth muscle in the tenth order bronchi, then very small subdivisions of the lung can be varying their ventilation as a function of the local P_{CO_2}. The latter will be a function of local blood flow. For the lung as a whole, the role of blood flow can be seen with the beginning and end of total bypass. Patterson and Sullivan[7] have shown that it also applies to the reduced pulmonary blood flow of hemorrhagic shock. The hypocapnic changes in mechanics are accompanied by a reduction in arterial P_{O_2},[3] suggesting that pulmonary capillary blood flow is not redistributed in proportion to the alveolar ventilation. We[4] have confirmed the demonstration of Prys-Roberts and associates[10] that this is P_{CO_2} dependent in anesthetized man. Breivik and associates[2] have reported that correction of hypocapnia by the addition of CO_2 to inspired gas produces a similar result in conscious man.

Powers and associates[9] have made the interesting observation that post-traumatic respiratory insufficiency is accompanied by a severe reduction in FRC. This could be improved by IPPB or IPPB and PEEP with correction of the severe reduction in dynamic compliance. The addition of PEEP was not accompanied by the expected increase in right atrial pressure. The data were not given to determine whether improvement in dynamic compliance by the use of PEEP decreased airway pressure sufficiently to compensate for the increase with PEEP. This might be expected from the increase in FRC. Powers has discontinued the measurement of dynamic compliance since it is so difficult to interpret its physiological significance. This attitude is valid if dynamic compliance is being equated with elastic properties of the lung. However, dynamic compliance has its own physiological significance since it defines the pressure required to achieve a given tidal volume. If this pressure is not provided, neither is the ventilation. Furthermore, therapy which is improving dynamic compliance is probably reversing the basic abnormality of lung function.

Our studies during total cardiopulmonary bypass confirm reports of others[3, 5-8, 11, 12] concerning the role of CO_2 in the local regulation of airway resistance. The changes in airway resistance impose changes in dynamic compliance as a function of the local RC or time constant. The response occurred in every patient and could be repeated in the same patient. There is suggestive evidence that airway closure occurs in the hypocapnic areas. Sighs temporarily reopen these airways but in the absence of CO_2 closure recurs rapidly. Pulmonary capillary blood flow is not evenly distributed. If the regional $\dot{V}_A/\dot{Q}_C$ is high, the local CO_2 may fall sufficiently to bring these mechanisms into play. If the over-all ventilation is excessive, as frequently occurs with the use of respirators, the required degree of regional hypocapnia will be even easier to achieve. The addition of CO_2 to the inspired gas will prevent the resistance-induced changes. Normocapnia will not prevent the airway closure of monotonous ventilation[1] but it will permit sighs to be effective in reopening these areas for more than one breath.

Our data show that the use of ventilation with maintainance of normal airway CO_2 and frequent sighs during bypass is associated with a significantly better dynamic compliance in the immediate post-bypass period. There is a strong trend toward a similar relationship between CO_2 and resistance, but the variability is sufficiently great that the changes are not statistically significant. The post-bypass values are probably not directly comparable to the pre-bypass values, since arterial and end-expiratory P_{CO_2} were higher despite the same ventilation. This elevation was variable and may be the basis for the variation in resistance. There was no correlation between the compliance or resistance and the subsequent clinical course of the patient.

Pulmonary gas exchange is a function of the $\dot{V}_A/\dot{Q}_C$ relationship. Pulmonary mechanics can modify the distribution of alveolar ventilation and, unless pulmonary capillary blood flow is similarly redistributed, a $\dot{V}_A/\dot{Q}_C$ mismatch will result. Certainly measures which minimize the maldistribution of alveolar ventilation will permit the ratio to be optimum. It may become necessary to include control of airway P_{CO_2} as part of the therapeutic use of assisted or controlled ventilation to optimize the distribution of alveolar ventilation.

REFERENCES

1. Bendixen, H. H., Hedley-Whyte, J., and Laver, M. G.: Impaired oxygenation in surgical patients during general anesthesia with controlled ventilation. A concept of atelectasis, N. Engl. J. Med. **269:** 991, 1963.
2. Breivik, H., Grenvik, A., Millen, E., and Satur, P.: Normalizing low arterial CO_2 tension during mechanical ventilation, Chest **63:** 525, 1973.
3. Monkon, W., and Patterson, R. W.: Ventilation-perfusion inequalities resulting from hypocapnic changes in lung mechanics, J. Thorac. Cardiovasc. Surg. **63:** 577, 1972.
4. Neville, J. F., and Israel, J.: Unpublished data.
5. Patterson, R. W.: Time-dependent carbon dioxide-induced changes in dynamic lung compliance, J. Thorac. Cardiovasc. Surg. **62:** 645, 1971.
6. Patterson, R. W.: Role of carbon dioxide in changes in lung mechanics after protamine administration, Anesth. Analg. Curr. Res. **51:** 733, 1972.
7. Patterson, R. W., and Sullivan, S. F.: The interrelationship between lung compliance and airway carbon dioxide concentration during hemorrhagic shock, J. Trauma **13:** 238, 1973.
8. Patterson, R. W., Sullivan, S. F., Malm, J. R., and Brownian, F. O., Jr.: Comparison of effects of airway versus systemic carbon dioxide tension on human airway mechanics, J. Thorac. Cardiovasc. Surg. **58:** 209, 1969.
9. Powers, S. R., Jr., et al.: Studies of pulmonary insufficiency in non-thoracic trauma, J. Trauma **12:** 1, 1961.
10. Prys-Roberts, C., et al.: Hemodynamics and alveolar-arterial P_{O_2} differences at varying Pa_{CO_2} in anesthetized man, J. Appl. Physiol. **25:** 80, 1968.
11. Severinghaus, J. W., Swenson, E. W., Finley, T. N., Lategzula, M. T., and Williams, J.: Unilateral hypoventilation produced in dogs by occluding one pulmonary artery, J. Appl. Physiol. **16:** 53, 1961.
12. Swenson, E. W., Finley, T. N., and Grezman, S. V.: Unilateral hypoventilation in man during temporary occlusion of one pulmonary artery, J. Clin. Invest. **40:** 828, 1961.

DISCUSSION

Dr. Eric W. Fonkalsrud (Los Angeles, Calif.). One point that has come from some of the lung preservation studies in the past is the fact that expansion of the lung is quite helpful. Studies by Dr. Veith and others have shown that continued expansion is better than normal intermittent expansion, and this would probably result in a reduced CO_2 in the alveoli. During the past few years, it has seemed that with the addition of PEEP one might even have better results during periods of lung ischemia.

I wonder if you have any suggestions from your studies that during cardiopulmonary bypass you might have improved compliance in the lung if you continue ventilation, but add an end-expiratory pressure of 5 to 10 cm., which has apparently produced some better results with the lung preservation studies?

Dr. J. R. Neville, Jr. (closing). We do not have any definite answers to your question. We are going to look at the use of A/A gradients as perhaps a more sensitive index of lung function, since the mechanical effects which were demonstrated here probably would be reflected also, and perhaps more sensitively in terms of A/A gradient effect. I suspect that this will improve things, and there is an implication, in part from the effect of the size, that the use of PEEP would probably obviate some of these airway closures.

Mechanisms of oxygen inhibition of pulmonary surfactant synthesis

Helena Gilder, M.D., *and* **Charles K. McSherry, M.D.,** *New York, N. Y.*

Oxygen under high pressure produces toxic effects on lung by damage to the alveolar lining. Previous work has revealed that the toxicity is due, in part at least, to the effect of oxygen on lung surfactant synthesis and/or excretion. The enzymes involved in the synthesis of dipalmitoyl lecithin, the principal component of surfactant, have been studied in lung preparations from normal rabbits and rabbits exposed to 100 percent oxygen at 3 atmospheres for 3 hours (OHP) using labelled precursors. Choline incorporation into the lecithin of lung slices was inhibited by OHP. The enzyme which transfers fatty acids to lysolecithin was also depressed in lung homogenates and in subcellular fractions. In efforts to determine the physiological importance of the enzyme systems, experiments were carried out in rats injected with the radioactive precursors, choline and palmitic acid. The half-life of palmitic acid-labelled lecithin and, to a lesser degree, that of choline-labelled lecithin were increased. The studies suggest that acylation is important in the production of surfactant, and that OHP damages the lung by its effect on this enzyme system. The analysis of the specific activity of radioactive lecithin in the alveolar fluid of these rats confirms that lecithin excretion is reduced in OHP exposed animals. It suggests that, in addition to inhibition of several enzyme systems, there may also be inhibition of the transport of surfactant to the alveoli.

From the Department of Surgery and Biochemistry, Cornell University Medical College, New York, N. Y.

LECITHIN (PHOSPHATIDYL CHOLINE) is a major phospholipid in living organisms and because of its dipolarity has a unique role in cell membranes where it functions as a bridge between polar compounds such as proteins and the nonpolar lipids. Besides these general properties which it shares with other phospholipids, lecithin has a unique role in the normal respiration of mammalian lung, where it functions as a surface-active agent. Surfactant is produced by specialized cells in the alveolar membrane, the great alveolar cells type II or granular macrophages. It is bound to a protein and is secreted onto the surface of the alveoli where it reduces the tension of the surface film and prevents collapse of the alveoli. Seventy-five percent of surfactant is phospholipid, of which 50 percent is dipalmitoyl phosphatidyl choline.[1, 6, 15, 16] Exposure to oxygen at high concentrations, under normal or hyperbaric pressure, reduces the synthesis of lecithin and the total amount of pulmonary surface active lipids, and may be responsible for part or all of the pulmonary toxic effects of oxygen.[3, 13, 14, 16]

This study was supported by the Office of Naval Research, Contract N 00014-70-A-0412-0001.

Presented at the Thirty-fifth Annual Meeting of the Society of University Surgeons, St. Louis, Mo., Feb. 14-16, 1974.

Reprint requests: Charles K. McSherry, M.D., 525 E. 68th St., New York, N. Y., 10021.

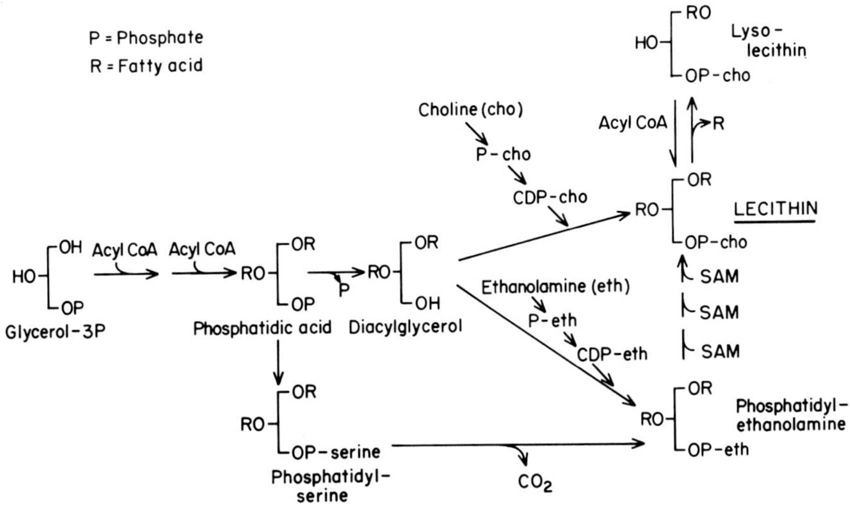

Fig. 1. Metabolic pathways in the biosynthesis of phosphatidyl choline (lecithin).

The possible pathways of lecithin synthesis are depicted in Fig. 1. The pathway which culminates in the incorporation of phosphoryl choline, via the intermediate cytidine diphosphocholine into the diglyceride, appears to be the major one in lung lecithin synthesis.[9] In the liver, on the other hand, a significant amount of lecithin is formed via a comparable route in which phosphatidyl ethanolamine is produced, followed by the methylation of the ethanolamine moiety to form phosphatidyl choline; this is believed to be a major source of endogenous free choline.

The present study deals with lecithin synthesis in lung by two multistep pathways. The one transfers choline to the diglyceride to form lecithin. The other incorporates palmitic acid into lecithin either de novo via phosphatidic acid and diglyeride, or by a monoacyl-diacyl lecithin cycle which introduces a specific fatty acid into the preformed lecithin. This occurs in two enzymatic steps involving a phospholipase and an acyl transferase.[10] This latter reaction might be particularly important in the production of lung surfactant in that it can modify the nonspecific or membrane lecithin which is rich in unsaturated fatty acids and produce the dipalmitoyl lecithin needed in surfactant by transferring palmitic acid directly to the preformed monoacyl derivative lysolecithin.

The following experiments seek to determine the relative importance of these two multienzyme systems in the production of lung surfactant. They demonstrate that these systems measured in vitro are inhibited by prior exposure of the animal to oxygen at hyperbaric pressure. In addition, in vivo studies of lecithin turnover have demonstrated the biological importance of the two series of reactions in the synthesis of lung lecithin and lung surfactant lecithin, and the degree to which these reactions are affected by hyperbaric oxygen.

MATERIALS AND METHODS

The enzyme studies were performed with New Zealand white rabbits. Experiments consisted of studies of paired rabbits, one of each pair serving as a control while the other was exposed to 100 percent oxygen at 3 atmospheres absolute for 3 hours followed by 45 minutes of decompression (OHP). At the conclusion of the oxygen exposure, both control and experimental animals were killed with intravenous sodium pentobarbital. The lungs were weighed, inflated with air, and inspected for gross morphologic changes.

Choline incorporation into lung lecithin was measured in 200 mg. portions of lung sliced with a Stadie-Riggs microtome. Slices were incubated in Krebs-Ringer phosphate (KRP) buffer (pH 7.2) containing 1.4 mM.

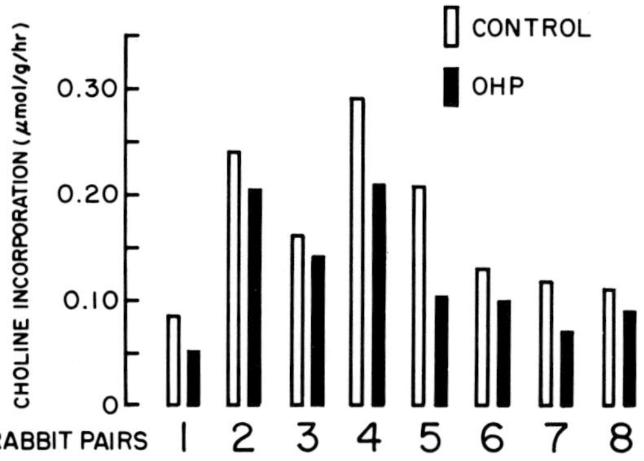

Fig. 2. The incorporation of ^{14}C-labelled choline into the lecithin of rabbit lung slices. Animals exposed to 100 percent oxygen at 3 atmospheres for 3 hours (OHP) had reduced incorporation of ^{14}C choline.

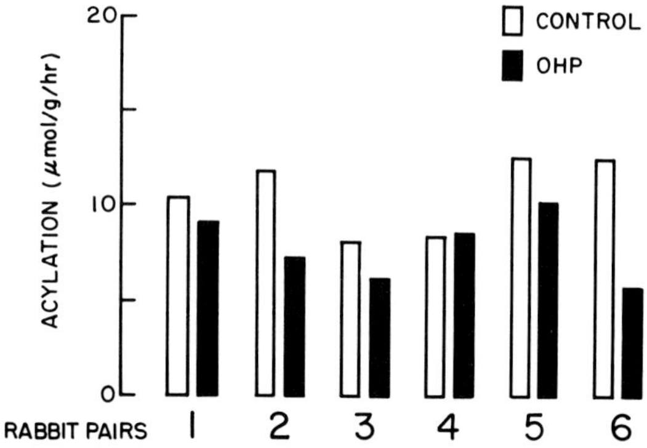

Fig. 3. The incorporation of ^{14}C-labelled palmitic acid into the lecithin of lung homogenates by the acylation of lysolecithin. Acylation activity was reduced by OHP in five of the six animals studied.

of choline and approximately 0.1×10^6 c.p.m. of choline-methyl-^{14}C per milliliter for one hour.* Slices were killed with HCl, and lipids extracted by grinding with chloroform:methanol (2:1).

Transacylation was measured in whole lung homogenates and in subcellular fractions of lung.[4] For homogenates, lung was ground with nine parts of KRP buffer in a Potter grinder with a Teflon plunger. For the organelles, lung was ground in 0.32M sucrose containing 2 mM. Mg Cl_2 (pH 7.4). After centrifuging off the unfragmented cells at low speeds, the mitochrondrial fraction was centrifuged, resuspended, and centrifuged again at 10,000 r.p.m. (12,000 g) for 20 minutes in a Sorvall RC 2-B refrigerated centrifuge. The post-mitochondrial supernatant was sedimented at 20,000 r.p.m. (50,000 g) for 2 hours to yield a heavy microsomal fraction. The post-microsomal supernatant containing soluble cytoplasm and small endoplasmic reticulum particles had minimal transacylation activity and was discarded. Mitochondrial and microsomal fractions were suspended in KRP buffer to 2 times the weight of the original lung. Transacylation was measured in 0.2 ml. aliquots of the homogenates and subcellular preparations in a total volume of one ml. in the presence of 0.2 mM. lysolecithin, 1.6 mM. palmitic acid complexed to albumin, 40 mM. fluoride, 10 mM. ATP, 21 mM. magnesium, 0.02 mM. coenzyme A, and about 0.1×10^6 c.p.m. of palmitic acid-1-^{14}C complexed to albumin.[3] Tubes were incubated at 37° C. for 30 minutes and inactivated by the addition of 5 ml. of chloroform:methanol (2:1).

Total lipid in all samples was extracted and purified by the Folch procedure.[2] Lecithin was isolated by thin-layer chromatography (TLC) on plastic-backed silica gel chromatograms. The lecithin spot was cut out and dropped, plastic and all, into vials for liquid scintillation counting in toluene scintillator fluid. Duplicate TLC samples of lecithin were analyzed for total phospholipid. The specific activity of the precursor (choline or palmitic acid), calculated in terms of c.p.m. per μmole of phospholipid in the incubate, and the radioactivity of the lecithin produced were used to determine the μmoles of lecithin synthesized per gram of lung per hour for the homogenates, and per gram of protein per hour for the organelles.

In vivo lecithin synthesis was studied in groups of up to 20 rats, weighing between 150 and 200 Gm., caged individually and observed at least one week before the experiment to ascertain uniform size and weight gain. After an overnight fast, they were given an accurately measured amount of two radio-

*Radioactive precursors were purchased from New England Nuclear and were checked for purity with thin-layer chromatography.

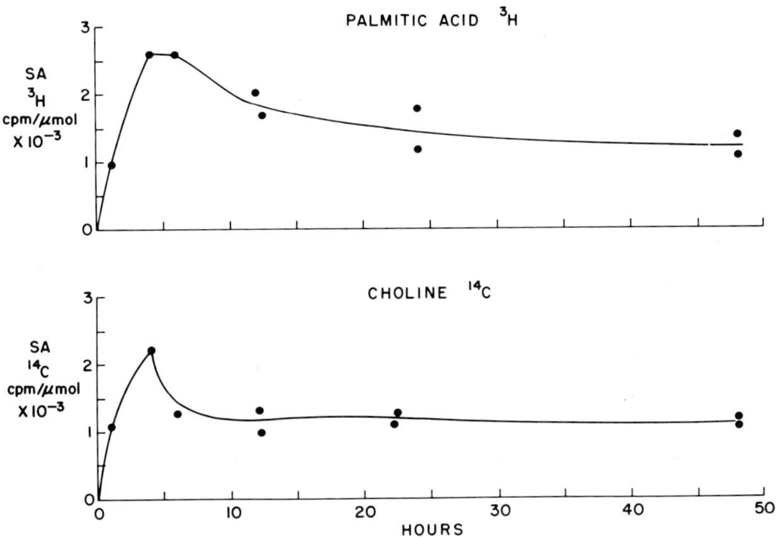

Fig. 4. The specific activity (SA) of lung lecithin as a function of time after the injection of ^{3}H-palmitic acid and ^{14}C-choline into rats. Each point represents the mean determination of two lung samples from each rat.

active precursors, choline-methyl-^{14}C and palmitic acid-9,10-^{3}H complexed to albumin, in 0.5 ml. of water via the tail vein. About half of the rats were subjected to OHP. Rats from the two groups were killed with intraperitoneal pentobarbital at intervals, from 4 hours to 48 hours after the injection of the radioactive precursors. The rats were exsanguinated from the heart, the lungs removed with trachea, weighed, and inflated for inspection of morphologic changes. Portions of 200 to 300 mg. of the right lung were accurately weighed and ground in a Virtis blendor with chloroform: methanol (2:1) and the lipids extracted by the Folch procedure.[2] The left bronchus was cannulated with a stiff plastic tube and the lung lavaged with three washings of 2 ml. each of saline. Lipids were extracted from this fluid. The radioactivity of the parenchymal and alveolar fluid lecithin, extracted as above, was measured in a two channel liquid scintillation counter with settings such that both isotopes could be calculated in the separate channels using a correction in the ^{3}H channel for the ^{14}C counts therein. Phospholipid was determined on the lecithin isolated from duplicate TLC chromatograms by the phosphorus method of Griswold[7] and more recently by the technique of Raheja[17] which allows determination of phospholipid extracted from silica directly without digestion. Protein concentrations in subcellular fractions was determined by the method of Lowry[11] using crystalline bovine albumin as a standard.

RESULTS

Lung slices actively incorporated radioactive choline into lecithin if sufficient carrier choline was added. The concentration of choline required for one-half maximum activity (Km) was 0.2 mM. In these experiments 1.4 mM. choline was utilized. Fig. 2 depicts the results obtained from the study of choline incorporation into lung slices on eight pairs of rabbits, one of each pair having been exposed to OHP immediately prior to study. There was a considerable variation in the level of synthesis from one pair to the other possibly due to unknown variables in the enzymatic assay from day to day or to the condition of the rabbits. However, there was a consistent reduction of activity in the lungs of OHP treated animals. The mean for the control animals was 0.17 ± 0.07 μmole per Gm. per hour, and for the oxygen exposed group 0.12 ± 0.06 μmole ($p < 0.01$).

Acylation activity was measure in six pairs

Table I. *Acylation by lung homogenates and organelles of normal and OHP exposed rabbits*

	No. of pairs	*μmole per milligrams of protein*		
		Normal	*OHP*	*P value*
Homogenate	6	0.18 ± 0.05	0.13 ± 0.04	$P < 0.05$
Mitochondrial fraction	6	0.47 ± 0.11	0.44 ± 0.12	NS
Microsomal fraction	6	0.51 ± 0.25	0.44 ± 0.25	$P < 0.05$

Table II. *Half-life of lung lecithin labelled with ^{14}C-choline and ^{3}H-palmitic acid*

Rat group No.	*Half-life in hours*	
	Precursor:choline	*Precursor:palmitic acid*
1	45	28
2	48	22
3	38	23
4	44	28
Mean	44	25

of rabbits and the results are depicted in Fig. 3. There is a significant difference between the lungs of the control animals and those of the animals exposed to OHP ($P = 0.05$). The mean acylation of the controls was 11.8 ± 1.8 μmole per Gm. per hour, and for the oxygen exposed animals 9.4 ± 2.8 (S.D.).

The level of transacylation activity of the organelles reveals that the enzyme system is present in approximately equal amounts in the mitochondrial and microsomal fractions when calculated in terms of lung protein (Table I). While oxygen exposure resulted in a decrease of acylation activity in most of the mitochondrial preparations, it was inconsistent and the differences were not significant. However, in the six pairs of lung microsomal samples there was a significant difference ($P < 0.05$) between control and oxygen exposed animals.

One cannot assume that the level of activity of enzyme systems in vivo are comparable to that in vitro. It is particularly unlikely that acylation occurs at the same rate as it does in the in vitro experiments where we have added unphysiological amounts of lysolecithin to enhance the acylation reaction. The in vivo studies were designed to determine the physiological importance of the two pathways in lung lecithin synthesis. Fig. 4 depicts the results obtained in one of the experiments in which the two lecithin precursors were injected intravenously into a group of rats. The specific activity (SA) of lung lecithin, calculated in terms of c.p.m. per μmole of lecithin is plotted against the hours after the isotope injection. The SA of lecithin tagged with choline-^{14}C rose to a peak at one to 4 hours. After 6 hours the radioactivity in lung fell off at an exponential rate. On the other hand, the SA of lecithin containing palmitic acid-^{3}H rose to a peak at four to eight hours and the disappearance curve plotted exponentially became a straight line at 10 to 12 hours. Table II summarizes the data on the half-life of lecithin in the lungs of four groups of normal animals as determined from the final first order portion of each curve by computer analysis. Lecithin labelled with palmitic acid had a mean half-life of 44 hours. In three experiments the palmitic acid-labelled lecithin of lungs of rats exposed to OHP turned over consistently more slowly than did that of the normal controls implying a reduced synthesis of this lecithin. Choline lecithin synthesis, on the other hand, was reduced to a lesser degree and in only two of the three experiments. Fig. 5 illustrates one of these experiments. The half-life of palmitic acid-labelled lecithin was prolonged by 4.5 times in this experiment, while that of choline-labelled lecithin was essentially unchanged.

The above experiments do not distinguish between whole lung lecithin and surfactant lecithin. The alveolar fluid was therefore studied in an attempt to estimate the quantitative importance of the fatty acid pathway in surfactant lecithin synthesis as distinct from whole lung lecithin synthesis. The latter

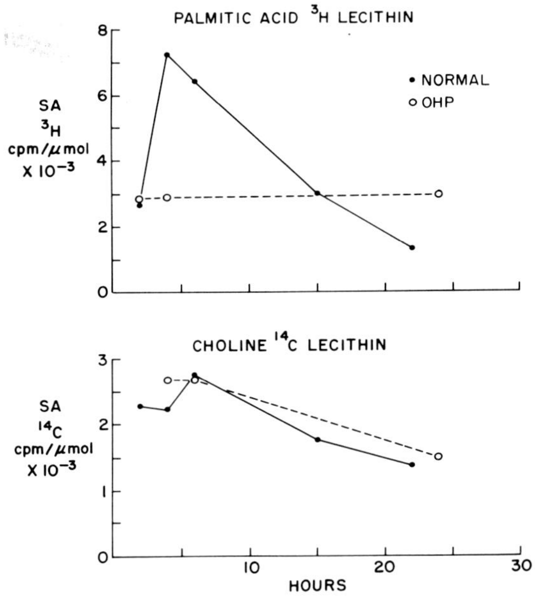

Fig. 5. Specific activity (SA) of lung lecithin after injection of radioactive precursors into normal and OHP-exposed rats. Each point represents the mean of duplicate determinations on each of two rats. OHP modified the disappearance curve of ^3H-palmitic acid lecithin but not of ^{14}C-choline lecithin.

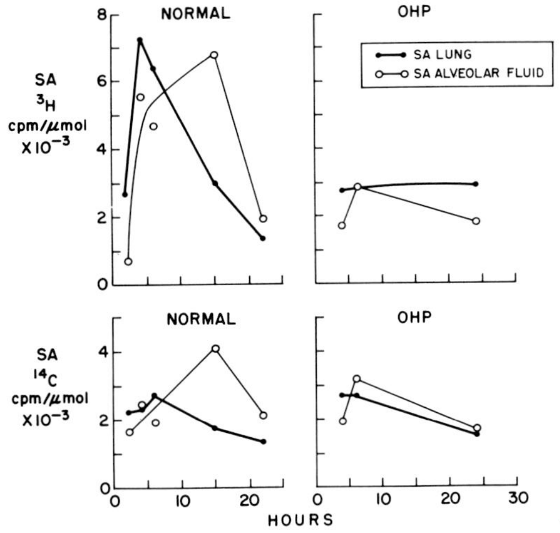

Fig. 6. Specific activity (SA) of the lecithin of lung and alveolar fluid after the injection of ^3H-palmitic acid and ^{14}C-choline into normal and OHP-exposed rats. With both precursors alveolar fluid SA was markedly reduced.

pathway includes de novo synthesis by acylation of glycerol-3-phosphate as well as the acylation of preformed lecithin. The SA of lung and alveolar fluid are plotted together in Fig. 6. The peak SA of whole lung lecithin from both precursors occurred 3 to 6 hours after injection, whereas the peak of the corresponding lecithin SA in alveolar fluid occurred at 15 hours and remained above that of the whole lung well beyond 24 hours. It is presumed that this is due to a delay in the breakdown of alveolar fluid lecithin after excretion into the alveoli where it is insulated from catabolic processes within the cell. Fig. 6 depicts the data on the six rats exposed to OHP in the same experiment. Here and in Fig. 7, where the ratio of alveolar SA to lung lecithin SA is plotted, the elevation of the alveolar lecithin SA above that of whole lung SA is entirely absent in the curves representing both of the precursors. This could be interpreted as a simple reduction of the surfactant lecithin synthesis which prevented excessive accumulation of high SA lecithin in the alveoli. It could also mean that surfactant is destroyed more rapidly in the OHP rats because it is abnormal. However, the half-life of alveolar lecithin synthesis from both radioactive precursors was unchanged by exposure to OHP; therefore, it would appear that OHP inhibited surfactant lecithin production and, possibly, its transport into the alveolar lumen, but did not alter its physiological function or chemical form.

DISCUSSION

These experiments reveal that OHP inhibited two different pathways of lecithin synthesis. The pathway that incorporates choline into lecithin in lung slices was strongly inhibited. The inhibition by OHP of this pathway in vivo was neither as marked nor as consistent. OHP inhibited the incorporation of palmitic acid into the lecithin of lung slices[3] as well as the acylation of preformed lecithin. In contrast to the choline pathway, the inhibitory effect of OHP on lecithin synthesis from palmitic acid in vivo was marked. Still to be determined however is whether the in vivo inhibition in the latter case is due to its effect on acylation alone, or to an effect on the over-all incorporation of fatty acid in all of the acylation steps of the pathway.

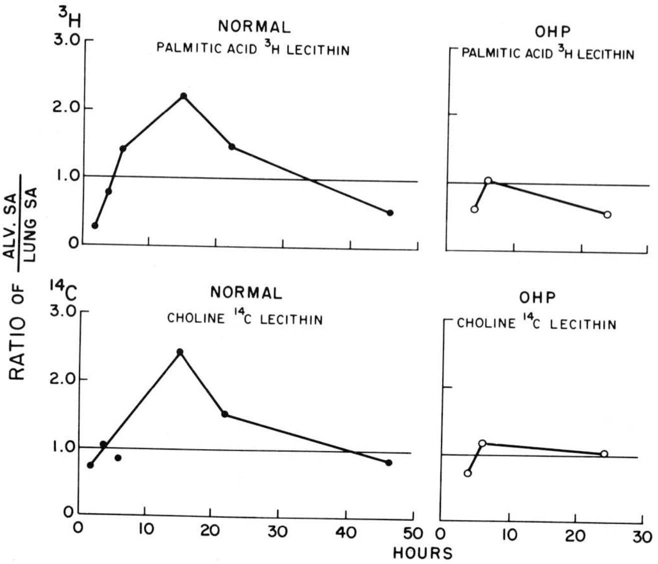

Fig. 7. The ratio of the specific activities of lung lecithin to alveolar lecithin in normal and OHP exposed rats. OHP reduced the ratios to near unity indicating a reduced excretion of surfactant.

Phospholipids are synthesized in the rough endoplasmic reticulum (RER).[12] Mitochondrial lecithin is believed to originate in the RER and to be transferred intact to the mitochondrial membrane by an active process requiring a soluble cell fraction.[19, 20] The production and secretion of surfactant by lung cells may be analogous to the production of chylomicra by the intestinal cell.[8] In this process the lipids, synthesized in the RER, combine in the smooth endoplasmic reticulum and Golgi apparatus with associated proteins to form liposomes which are then evacuated from the cell. In the lung, organelles known as lamellar bodies are specialized multivesicular bodies, derived from the Golgi apparatus in which surfactant collects before excretion into the alveoli.

The acylation activity appears to be an important one in lung because it is a means of enriching lecithin with the particular fatty acid required for surfactant, namely palmitic acid, without requiring synthesis of the whole molecule. Our studies reveal that acylation occurs in both mitochondrial and microsomal fractions and that the microsomal acylation activity is significantly affected by OHP.

Total lecithin in terms of μmole per Gm. of protein is increased in lung mitochondria in lungs from animals exposed to OHP.[5] This is in keeping with the marked hypertrophy of lung mitochondria demonstrated by Rosenbaum[18] in chronic oxygen toxicity. It is possible that some of the toxicity observed in the present experiments is due to the diversion of lecithin into mitochondrial membranes at the expense of that normally available for surfactant. Reduced acylation activity may be the result of a decreased amount of available substrate as well as an inhibition of the enzyme itself.

The authors are grateful to Dr. Patrick Cahill for the computer program used in the analysis of the disappearance curves. Skillful technical assistance was provided by Mrs. Miroslava Valcic.

REFERENCES

1. Clements, J. A.: The alveolar lining, *in* de Reuch, A. V. S., and Porter, R., editors: Development of the lung, Ciba Foundation Symposium, 1967.
2. Folch, J., Lees, M., and Stanley, G. H. S.: A simple method for isolation and purification of total lipides from animal tissues, J. Biol. Chem. **226:** 497, 1957.
3. Gilder, H., and McSherry, C. K.: An improved method for measuring the incorporation of palmitic acid into lung lecithin, Am. Rev. Respir. Dis. **106:** 556, 1972.
4. Gilder, H., and McSherry, C. K.: The effects of oxygen on pulmonary phospholipid synthe-

sis, *in* Fifth synposium on underwater physiology. In press.
5. Gilder, H., and McSherry, C. K.: Pulmonary surfactant synthesis and the effect of high oxygen tensions, *in* Proceedings of the fifth international congress on hyperbaric medicine, 1973. In press.
6. Gluck, L., Landowne, R. A., and Kulovich, M. V.: Biochemical development of surface activity in mammalian lung. 3. Structural changes in lung lecithin during development of the rabbit fetus and newborn, Pediatr. Res. **4:** 352, 1970.
7. Griswold, B. L., Humoller, F. L., and McIntyre, A. R.: Inorganic phosphates and phosphate esters in tissue extracts, Anal. Chem. **23:** 192, 1951.
8. Higgins, J. A., and Barrett, R. J.: Fine structural localization of acyltransferases, J. Cell. Biol. **50:** 102, 1971.
9. Kennedy, E. P., and Weiss, S. B.: The function of cytidine coenzymes in the biosynthesis of phospholipids, J. Biol. Chem. **222:** 193, 1956.
10. Lands, W. E. M., Blank, M. L., Nutter, J. L., and Privett, O. S.: A comparison of acyltransferase activities in vitro with the distribution of fatty acids in lecithins and triglycerides in vivo, Lipids **1:** 224, 1966.
11. Lowry, O. H., Rosebrough, N. J., Farr, A. L., and Randall, R. J.: Protein measurement with the Folin phenol reagent, J. Biol. Chem. **193:** 265, 1951.
12. McMurray, W. C., and Dawson, R. M. C.: Phospholipid exchange reactions within the liver cell, Biochem. J. **112:** 91, 1969.
13. McSherry, C. K., and Gilder, H.: Pulmonary oxygen toxicity and surfactant, *in* Wada, J., and Iwa, T., editors: Proceedings of the fourth international congress on hyperbaric medicine, Tokyo, 1970, Igaku Shoin Ltd., p. 10.
14. Morgan, T. E.: Pulmonary surfactant, N. Engl. J. Med. **284:** 1185, 1971.
15. Morgan, T. E., Finley, T. N., and Fialkow, H.: Comparison of the composition and surface activity of "alveolar" and whole lung lipids in the dog, Biochim. Biophys. Acta **106:** 403, 1965.
16. Norman, J. N., MacIntyre, J., Ross, R. R., and Smith, G.: Etiological studies of pulmonary oxygen poisoning, Am. J. Physiol. **220:** 492, 1971.
17. Raheja, R. K., Kaur, C., Singh, A., and Bhatia, I. S.: New colorimetric method for the quantitative estimation of phospholipids without digestion, J. Lipid Res. **14:** 695, 1973.
18. Rosenbaum, R. M., Wittner, M., Lenger, M.: Mitochondrial and other ultrastructural changes in great alveolar cells of oxygen-adapted and poisoned rats, Lab. Invest. **20:** 516, 1969.
19. Wilgram, G. F., and Kennedy, E. P.: Intracellular distributions of some enzymes catalyzing reactions in the biosynthesis of complex lipids, J. Biol. Chem. **238:** 2615, 1963.
20. Wirtz, K. W. A., and Zilversmit, D. B.: Exchange of phospholipids between liver mitochondria and microsomes in vitro, J. Biol. Chem. **243:** 3596, 1968.

DISCUSSION

Dr. Richard E. Wilson (Boston, Mass.). Could you give us any idea of the time course of this suppression of activity? In other words, how soon after the oxygen toxicity, or oxygen concentration, is raised do you begin to see reduction in production or release of lecithin from the cell?

Dr. Helena Gilder (closing). We do not really have that information for you. We have the animals in a pressure chamber for 3 hours at 3 atmospheres, so that we do not have any information during that time.

Effect of immunosuppression and lung transplantation upon surfactant

John A. Drews, M.D., Donald F. Tierney, M.D., *and* **John R. Benfield, M.D.,**
Los Angeles, Calif.

Previous studies of surfactant after lung grafting in dogs gave contradictory data, probably because they relied upon surface-tension measurements of lung extracts. We studied the loss of radioactive-labelled dipalmitoyl lecithin (DPL), a quantitative indicator of surfactant, after allografting and after reimplantation. To label the total lipid fraction and its DPL component, 1-^{14}C-palmitate was injected into donor dogs, and retention of the label in the grafted lungs was determined from serial lung biopsies. Five normal dogs, 5 immunosuppressed normals, 10 reimplant recipients, and 8 immunosuppressed lung allograft recipients were studied. The decrease in radioactivity in the controls and in the reimplanted lungs was essentially the same. After allografting, however, the radioactivity (decompositions per minute per milligram of DNA) was significantly less than in the controls. We conclude that neither immunosuppression nor lung autografting changes the turnover rate of DPL, a quantitative indicator of surfactant. Allograft rejection, as early as the second postoperative day, is associated with increased DPL turnover and loss of the initial surfactant.

From the Departments of Surgery and Medicine, Harbor General Hospital, Torrance, Calif., and the UCLA School of Medicine, Los Angeles, Calif.

The pulmonary alveolar surfaces are coated with a surface-active material that reduces surface tension as the alveolar size decreases.[13, 15] Hence, alveoli do not collapse despite relatively low intra-alveolar pressures. A deficiency in the pulmonary surfactant system could affect the rate of recovery after lung allografting, since decreased surfactant could predispose to such complications as pulmonary edema, atelectasis, and pneumonia.

This study was supported in part by Research Grants No. HL 13077 & HL 14474 from the National Heart & Lung Institute, National Institutes of Health.

Presented at the Thirty-fifth Annual Meeting of the Society of University Surgeons, St. Louis, Mo., Feb. 14-16, 1974.

Reprint requests: Dr. John R. Benfield, Harbor General Hospital, Box 250, 1000 W. Carson St., Torrance, Calif. 90509.

Previous studies of surfactant after lung grafting have given contradictory data.[17, 18] While all investigators have agreed that surfactant is decreased following allografting, the controversy has centered on changes in surfactant following reimplantation. The work of others has recently been reviewed.[3] The variable results can be explained at least partially by the fact that these studies measured surface tension of lung extracts as an index of the surfactant.[1, 4] It is now known that the surface tension can be altered by disease or even by the presence of blood or other inhibiting substances.[6, 16]

Fortunately, there are quantitative methods for assessing the surfactant system. The surface-active material in lungs is believed to be a complex mixture of lipids, proteins, and carbohydrates, of which the major surface-active component is the phospholipid dipalmitoyl lecithin (DPL). Turnover or loss of DPL can be estimated by injecting albumin-bound 1-^{14}C-palmitate and by determining the loss of ^{14}C-DPL from the lungs.[19] To separate the possible effects of denervation as compared to rejection, we studied the loss of radioactive-labelled DPL in reimplanted and transplanted lungs following 1-^{14}C-palmitate injection.

METHOD

We injected into the veins of mongrel dogs 100 μc of 1-^{14}C-palmitate* 16 hours prior to operation. The radio-labelled palmitate was bound to bovine serum albumin by dissolving it in hot, alkaline water (pH $>$ 8.0), and then mixing it with a 5 percent albumin solution. It is known that about 2 percent of the radioactive dose appears in the lungs and that it is incorporated into the highly surface-active phospholipids within 60 minutes.[15] Sixteen hours after injection, baseline radioactivity was obtained by taking biopsies of the right lung immediately prior to left lung autografting or allografting. In order to follow the relative loss of surfactant, we determined the loss of radioactivity after open biopsy of the grafted left lungs on days 2, 7 and 13.

Preliminary studies were done in six dogs to answer certain questions basic to our experimental design. Two dogs had multiple biopsies from different parts of the lungs after injection of the labelled palmitate in order to evaluate the possibility of selective labelling of dependent portions of the lungs because of the effects of gravity or position of the dogs. Instead of preliminary injection of 1-^{14}C-palmitate, two dogs were injected following excision of the left lung and prior to reimplantation so as to determine the extent of recirculation of the labelled palmitate. Two additional dogs had whole lung DNA determinations to evaluate the extent of DNA changes in the lung associated with the transplant response.

The lung tissue from each biopsy (about 1 Gm.) was extracted overnight in 2:1 chloroform:methanol, and washed according to the method of Folch and associates,[7] to obtain total lipids. The extracts were then separated into neutral fats and phospholipids with silicic acid columns after removing an aliquot for determining radioactivity. To separate the saturated from the unsaturated phospholipids, we prepared mercuric acetate adducts by a modification of Mangold's method.[12] Thin-layer chromatography was used to recover the saturated lecithin fraction, or DPL. Gas-liquid chromatography was utilized to confirm this fraction to be greater than 80 percent palmitate. Phosphorus determinations to quantitate the DPL were done using a colorimetric method.[2] Determinations of radioactivity were done with a liquid scintillation counter.* Corrections for efficiency of counting were made by using an external standard. DNA determinations were made to reduce error secondary to increased weight of the lungs following reimplantation or transplantation.[5] The method was a modification of that described by Schneider.[14] Radioactivity was then expressed in decompositions per minute per milligram of DNA.

All biopsies were examined by light microscopy in addition to being subjected to the lipid and DNA analyses that were described above.

Four experimental groups were studied: (1) normal dogs; (2) immunosuppressed normal dogs treated with azathioprine 3.5 mg. per kilogram per day and methyl prednisolone 2.0 mg. per kilogram per day commencing 2 days before injection and continued until the animals were killed; (3) left lung reimplant or lung autografted recipients; and (4) left lung allograft recipients from unmatched randomly chosen donors. Immunosuppressive regimens in this group were identical to those of Group (2). All animals received 500,000 units of penicillin and 500 mg. of streptomycin every day for 7 days.

RESULTS

Our preliminary studies showed no significant difference in specific activity of lung

*Amersham/Searle Corp.

*Packard Instrument Co., Model 3320

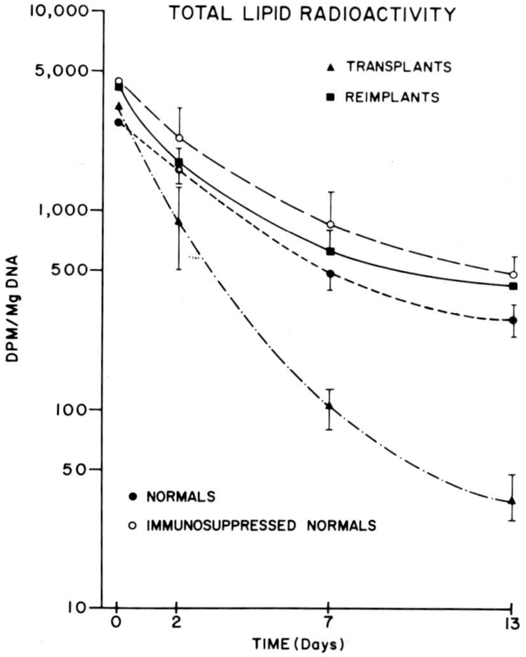

Fig. 1A. Total lipid radioactivity in DPM per milligram of DNA. There was no significant difference between controls and lung reimplants; after allografting, surfactant turnover was signicantly increased as compared to controls ($P < 0.025$, day 2; $P < 0.001$, day 7).

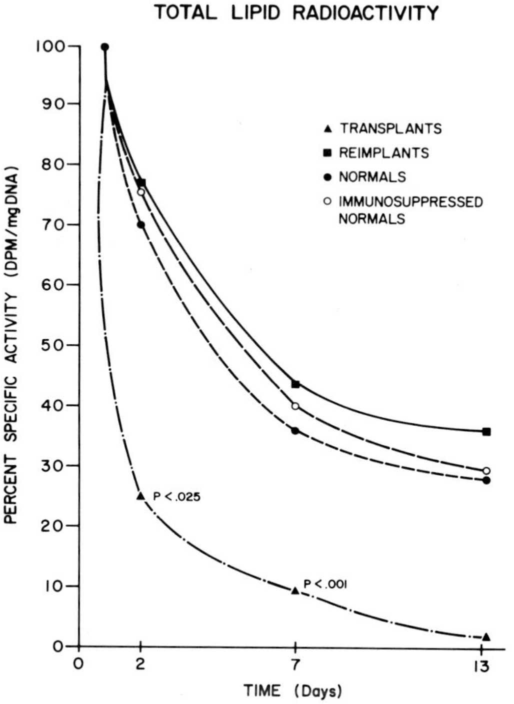

Fig. 1B. Total lipid radioactivity expressed as percent of baseline values per milligram of DNA. Surfactant turnover was significantly increased in allografts at postoperative days 2 and 7 as compared to controls.

specimens taken from all lobes of the lung, indicating no effect of position of the dogs or gravity upon selective labelling of dependent portions of the lungs. There was also negligible radioactivity noted in serial biopsies of the lungs from the dogs which were injected after left lung excision and prior to reimplantation. This ruled out significant recirculation of the labelled palmitate, in that essentially none was found in the lung which had been extracorporeal when the isotope was injected. Furthermore, whole-lung DNA determination following lung transplantation indicated some increase in DNA associated with the allograft response.

Five normal dogs, five immunosuppressed normals, ten reimplants, and eight transplants were studied. All of the normal dogs survived four successive thoracotomies, while of the original ten reimplants, eight survived to 7 days, and four were alive at 13 days. Of the eight transplants, seven survived to 7 days, but only two lived for 13 days.

Specific activities of the total lipid fractions of the four groups of experimental animals are seen in Fig. 1*A*. The decrease of radioactivity was essentially the same in the control lungs and the reimplants. However, after allografting, the radioactivity (DPM per milligram of DNA) was significantly less than controls ($P < 0.025$, day 2; $P < 0.001$, day 7). As shown in Fig. 1*B,* these data are even more clearly illustrated when expressed as percents of baseline radioactivity rather than in absolute values. We chose to use percent of radioactivity, because the initial absolute values of the four groups of dogs were somewhat different because of variances in dog weights.

Specific activities of the DPL fractions of the four groups of experimental animals are seen in Fig. 2. Again, significantly less radioactivity was seen following lung allografting

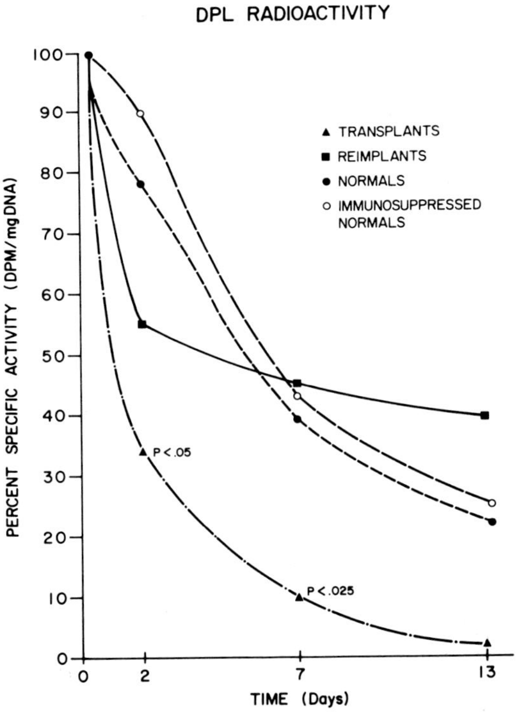

Fig. 2. DPL radioactivity expressed as percent of baseline values per milligram of DNA. Surfacant turnover was significantly increased in allografts at days 2 and 7 as compared to controls.

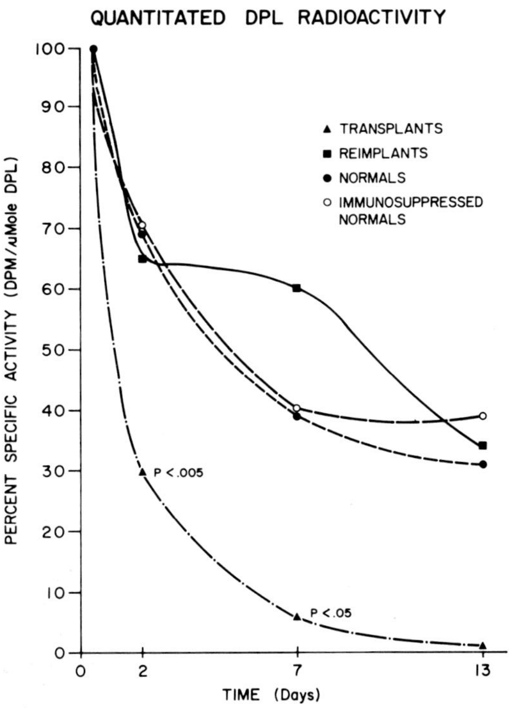

Fig. 3. Quantitated DPL radioactivity expressed as percent of baseline values per micromole of DPL. Surfacant turnover was significantly increased in allografts at days 2 and 7, as compared to controls.

as compared to autografts and controls ($P < 0.05$, day 2; $P < 0.025$, day 7). When the DPL was quantitated by phosphorus determinations and specific activity expressed as decompositions per minute per micromole of DPL (Fig. 3), the same relationships were observed ($P < 0.005$, day 2; $P < 0.05$, day 7).

Tangential to the main purpose of these experiments, after the ratios of DPL per DNA of the four experimental groups had been calculated and compared, was that no significant difference among the four groups was noted and that the ratios remained constant from 0 to 7 days (Fig. 4). In addition, the average half-life of labelled DPL in the allografts was 1.8 days, while the half-life of labelled DPL in the autographs and controls was 5.5 days. The significance of these observations will be described in the discussion.

Evidence of early rejection (Fig. 5) was seen in seven biopsies of the transplant recipients while ten showed no such changes.

In summary, allografts, as early as the second postoperative day and continuing until the seventh day, demonstrated significant increased loss of labelled total lipid and DPL when compared to autografts and controls. These increased losses of radioactivity apparently persisted until 13 days after transplantation, but because of the fact that only two allograft recipients reached this point of the experiment, statistical analysis would be meaningless.

DISCUSSION

When lung tissue extracts or endobronchial lavage fluids are spread over the surface of normal saline, and the surface film is compressed into a constantly decreasing area, the surface tension (dynes per centimeter) is plotted against the area of the film. Measurements of this type have been assumed to be

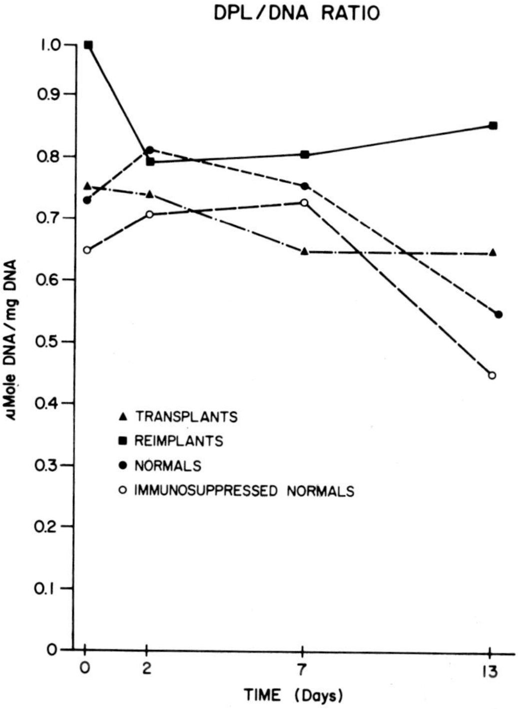

Fig. 4. DPL to DNA ratios expressed as micromoles of DPL to milligram of DNA. No significant difference among the four groups was noted and the ratios remained constant.

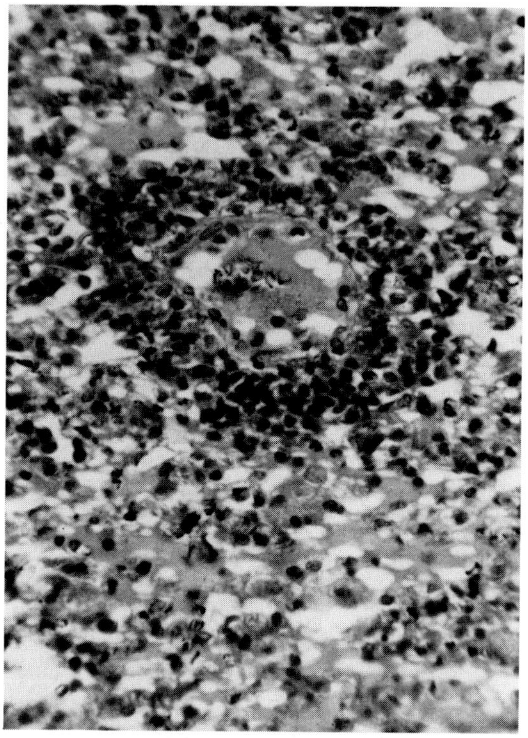

Fig. 5. Mononuclear cell perivascular cuffing, characteristic of early rejection in lung allografts. (Hematoxylin and Eosin stain; ×450.)

indicators of surfactant, but we now know that abnormalities may only reflect inhibition by blood or other substances associated with the allograft response or naturally occurring diseases. In fact, allografted lung extracts have been shown to inhibit normal lung extracts.[6] Because of this, we felt a quantitative study of surfactant, following lung allografting, was important.

While the mechanism for the loss of surfactant as part of the allograft response is not known, there are some noteworthy morphologic correlations with previous electron microscopic findings.[8, 11] The Type II alveolar cells are generally agreed to play an important role in the surfactant system.[13] Their lamellar inclusion bodies are thought to have secretory function.[10] Early in rejection there is proliferation of Type II alveolar cells, but their lamellar inclusion bodies show vacuolization, fraying, and membrane disruption. Later, during rejection, and preterminally, there is a relative decrease in the number of Type II alveolar cells. Therefore, the hypothesis that disrupted lamellar inclusion bodies during the early allograft response are the morphologic correlate of changes in surfactant production is reasonable. The relative increase in the number of Type II cells during the early phases of rejection could be the histological manifestation of a compensatory effort, and the subsequent decrease in the number of these cells during the preterminal phase of the allograft response could reflect a failure of this compensatory mechanism.

It is of theoretical interest to consider whether our data reflect surfactant loss or turnover. Clearly, these alternative mechanisms could yield the same results by the methods of study we employed. We related the radioactivity in the lung biopsies to DNA, which is an indicator of lung tissue mass. We calculated the ratios of micromoles of

DPL to milligrams of DNA in all four experimental groups and found no significant differences among them. In fact, the ratios remained constant from 0 to 7 days in each group. Therefore, one of three of the following things happened: (1) there was no change in the quantity of DPL or DNA after transplantation; (2) DPL and DNA both decreased in equal amounts following lung transplantation; (3) DPL and DNA both increased after lung transplantation. In our preliminary studies, we observed a relative increase in whole lung DNA following allografting, and others have noted an unexplained increase in dry weight as part of the reimplantation response.[5] Since DPL/DNA ratios remain constant, the third alternative seems most likely. DPL probably increased concomitantly with the rise in DNA, and our measurements, therefore, most likely reflect an increased surfactant turnover, or synthesis. This can correlate with Type II alveolar cell proliferation in early rejection, on which we commented earlier. With the calculated half-life of normal DPL (5.5 days) and that of DPL in lung allografts (1.8 days), a turnover rate in allografts more than 3 times as great as that of the autografts and normal controls is found. Since we know that labelled surface active material can be recovered from bronchial washings, it should be possible to further test this hypothesis and, ultimately, perhaps, to measure surfactant turnover as an indicator of allograft rejection.

Potentially the most exciting observation we made in this study was that the increased surfactant turnover preceded microscopic evidence of rejection in more than half of the transplant biopsy specimens. We have already alluded to the possibility that measurements of the surfactant system may prove to be of practical value in differentiating rejection from infection. The fact that King and his group[9] have recently developed a radioimmunoassay of pulmonary surface-active material which is applicable to both lung tissue and endobronchial lavage fluid adds realism to this concept. It is conceivable to us that surfactant assays of endobronchial washings may become an important guide to immunotherapy of future lung transplant recipients.

We have concluded that lung allografting causes a decrease in labelled DPL, a quantitative indicator of surfactant. This alteration probably reflects increased surfactant turnover. It is not due to denervation and it is not a consequence of immunosuppression, since neither reimplant recipients nor the immunosuppressed controls differed from normals. We have interpreted this change in the surfactant system to be a manifestation of graft rejection.

We wish to thank Edwin Shors, B.S., Betty Hayakawa, M.S., and Thomas Jensen, B.S., for loyal and constructive technical assistance throughout the study. Without their contributions, this work would not have been possible.

REFERENCES

1. Abrams, M. E.: Isolation and quantitative estimation of pulmonary surface-active lipoprotein, J. Appl. Physiol. **21:** 718, 1966.
2. Bartlett, G. R.: Phosphorus assay in column chromatography, J. Biol. Chem. **234:** 466, 1959.
3. Benfield, J. R., Drews, J. A., and Shors, E.: Lung grafting and surfactant, Angiology. In press.
4. Clements, J. A.: Surface tension of lung extracts, Proc. Soc. Exp. Biol. Med. **95:** 170, 1957.
5. Cowan, G. S., Jr., Edmunds, L. H., Jr., and Erdmann, A. J., III: Analysis of weight gain in reimplanted dog lungs, Surg. Forum. **24:** 269, 1973.
6. Drews, J. A., Tierney, D. F., and Benfield, J. R.: Unpublished data.
7. Folch, J., Lees, M., and Sloane-Stanley, G. H.: A simple method for the isolation and purification of total lipid from animal tissues, J. Biol. Chem. **226:** 497, 1957.
8. Gondos, B., White, P., and Benfield, J. R.: Ultrastructural alterations in canine lung allografts, Am. J. Pathol. **64:** 373, 1971.
9. King, R. J., Gikas, E., Ruch, J., and Clements, J. A.: The radioimmunoassay of pulmonary surface active material in sheep lung, Physiologist **16:** 364, 1973.
10. Klaus, M. H., Reiss, O. K., Tooley, W. A., Piel, C., and Clements, J. A.: Alveolar epithelial cell mitochondria as source of the

surface-active lung lining, Science **137:** 750, 1962.

11. Kondo, Y., Turner, D., Lockard, V. G., Hallford, C., and Hardy, J. D.: Scanning electron microscopy of canine lung transplants, J. Thorac. Cardiovasc. Surg. **65:** 940, 1973.
12. Mangold, H. K. *In* Stahl, E., editor: Thin-layer chromatography; a laboratory handbook, New York, 1965, Academic Press, Inc., p. 137.
13. Morgan, T. E.: Pulmonary surfactant, N. Engl. J. Med. **284:** 1185, 1971.
14. Schneider, W. C.: Determination of nucleic acids in tissues by pentose analysis, J. Biol. Chem. **161:** 293, 1945.
15. Tierney, D. F.: Lung metabolism and biochemistry, Annu. Rev. Physiol. 1974. In press.
16. Tierney, D. F., and Johnson, R. P.: Altered surface tension of lung extracts and lung mechanics, J. Appl. Physiol. **20:** 1253, 1965.
17. Trimble, A. S., Kim, J. P., Bharadwaj, B., Bedard, P., and Wells, C.: Changes in alveolar surfactant after lung reimplantation, J. Thorac. Cardiovasc. Surg. **52:** 271, 1966.
18. Waldhausen, J. A., Giammona, S. T., Kilman, J. W., and Daly, W. J.: Effect of transplantation of canine lung on pulmonary compliance and surfactant, J. A. M. A. **191:** 130, 1965.
19. Young, S. L., and Tierney, D. F.: Dipalmitoyl lecithin secretion and metabolism by the rat lung, Am. J. Physiol. **222:** 1539, 1972.

DISCUSSION

Dr. John A. Waldhausen (Hershey, Pa.). This study clearly confirms our earlier study, which was done on surfactant in the Wilhelmy balance. It definitively makes it evident that reimplanting the lung has no effect on surfactant. I think this probably is what one should expect, in that the alveolus is not innervated. The alveolar cell has very little to do with the nervous system; and the bronchial arteries, of course, supply the bronchi.

Of real interest to me was the fact that the surfactant, or, at least, the radioactivity of the palmitate, was decreased before you could see histologic changes. Have you used this method as a monitor, perhaps, to see how well you are using your immunosuppression in your allografts?

Dr. Watts R. Webb (Syracuse, N. Y.). In looking at the allografted lungs with the microcirculatory studies, one can see changes in the pulmonary microcirculation within a few hours in the non-immunosuppressed animal. If you have a xenograft, of course, you see these microcirculatory changes in capillary flow, sludging in the capillaries, within even a few minutes. In the allografted lung it occurs within a few hours, so I would think at that point you should see surfactant changes and other fine indices of pulmonary damage.

Do you have any idea from these studies of the rate of incorporation, or turnover? Some of our studies a few years ago with Dr. Sam Giamone indicated a turnover surfactant incorporation of the radioactive carbon within approximately 90 minutes, although most people have taken, I think, 12 to 14 hours as the half-life.

Dr. Eric W. Fonkalsrud (Los Angeles, Calif.). I take it that these were mongrel dogs. Have you done any of these experiments on closely inbred species, such as the beagles which were used in Cooperstown, which might minimize the rejection process? You might get some idea as to whether or not it is rejection or lung ischemia that causes these problems.

Some of these studies with lung preservation, in which the lung has been rendered ischemic for periods up to 10 to 12 hours, show that one gets rather marked changes in surface tension and in the production of surfactant in the dog in which the lung has not been removed or the nerves altered in any way, suggesting that you might see the changes that you have described not only with transplantation, but also with just lung ischemia.

Have you had any occasion to compare the changes in your surface tension with changes in lung scans, which have also been used to detect early rejection?

Dr. Helena Gilder (New York, N. Y.). I was wondering about the time when you injected the isotope and when you took your first samples.

As I see it, what you are studying is the surfactant synthesis at the time of injection the slug of isotope, so that what you are measuring is the total amount of lecithin that is being synthesized and broken down then. The crucial time is in the first few minutes, when a large quantity of radioactive palmitic acid is present in the body; after that period of time I would think that what you were measuring was the disappearance of a rather small amount of lecithin. Your disappearance curves are actually dependent on the amount of lecithin that you had at the early part of the injection.

Dr. John Drews (closing). We have not monitored rejection with surfactant, although this is a distinct possibility that we raised in our manuscript. Dr. Clements in San Francisco has developed a radioimmune assay for monitoring the surfactant of endobronchial washings, or of lung tissue.

We did not use nonimmunosuppressed animals mainly because of the high mortality rate of serial thoracotomies in these animals. The rate of incorporation of the injected palmitate has been shown to be within 30 to 60 minutes by Dr. Tierney of our institution. The half-life of palmitate in rats, as shown by Dr. Gilder and by Dr. Tierney in some of their previous work, has been in the range of 16, 18, and 22 hours. In dogs, we have shown the half-life to be as long as 5½ days in normals and 1.8 days in the allografts, or more than 3 times as great.

We have not used any of these studies with inbred beagles. I feel certain, however, that our data were not due to lung ischemia. That is why we used the controls; we took only well-perfused, well-ventilated lung tissue at the time of each biopsy.

It is true the palmitate is incorporated at the end of about 60 minutes. We injected 16 hours ahead of time and feel that we were measuring the turnover, rather than the actual loss of DPL. We found that the half-life in normals is 5½ days in dogs, and 1.8 days in the allografts.

Immunologic injury induced by ex vivo perfusion of canine renal autografts

R. S. Filo, Commander (MC) USNR, L. G. Dickson, Captain (MC) USN, E. A. Suba, *and* **K. W. Sell, Captain (MC) USN,** *Bethesda, Md.*

Ex vivo perfusion with cryoprecipitated plasma is commonly employed for cadaver renal preservation in many transplantation centers. Using this technique for perfusion, specifically sensitized canine homologous plasma was able to induce a broad spectrum of immunologic damage in canine renal autografts. The degree of immunologic injury for these kidneys was documented both functionally and histologically and correlated with the cytotoxic antibody titer of the perfusate. The mechanism of injury appeared to be related to the deposition of immunoglobulin throughout the renal parenchyma during perfusion, which, in turn, resulted in complement fixation and tissue injury only after reimplantation. Because of this delayed response in the recognition of tissue injury, the causative agent, i.e., the plasma perfusate, can go unrecognized. It is recommended that the plasma perfusate undergo a dilutional cross-match against potential donor cells prior to perfusion.

From the Transplantation Division, Department of Clinical Medical Sciences, Naval Medical Research Institute, Bethesda, Md.

ORGAN PRESERVATION of some type has become a necessary part of all cadaver renal transplantation programs involved in the regional and national sharing of kidneys. At present, there are two methods commonly employed. The first technique has been advocated by Collins,[8] and consists of simple cold storage in an ice and intracellular (high potassium) fluid milieu.

The second technique, and the one more commonly used, is that of ex vivo continuous perfusion with cryoprecipitated plasma, first successfully employed by Belzer and Kountz.[2] Using this technique, human kidneys can be preserved for up to 72 hours with good function after reimplantation. This type of preservation has also been demonstrated to be superior for kidneys which have been subjected to hypotension or warm ischemia.[12, 17] In addition, some assessment of graft viability can be made by the kidney perfusion characteristics.

Although considerable attention has been given to the relative merits of various artificial perfusates for ex vivo organ perfusion, cryoprecipitated plasma has given the best results experimentally and is generally accepted as the standard by which all others

This study was supported by the Bureau of Medicine and Surgery Work Unit No. MF51.524.013.1005.

The experiments reported herein were conducted according to the principles outlined in the Animal Welfare Act (PL 89-544, as amended) and followed the guidelines prescribed in DHEW Publication No. (NIH) 72-23, formerly PHS Publication No. 1024, "Guide for Laboratory Animal Facilities and Care."

The opinions or assertions contained herein are the private ones of the authors and are not to be construed as official or reflecting the views of the Navy Department or the naval service at large.

Presented at the Thirty-fifth Annual Meeting of the Society of University Surgeons, St. Louis, Mo., Feb. 14-16, 1974.

Reprint requests: R. S. Filo, Commander, (MC) USNR, Department of Surgery, Indiana University School of Medicine, 1100 W. Michigan St., Indianapolis, Ind. 46202.

are measured. In suggesting purified plasma protein fraction (PPF) for use as a perfusate, Johnson[13] has emphasized the several disadvantages of using plasma, i.e., the presence of lipoprotein requiring cryoprecipitation for preparation, the inconvenience with storage, the expense and small risk of hepatitis. Recent experience in this laboratory would suggest that still another problem with the use of cryoprecipitated plasma for perfusion, heretofore not considered, is its possible role in inducing immunologic damage to the kidney.

Several studies have pointed out that hyperacute or accelerated allograft rejection can occur in the face of a negative cross-match.[7, 19] There can be no disagreement with the concept that present screening techniques are inadequate for detecting the pre-sensitized state. However, little attention has been given to the possible role of humeral antibodies in the plasma perfusate as an additional mechanism whereby immune injury can be inflicted upon the kidney. Such a mechanism could be equally important in understanding the unexplained hyperacute or accelerated graft rejection seen clinically.

It was the purpose of this study to investigate the role of cytotoxic antibody in the plasma perfusate in causing immune injury of canine renal autografts.

MATERIALS AND METHODS

Animals and surgical technique. Twelve adult male mongrel dogs (18 to 25 kilograms) were used as renal autograft models. All animals were anesthetized with sodium pentothal for induction, followed by endotracheal administration of halothane, nitrous oxide, and oxygen. Hydration was maintained during surgery with a continuous intravenous infusion of Ringer's lactate solution at a rate of 20 c.c. per kilogram per hour for each dog. Through a midline abdominal incision, the left kidney (unless it possessed a double renal artery) was surgically isolated using the "no touch technique." Thirty minutes prior to removal, the animals were systemically heparinized (1.5 mg. per kilogram) and given an intravenous bolus of 12.5 Gm. of mannitol to initiate an osmotic diuresis. At the time of surgical removal for perfusion, all kidneys were excreting urine at a rate of at least 3 ml. per minute. Upon removal, the renal artery was cannulated, and the kidney flushed with cold Ringer's lactate solution (hydrostatic pressure 1 M.) until the renal vein effluent became clear. The kidney was then placed on the perfusion apparatus and maintained for four hours. The warm ischemic periods for kidneys were never more than 10 minutes for any experiment.

After the four-hour perfusion preservation, the dogs were reanesthetized as before and the autologous kidney grafted into the neck, using the internal carotid artery and external jugular vein as the vascular pedicle. The vascular anastomoses were always completed within 30 minutes. The ureter was brought through a subcutaneous tunnel and a cutaneous ureterostomy constructed. Contralateral nephrectomy was performed at this time in all animals.

Perfusion techniques and perfusate. The renal perfusion techniques and preparation of the cryoprecipitated plasma perfusate were similar to those reported by Belzer.[1] The perfusion periods were four hours in duration. The perfusion pressure was initially set at 60 mm. Hg systolic and permitted to seek its own level during the course of the experiment. The kidney temperature was maintained between 8° to 10° C. Perfusate pH was maintained between 7.3 and 7.5 by manipulation of CO_2 partial pressure. Oxygen partial pressure was 200 to 250 mm. Hg.

All of the plasma perfusate was obtained by plasmaphoresis of each dog on four separate occasions prior to the perfusion experiment. For each plasmaphoresis, 500 c.c. of whole blood was collected from the dog while under light pentobarbital anesthesia (25 mg. per kilogram) into a standard ACD-transfer pack. Following centrifugation at 3,500 r.p.m. for six minutes, the plasma was separated from the R.B.C.'s and stored at –20° C., and the R.B.C.'s were reinfused into the donor dog with an equal volume of saline. This furnished 800 to 1,000 ml. of plasma perfusate for each graft-perfusion study.

The specifically sensitized plasma was produced by skin grafting donor dogs three to five weeks prior to the plasmaphoresis. This technique yielded sensitized homologous plasma which demonstrated cytotoxic antibody titers that ranged from $\frac{1}{32}$ to $\frac{1}{1,024}$.

Twenty-four hours or less from the time of use, the individual autologous or homologous plasma units were thawed at 4° to 8° C., pooled, and the cryoprecipitate removed by centrifugation and filtering. Immediately prior to use, the plasma perfusate was corrected for the proper electrolyte balance and osmolarity by the addition of water, KCl, glucose, magnesium sulfate, insulin, hydrocortisone, penicillin, phenosulfonphthalein, and mannitol in the prescribed amounts.[1]

Six kidneys (Group I) were perfused with the autologous plasma and six other kidneys (Group II) were perfused with the specifically sensitized homologous plasma prior to autografting. Data from another series of six kidney perfusion experiments from this laboratory have been included for comparison. These canine kidneys (Group III) underwent the exact same protocol as the present study with the exception that a commercial-pooled homologous canine plasma* was used as the perfusate.

Cytotoxic antibody and immunofluorescent technique. Lymphocytotoxic antibody titers were determined, using a modified technique of Mittal and associates[16] on both plasma and serum in undiluted and diluted samples. The end point was read as 80 percent of the cells killed. Cytotoxic antibody cross-matches were performed on the autologous plasma and cells for controls. The specifically sensitized homologous plasma was cross-matched against the cells of the donor dog and antibody titers determined prior to pooling of the plasma perfusate, after pooling, cryoprecipitation, and addition of additives, and serially at hourly intervals during the perfusion.

The indirect immunofluorescent technique of Coons and Kaplan[9] was used. Serial biopsies of the dog kidneys were made prior to perfusion, during perfusion, and after reimplantation to serve as tissue substrate. Sections 4 to 6μ thick were cut from frozen tissue blocks (−20° C.) and were dehydrated for 10 minutes in acetone before sequential treatment with specific antisera.

The unconjugated rabbit anti-dog gamma globulin, β_1C, and fibrinogen sera were commercially prepared.* The specificity of the reagents was verified in our laboratory by immunoelectrophoresis and gel diffusion techniques. Monospecific fluorescene-conjugated and unconjugated goat-antirabbit-immunoglobulin was prepared in our laboratory as described by The and Feltkamp.[18] Slides were examined with a Leitz–Orthomat microscope system.

Laboratory testing. Blood samples for baseline and serial blood urea nitrogen levels were obtained on days one, two, four, eight, and 14, after autografting. Open renal biopsies were performed at 15, 30, and 60 minutes, as well as at the times outlined for renal function tests. Regular histology and immunofluorescent studies were performed. Kidneys which failed to produce any urine during the first 24 hours after reimplantation were removed for histologic study at that time.

RESULTS

Renal function. All 12 animals survived the surgical procedures without technical difficulties.

Control animals (Group I). The six dogs in the control group whose kidneys were perfused with autologous plasma demonstrated immediate production of clear urine upon release of the vascular clamps. A very mild and transient depression of renal function was observed in this group (Fig. 1). A mean maximum rise in BUN of 36 ± 2.4 mg. percent occurred on the second day post-reimplantation and returned to normal levels by the seventh day after autografting.

Experimental animals (Group II). The six dogs in the experimental group whose kidneys were perfused with sensitized homol-

*St. Louis Serum Co., East St. Louis, Ill.

*Cappel Laboratories, Downington, Pa.

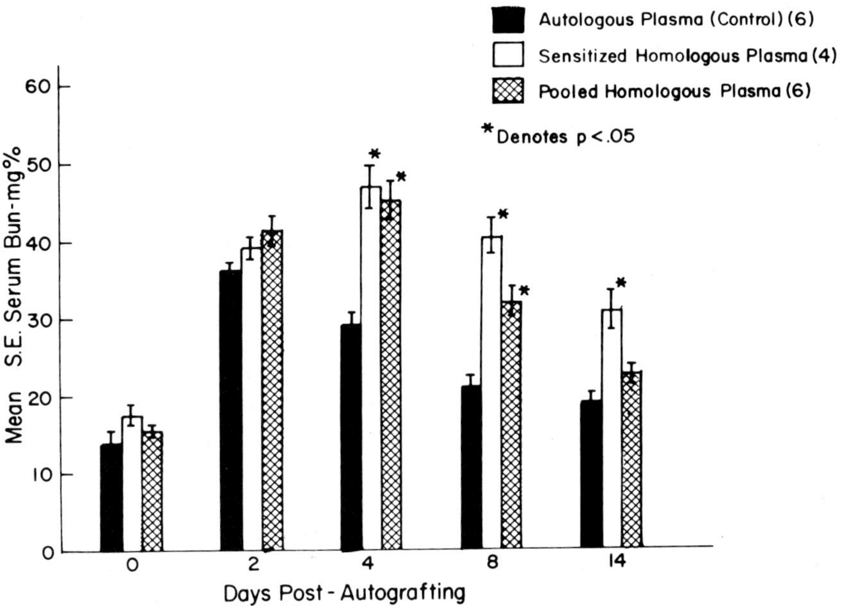

Fig. 1. Serial mean ± S.E. of blood urea nitrogen as an indicator of in vivo renal function after autografting. Group I (n = 6), depicted by the solid bars, are the control animals whose kidneys were perfused with autologous plasma; Group II (n = 4, 2 dogs excluded because of hyperacute rejection), depicted by the open bars, are the experimental animals whose kidneys were perfused with sensitized homologous plasma; Group III (N = 6), depicted by the cross-hatched bars, are animals whose kidneys had been perfused with commercial-pooled homologous plasma in another study. *Denotes statistically significant differences from the control animals at $p < 0.05$ by the Student t test.

ogous plasma demonstrated a broad spectrum of depression in renal function after reimplantation. All the animals in this group appeared to have at least some renal injury, as manifested by renal function studies when compared with controls. Two of the six animals in this group had kidneys which were removed after 24 hours because of anuria, poor blood flow, and a clinical diagnosis of "hyperacute rejection." In both of these dogs (C-64, C-92), immediately after the release of the vascular clamps, the kidneys filled with blood, became a bright pink color, demonstrated good turgor, and excreted clear urine. Over the next five to 10 minutes the kidney became soft, mottled and bluish in color, indicative of poor renal blood flow. Biopsies taken at this time bled poorly. Urine which initially had been clear became grossly bloody and in the case of C-64, by 30 minutes after reimplantation, there was complete cessation of urine flow. Dog C-92 continued to make small amounts of bloody

Table I. *Relationship of post autograft renal function to perfusate antibody titer*

Dog No.	Cytotoxic antibody titer in perfusate: Pre-perfusion	Cytotoxic antibody titer in perfusate: Post-perfusion	Maximum BUN (mg./100 ml.)
A-80	1/32	0	51
D-02	1/32	1/2	36
F-34	1/64	1/4	42
C-93	1/128	1/16	60
C-64	1/512	*	†
C-92	1/1,024	1/128	†

*Cytotoxic titers could not be determined because of nonviable donor cells.

†"Hyperacute rejection." Kidney removed at 24 hours because of nonfunction.

urine for several hours post reimplantation. At the time of repeat biopsy at 24 hours, both of these kidneys were removed because of nonfunction.

The other four dogs in this group had far more subtle changes of renal injury. There were no gross signs of renal injury at the time of reimplantation, although these kid-

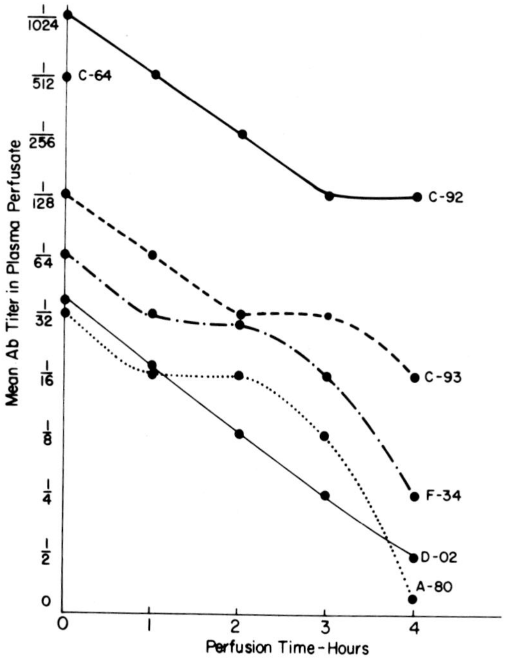

Fig. 2. Serial changes in the sensitized plasma perfusate lymphocytotoxic antibody titer during the ex vivo perfusion of the six experimental kidneys. *Note:* Serial cytotoxic titers could not be determined because of nonviable donor cells in the case of C-64.

neys tended not to excrete urine as soon as the controls. The serial mean BUN's (Fig. 1) of these remaining four dogs was found to be significantly elevated ($p < 0.05$) over the controls on the fourth, eighth, and fourteenth day after autografting.

Previous study animals (Group III). When compared with the present control dogs (Group I), whose kidneys were perfused with autologous plasma, the post-autograft renal function in kidneys perfused with pooled homologous plasma (Group III) was significantly worse ($p < 0.05$) at day four, and day nine, and comparable to the function seen in the dogs whose kidneys were perfused with the lower titer specifically sensitized plasma (Fig. 1). Cytotoxic antibody titers of random samples of this pool homologous plasma were significantly elevated about 10 percent of the time.

The wide variability of post-autograft renal function seemed to be related to the cytotoxic antibody titer of the plasma perfusate (Table I). Both kidneys which failed to function post-reimplantation were perfused with the plasma containing the highest antibody titers, i.e., $1/512$ and $1/1,024$ respectively. The remaining kidneys, which were perfused with antibody titers of $1/32$ to $1/128$, demonstrated much less severe depression of renal function as measured by the maximum elevation of the BUN.

Except in the two instances of "hyperacute rejection," where the kidneys were removed at 24 hours, renal function returned to normal in all the remaining dogs over a two to three week period.

Ex vivo perfusion parameters. The usual hemodynamic parameters used for ascertaining the well-being of the perfused kidney were of no help in indicating that any significant renal injury had occurred during the four hour perfusion. There was no significant rise in perfusion pressure in either group. Mean renal perfusate flows remained excellent in both groups and were not significantly different at four hours, i.e., $0.91 \pm .30$ c.c. per gram per minute for the controls and $0.86 \pm .27$ c.c. per gram per minute for the experimental group. In addition, there was no difference in percent weight gain of the perfused kidneys for either group, both gaining about 6 percent during the perfusion period.

The plasma perfusate cytotoxic antibody titers were always negative if the antibody screen was performed on the undiluted plasma. Further studies demonstrated that there was insufficient Ca^{++} present in the ACD-plasma samples to permit full activity of the rabbit complement to cause cell death; hence, the false-negative results. One to one dilution of the plasma sample with buffer, or conversion of the plasma samples to serum by the addition of 0.05 M CaCl, enabled the accurate determination of the cytotoxic antibody titer of the sensitized plasma.

The range of the initial titers of the plasma perfusate obtained from the sensitized dogs ranged from $1/32$ to $1/1,024$ (Table I). Cryoprecipitation and addition of the additives prior to perfusion had no significant effect on the antibody titer. Serial antibody titers

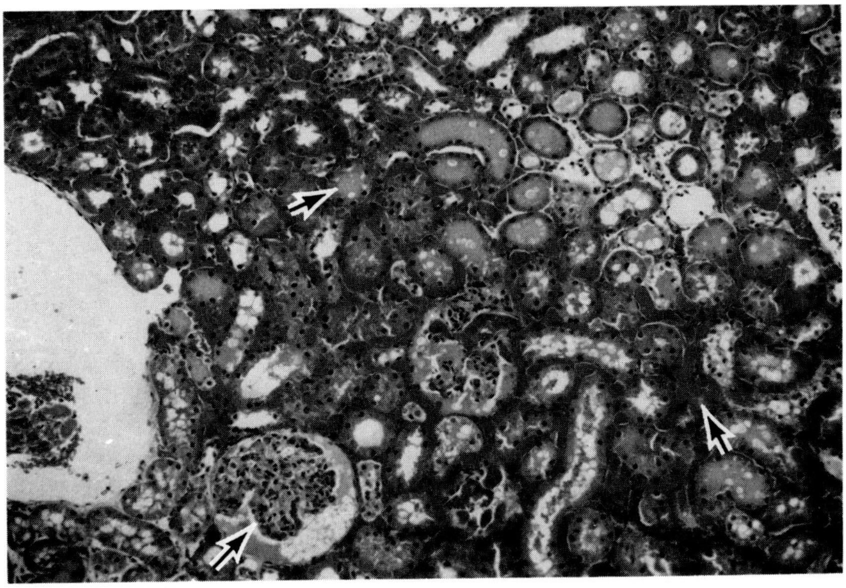

Fig. 3. Photomicrograph of hematoxylin-eosin stained 60 minute biopsy of kidney C-64. Kidney did not function after reimplantation. Arrows indicate typically engorged glomerulus, occluded tubules, and peritubular interstitial edema and hemorrhage (×50).

performed on the sensitized plasma perfusate at hourly intervals during the renal perfusion run showed a drop in the antibody titer from three to four tubes in every case (Fig. 2). In a separate experiment, perfusion of a kidney, which did not possess specific antigens for the cytotoxic antibody present in the perfusate, caused no drop in antibody titer.

Unlike the cytotoxic antibody titers, the in vitro complement activity of the plasma perfusate did not change over the four hour period.

Histology. In general, the histologic and immunofluorescent studies seemed to correlate with the degree of depression of renal function. Histology of control kidneys generally demonstrated a well-preserved architecture with normal glomeruli, mildly hydropic tubular epithelium, and a mild inflammatory response composed of lymphocytes. The presence of polymorphic neutrophils found so frequently in the kidneys perfused with sensitized plasma was noticeably absent in the control kidneys.

The two kidneys which failed to function (C-64, C-92) demonstrated histologically the most severe renal injury, as illustrated by the 24 hour biopsies. Fig. 3 shows a low-powered view of kidney C-64. It shows a generalized inflammatory infiltrate composed of neutrophils and mononuclear cells. The interstitium contain large confluenct areas of severe engorgement of nearly all the vascular spaces and interstitial hemorrhage and edema. The glomeruli show widespread capillary engorgement, endothelial swelling, and distention of the urinary spaces with granular, homogenous, eosinophilic material. Tubular epithelium is severely hydropic and many of the tubules are occluded with an eosinophilic material similar to that found in the glomeruli. Fig. 4 shows a comparable view of kidney C-92 with a similar diffuse inflammatory infiltrate but somewhat less peritubular interstitial hemorrhage. In addition, a large, partially organized thrombus is present in an artery in the center of the field.

In kidneys that exhibited only mild depression of renal function, the histologic studies tended to demonstrate a more focal but qualitatively similar injury. The injury was characterized by an inflammatory cellular infiltrate, composed of polymorphic neutrophils and lymphocytes, often with some plasmacytoid differentiation (Fig. 5). This cellular infiltrate was most frequently found

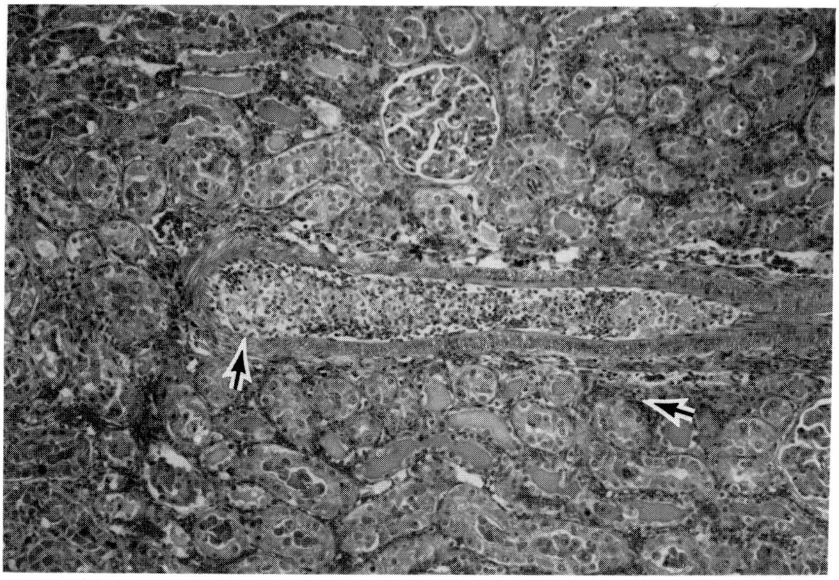

Fig. 4. Photomicrograph of hematoxylin-eosin stained 24 hour biopsy of kidney C-92. Kidney functioned only a few hours after reimplantation. Arrows indicate interstitial hemorrhage and partially organized thrombus in a major arterial (×50).

in a perivascular and periglomerular location. In addition, the glomeruli showed endothelial swelling, lobulation of the capillary tuft, mesangial proliferation, and thickening of Bowman's capsule, as well as cellular infiltration (Fig. 6). The interstitium was generally edematous and had variable inflammatory infiltrate. Tubular epithelium was severely hydropic and frequently had areas of necrobrosis and coagulation necrosis. Interstitial blood vessels were often occluded, with secondary to severe endothelial swelling and thrombus formation.

The timing of events was remarkably similar in those kidneys which continued to function. Serial biopsies indicated a rather rapid onset, in that, by 60 minutes after reimplantation, there was always P.M.N. infiltration in the injured kidneys. The histologic changes continued to progress through the first 48 hours, at which time they generally peaked. There was a plateau lasting another two days, followed by the slow resolution of the changes over the next 10 to 14 days.

Immunofluorescent studies. All reagent sera were demonstrated to be substrate-specific by the development of single precipitant lines with Ouchterlony immuno-gel diffusion technique. Controls using normal dog serum and the unconjugated serum prior to fluorescent staining gave the appropriate negative results, indicating that the observations made were the result of antigen-antibody interaction with the secondary fixation of complement (β_1C).

Control kidneys perfused with autologous nonsensitized plasma never demonstrated significant binding of dog IgG, β_1C, or fibrin by fluorescent staining.

All kidneys perfused with the sensitized homologous plasma demonstrated a generalized linear deposition of dog IgG along the endothelial surfaces, in glomeruli, vasculature, and the peritubular areas after the four hour perfusion period but prior to reimplantation (Fig. 7). There was negligible deposition of β_1C or fibrin at this stage.

After reimplantation the two kidneys which failed to function showed abundant and linear deposition of β_1C and fibrin in a pattern similar to that seen for the IgG. The heaviest areas of complement fixation seemed

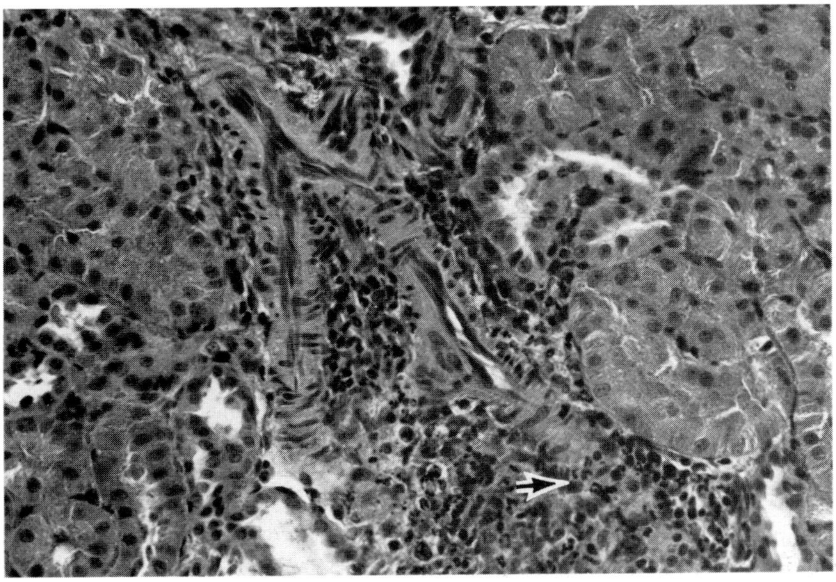

Fig. 5. Photomicrograph of hematoxylin-eosin stained 48 hour biopsy of kidney C-93. Kidney demonstrated reversible depression of function. Arrow indicates typical perivascular infiltration with PMN's and lymphocytes (×125).

to correlate where the greatest degree of hemorrhage and injury was observed on the regular histologic sections.

Those kidneys which demonstrated milder depression of physiologic function had a similar linear deposition of IgG but stained less brightly than the severely injured kidneys. In addition, these kidneys showed much less and frequently more focal deposition of β_1C on fluorescent staining. There appeared to be gradual elution of IgG from the membrane surfaces during the two week post-grafting period. The complement deposition was somewhat slower to dissipate, took on a more granular pattern, but continued to stain brightly on fluorescent staining (Fig. 8).

DISCUSSION

Little attention has been given to the immunologic potential of cryoprecipitated plasma as currently used for organ perfusion. While studies have demonstrated that cryoprecipitation will remove immune complexes,[10] the immunoglobulins and complement are unaffected by this step. Hence, under the proper conditions, the immunoglobulins of cryoprecipitated plasma have the immunologic potential to cause a complete antigen-antibody reaction with the fixation of complement and tissue injury.

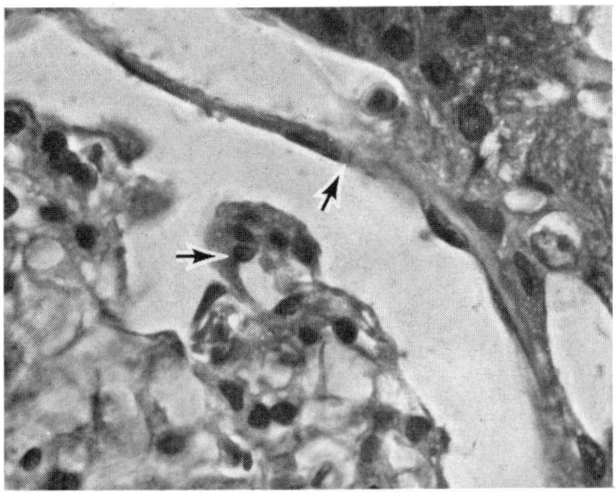

Fig. 6. Photomicrograph of hematoxylin-eosin stain of eight day biopsy of kidney A-80. Typically this endothelial swelling, mesangial proliferation, and cellular infiltration were associated with reversible depression of renal function. Arrows indicate thickening of Bowman's Capsule and lymphocytic infiltrate (×1,200).

Complement present in the plasma per-

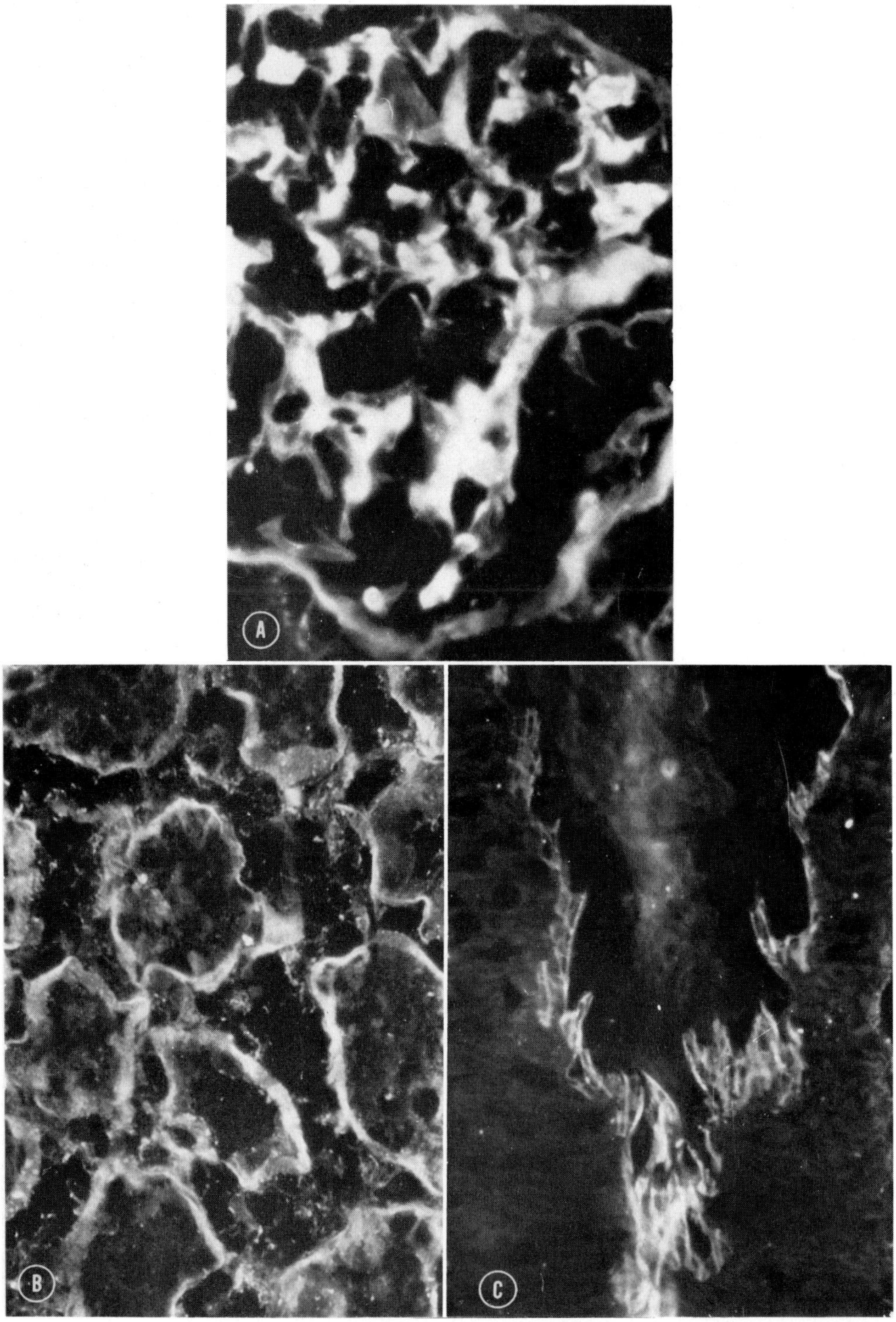

Fig. 7. Photomicrographs showing immunofluorescent staining pattern of kidney C-92 after four hours perfusion with sensitized plasma. *A,* IgG deposition in a linear pattern of glomerulus; *B,* peritubular deposition of IgG; *C,* IgG staining on endothelial surface of a blood vessel. The early pattern of β_1C deposition was similar after reimplantation (×400).

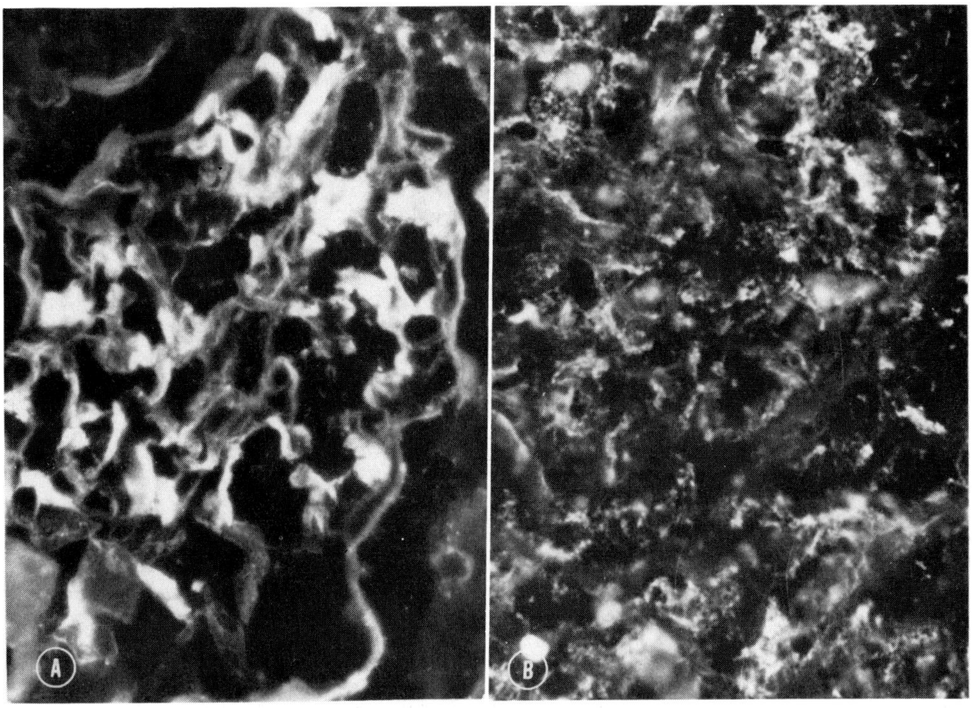

Fig. 8. Photomicrograph of immunofluorescent staining pattern of β_1C in kidney A-80; *A.* four day biopsy showing a more lumpy deposition of β_1C in a glomerulus; and *B.* seven day biopsy showing a granular deposition remaining in peritubular areas (×400).

fusate is fully active after conversion to serum at 37° C. It remains inactive in the ACD-plasma perfusate because of the calcium deficient state provided by the citrate-binding of calcium as well as the lower perfusion temperature of 8° to 10° C. This inhibition of complement during the perfusion could account for the lack of discernible differences in the perfusion hemodynamic of the kidneys perfused with unsensitized or sensitized plasma. Even though immunoglobulin was binding with the kidney antigens during perfusion with the sensitized plasma, under these conditions complement fixation could not occur. Linn[15] has shown that in a xenogenic system there are marked changes in renal perfusion hemodynamics, i.e., increased vascular resistance and cessation of perfusate flow, when complement is active. Under the conditions used for renal preservation by perfusion complement, fixation does not occur and, hence, the immunologic injury is not manifested until the kidney is reimplanted. Because of this delayed response, the causative agent, the plasma perfusate, can go unrecognized.

Other investigators have found "sensitization" of renal autografts after short periods of in vivo storage. Clark and associates[5] reported the immediate or "hyperacute" rejection of canine autografts which had been allobanked in specifically presensitized dogs whose cellular immune system had been rendered incompetent by irradiation. Benjamin and Sell[3] found that a much milder and reversible form of rejection occurred in monkey autografts that had been xenobanked in irradiated baboons. Hence, there is some evidence to support our findings of a variable immune response to such a "sensitized" kidney.

We found that high titers of cytotoxic antibody in the plasma perfusate were associated with an obvious "hyperacute" rejection of the autograft upon reimplantation; whereas perfusion with the lower titer plasma resulted in much more subtle injury, which might be very difficult to diagnose during the immediate post-transplant period in a clinical setting. In this experimental setting the immunologic injury induced in autografts by the lower antibody titer perfusate was entirely reversible. This may not be the case for allografts undergoing a similar type injury since the immunologic environment for an allograft continues to remain hostile after reimplantation, which is not the case for an autograft. Although the immune injury secondary to perfusion "sensitization" might in itself not be severe, such injury could potentiate further immunologic damage by increased exposure of antigenic surfaces in the allograft. Braun[4] has reported such an increase in antigen expression of kidney cells after treatment with trypsin or tissue injury.

The mechanism of immune injury in the case of hyperacute rejection seems evident in plasma perfusate containing high titers of cytotoxic antibody. Low titer cytotoxic antibodies, as well as other noncytotoxic antibodies present in plasma, could be equally important in inducing immune injury in renal allografts. Lindquist and Osterland[14] have demonstrated a vascular endothelial antibody in nearly 20 percent of normal subjects, increased in certain disease states, and have shown that, under the appropriate conditions, this antibody can induce immune injury. Furthermore, the work of Cochrane and his co-workers[6] suggests still another possible mechanism of immune injury by the formation of local immune complexes in the kidney, with subsequent release of vasoactive amines causing changes in vascular permeability. In that same laboratory Henson[11] has demonstrated the importance of interaction of neutrophils with immune complexes in producing tissue injury. In addition, he has shown that nonphagocytosable immune complexes deposited along surface membranes in vivo are many times more potent in stimulating immune tissue injury than when free in the circulatory blood. In the light of this information, the significance of the neutrophilic infiltrate and deposition of IgG and complement in the reversibly injured kidneys of this study takes on further meaning in suggesting a possible mechanism of injury.

This study demonstrates that perfusion of a kidney with cryoprecipitated plasma containing allogenic antibody can result in immune injury to that kidney. The clinical significance of such an observation is still not fully understood. It would seem prudent at this point to recommend that all plasma perfusate be screened for cytotoxic antibody against the cells of the potential kidney donor. It should be emphasized that this ACD-plasma cross-match must be performed only after dilution of the plasma or the conversion of the plasma to serum, since falsely negative results are obtained on the full-strength plasma. This cross-match of the perfusate and donor cells adds one additional logistical problem to the complexity of steps now necessary in the preparations for organ perfusion. A satisfactory alternative might be to screen all potential plasma perfusate against a random panel of cells containing most of the known HL-A antigens, and to use only those units of plasma which are free of any cytotoxic antibody. Using pooled plasma in hopes of diluting out the damaging antibodies does not seem to be a satisfactory answer. As suggested in this study, pooled, homologous, canine plasma containing low titers of antibody appeared to have the potential to induce at least some injury.

While the significance of other noncytotoxic antibodies in perfusate needs further delineation as to their immune injury potential, it seems that the ideal perfusate, from the standpoint of the most limited potential in causing any immune injury, would be one that is free of immunoglobulins and complement. The purified plasma protein fraction (PPF) recommended by Johnson and associates[13] can offer this advantage. Whether PPF is comparable to cryoprecipitated plasma for renal preservation from other standpoints remains less clear.

REFERENCES

1. Belzer, F. O., Ashby, B. S., and Dumphy, J. E.: Twenty four hour and seventy two hour preservation of canine kidneys, Lancet **2:** 526, 1967.
2. Belzer, F. O., and Kountz, S. L.: Preservation and transplantation of human cadaver kidneys: A two year experience, Ann. Surg. **172:** 394, 1970.
3. Benjamin, J., and Sell, K. W.: Xenogeneic renal preservation for transplantation in primates, Transplant. Proc. **17:** 164, 1974.
4. Braun, W. E., Magnusson, M., Nakamoto, S., Popowniak, K. L., and Kiser, W. S.: Intraoperative blood transfusion and hyperacute renal allograft rejection in a presensitized recipient, Transfusion **12:** 348, 1972.
5. Clark, D. S., Foker, J. E., Good, R. A., and Varco, R. L.: Humoral factors in canine renal allograft rejection, Lancet **1:** 8, 1968.
6. Cochrane, C. G.: Mechanisms involved in the deposition of immune complexes in tissues, J. Exp. Med. **134:** 75, 1971.
7. Colberg, J. E., McGraph, P., Cress, H., Lempert, N., and Eckert, C.: The cross-match profile and other extended cross-match methods and clinical transplantation, Arch. Surg. **105:** 237, 1972.
8. Collins, G. M., Bravo-Shugarman, M., and Terasaki, P. I.: Kidney preservation for transplantation, Lancet **2:** 1219, 1969.
9. Coons, A. H., and Kaplan, N. H.: Localization of antigen in tissue cells: Improvements in a method for the detection of antigen by means of fluorescent antibody, J. Exp. Med. **91:** 1, 1950.
10. Griswold, W. R., Hsu, K. C., and McIntosh, R. N.: Cryoprecipitates and immune complexes: Decrease in antibody bound I131 labeled B.S.A. antigen after cryoprecipitation in rabbit serum, Proc. Soc. Exp. Biol. Med. **142:** 1292, 1973.
11. Henson, P.: Interaction of cells with immune complexes: Adherence, release of constituents and tissue injury, *in* Branca, N., et al.: Immune complexes and the pathogenesis of disease, Madison Ave., New York, N. Y., 1973, MSS Information Corp., p. 199.
12. Johnson, R. W. G.: The effect of ischemic injury on kidneys preserved for twenty four hours before transplantation, Br. J. Surg. **59:** 769, 1972.
13. Johnson, R. W. G., Anderson, N., Flear, C. T. G., Murray, S. G. H., Taylor, R. N., and Swinney, J.: Evaluation of a new perfusion solution for kidney preservation, Transplanatation **13:** 270, 1972.
14. Lindqvist, K. J., and Osterland, C. K.: Human antibodies to vascular endothelium *in* Branca, N., et al.: Immune complexes in the pathogenesis of various diseases, Madison Ave., New York, N. Y., 1973, MSS Information Corp., p. 150.
15. Linn, B. S., Jensen, J. A., Pardo, V., Davies, D., and Franklin, L.: Relationships between structural and functional changes in rejecting renal xenografts, Transplant. Proc. **3:** 527, 1971.
16. Mittal, K. K., Mickey, M. R., Singal, D. P., and Terasaki, P. I.: Serotyping for homotransplantation, Transplantation **6:** 913, 1968.
17. Santiago-Delpin, E. A., Moberg, A. W., Mozes, M. F., Champos, R. A., Mason, R. Z., and Najarian, J. S.: Comparative analysis of perfusion and non-perfusion methods for renal preservation, SURGERY **72:** 793, 1972.
18. The, T. H. and Feltkamp, T. E. W.: Conjugation of fluorescein isothiocyanate to antibodies. II. A reproducible method, Immunology **18:** 875, 1970.
19. Williams, G. M., De Planque, B., Lower, R., and Hume, D.: Antibodies and human transplant rejection, Ann. Surg. **170:** 603, 1969.

DISCUSSION

Dr. Joshua Miller (St. Louis Park, Minn.). I think that the model is one that can be used for an autoimmune disease, and it might also be used for the amelioration of rejection in terms of perfusion with either fat fragments or blocking antibodies.

In your determination of thyroplastic antibodies pre- and post-perfusion, I wonder whether you have just run your perfusate through for four hours without kidneys, to see whether you got adsorption, inasmuch as antibody is a rather sticky substance, and it might well have stuck to the membranes of your perfusion system?

Dr. Nicholas A. Halasz (San Diego, Calif.). We really should look at the continuing use of plasma with some question. I think all of us have experienced an increasing incidence of viral problems in our patients.

It is worth rementioning that in working with dogs and in using albumin rather than plasma in organ perfusion and in using human albumin, we have been able to show that at 48 and 72 hour perfusions without ischemia, and 48 hour perfusions with 20 minute warm ischemia periods, there is no difference in terms of the rate of improvement of creatinine after implantation whether you use plasma or cryoprecipitated dog albumin. And we now have done eight human kidney perfusions, of which six kidneys worked immediately without need for dialysis.

I think albumin is useful. I think I would give a warning, though, that some batches, and particularly some manufacturers' albumin, do not work as well as others. I do not know the reason for this. It is not fatty acids, because we have done some of these studies with fatty acid–poor albumin, and they worked just as well as the albumin with normal fatty acids. But I think the dog experience can be transferred to the human. If albumin works in dogs, it can be used in humans just as satisfactorily.

Dr. J. Wesley Alexander (Cincinnati, Ohio). For some time many of us have been working with kidney perfusion and reimplanting them, and have been a little perplexed in that occasionally we have kidneys that seem to perfuse very well that do not work so well after reimplantation.

About four months ago we had an experience with a set of kidneys that had excellent perfusion, both of which had hyperacute rejection in the absence of antibodies that were detectable in the recipient, and we suspected that this might be the case, and did try and test the perfusate for the presence of cytotoxic antibodies during the post-perfusion period. I think that the demonstration that Dr. Filo has shown, that antibody is consumed or absorbed in the kidneys during the perfusion, would explain the absence of cytotoxic antibody in that perfusate when examined at a later time. Since then we have routinely run screens for cytotoxic antibody in the perfusate, which I think now is a critical component of the perfusion program.

Dr. Paul Richard Schloerb (Kansas City, Kan.) Why not hypothermic preservation itself? The work of Sachs at UCLA has shown that the dog kidney can be maintained nicely for 72 hours. We have been investigating the use of a zero chloride, hypertonic potassium sulfate type of perfusate and have easily gotten preservation of the dog kidney with life-sustaining normal function after 48 hours with simple keep-it-in-the-icebox type of perfusion. So I wonder if we are asking the right questions.

Dr. Alan G. Birtch (Springfield, Ill.). Since you stressed the fact that these kidneys did not change on perfusion, I wonder whether you have done any additional work in adding a little complement to that system to see whether or not you can bring out the change while they are on perfusion?

President Kountz: I would like to ask if you have any evidence that perfusion itself, over and above the plasma, might cause predisposing immunological injury?

Dr. R. S. Filo (closing). We saw no significant drop in antibody titer with just the membrane and the tubing conduit system itself. In addition to this, kidneys that did not express target antigen, as demonstrated in our lymphocytic toxic tests, were perfused as essentially neutral kidney, and this did not absorb the antibody either.

R. W. Johnson in Great Britain has been proposing a purified plasma protein fraction for perfusion. Several laboratories in the United States have also been proposing this, as well as the albumin substitutes.

The literature that is available so far would show that when there is any ischemic injury in a heart-beating cadaver, or when there is no warm ischemic time in an ideal kidney, the intracellular milieu, hypothermic perfusion is perfectly adequate for short periods of time. Dr. Alexander, Dr. Miller, and other people have demonstrated that when there is ischemic injury to the kidney, some type of perfusion is superior. Whether this is with an albumin solution or a purified protein fraction or a plasma solution that has had immune potential removed by the removal of complement and IgG, I do not know the answer to that yet.

We have done the experiments with addition of complement. The complement is there, I'd like to reemphasize, and it's perfectly active. The problem is, at 10° C., complement is not very effective. In vitro lymphocytoxic testing has to be done at 37° C. in order to get accurate results. Complement is very inactive at low temperatures, and there are numerous investigators who have done temperature curves showing this. IgG is sticky at low temperatures, and does bind; so that's not the problem.

Dr. Lynn demonstrated this in a xenogeneic system by perfusing animal kidneys in a dog-pig model at 37° C., using serum that had been sensitized, as opposed to plasma, and observed hyperacute rejection on the perfusion run, almost the exact clinical corollary in an acellular perfusate. Others have used this as a model to study hyperacute rejection in vitro.

We purposely chose the four hour perfusion period to eliminate the mechanical damage that perfusion itself may do. I feel that, perhaps, a twenty-four hour perfusion with an antibody in the low cytotoxic group may provide even more injury to the kidney with subsequent damage, in addition to the mechanical injury.

Clinically the injury that was induced in an autograft model was reversible, as we saw in four of the six dogs. In an allograft model, where the environment remains hostile after one reimplants a kidney, this injury could be even more potentially dangerous, in that Dr. Pierce, Dr. Williams and other investigators have shown that cells, kidney cells in particular that have been partially damaged, express more antigenicity, and, therefore, may make the "accelerated" rejection type of phenomenon more possible.

The kidney cell crossmatch in retransplantation

James C. Pierce, M.D., Ph.D., *and* **Hyung M. Lee, M.D.,** *Richmond, Va.*

A sensitive crossmatch that employs kidney cells and the immune adherence or mixed agglutination techniques has been devised and applied prospectively together with a lymphocytotoxicity crossmatch to the selection of cadaver kidneys for retransplantation in 11 consecutive patients. All of these recipients had rejected one or more previous transplants—in four cases by hyperacute rejection—and seven had cytotoxic antibodies (8 to 56 per cent). The functional survival rate of these cadaver kidney retransplants was 82 percent at nine months and patient survival was 100 percent. Current serum creatinines range from 0.8 to 1.8 mg. per 100 ml. These results contrast with 30 previous cadaver kidney retransplants for which the nine-month graft survival was 41 percent and patient survival 70 percent. The discontinuance of azathioprine before removal of a rejected transplant adversely affected the survival of a subsequent transplant and contributed to the poor results seen in the earlier group. Three retransplants from living related donors have excellent function at six months to nine years. The prospective kidney cell crossmatch is a promising technique for the improvement of cadaver kidney survival in highly immunized recipients who have rejected previous transplants. Azathioprine or other immunosuppressive therapy should be continued until a rejected transplant is removed in order to avoid sensitization to a subsequent transplant.

From the Departments of Surgery and Microbiology, Medical College of Virginia, Virginia Commonwealth University.

Although second transplants from living related donors (LRD) have a functional survival rate which is virtually the same as that of first transplants, second transplants from cadaver donors (CD) have had a significantly lower survival rate than that of first transplants.[24] When the recipients were highly immunized, as evidenced by cytotoxic antibodies against random panels of third-party donors[17] or hyperacute or acute rejection of a previous transplant,[15] the one-year survival rate of CD retransplants was reduced to 35 percent or less, even though the donor's specific lymphocyte crossmatch was negative. This study was undertaken to evaluate the use of kidney cell crossmatch in addition to a lymphocytotoxicity crossmatch for the selection of CD kidneys for retransplantation into a group of high-risk recipients.

This investigation was supported in part by Contract Ph-43-68-659 and Grant HE 08203 from the National Institutes of Health.

Presented at the Thirty-fifth Annual Meeting of the Society of University Surgeons, St. Louis, Mo., Feb. 14-16, 1974.

Reprint address: Dr. James C. Pierce, MCV Station, Box 95, Richmond, Va. 23298.

METHODS

Kidney cell crossmatch techniques. A wedge biopsy of the kidney, approximately 100 mg. in weight, was taken just prior

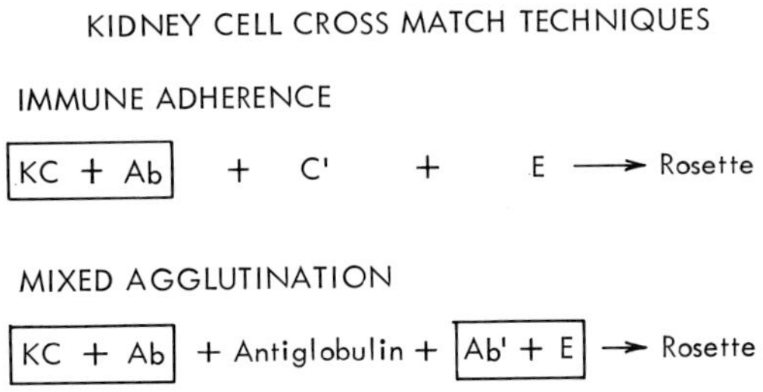

Fig. 1. In the immune adherence reaction antibody *(Ab)* bound to antigens on the surface of kidney cells *(KC)* binds and activates complement components *(C')*. These cause the adherence of primate erythrocytes *(E)*. In the mixed agglutination reaction antibody bound to kidney cells combines with an antiglobulin molecule which causes antibody-coated erythrocytes to adhere to the kidney cells. In both tests the formation of a rosette—a kidney cell encircled by erythrocytes—is the detector system.

to placement of the kidney on a pulsatile flow preservation apparatus and minced into 1 mm. cubes. It was incubated for 40 to 60 minutes at 37° C. in MEM, trypsinized (0.25 percent) for 20 minutes, and suspended in Eagle's minimal essential media (MEM) with 1 percent gelatin at a concentration of approximately 130 cells per cubic millimeter.

An immune adherence reaction was then carried out by incubating the cell suspension with a mixture of antisera, guinea pig complement, and indicator erythrocytes for 90 minutes at 37° C. on a serological ring slide, as has been previously described.[21] The reaction was read with an inverted phase microscope. A reaction was considered to be positive when 10 percent or more of the kidney cells had two or more adherent erythrocytes (Fig. 1).

The mixed agglutination test was performed by incubating kidney cells with antisera for 30 minutes at room temperature. The cells were washed three times, incubated with goat anti–human IgG for 15 minutes, washed three times, and then mixed with human erythrocytes coated with anti-rh IgG. The reaction was read on a serological ring slide after incubating for 20 minutes at room temperature with intermittent agitation. A reaction was classified as positive when 10 percent or more of the cells had two or more adherent erythrocytes (Fig. 1).

Lymphocytotoxicity techniques. Prospective crossmatches by microlymphocytotoxicity methods have been done since 1967. Since 1970, these crossmatches have been carried out on serial dilutions of recipient's serum from neat to 1:32 in duplicate by two different methods of microlymphocytotoxicity.[1, 13] Testing for preformed antibodies was done with a panel of lymphocytes from at least 40 donors. It was concluded that cytotoxins were present when 5 percent or more of the reactions were positive.

Clinical management. When the initial transplant failed, transplant nephrectomy was carried out as soon as practicable. Although abscess formation at the site of transplant nephrectomy was a frequent complication early in the series,[14] this has not occurred since we have begun to drain the nephrectomy site with a suction catheter. Details of clinical management have been previously described.[9, 10]

Statistical methods. The survey undertaken was retrospective with limited numbers of observations and several possible factors of importance were involved. The potential confounding of the effects of these factors was recognized.

For each factor analyzed it was decided to test the difference in hyperacute rejection rates, the difference in the over-all nine-month survival rates, and the difference in the nine-month survival rates deleting the hyperacute rejections. For a given factor, the first and third of these tests are independent and the second is a composite of the first and third.

In order to make the tests performed consistent with the actuarial method for analyzing survival data, the "effective number" exposed to the risk of failure was computed which gave partial survival credit to retransplant patients who were withdrawn functioning in the time interval under consideration. Fisher's Exact Test was used for performing the tests of significance because the small sample sizes precluded the use of more commonly used t or chi-square tests. Fisher's

Table I. *Clinical data on recipients of cadaver kidney retransplants selected by kidney cell crossmatch*

Pt. No.	Age (yr.), sex	Previous transplants: Source	Previous transplants: Function (mo.)	Previous transplants: Cause of failure	Interval between transplants (mo.)	Highest pre-transplant cytotoxic antibody %	Retransplants: Function (mo.)	Retransplants: Present serum creatinine (mg./100 ml.)
74	43 M	C*	52	CR†	5	46	41	1.7
185	20 M	F	0	HA	17	26	25	1.8
149	43 F	C	5	CR	2	2	34	1.2
120	22 M	B	31	CR	19	2	18	1.0
125	26 F	C	2	Infection	3			
		C	0	HA	2			
		C	0	AR	31	52	18	0.8
145	41 F	B	0	HA	26	34	18	1.4
192	30 M	C	0	HA	13	2	0	HA
146	23 M	F	0	AR	29	29	0	ATN, AR, Infection
166	47 F	Son	0	AR	17	56	11	1.1
181	36 M	C	10	CR	8	8	10	1.6
188	35 M	B	1.3	AR	10	2	2	1.2

*C, Cadaver; F, father; B, brother.
†CR, Chronic rejection; HA, hyperacute rejection; AR, acute rejection.

Exact Test requires integer values in all categories, i.e., is potentially incompatible with the "effective numbers" of the acturial method. This problem was handled by rounding down the "effective number" to the next lowest integer value. It should be noted that this approximation did not occur in comparing hyperacute rejection rates, that there was only one functioning retransplant in the study in the 0 to 9 month period (i.e., the use of "effective numbers" applies to only one case in the analysis of this particular data set), and that the rounding-down procedure was a conservative one.

RESULTS

The patients in which the CD kidney retransplant was selected by kidney cell crossmatch were an immunologically unfavorable group (Table I). Only two of the recipients were favorable candidates in that their previous grafts had undergone chronic rejection and they lacked significant amounts of cytotoxic antibodies. The recipients of 30 previous cadaver kidney transplants were likewise highly immunized. In nine of them previous kidneys had undergone hyperacute rejection and in three additional cases previous kidneys had undergone acute rejection. Also, 15 out of 19 patients studied had cytotoxins against a random panel of lymphocytes. The three LRD recipients were a more favorable group. Two had lost their first kidneys due to chronic rejection and one due to a combination of severe acute tubular necrosis and chronic rejection. One of these patients had antibodies against 6 percent of the random panel, one against 1 percent, and no pretransplant serum was available for analysis from the third.

In the kidney cell crossmatch group of 11 patients, the average number of HL-A antigens matched was 1.1 and ranged from 0 to 2 antigens. Of the LRD transplants, two were one haplo-type matches and one received a transplant from an HL-A identical sibling.

One of the patients in the kidney cell crossmatch group (No. 181) received a second transplant which shared two antigens present in the first transplant and absent in the recipient. One patient in the earlier CD

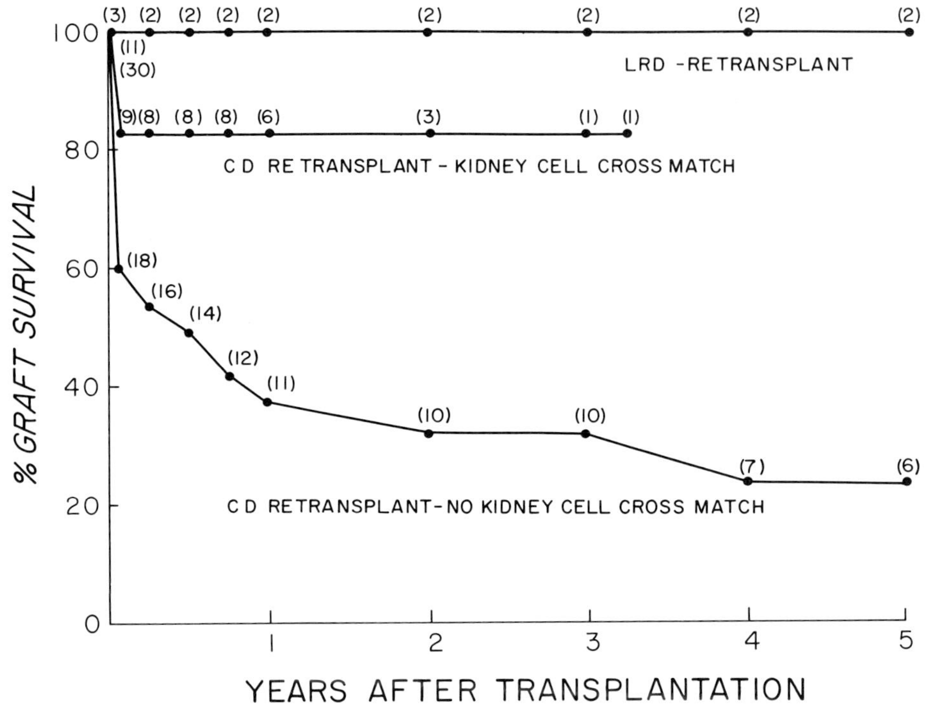

Fig. 2. Effect of selection by the kidney cell crossmatch on cadaver donor (CD) kidney survival computed by actuarial methods. There was a significant difference between the group selected by the kidney cell crossmatch and the group without with respect to the incidence of hyperacute rejection ($p = 0.011$) and the graft survival rates at nine months ($p = 0.028$). Survival of living related donor *(LRD)* retransplants was 100 percent. Numbers in parentheses refer to numbers of grafts surviving at time points.

kidney transplant group received a kidney which shared one antigen with the previous transplant and absent in the recipient. This patient continues to have excellent function more than five years after retransplantation.

Of the 11 CD retransplants selected by kidney cell crossmatch, nine continue to function from two months to three years following transplantation (Fig. 2). One kidney was lost because of hyperacute rejection in a recipient whose first kidney was also lost from hyperacute rejection. A CD transplant in a second recipient (No. 146) functioned so poorly that the patient continued to require dialysis after transplantation. One month following transplantation, the kidney began to open up, with urine outputs ranging from 244 to 547 ml. over the next 10 days, but then deteriorated when it was necessary to ligate one of the two renal arteries and the external iliac artery because of hemorrhage secondary to infection. The courses of two other patients were complicated by the development of steroid diabetes and in one patient the ureter had to be reimplanted into the bladder on the day following transplantation. All patients continue to survive and, in nine patients with functioning grafts, the serum creatinine ranges from 0.8 to 1.8 mg. per 100 ml. In the previous CD kidney retransplant group, there were 11 instances of hyperacute rejection and six kidneys underwent acute rejection during the first year following transplantation. Six of the 22 recipients continue to live and all of these have functioning CD kidney retransplants from four to nine years following transplantation. All three of the recipients of LRD kidney retransplants continue to survive with functioning transplants from six

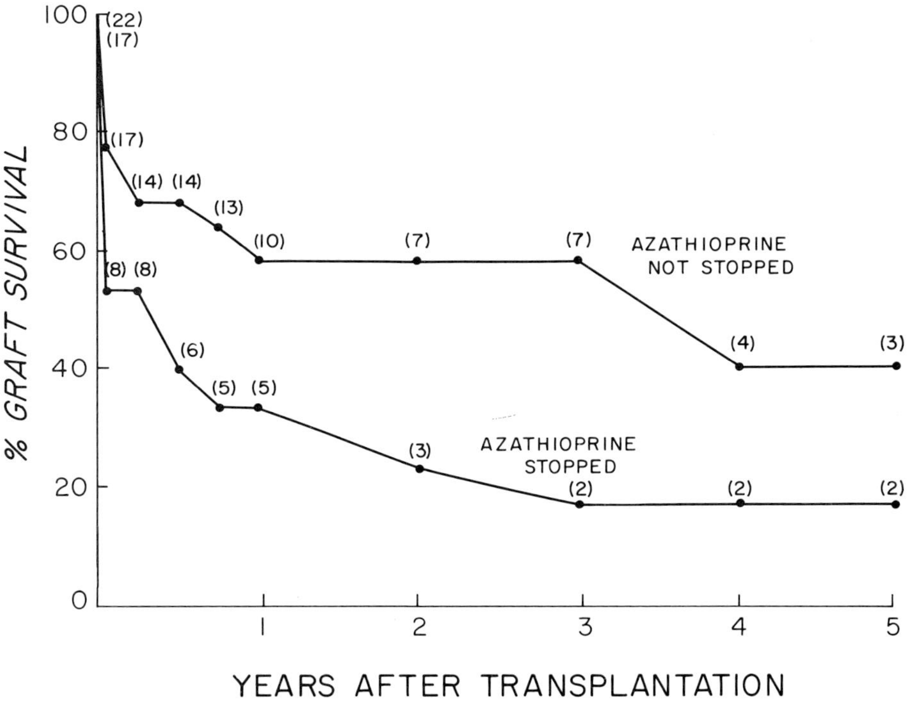

Fig. 3. Effect of discontinuance of azathioprine before removal of the previous kidney transplant upon the subsequent cadaver donor transplant survival computed by actuarial methods. There was a significant difference between the two groups with respect to the incidence of hyperacute rejection ($p = 0.011$) and the graft survival rate at nine months. ($p < 0.047$). Numbers in parentheses refer to numbers of grafts surviving at time points.

months to nine years after transplantation. The serum creatinines in this group range from 1.0 to 1.3 mg. per 100 ml.

The effect of the kidney cell crossmatch was particularly significant in recipients of retransplanted kidneys who had cytotoxic antibodies. The nine-month survival rate in the kidney cell crossmatch group was 86 percent, compared with 20 percent for those without a kidney cell crossmatch. This was significant ($p = 0.012$).

The discontinuance of azathioprine prior to removal of a transplanted kidney had an adverse effect on the survival of the subsequent transplant (Fig. 3). The one-year survival of 17 CD retransplants was only 33 percent when azathioprine had been discontinued before removal of the previous transplant; it was 58 percent when azathioprine had been continued up to the time of removal of the previous transplant. Azathioprine was discontinued a median of 14 days prior to removal of the kidney, with a range of 3 to 196 days. In the group of kidneys selected by kidney cell crossmatch, azathioprine was discontinued while the previous kidney was still in place in two patients.

Azathioprine had been discontinued prior to removal of the previous transplant for 16 of the 28 CD kidney retransplants in the earlier group and in none of the 3 recipients who received LRD kidney retransplants. Data on two patients who received their initial transplants at other centers was not available.

Splenectomy was carried out prior to the second CD transplant in 16 recipients whose kidneys had a one-year survival rate of 69 percent as compared with a functional survival rate of 36 percent in 17 second CD kidneys for which splenectomy was not per-

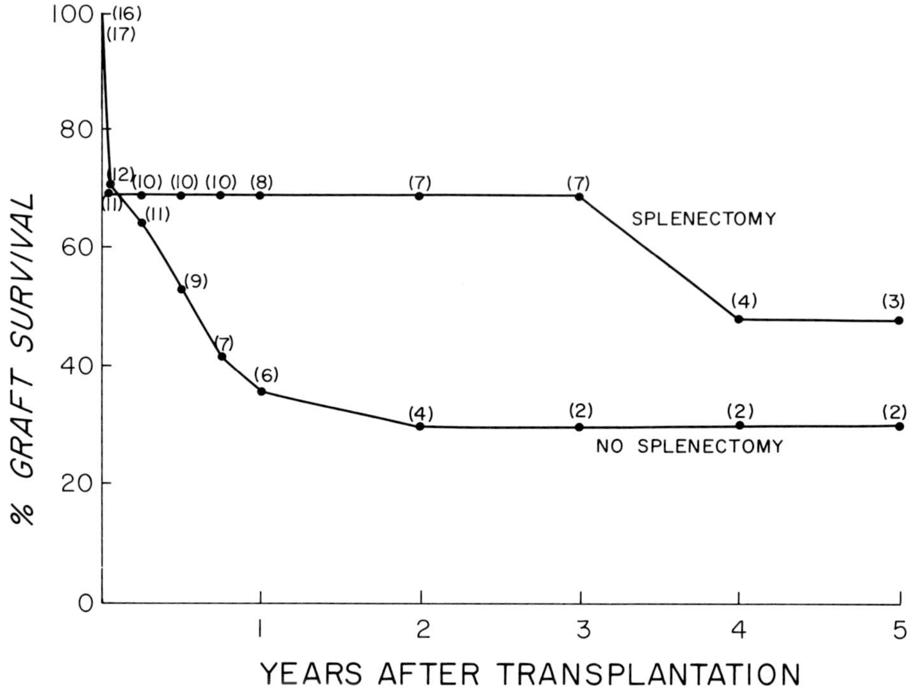

Fig. 4. Effect of splenectomy on the survival of second cadaver kidneys computed by actuarial methods. There was no significant difference between the two groups with respect to the incidence of hyperacute rejection or at individual times points but the difference in survival rates excluding hyperacute rejections from 0 to 9 months approached significance ($p < 0.060$). Numbers in parentheses refer to numbers of grafts surviving at time points.

formed (Fig. 4). Splenectomy was performed prior to retransplantation in eight of the recipients of CD kidneys selected by kidney cell crossmatch and before 13 of the 30 CD kidney transplants performed previously and prior to retransplantation in one of the LRD kidney recipients.

Nine of the recipients in the kidney cell crossmatch group received ALG; only seven of the previous CD kidney retransplant recipients were treated with it. The one-year graft survival rates were 62 percent for the ALG group and 40 percent for the group without ALG, but there was no significant difference between the survival curves of the two groups at any time point. None of the LRD retransplant recipients received ALG.

DISCUSSION

As a result of early experience with retransplantation, it was suggested by some workers[7] that retransplantation should not be undertaken if the initial graft failed because of rejection, but only in the circumstance where it was a technical failure. Hume and associates,[10] however, reported successful retransplantation in patients who had rejected an initial transplant. It is now widely accepted that retransplantation may be undertaken even when the initial graft failed because of rejection. More recently it has been reported that retransplantation with CD kidneys was particularly likely to fail when the recipient had cytotoxic antibodies or when the initial transplant had failed because of hyperacute or acute rejection. Opelz and Terasaki[17] found that the one-year graft survival rate for CD kidney retransplants was only 35 percent when the recipient had cytotoxins, whereas it was 64 percent in recipients who lacked cytotoxins. Opelz, Mickey, and Terasaki[15] found that when the first graft was rejected hyperacutely only 27 percent of second CD grafts survived for one year.

When grafts were rejected acutely, between one and three months following transplantation, the one-year survival of subsequent CD kidney grafts was reduced to 28 percent. In contrast to these poor results, the one-year graft survival in recipients without cytotoxins whose first graft was rejected after more than three months was 77 percent. The one-year graft survival rate of 82 percent in 11 recipients of CD kidney retransplants reported here is remarkable because nine of them were in the high immunological risk group according to the criteria cited above. Factors which may have contributed to this improved success rate include the employment of a kidney cell crossmatch, the continuance of azathioprine therapy until removal of the previous rejected kidneys, pretransplant splenectomy, and the use of antilymphocyte globulin.

The use of the kidney cell crossmatch technique was suggested by the retrospective observations of Williams and associates[25] that antibody directed against kidney cells could be identified in pretransplant samples of patient's serum when hyperacute rejection of a kidney transplant had occurred in the face of a negative pretransplant microlymphocytotoxicity crossmatch. With the development of an effective means of kidney preservation on a pulsatile flow apparatus with cryoprecipitated plasma by Belzer and Kountz,[2] an opportunity to apply these methods to the clinical selection of recipients for kidney transplants presented itself. A kidney cell crossmatch technique was devised which used the immune adherence technique.[21] In the meantime efforts were continued to develop a method of detection of antibody against a suspension of individual kidney cells by the mixed agglutination technique which would not require propagation of the cells in tissue culture. This succeeded and comparisons with the immune adherence technique have indicated that it is more sensitive, more reproducible, and easier to perform.

If the use of the kidney cell crossmatch technique in addition to the lymphocytotoxicity technique results in a more sensitive detection of preformed antibody directed against a donor kidney, it would be expected to improve the survival rate of retransplanted cadaver kidneys by reducing the incidence of hyperacute rejection as reported here and by Kountz and associates.[11] In addition, certain observations suggest that it might reduce the incidence of acute rejection as well. Lucas and associates[12] were able to detect low levels of antibody which were not detectable by cytotoxicity assays by means of the inhibition of binding of radiolabeled anti–HL-A IgG. Intermediate titers of antibody were associated with accelerated rejection and lower levels were associated with mild impairment of renal function. Sterling and associates[22] observed a correlation between deposits of IgG, β_1C, and fibrinogen on one-hour renal biopsies and the subsequent course of the transplant.

The discontinuance of azathioprine after a previous transplant had been rejected but not yet removed appeared to affect the survival of a subsequent transplant adversely, and this was statistically significant. The observation in rabbits[4] that 6-mercaptopurine, an analogue of azathioprine, augmented antibody response if given prior to challenge with an antigen suggests that discontinuance of azathioprine during rejection might have augmented the sensitization of the recipient to all of the HL-A antigens present on the kidney which he lacked and thereby contributed to the very high incidence of acute humoral rejection which was observed earlier in our series.[19] Also, Cleveland and associates[5] found that when dogs were treated with azathioprine during the course of a primary kidney transplant, a second kidney from the same donor underwent primary rather than accelerated rejection. It is our current practice to continue azathioprine and prednisone up until the time that the transplant is removed whenever the patient's clinical condition permits. Gustafsson and associates[8] reported that they continue to give immunosuppressive therapy after rejection of a transplant, but if it has failed late from chronic rejection and is extraperitoneal in location, it is often left in place after retransplantation. Kountz and associates[11] said that they often remove the initial transplant when it is functioning poorly because of repeated rejection and replace it with a second transplant while continuing the immunosuppressive therapy.

Splenectomy may also have contributed to the improved survival of the kidney cell crossmatch group of cadaver retransplants. In an earlier analysis of our experience we observed that, while splenectomy did not have a beneficial effect on survival of first transplants, it appeared to improve the survival of second transplants.[20] Unless splenectomy is performed prior to immunization of the recipient by blood transfusions, pregnancies, or transplants, it is unlikely to have any effect on hyperacute rejection. In our series it appears to improve the survival of CD retransplants during the initial months following transplantation and this verges on statistical significance. Opelz and Terasaki,[18] as the result of the study of data collected from a number of centers, have concluded that splenectomy does not have a beneficial effect upon the survival of first transplants, second cadaver transplants, or cadaver transplants in recipients with cytotoxic antibodies. It is possible that the apparent improvement in our splenectomized group of retransplant cadaver kidney recipients was not due to splenectomy but rather to the use of a kidney cell crossmatch or some other factor. Nevertheless, we still employ splenectomy after the failure of the first transplant except in recipients of living related donor retransplants and in recipients who lack cytotoxic antibodies.

Opelz, Mickey, and Terasaki[16] have proposed that kidney transplant recipients may be responders or nonresponders to HL-A antigens. Nonresponders fail to make cytotoxins even after long periods of dialysis and have excellent transplant courses; responders make cytotoxins and tend to reject their kidney transplants. Some transplant surgeons have avoided transplantation in patients with cytotoxins because they felt that a poor outcome was likely.[26] The experience reported here with the retransplantation of cadaver kidneys suggests that even highly immunized responders who have rejected previous transplants will tolerate subsequent cadaver kidneys with good function. It is of interest that this can be achieved without matches for three and four HL-A antigens. The Minnesota group has also recently reported no difference in the survival of kidney transplants in patients with and without cytotoxins.[3]

As more and more patients receive kidney transplants, the need for retransplantation will grow. Of our first 200 patients, 18 percent received two or more kidneys. Kountz and associates[11] have estimated that 20 percent of their patients will need retransplantation. Although a few patients find dialysis preferable to transplantation, most patients after the loss of a kidney look forward to receiving another one. This is probably because it affords them the best opportunity for rehabilitation.[23] The ACS-NIH Transplant Registry[24] cites one-year cadaver kidney functional survival rates of 37.3 and 35.7 percent, but these figures are biased by the inclusion of bad results from earlier experience. In the small series of recent cases reported here, the one-year functional survival rate for cadaver kidney retransplants was 82 percent. Kountz and associates[11] reported that in their most recent experience retransplants of cadaver kidneys had the same survival rates as first cadaver kidneys, i.e., 67 percent. Fine and associates[6] reported that 11 of 13 of cadaver kidney retransplants in children were functioning from three to 36 months after transplantation. Four of those recipients had cytotoxic antibodies. We conclude that current results from retransplantation with cadaver kidneys are considerably improved over those reflected in the Transplant Registry.

The authors wish to acknowledge the inspiration and participation of the late David M. Hume, M.D., in the work presented here. Particular thanks are due Walter Cummings, Ph.D., for his assistance with the statistical analysis.

REFERENCES

1. Amos, B., Cabrera, G., Bias, W. B., MacQueen, J. M., Lancaster, S. L. Southworth, J. G., and Ward, F. E.: The inheritance of human leukocyte antigens. III. The organization of specificities, *in* Terasaki, P. I., editor: Histocompatibility testing, Copenhagen, 1970, Ejnar Munksgaard Forlag, p. 259.
2. Belzer, F. O., and Kountz, S. L.: Preservation and transplantation of human cadaver kidneys: A two year experience, Ann. Surg. **172:** 394, 1970.
3. Callender C. O., Simmons, R. L., Yunis, E. DeShazo, M.D., Toledo-Pereyra, L. H., and Najarian, J. S.: Failure of lymphocytotoxic antibodies to correlate with renal allograft rejection, *in* Abstracts, American Society of Nephrology, p. 18, 1973.
4. Chanmougan, D., and Schwarz, R.S.: Enhancement of antibody synthesis by 6-mercaptopurine, J. Exp. Med. **124:** 363, 1966.
5. Cleveland, R. J., Kauffman, H. M., Graham, W. H., and Hume, D. M.: Prolongation of renal homograft survival by inhibition of the afferent arc of the immune response, Surg. Forum **16:** 269, 1965.
6. Fine, R. N., Korsch, B. M., Riddell, H., Stiles, Q. R., Edelbrock, H. H., Brennan, L. P., Heuser, E., and Grushkin, C. M.: Second renal transplants in children, SURGERY **73:** 1, 1973.
7. Gifford, R. W., Deodhar, S. D., Stewart, B. H., Nakamoto, S., Shibagaki, M., and Kolff, W. J.: Retransplantation after failure of first renal homografts, J. A. M. A. **199:** 799, 1967.
8. Gustafsson, A., Groth, C. G., Halgrimson, C. G., Penn, I., and Starzl, T. E.: The fate of failed homografts retained after retransplantation, Surg. Gynecol. Obstet. **137:** 40, 1973.
9. Hume, D. M., Magee, J. H., Prout, G. R., Jr., Kaufman, H. M., Jr., Cleveland, R. H., Bower, J. D., and Lee, H. M.: Studies of renal homotransplantation in man, Ann. N. Y. Acad. Sci. **120:** 578, 1964.
10. Hume, D. M., Lee, H. M., Williams, G. M., White, H. J. O., Ferré, J., Wolf, J. S., Prout, G. R., Jr., Slapak, M., O'Brien, J. Kilpatrick, S. S., Kauffman, H. M., Jr., and Cleveland, R. J.: Comparative results of cadaver and related donor renal homografts in man, and the immunologic implications of the outcome of second and paired transplants, Ann. Surg. **164:** 352, 1966.
11. Kountz, S. L., Thibault, P. M., Endo, T., Margules, R., and Belzer, F. O.: Results of immediate and delayed retransplantation, Transplant. Proc. **4:** 735, 1972.
12. Lucas, Z. J., Coplon, N., Kempson, R., and Cohn, R.: Early renal transplant failure associated with subliminal sensitization, Transplantation **10:** 522, 1970.
13. Mittal, K. K., Mickey, M. R., Singal, D. P., and Terasaki, P. I.: Serotyping of homotransplantation. XVIII. Refinement of micro-droplet lymphocyte cytotoxicity test, Transplantation **6:** 913, 1968.
14. Moore, T. C., and Hume, D. M.: The period and nature of hazard in clinical renal transplantation. I. The hazard to patient survival, Ann. Surg. **170:** 1, 1969.
15. Opelz, G., Mickey, M. R., and Terasaki, P. I.: Prolonged survival of second human kidney transplants, Science **178:** 617, 1972.
16. Opelz, G., Mickey, M. R., and Terasaki, P. I.: Identification of unresponsive kidney-transplant recipients, Lancet **1:** 868, 1972.
17. Opelz, G., and Terasaki, P. I.: Second kidney transplants and presensitization, Transplant. Proc. **4:** 743, 1972.
18. Opelz, G., and Terasaki, P. I.: Effect of splenectomy on human renal transplants, Transplantation **15:** 605, 1973.
19. Pierce, J. C., Cobb, G. W., and Hume, D. M.: Relevance of HL-A antigens to acute humoral rejection of multiple renal allotransplants, N. Engl. J. Med. **285:** 142, 1971.
20. Pierce, J. C., and Hume, D. M.: The effect of splenectomy on the survival of first and second renal homotransplants in man, Surg. Gynecol. Obstet. **127:** 1300, 1968.
21. Pierce, J. C., and Hume, D. M.: Cross-matching for organ transplantation. I. The use of kidney cells and immune adherence, Transplant. Proc. **3:** 127, 1971.
22. Sterling, W. A., Bryant, C. P., Ohanian, S. H., Pierce, J. C., Lee, H. M., Hume, D. M., Weymouth, R. J., and Seibel, H. R.: Evaluation of renal transplant recipients by immunofluorescent microscopy, Surg. Forum **22:** 263, 1972.
23. Sterling, W. A., Pierce, J. C., Lee, H. M., and Hume, D. M.: Rehabilitation of retransplant patients, Transplant. Proc. **4:** 751, 1972.
24. U. S. Kidney Transplant Fact Book: Information from ACS/NIH Registry, 1972, U. S. Department of Health, Education and Welfare, DHEW Publication No. (NIH) 73-335, p. 14.
25. Williams, G. M., DePlanque, B., Lower R. R., and Hume, D. M.: Antibodies and human transplant rejection, Ann. Surg. **170:** 603, 1969.
26. Wilson, R. E., Carpenter, C. B., Birtch, A. G., Murray, J. E., and Merrill, J. P.: Peter Bent Brigham Hospital experience with controlled

clinical trial of anti-lymphocyte globulin for human renal allografts, *in* ALG therapy and standardization workshop, Behring Institute Research Communications, No. 51, Behringwerke AG, Marburg, p. 129, 1972.

DISCUSSION

Dr. Jerry C. Rosenberg (Detroit, Mich.). Relative to the use of kidney cells, do you think you have to use kidney cells? Do you think that the immune adherence assay or the mixed agglutination reaction may not be just as effective with lymphocytes? Did you simultaneously use lymphocytes as the target cell, rather than kidney cells? The increased sensitivity may not require the use of kidney cells. Does that produce any problems? Does that subsequently produce a site of bleeding, or perhaps blow out a urine leak after transplantation?

Did you utilize the newer complement-dependent assays, the flicking technique, and washing off anticomplementary materials from lymphocytes, and compare your assay (the mixed agglutination assay) with the lymphocytotoxicity test?

Dr. Jeremiah George Turcotte (Ann Arbor, Mich). In the discussion you brought up the problem about patients who do have a high percentage of reaction to a high percentage of cells in the panel that are considered cytotoxic antibodies. Have you actually put your more sensitive test to the test clinically—that is, selected kidneys with a negative crossmatch by your most sensitive test?

I think this is a very important issue, because in Terasaki's own registry two thirds of all patients have a positive cytotoxic antibody panel. We have experience with two patients now reacting against more than 80 percent of the panel range of cells, in which we identified which HL-A antigens are reacting to and selected a kidney that did not have those antigens and also had a negative crossmatch by two or three different methods. Both those kidneys functioned well.

Dr. Richard E. Wilson (Boston, Mass.). We have tried to use an ATG crossmatch to increase the sensitivity of the standard crossmatch and have selected patients who are positive to a panel with this basis. It has not worked, and so I think this is very important. Have you tried this in first transplant patients? How long does this take to do from the time you get the biopsy till the study is completed?

Dr. G. Melville Williams (Baltimore, Md.). I have been trying to work out a technique for producing a valid assay in fresh kidney cells for seven years, and sometimes it works and sometimes it doesn't. In those cases that were shown, what is the consistency? In other words, can he get good cell preps invariably and invariably have negative controls and positive controls, and everything smooth, or does it sort of work on Tuesday and not on Friday?

President Kountz. Have you encountered a patient in whom, after transplant rejection of an unrelated transplant that has been matched for all four HL-A factors, you have found a positive crossmatch against kidney cells, suggesting there is indeed a kidney-specific antigen to which the patient was sensitized?

Dr. James C. Pierce (closing). We have tried the mixed agglutination test with lymphocytes, and there are two problems. One, of course, is that the lymphocyte has immunoglobulins on it, and that leads to a problem with background. It appears to be less sensitive with lymphocytes than with kidney cells where we have taken kidney cells and lymphocytes from the same donor and used sera that were very sensitive with kidney cells.

We have not given up on that problem, but we have not been able at this point to resolve it. You can do the immune adherence with lymphocytes, but in my view this is a more cumbersome and less sensitive test, and we are now less interested in that test than we are in the mixed agglutination.

With regard to the biopsy, we have done hundreds of these biopsies, not only for this test but also for examination of the kidney, and we have never had any significant problems with them. So I do not think that that really is a major problem.

With regard to the new, more sensitive lymphocytotoxicity tests, we have run laboratory comparisons between sera against kidney cells and against a variety of tests. We found that the mixed agglutination test is much more sensitive (about twice as sensitive) than the most sensitive of these other tests. And I mean by that the Amos three-flick or three-wash technique and the Terasaki long-incubation techniques.

We have selected kidneys for patients who have high percentages of antibodies; in this group of patients six had antibodies against 23 percent or more of a random panel. In our first cadaver kidney group we had a number of patients who had antibodies against more than 40 percent of a random panel. We did one patient who had 99 percent, and the kidney did all right for several weeks. This was performed at the McGuire Veterans Hospital by Dr. Wolf, and, tragically, the patient died from a heart attack, so that long-term follow-up in that instance was not possible.

We have compared our method with the antiglobulin-augmented lymphocytoxicity test, and it is about twice as sensitive. In fact, we find with the antiglobulin we are using that the antiglobulin-augmented test is no more sensitive than if one just washes the cells three times.

The time for the test is six to eight hours. In

regard to Dr. Williams' very insightful question, the answer is that the cell prep is a problem. It was more of a problem earlier in our experience that it has been more recently. There are two factors that I think are helpful there. One is the realization that trypsin adheres to cell surfaces, and that there are factors in serum which neutralize that; therefore, it is essential to wash the kidney cells with serum-containing media, and to wash them several times to completely get rid of the trypsin. That is an advantage of the immunoglobulin test over the other tests; it is performed at room temperature, and does not require 37°, as immune adherence does. Incubation can wipe the antigens off, or damage the cells and give false-positive results. The second point, of course, is just filtering the cells to get rid of cell debris which competes for antibody.

We have been looking for HL-A identical patients who have lost their kidneys to test exactly this hypothesis, Dr. Kountz. In one patient there was no evidence of antibody at any time during the patient's course; and with the antiglobulin test we can detect the antibodies early in the course of such a patient, while the kidney is in and while it is functioning. In the second patient, who lost also an HL-A identical kidney, we found 10 percent, just at the minimum level of sensitivity; the problem was that this same level of antibody was present prior to the transplant and during the transplant. One would like to see an augmented response with challenge.

Passive enhancement of canine renal allografts with polyspecific $F(ab')_2$ fragments

Simon F. G. Wren, M.D., Antonio C. P. Martins, M.D., Ulrich Von Haefen, M.D., George J. Busch, M.D., Gordon E. Katske, M.D., Thomas L. Koppenheffer, Ph.D., Thongdee Shaipanich, M.D., *and* **Richard E. Wilson, M.D.,** *Boston, Mass.*

The use of polyspecific $F(ab')_2$ fragments, derived from allogeneic hyperimmune serum, has been investigated as a method for achieving passive enhancement of canine renal allografts. Nine groups of dogs were studied, with variations in $F(ab')_2$ and IgG dosages, routes of administration, and minimal immunosuppressive drug therapy. Significant prolonged survival was achieved only with ex vivo renal perfusion and intravenous administration to the recipient of $F(ab')_2$ fragments combined with suboptimal azathioprine and prednisolone therapy. Drug therapy alone, $F(ab')_2$ perfusion alone, combined $F(ab')_2$ perfusion and intravenous administration without immunosuppressive drugs or IgG therapy all failed to prolong survival of the transplanted animals. When lower doses of $F(ab')_2$ fragments (400 mg.) were given in the same protocol that was successful with 1,900 mg., some prolongation of host survival was achieved but not to a significant degree. Antigen matching was not a controlling feature in successful graft prolongation. $F(ab')_2$ fragments were capable of inhibiting the complement-mediated cytotoxicity of the whole hyperimmune serum at every dilution studied, shifting the endpoint of cell death by three dilutions. Transplant results presented for an additional group of eight dogs indicated that in vitro inhibition by polyspecific $F(ab')_2$ of cytotoxicity against specific donor cells by the immune serum may represent a technique for selecting appropriate donor-recipient pairs to achieve a higher success rate with this form of passive enhancement.

From the Departments of Surgery and Pathology of Harvard Medical School at the Peter Bent Brigham Hospital, Boston, Mass.

PASSIVE administration of monospecific immune serum to inbred rats will prolong survival of renal allografts[4, 16] as will the use of $F(ab')_2$ fragments of an immune serum that has been raised against the specific organ being trnasplanted[12] or against spleen cells.[13]

This work was supported in part by grants from the National Institutes of Health, The Atomic Energy Commission, and The Hartford Foudation, Inc.

Presented at the Thirty-fifth Annual Meeting of the Society of University Surgeons, St. Louis, Mo., Feb. 14-16, 1974.

Reprint address: Richard E. Wilson, M.D., Peter Bent Brigham Hospital, 721 Huntington Ave., Boston, Mass. 02115.

Active enhancement in inbred strains with whole cells[10, 16] and soluble antigen[8, 17] is also an effective method of extending survival of renal allografts.

Enhancement in outbred animals, such as the dog, is more difficult to achieve. Pretreatment with subcellular specific antigen, when combined with suboptimal immunosuppression, can be highly effective in certain dosage schedules[5, 18] but polyspecific subcellular antigen therapy has been ineffective.[15] Treatment with donor-specific whole cells has permitted graft prolongation when combined with drugs.[11]

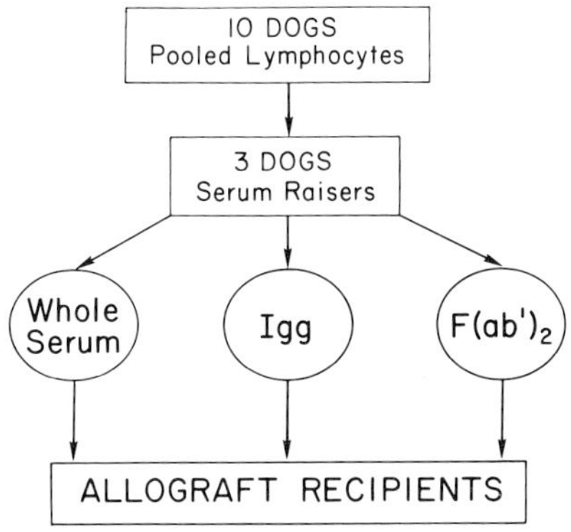

Fig. 1. General scheme for the production of polyspecific antiserum. The immune serum was consistently cytotoxic to all canine lymphocytes tested.

Table I. *Identification of experimental groups*

Group No.	*Method of administration*	*Serum fraction*	*Suboptimal immuno-suppression**
I	0	0	+
II, IV	Renal perfusion + intravenously	F(ab′)$_2$	0
III, V	Renal perfusion + intravenously	F(ab′)$_2$	+
VI	Intravenously	IgG	0
VII	Intravenously	IgG	+
VIII	Renal perfusion	F(ab′)$_2$	+
IX	Intravenously	F(ab′)$_2$	+

*Azathioprine, 2 mg per kilogram per day. Methylprednisolone, 1 mg per kilogram per day.

Passive enhancement has met with little success in dogs. Therapy with donor-specific homologous and heterologous F(ab′)$_2$ fragments raised to kidney and perfused directly into the kidney failed[19]; polyspecific heterologous and homologous F(ab′)$_2$ fragments raised to kidney, skin, and leukocytes produced minimal graft prolongation.[1] In neither of these studies was immunosuppression included in the treatment protocol. Myburgh and Smith[9] have performed liver transplants in baboons and have reported excellent prolongation of survival using polyspecific serum in its original hyperimmune state. The use of a polyspecific serum in clinical renal transplantation has much to commend it; its availability, its wide range of alloantibody representation, the ability to use it for cadaver as well as living donor recipients, and the advantages of passive over active immunization. The use of F(ab′)$_2$ fragments from such a serum removes a major disadvantage of the whole serum—i.e., its cytotoxicity and its potential destructive effect on a renal graft. This experiment was designed to test the in vivo action of polyspecific F(ab′)$_2$ fragments and IgG on the survival of canine renal allografts and their ability to inhibit, in vitro, a standard microplate cytotoxic assay.

MATERIALS AND METHODS

Experimental design. Fig. 1 shows the general scheme of the protocol by which the polyspecific serum was raised. Three outbred mongrel dogs were immunized with pooled peripheral lymphocytes of another 10 dogs. The initial injection was intradermal, with Freund's complete adjuvant, and three subsequent weekly injections were made subcutaneously without Freund's adjuvant. Booster injections were given as needed to raise more serum. These dogs were subjected to plasmapheresis and the IgG and F(ab′)$_2$ fragments processed from the serum. Table I shows the methods of administration of F(ab′)$_2$ and IgG to the various groups of dogs with or without suboptimal immunosuppression. The IgG was given only intravenously; the F(ab′)$_2$ was given by perfusion into the kidney at the time of transplantation, or intravenously after transplant, and by combining both perfusion and intravenous administration. Renal perfusion was carried out with the use of an oxygenated, salt-containing Dextran solution[6] as a perfusate (volume 75 ml.), buffered during the course of a one-hour perfusion at a pH of 7.3 to 7.5 with Tris HCl. The perfusion was pulsatile and carried out at a temperature of 19 to 20° C. and a pressure of 40 to 60 mm. Hg.

Dogs were subjected to transplantation and bilateral nephrectomy in the usual manner; the blood urea nitrogen level (BUN) was determined twice weekly. A number of in vitro studies were performed: (1) each donor and recipient underwent serotyping; (2) the F(ab′)$_2$ and whole serum were tested for

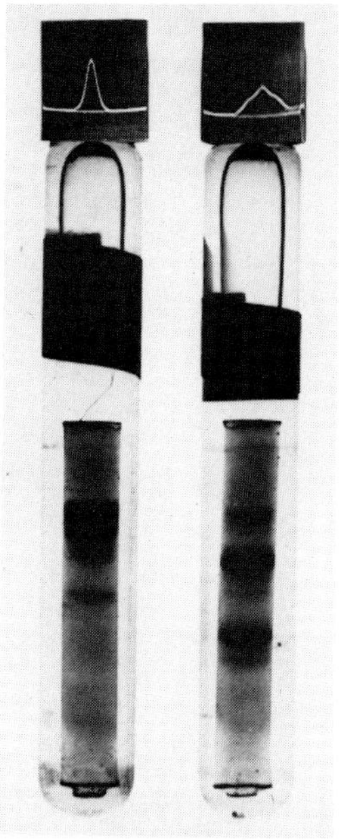

Fig. 2. SDS disc gel electrophoresis, with the corresponding ultracentrifugal analysis, of the purified IgG on the left and $F(ab')_2$ fragments on the right.

their ability to lyse lymphocytes in a microplate cytotoxicity assay; (3) the $F(ab')_2$ was tested for its capability to inhibit the cytotoxicity of a whole polyspecific serum on random dog lymphocytes; (4) in selected donor-recipient combinations the $F(ab')_2$ was tested for its ability to block cytotoxicity of polyspecific serum on specific donor lymphocytes, in an attempt to correlate this with graft survival; and (5) the $F(ab')_2$ was tested at various times during the course of the one-hour renal perfusion to identify the loss of cytotoxic-inhibiting activity.

$F(ab')_2$ production. Whole serum was decomplemented and precipitated with cold, 40 percent supersaturated $(NH_4)_2SO_4$. The resultant globulin was further purified by chromatography with a DE52 cellulose column and eluted with 0.075M Tris HCl buffer. The resultant eluate contained the purified IgG. This IgG was digested for 24 hours with pepsin at pH 4.0 at a pepsin:protein ratio of 1:40. The $F(ab')_2$ obtained was dialyzed against phosphate-buffered saline, pH 7.2, and stored at –20° C.

Ultracentrifugal analysis (Fig. 2) and sodium dodecyl sulfate (SDS) disc gel electrophoresis of the purified IgG showed a major peak at 6.3 S with no contamination; analysis of the $F(ab')_2$ fragment showed a major peak at 5 S with two minor peaks, one faster and one slower moving.

Cytotoxic antibody. This was measured by a microplate modification of the method of Ballantyne and Stetson[2] with 1×10^7 random lymphocytes per milliliter as the target cell concentration. Fresh frozen rabbit serum, diluted 1:2 with phosphate-buffered saline, served as the complement source; 25 percent cell death was selected as the endpoint. Lymphocytes were treated with 0.83 percent NH_4Cl buffered with Tris-HCl, pH 7.2,[3] to remove the red cells. Complement-dependent cytotoxic assays were performed against peripheral lymphocytes of donor-recipient pairs in most combinations used in these experiments.

Cytotoxic inhibition. This was carried out in the same manner as the cytotoxic antibody test except that prior to the addition of the cells to the microtiter wells, they were incubated at room temperature for 15 minutes in the $F(ab')_2$ solution (conentration 10 to 15 mg. per milliliter). The percent inhibition was calculated by the formula:

$$100\left(1 - \frac{\text{no. of cells killed with } F(ab')_2 + \text{serum}}{\text{no. of cells killed with serum}}\right) = \%\ \text{inhibition}$$

Canine serotyping. The dogs were typed with eight sera available in our laboratory and previously described.[14] These were raised in litter mates; four sera obtained in our laboratory and four sera courtesy of Dr. E. D. Thomas, Seattle, Wash. At least four major antigenic determinants are thought to be identified by these eight sera.

RESULTS

Cytotoxicity and cytotoxic inhibition. Fig. 3 demonstrates the cytotoxicity of the polyspecific serum both alone and when $F(ab')_2$ was present with the serum in varying dilutions. The $F(ab')_2$ fragments were capable

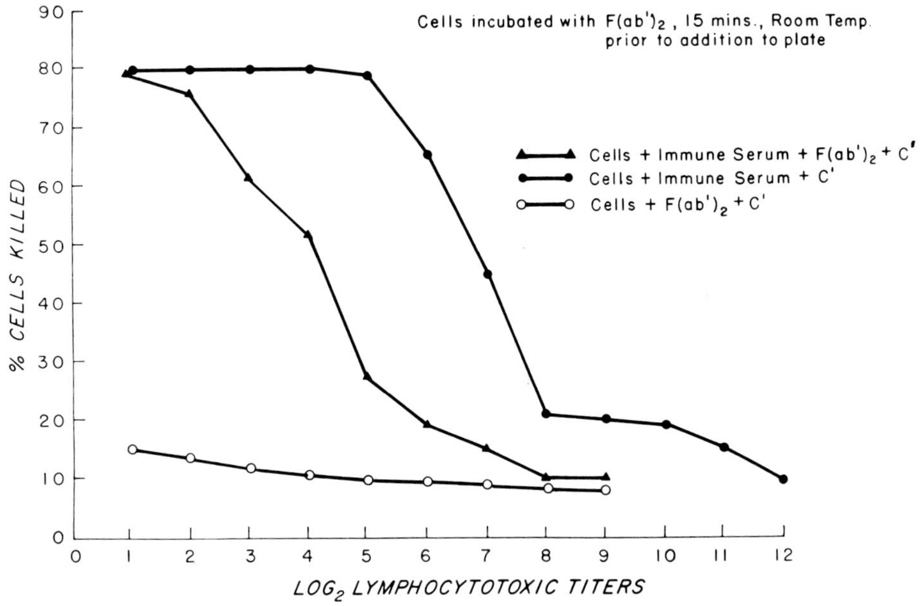

Fig. 3. Curves of percent cell death plotted against $\log_2$ dilution for $F(ab')_2$ alone, $F(ab')_2$ + whole serum, and serum alone.

Table II. *Treatment schedules and results in the experimental groups*

Group No.	No. of dogs	$F(ab')_2$, by perfusion (mg.)	$F(ab')_2$ intravenously (mg.)	Total $F(ab')_2$ (mg.)	IgG intravenously (mg.)	IgG total (mg.)	Suboptimal immunosuppression drugs*	Mean survival time (days ± S.D.)
I	10	—	—	—	—	—	+	9.3 ± 6.3
II	6	150	50 × 5 days	400	—	—	0	10.8 ± 1.2
III	8	150	50 × 5 days	400	—	—	+	29.3 ± 30†
IV	6	400	100 × 5 days + 50 × 20 days	1,900	—	—	0	11.3 ± 1.5
V	8	400	100 × 5 days + 50 × 20 days	1,900	—	—	+	32.0 ± 30‡
VI	5	—	—	—	100 × 6 days	600	0	11.4 ± 3.6
VII	8	—	—	—	100 × 6 days	600	+	14.1 ± 6.5
VIII	5	400	—	400	—	—	+	11.8 ± 2.49
IX	5	—	200 × 1 day + 50 × 4 days	400	—	—	+	14.2 ± 6.1

*Azathioprine, 2 mg. per kilogram per day. Methylprednisolone, 1 mg. per kilogram per day.
†p = 0.06.
‡p = 0.03.

of inhibiting the cytotoxicity of whole polyspecific serum at every dilution. The arbitrary endpoint of 25 percent cell death was shifted by three dilutions; from a serum dilution of $\log_2$ titer of 8 to a $\log_2$ titer of 5. The cytotoxicity of $F(ab')_2$ alone is represented by the lower curve in Fig. 3 and is by definition "0" since at no dilution was there greater than 25 percent cell death. No batch of $F(ab')_2$ with a measured cytotoxicity greater than $\log_2$ titer of 1 was utilized.

Survival. Table II shows the results of renal transplantation in the various treatment groups with their respective dosages and methods of administration for $F(ab')_2$, IgG, azathioprine, and prednisone. The mean survival times have been calculated for each group and probability levels are given when

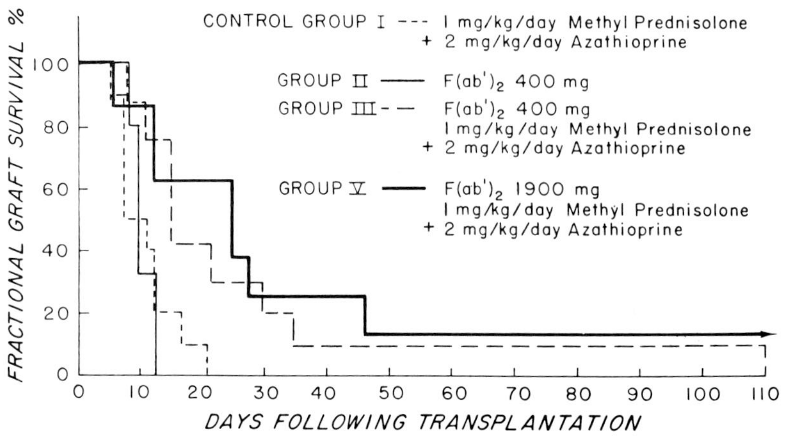

Fig. 4. Cumulative survival curves for Groups I, II, III, and V. Group V dogs showed the only significantly prolonged mean survival time.

they are at, or approach, significance. Group I dogs, treated with drugs alone, served as controls; mean survival time (MST) was 9.3 ± 6.3 days. Dogs in Groups II and IV were treated with $F(ab')_2$ in low doses (total 400 mg.) or high doses (total 1,900 mg.), respectively, by combined perfusion and intravenous therapy but without immunosuppression. Their survival was not prolonged. Groups III and V dogs received the same doses of $F(ab')_2$ administered in the same manner but combined with minimal immunosuppression. The MST in the low-dose $F(ab')_2$ Group III appears to be increased (29.3 ± 30 days) but not quite to significant levels ($p = 0.06$). The individual survival times for those dogs in Group III were 9, 14, 14, 15, 21, 29, 35, and 120 days. The MST in the high-dose $F(ab')_2$ group was significantly increased to 32.0 ± 30 days, with a significance level of $p = 0.03$. The individual survival times for the dogs in Group V were 9, 11, 13, 25, 25, 27, 46, and 250 days (still alive). Dogs in Group IX, receiving intravenous $F(ab')_2$ (400 mg.) over five days as well as minimal immunosuppression, represent an incomplete experimental group at the time of writing. Of five dogs, three showed no prolongation (5, 13, and 14 days), but two dogs are alive at 20 and 21 days, respectively, with BUN values at 17 and 48 mg. per 100 ml., and represent prolonged survivors. The remaining groups, given IgG intravenously either without (Group VI) or with (Group VII) immunosuppression, as well as those treated with 400 mg. of $F(ab')_2$ by perfusion alone (Group VIII), all failed to show any significant prolongation of survival.

In Fig. 4, the cumulative survival curves for Groups I, II, III, and V are plotted. In Group V, which has the only significant survival prolongation, 50 percent of the dogs survived for more than 20 days. The one long survivor in Group III had immunosuppressive therapy halved at 80 days and stopped at 100 days; the kidney rejected and death occurred at 120 days. The longest surviving dog in Group V, now at 250 days, had immunosuppression halved at day 120 but not stopped.

Cytotoxic inhibition studies. Fig. 5 shows the inhibitory effect of $F(ab')_2$ on the cytotoxicity of whole polyspecific serum, with specific donor lymphocytes as the target cells. These specific dogs were used as donors of renal allografts treated with this $F(ab')_2$. For each curve, a graft survival value is stated for the recipient. There are curves for eight dogs, five of which show more inhibition at the lower dilutions and a greater maximum inhibition at the higher dilution (> 80 percent), compared with the three remaining curves. Survival figures for the former five dogs show that four of five recipients survived 20 days or longer (11, 20, 21, 30, and 35

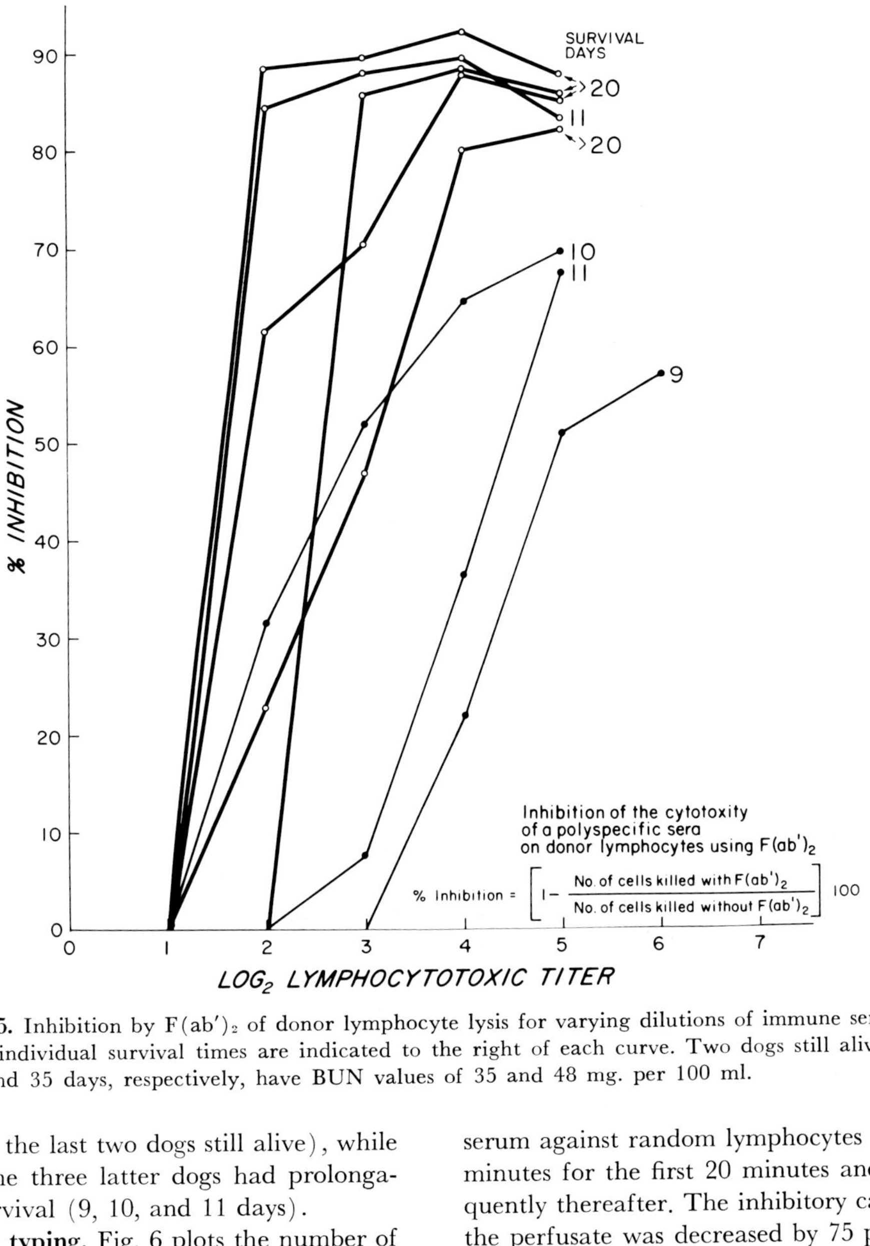

Fig. 5. Inhibition by $F(ab')_2$ of donor lymphocyte lysis for varying dilutions of immune serum. The individual survival times are indicated to the right of each curve. Two dogs still alive at 30 and 35 days, respectively, have BUN values of 35 and 48 mg. per 100 ml.

days, with the last two dogs still alive), while none of the three latter dogs had prolongation of survival (9, 10, and 11 days).

Antigen typing. Fig. 6 plots the number of antigen mismatches in any donor-recipient combination compared to the survival of that recipient in Groups III and V dogs; no correlation between these two factors can be seen. In fact, the only fully antigen-matched pair in the group did not have prolonged survival.

Removal of cytotoxic inhibition following perfusion through the kidney. During renal perfusion, an aliquot of the perfusate was tested for inhibition of cytotoxicity of whole serum against random lymphocytes every five minutes for the first 20 minutes and less frequently thereafter. The inhibitory capacity of the perfusate was decreased by 75 percent at 20 minutes and was totally absent after 30 minutes.

DISCUSSION

The survival data for the groups of dogs shown have demonstrated a number of points. The use of minimal or suboptimal immunosuppression is a necessary part of the treatment, at least at the $F(ab')_2$ dosage level used. This corroborates previous work[18] with active enhancement and also implies that

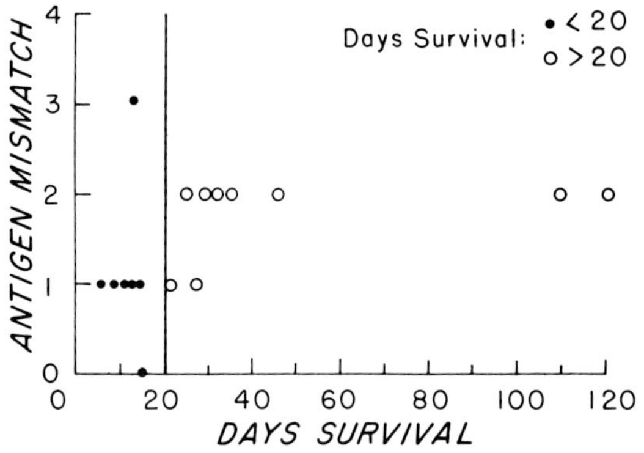

Fig. 6. No correlation exists between the number of antigen mismatches and recipient survival.

there is some synergism[11] between chemical immunosuppression and the polyspecific $F(ab')_2$. It is apparent from these data that $F(ab')_2$ fragments alone at either high or low dosages were completely ineffective in prolonging allograft survival. When immunosuppressive drugs were added, however, there was a dose-response effect for the $F(ab')_2$ fragments. It would seem that in this species and with this organ graft, it is necessary to minimally suppress the general host response. Indeed, additional studies in some of the recipients have shown that the cytotoxic antibody response to donor cells was reduced in the first two weeks, when drugs were used as part of the treatment.

Perfusion of the $F(ab')_2$ fragments through the kidney may be a necessary part of the treatment. Some of the dogs in the group with intravenous therapy alone appeared to show prolongation of survival, however, but this will probably not be significant for the group as a whole once the number is enlarged. The major feature of these data is the suggestion of synergism between renal perfusion and intravenous therapy, since the only prolongation of graft survival was observed after administration of $F(ab')_2$ both into the kidney and the host. These studies, in a sense, have been pilot projects using high and low doses of $F(ab')_2$ in various ways. The present indications of success point the way toward more investigation with intervening $F(ab')_2$ doses given intravenously either alone or in combination with perfusion and with variations in the immunosuppressive drug regimen.

The implications of a $F(ab')_2$ "blocking" assay for predicting allograft survival by determining the inhibition of cytotoxicity of whole immune serum against donor lymphocytes may be important, but the data are preliminary and too few to analyze fully. These studies are suggestive, however, of a number of points. (1) There would seem to be some correlation between the degree of inhibition and individual graft survival, the interpretation being that the greater the inhibition, the more complete the representation of alloantibody in the polyspecific $F(ab')_2$ for the alloantigens in the individual donors. This results in more efficient suppression of the immune response. (2) The range of antibody in the polyspecific $F(ab')_2$ must be as broad as possible in order that all alloantigens in the graft are covered. This has been shown in inbred strains.[7] (3) At least part of the action of the $F(ab')_2$ is peripheral in nature since this in vitro model presumably identifies the covering of antigenic sites. This point is supported by the fact that the allograft probably must be perfused to obtain adequate prolongation.

The appearance of a recipient with poor survival but good donor inhibition is not too surprising, and will probably recur as the group is expanded. Reasons for this might be that this model does not take into account inhibition of cell-mediated immunity, inhibition of the central arc of the immune response, and recipient histocompatibility differences. This latter point is in part negated by the findings shown in Fig. 6, where the number of antigen mismatches present in any donor-recipient combination does not play a major role in graft survival.

These experimental findings demonstrate that the $F(ab')_2$ fragments of a polyspecific antiserum can be an effective method of immunosuppression when combined with suboptimal doses of azathioprine and prednisolone. They leave unanswered, however, a number of questions, among which are: (1) the range of specificity required for an effective polyspecific serum, (2) how to measure whether a particular serum has an adequate range of specificity for a given donor, and (3) the correlation of this range of alloantibody specificity with significant allograft survival.

REFERENCES

1. Abouna, G. M., Garver, F. A., Kogure, H., DeLong, T. G., and Andres, G. A.: Survival of canine renal allografts after treatment with polyspecific $F(ab')_2$ fragments, Surg. Forum **24:** 318, 1973.
2. Ballantyne, D. L., Jr., and Stetson, C. A., Jr.: Serologic reactions to skin homografts of various sizes in the rat, Ann. N. Y. Acad. Sci. **120:** 7, 1964.
3. Boyle, W.: An extension of the ^{51}Cr-release assay for the estimation of mouse cytotoxins, Transplantation **6:** 761, 1968.
4. French, M. E., and Batchelor, J. R.: Immunological enhancement of rat kidney grafts, Lancet **2:** 1103, 1969.
5. Halasz, N. A., Miller, S. H., and Romoro, J. L.: Tolerance, enhancement and prolonged survival of organ transplants, Ann. Surg. **176:** 538, 1972.
6. Herrmann, T. J., and Turcotte, J. G.: Preservation of canine kidneys by hypothermia and low flow perfusion with bloodless perfusate, Arch. Surg. **98:** 121, 1969.
7. Jeekel, J. J., McKenzie, I. F. C., and Winn, H. J.: Immunological enhancement of skin grafts in the mouse, J. Immunol. **108:** 1017, 1972.
8. Kim, J. P., Shaipanich, T., Sells, R. A., Maggs, P., Lukl, P., and Wilson, R. E.: Transplantation **13:** 322, 1972.
9. Myburgh, J. A., and Smith, J. A.: Passive and active enhancement in baboon liver allografting, Transplantation **14:** 227, 1972.
10. Ockner, S. A., Guttmann, R. D., and Lindquist, R. R.: Renal transplantation in the inbred rat. XIV. Mechanism of the modified rejection produced by bone marrow cell pretreatment, Transplantation **9:** 39, 1970.
11. Rivard, J. Y., Beaudoin, J. G., and Guttmann, R. D.: Prolonged survival of canine renal allografts by pretreatment with viable lymphoid cells, Transplantation **16:** 88, 1973.
12. Shaipanich, T. D., Vanwijck, R. R., Kim, J. P., Lukl, P., Busch, G. J., and Wilson, R. E.: Enhancement of rat renal allografts with $F(ab')_2$ fragment of donor-specific antikidney serum, SURGERY **70:** 113, 1971.
13. Shaipanich, T., Wren, S., Von Haefen, U., Koppenheffer, T., Busch, G., and Wilson, R. E.: Evaluation of organ specificity in renal allograft enhancement with $F(ab')_2$ fragments, Transplant. Proc. **5:** 581, 1973.
14. Simonian, S. J., and Murray, J. E.: Further analysis of the mechanism of prolonged survival of canine renal allografts, Transplant. Proc. **3:** 470, 1971.
15. Stephens, F. O., Cochnun, K. C., Scott, D. F., Price, D. C., and Belzer, F. O.: Attempted renal allograft enhancement by pooled kidney antigen pretreatment, Ann. Surg. **175:** 41, 1972.
16. Stuart, F. P., Saitoh, T., Fitch, F. W., and Spargo, B. H.: Immunologic enhancement of renal allografts in the rat, SURGERY **64:** 17, 1968.
17. Von Haefen, U., Wren, S. F. G., Shaipanich, T., Martins, A. C. P., Busch, G. J., and Wilson, R. E.: Active enhancement of rat renal allografts with papain-released specific antigens, Transplantation **16:** 295, 1973.
18. Wilson, R. E., Rippin, A., Dagher, R. K., Kinneart, P., and Busch, G. J.: Prolonged canine renal allograft survival after pretreatment with solubilized antigen, Transplantation **7:** 360, 1969.
19. Yonemoto, R. H., Deliman, R. M., DuSold, W. D., and Hamilton, T.: Inhibition of renal allograft rejection: Instances in dogs with specific enhancing immunoglobulin and its proteolytic fragments, Arch. Surg. **107:** 390, 1973.

DISCUSSION

Dr. John S. Najarian (Minneapolis, Minn.). The fact that we could get polyspecific antisera of this sort—that is, a $F(ab')_2$ fragment—I think has great clinical potential. Have you had an opportunity to check where this path is with the specific antisera by fluorescence or the like, to see if it is, in fact, coating the kidney? Is it working on the efferent arc as an overcoat over the antigens and protecting them against the cytotoxicity of the particular recipient? If it is working that way, and there is some suggestion that it may be, considering that when you deal with intravenous administration it works less well, or not at all (you had to perfuse it, and then go intravenously) we have to assume that it is working on the efferent side.

Did you work with any sensitized animals? If this were to be used as a practical technique, it would seem that the most likely possibility would be in the sensitized individual, where you are trying to avoid an immediate reaction or an acute reaction. If you expect it to work as an immunosuppressant for a time, I would guess, if the $F(ab')_2$ itself was really coated to the kidney, or to the endothelium of the kidney, that it would come off rather rapidly with time, and the kidney would then become exposed to the immunological assault at a later date. Do you know where it is? And if you do know where it is, have you tried it in sensitized animals?

Dr. Andrew M. Munster (Charleston, S. C.). We have been working on the enhancement with the $F(ab')_2$ fragments of skin allografts in the burned rat as a method of skin transplantation. Dr. Najarian alluded to the labeling of the target organ, and we have failed to do this with immunofluorescent label. However, when we tried I^{125} labeling, the skin lit up beautifully. This is a much more sensitive technique; and until now there has been some question as to whether skin can be labeled; it cannot be reliably labeled with immunofluorescence, but it can be labeled with iodine. We had also shown that the humoral antibody response to bacterial challenge in the enhanced rat remains normal, and I wonder, in the context of added immunosuppression, whether with other agents this would still hold true.

I was confused about whether your $F(ab')_2$ was cytotoxic or not. I seem to remember there was a contradiction in one of the slides, whether the $F(ab')_2$ by itself was cytotoxic or not.

Dr. Frank P. Stuart (Chicago, Ill.). We have found that the polyspecific $F(ab')_2$ in rabbit kidney transplants is about as effective as what Dr. Wilson and his group have shown with the dog. We would agree, I think, with Dr. Najarian's comments that $F(ab')_2$ probably acts peripherally. We think that if intact gamma G is infused intravenously after a loading dose, or protecting dose, of the $F(ab')_2$ fragments, we may be seeing a central suppressive mechanism. At least, the over-all survival is improved, and it may be that it's necessary to have the FC piece to do whatever has to be done in the central site.

Dr. Israel Penn (Denver, Colo.). At what temperature is the perfusion performed? This may be an important matter considering at what temperature the $F(ab')_2$ fragments will bind with kidney tissue.

If I remember correctly, in similar studies that you presented several years ago, you found that the $F(ab')_2$ bound to endothelium in an irregular fashion. If you got a binding in an irregular fashion, why should it protect the kidney at all?

Dr. S. F. G. Wren (closing). We have not, in fact, done any studies in the dog, but in the rat kidney model, where all of this started, we did do some. We investigated radioactive uptake of the $F(ab')_2$ in an inbred rat strain and found that there was a small but specific uptake of $F(ab')_2$ in the kidney. We aslo did immunofluorescent studies, and showed a small and spotty uptake in the kidney.

In answer to the question whether we have used this in the sensitized animal, yes, we have, and we're doing it right now. Dr. Mutashabal started this work, and Dr. Antonio Martins has continued it. I can tell you that in a monospecific donor-recipient $F(ab')_2$ situation, in which the recipient is sensitized to the donor, and the recipient makes his own $F(ab')_2$—in these situations and when heavy doses of standard drug therapy are given, you can get survival in the monkey model to 25 days. I think this is a pretty remarkable survival, with normal renal function out to about two weeks. With the original control it was about five minutes. There was absolutely no evidence of hyperacute rejection at all.

We measured the cytotoxic antibody response of the recipient to donor lymphocytes and did not find too much. The only thing we did find was that when you place the animal on suboptimal doses of immunosuppression, the humoral antibody response is reduced in the first two weeks.

We have made many, many batches of $F(ab')_2$. The curve I showed you was for a batch of $F(ab')_2$ in which there was no cytotoxicity. We generally do not like to let the $F(ab')_2$ have a cytotoxicity of greater than the first well. If we find this, we do not use it.

The FC fragment is important to the molecule. I think this has been shown in in vitro studies; particularly, Sinclair and Chan have shown it; it would be nice to use the whole antibody, because the binding of the whole antibody would unquestionably be better than the $F(ab')_2$ fragment. But as you can see, the whole antibody —anyway, in this model, and at this dosage level— is not effective.

We spent a long time on the perfusate characteristics in autograft models. We used a dextran containing perfusate, particularly, because we did not want any homologous or heterologous protein around to perhaps interfere with uptake of the $F(ab')_2$ fragment. We used a room temperature of 19 to 20° C., because we thought this would be a more physiological temperature at which $F(ab')_2$ would be taken up. We have no further information about that. We used physiological pH's, and I think this is most important too, that during the one-hour perfusion you should make sure that the pH stays between 7.3 and 7.5. Otherwise, you do not get a good functioning kidney—in our system, anyway.

Renal allograft prolongation using phytomitogens to mask graft antigens

Luis H. Toledo-Pereyra, M.D., Prasanta K. Ray, Ph.D.,* Clive O. Callender, M.D., John S. Najarian, M.D.,** *and* **Richard L. Simmons, M.D.,** *Minneapolis, Minn.*

Mongrel dog kidneys were allografted to unrelated nephrectomized recipients which were then treated with subimmunosuppressive doses of azathioprine (2.5 mg. per kilogram per day). Dog kidneys treated in vitro with perfusates containing concanavalin A (ConA) or phytohemagglutinin-P (PHA) survived as long as 60 days (mean 39.8 ± 4.3) after transplanation, whereas normal kidneys survived less than 16 days. The optimal prolongation was achieved by perfusing the kidneys with 500 ml. of Ringer's lactate containing 25 mg. per liter ConA, at 4° C. Lesser effects were achieved with higher or lower concentrations of ConA, or with perfusions carried out at 25° C. Most evidence suggests that ConA and PHA bind to cell surfaces and interfere with the perception of the graft antigens by the host.

From the Department of Surgery, University of Minnesota, Minneapolis, Minn.

PROLONGATION OF ORGAN allografts has generally required the use of systemic immunosuppressive agents in order to modify host reactivity to the histocompatibility antigens on the graft. Introduction of the graft antigens at time of maximal immunologic unresponsiveness may lead to a state of partial immunologic tolerance to graft antigen. The opposite approach, that of altering the grafted tissue so that the histocompatibility antigens of the tissue are masked, and thus not recognized by the host, has received comparatively little attention.[4, 5, 8, 9, 10, 14, 22, 23, 24, 25, 38] We have previously demonstrated that the plant lectins concanavalin A (ConA) and phytohemagglutinin-M (PHA) mask strong histocompatibility antigens on mouse lymphoid cells when these agents are bound to the cell surfaces.[40] The maximum obliteration of the antigen was seen at concentrations of ConA greater than 25 μg per milliliter and of PHA greater than 500 μg per milliliter. Similarly we have shown that perfusing kidney grafts with antilymphocyte globulin (ALG) led to prolongation of such kidneys in mildly immunosuppressed dogs.[8, 9] These results suggest that antigen modification might supplement modest levels of immunosuppression in the prolongation of renal allografts. The present study was designed to determine if ConA or PHA would mask the histocompatibility antigens on kidney grafts and allow for their prolongation in moderately immunosuppressed dogs.

This study was supported in part by United States Public Health Service grants No. AM 13083 and No. CA 11605 and grant No. DRG 1186 from the Damon Runyon Memorial Fund for Cancer Research.

Reprint requests: Richard L. Simmons, M.D., Box 185, Mayo Memorial Building, University of Minnesota, Minneapolis, Minn. 55455.

Presented at the Thirty-fifth Annual Meeting of the Society of University Surgeons, St. Louis, Mo., Feb. 14-16, 1974.

*Current address: Bhabha Atomic Research Center, Trombay/Bombay, India.

**Current address: Transplant Service, Howard University, Washington, D. C.

Table I. *Effect of renal allograft pretreatment on rejection and survival of recipient dogs*

Group	*Graft treatment*	*Recipient treatment*	*Mean onset of rejection (days ± SE)*	*p values*	*Mean survival (days ± SE)*	*p values*
I	Ringer's	None	6.8 ± 0.5	—	11.0 ± 0.7	—
II	Ringer's	Azathioprine†	8.5 ± 0.7	*	12.5 ± 0.7	*
III	ConA (25 mg./L.) in Ringer's	None	8.5 ± 0.9	> 0.5	12.8 ± 0.8	> 0.5
IV	ConA (12.5 mg./L.) in Ringer's	Azathioprine†	19.8 ± 4.8	< 0.05	26.6 ± 5.7	< 0.05
V	ConA (25 mg./L.) in Ringer's	Azathioprine†	34.3 ± 5.6	< 0.001	39.8 ± 4.3	< 0.001
VI	ConA (50 mg./L.) in Ringer's	Azathioprine†	22.2 ± 2.5	< 0.001	27.7 ± 2.8	< 0.001
VII	ConA (25 mg./L.) followed by Ringer's flush	Azathioprine†	10.1 ± 1.0	> 0.1	15.1 ± 1.5	> 0.1
VIII	ConA (25 mg./L. 25° C.) in Ringer's	Azathioprine†	9.7 ± 1.0	> 0.2	19.6 ± 2.2	> 0.05
IX	Ringer's	ConA (2.5 mg.) into renal artery + azathioprine†	7.8 ± 1.2	> 0.5	11.5 ± 1.3	> 0.2
X	ConA (5 mg./L.) in Ringer's	ConA (5 mg.) IV: no azathioprine	8.3 ± 1.0	> 0.5	14.1 ± 1.2	> 0.2
XI	PHA (10 mg./L.) in plasma	Azathioprine†	8.2 ± 1.0	> 0.8	13.1 ± 0.9	> 0.5
XII	PHA (20 mg./L.) in plasma	Azathioprine†	7.1 ± 0.8	> 0.1	12.0 ± 0.8	> 0.2
XIII	PHA (160 mg./L.) in Ringer's	Azathioprine†	17.9 ± 6.5	> 0.2	25.6 ± 5.9	< 0.05

*All p values compared to azathioprine control group (II).

†Azathioprine (5.0 mg. per kilogram per day for 3 days, then 2.5 mg. per kilogram until death.

MATERIALS AND METHODS

One hundred and four dogs, weighing 16 to 23 kilograms, received unrelated kidneys by standard operative techniques. After opening the vascular clamps, 20 mg. of furosemide was given intravenously. Immediate bilateral nephrectomy was then performed. Serum creatinines were recorded daily. The onset of rejection was defined as the day on which the creatinine was elevated 2.0 mg. percent above normal. Postmortem examinations with kidney histology were performed in all cases.

The dogs were randomly divided into 13 groups of eight dogs each (Table I). Most recipient dogs were given azathioprine, 5.0 mg. per kilogram per day for 3 days, then 2.5 mg. per kilogram until death. Three groups of dogs (Groups I, III, X) were not given azathioprine. Immediately after nephrectomy, the kidneys of most groups (Table I) were flushed with Ringer's lactate solution (500 ml., 4° C., procaine 1 Gm. per liter, heparin 10,000 U. per liter) containing various concentrations of plant lectins* in solution. The kidneys of Groups I, II, and IX were flushed with the regular perfusate without lectins. The kidneys in Group VII were perfused with 500 ml. of Ringer's containing ConA (25 mg. per liter), and then perfused a second time with Ringer's without ConA. The kidneys of Group VIII were flushed at 25° C. ConA (2.5 mg.) was infused intra-arterially into the renal arteries immediately after transplantation of the kidneys in Group IX. Animals in Group X were given 25 mg. per liter ConA in the perfusate but 5 mg. was given intravenously after grafting. Groups

*Concanavalin A, Calbiochem, San Diego, Calif., and phytohemagglutinin-P, Difco Laboratories, Detroit, Mich.

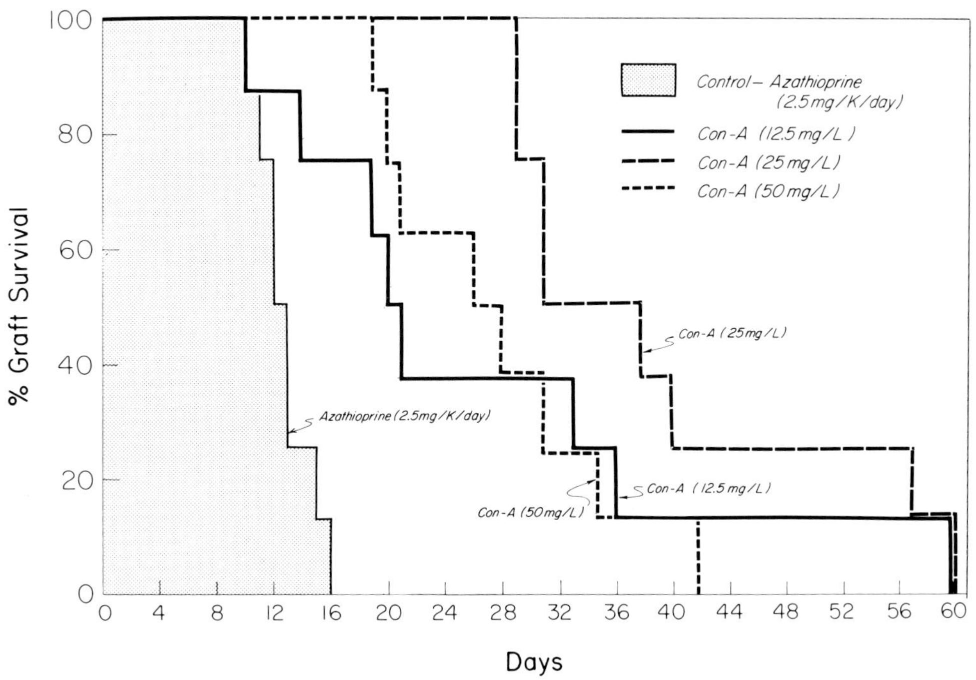

Fig. 1. Cumulative survival of dogs receiving renal allografts perfused in vitro with ConA in Ringer's lactate. The data here include experimental Groups II, IV, V, and VI.

XI and XII received kidneys that were given PHA during hypothermic pulsatile perfusion (7° C., pH 7.4, Po_2 200 mm. Hg, pulse rate 60 per minute systolic pressure 60 mm. Hg) with pooled dog cryoprecipitated plasma for 24 hours and one hour, respectively. Animals in Group XIII were given PHA (160 mg. per liter) in the regular perfusate.

Ten additional dogs, with obvious technical problems such as anesthesia complications, postoperative hemorrhage, or ureteral leakage, and those that died in the first five days after transplantation from other nonrelated causes, such as distemper and intussusception, were immediately excluded from analysis.

RESULTS

The rejection time and survival of the recipients of all renal allografts are summarized in Table I and Figs. 1 and 2. Dogs given normal kidneys rejected them in less than two weeks even if azathioprine (2.5 mg. per kilogram per day) was given.

Concanavalin A (ConA) treated kidneys. Kidneys perfused with ConA in concentrations greater than 12.5 mg. per liter survived for more prolonged periods in dogs given azathioprine (Groups IV, V, VI) but not in dogs which were not given azathioprine (Group III). The optimal concentration of ConA was 25 mg. per liter (Group V), higher or lower concentrations having less effect (Groups IV, VI). If the kidneys were perfused with 500 ml. of Ringer's lactate after optimal ConA perfusion (Group VII) little prolongation was seen. Similarly, optimal concentrations of ConA have less effect if the perfusion was carried out at 25° C. (Group VIII) rather than 4° C. (Group V).

Two control groups were designed to test if the systemic effect of ConA remaining unbound in the kidney was responsible for the prolongation. Systemic ConA (5 mg. intravenously) in dogs which had not received azathioprine, or 2.5 mg. into the renal artery of dogs given azathioprine had no perceptible immunosuppressive effect (Groups IX, X).

Phytohemagglutinin-P (PHA) treated kidneys. PHA in a concentration of 160 mg.

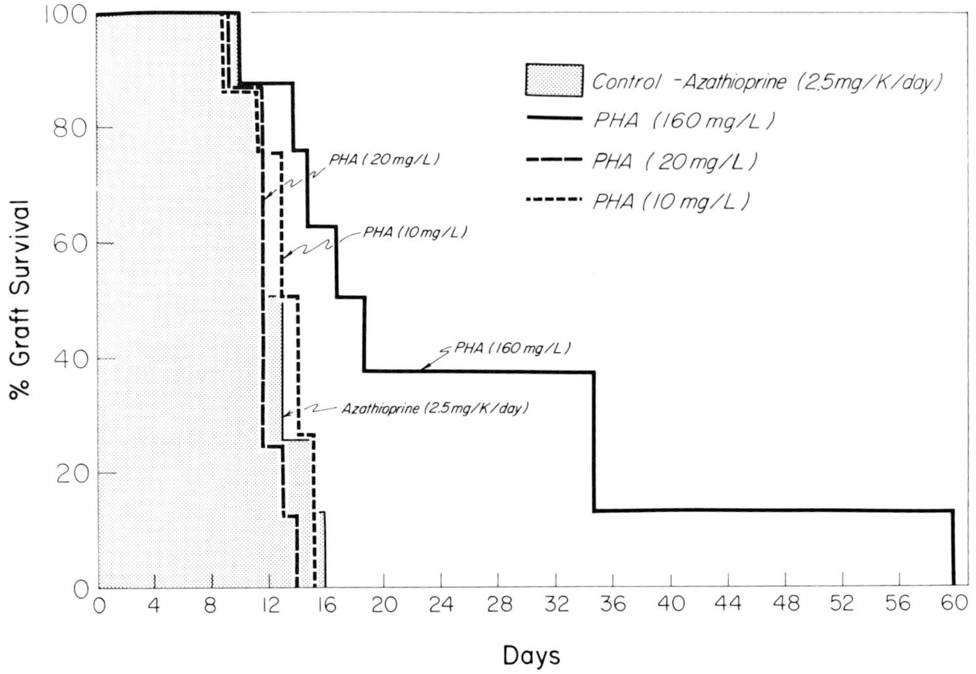

Fig. 2. Cumulative survival of dogs receiving renal allografts perfused in vitro with PHA in Ringer's lactate. The data here include experimental Groups II, XI, XII, and XIII.

per liter in Ringer's lactate (Group XIII) had a similar effect as ConA. Lesser amounts of PHA in cryoprecipitated plasma perfusate had no effect on graft prolongation (Group XI, XII).

DISCUSSION

The present experiments demonstrate that perfusion of dog kidneys at 4° C. with varying concentrations of concanavalin A (ConA) or phytohemagglutinin-P (PHA) will allow moderately immunosuppressed dogs to maintain these grafts for significant periods of time. Ultimate rejection always occurred but occasional survival as long as 60 days was seen. The doses of azathioprine utilized were not sufficient to produce prolonged survival of kidney grafts by themselves. Similarly, perfusion of kidneys with the optimal concentration of ConA had no effect on dogs that did not receive some systemic immunosuppression. The synergistic effect of minimal immunosuppression and alteration of graft has previously been reported.[8, 9] We showed that the in vitro perfusion of kidney allografts with goat antidog lymphocyte globulin would lead to prolonged survival of dog kidneys, only if the dogs also received subimmunosuppressive doses of azathioprine.[8, 9] Neither immunosuppression alone nor treatment of the kidneys with ALG alone achieved graft prolongation. It is likely that all experiments designed to investigate reductions in graft immunogenicity may require the use of some host immunosuppression, since total ablation of graft immunogenicity may be impossible to achieve. This finding may help to explain the failure to obtain satisfactory results with previous attempts to reduce graft immunogenicity.[1, 10, 14, 18, 19, 26, 43]

ConA and PHA were chosen for these experiments because of their ability to bind firmly to tissues. ConA reacts with neutral polysaccharides.[17] It can bind specifically to the C^3, C^4, and C^6 hydroxyl positions on terminal glucopyranose or mannopyranose residues of highly branched polysaccharides.[16] ConA also reacts with mucopolysaccharides,[12] galactan sulfate,[27] glycoproteins,[16] and bacterial lipopolysaccharides.[16] For PHA very little information is available in this regard. PHA has been found to bind with nuclei,[29, 30] cytoplasm,[13] or cell surface.[47] N-acetyl galactosamine has been suggested to be the constituent of the PHA-combining sites on the cell.[6] Other sugars, such as D-glucose, N-acetyl glucosamine, D-galactose, and D-mannose, cannot react with PHA, and D-L-fucose has little tendency to do so.[6]

Thus, both ConA and PHA interact with chemical groupings on the cell surface.[30, 47] We have previously shown that both ConA and PHA bound to mouse lymphoid cells will prevent the lysis of these cells by antibody and complement.[40] In addition, ConA and PHA on the surface of mouse lymphocytes will interfere with the binding of anti-H-2 specific antibody to those cells as measured by antibody absorption experiments.[40] Thus by analogy, one could expect that ConA and PHA act to mask the immunogenicity of graft antigents by the same mechanism, i.e., by binding to the cell surfaces and interfering with the perception of the antigens on the graft by immune lymphocytes or by antibodies.[21, 39] It is possible, of course, that ConA acts by damaging passenger leukocytes so that the immunogenicity in passenger leukocytes is destroyed,[3, 46, 48] but other methods of reducing passenger leukocytes have not always been as effective.[15]

It is not clear from these experiments or our previous ones[40] whether these lectins bind to (1) chemical groupings responsible for strong histocompatibility antigens, (2) chemical groupings which are not related to histocompatibility antigenicity but disarrange the cell surface so that the histocompatibility antigenic groupings are distorted, or (3) nonantigenic groupings leading to stearic interference with the interaction of antigen and receptors for these antigens on immunoreactive cells. Neither do we know if agglutinin-binding on cell surfaces might induce the cooperative phenomena in cell membranes initiating either trans (allosteric) or cis effect on the membrane as proposed by Singer and Nicolson[44] in their fluid mosaic model of the structure of cell membranes. Either of these effects might result in a conformational rearrangement of the membrane structure, and thereby change the functional property of the histocompatibility antigens. There is evidence to suggest that subsequent to binding on the cell surface, lectins may, in fact, be internalized by pinocytosis.[37, 41] Then a major conformational change might be expected during pinocytosis following the dynamic fluid character of the cell membrane components.[44]

It is clear that these lectins[2, 7, 12, 20, 27, 31, 32, 34, 45] bind with carbohydrate molecules. Although Reisfeld and Kahan[42] have reported that most of the antigenic determinants of human alloantigens are polypeptide in nature, they admit that it is impossible to rule out that either lipid or carbohydrate moieties express a specific alloantigenic specificity or that they confer a unique protein configuration that determines such a specificity. It appears from the present study that the carbohydrate receptors for ConA and PHA are in some way related or linked to histocompatibility antigens which are recognized by specific alloantibody on the cell surface.

Several aspects of this experiment may ultimately shed light on the mechanism of antigen masking by plant lectins. Apparently, washing out the ConA with normal Ringer's lactate removes it, so that the ConA must be bound weakly to cell surfaces. This effect does not seem to be due to the ConA itself acting as an immunosuppressant[28] in the recipient dog, since ConA given intra-arterially into the renal artery, or intravenously in amounts that might be found in the kidney after perfusion do not seem to prolong graft survival. In support of this hypothesis is the fact that ConA at 50 mg. per liter is less effective than 25 mg. per liter. If the ConA remaining unbound within the kidney acted synergistically with azathioprine as a systemic immunosuppressive one would expect that the higher concentration of ConA would be more effective than the lesser one. Nevertheless, the failure of ConA to remain bound to the kidney and achieve its masking effect after washing out with Ringer's lactate is puzzling.

One possible mechanism is suggested by consideration of the behavior of polyvalent lectins like ConA and PHA on cell surfaces. When lectins bind to cell surfaces at room temperature, the lectins are found in clusters on the cell membrane.[35] When lectins bind at 4° C., they are more evenly distributed; when the cells are warmed, clustering takes place presumably due to the fluid nature of the cell membrane.[35] One can hypothesize that clustered ConA on kidney cell surfaces will not mask antigens since perfusion of kidneys with ConA at 25° C. will not prolong their survival. The ConA apparently needs to be evenly distributed on cell surfaces to mask antigens. Failure to observe clustering on cell surfaces in the cold may reflect not only the "frozen" status of the cell membrane at 4° C., but also a relatively lower binding affirmity of ConA to cell surfaces in the cold so that multiple membrane receptor sites are not pulled together and ConA is easy to wash off.

Why, then, does transplantation into a warm recipient not interfere with antigen masking? ConA is a polyvalent material which can bind to many types of glucoproteins including those in blood.[11, 33, 36] We can speculate that rapid warming in the presence of host blood succeeds in binding protein to the evenly distributed ConA on the graft cell surfaces. Such binding may not only insure even distribution of the ConA on the surface but may also further mask the antigens by ConA-protein complexes. These speculations are currently under investigation.

REFERENCES

1. Abbott, W. M., and Pappas, A. M.: Comparative studies on fresh and preserved skin: Fundamental biological differences in behavior as grafts, Ann. Surg. **172:** 781, 1970.
2. Aub, J. C., Sanford, B. H., and Cote, M. N.: Studies on reactivity of tumor and normal cells to a wheat germ agglutinin, Proc. Natl. Acad. Sci. **54:** 396, 1965.
3. Billingham, R. E.: The passenger cell concept in transplantation immunity, Cell. Immunol. **2:** 1, 1971.
4. Billingham, R. E., Krohn, P. L., and Medawar, P. B.: Effect of locally applied cortisone acetate on survival of skin homografts in rabbits, Br. Med. J. **2:** 1049, 1951.
5. Bonmassar, E., Francisconi, G., and Manzoni, S. C.: Chemical deletion of histocompatibility antigens—Homograft survival of rat skin treated with urethan in vitro, Nature **209:** 1141, 1966.
6. Borberg, H., Woodruff, J., Hirschhorn, R., Gesner, B., Miescher, P., and Silber, R.: Phytohemagglutinin: Inhibition of the agglutinating activity by N-acetyl-D-galactosamine, Science **154:** 1019, 1966.
7. Burger, M. M., and Goldberg, A. R.: Identification of a tumor-specific determinant on neoplastic cell surfaces, Proc. Natl. Acad. Sci. **57:** 359, 1967.
8. Callender, C. O., Simmons, R. L., Toledo-Pereyra, L. H., Santiago-Delpin, E. A., and Najarian, J. S.: Prolongation of kidney allografts perfused by ALG in vitro, Transplantation **16:** 377, 1973.
9. Callender, C. O., Santiago, E. A., Sutherland, D., Howard, R. J., Toledo-Pereyra, L. H., Olsen, L., Condie, R., Simmons, R. L., and Najarian, J. S.: Renal allograft prolongation after graft perfusion with heterologous ALG, Surg. Forum **XXIV:** 306, 1973.
10. Callender, C. O., Sutherland, D. E. R., Howard, R. J., Toledo-Pereyra, L. H., and Najarian, J. S.: Failure of pepsin-digested donor-specific alloantibody to prolong renal allograft survival in dogs, Immunol. Comm. Submitted for publication.
11. Chase, P. S.: The effect of human serum fractions on phytohemagglutin- and concanavalin A-stimulated human lymphocyte cultures, Cell. Immunol. **5:** 544, 1972.
12. Cifonelli, J. A., Montgomery, R., and Smith, F.: The reaction of concanavalinA with mucopolysaccharides, J. Am. Chem. Soc. **78:** 2488, 1956.
13. Conrad, R. A.: Autoradiography of leukocytes cultured with tritiated bean extract, Nature **214:** 709, 1967.
14. Dukes, C. D., and Blocker, T. G.: Studies on the survival of skin homografts. I. Prolongation of life of full-thickness grafts by the action of streptokinase-streptodornase, Ann. Surg. **136:** 999, 1952.
15. Freeman, J. S., Chamberlain, E. C., Reemtsma, K., and Steinmuller, D.: Prolongation of rat heart allografts by donor pretreatment with immunosuppressive agents, Transplant Proc. **3:** 580, 1971.
16. Goldstein, I. J., and Iyer, R. N.: Interaction of concanavalin A, a phytohemagglutinin with model substrates, Biochim. Biophys. Acta **121:** 197, 1966.
17. Goldstein, I. J., Hollerman, C. E., and Smith, E. E.: Protein-carbohydrate interaction. II. Inhibition studies on the interaction of con-

canavalin A with polysaccharides, Biochemistry **4:** 876, 1965.
18. Grillo, H. C., and McKhann, C. F.: The acceptance and evolution of dermal homografts freed of viable cells, Transplantation **2:** 48, 1964.
19. Hellmann, K., and Duke, D. I.: In vitro alteration of skin graft antigenicity, Transplantation **5:** 184, 1967.
20. Inbar, M., and Sachs, L.: Interaction of the carbohydrate-binding protein concanavalin A with normal and transformed cells, Proc. Natl. Acad. Sci. **63:** 1418, 1969.
21. Jannosy, G., and Greaves, M. F.: Lymphocyte activation. I. Response of T and B lymphocytes to phytomitogens, Clin. Exp. Immunol. **9:** 483, 1971.
22. Jolley, W. B., Hinshaw, D. B., and Peterson, M.: The effect of RNA on homograft survival, Surg. Forum **12:** 99, 1961.
23. Klaue, P., and Jolley, W. B.: Prolongation of rabbit skin allograft survival following treatment of the skin with electrophoresis prior to transplantation, Transplantation **11:** 30, 1971.
24. Klaue, P., and Jolley, W. B.: The comparative effectiveness of corticosteroids applied topically as pretreatment of rabbit skin allografts, Surgery **70:** 718, 1971.
25. Klaue, P., and Jolley, W. B.: Prolonged survival of rabbit skin allografts after treatment with locally applied triamcinolone acetonide in combination with small doses of systemic immunosuppressives, Transplantation **13:** 53, 1972.
26. Lemperle, G.: Prolonged survival of skin allografts after incubation with recipient DNA or RNA, J. Surg. Res. **8:** 511, 1968.
27. Manners, D. J., and Wright, A. J.: Alpha-1, 4-glucosans. Part XIV: The interaction of concanavalin A with glycogen, J. Chem. Soc. (London) 4592, 1962.
28. Markowitz, H., Person, D. A., Gitnick, G., and Ritts, R. E., Jr.: Immunosuppressive activity of concanavalin A, Science **163:** 476, 1969.
29. Michalowski, A., Jasinska, J., Brzosko, W. J., and Nowaslawski, A.: Cellular localization of the mitogenic principle of phytothemagglutinin in leucocyte cultures, Exp. Cell Res. **34:** 417, 1964.
30. Michalowski, A., Jasinska, J., Brzosko, W. J., and Nowoslawski, A.: Studies on phytohemagglutinin. II. Cellular localization of phytohemagglutinin in white blood cell cultures with immunohistochemical methods, Exp. Med. Microbiol. **17:** 197, 1965.
31. Moscona, A. A.: Embryonic and neoplastic cell surfaces: Availability of receptor for concanavalin A and wheat germ agglutinin, Science **171:** 905, 1971.
32. Nakamura, S., and Suzuno, R.: Crystallization of concanavalins A and B and canavalin from Japanese jack beans, Arch. Biochem. Biophys. **111:** 499, 1965.
33. Nakamura, S., Tanaka, K., and Murakawa, S.: Specific protein of legumes which reacts with animal proteins, Nature **188:** 144, 1960.
34. Naspitz, C. K., and Richter, M.: The action of phytohemagglutinin in vivo and in vitro, a review, Progr. Allergy **12:** 1, 1968.
35. Nicolson, G. L.: Temperature-dependent mobility of concanavalin A sites on tumour cell surface, Nature (New Biol.) **243:** 218, 1973.
36. Novogrodosky, A., Biniaminov, M., Ramot, B., and Katchalski, E.: Binding of concanavalin A to rat, normal human, and chronic lymphatic leukemia lymphocytes, Blood **40:** 311, 1972.
37. Pauli, R. M., DeSalle, L., Higgins, P., Henderson, E., Norin, A., and Strauss, B.: Proliferation of stimulated human peripheral blood lymphocytes: Preferential incorporation of concanavalin A by stimulated cells and mitogenic activity, J. Immunol. **111:** 424, 1973.
38. Raju, M. D., Grogan, J. B., and Hardy, J. D.: Prolonged survival of skin allografts exposed to heterologous antilymphocyte serum in vitro, J. Surg. Res. **9:** 327, 1969.
39. Ray, P. K., Jeitz, L., Sarquis, L., and Simmons, R. L.: Mechanisms of increased immunogenicity of cells treated with concanavalin, Fed. Proc. **31:** 234, 1972.
40. Ray, P. K., and Simmons, R. L.: Masking of cellular histocompatibility antigens with phytomitogens, J. Immunol. **110:** 1693, 1973.
41. Razavi, L.: Cytoplasmic localization of phytohemagglutinin in peripheral white cells, Nature **210:** 444, 1966.
42. Reisfeld, R. A., and Kahan, B. D.: Transplantation antigens, Adv. Immunol. **12:** 117, 1970.
43. Silverstein, P., Raulston, G. L., Walker, H., Foley, F. D., and Pruitt, B. A.: Evaluation of formalin-fixed skin as a temporary dressing for granulating wounds, Surg. Forum **22:** 60, 1971.
44. Singer, S. J. and Nicolson, G. L.: The fluid mosaic model of the structure of cell membranes, Science **175:** 720, 1972.
45. Steck, T. L., and Wallach, D. F. H.: The binding of kidney-bean phytohemagglutinin by Ehrlich ascites carcinoma, Biochim. Biophys. Acta **97:** 510, 1965.
46. Steinmuller, D., and Hart, E. A.: Passenger leukocytes and induction of allograft immunity, Transplant. Proc. **3:** 673, 1971.
47. Vassar, P. S., and Culling, C. F. A.: Cell surface effects of phytohemagglutinin, Nature **202:** 610, 1964.
48. Warden, G., Reemtsma, K., and Steinmuller,

D.: Survival of rat heart allografts irradiated in vitro, Surg. Forum XXII: 252, 1917.

DISCUSSION

Dr. Charles F. Zukoski (Tucson, Ariz.). I know that lymphocytes will cap when they are exposed to these drugs, or agents, but is this also true for kidney cells? Or, are you postulating that the agents are acting on the endothelial cell in the kidney?

You note that lysolecithin acetyltransferase is activated maximally with ConA on lymphocytes within 30 minutes in cold cells of 0° C., and that it is an irreversible reaction that takes place. One of the things that bothers me considerably is the understanding that you have concerning the warm (why it does not work there) when you can put it on in the cold, and then flush it off immediately. I would think it would stay attached to the cells longer than that.

Dr. Frank P. Stuart (Chicago, Ill.). Do you know whether or not treating allogeneic cells in the cold with ConA changes their immunogenicity?

Dr. Thomas Blanke (St. Louis, Mo.). What did agglutination of the cells by the ConA have to do with the decreased antibody binding?

Dr. Luis H. Toledo-Pereyra (Closing). We postulated that the ConA in the kidney cells is masking the graft antigenicity of those cells in the kidney itself. We are doing radioactive and immunofluorescent studies now to further study ConA and to determine to what it is binding in the kidney.

We did not think that the ConA was acting peripherally or systemically. We thought it was acting locally, as I mentioned before.

In our preliminary in vitro studies with mouse lymphocyte cells, we have not determined whether or not the temperature will modify the response of those cells to the PHA and ConA. We are doing some in vitro experiments in mouse lymphoid cells at 4°, 25°, and 37° C., to determine that question.

Functional characterization of blocking antibody after human renal transplantation

Joshua Miller, M.D., Judith Lifton, Faye Rood, George Kyriakides, M.D., Kazimiera Y. Gajl-Peczalska, M.D., Edmond J. Yunis, M.D., *and* **Brack G. Hattler, Jr., M.D.,**
Minneapolis, Minn., and Tucson, Ariz.

The site of action and specificity of blocking IgG have now been examined in five recipients one year after transplantation, using a panel of 30 responding and stimulating cell combinations, in which lymphocytes of each specific donor were included as well. The strongest blocking occurred using IgG specific for donor lymphocytes, but blocking also occurred reproducibly with certain other cell combinations. This did **not** correlate with HLA antigens in common between donor cells and these other cell combinations. Blocking IgG was not cytotoxic for donor or other lymphocytes, using cytotoxicity tests of magnified sensitivity, i.e., heterologous, antihuman globulin. Moreover, recipient-blocking IgG, incubated with donor cells, did not block cytotoxic reactions using known monospecific HLA antisera directed against HLA donor determinants not present in the recipient. Binding of blocking IgG could only minimally be demonstrated by immunofluorescence, possibly due to its low density and avidity on the cell membrane, as contrasted with anti-HLA antibody (strongly positive). Therefore, blocking IgG is not directed against HLA determinants but against other determinants found thus far at random in an outbred human population, i.e., phenotypes of either special MLC genotypes closely linked with HLA subloci, or "minor" histocompatibility genotypes heretofore unable to be serologically classified.

From the Department of Surgery, University of Minnesota School of Medicine, Minneapolis, Minn., and the Department of Surgery, University of Arizona School of Medicine, Tucson, Ariz.

THERE HAVE BEEN several recent reports stating that serum obtained from human or animal subjects immunized by transplantation has in vitro activity other than its cytotoxicity properties.[2, 5, 6, 17, 21, 23, 25, 28] We have demonstrated that human and canine whole (undigested) immunoglobulin G (IgG), as well as the $(Fab')_2$ pepsin digested fragments obtained after renal allotransplantation, will, under certain conditions, block or inhibit unidirectional mixed lymphocyte reactions (MLC) in which donor lymphocytes are present either as stimulating or responding cells.[8, 10, 18] Other investigators have demonstrated that antibodies presumably directed against transplantation antigens will also block tuberculin responses in vitro.[3, 4] We have also seen this when using canine IgG, obtained four to six months after renal transplant rejection, which inhibited responses to phytohemagglutinin (PHA-P) and tuberculin in the absence of cytotoxicity.

In our experiments thus far in human subjects, conditions accompanying the develop-

Presented at the Thirty-fifth Annual Meeting of the Society of University Surgeons, St. Louis, Mo., Feb. 14-16, 1974.

Reprint requests: Joshua Miller, M.D., Department of Surgery, University of Minnesota School of Medicine, Minneapolis, Minn. 55455.

ment of MLC-blocking antibody after renal transplantation appear to demonstrate: (1) minimal to moderate MLC reactivity of the recipient responding against the donor preoperatively; (2) the absence of rejection episodes; (3) the absence on biopsy of evidence of either cellular or humoral rejection; (4) an interval of about three months after transplantation before the emergence of blocking; and (5) persistence, essentially unaltered, of recipient-responding cell MLC reactivity after transplant.

The present work is a further attempt to functionally characterize post-transplant blocking IgG, with respect to specificity, avidity, target site, and mechanism of action. Qualitative differences are demonstrated in these parameters between the MLC-blocking immunoglobulin moiety and cytotoxic antibody.

MATERIALS AND METHODS

Five related, human, donor-recipient combinations and unrelated, indifferent subjects were studied preoperatively from several weeks before renal transplantation until one year postoperatively. Each transplant recipient was treated intravenously with 20 mg. per kilogram of body weight of horse anti-human lymphoblast globulin daily for 14 days after transplantation, as previously described,[24] in addition to treatment with Imuran and Medral. In each case there was good renal function (creatinine clearance of over 60 ml. per minute) at one year without evidence of rejection or overt illness. For each donor-recipient pair a designated indifferent subject was utilized throughout the period of study. Mixed lymphocyte cultures were obtained at one month and three days prior to transplantation, weekly for four weeks postoperatively, and at one to three month intervals thereafter in each group. Combinations of stimulating and responding cells were as follows: Recipient responding plus recipient stimulating (R + Rx); recipient responding plus donor stimulating (R + Dx); recipient responding plus indifferent stimulating (R + Ix); donor responding plus donor stimulating (D + Dx); donor responding plus recipient stimulating (D + Rx); donor responding plus indifferent stimulating (D + Ix); indifferent responding plus indifferent stimulating (I + Ix); indifferent responding plus recipient stimulating (I + Rx); indifferent responding plus donor stimulating (I + Dx). All stimulating cells (Rx, Dx, and Ix) were inactivated with 1,500 rads x-irradiation.

At intervals pre- and post-operatively, recipient serum was obtained and IgG derived by saturated ammonium sulfate precipitation of globulins followed by DEAE column chromatography.[22]

Mixed lymphocyte cultures were performed in duplicate or triplicate on lymphocytes separated by Ficol-Hypaque density gradients. Methodology for separation procedure, as well as culture conditions, have been previously described for 2 ml. macrocultures.[18, 19] Two concentrations of IgG, 2 and 0.5 mg., were added per culture.

Immunofluorescence of lymphocyte preparations was performed with goat anti–human IgG, using a modification of the method of Pernis and colleagues.[7] Responses to PHA were tested by adding 40 μg of PHA-P (Difco) per culture. Tritiated thymidine was added 16 hours before culture termination, and uptake in counts per minute (c.p.m.) was measured at three, five, seven, and nine days after culture preparation by washing, solubilization, and liquid scintillation counting.[18]

Microcytotoxicity tests and HLA haplotyping of families of recipients and donors were performed according to the methods of Amos,[1, 14] as modified by one of us (E.J.Y.). A microcytotoxicity test using goat anti–human IgG, previously shown to be several times more sensitive than the standard test,[13] was also used.

The antibody-mediated, cellular-immune lysis assay described by Moller,[20] modified, and called ABCIL by Kovithavongs and associates,[15] was used to test each recipient serum. Postitive control sera were anti-HLA sera collected by one of us (E. J. Y.), directed against specificities possessed by the donor and not by the recipient. Ten million target cells in a resuspended pellet were incu-

Table IA. *MLC inhibition by blocking IgG and HLA phenotype Pretransplant*

Group No.		Initials	HLA type: Locus 1	HLA type: Locus 2	Plasma	Responding cells	Stimulating cells: Rx	Stimulating cells: Dx	Stimulating cells: Ix
1	R	H. F.	2,—	7,—*		R	**423**	2,495	7,256
	D	W. F.	1,2	7,—†	R	D	5,481	**1,047**	10,529
	I	F. R.	2,11	7,8		I	7,908	9,999	**1,430**
						R	**621**	1,895	7,806
					I	D	4,991	**986**	11,259
						I	9,507	9,609	**1,028**
2	R	S. H.	2,11	5,W10		R	**386**	365	12,504
	D	C. B.	2,11	5,W10	R	D	210	**257**	10,371
	I	J. L.	1,10	8,W27		I	18,148	16,295	**907**
						R	**497**	574	10,319
					I	D	1,126	**1,040**	9,698
						I	18,517	16,007	**1,314**
3	R	B. W.	2,3	W5,W10		R	**908**	8,727	8,745
	D	D. M.	2,1	8,W10	R	D	13,277	**700**	12,042
	I	B. H.	2,3	4,W27		I	6,508	10,794	**587**
						R	**1,566**	12,847	10,174
					I	D	9,700	**566**	6,233
						I	10,082	8,835	**1,064**
4	R	J. M.	3,W19	8,W5		R	**378**	4,337	7,408
	D	B. M.	2,3	W5,W15	R	D	12,898	**629**	18,358
	I	E. A.	2,3	12,W15		I	11,887	15,184	**599**
						R	**665**	6,250	12,065
					I	D	19,744	**612**	10,691
						I	22,107	13,816	**1,911**
5	R	B. B.	1,3	7,8		R	**401**	6,414	9,575
	D	R. B.	3,9	7,W27	R	D	4,590	**425**	8,392
	I	J. L.	1,10	8,W27		I	8,958	9,253	**590**
						R	**494**	7,209	10,250
					I	D	9,861	**863**	10,243
						I	8,846	9,347	**888**

*Homozygous for HLA-2 and 7.
†Homozygous for HLA-7.

bated with 50 μCi of ^{51}Cr at 37° C. for one hour, washed four times, and 5×10^5 cells resuspended with 2×10^6 effector cells in 1 ml. of RPMI 1640 containing 10 percent calf serum. Test serum (0.1 ml.) was added and the suspension incubated for four hours at 37° C. in 8 percent CO_2 and high humidity. Cold medium (1 ml.) was then added and the cells were centrifuged for 10 minutes at 2,500 r.p.m. at 4° C. The decanted supernate and the cell pellet were counted in a gamma counter. The results are expressed as percentage of chromium release, i.e., (counts in supernatant/counts in cell pellet plus supernatant) $\times$ 100.

Recipient IgG and human cytotoxic sera were tested in the discriminatory mixed lymphocyte culture (D MLC), previously described,[17] to differentiate between cytotoxic serum and blocking antibody. In this test, responding and stimulating cells were initially combined in the presence of test antibody, i.e., cytotoxic or blocking. After 48 hours the cultures were washed and new stimulating cells were then added, this time in the presence of normal IgG or serum. In controls the order of addition of the test serum was reversed so that it was added at 48 hours after washing cells originally incubated with normal serum. Other controls included the addi-

Table IB. *MLC inhibition by blocking IgG and HLA phenotype*
One year posttransplant

Group No.	Plasma	Resp. cells	*Stimula* No IgG Rx	No IgG Dx	No IgG Ix	Cultured with preop. IgG‡ Rx	Cultured with preop. IgG‡ Dx	Cultured with preop. IgG‡ Ix	Cultured with postop. IgG No. 1‡ Rx	Cultured with postop. IgG No. 1‡ Dx	Cultured with postop. IgG No. 1‡ Ix
1†	R	R	**211**	171*	2,203*						
		D	1,142*	**109**	541*						
		I	3,382*	199*	**258**						
	I	R	**309**	1,826	5,358	**185**	1,880	4,984	**147**	240*	3,551
		D	4,100	**190**	6,915	3,954	**859**	9,180	1,748*	**100**	1,866*
		I	7,361	5,013	**1,040**	4,734	7,996	**1,042**	4,397	1,680*	**633**
2	R	R	**1,052**	1,118	12,124						
		D	1,110	**1,499**	9,949						
		I	23,899	19,399	**1,454**						
	I	R	**1,454**	1,089	17,654	**876**	925	9,666	**1,519**	1,203	4,014*
		D	1,872	**1,778**	13,002	974	**888**	8,158	889	**810**	2,092*
		I	23,484	22,431	**1,818**	13,245	13,525	**1,194**	2,734*	6,281*	**741**
3	R	R	**116**	200*	443*						
		D	696*	**1,373**	1,082*						
		I	2,198*	2,102*	**173**						
	I	R	**1,062**	6,519	10,860	**362**	5,930	11,217	**353**	453*	472*
		D	4,907	**1,116**	7,043	8,631	**791**	11,482	478*	**798**	2,153*
		I	8,043	9,246	**972**	7,014	8,776	**1,217**	490*	707*	**595**
4	R	R	**315**	2,884	9,976						
		D	6,915	**336**	9,905						
		I	10,588	8,853	**1,020**						
	I	R	**969**	4,007	6,235	**817**	3,078	9,008	**439**	653*	6,510
		D	8,272	**910**	7,654	7,573	**852**	11,923	2,781*	**404**	3,897*
		I	9,040	9,207	**1,239**	12,631	12,274	**1,391**	5,630*	4,461*	**585**
5	R	R	**1,472**	3,648*	7,223*						
		D	3,119	**1,865**	2,791*						
		I	6,509*	2,702*	**1,672**						
	I	R	**1,354**	7,509	14,158	**107**	5,948	8,511	**501**	5,428	8,691
		D	12,170	**760**	10,068	8,857	**687**	13,532	1,083*	**573**	8,637
		I	12,386	13,690	**680**	9,073	12,183	**437**	3,804*	10,789	**557**

*Blocking effect.
†For HLA phenotype, see Table I*A*.
‡All cultures were prepared in I plasma.

tion of normal serum, test serum, or IgG in both the first and second stages. Tritiated thymidine uptake was measured at three, five, and seven days after the second stage was prepared.

Additionally, lymphocytes of indifferent individuals were placed in culture for one, two, three, and four weeks. Serum-supplemented medium was replenished weekly. At each of these weekly time intervals, the cultured cells were used as responding and stimulating cells combined with fresh indifferent lymphocytes in MLC, and also as responding cells stimulated by PHA-P. These results were compared with those using fresh cells obtained from the donor of the cultured cells tested at the same time. Blocking IgG in concentrations of 2 and 0.5 mg. was added to the preparations of fresh and cultured lymphocyte combinations.

RESULTS

Of 31 renal transplants serially followed for one year using the MLC test, five donor-recipient-indifferent groups are described in this study in detail. These five combinations were chosen because there was no significant difference in cultures tested in the recipient, preoperative, uremic plasma and IgG, as

...ing cells											
Cultured with postop. IgG No. 2‡			*Cultured with postop. IgG No. 3‡*			*Cultured with postop. IgG No. 4‡*			*Cultured with postop. IgG No. 5‡*		
Rx	*Dx*	*Ix*	*Rx*	*Dx*	*Ix*	*Rx*	*Dx*	*Ix*	*Rx*	*Dx*	*Ix*
184	1,688	5,605	**204**	1,273	4,093	**171**	1,378	3,822	**175**	440*	3,406
4,078	**1,107**	10,030	4,405	**823**	8,752	5,092	**1,076**	10,387	3,607	**948**	10,892
4,855	6,590	**1,016**	4,568	6,918	**1,023**	4,472	4,915	**1,040**	4,568	3,839	**1,036**
730	1,059	9,354	**759**	935	8,329	**766**	567	7,361	**977**	849	4,172*
826	**791**	9,564	943	**892**	7,269	647	**770**	9,650	1,074	**1,093**	4,144*
5,607	12,190	**1,206**	15,469	12,263	**956**	17,417	14,275	**1,047**	14,692	10,958	**1,258**
1,011	8,624	15,514	**1,082**	9,068	13,740	**1,397**	8,921	18,770	**940**	10,101	10,232
2,861	**1,093**	8,381	10,896	**987**	4,352*	8,324	**1,118**	17,924	5,013*	**1,078**	6,752*
9,617	8,577	**1,240**	11,206	6,352	**892**	14,350	10,262	**1,490**	9,501	4,163*	**892**
530	3,607	7,143	**523**	3,338	8,045	**1,251**	2,238	5,667	**916**	1,093	2,060
5,655	**934**	8,336	7,418	**447**	8,237	7,242	**1,085**	6,307	2,774*	**377**	4,951
9,805	10,165	**1,469**	9,545	8,396	**1,019**	8,308	9,531	**1,455**	5,685	7,943	**731**
908	6,884	8,545	**910**	4,001	7,065	**885**	4,875	8,936	**923**	2,948*	6,511
,879	**1,241**	10,118	10,785	**575**	12,093	7,318	**758**	14,816	3,857*	**687**	4,532*
,911	14,252	**1,338**	7,968	9,997	**642**	8,879	14,726	**583**	5,077	4,183*	**427**

compared with cultures prepared in indifferent plasma. Immunoglobulin G, obtained preoperatively from each recipient, was tested in 30 MLC combinations (Table I), and compared with IgG obtained one year after transplant. It was found that recipients of groups No. 1 and 5 at one year after transplant developed MLC serum-blocking factor de novo. These two recipients differed from their donors by one haplotype. However, although cross-reacting inhibition occurred, neither the presence nor the magnitude of the inhibition was related to specific HLA determinants. Recipient No. 2 was HLA-identical and MLC-unresponsive when tested against his donor. No blocking factor developed in his serum or IgG. Each of the other pairs had one haplotype difference. Recipient No. 3 developed a serum-inhibitory factor one year postoperatively, but it was not significantly present in the IgG fraction of his serum. This patient demonstrated a strong MLC response against the donor (one haplotype difference) preoperatively. In no case were there any significant differences between cellular reactivity preoperatively and one year postoperatively. The recipient of group No. 4, with moderate pretransplant and post-

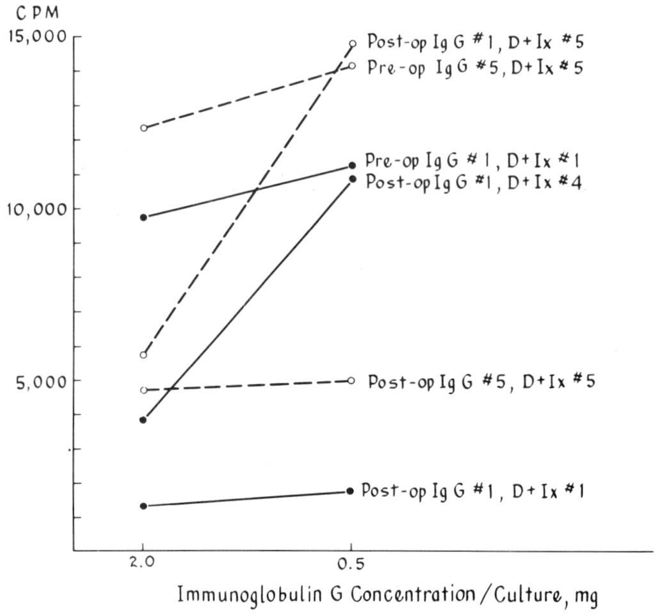

Fig. 1. Effect of 2 and 0.5 mg. of specific and nonspecific blocking IgG on D + Ix combinations. Both concentrations block only with the specific donor cells.

Table II. *Postoperative IgG (2 mg. per culture) inhibition of PHA reactivity by blocking antibody*

	IgG No. 1		*IgG No. 2*		*IgG No. 3*		*IgG No. 4*		*IgG No. 5*		*No IgG*	
Cell donor	*Control*	*PHA*	*Control*	*PHA*	*Control*	*PHA*	*Control*	*PHA*	*Control*	*PHA*	*Control*	*PHA*
D. M.*	340	5,222‡	400	11,800	418	10,850	263	12,117	593	4,797‡	309	10,212
W. F.†	440	5,133‡	318	10,928	166	13,611	283	12,368	326	11,529	179	10,145
H. F.§	383	10,016	436	11,816	119	10,004	318	11,016	289	4,055‡	282	12,095

*Donor No. 3, see Table I.
†Donor No. 1, see Table I.
‡PHA response inhibited by immunoglobulin.
§Recipient No. 1, see Table I.

transplant reactivity against her donor, had not developed blocking antibody. Other recipients with similar residual MLC reactivity have also developed blocking IgG postoperatively, but are not included in this study because of inadequate characterization. Postoperative immunoglobulin G of recipients Nos. 1 and 5 not only blocked MLC reactions (Table I) and PHA reactions (Table II) of their respective donors, but also cross-inhibited these reactions involving unrelated donors, recipients, and indifferent individuals. By contrast, no blocking of MLC or PHA reactivity was seen using preoperative IgG (not shown in Table II). Inhibition of PHA responses by blocking IgG was limited to a twofold drop in reactivity, even in combination with specific donor cells, whereas MLC reactivity, using specific donor cells, was reduced as much as tenfold. The MLC and PHA cross-reacting, inhibitory activity of the blocking IgG of recipients Nos. 1 and 5 did not correlate with HLA antigens in common between donors Nos. 1 and 5 and individuals of other combinations in which inhibition occurred. For example, in Table I, donor-HLA determinants not present in recipient No. 5 were HLA-9 and W-27. Yet, postoperatively, IgG of recipient No. 5 blocked reactivity of R and D of recipient-

Table III. *Cytotoxic and ABCIL effects of blocking IgG No. one on donor No. one cells*

	Donor cells + anti-HLA-1 serum	Donor cells + recipient No. 1 IgG* (blocking)	Donor No. 1 cells absorbed with recipient No. 1 IgG‖ + anti-HLA-1	Donor cells + recipient No. 1 IgG + heterologous goat anti–human IgG
Cytotoxic titer	1:8	0̄	1:8	0̄
ABCIL reaction†	21 percent‡	3 percent§	—	—

*Serum was used rather than IgG in the ABCIL reaction.
†Effector cells were normal indifferent cells without the HLA-1 determinants.
‡Percent experimental ^{51}Cr release.
§Not significant ^{51}Cr release.
‖Absorbed at 37° C. or room temperature for one hour.

Table IV. *D MLC assay of blocking activity using D + Ix cell combination Group No. 1*

Culture additives		Days after second stage D MLC preparation		
First stage	Second stage	Three	Five	Seven
R serum*	Normal serum†	699§	5,020	9,115
Cytotoxic serum‡	Normal serum	656	2,005	3,091
Cytotoxic serum 1:16 dilution	Normal serum	1,941	8,039	10,759
Normal serum	Cytotoxic serum	971	2,485	4,300
Normal serum	Cytotoxic serum 1:16 dilution	1,986	12,673	11,378
Normal serum	R serum	1,807	9,416	8,628
Normal serum	Normal serum	1,998	8,454	9,194

*Blocking MLC activity 1 year post-transplant.
†Indifferent (I of group No. 1).
‡Anti HLA-1 (see Table I)—donor HLA determinant not present on recipient cells.
§CPM of duplicate or triplicate cultures of D + Ix.

combinations Nos. 1 and 4 lacking the common HLA specificities. Conversely, donor specificity HLA-1 was not present in recipient No. 1. However, IgG of recipient No. 1 did not block several R, D, and I combinations of group No. 5, in which R and I cells contained the common HLA-1 determinant.

Using two concentrations of IgG, 2 and 0.5 mg. per culture (Fig. 1), it was seen that inhibition by IgG directed against a specific donor was present with both concentrations, while inhibition in nonspecific combinations was usually only present at 2 mg. per culture.

In each case blocking IgG tested in routine and enhanced microcytotoxicity tests (i.e., using heterologous goat anti–human IgG) was not cytotoxic against either the specific donor or the non-specific indifferent cells which were inhibited in culture. Table III indicates this test in group one. Preincubation of these cells, with blocking IgG in concentrations that inhibited MLC reactivity (2 mg. per 1.2 million cells), or in a concentration ten times as strong, did not decrease the titer of anti-HLA sera directed against donor-HLA determinants not present in the recipient. Additionally, although anti-HLA-1 serum normally demonstrated ABCIL activity against the donor cells, no ABCIL activity was seen using blocking antiserum. ABCIL activity was absent in each of the five recipients studied. Similar results were observed for cytotoxicity and absorption studies.

Blocking serum was then tested using the D MLC assay. This further demonstrated its low avidity and the absence of cytotoxicity, differentiating it from HLA cytotoxic antibody (Table IV). While recipient No. 1's serum initially inhibited reactivity of D + Ix

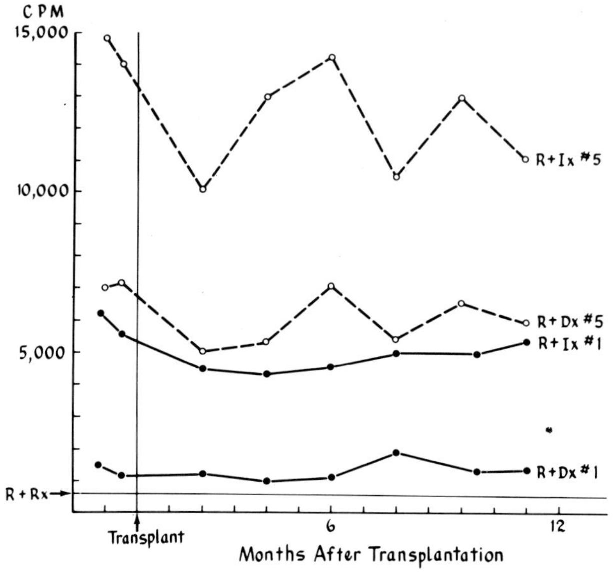

Fig. 2*A*. Mixed lymphocyte culture reactivity of recipients Nos. 1 and 5 against their specific donors, as well as indifferent individuals followed for one year after transplantation. No significant change was seen.

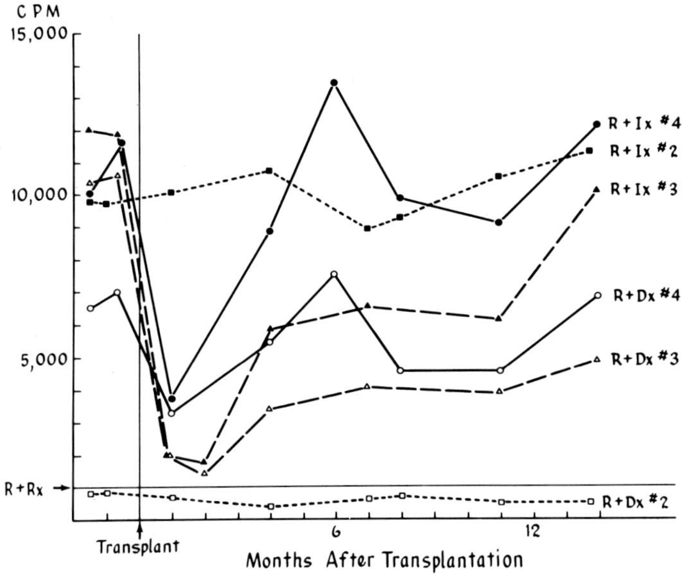

Fig. 2*B*. Mixed lymphocyte culture reactivity of recipients Nos. 2, 3, and 4 against their specific donors, as well as indifferent individuals. Note the marked inhibition in reactivity during the first few weeks after transplantation in Nos. 3 and 4 as contrasted with No. 2 (HLA and MLC identical).

of recipient No. 1, if added during the recognition phase of the MLC (first stage), reactivity returned to normal by seven days, after the second stage was prepared. By contrast, cytotoxic serum added at the first stage inhibited reactivity equally throughout culture period. If blocking serum was added at the second stage, no significant inhibition was seen, while cytotoxic serum would inhibit at this stage as well. A dilution of cytotoxic serum (1:16), which was just below threshold for cytotoxicity (Table III), caused no

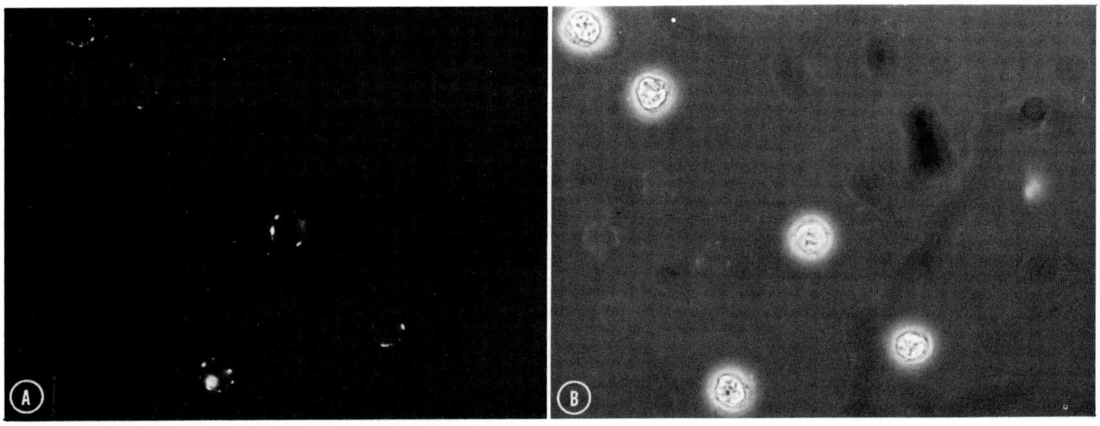

Fig. 3. *A,* Donor lymphocytes incubated with anti-HLA serum and then stained with anti-human IgG labeled with fluorescein isothiocyanate. Note that all cells are stained when compared with *B,* taken from the same field in phase-contrast.

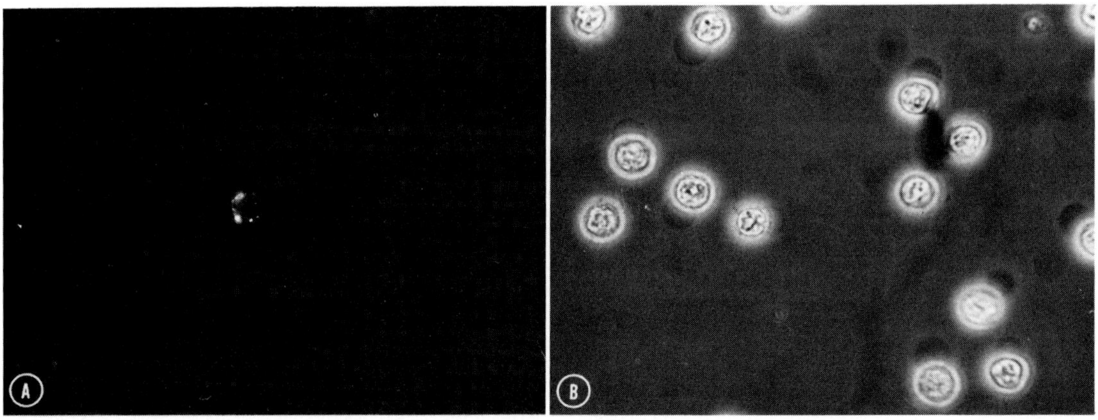

Fig. 4. *A,* Donor lymphocytes incubated with recipient IgG and then stained with fluoresceinated anti-human IgG serum. Only one of 15 cells shows surface-associated IgG when compared with *B,* taken from the same field in phase-contrast.

MLC inhibition at either stage of the D MLC. This observation further argues against MLC inhibition caused by blocking IgG being due merely to cytotoxic antibody present at concentrations lower than those detectable using microcytotoxicity tests.

There was no evidence that clinically or immunologically pointed to the appearance of inhibitory IgG. There was, however, a marked difference in the pattern of MLC reactivity of recipients who developed blocking IgG, versus those who did not develop it (Figs. 2*A* and 2*B*). There was an early depression in reactivity of recipients Nos. 3 and 4, which, in the past, in the absence of ALG treatment, usually correlated with rejection episodes. These recipients, however, did not show clinical rejection. Reactivity of recipients Nos. 1 and 5, who developed blocking IgG, did not show the pattern of early decrease in responsiveness.

Immunofluorescent tests comparing the effect of HLA antisera and blocking IgG failed to demonstrate any significantly greater binding of blocking IgG than non-specific binding of pre-operative IgG to lymphocytes (minimal). By contrast, anti-HLA antibody specific to donor determinants not present in the recipient could be easily demonstrated by this technique (Figs. 3*A,* 3*B,* 4*A,* and 4*B*). It

Table V. *Inhibition of PHA response of fresh vs. cultured cells by blocking IgG*

Weeks in culture	PHA response					
	Fresh cells			Cultured cells		
	No PHA	PHA	PHA + IgG	No PHA	PHA	PHA + IgG
1	621	15,950	—	580	28,528	—
2	916	22,935	9,818	476	28,497	28,089
3	208	16,029	10,075	457	26,492	28,688
4	299	16,895	—	680	33,125	—

*F = fresh cells, lymphocytes separated from whole blood and prepared in culture that day; C = cultured cells, lymphocytes vidual; and x = x-irradiated.

could, therefore, be concluded thus far that the binding site for blocking IgG on the cell membrane is not the same as that for anti-HLA antibodies.

In order to positively characterize the cell surface target site of blocking IgG, a finding recently described by ourselves,[11] using lymphocytes in culture, was applied. In an attempt to explain the work of Summerlin and associates,[26] in which tissues in culture sequentially lost transplantation immunogenicity, we have recently found that cultured lymphocytes lost stimulating and responding properties in MLC over a 28 day period (Table V), but maintained normal responsiveness to PHA during this period. A possible explanation for this is the loss of transplantation antigens. However, HLA phenotypes were qualitatively and quantitatively equivalent in cultured and fresh cells of the same phenotype. Since blocking IgG inhibited PHA responsiveness in selected individuals, PHA responsiveness of fresh and cultured cells of several of these subjects was compared. Inhibition by IgG occurred in cultures using fresh lymphocytes but not with cultured lymphocytes, indicating that the absence, not of HLA antigens, but of MLC reactive sites on the cultured cells was responsible for the loss of blocking activity, or, conversely, blocking IgG was specifically directed against MLC reactive sites and not against HLA antigens.

DISCUSSION

Previously, several patients were studied after renal transplantation, who had developed blocking factors in serum.[9, 23] The significance of these factors in influencing the acceptance of the allograft has been vague. Our first description of the de novo development of MLC blocking IgG in a transplant patient was associated with a totally benign, immunological course post-transplantation and long-term biopsies, which were devoid of rejection criteria.[8] The non-cytotoxic D MLC positive IgG, which has developed in the present patients, fits these criteria. With the further characterization of this IgG, generalizations about the immunological preconditions associated with its development might be tentatively discussed:

1. Blocking, thus far, has not been observed to evolve in HLA- and MLC-identical combinations. However, this may only be a matter of test sensitivity since minor histocompatibility loci in mice have been difficult to work with until recently in demonstrating humoral immunity.[27] Enhancement, however, may be most effective in this latter setting, as it has been in the rat species,[12] in which histocompatibility between many strains is not as marked. The fact that in two instances, herein described, MLC blockade was a serological method of differentiating MLC-identical individuals reacting against the same indifferent individual indicates that minor histocompatibility factors in humans may yet be differentiated and that, perhaps, blocking factors may even be present in this setting.

2. Blocking IgG has not been demonstrated as yet in strongly reactive MLC combinations. Several of these related donor-recipient pairs have had rejection and kidney loss occur together with the development of cytotoxic antibody. However, this does not mean that

MLC* response						
F + Fx	F + Ix	C + Cx	C + Ix	I + Ix	I + Fx	I + Cx
1,169	11,925	1,818	13,765	1,195	18,445	14,021
1,052	14,545	1,451	951	1,946	14,218	6,580
1,380	16,890	840	688	1,887	16,385	4,309
1,897	17,777	1,633	1,211	2,082	16,692	4,871

ured for 1, 2, 3, and 4 weeks respectively, and F and C are from the same donor; I = fresh lymphocytes of an indifferent indi-

cytotoxic and blocking antibodies are mutually exclusive, but merely that, in the presence of HLA-induced cytotoxicity, blocking by non-HLA antibodies is difficult to demonstrate. On the other hand, this may well be possible by suitable absorption experiments and the use of the D MLC in the future.

3. The immunological pre-condition that has been associated with the development of MLC blockade (albeit only using tests with the current magnitude of sensitivity) has been HLA non-identity but minimal MLC responsiveness before transplantation. Again, this may merely mean that this is the unique combination, i.e., where HLA cytotoxicity does not develop and where antigen persistence in the form of prolonged acceptance of the allograft is present, in which current tests can thus far detect it.

We have previously described a pattern of MLC inhibition, both in man and dogs, in cultures prepared in indifferent sera, that was associated with rejection and had its onset before clinical rejection could be detected.[16] We proposed that this was due to the entrapment of MLC-reactive cells in the rejecting organ. Several of our present patients have shown this pattern in a series treated with anti-lymphocyte globulin, but have shown no clinical evidence of rejection. We would speculate that ALG has aborted rejection in these patients but has not fully prevented entrapment from occurring. At the time of this writing (six months to two years), these patients have shown no evidence of clinical rejection and MLC reactivity has returned to the strong pretransplant values.

It should also be noted that in this study blocking IgG failed to block HLA cytotoxicity in vitro. This may or may not have in vivo correlation and should be investigated in enhancement experiments.

We think the present work is indicative of a potential for the development of a serology exclusively for non-HLA specificities, using sera or immunoglobulin collected from patients with D MLC positive blocking that has developed after renal transplantation. Speculatively, families might be genotyped with these sera in a manner similar to HLA serological classification. Blocking might then, perhaps, be utilized in clinical therapy as well when cross-reacting antigenicity is defined.

REFERENCES

1. Amos, D. G., Barber, H., Bayler, W., MacQueen, M., and Tiilikainen, A.: A simple microcytotoxicity test, Transplantation 7: 220, 1969.
2. Batchelor, J. R., Ellis, F., French, M. E., Bewick, M., Cameron, J. S., and Ogg, C. S.: Immunological enhancement of human kidney graft, Lancet 2: 1007, 1970.
3. Ceppellini, R., Bonnard, G. D., Coppo, F., Miggiano, V. C., Pospisil, M., Curtoni, E. S., and Pellegrino, M.: Mixed leukocyte cultures and HLA antigens. I. Reactivity of young fetuses, newborns, and mothers at delivery, Transplant. Proc. 3: 58, 1971.
4. Ceppellini, R., et al.: II. Inhibition by anti-HL-A sera, Transplant. Proc. 3: 63, 1971.
5. Cruse, J. M., Germany, W. W., and Dulaney, A. D.: Effects of immune serum and spleen cells on C3Hj/He tumor graft survival in Tennessee swiss mice, Lab. Invest. 14: 1554, 1965.
6. French, M. E., and Batchelor, J. R.: Immunological enhancement of rat kidney grafts, Lancet 2: 1103, 1969.
7. Gajl-Peczalska, K. J., Park, B. H., Biggar,

W. D., and Good, R. A.: B and T lymphocytes in primary immunodeficiency disease in man, J. Clin. Invest. **52**: 919, 1973.
8. Hattler, B. G., Jr., and Miller, J.: Blocking antibody in the sera and on the kidneys of successful human transplants, Transplant. Proc. **5**: 655, 1973.
9. Hattler, B. G., Jr., Karesh, C., and Miller, J.: Inhibition of the mixed lymphocyte culture response by antibody following successful human renal transplantation, Tissue Antigens **1**: 270, 1971.
10. Hattler, B. G., Jr., Davis, M., Soehnlen, B., and Miller, J.: Prospective in vitro prediction of enhancement of canine renal allografts, SURGERY **74**: 163, 1973.
11. Hattler, B. G., Jr., Rood, F., Lifton, J., Soehnlen, B., and Miller, J.: Diminished stimulatory capability of lymphocytes in mixed lymphocyte cultures following in vitro cultivations, Clin. Res. (abst.) 1974.
12. Hildemann, W. H., and Mullen, Y.: The weaker the histoincompatibility, the greater the effectiveness of specific immunoblocking antibodies: A new immunogenetic rule of transplantation, Transplant. Proc. **5**: 617, 1973.
13. Johnson, A. H., Rossen, R. D., and Butler, W. T.: Detection of allo-antibodies using a sensitive antiglobulin microcytotoxicity test: Identification of low levels of preformed antibodies in accelerated allograft rejection, Tissue Antigens **2**: 45, 1972.
14. Karger, S., AG: Proceedings of the ninth congress of the European society of hematology, 1963, p. 1132.
15. Kovithavongs, T., McConnachie, P. R., Dossetor, J. B.: Immunity to tissue sensitisation, HLA and non HLA, as detected by the antibody-mediated cell-dependent immune lympholysis system. I. Parous women, Transplantation **17**: 453, 1974.
16. Miller, J., and Hattler, B. G., Jr.: Reactivity of lymphocytes in mixed culture in response to human renal transplantation, SURGERY **72**: 220, 1972.
17. Miller, J., Hattler, B. G., Jr., and Johnson, M. C.: Cellular and humoral factors governing canine mixed lymphocyte cultures after renal transplantation. III. Antibody, Transplantation **14**: 57, 1972.
18. Miller, J., Hattler, B. G., Davis, M., and Johnson, M. C.: Cellular and humoral factors governing canine mixed lymphocyte cultures after renal transplantation. I. Antibody, Transplantation **12**: 65, 1971.
19. Miller, J., Rood, F., Lifton, J., and Hattler, B. G., Jr.: Cellular and humoral factors governing canine mixed lymphocyte cultures after renal transplantation. IV. Second set transplants and cytophilic antibody, Transplantation **16**: 142, 1973.
20. Moller, E.: Contact-induced cytotoxicity by lymphoid cells containing foreign isoantigens, Science **147**: 873, 1965.
21. Mullen, Y., and Hildemann, W. H.: Kidney transplantation genetics and enhancement in rats, Transplant. Proc. **3**: 669, 1971.
22. Peterson, E. A., and Sober, H. A.: Chromatography of proteins. I. Cellular ion-exchange adsorbents, J. Am. Chem. Soc. **78**: 751, 1956.
23. Quadracci, L. J., Hellstrom, I. E., Striker, G. E., Marchioro, T. M., and Hellstrom, K. E.: Immune mechanisms in human recipients of renal allografts, Cell. Immunol. **1**: 561, 1971.
24. Simmons, R. L., Condie, R., and Najarian, J. S.: Antilymphoblast globulin for renal allograft prolongation, Transplant. Proc. **4**: 487, 1972.
25. Stuart, F. P., Saitoh, R., and Fitch, F. W.: Rejection of renal allografts: Specific immunologic suppression, Science **160**: 1463, 1968.
26. Summerlin, W. T., Broutbar, C., Foanes, R. B., Payne, R., Stutman, O., Hayflick, L., and Good, R. A.: Acceptance of phenotypically differing cultured skin in man and mice, Transplant. Proc. **5**: 707, 1973.
27. Voisin, G. A.: Immunological facilitation, a broadening of the concept of the enhancement phenomenon, Prog. Allergy **15**: 328, 1971.
28. Wilson, R. E., Maggs, P. R., Vanwijck, R., Shaipanich, T., Holl-Allen, R. T. J., Lukl, P., and Simonian, S. J.: Active enhancement of renal allografts in dog and rat by subcellular antigen, Transplant. Proc. **3**: 705, 1971.

DISCUSSION

Dr. George L. Irvin, III (Miami, Fla.). I would like to ask if you tried to characterize your IgG a little more in regard to the sulf-S's, forcing them into two systems. It has been shown by several people that 7-S gamma-2 is the enhancing antibody and that it also has cytotoxic ability with exogenous complement. Have the authors looked at any of the subclasses of IgG that they are talking about?

Dr. Frank P. Stuart (Chicago, Ill.). McKern and Fitch, in our laboratory, have recently been able to show the occurrence of anti-idiotypic or, antireceptor, antibody against the immunoglobulin sites or antigen recognition sites on lymphocytes. This antireceptor antibody can be isolated; it appears within the first several weeks after transplant, persists for a long time, and does specifically block the response of the responding cells in mixed lymphocyte culture.

Dr. Richard E. Wilson (Boston, Mass.). Can

you explain how loss of MLC reactivity of cultured cells, but not loss of HL-A activity, could explain inability to reject a cultured graft? I am not quite sure that I can understand why that would explain Summerlin's work.

President Kountz. I would like to ask your feelings regarding the predictability of graft survival using HL-A and MLC. Do you now feel that MLC might be more important?

Dr. Joshua Miller (closing). We have not attempted to further classify blocking IgG in humans, other than to say that it is an IgG; but it would probably go into the IgG subclass that contains other enhancing antibodies.

It may well be that enhancing antibody may be an antirecognition site antibody. It is a little bit puzzling to try and picture how the donor cell, or the donor antigen, or the donor cell membrane components can stimulate the recipient to make an antirecognition antibody against donor cell components. Most of the antirecognition work has been done using a heterologous species as an immunizing substrate. However, I think that the one concept that might emerge is that the antibody that we are dealing with, and antibodies that have been described in other in vitro enhancing type systems, may affect a cell membrane in a steric way, so that it is unable to respond to a normal immunological stimulus, either in vivo or in vitro. This has been shown by many investigators, first, possibly, by Cepellini; the work, possibly, of Quadracci and Hellstrom is along the same conceptual line.

We're trying to repeat Summerlin's work on skin grafting and have not been able to as yet. But I think that one might think of this as a phase of deletion. Perhaps, with further culturing, we might lose both PHA responsiveness and HL-A antibodies and perhaps, eventually, have our cells turn into fibroblasts.

But we do know, however—I think your point is well taken—there are many lymphoid cell lines that have continued in culture for long periods of time with perpetuation of HL-A antigens. The question is quantitatively, are all antigens continued? Further, is the HL-A system the system that is involved in graft rejection? I don't know the answer, certainly, to this, but I do think that what we describe is a system where we can predict that enhancement or some humoral factor will eventually occur. If we have a low MLC response preoperatively, then perhaps we will see this enhancing factor developing in the postoperative period. And this does not appear to be a damaging antibody; so, to that extent I think the MLC is better than HL-A in determining results preoperatively.

Tolerance to myocardial tissue allografts by pretreatment with cross-reactive streptococcal membrane antigen

Robert J. Ellis, M.D., John B. Zabriskie, M.D., *and* **Paul A. Ebert, M.D.,** *New York, N. Y.*

Induction of immune paralysis to myocardial tissue allografts was accomplished using Type 6 streptococcal membrane (STM) pretreatment. This antigen is known to be cross-reactive with cardiac tissue. C57/B16 mouse hearts were grafted across an H_2 barrier to Balb C mice as free grafts. ECG activity, histological studies, and direct lymphocyte migration inhibition (LMI) were used to detect rejection. In 10/12 Balb C mice pretreated with 500 μg of STM one week prior to allografting of myocardial tissue, no evidence of rejection was found at 10 days. No other immunosuppressive agents were used for this study. Direct LMI in the pretreated group was 8 ± 3 percent as compared with an untreated group of myocardial tissue allografted mice, where LMI was 30 ± 2 percent in 11 Balb C mice ($p < 0.01$). ECG evidence of graft function was present at 10 days in the pretreated group, and no ECG evidence of graft function was found in the untreated group. Pretreatment with STM results in a cross-reactivity that produced tolerance to allografted myocardial tissue in mice.

From the Department of Surgery, The New York Hospital–Cornell Medical Center and The Rockefeller University, New York, N. Y.

CONTROL OF THE rejection process by organ-specific induction of tolerance is the ultimate goal of transplantation. Among the methods used to achieve organ-specific tolerance has been the injection of tolerance-inducing doses of donor antigen prior to organ transplantation. Many investigators have demonstrated prolonged graft survival in animals using pooled antigen, such as spleen or liver obtained from isogeneic hosts prior to kidney transplantation.[8, 10] Although these techniques have been successful, they are limited by the practicability of obtaining and processing pooled, cadaveric, organ-specific antigen prior to clinical transplantation.

This study was supported in part by United States Public Health Service grant No. HL 03919.

Presented at the Thirty-fifth Annual Meeting of the Society of University Surgeons, St. Louis, Mo., Feb. 14-16, 1974.

In view of the limitations on easily obtaining homologous or autologous donor antigen, our investigative approach led us to search for other antigens capable of inducing tolerance. The possibility that Group A streptococcal membranes might serve as a useful source of pooled antigen for induction of tolerance was based on previous observations. First, Zabriskie and associates[11] have demonstrated the cross-reactivity between strains of Group A streptococcus, kidney, and heart tissue. Second, Rapaport[7] immunized a series of dogs with streptococcal membrane (STM) and challenged the animals with renal transplants. This prior sensitization to STM resulted in a hyperacute rejection of the kidney grafts indicating a common antigenicity between STM and renal tissue. Third, we have demonstrated that by using STM as an antigen, detection of kidney rejection could be performed clinically using the in vitro assay of direct leukocyte migration.[1]

In view of this established cross-reactivity between Group A streptococcus and renal and cardiac tissue, it was thought that tolerance induced to STM could be used to prolong myocardial tissue allografts. The present report demonstrates that, under proper conditions, both cellular and humoral tolerance to streptococcal membrane antigens can be induced in mice. Animals made tolerant to these streptococcal antigens had prolonged survival of myocardial tissue allografts, whereas nonimmunized animals rejected the grafts in a normal fashion.

METHODS AND MATERIALS

Preparation of streptococcal membrane. Type 6 (S43/192/2) Group A streptococci obtained from R. Lancefield were grown in Todd Hewitt broth, harvested during the logarithmic growth phase, washed in saline, and incubated for 60 minutes at 37° C. with Group C phage-associated lysin in 4 percent NaCl.[4] The phage-associated lysin acts as an amidase, breaking the peptide bond in the mucopeptide layer of the cell wall. Following a hypertonic wash in 4 percent NaCl, the protoplasts and cell walls were centrifuged at 5,000 G for 30 minutes at 4° C. The protoplasts were then taken up in a magnesium-activated DNAase and RNAase mixture in distilled water. This hypotonic solution produced osmotic disruption of the protoplasts with resultant release and enzymatic degradation of the cytoplasmic components. After 30 minutes of incubation, the suspension was centrifuged at 37,000 G for 60 minutes at 4° C. to separate the pure membrane fraction. Dialysis over 24 hours in repeated changes of isotonic saline was then accomplished and protein determination of the membrane fraction was obtained. The membrane material was frozen at −70° C. in a Revco Freezer in 1 mg. per 100 ml. aliquots. A more detailed description of the purification and isolation of STM has been previously published.[12]

Induction of immunity and immune paralysis. Balb C female mice (20 to 25 gm. weight/Jackson Laboratory) were used in the immunization and tolerance-induction studies. Several routes of immunization were compared with each other in their ability to produce both a cellular and humoral response. The immunization methods consisted of the following: (1) injection of 2.5 mg. STM in 0.5 c.c. of incomplete Freund's adjuvant into both foot pads of six mice; (2) 10 μg STM per 0.5 c.c. saline injected into 13 Balb C mice intravenously via the tail vein; and (3) 500 μg STM per 0.5 c.c. saline injected intraperitoneally over three weeks at one injection per week. Cellular reactivity was measured at two weeks after method 1, at the end one week after method 2, and seven days after the last peritoneal injection in method 3.

Immune paralysis was attempted in Balb C mice by using various doses of STM injected intravenously. Doses of 50 μg to 1 Gm. per 0.5 c.c. of saline were used. Both cell-mediated and humoral responses were measured at one and two weeks after injection.

Measurement of cell and humoral-mediated immunity. Cell-mediated immunity was measured by using the direct lymphocyte migration assay described by Falk.[2] Briefly following the death of Balb C mice by cervical dislocation, spleen cell suspensions were diluted with RPMI 1640 and then centrifuged at 1,000 rpm for 10 minutes. The cell pellet was then treated with 0.85 percent NH_4Cl for lysis of red cells and again centrifuged at 1,000 rpm for 10 minutes. The cells were then washed with saline and centrifuged for 10 minutes, after which the cells were diluted to a concentration of 60×10^6 cells per cubic centimeter in 10 percent fetal calf serum in RPMI 1640 solution.

Streptococcal membranes were diluted in 10 percent FCS/RPMI to a concentration of 10 μg per cubic centimeter. Lymphocyte suspensions were made in 75 mm. capillary tubes* and sealed at one end. The capillaries were then centrifuged at 1,000 rpm for 10 minutes and cut at the fluid-cell interface. The cell pellet end of the capillary

*Sherwood Plastics.

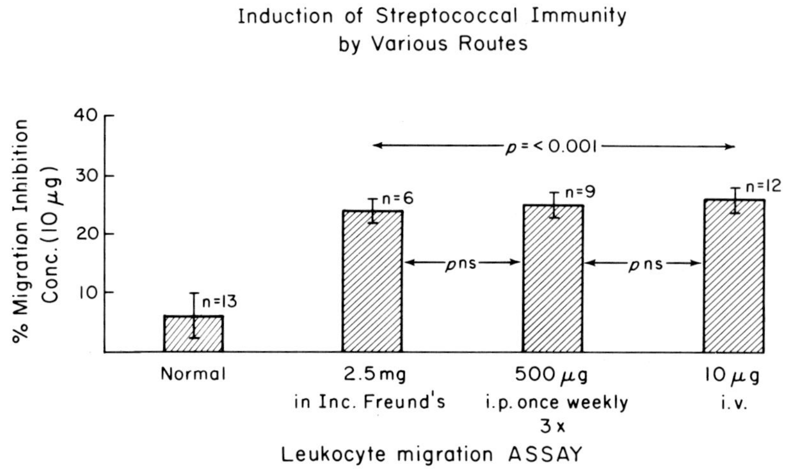

Fig. 1. A comparison of the leukocyte migration inhibition values in normal Balb C mice, immunized by three different methods of injection. Spleen cell suspensions were tested against 10 μg per cubic centimeter of streptococcal membranes in all experiments.

tube was placed in a microchamber planchette, and the tissue media added to the planchette in which appropriate dilutions of the antigen had been added. While several concentrations of membrane antigens were tried, 10 μg per cubic centimeter of membranes was selected as the optimal concentration. In the experiments described below, this concentration of antigen was used for all tests. There was a control run for each mouse's lymphocytes. All experiments were carried out in triplicate. The planchettes were sealed with coverslips and placed in an incubator at 37° C. for 24 hours. Using a standard photographic enlarger, the fans were projected on tracing paper, drawn, cut out, and weighed. The formula for migration index was:

$$\frac{\text{Weight of fans with antigen}}{\text{Weight of fans without antigen}} \times 100 \text{ percent}$$

The Migration Inhibition Index was 100 percent – Migration Index percent.

Humoral-mediated immunity was qualitatively determined by the presence of heart-reactive antibody in the serum samples collected from the retro-orbital sinus of the mice prior to death. This antibody was determined by indirect fluorescent microscopy. Briefly, a normal Balb C heart was frozen at –70° C. from which frozen sections 4 μ thick were cut on a cryostat. The cardiac sections were fixed to the glass slides with acetone for one minute. The slides were then washed for 5 minutes with 0.01M phosphate-buffered saline pH 0.5 (PBS). Serum from immunized mice was layered on the sections of heart tissue in controlled humidity for 25 minutes. The sections were then washed with PBS. Next, the slides were layered with rabbit anti–mouse fluoresceinated IgG* and 25 minutes later were again washed for 5 minutes with PBS. The slides were covered with a 1:1 ratio of glycerol:PBS solution and coverslips applied. With the use of a Zeiss fluorescent microscope equipped with BG12+OG9 filters, the slides were examined for the presence of mouse IgG bound to the cardiac fibers.

Cardiac transplantation. Using the technique described by Fulmer,[5] newborn C57 B16 mouse ventricles were transplanted into adult Balb C mice as free grafts in the subcutaneous tissue of the Balb C ear under ether anesthesia. These two inbred strains differed at a major histocompatible locus (2k) and resulted in a first set rejection.

Detection of rejection. Electrocardiographic voltage patterns were recorded using a Hewlitt-Packard recorder with a DC channel which had been modified to measure activity of the transplanted heart. Pins cor-

*Melloy Lab.

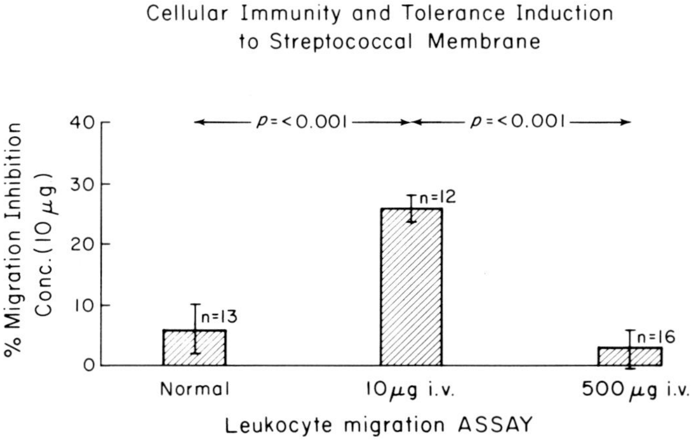

Fig. 2. A comparison of the migration values in Balb C mice immunized with 500 μg intravenously, as compared with mice given 10 μg per cubic centimeter intravenously. Note the absence of immune response in mice injected with high doses of antigen as compared with the strong immune response in mice injected with low doses of antigen.

responding to the limb leads of a normal ECG were placed in respective positions around the heart graft in the ear and, with the sensitivity turned to maximum and recording at 10 mm. per second, a rhythm strip on lead II was recorded.

After the mice were killed, the ears with the transplanted ventricle were removed and placed in a 10 percent formalin solution. Histological sections were made serially with standard hematoxylin and eosin stains.

RESULTS

Immunization studies. In Fig. 1 a comparison of cell-mediated immunity by the three routes was made as measured by the direct lymphocyte migration assay. All three groups of animals had similar responses in the in vitro assay. The migration-inhibition index was approximately 26 percent (S.E. ± 2 percent) in all three groups of animals and the results were not statistically different. In comparison to a group of 13 normal Balb C mice that were not injected with STM, there was a significant difference in the migration-inhibition index. The unimmunized group of mice had an index of 6 percent (S.E. ± 4 percent), indicating a strong cellular-immune response in the immunized group ($p < 0.01$). All three groups produced heart-reactive antibody, as detected by indirect fluorescent microscopy. The most intense binding of antibody was seen in animals that had been immunized with three weekly intraperitoneal injections of streptococcal membranes.

Immune paralysis. Cell-mediated immunity was not produced in a group of 16 Balb C mice that were injected intravenously with 500 μg STM per 0.5 c.c. of saline and assayed one week following injection. The same time interval after injection of 10 μg STM per 0.5 c.c. of saline, however, resulted in a cellular immune response (Fig. 2). The migration-inhibition index was 3 percent (S.E. ± 3 percent) in the group which received 500 μg STM per 0.5 c.c. of saline intravenously. This was not statistically different from a group of mice not injected with STM, but it was statistically different from a group of mice receiving 10 μg STM per 0.5 c.c. intravenously. No heart-reactive antibody was detected in the group receiving the large intravenous dose.

To determine if the dose used to produce unresponsiveness was a tolerizing dose of STM, Balb C mice were injected with 500 μg STM per 0.5 c.c. of saline intravenously, and one week later given 10 μg STM per 0.5 c.c. of saline intravenously, a dose which produced immunization. Fig. 3 summarizes the results in the three groups of mice. The two control groups responded as predicted earlier, in that the groups of five mice re-

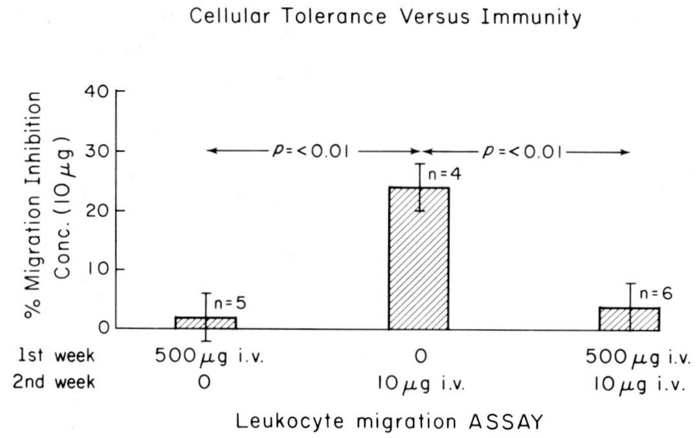

Fig. 3. Leukocyte migration values in groups of Balb C mice injected with low and high doses of streptococcal antigen. Animals previously injected with high doses of antigen blocked the expected immune response to a subsequent challenging dose of antigen.

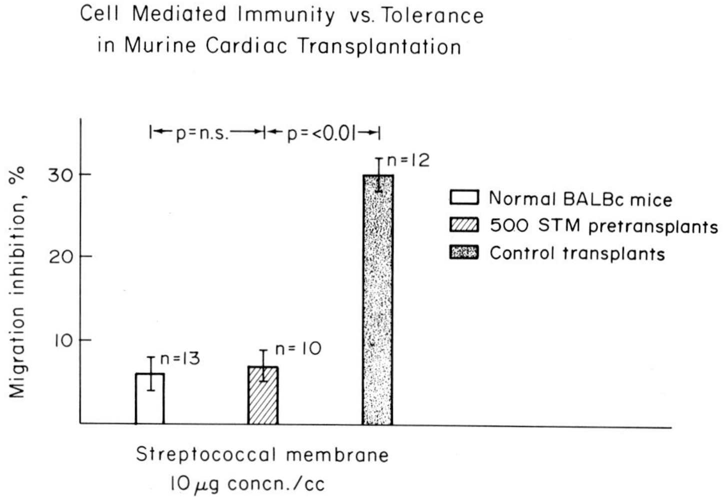

Fig. 4. Leukocyte migration values in groups of Balb C mice indicating that pretreatment of mice with STM resulted in blocking of the expected cellular response to myocardial tissue allografts, as seen in the control transplants.

ceiving only 500 μg STM per 0.5 c.c. of saline had a migration-inhibition index of 2 percent (S.E. ± 4 percent), while the control group of four mice receiving 10 μg STM per 0.5 c.c. of saline had a migration-inhibition index of 25 percent (S.E. ± 4 percent). In the group receiving both doses one week apart, it was evident that the 500 μg STM per 0.5 c.c. of saline given intravenously blocked the expected imune response with a migration-inhibition index of 3 percent (S.E. ± 4 percent) in the six mice. This migration-inhibition index was not statistically different from the control uninjected Balb C mice (MI = 6 percent ± 7 percent).

Tolerance to cardiac allografts. Since the experiments indicated that tolerance to STM could be produced in Balb C mice, myocardial tissue allografts were planned in animals pretreated with STM. A group of 12 Balb C mice were given 500 μg STM per 0.5 c.c. of saline intravenously 7 days prior to cardiac transplantation. A group of 13 Balb C mice that were transplanted, but did not receive pretreatment with STM, served as controls. Electrocardiograms were taken 10

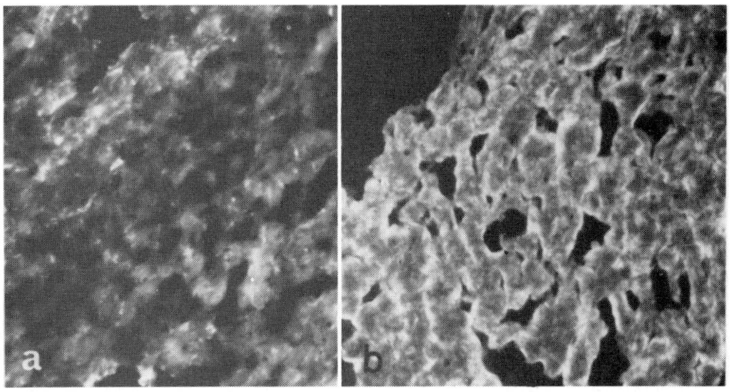

Fig. 5. The left side of this photomicrograph reveals the immunofluorescent staining pattern characteristic of heart-reactive antibody present in the series of the control-transplant group of mice (×320). The right side of the photograph reveals the absence of this antibody in animals pretreated with 500 μg per cubic centimeter of STM.

days following cardiac transplantation in both groups. Ten days after cardiac implantation, the mice were killed and direct lymphocyte-migration assays and heart-reactive antibody titers were performed on both groups of mice.

In Fig. 4 it can be seen that 10/12 animals pretreated with streptococcal membrane antigens (lined bar) had a migration-inhibition index of 8 percent (S.E. ± 3 percent). These values were not significantly different from the values (6 percent ± 2 percent) obtained in nonimmunized control mice (open bar). In contrast, the control transplants responded to the streptococcal antigens with a significant migration inhibition index of 30 percent (S.E. ± 2 percent). Thus, it appears that cellular immunity to cardiac tissue was blocked by pretreatment of the Balb C mice with 500 μg STM. In addition, heart-reactive antibody was absent in the pretreated group but present in the control transplant group as seen in Fig. 5.

Fig. 6 demonstrates that electrocardiographic activity was present in all 10/12 pretreated mice and not present in the control transplant group. A histological examination of the cardiac allografts was performed in both groups of mice. As illustrated in Fig. 7*B*, extensive destruction and lymphocytic infiltration were seen in the control tissue, indicative of active rejection. Fig. 7*A* indicates that there was no destruction or

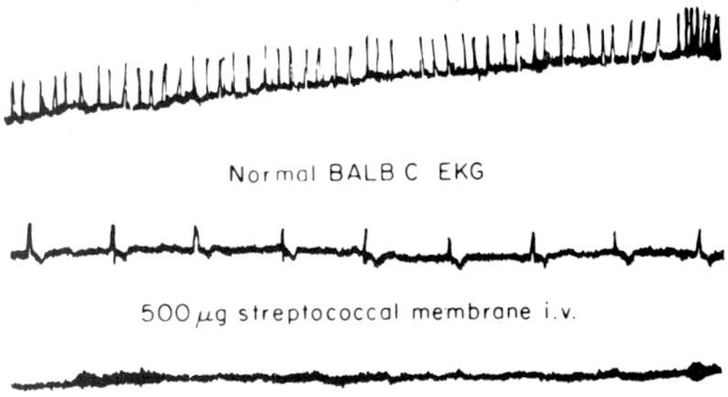

Fig. 6. Electrographic patterns demonstrating functional integrity of the cardiac allograft in pretreated Balb C mice and the lack of functional ECG patterns in the cardiac allograft in untreated mice.

lymphocytic infiltration in the cardiac allografts of the pretreated group. In the remaining 2/12 Balb C mice pretreated with STM, it was noted that STM had been extravasated into the tail upon injection. Both grafts demonstrated evidence of rejection histologically.

DISCUSSION

Tolerance or immune unresponsiveness was induced in Balb C mice receiving myocardial tissue allografts from newborn C57 B16 mice when pretreated with 500 μg STM one week prior to transplantation. The evidence for tolerance and prolonged survival of the graft had been obtained from several lines of investigation. First, functional integrity of the graft was detected by the continuance of normal ECG voltage patterns,

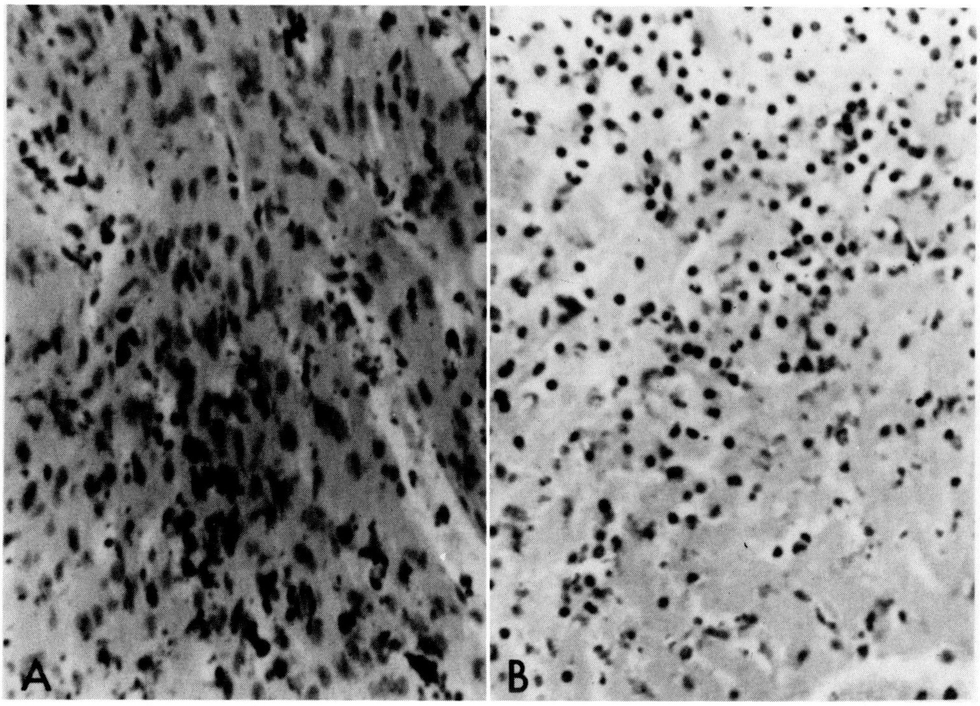

Fig. 7. Histological pattern of allografted myocardial tissue 10 days following transplantation. *A*, Section of allografted myocardial tissue in an STM pretreated Balb C mouse. Note the normal cardiac fibers with distinct nuclei. There is no lymphocytic infiltration or destruction of cardiac fibers (×45). *B*, Section of allografted myocardial tissue in an untreated Balb C mouse. Note the destruction of cardiac fibers with loss of nuclei. There is extensive lymphocytic infiltration with edema separating the destroyed cardiac fibers (×45).

and histological examination of the tissues revealed an intact cardiac transplant in the tolerant mice. Second, at the cellular level, spleen cell suspensions obtained from pretreated mice failed to respond to the immunizing antigen either before or after cardiac implantation. Finally, humoral antibodies were never detected in pretreated animals. Thus, tolerance and prolonged integrity, as well as a lack of cellular and humoral immunity, were evident in all animals pretreated with streptococcal membrane antigens.

Since both sarcolemmal and streptococcal membrane structures share common antigenic determinants, it has been possible to induce tolerance to cardiac allografts in mice. This concept was further strengthened by glycoprotein-structured studies performed by Fayolee and associates,[3] in which the amino acid sequences of both streptococcal membrane antigens and glycoprotein isolated from mouse and human cardiac tissue were found to be quite similar.

The exact mechanism whereby administration of a heterologous antigen results in tolerance and prolonged survival to allografts remains unclear. The experiments of Weigle[9] that demonstrated that tolerance to BSA could not be broken when challenged with antigenically similar albumins support our hypothesis of shared antigenicity being responsible for induction of tolerance. In addition, the large amounts of antigen used in these experiments may be a crucial factor in the induction. For example, Paul and associates[6] demonstrated that, depending on the quantity of tolerizing antigen used, tolerance would not be broken when quantities 100 times the normal tolerizing dose were used. This implied that the doses of tolerizing antigen regulated the specificity and breadth of tolerance which was maintained when challenged by cross-reactive antigens. It is quite possible that the large dose of STM used in these experiments did produce enough of an unresponsive state to be carried over to the myocardial tissue transplant.

It is conceivable, however, that several mechanisms are operative. For example, the large doses of antigen used may have effectively blocked all immune responses to both the autologous antigents (STM) as well as the heterologous cardiac antigens. Second, the nature of the membrane antigens may result in the coating of all immunocompetent cells. This concept is strengthened by the recent work of Rapaport and his associates[7] in which small molecular weight-fragments of these membranes bound firmly to the majority of human lymphocytes.

Several questions are raised by this phenomenon: How long can the unresponsive state last? Will new immunocompetent cells be produced and result in subsequent rejection? Can this mode of therapy be used in conjunction with a limited immunosuppressive regimen to induce a lasting state of tolerance? Further investigation is needed not only to answer these questions but also to investigate what role STM pretreatment may play in vascularized grafts. Specifically, can this phenomenon be duplicated in larger animals receiving either kidney or cardiac allografts where other functional parameters can be monitored?

It is our feeling that the use of cross-reactive streptococcal membrane pretreatment offers a unique way of altering the recipient's response to allografted myocardial tissue, and enables tolerance induction to occur prior to graft transplantation because of the readily available source of pooled streptococcal membrane.

REFERENCES

1. Ellis, R., Read, S., and Zabriskie, J. B.: Leukocyte migration: A cellular index of renal allograft function, Surg. Forum **22:** 285, 1971.
2. Falk, R., Colliste, L., and Moller, G.: In vitro correlation of transplantation immunity: The release of substances by immune lymphocytes confronted with specific antigens, SURGERY **66:** 5, 1969.
3. Fayolee, L., Deroriette, S., and Zabriskie, J. B.: Homology of amino acid composition of structural glycoproteins, transplantation antigens, cell wall glycoproteins and streptococcal A. cell membrane, Transplant. Proc. **4:** 415, 1972.
4. Fischetti, V., Gotschlich, E., and Bernheimer, A.: Purification and physical properties of Group C streptococcal phage-associated lysin, J. Exp. Med. **133:** 1105, 1971.
5. Fulmer, R., Cramer, A., and Liehet, P.: Transplantation of cardiac tissue into the mouse ear, Am. J. Anat. **113:** 273, 1963.
6. Paul, W., Thorbecke, J., Siṣkind, G., and Benacerraf, B.: The effect of dose in tolerance induction on the subsequent response to a cross-reactive antigen, J. Immunol. **17:** 85, 1969.
7. Rapaport, F., Bachvaroff, R., and Markowitz, A.: Lymphocyte surface effects of soluble extracts of streptococcal membranes, J. Immunol. **110:** 1058, 1973.
8. Stuart, F. P., Soitoh, T., and Fitch, F.: Immunologic enhancement of renal allografts in the rat, SURGERY **64:** 17, 1968.
9. Weigle, W.: Immune response of rabbits tolerant to bovine serum albumin to the injection of other heterologous serum albumins, J. Exp. Med. **114:** 111, 1961.
10. Wilson, R. E., Rippin, A., Dagher, R., and Kinneart, P.: Prolonged canine renal allograft survival after pretreatment with solubilized antigen, Transplantation **7:** 300, 1969.
11. Zabriskie, J. B.: The relationship of streptococcal cross-reactive antigens to rheumatic fever, Transplant. Proc. **1:** 968, 1969.
12. Zabriskie, J. B., and Freimer, G.: An immunological relationship between Group A streptococcus and mammalian muscle, J. Exp. Med. **124:** 661, 1966.
13. Zabriskie, J. B., Read, S., Ellis, R., Markowitz, A., and Rapaport, F.: Studies in human and experimental renal transplantation, Transplant. Proc. **4:** 259, 1972.

DISCUSSION

Dr. Richard E. Wilson (Boston, Mass.). Is there an antibody against the cardiac muscle in the animals into which you put the transplant?

Dr. Robert J. Ellis (closing). The slide that I showed demonstrating the immunofluorescence was from the group that were pretreated, demonstrating no antibody. The group that served as the control demonstrated that intense staining pattern.

Prolongation of rat cardiac allograft survival by a new immunosuppressant: Chicken anti–rat lymphocyte globulin

R. E. Morris, B.A., S. G. Souther, M.D., E. Dong, Jr., M.D., L. M. Vistnes, M.D., *and* **N. E. Shumway, M.D.,** *Stanford, Calif.*

Chickens were immunized with lymphocytes either syngeneic or allogeneic to cardiac donor strain rats to elicit preparations of either "donor-specific" or "donor-nonspecific" chicken anti–rat lymphocyte globulin (CARLG). Both preparations were effective in prolonging the survival of Buffalo or Brown Norway hearts in Lewis recipients ($p < 0.01$), indicating that specific anti-donor alloantibody is not required for the immunosuppressive effects of CARLG. These data eliminate classical allo-specific immunological enhancement as a mode of action of CARLG. CARLG also differs in its mode of immunosuppressive actions from heterologous mammalian ALG in that: (1) CARLG is not cytotoxic to rat lymphocytes using rat serum as a complement source; (2) CARLG does not opsonize lymphocytes; (3) CARLG produces neither peripheral lymphopenia nor central lymphoid depletion; (4) CARLG does not depress the primary humoral response; (5) CARLG is not a nonspecific anti-inflammatory agent; (6) CARLG does not suppress the delayed hypersensitivity response to human red blood cells. These findings suggest that CARLG is a unique immunosuppressant. The mechanisms of action responsible for its immunosuppressive effects differ from those of both allo-specific immunological enhancement and heterologous mammalian ALG.

From the Department of Cardiovascular Surgery and Division of Plastic and Reconstructive Surgery, Department of Surgery, Stanford University School of Medicine, Stanford, Calif.

FREEDOM FROM rejection in human allograft recipients without concomitant predisposition to infections and neoplasms has been only partially achieved with the current nonspecific immunosuppressants. Moreover, it is generally considered that limits are being reached in the expertise required to manipulate these immunosuppressants more effectively. Application of passive immunological enhancement to attain prolongation of survival of rat kidney allografts has introduced a modality that specifically suppresses allograft rejection.[7, 23] There are several possible reasons why there has been neither prevalent use nor convincing clinical application of this concept. (1) The rejection of rodent kidney allografts is comparatively easy to suppress.[5, 27] The privileged nature of this system is aided by the prevalent use of semi-allogeneic donors.[3, 23] (2) Allograft enhancement by whole, unmodified rat alloantibody may be used without risk of hyperacute rejection. This may be related to the relatively ineffective fixation of rat complement by rat alloantibody binding to the donor organ.[8] (3) The production of homologous donor-

Supported by research grants from the National Heart and Lung Institute (HL 08696), and National Institutes of Health Medical Scientist Training Program Grant GM 01922.

Presented at the Thirty-fifth Annual Meeting of the Society of University Surgeons, St. Louis, Mo., Feb. 14-16, 1974.

Reprint requests: R. E. Morris, Department of Cardiovascular Surgery, A206, Stanford University Medical Center, Stanford, Calif. 94305.

specific alloantibodies required for immunological enhancement, so easily obtained with inbred strains of rats, would be difficult in an outbred human population whose transplantation antigens are incompletely delineated, and where serious logistic and ethical considerations exist concerning the source and availability of such antibodies.

This report introduces chicken anti–rat lymphocyte globulin (CARLG) as a new heterologous immunosuppressant that appears to inhibit specifically allograft rejection. Evidence is presented that: (1) significant prolongation of survival of Buffalo and Brown Norway cardiac allografts to Lewis recipients is achieved with CARLG; (2) specific anti-donor alloantibody is not required for immunosuppression by CARLG; (3) CARLG neither binds rat complement nor has the same mechanisms of action as heterologous mammalian ALG (HMALG); (4) CARLG apparently suppresses specifically only the graft rejection reaction. These unique features of CARLG may provide direct clinical application previously not possible with other specific immunosuppressants.

METHODS AND MATERIALS

Animals. Male Lewis (LEW; AgB^1), Buffalo (BUF; AgB^6), and Fischer rats (180 to 210 grams) were obtained from Simonsen Laboratories, Gilroy, Calif. Brown Norway (BN; AgB^3) rats were purchased from Microbiological Associates, Inc., Walkersville, Md.

Transplantation and evaluation of graft function. Heterotopic (abdominal) transplantation of BUF or BN hearts into LEW recipients essentially followed the microvascular technique of Ono and Lindsey.[19] Cardiac function after transplant was evaluated daily by either palpation or electrocardiographic activity. Complete rejection was operationally defined as the first day on which ECG activity was isoelectric.

Globulin preparations. CARLG was prepared by injecting 1 to 2 × 10^8 lymph node lymphocytes from BUF, LEW, or BN rats intravenously into adult White Leghorn roosters on days 0, 14, and 21. The roosters were fasted for 48 hours prior to exsanguination on day 28. The plasma was decomplemented for 30 minutes at 56° C., absorbed with rat erythrocytes, subjected to two 40 percent $(NH_4)_2SO_4$ precipitations, dialyzed against phosphate-buffered saline, adjusted to a gamma globulin content of 25 mg. per milliliter, and stored at –70° C. After thawing, the CARLG was prepared for use by ultracentrifugation and Millipore filtration. The composition of the CARLG was 80 percent gamma and 20 percent beta globulin. Unless stated otherwise, the CARLG was always administered intravenously and whenever doses are reported, they refer to milligrams of gamma globulin per kilogram. The above purification steps were followed during the preparation of normal chicken globulin (NCG) obtained from unimmunized chickens. Rabbit anti–rat lymphocyte globulin (RARLG, Lot No. 13163) and normal rabbit globulin (NRG) were purchased from Microbiological Associates. Horse anti–rat thymocyte gamma globulin (HARTGG) was a gift from Upjohn, Kalamazoo, Mich.

Assays of antibody activity. Hemagglutination (HA) and an antibody-mediated cytotoxicity assay with ^{51}Cr release were performed by standard techniques.[12] The mixed agglutination assay (MAT) was performed essentially as originally described.[9]

Lymphocyte opsonization assay. LEW lymph node lymphocytes were prepared and labeled with $Na_2{}^{51}CrO_4$ (New England Nuclear, Boston, Mass.) essentially as described by Heslop and Hardy.[10] The labeled, washed lymphocytes were then dispersed at a concentration of 10^8 lymphocytes per milliliter in Eagle's Minimum Essential Medium (MEM) into tubes containing 0.5 mg. per milliliter final concentration of either RARLG, NRG, CARLG, or NCG and incubated for 30 minutes at 37° C. These cells were washed three times in MEM and 5 × 10^7 of the variously treated lymphocytes were injected intravenously into each of the LEW rats in the four groups (five rats per group). Four hours after injection all rats were exsanguinated and the livers and spleens were removed. The relative amounts of ac-

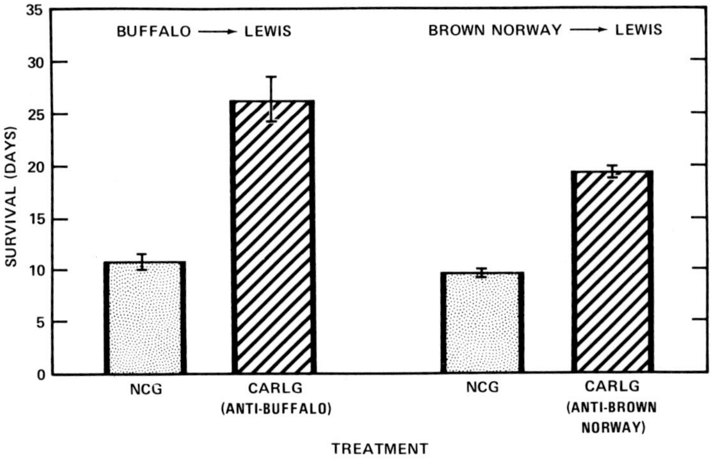

Fig. 1. Prolongation of rat cardiac allograft survival by "anti-donor" CARLG (group means ± S.E.). Recipients were treated with CARLG made with lymphocytes syngeneic to the cardiac donor strain.

tivity were determined in a Gamma Counter (Picker Auto Gamma II). Liver:spleen ^{51}Cr uptake ratios were derived by dividing the counts per minute in the liver by the counts per minute in the spleen for each rat.

Hematological and histological studies. Total white blood cell counts from tail vein blood were determined by a Coulter Counter and the absolute lymphocyte count derived from Wright-Giemsa–stained smears. Tissues for histology were fixed in 10 percent buffered formalin and the sections stained with hematoxylin and eosin.

Humoral response to sheep red blood cells (SRBC). Five groups of LEW rats, with from four to eight LEW rats per group, were studied. All rats in each group were injected intraperitoneally on days –3, –2, and –1 with either various globulin preparations or saline. On day 0, all rats received a 1 ml. intraperitoneal injection of 10 percent washed SRBC in normal saline. On day +7, all rats were bled and the serum was titered for anti-SRBC HA activity.

Anti-inflammatory study. These studies were performed by Dr. E. M. Glenn at Upjohn by injecting 40 mg. per kilogram of either CARLG, NCG, or HARTGG into rats subcutaneously at 4:00 P.M. and at 8:00 A.M. Carrageenan (0.1 ml. of 0.5 percent solution in saline) was injected into the right hind paws of nine rats per dosage group; five hours later paws were removed and differences (in milligrams) between injected and noninjected paws were calculated as edema per 100 Gm. of final body weight.

Student's t test was used to determine statistically significant values in these studies.

RESULTS

Survival of cardiac allografts. Previous preliminary work demonstrated the efficacy of a two-week course of CARLG ("anti-BN") at a dose level of 60 to 120 mg. per kilogram on the prolongation of survival of rat renal allografts.[17] All recipients of cardiac allografts in this paper were treated daily for one week with 300 mg. per kilogram of CARLG. A subsequent dose-response study indicated that a dose of 175 mg. per kilogram was an equally effective immunosuppressant dose.[18] NCG-treated rats were also treated daily for one week at a dose of 175 mg. per kilogram. Fig. 1 illustrates significant ($P < 0.01$) prolongation of survival in both the BUF and BN to LEW combinations compared to NCG-treated controls (five to seven rats per group). Fig. 2 demonstrates that significant ($P < 0.01$) prolongation of survival of rat cardiac allografts (four to six rats per group) can be obtained by CARLG preparations that do not contain specific anti-donor alloantibodies. In addition, a preparation of "anti-BN" CARLG was rendered

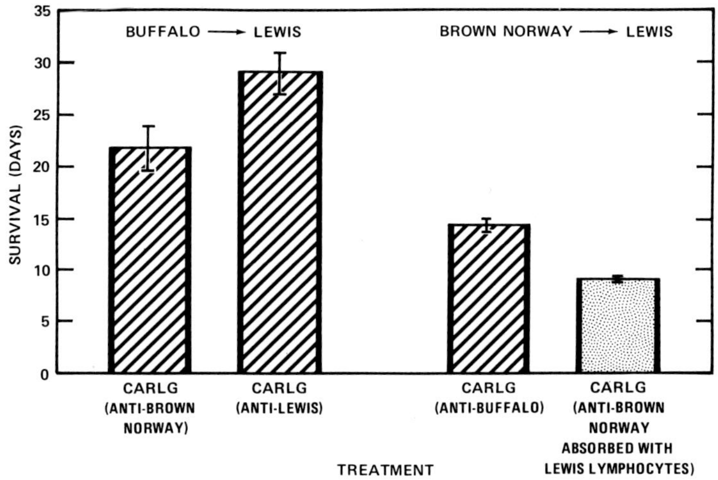

Fig. 2. Prolongation of rat cardiac allograft survival: No requirement for anti-donor alloantibody (group means ± S.E.). Recipients were treated with CARLG made with lymphocytes allogeneic to the cardiac donor. In one case, an "anti-donor" CARLG, absorbed with recipient membranes and cells, was rendered incapable of prolonging graft survival.

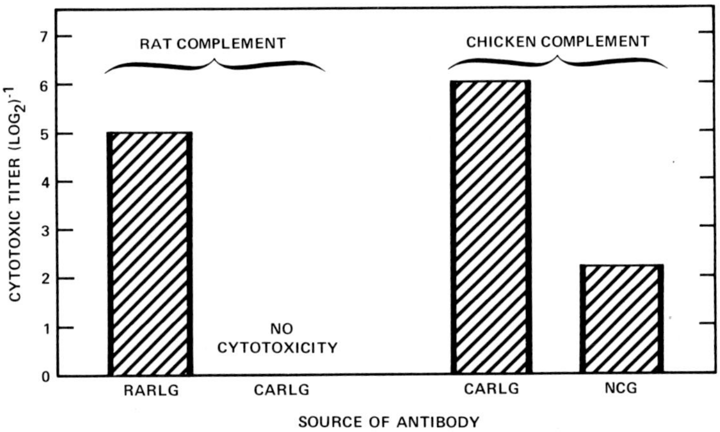

Fig. 3. Effect of the antibody source and the complement source on the cytotoxicity titer as quantitated by ^{51}Cr release from rat lymphocytes.

completely ineffective after it had been absorbed with cells from LEW lymph nodes and spleens as well as a LEW liver membrane preparation.

Antibody activity. Fig. 3 confirms other studies indicating that chicken antibody is incapable of binding mammalian complement.[20] In this case CARLG, which was cytotoxic to BN lymphocytes in the presence of chicken complement, lost all cytotoxic activity when rat serum was replaced as the complement source. Cytotoxicity mediated by RARLG and rat complement was included as a positive control for the source of rat complement.

Mixed agglutination titers were obtained for the one lot of RARLG used in all experiments as well as for all CARLG preparations. All samples were normalized to a concentration of 10 mg. per milliliter before beginning doubling dilutions. The RARLG MAT was 1:3,200 and 1:51,200 for CARLG. These values demonstrate the much higher specific activity of CARLG which should be considered when RARLG and CARLG are compared in the following studies.

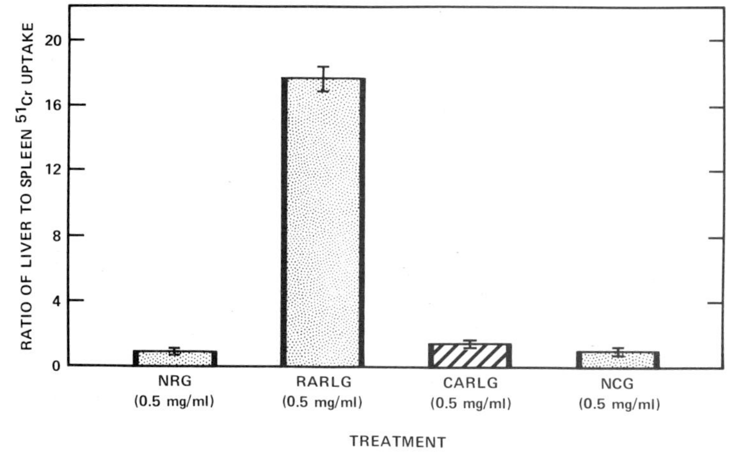

Fig. 4. Effect of preincubation with various globulin preparations on the subsequent in vivo distribution of ^{51}Cr labeled lymphocytes as quantitated by the liver to spleen ^{51}Cr uptake ratios (group means ± S.E.).

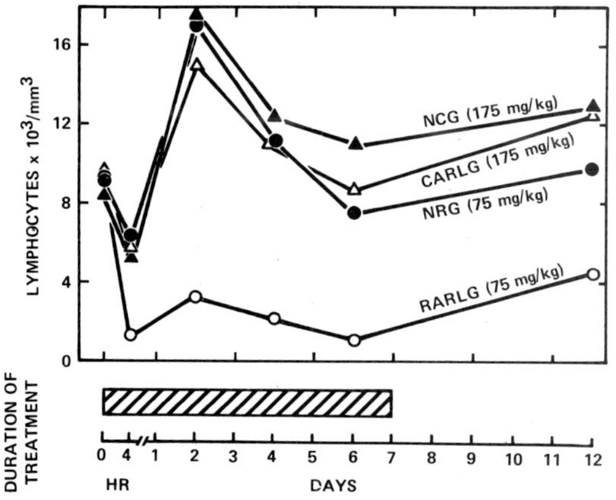

Fig. 5. Means of peripheral absolute lymphocyte counts for groups of rats treated with various globulin preparations.

Lymphocyte opsonization assay. This assay has been accurate in estimating the immunosuppressive potency of HMALG.[16] Fig. 4 illustrates that preincubation of lymphocytes with CARLG does not deviate lymphocytes to the liver to any greater degree than NRG or NCG, in contrast to RARLG. Neither CARLG nor the Fab fragments of rabbit anti–mouse lymphocyte globulin are effective opsonins because effective opsonization requires complement activation and/or a functional Fc piece.[2, 25]

Hematology and histology. Groups of Fischer rats (five rats per group) were treated with various globulin preparations daily for one week and their absolute lymphocyte counts followed. Fig. 5 illustrates the means of the absolute lymphocyte counts for each group. Two rats from each group were killed eight days after initiating treatment and lymph nodes and spleens were removed for histological examination. As expected, RARLG resulted in profound lymphopenia and depletion of the paracortical and periarteriolar areas of lymph nodes and spleens, respectively. However, since CARLG is unable to bind mammalian complement, no lymphopenia secondary to lymphocytotoxicity or opsonization can occur. For these reasons the peripheral lymphocyte levels in CARLG-treated rats did not differ from those in NCG- or NRG-treated animals. Histologic examination revealed neither lymph node paracortical nor splenic periarteriolar lymphoid depletion in CARLG-treated animals. Similar results have been obtained with antilymphocyte antibody fragments[1] and with duck anti–mouse lymphocyte serum.[24]

Primary humoral response. Consistent with the results of other studies,[4] pretreatment of rats with RARLG considerably impaired the primary response to SRBC (Fig. 6). This effect is believed to be subsequent to the elimination of thymus-derived (T) cells by the RARLG which are important collaborators in the primary antibody re-

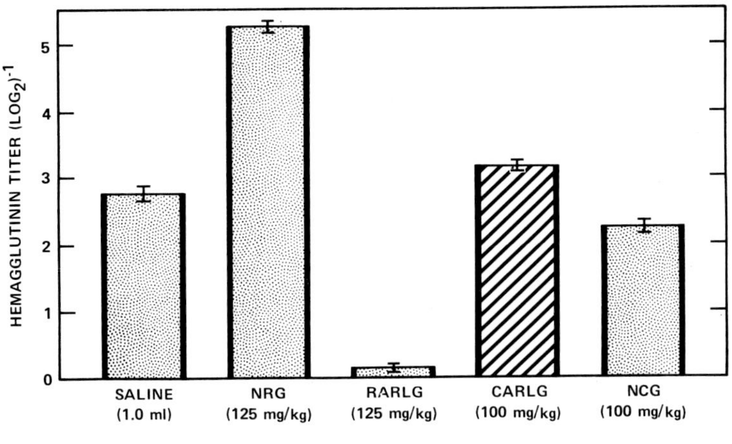

Fig. 6. Effect of pretreatment with saline and various globulin preparations on the primary antibody response to SRBC as quantitated by anti-SRBC HA titers (group means ± S.E.).

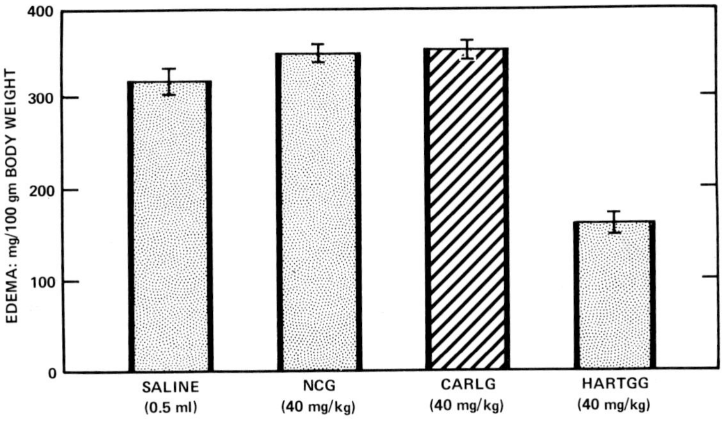

Fig. 7. Anti-inflammatory effects of saline and various globulin preparations as quantitated by hind paw edema values (group means ± S.E.).

sponse to a T-cell–dependent antigen.[15] Anti-SRBC HA titers of CARLG rats were not significantly reduced below saline and NCG control levels, suggesting that CARLG eliminates neither quantitatively nor functionally cells responsible for, or collaborating in, the primary humoral response to SRBC.

Anti-inflammatory effects. The anti-inflammatory effect of HMALG has been postulated by others as one of the nonspecific components comprising its immunosuppressive effects.[26] As illustrated in Fig. 7, the acute anti-inflammatory effect of HARTGG was not shared by CARLG.

DISCUSSION

Continued progress in the field of clinical organ transplantation demands the development of specific suppression of allograft rejection. The demonstration that survival of rat kidney allografts could be prolonged by passively administered homologous, specific anti-donor alloantibody has generated optimism regarding the clinical utility of specific immunological enhancement. However, because of the privileged nature of the initial experimental systems, direct human application has not been attained. Before specific immunological enhancement can be applied clinically, two criteria should be met. First, the availability of enhancing antibody should not be limited by ethical constraints or logistic problems inherent in the production of homologous antisera. Second, to avoid hyperacute rejection, the enhancing antibody must be incapable of activating the recipient's complement system. A source of heterologous, non–complement-binding antibody is required. The classical definition of immunological enhancement is "the enhanced or prolonged growth of allografts due to the presence in the graft recipient of alloantibody, directed against the specific alloantigens of the graft donor."[22] Therefore, to be an "enhancing antibody," the heterologous source must contain specific alloantibodies to all relevant donor alloantigens.[11]

Previous studies demonstrated the inability of chicken antibody to activate the mammalian complement system.[20] We originally hypothesized that CARLG might be an ideal source of heterologous enhancing antibody. Results from preliminary experiments substantiated this hypothesis.[17] CARLG made with BN lymphocytes as the immunogen produced survival of LBN F_1 hybrid or BN kidneys in LEW recipients. Prolongation of the survival of rat cardiac allografts is less easily achieved than rat renal allograft survival. In order to evaluate more critically the immunosuppressive capabilities of CARLG, the rat cardiac allograft model has been adopted. Significant prolongation of survival of BUF hearts in LEW rats was attained by recipient treatment with an "anti-BUF" CARLG. Similarly, an "anti-BN" CARLG significantly prolonged survival of BN hearts in LEW recipients. Moreover, "anti-BN" and "anti-LEW" CARLG resulted in significantly prolonged survival of BUF hearts in LEW recipients. Similarly, "anti-BUF" CARLG prolonged survival of BN hearts in LEW recipients. In vitro studies demonstrated that successive absorptions of "anti-BN" CARLG by LEW lymphocytes eliminated the antibody activity of the absorbed CARLG. This was assayed in a two-stage cytotoxicity test using BN lymphocytes and chicken complement.[18] In addition, when an "anti-BN" CARLG was absorbed extensively with LEW liver membranes and cells from LEW lymph nodes and spleens, its immunosuppressive effectiveness was abolished. It is clear from these results that CARLG does not rely on specific anti-donor alloantibodies for its immunosuppressive effects. Therefore, allo-specific immunological enhancement is not the mechanism of action of CARLG.

There are several clinical advantages associated with an immunosuppressant that does not rely on the presence of specific anti-donor alloantibodies, especially since the biological and genetic characteristics of human transplantation antigens are so poorly understood. However, the alloantigenic nonspecificity of current immunosuppressants is associated with undesirable side effects which are secondary to a nonspecific suppression of the immune response.

The mechanisms of action of HMALG are such that specific anti-donor alloantibodies are not required for the nonspecific depression of the immune response by HMALG.[13] It therefore becomes important to determine whether CARLG shares mechanisms of action similar to those of HMALG. Such studies would aid in the definition of the specificity of the suppression of the immune response by CARLG. It is believed that the immunosuppressive action of HMALG is due to depletion of circulating lymphocytes[14] by their opsonization and subsequent phagocytosis by the reticuloendothelial system (RE) of the liver.[25] These RE cells are able to phagocytose lymphocytes via a Fc receptor or a complement receptor once ALG has bound to the lymphocytes and activated the complement system. Direct lymphocytolysis by activation of the entire complement sequence also plays a role, although it is not essential.[2] The following characteristics of HMALG can be related to its mechanism of action. (1) HMALG requires a biologically active Fc piece to activate the recipient's complement system.[1, 2] (2) Secondary to opsonization, HMALG treatment results in a deviation of recirculating lymphocytes from lymphoid tissues to the liver as quantitated by increased liver:spleen ^{51}Cr lymphocyte ratios.[16] (3) HMALG produces profound lymphopenia and central lymphoid depletion.[24] (4) Reduction of recirculating lymphocytes by HMALG reduces the primary antibody response to "T-cell–dependent" antigens such as SRBC.[4, 15] (5) For several reasons, including possibly complement consumption and antagonism to certain pharmacologic mediators, HMALG demonstrates anti-inflammatory activity.[26] (6) The depression of delayed hypersensitivity responses by HMALG is most probably due to its lymphopenic and anti-inflammatory effects.[6]

The data presented here indicate that: (1) CARLG does not activate rat complement in an antibody-mediated lymphocytotoxicity assay; (2) CARLG does not redistribute lymphocytes from lymphoid tissues to the liver as measured by liver:spleen ^{51}Cr lymphocyte uptake ratios; (3) CARLG produces neither peripheral lymphopenia nor central lymphoid depletion; (4) CARLG does not reduce the primary humoral response to SRBC; (5) CARLG is not an anti-inflammatory agent as evidenced by its inability to suppress an inflammatory response induced by carrageenan. Recent experiments demonstrate that RARLG (100 mg. per kilogram) abrogates the delayed hypersensitivity response to human red blood cells, while CARLG (200 mg. per kilogram) does not.[18] We conclude that the immunosuppressive effects of CARLG cannot be due to the same mechanisms of action responsible for immunosuppression by HMALG.

This report has demonstrated that CARLG is a unique immunosuppressant. Its mechanisms of action can be differentiated both from allo-specific immunological enhancement and HMALG. It does not rely on specific anti-donor alloantibodies for its immunosuppressive effects, yet its immunosuppressive actions appear at this time to be limited to the allograft rejection reaction. Ongoing investigations will allow us to define more accurately the specificity of action of CARLG and to formulate hypotheses concerning its mechanisms of action.

We wish to acknowledge the technical assistance of Miss Geraldine Holland and Edward So and the helpful discussion of this manuscript with Dr. Lyle David.

REFERENCES

1. Anderson, N. F., James, K., and Woodruff, M. F. A.: Effect of antilymphocytic antibody and antibody fragments on skin-homograft survival and the blood-lymphocyte count in rats, Lancet **1:** 1126, 1967.
2. Barth, R. F., and Carroll, G. F.: Immunosuppressive effects of antilymphocyte serum in complement-deficient mice: Evidence that immune cytolysis is not essential for ALS activity, J. Immunol. **104:** 522, 1970.
3. Batchelor, J. R., Fabre, J., and Morris, P. J.: Passive enhancement of kidney allografts. Potentiation with antithymocyte serum, Transplantation **13:** 610, 1972.
4. Baum, J., Liebermann, G., and Frenkel, P.: The effect of immunologically induced lymphopenia on antibody formation, J. Immunol. **102:** 187, 1969.
5. Corry, R. J., Winn, H. J., and Russell, P. S.: Heart transplantation in congenic strains of mice, Transplant. Proc. **5:** 733, 1973.
6. Flax, M. H., and Waksman, B. H.: Delayed cutaneous reactions in the rat, J. Immunol. **89:** 496, 1962.
7. French, M. E., and Batchelor, J. R.: Immunological enhancement of rat kidney grafts, Lancet **2:** 1103, 1969.
8. French, M. E.: The early effects of alloantibody and complement on rat kidney allografts, Transplantation **13:** 447, 1972.
9. Gozzo, J. J., Wood, M. L., Pompei, R., and Monaco, A. P.: A new in vitro assay for immunosuppressive potency of antilymphocyte serum, Transplant. Proc. **4:** 481, 1972.
10. Heslop, B. F., and Hardy, B. E.: The distribution of ^{51}Cr-labelled syngeneic and allogeneic lymph node cells in the rat, Transplantation **11:** 128, 1971.
11. Jeekel, J. J., McKenzie, I. F. C., and Winn, H. J.: Immunological enhancement of skin grafts in the mouse, J. Immunol. **108:** 1017, 1972.
12. Kaliss, N.: Micromethod for assaying immune cytolysis by the release of ^{51}Cr, Transplantation **8:** 526, 1969.
13. Lance, E. M.: The selective action of antilymphocyte serum on recirculating lymphocytes: A review of the evidence and alternatives, Clin. Exp. Immunol. **6:** 789, 1970.
14. Lance, E. M.: The effects of chronic ALS administration in mice, *in* Dausset, J., Hamburger, J., and Mathé, G., editors: Advance in transplantation, Copenhagen, 1968, Ejnar Munksgaard Forlag, p. 107.
15. Martin, W. J., and Miller, J. F. A. P.: Cell

to cell interaction in the immune response. IV. Site of action of antilymphocyte globulin, J. Exp. Med. **128:** 855, 1969.
16. Miller, W. J.: Assay for the immunosuppressive capacity of antilymphocyte serum. II. Nature and specificity of opsonizing antibody, J. Immunol. **103:** 990, 1969.
17. Morris, R. E., Enomoto, K., Kay, G. L., Dong, E., Jr., and Shumway, N. E.: Prolongation of rat renal allograft survival by chicken antirat lymphocyte globulin, Transplant. Proc. **5:** 535, 1973.
18. Morris, R. E.: Unpublished results.
19. Ono, K., and Lindsey, E. S.: Improved technique of heart transplantation in rats, J. Thorac. Cardiovasc. Surg. **57:** 225, 1969.
20. Rose, E. M., and Orlans, E.: Fowl antibody. III. Its hemolytic activity with complements of various species and some properties of fowl complement, Immunology **5:** 633, 1962.
21. Shaipanich, T., Vanwijck, R. R., Kim, J., Lukl, P., Busch, G. J., and Wilson, R. E.: Enhancement of rat renal allografts with $F(ab')_2$ fragment of donor-specific antikidney serum, Surgery **70:** 113, 1971.
22. Snell, G. D.: Immunologic enhancement, Surg. Gynecol. Obstet. **130:** 1109, 1970.
23. Stuart, F. P., Saitoh, T., Fitch, F. W., and Spargo, B. H.: Immunologic enhancement of renal allografts in the rat, Surgery **64:** 17, 1968.
24. Taub, R. N., and Lance, E. M.: Histopathological effects in mice of heterologous antilymphocyte serum, J. Exp. Med. **128:** 1281, 1968.
25. Tyler, R. W., Everett, N. B., and Schwarz, R. M.: Effect of antilymphocyte serum on rat lymphocytes, J. Immunol. **102:** 179, 1969.
26. Turk, J. L.: Pathological effects and mode of action of antilymphocyte serum treatment, Fed. Proc. **29:** 136, 1970.
27. van Bekkum, D. W., Heystek, G. A., and Marquet, R. L.: Effects of immunosuppressive treatment on rejection of heart allografts in rats, Transplantation **8:** 678, 1969.

DISCUSSION

Dr. Joshua Miller (St. Louis Park, Minn.). A few years ago we did demonstrate in a heterologous system in mice that ALG did appear to have an enhancing, or antidonor, specificity if you slanted your experiment in the right direction. I am not sure that you can rule out this possibility with the experiments that you presented, because it is difficult for a widely dispersed species to be able to pick up donor antigens, to be sure. Just the fact that you have antispecies antibodies may well be protecting your graft, since it is neovascularized, and perhaps other things, that may cause antibodies to stick to it. This may well be one of the mechanisms of ALG reaction. We certainly cannot as yet correlate in vitro functions of ALG with its in vivo functions.

I am not sure either that the fact that you do not demonstrate complement dependency in the systems that you use means that chicken ALG cannot utilize mammalian complement. Perhaps through alternative pathways—you have to slant your experiments in order to be able to absolutely rule these things out. When you make a negative statement, it is difficult to say that it might not occur under some circumstances. And it may well be that perhaps the poor utilization of mammalian complement may be a beneficial effect in the use of differing antilymphocyte globulin or antirat globulin, because then if antibodies do stick onto your graft, it might not be destroyed as rapidly.

President Kountz. Is the chicken unique in the phylogenetic kingdom in that it does not produce an antibody that does not activate complement?

Dr. Nicholas A. Halasz (San Diego, Calif.). Have you looked at all at chicken anti–other-than-lymphocyte antibody—in other words, chicken antimuscle, or antikidney antibody—to see whether a similar effect was obtained? You are basically postulating that this is not antilymphocyte directed antibody, and maybe the chicken produces some peculiar antibody, not complement, or partly independent of complement, that has this peculiar effect you describe.

Dr. G. Melville Williams (Baltimore, Md.). Looking at the blocking factors that can be present in serum raises whole new questions about what may be the most significant histocompatibility situation in experimental animals and man. For example, if one looks at blocking in microcytotoxicity assays—the material that Dr. Parks presented yesterday—one could not make any sense out of why a transplant serum with known specificity to recipient and donor should actually block some microcytotoxicity reactions. These reactions, also by typing, should not have been blocked by a particular serum; yet the serum was not nonspecific. In other words, it did not block all reactions. It blocked some: two out of five.

We go from that type of specificity, which we do not understand in HL-A terms, to the IRA, which is utterly nonspecific, to the type of factors that Dr. Miller and his group have been describing, which also have specificity, but perhaps are not always explained on the basis of HL-A compatibility. I wonder if you could enlarge on what your ideas are on how this works, because I think this is a very important area of transplant immunology now.

Dr. R. E. Morris (closing). Some work reported at Federation meetings a few years ago showed that the C-1 fragment of mammalian complement was the component that was incapable of binding to the FC fragment of chicken—ALG or chicken—globulin. If these investigators were able to bind the chicken C-1 component to the chicken immunoglobulin, the rest of the complement sequence derived from mammals was able to become activated.

We have done successive absorption studies using the two-stage cytotoxic test to determine whether or not there was any residual cytotoxic activity, for example, in a chicken anti–Brown Norway ALG after absorption with Lewis lymphocytes titered against Brown Norway lymphocytes. We were always unable to find any residual specific anti–Brown Norway activity.

A group in Michigan has injected chickens with soluble H-2 purified antigens, and have been able to determine that the chicken was unable to produce a specific anti-H-2 antibody. They again did this by absorption studies.

Many persons here are familiar with the fact that other animals, such as rabbits, are able to produce specific anti-HL-A antibodies if injected with purified HL-A antigen. The fact that the chicken does not produce antibodies of alloantigenic specificity may be due to the phylogenetic distance of the chicken from mammals.

When I say it is not alloantigen specific, I do not mean that it may be completely nonspecific, but there may be an overlap in the antibodies produced. In other words, they may be overlapping both species and alloantigens in their specificity.

We produced serum only against lymphocytes, and there are some planned attempts in our laboratory to produce it against heart extracts to determine whether or not the importance of organ specific antigens would perhaps augment its immunosuppressive effect.

Work has been done with the duck, and that has been shown to be incapable of binding mammalian complement. In fact, some of the studies that were presented here with this chicken ALG were done by Lance, in which he looked for the ability of duck ALG to suppress the peripheral lymphocyte count and destroy the peripheral lymphoid tissue. His results were similar to those detailed in this report.

Dr. Williams' question is most difficult to answer. When I mentioned mechanism of action, I was referring to the mechanism of action of blocking of cellular immunity, rather than humoral immunity. There is a big difference. I believe that the cellular immune response is basically a carrier-dependent response, rather than a hapten-dependent response. I think if we look at transplantation antigens as a combination of carrier and hapten, wherein the species backbone of the antigen is the carrier, and the amino acid sequences peculiar to that particular strain or person are the haptens, then we can get an idea of how the chicken ALG works, if it in itself is a carrier-specific antibody. This presupposes that T-cells, which are the initiators of graft rejection, are carrier specific. If you can develop an antibody that is anticarrier, then you may be able to block the T-cell mediation of rejection. However, if it is anticarrier, it does not necessarily block the haptenic groups on the transplantation antigen, which is what you are talking about in a humoral immune response. The previous work in enhancement has mainly been involved with an antihapten antibody, because the enhancing antibodies are produced homologously. In other words, it has been rat anti–rat, and a rat is not going to produce an anti–rat-species antibody. It will produce anti-AGB^1 or AGB^2, which will then block the rejection response when given passively in a rat renal allograft system.

Effects of pulmonary embolism on regional myocardial blood flow

H. Newland Oldham, Jr., M.D., Jimmy L. Cox, M.D., Harvey I. Pass, B.A., Andrew S. Wechsler, M.D., *and* **David C. Sabiston, Jr., M.D.,** *Durham, N. C.*

The effects of autologous pulmonary embolism and pulmonary artery constriction on regional myocardial blood flow and ventricular hemodynamics were evaluated in 15 trained, awake, spontaneously breathing dogs. RV and LV myocardial blood flows were measured by 8 to 10μ radioactive microspheres. Tension-time index and minute work were calculated for each ventricle to indicate hemodynamic load. Control measurements were compared with those obtained following pulmonary artery constriction and after pulmonary embolism at equal levels of increased afterload. Arterial blood pressure, heart rate, and arterial Po_2 were unchanged throughout the study. Control RV myocardial flow averaged 59 percent of LV myocardial flow. Both pulmonary artery constriction and embolism produced a twofold increase in blood flow to the RV myocardium without corresponding changes in LV myocardial flow. Indices of RV hemodynamic load significantly increased during constriction and embolism without changes in LV values. Both interventions were accompanied by parallel decreases in RV coronary vascular resistance. These data indicate that the compensated RV responds to increased regional work load following either pulmonary artery constriction or pulmonary embolism by local autoregulation producing an increase in RV myocardial blood flow independent of LV hemodynamics or myocardial blood flow.

From the Department of Surgery, Duke University Medical Center, Durham, N. C.

ACUTE PULMONARY embolism may produce profound changes in systemic, pulmonary, and coronary hemodynamics with resultant effects on cardiac performance. Myocardial ischemia has been incriminated as one of the consequences of pulmonary embolism and was originally proposed by Virchow[26] as a cause of sudden death following pulmonary embolism. The mechanism later postulated was that of a pulmonocoronary reflex that decreased coronary blood flow by spasm or constriction of the coronary vessels.[7] Experimental efforts to document the presence of such a reflex have been largely unsuccessful, and most recent studies have reported coronary vasodilatation in response to pulmonary embolism.[12, 15, 21, 23-25] Explanations offered for this coronary vasodilatation have included hypoxemia, tachycardia, increased myocardial oxygen requirements, and reflex changes secondary to pulmonary embolism. Attempts to differentiate the effects of experimental emboli on right ventricular (RV) and left ventricular (LV) myocardial blood flow have produced equally conflicting results. It is difficult to compare data in published reports due to differences in animal

Supported by National Institutes of Health Grant HL 09315.

Presented at the Thirty-fifth Annual Meeting of the Society of University Surgeons, St. Louis, Mo., Feb. 14-16, 1974.

Reprint address: H. Newland Oldham, Jr., M.D., Department of Surgery, Duke University Medical Center, Durham, N. C. 27710.

models, changes in hemodynamic determinants of coronary blood flow, and variations in anesthetic agents. The conclusions also have been influenced by the different techniques used for measurement of coronary artery inflow, coronary sinus outflow, or myocardial blood flow, and the various materials and methods used to produce experimental pulmonary emboli.

The present study was designed to control the known systemic determinants of myocardial blood flow and to compare the effects of pulmonary embolism and pulmonary artery constriction on regional myocardial blood flow and ventricular hemodynamic changes. Intact, awake animals were utilized and the experiment was performed during a compensated state following sublethal autologous embolism, rather than during a state of circulatory collapse following massive embolism.

METHODS

Studies were performed in 15 awake, trained dogs weighing between 16 and 22 kilograms. Approximately three weeks prior to study, a sterile left thoracotomy was performed on each animal with sodium pentobarbital anesthesia. Polyethylene catheters were inserted into the left atrium and RV. Pacing wires were sutured to the right atrium and an adjustable occluding snare was positioned around the main pulmonary artery. The opposite end of each of these devices was secured in a subcutaneous position for later use. After recovery, each animal was trained to lie quietly for several hours on a padded table while breathing 100 percent oxygen from a clear plastic head tent. The day prior to study, all catheter tips and wires were exposed with the use of local anesthesia. An additional catheter was inserted into the femoral artery, and 100 ml. of autologous blood were removed for thrombus formation. The jugular vein was isolated and cannulated with a large-bore connector and all incisions were closed. On the day of the final study, each dog was given 15 mg. of morphine sulfate intravenously, one and a half hours before the experiment. The incisions were reopened without local anesthesia and the catheters and wires extracted and connected. The animals were fully conscious and spontaneously breathed 100 percent oxygen throughout the study. During the remaining approximately two hours of the procedure, most animals were calm and seemingly unaffected by the interventions, including pulmonary embolism.

Regional and transmural myocardial blood flows were quantitated with suspensions of radioactive microspheres, 8 to 10 μ in diameter, labeled with 141-cerium, 51-chromium, 85-strontium, or 46-scandium.[8] Between 400,000 and 800,000 microspheres were injected through the left atrial catheter for each measurement of blood flow. Constant withdrawal of femoral artery blood for two minutes beginning immediately prior to microsphere injection provided a reference sample allowing calculation of myocardial blood flow in milliliters per 100 Gm. per minute.[4] After all interventions were completed, each animal was killed and the heart and lungs were removed. Full-thickness samples of the free wall of the LV and RV were excised and trimmed and each sample was divided into an outer half or subepicardial layer and an inner half or subendocardial layer. Samples of blood and myocardium were analyzed for radioactivity in duplicate with a well scintillation counter, and appropriate corrections were made for overlaps of emitted radioactivity of each sample.[19]

Pulmonary emboli were prepared from autologous whole blood clots obtained from each animal 24 hours before the study. Blood was placed in a section of three-eighths inch diameter Tygon tubing and stored overnight. At the time of embolization, this tubing was connected to the jugular vein cannula for thrombus injection. Each animal received between 1.5 and 4 ml. per kilogram of autologous thrombus. After death the lungs were examined and the distribution of embolized material was recorded.

Measurements were obtained in each animal during four periods designated as control 1 (C1), snare (S), control 2 (C2), and pulmonary embolism (E). Data obtained included simultaneous recording of left atrial,

Table I. *Summary of results after pulmonary artery constriction and pulmonary embolism*

	First control period*	*Pulmonary artery constriction*	*Second control period*	*Pulmonary embolism*
Heart beats/min. (14)†	127 ± 8‡	133 ± 8	128 ± 6	136 ± 5
Mean aortic pressure, mm. Hg (14)	110 ± 3	114 ± 4	111 ± 4	116 ± 5
RV systolic pressure, mm. Hg (14)	37 ± 2	62 ± 2§	35 ± 2	56 ± 2§
RV diastolic pressure, mm. Hg (12)	2.8 ± 0.8	6.2 ± 0.7§	1.9 ± 0.6	5.8 ± 0.7§
RV/LV systolic pressure ratio (14)	0.25 ± 0.01	0.42 ± 0.02§	0.24 ± 0.01	0.37 ± 0.02§
pH, units (13)	7.37 ± 0.02	7.36 ± 0.03	7.34 ± 0.02	7.36 ± 0.03
Po_2, mm. Hg (13)	425 ± 24	406 ± 38	434 ± 28	427 ± 32
Pco_2, mm. Hg (13)	32 ± 2	31 ± 2	33 ± 2	33 ± 2
Cardiac output, L./min. (11)	3.8 ± 0.4	3.3 ± 0.3	3.9 ± 0.4	3.2 ± 0.3
LV blood flow, ml./100 Gm./min. (12)	113 ± 12	137 ± 8‖	115 ± 12	119 ± 9
RV blood flow, ml./100 Gm./min. (13)	65 ± 5	117 ± 10§	65 ± 6	110 ± 10§
RV/LV myocardial flow ratio (12)	0.59 ± 0.03	0.86 ± 0.07§	0.58 ± 0.06	0.94 ± 0.07§
LV endo/epi flow ratio (12)	1.22 ± 0.05	1.24 ± 0.04	1.19 ± 0.06	1.12 ± 0.05
RV endo/epi flow ratio (13)	1.10 ± 0.06	1.17 ± 0.05	1.14 ± 0.05	1.12 ± 0.05
LV TTI, mm. Hg sec./min. (12)	2,990 ± 200	2,840 ± 200	2,790 ± 200	2,870 ± 150
RV TTI, mm. Hg sec./min. (12)	525 ± 30	1,272 ± 69§	508 ± 31	1,221 ± 69§
RV/LV TTI ratio (12)	0.18 ± 0.01	0.47 ± 0.03§	0.19 ± 0.01	0.43 ± 0.03§
LV minute work, Kg. M./min. (11)	7.04 ± 0.78	6.18 ± 0.61	7.06 ± 0.76	6.08 ± 0.57
RV minute work, Kg. M./min. (11)	1.19 ± 0.16	1.95 ± 0.15§	1.22 ± 0.16	1.91 ± 0.17§
RV/LV minute work ratio (11)	0.17 ± 0.01	0.33 ± 0.01§	0.17 ± 0.01	0.32 ± 0.01§
RV coronary driving force, mm. Hg (11)	92 ± 4	83 ± 4	91 ± 4	86 ± 5
RV coronary vascular resistance, mm. Hg/ml./100 Gm./min. (11)	1.72 ± 0.16	1.03 ± 0.12§	1.70 ± 0.18	1.05 ± 0.11§

*Values obtained during the first control period did not differ statistically from those in the second control period.
†Number in parentheses indicates number of animals for that determination.
‡Values expressed as mean ± S.E.M.
§$P < 0.01$ compared to preceding control value.
‖$P < 0.05$ compared to preceding control value.

central aortic, and RV pressures and the ECG; determinations of arterial pH, Po_2, and Pco_2; measurements of cardiac output; and determinations of regional myocardial blood flow. Heart rate was controlled by electrical pacing at approximately 130 beats per minute for the entire study. After the first control measurements were obtained, the pulmonary artery was gradually constricted by the implanted snare, over a five-minute period, until a stable twofold increase in RV systolic pressure was reached. Repeat measurements were then obtained. Following release of the snare and a 20 minute period of stabilization, a second group of control measurements was made. Increments of autologous clot then were injected over a 5 to 10 minute period until a stable level of RV pressure was reached which approximated the RV systolic pressure produced by the previous pulmonary

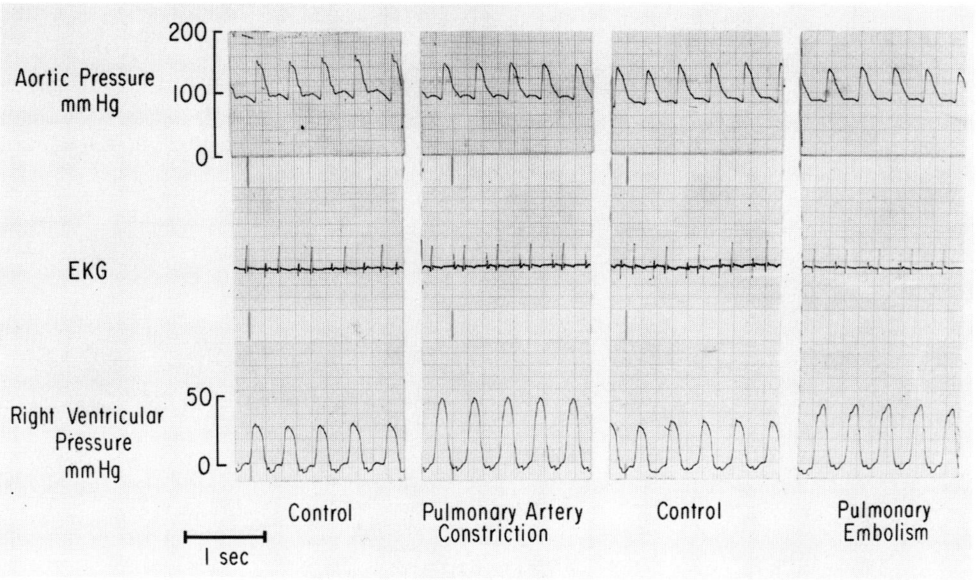

Fig. 1. Simultaneous recording of aortic blood pressure, ECG, and RV pressure during the control periods and following pulmonary artery constriction and pulmonary embolism.

artrey constriction. After an additional 10 minute period the final measurements were recorded.

Measured and calculated data for the four study periods were examined for statistically significant differences between the first control period vs. pulmonary artery constriction, the second control vs. pulmonary embolism, and the first vs. second control with Student's t test for paired data. The hemodynamic load for each ventricle was estimated by calculated values of tension-time index (mean systolic ventricular pressure × systolic time per minute) and minute work ([mean systolic ventricular pressure minus end diastolic or atrial pressure] × cardiac output × 0.0136). Cardiac output was determined by the indicator dilution method, using the average of two determinations. Coronary vascular resistance for the RV was calculated as the difference between mean aortic pressure and RV end-diastolic pressure, divided by RV myocardial blood flow. Coronary driving force for RV was measured as the mean difference between phasic recordings of aortic and RV pressure.[6] This value was derived once for each animal but multiple values were calculated from the formula: Driving force = mean aortic pressure − ½ RV systolic pressure. The average difference between the calculated and measured values of coronary driving force was 7 mm. Hg.

RESULTS

Data were obtained for analysis from 14 of the animals; one preparation was eliminated because of failure of the pulmonary artery snare. The measured and calculated values are summarized in Table I and the number of observations available for each determination is indicated. There were no statistically significant differences between any of the observations comparing the first and second control periods. The major changes noted following either pulmonary artery constriction or pulmonary embolism were significant alterations in RV hemodynamics and RV myocardial blood flow during a time of relative LV and systemic stability. Heart rate remained unchanged during pacing although pacing in some instances varied intermittently with respiration. Mean aortic pressure did not change and the ratio of RV/LV systolic pressure increased proportional to the increase in RV systolic pressure after pulmonary artery constriction or embolism (Fig. 1). During the interventions, no significant changes occurred in cardiac output or arterial pH, Po_2, or Pco_2.

Increased RV pressure from either pul-

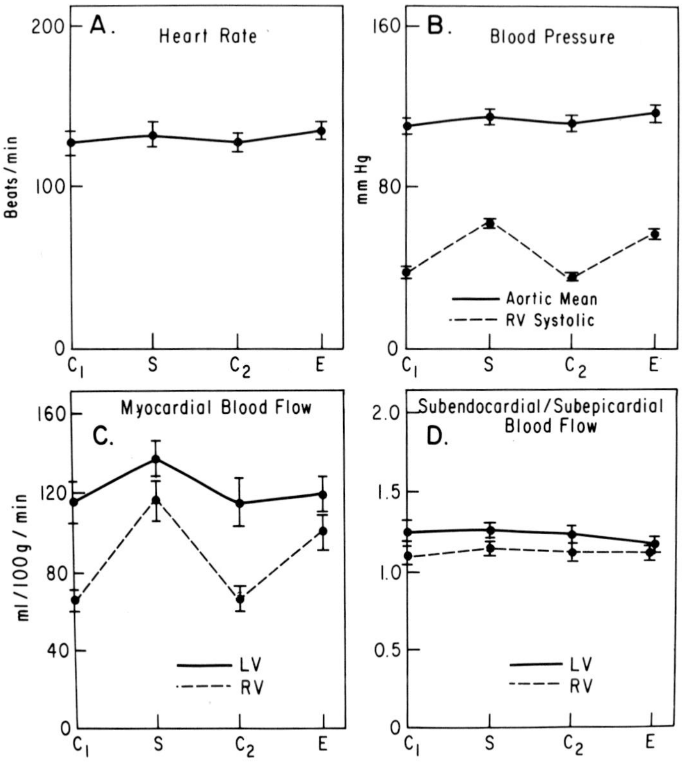

Fig. 2. *(A)* Changes in heart rate. *(B)* Aortic and RV blood pressure. *(C)* RV and LV myocardial blood flow. *(D)* Transmural distribution of RV and LV myocardial blood flow.

monary artery constriction or embolism was accompanied by a twofold increase in RV myocardial blood flow. At the same time there was a modest increase ($p < 0.05$) in LV myocardial blood flow during pulmonary artery constriction, but no significant change following embolism. Measurements of transmural distribution of myocardial blood flow indicated a slightly higher proportion of blood delivered to the subendocardial layer of both RV and LV during the control periods, which agrees with the distribution reported by Neill and associates[18] using similar methods in awake dogs. There was no significant change in transmural distribution of flow in either ventricle following constriction or embolism (Fig. 2). The absolute values of RV myocardial blood flow obtained during control, constriction, and embolism were related to the respective level of systolic RV pressure with a correlation coefficient of 0.68 (Fig. 3). Other comparisons included a similar correlation between RV flow and RV tension-time index (TTI) ($r = 0.62$), but a lesser degree of correlation between RV flow and RV minute work ($r = 0.43$). In each comparison, the changes between the first control and pulmonary artery constriction were of the same direction and magnitude as those between the second control and pulmonary embolism (Fig. 3).

Although systemic or LV hemodynamic and myocardial blood flow values were essentially unchanged throughout the experiment, there were variations between the individual measurements. The influences of these LV variations on RV function and blood flow were minimized by expressing the data as ratios of RV/LV. Examination of these data indicated that the closest correlation existed between the RV/LV TTI and the ratio of RV and LV systolic pressure ($r = 0.71$). Comparison of the changes in RV/LV myocardial blood flow and indices of ventricular hemodynamic load demonstrated parallel changes in RV/LV systolic pressure, RV/LV

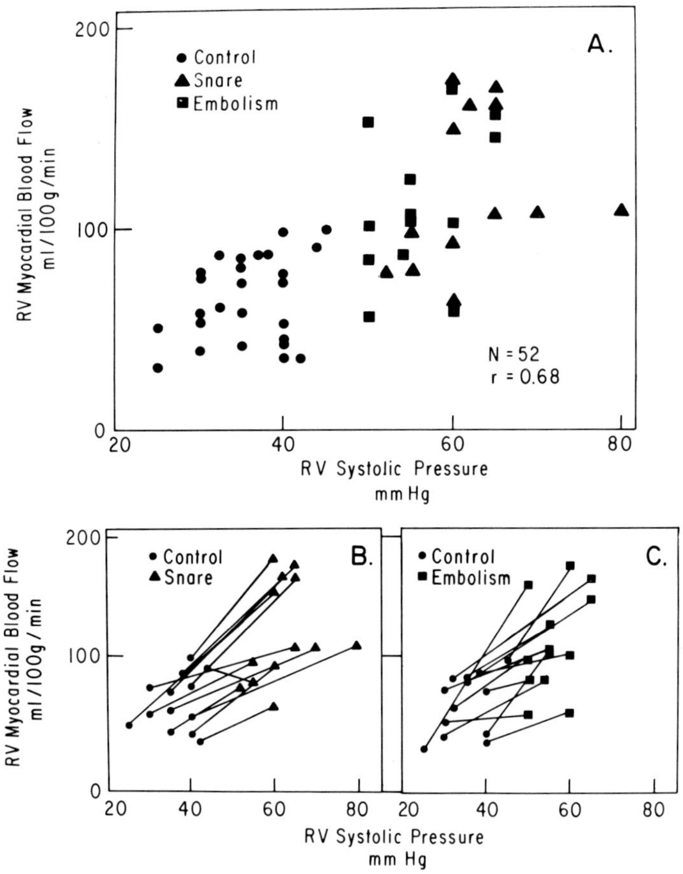

Fig. 3. *(A)* Comparison of RV myocardial blood flow and RV ventricular systolic pressure for all observations. *(B)* Changes in these values are indicated following pulmonary artery constriction. *(C)* Changes in these values after pulmonary embolism.

TTI, and RV/LV minute work following both pulmonary artery constriction and pulmonary embolism (Fig. 4).

Both pulmonary artery constriction and pulmonary embolism were accompanied by a significant increase in both the magnitude of RV systolic pressure and the duration of the RV systolic time interval. The average difference between the phasic recordings of aortic pressure and RV pressure was decreased by only 9 mm. Hg following constriction and 5 mm. following embolism (p = NS). These directional changes indicate a small reduction of coronary driving force, but the lack of statistical significance is primarily due to the absence of any changes in aortic blood pressure after constriction or embolism. In contrast, a significant decrease in the calculated values of coronary vascular resistance expressed in terms of RV myocardial blood flow was present following both pulmonary artery constriction and pulmonary embolism (Fig. 4).

Examination of the heart and lungs confirmed the presence of multiple large thrombi within the pulmonary arteries of each animal. These were located primarily in the main and first-order pulmonary arteries, with only a few fragmented smaller clots in the peripheral pulmonary vessels. Eleven of the 14 specimens had emboli in both right and left lungs and three were distributed unilaterally. In contrast to the stable systemic hemodynamics and arterial blood oxygen tensions observed during pulmonary embolism, the degree of pulmonary artery occlusion was rather ex-

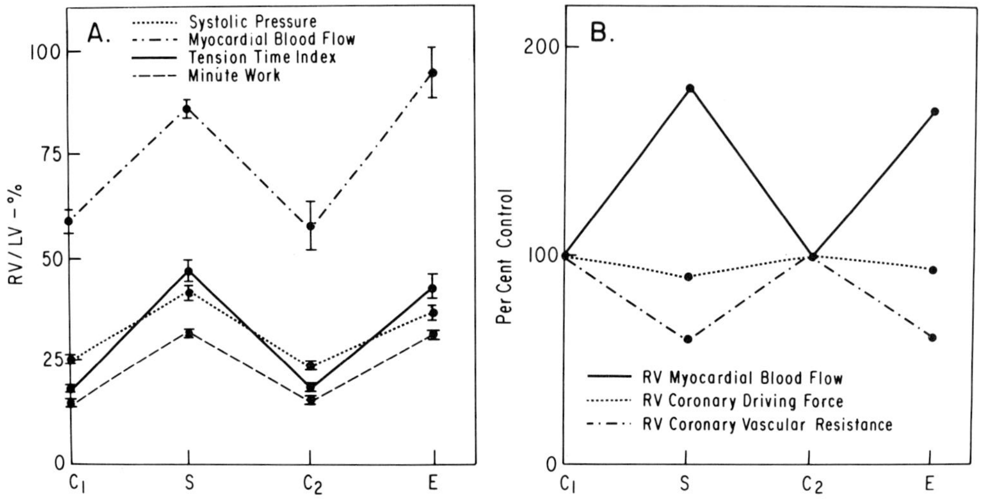

Fig. 4. *(A)* Changes in myocardial blood flow and indices of ventricular load with RV measurements expressed as percent of LV values. *(B)* Changes in RV myocardial blood flow, coronary driving force, and coronary vascular resistance expressed as percent of control measurements.

tensive, with an average of three totally obstructed lobar arteries and multiple arteries with partial occlusion present in each dog.

DISCUSSION

The major effects of acute pulmonary embolism in this experimental preparation were an increase in hemodynamic load on the RV and a proportional increase in RV myocardial blood flow. These observations were made during a stable period following autologous pulmonary embolization designed to increase the afterload on the right ventricle, but not to cause acute RV failure or cardiovascular collapse. In this setting there were surprisingly few systemic hemodynamic changes and no corresponding changes in left ventricular work load or myocardial blood flow. The response of the stressed but compensated RV to increasing regional myocardial demands was therefore local autoregulation of blood flow allowing an increase in myocardial oxygen delivery. The twofold increase in RV myocardial blood flow was delivered equally to the subendocardial and subepicardial layers with no evidence of relative underperfusion of the RV subendocardium. Although the elevated RV pressure tended to increase extravascular compression of the RV intramyocardial vessels, the measured right coronary driving force or difference between the aortic and RV pressure was not significantly reduced due to maintenance of a stable aortic pressure. The striking similarity between the changes produced by pulmonary artery constriction and pulmonary embolization indicated that the observations in this model were primarily in response to mechanical obstruction of the pulmonary artery rather than due to the effects of a humoral substance released from either the thrombus or lung tissue receiving the embolism.

Early experimental studies by Gregg[10] and by Katz and associates[14] concerning the effects of pulmonary artery constriction on coronary artery flow indicated that an increased RV load would decrease the driving force for the right coronary artery and also decrease its flow. Gregg and associates,[11] however, later demonstrated that an increase in RV work load could produce up to a 200 percent increase in right coronary artery inflow with only a small change in the left circumflex coronary artery inflow. Hackel and associates,[13] using the nitrous oxide coronary sinus technique, demonstrated no change in coronary outflow predominantly from the LV following experimental pulmonary embolism and concluded that there was no support for the so-called pulmono-coronary reflex. It became apparent that pulmonary artery constriction or pulmonary embolism might not produce the same changes in coronary flow to the RV and LV. The work of Love and O'Meallie,[15] using rubidium uptake, indicated a marked increase in RV myocardial flow with only a modest change in that of the LV following both pulmonary embolism and pulmonary artery constriction. Using a similar method of blood flow determination, Guzman and associates[12] showed an increase in myocardial blood flow in both ventricles. By measuring regional hydrogen clearance, Aukland and associates[1] reported that constriction of either the aorta or the pulmonary artery predominantly affected the respective ventricle and suggested that the concept of myocardial wall tension as a primary determinant of myocardial blood flow was valid for the RV as well as the LV. Their study also indicated that changes in RV geometry had little influence on RV blood flow in the absence of acute terminal dilatation.

A recent study performed by Fixler and associates[9] utilized radioactive microspheres to measure regional changes in myocardial blood flow following pulmonary artery obstruction. He concluded that mild increases in RV load were accompanied by an increase in myocardial blood flow, but that after a certain level of RV strain, no further vasodilatation occurred and myocardial flow was primarily determined by the coronary driving pressure. In his study, RV decompensation occurred at a relatively low level of RV hypertension, primarily due to a significant reduction in central aortic blood pressure. In a later report, using the same method, Monroe and associates[17] were able to show an almost linear relationship between increasing RV pressure and RV myocardial blood flow ($r = 0.78$), even at very high levels of RV pressure.

Bloor and associates[2] have recently emphasized the importance of using awake, trained animals in evaluating the hemodynamic changes following experimental pulmonary embolism and were able to produce significant changes in RV hemodynamics without the frequently observed tachycardia and hypotension. Vatner and Van Citters[25] subsequently reported a similar study performed in an awake dog model with chronically implanted flow probes and described an increase in left circumflex coronary artery inflow following pulmonary embolism. They noted that this increase in left coronary artery flow following an increase in RV pressure could have been due to the associated increase in heart rate or due to that portion of flow through the circumflex coronary artery supplying the canine RV.

It is important to emphasize the physiological sequences following an increase in RV afterload. The increased RV cavitary pressure is a primary determinant of RV wall tension and, therefore, of RV myocardial oxygen consumption. The local response to this increased load is one of autoregulation producing vasodilatation with an increase in myocardial blood flow. At the same time, this increase in wall tension increases the compressive force on intramyocardial vessels and increases extravascular resistance to flow or conversely decreases the coronary driving force. This resistance to flow becomes important only when the demands for increased blood flow exceed the limits of autoregulation. At this point, RV myocardial flow becomes proportional to the coronary driving force and thus may be influenced by changes in either the RV systolic pressure or the central aortic pressure. Caution must therefore be exercised in relating changes in RV myocardial flow to RV pressure unless the aortic pressure remains constant.

These concepts may be applicable to the clinical problem of RV failure following acute pulmonary embolism. Early work by Salisbury[20] and more recent experiments by Brooks and associates[3] and by Spotnitz and associates[22] have shown that when RV myocardial blood flow is limited, any increase in RV afterload is more likely to produce RV decompensation. Maneuvers that increase the driving force for the right coronary artery in this situation are capable of reversing this RV failure. Thus, pharmacologic agents that increase central aortic blood pressure with improvement of right coronary artery perfusion pressure may be effective in restoring the contracility of the RV. Conversely, agents that increase myocardial oxygen requirements or decrease systemic vascular resistance and aortic blood pressure may adversely influence RV performance. Spotnitz and associates[22] also reported the experimental use of counter-pulsation of the pulmonary artery as a means for reducing the systolic work load of the RV. The role of intra-aortic balloon pumping in the treatment of RV failure due to pulmonary emoblism has not been established. The diastolic augmentation produced by this form of circulatory assist would increase the driving force for RV myocardial blood flow, but the systolic unloading would reduce the important systolic component of RV myocardial blood flow. The net result of these two opposing influences in this setting has not been determined.

In conclusion, it should be emphasized that the present experiments were performed in dogs with normal hearts, capable of extreme degrees of coronary artery vasodilatation. While the majority of patients with pulmonary embolism do not have pre-existing cardiac disease, the response of those patients with prior cardiopulmonary involvement may well be different in view of evidence that such factors as coronary atherosclerosis or myocardial hypertrophy may limit the ability of the myocardium to increase its blood supply by autoregulation.[5, 16]

REFERENCES

1. Aukland, K., Kiil, F., and Kjekshus, J.: Relationship between ventricular pressures and right and left myocardial blood flow, Acta Physiol. Scand. **70:** 116, 1967.
2. Bloor, C. M., Sobel, B. E., and Henry, P. D.: Autologous pulmonary embolism in the intact, unanesthetized dog, J. Appl. Physiol. **29:** 670, 1970.
3. Brooks, H., Kirk, E. S., Vokonas, P. S., Urschel, C. W., and Sonnenblick, E. H.: Performance of the right ventricle under stress: Relation to right coronary flow, J. Clin. Invest. **50:** 2176, 1971.
4. Buckberg, G. D., Luck, J. C., Payne, B. D., Hoffman, J. I. E., Archie, J. P., and Fixler, D. E.: Some sources of error in measuring regional blood flow with radioactive microspheres, J. Appl. Physiol. **31:** 598, 1971.
5. Carlson, E. L., Cant, J. R., and Sparks, H. V.: Coronary blood flow of unanesthetized dogs with experimental coronary artery disease, Cardiovasc. Res. **7:** 789, 1973.
6. Cross, C. E.: Right ventricular pressure and coronary flow, Am. J. Physiol. **202:** 12, 1962.
7. Dack, S., Master, A. M., Horn, H., Grishman, A., and Field, L. E.: Acute coronary insufficiency due to pulmonary embolism, Am. J. Med. **7:** 464, 1949.
8. Domenech, R. J., Hoffman, J. I. E., Noble, M. I. M., Saunders, K. B., Henson, J. R., and Subijanto, S.: Total and regional coronary blood flow measured by radioactive microspheres in conscious and anesthetized dogs, Circ. Res. **25:** 581, 1969.
9. Fixler, D. E., Archie, J. P., Ullyot, D. J., Buckberg, G. D., and Hoffman, J. I. E.: Effects of acute right ventricular systolic hypertension on regional myocardial blood flow in anesthetized dogs, Am. Heart J. **85:** 491, 1973.
10. Gregg, D. E.: Phasic blood flow and its determinants in the right coronary artery, Am. J. Physiol. **119:** 580, 1937.
11. Gregg, D. E., Pritchard, W. H., Shipley, R. E., and Wearn, J. T.: Augmentation of blood flow in the coronary arteries with elevation of right ventricular pressure, Am. J. Physiol. **139:** 726, 1943.
12. Guzman, S. V., Chavez, F. R., and Imperial, E. S.: Myocardial blood flow after experimental pulmonary embolism in the intact dog, Am. Heart J. **68:** 66, 1964.
13. Hackel, D. B., Kinney, T. D., and Goodale, W. T.: Cardiovascular effects of pulmonary embolization in intact dogs studied by venous catheterization of the coronary sinus, Am. J. Physiol. **176:** 135, 1954.
14. Katz, L. N., Jochim, K., and Bohning, A.: The effect of the extravascular support of the ventricles on the flow in the coronary vessels, Am. J. Physiol. **122:** 236, 1938.
15. Love, W. D., and O'Meallie, L. P.: Increase in coronary blood flow to the right atrium and ventricle in response to an acute increase in hemodynamic load, J. Lab. Clin. Med. **62:** 72, 1963.
16. Marchetti, G. V., Merlo, L., Noseda, V., and Visioli, O.: Myocardial blood flow in experimental cardiac hypertrophy in dogs, Cardiovasc. Res. **7:** 519, 1973.
17. Monroe, G. A., Knapp, R. S., II, Fixler, D. E., and Mullins, C. B.: Effect of acute pulmonary arterial obseruction on right ventricular volume and coronary flow in closed chest, anesthetized dogs, Circulation **5-8** (Suppl. IV): 197, 1973.
18. Neill, W. A., Phelps, N. C., Oxendine, J. M.,

Mahler, D. J., and Sim, D. N.: Effect of heart rate on coronary blood flow distribution in dogs, Am. J. Cardiol. **32:** 306, 1972.
19. Rudolph, A. M., and Heymann, M. A.: Circulation of the fetus in utero; Methods for studying distribution of blood flow, cardiac output and organ blood flow, Circ. Res. **21:** 163, 1967.
20. Salisbury, P. F.: Coronary artery pressure and strength of right ventricular contraction, Circ. Res. **3:** 633, 1955.
21. Sharma, G. V. R. K., Wrenn, C. E., Godin, P. F., O'Neil, D. M., and Sasahara, A. A.: Regional and transmural myocardial blood flow distribution in experimental pulmonary embolism, Circulation **45-46** (Suppl. II): 57, 1972.
22. Spotnitz, H. M., Berman, M. A., and Epstein, S. E.: Pathophysiology and experimental treatment of acute pulmonary embolism, Am. Heart J. **82:** 511, 1971.
23. Stein, P. D., Alshabkhoun, S., Hawkins, H. F., Hyland, J. W., and Jarrett, C. E.: Right coronary blood flow in acute pulmonary embolism, Am. Heart J. **77:** 356, 1969.
24. Symbas, P. N., and Bonanno, J. A.: Coronary blood flow in acute experimental pulmonary embolization, J. Surg. Res. **10:** 377, 1970.
25. Vatner, S. F., and Van Citters, R. L.: Effects of acute pulmonary embolism on coronary dynamics in the conscious dog, Am. Heart J. **83:** 50, 1972.
26. Virchow, R.: *Quoted by* Dack et al.[7]

DISCUSSION

Dr. Paul Allen Ebert (New York, N. Y.). It is all local vascular or metabolic response because of its increased flow, because in chronic states, if you increase the pressure load of the ventricle, most likely you are going to decrease flow, for a period of time, anyway. I wondered if you had thought of looking at it from a flowmeter to see whether or not you can document this right ventricular increase in the right coronary artery? Also, have you had any ideas as to whether, if you measure coronary sinus metabolic changes to see whether or not you are really getting an increased oxygen uptake, an A/V difference? Or is this just increase in A/V shunt within the ventricle that might not be delivering the oxygen, actually, to where it is needed?

Dr. Alexander S. Geha (St. Louis, Mo.). These data are similar to our findings with normal and hypertrophied left ventricular myocardium with stress increasing the hemodynamic load. In our work in this area we have found that the normal myocardium in the left ventricle responds to an increased load by increasing its ventricular myocardial coronary flow, but also increases its oxygen extraction, while the hypertrophied myocardium extracts, basically, the maximum amount of oxygen at rest, and responds to further stressing by an increase in coronary flow only.

Have you looked at oxygen extraction data?

Dr. H. Newland Oldham, Jr. (closing). Dr. Ebert, our study indicates that the increase in RV myocardial flow is primarily a local response to increasing energy requirements. We documented the increase in right coronary artery flow using electromagnetic flow probes in preliminary acute experiments. The chronic animals reported today did not have implanted flow probes, but RV flow was measured by microspheres. Other investigations have demonstrated absence of AV shunting in a wide variety of hemodynamic situations by this method. Had we used electromagnetic flow determinations an increase could well have been due to shunting, but by the microsphere method the increase represents nutritional blood flow delivered to the RV myocardium. Other workers have directly measured the RV oxygen uptake by cannulating the anterior cardiac vein rather than the coronary sinus. They have demonstrated an RV oxygen uptake in situations of increased RV load.

Dr. Geha, your comments are pertinent as our model was the normal dog without myocardial hypertrophy. Both hypertrophy and coronary artery disease limit local autoregulation. It would seem indicated to extend our work to a preparation with chronic right ventricular hypertrophy, and to determine not only myocardial blood flow but also oxygen extraction, as you suggest. Most investigators in the past have stated that myocardial oxygen uptake is increased by augmenting blood flow rather than by an increasing oxygen extraction. Your findings are interesting, indicating that both mechanisms are utilized by the nonhypertrophied dog heart.

The training of surgeons: How many, in what, and by whom?

Leonard D. Miller, M.D., *Philadelphia, Pa.,* **William B. Saxbe, Jr., M.D., M.P.H.,** *Boston, Mass.,* **Edward F. X. Hughes, M.D., M.P.H.,** *New York, N. Y.,* **Richard M. Bergland, M.D.,** *Hershey, Pa.,* **James A. O'Neill, Jr., M.D.,** *Nashville, Tenn.,* **Mark M. Ravitch, M.D.,** *Pittsburgh, Pa.,* **Bruce Barton, M.S.,** *Pittsburgh, Pa.,* **Frank C. Spencer, M.D.,** *New York, N. Y., and* **Francis D. Moore, M.D.,** *Boston, Mass.*

Introduction

Leonard D. Miller, M.D., *Philadelphia, Pa.*

From the University of Pennsylvania School of Medicine, Philadelphia, Pa.

AT A MOMENT in this country's history when there is increasing concern about the inevitable conflicts, in individuals and institutions, between private interest and the public good, American surgeons are completing what is surely one of the most definitive and broadly based self-examinations ever undertaken by a learned profession—the Study on Surgical Services for the United States (SOSSUS). A portion of this Study is an analysis of surgical manpower needs and distributional requirements for the next several decades. Dr. Francis D. Moore, one of the contributors to this symposium, has chaired the SOSSUS Committee on Academic Manpower that has been examining these and other questions. Some data, by no means complete, from the SOSSUS Study are presented here by Drs. Moore, Saxbe, and O'Neill. To its credit, the need to take stock of surgical resources and capabilities, in relation to the societal needs and demands, arose and was nurtured among the surgical community itself. One must fervently hope that, if controls on the training of surgeons are deemed necessary, these will also be generated and implemented, voluntarily, by surgical educators, themselves, before impending Congressional action is taken.

The results of the SOSSUS Study, under the admirable leadership of Dr. George D. Zuidema, are beginning to emerge at a crucial but, in a sense, an inopportune time for change in academic surgical services. Among the many complicating factors that impinge on an orderly, balanced plan for the delivery of surgical training and service are a proportional reduction in Federal funds and the increasing reluctance of third-party insurers to support medical education; a concomitant sharp rise, in recent years, in the contribution from private-practice income that academic surgeons make to their departmental budgets —income that now comprises well over one quarter of the average department's resources; an annual influx of foreign medical graduates, with widely divergent educational and linguistic backgrounds, that has doubled or tripled since the decade ending in 1971; an estimate that approximately one out of seven budgeted surgical faculty positions, in medical schools, remain unfilled, while the number of incoming medical students continues to escalate; an increasing tendency, on the part of community hospitals, to seek the intellectual advantages of affiliation with academic medical centers. Clearly, diminished resources, coupled with competing demands for time, stand in contradistinction to the heightened public expectation of the best in surgical care as every citizen's right. In large

Presented at the Thirty-fifth Annual Meeting of the Society of University Surgeons, St. Louis, Mo., Feb. 14-16, 1974.

Reprint address: Leonard D. Miller, M.D., 3400 Spruce St., Philadelphia, Pa. 19104.

measure, these documented trends serve as a further tribute to the continued dedication of surgical scholars and educators. A judicious reorganization of surgical training will have economic, as well as pedagogic consequences, perhaps for the better. There are no simplistic answers to the questions posed in the title of this Symposium, but for the opportunity to further the discussion, in print, we express our appreciation to the Editors of SURGERY.

William B. Saxbe, Jr., M.D., M.P.H., is currently finishing his chief surgical residency under the aegis of the Harvard Medical School. He has been a consultant for the SOSSUS Committee on Academic Manpower. Dr. Saxbe has not only thought long and hard about the problem of distribution of surgical care, he plans to do something about it. Following his residency he will begin work at a hospital in Ohio that previously has been without a trained surgeon. His paper personifies the product of our teaching, the surgical resident, humanizing instead of itemizing him as another bit of data on a computer print-out. In a unique contribution, he deals with the general surgical trainee's background, training, workload, operative experience, finances, "moonlighting," motivation, plans, and opinions.

Edward F. X. Hughes, M.D., M.P.H., is currently Assistant Professor in the Department of Community Medicine at the Mount Sinai School of Medicine and Research Associate at the National Bureau of Economic Research in New York City. He has been a consultant to the SOSSUS Committee on Organization, Financing, and Delivery of Surgical Care. In previous publications Dr. Hughes and his colleagues[1, 2] coined the term "hernia equivalent" as an index of the volume and complexity of operative experience in a well-studied group of general surgical residents and in a group of community surgeons in actual practice. Both studies suggested that, at least in terms of operative workloads, per se, in the circumscribed populations examined, there is not optimal utilization of surgical talent. This paper complements his prior work, in terms of the patterns and numerical growth of surgical specialists, and what this portends for the future.

Richard M. Bergland, M.D., is Chief of the Division of Neurosurgery at the Pennsylvania State University, M. S. Hershey Medical Center, and Head of the Continuing Education Program at that institution. Dr. Bergland has been an outspoken proponent of individual departmental action to regulate the output and quality of training of neurosurgeons. In a recent paper article entitled "Neurosurgery may die," Dr. Bergland[3] stated, "Evolution, after all, is not a matter for committee action. It follows in the wake of individuals strong enough to swim from the certain doom of a stagnating sea." In his paper, he describes his "residency without residents" as one stimulating "do-it-yourself" way of approaching the problem of internal regulation.

James A. O'Neill, Jr., M.D., is Professor of Surgery and Head of the Division of Pediatric Surgery at Vanderbilt University. At about the time of the inception of the SOSSUS Study, the American Pediatric Surgical Association began a separate study of manpower needs in its own subspecialty. This became united, with Dr. O'Neill's representation, with SOSSUS in 1972. Since there are less than 300 or so pediatric surgeons in the United States, Dr. O'Neill's paper describes a model study of a more circumscribed population that gives us insight into one method of approach to the problem; in a sense, it is a "mini-SOSSUS" study.

Frank C. Spencer, M.D., is George David Stewart Professor and Chairman of the Department of Surgery at New York University. His paper concerns itself with the pivotal problem of how American Surgery can assert its own manpower controls, flexible enough to allow for changing needs and individual freedom before the Government imposes them upon us. He also addresses the question of the foreign medical graduate's role in American training programs.

Francis D. Moore, M.D., is Moseley Professor of Surgery at Harvard and is currently serving as Chairman of the SOSSUS Committee on Academic Manpower. His summary of some of the salient points of this symposium includes the perplexing problems of distribution of surgical care and the organizational steps that might be taken to initiate a reasonable internal regulatory plan.

It must be emphasized that this symposium is neither a sufficient preview nor, certainly, a substitute for the results of the SOSSUS Study which is yet to come. The conclusions drawn from these presentations are by no means the last word—in point of fact, they are among the first in what will inevitably be a continuing, long-term commitment to answer the questions raised in the title thoughtfully enough to accommodate the best interests of the young surgeon and the community he or she serves. If these papers enhance the thinking process on these pressing, multifaceted problems, then the authors will consider their efforts eminently worthwhile.

REFERENCES

1. Hughes, E. F. X., Fuchs, V. R., Jacoby, J. E., and Lewit, E. M.: Surgical work loads in a community practice, SURGERY **71:** 315, 1972.
2. Hughes, E. F. X., Lewit, E. M., and Rand, E. H.: Operative work loads in one hospital's general surgical residency program, N. Engl. J. Med. **289:** 660, 1973.
3. Bergland, R. N.: Neurosurgery may die, N. Engl. J. Med. **288:** 1043, 1973.

The surgeon-in-training: A preview

William B. Saxbe, Jr., M.D., M.P.H., *Boston, Mass.*

From the West Roxbury VA Hospital, West Roxbury, Mass.

WITH THE BELIEF that the plans and opinions of the next generation of surgeons are crucial to the future of American surgery, a survey of surgical trainees was undertaken. The aim was to characterize them as to background, training, workload, operative experience, finances, moonlighting, motivation, plans, and opinions. This information provides a factual basis for rational planning as national needs for surgeons become clearer and mechanisms for coordination emerge.

An 80 item questionnaire was distributed to all of the surgical interns and residents in general surgery and the surgical specialties in 123 programs in 24 hospitals in 9 states. Table I gives the breakdown by specialty and the rates of response. The questionnaires were completed by 84 percent of the general surgical trainees and 63 percent of the surgical specialty residents. Responses were stratified, where appropriate, by specialty, year in training, hospital ownership, teaching status, region of the country, and whether the respondent was a foreign medical graduate (FMG). Table II gives the distribution of training programs by hospital ownership and teaching status.

The study has generated an enormous volume of data—approximately 2,000 tables on the first computer run, with some of the data yet to be processed. The purpose of this presentation is to give a small preliminary sampler of the data and to provide an idea of the questions asked and of the answers received.

Fig. 1 shows what type of internship was served by residents in the different specialties. The surprise here is the limited number of specialists who had straight surgical internships. We have similar data on the average length of general surgical residency which specialists had, ranging from less than a month for obstetric-gynecologic residents to 49 months for thoracic surgical residents.

Table III gives the composition of the average work week. The total ranged from 60 hours for ophthalmologists to 94 hours for surgical interns.

Table IV shows the average operative experience for the past year and indicates what proportion of the operations were done by the trainee, ranging from 27 percent in neurosurgery to 56 percent in thoracic surgery.

Table V shows how many trainees "moonlight," that is, seek outside employment to

Presented at the Thirty-fifth Annual Meeting of the Society of University Surgeons, St. Louis, Mo., Feb. 14-16, 1974.

Reprint address: William B. Saxbe, Jr., M.D., Department of Surgery, West Roxbury VA Hospital, West Roxbury, Mass. 02132.

Table I. *Sample population and responses*

Specialty	*No. of programs*	*No. of trainees*	*No. of responses*	*Percent of responses*
General surgery:	36	441	370	83.9
Interns	12	73	62	84.9
Residents	24	368	308	83.7
Surgical specialties:	87	641	404	63.0
Obstetrics-gynecology	14	164	84	51.2
Orthopedics	15	136	77	56.6
Neurosurgery	12	48	40	83.3
Ophthalmology	9	94	56	59.6
Thoracic surgery	9	27	18	66.7
Plastic surgery	8	24	22	91.6
Otolaryngology	8	68	49	72.1
Urology	11	74	57	73.1
Colorectal surgery	1	2	1	50.0
Total	123	1,082	774	71.5

Table II. *Types of training programs*

	No.
Hospital ownership:	
Private	65
City/county	12
State	40
Federal	6
Teaching status:	
Teaching*	76
Nonteaching	47

*Medical undergraduates present as clinical clerks.

Table III. *Weekly workload*

	Hours per week (mean)	
	General surgery	*Specialties*
Direct inpatient care	55	38
Indirect inpatient care	13	9
Outpatient care	8	15
Research	1.6	1.9
Teaching—with patients	3.0	2.7
Being taught—with patients	4.9	3.3
Teaching—didactic	0.5	0.7
Being taught—didactic	3.4	3.6
Administrative work	0.6	0.8
Total hours per week	91.3 ± 23	75.3 ± 25
Independent study	8	10
Paramedical work	13	10
On call* (additional)	41	41
Duplicated work†	11	9

*Applies to 52 percent.
†Applies to 39 percent.

increase income. Specialties with a long work week show lower rates. Moonlighting correlates positively with debt and years in training but negatively with marriage and number of children. Trainees admit that moonlighting interferes with their sleep and their family life but generally deny that it interferes with their efficiency in their primary work or their academic effort.

By asking a number of questions about what factors were important to trainees in choosing a type or a place of practice we were able to group them roughly into one of four categories according to primary motive: service, profit, the amenities, or academic achievement (see Table VI). This is, of course, the softest of soft data, but we were able to use the groupings in examining the answers to questions about plans and attitudes.

Nearly all trainees (98 percent) plan to seek certification but relatively few (22 percent) are in the Candidate Group of the American College of Surgeons.

Table VII shows how trainees expect to practice in the future. There is no major departure from present patterns of practice and the number of men interested in prepaid group practice (sometimes represented as the wave of the future) is quite small.

We asked: "Have financial considerations played a major role in your professional plans (type and location of residency and future

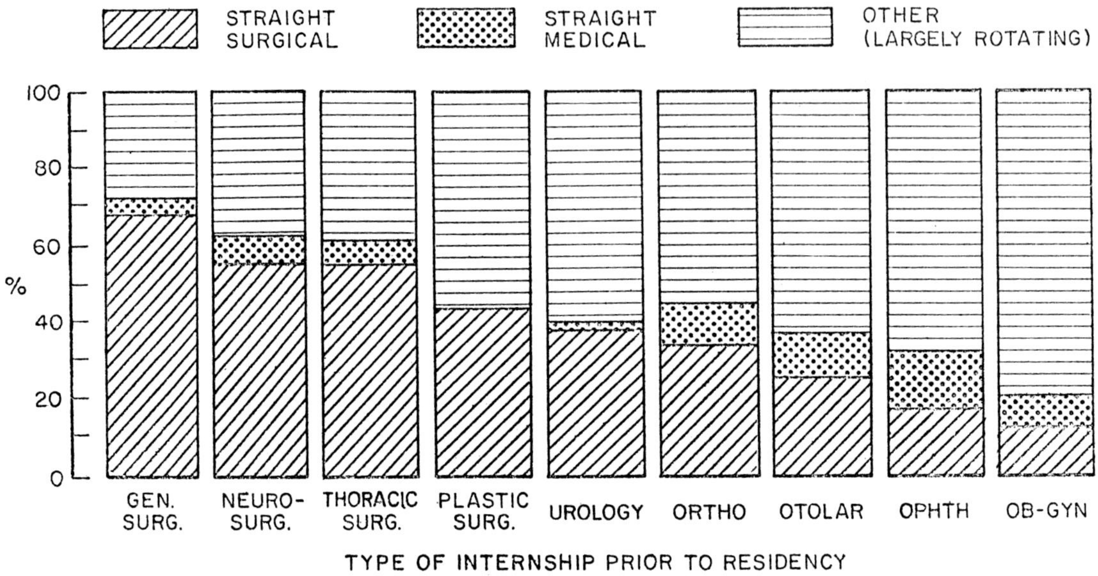

Fig. 1. Type of internship served. (Nonrespondents and those who served no internship omitted.)

Table IV. *Operative record for past year*

	Surg.	*Ob.-Gyn.*	*Ortho.*	*Neuro.*	*Ophth.*	*Thor.*	*Plast.*	*Otol.*	*Urol.*	*Mean*
As surgeon	89	113	106	54	57	162	195	118	104	90
As assistant	165	109	210	148	90	134	166	161	144	145
Total	254	222	316	202	147	296	361	289	248	235
Percent as surgeon	35.0	50.9	34.8	26.7	38.8	55.7	54.0	40.8	41.9	38.3

Table V. *Moonlighting*

	Yes		*No*	
	No.	*%*	*No.*	*%*
Intern	2	3.3	59	96.7
General surgery	102	33.4	203	66.6
Obstetrics-gynecology	46	56.8	35	43.2
Orthopedics	39	50.6	38	49.4
Neurosurgery	13	32.5	27	67.5
Ophthalmology	27	49.1	28	50.9
Thoracic	3	17.6	14	82.4
Plastic	9	40.9	13	59.1
Otolaryngology	25	54.3	21	45.7
Urology	33	58.9	23	41.1
Total	300	39.4	461	60.6

practice)?" Table VIII gives the responses: 76 percent said "no."

Similarly, we asked: "Have financial considerations caused you to defer marriage or children?" Table IX shows the answers: 74 percent said "no."

Table VI. *Primary motive*

	No.	*Percent*
Service	240	38.9
Profit	26	4.2
Amenities	108	17.5
Academic	34	5.5
Mixed	209	33.9
Total	617	100.0

Table VII. *Plans for type of practice*

	No.	*Percent*
Partnership	363	48.5
Fee-for-service group practice	140	18.7
Full-time teaching hospital	108	14.4
Solo	76	10.2
Prepaid group practice	16	2.1
Full-time nonteaching hospital	12	1.6
Government	5	0.7
Other	28	3.7
Total	748	100.0

Table VIII. *Effect of financial considerations on professional plans: Have financial considerations played a major role in your professional plans (type and location of residency and future practice)?*

	No.	Percent
Yes	189	24.5
No	581	75.5
Total	770	100.0

Table IX. *Effect of financial considerations on personal plans: Have financial considerations caused you to defer:*

	No.	Percent
Marriage	22	2.9
Children	140	18.4
Both	37	4.9
Neither	560	73.8
Total	759	100.0

Table X. *Present plans for location of practice*

	General surgery		Surgical specialties		Total	
	No.	%	No.	%	No.	%
Yes	251	67.8	300	74.3	551	71.2
No	119	32.2	104	25.7	223	28.8
Total	370	100	404	100	774	100

Table XI. *Present supply of surgeons in planned locality of practice*

	General surgery		Surgical specialties		Total	
	No.	%	No.	%	No.	%
Inadequate	62	24.7	94	31.3	156	28.2
About right	63	25.1	110	36.7	173	31.3
In excess	62	24.7	41	13.7	103	18.7
Don't know	64	25.5	55	18.3	119	21.6
Total	251	100.0	300	100.0	551	100.0

Table XII. *AMG/FMG vs. citizenship*

	AMG		FMG	
Citizenship	No.	%	No.	%
U. S. A.	664	99.7	13	12.1
Canada			8	7.5
Latin America			14	13.1
Europe	2	0.3	21	19.6
Mid-East			8	7.5
India/Pakistan/Ceylon			17	15.9
East Asia			21	19.6
Africa			2	1.9
Australia/New Zealand			3	2.8
Total	666		107	

Table XIII. *FMG plans for future location of practice*

	No.	%
United States	33	30.6
Home country	32	29.6
Uncertain	36	33.3
No reply	7	6.7
Total	108	100.0

Trainees were asked if they had in mind a site for eventual practice: a surprising 71 percent already did (Table X). Even more surprising is their information about the current supply of surgeons in their specialty in that site (Table XI): 75 percent of general surgical trainees, for example, are considering practice in a location where they may not be needed at this time, though age and population factors always make this a "soft" judgment.

Table XII gives the nationality and country of medical education of all trainees. A few American medical graduates are foreign citizens; a considerably larger group of FMG's are American citizens (12 percent). Table XIII shows where FMG's plan to go on completion of their training.

A large amount of information about the past, present, and future of surgeons-in-training has been compiled. At this stage it consists of an inventory rather than a blueprint for the future, but it gives us the means to make reasonable statements about the nature of surgical training and reasonable plans for its improvement. Much more extensive analysis of the data is required.

Among the very many conclusions which the resultant data permit are: (1) nearly all trainees plan to seek certification; (2) financial considerations play a relatively minor role in personal and professional plans; (3) the choice of a place for practice is largely independent of that place's need for a surgeon; and (4) the proportion of trainees whose primary motivation is academic is quite small.

The demand for surgical residents: Some preliminary observations

Edward F. X. Hughes, M.D., M.P.H.,
New York, N. Y.

From the Department of Community Medicine, Mount Sinai School of Medicine of the City University of New York, and the National Bureau of Economic Research, New York, N. Y.

THE INCREASINGLY articulated inability of Americans to gain access to primary care in the face of both substantial governmental support for the training of physicians and the escalating costs of health care is causing policy makers to look seriously at the process whereby future physicians are being trained.[12] Simultaneously, a trend that has distinguished American medicine in its quest for quality over the last quarter century—the thrust toward specialization—is being perceived, in its present dimensions, as contrary to the health needs of the American people. As a result, incentive systems specific to the production of primary-care physicians are being explored and considerable thought is being directed toward possible regulation of both the number and the specialty distribution of residents. The factors contributing to the trend toward specialization are multiple and complex. I would like to focus in a pre-

Supported by a United States Public Health Service research grant (5 PO1 HS 00451) from the Bureau of Health Services Research and Evaluation and Health Career Scientist Award No. 1786 from the Health Research Council of the City of New York.

The findings reported herein have not yet undergone the full critical review accorded the National Bureau's studies, including review by the Board of Directors.

Presented at the Thirty-fifth Annual Meeting of the Society of University Surgeons, St. Louis, Mo., Feb. 14-16, 1974.

Reprint address: Edward F. X. Hughes, M.D., National Bureau of Economic Research, 261 Madison Ave., New York, N. Y. 10016.

Table I. *Growth rates of approved residency positions offered by various specialties in the United States by selected intervals, 1940-73* (continuously compounded per annum)*

Residency positions offered	*Interval*			
	1940-50	*1950-60*	*1960-66*	*1966-73*
All surgical specialties:	13.9	4.8	3.0	3.2
General surgery	16.3	4.4	2.3	2.3
Neurosurgery	17.6	7.2	4.5	3.8
Obstetrics-gynecology	12.9	5.8	1.1†	2.4
Ophthalmology	11.9	4.6	5.9	4.1
Orthopedic surgery	13.9	4.6	4.6	6.1
Otolaryngology	4.3	2.8	7.5	4.4
Plastic surgery	20.5	10.8	7.8	8.4
Thoracic surgery	12.0	8.9	5.1	1.6
Urology	13.7	3.8	3.3	3.1
Colon and rectal surgery	‡	7.2	−4.4	8.7†
Nonsurgical specialties§	13.6	6.5	3.7	4.9
Family practice‖	‡	17.3	1.0†	13.3
All specialties	13.8	5.8	3.5	3.5
Graduating M.D.'s	0.9	1.9	1.2	2.4

*In the following equation: $\ln P_t = a + bt$, where P_t = number of positions offered in year t, was fit to annual data by a linear regression. In this specification, the estimated b is the correct estimate of the continuously compounded growth rate per annum.

†Not significant at the 0.05 level by t test.

‡None in 1940.

§Hospital-based specialities only: does not include Aerospace Medicine, General Preventive Medicine, Occupational Medicine, and Public Health.

‖Includes general practice.

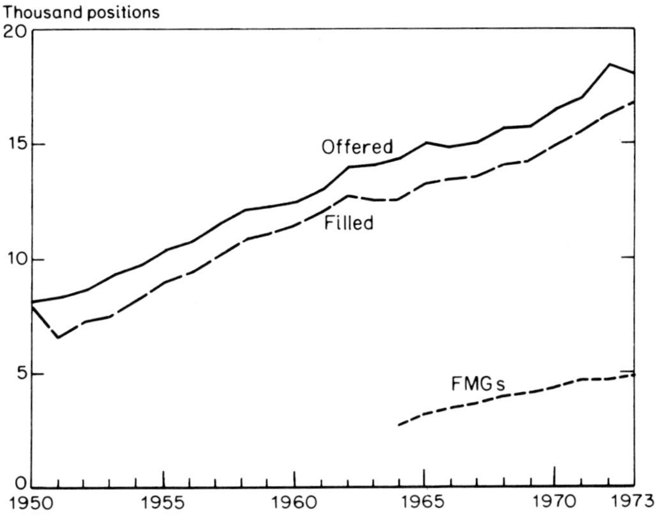

Fig. 1. Approved residency positions offered and filled by U. S. and Canadian medical graduates and FMG's, all surgical specialties, United States, 1950-1973. Data on the number of FMG's in approved residency programs by specialty were first published in 1964. Source: American Medical Association: Approved internships and residencies in the United States, J. A. M. A., annually 1950-1955; American Medical Association: Graduate medical education in the United States, J. A. M. A., annually 1956-1960, 1962; Nunemaker, J. C., Thompson, W. V., Adams, R. E., and Tracy, R.: Directory of approved internships and residencies, Chicago, 1961, American Medical Association; American Medical Association: Medical education in the United States, J. A. M. A., annually 1963-1969, 1971-1973; American Medical Association, Council on Medical Education: Unpublished 1970 data.

liminary fashion on one aspect of the trend toward specialization in surgery—the demand for surgical residents.

Since 1940, the quantity of surgical residents demanded in the United States—the number of approved surgical residency positions offered—has grown at a continuously compounded rate of 7 percent per annum and is now almost nine times what it was in 1940.* In that year, there were 2,030 approved surgical residency positions offered† and today there are 18,174.[2, 21] These surgical positions comprise 35.6 percent of all approved residency positions offered in the United States.[2] The period of most rapid growth in surgical positions offered occurred in the 1940's when they increased at a rate of 14 percent per annum (Table I). Both Pearse[16] and Rousselot[18] have commented on on the role of both World War II and the G.I. bill in contributing to this growth. Growth rates declined in the fifties to 5 percent per year and in the sixties to 3 percent a year. This decline is attributable in part to a growing base phenomenon, such that an increasing number of new positions must be added each year to maintain a steady growth rate. For example, almost the same number of new positions was added per year in the late sixties (414) as in the 1950's (431) even though the rate of growth in the sixties (2.6 percent per annum) was roughly half that of the fifties (4.8 percent per annum). Despite a decline of 376 positions offered in 1973, the mean number of new positions offered per year in the seventies has been 529, 28 percent in excess of the mean number of new positions offered in the previous four years. It remains to be seen whether the 1973

*Throughout this paper, growth rates are measured as continuously compounded rates per annum unless otherwise specified. These growth rates are estimated using annual data fit by linear regression to the equation: $\ln P_t = a + bt$, where P_t = number of positions offered in year t. In this specification, the estimated b is the correct estimate of the continuously compounded growth rate per annum.

†Figures include specialties of colon and rectal surgery, (general) surgery, neurological surgery, obstetrics and gynecology, ophthalmology, orthopedic surgery, otolaryngology, plastic surgery, thoracic surgery, and urology.

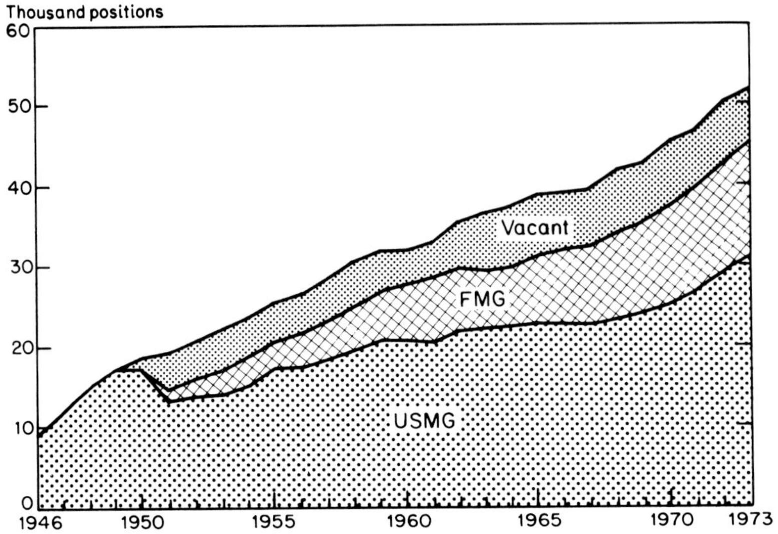

Fig. 2. Approved residency positions offered and filled by U. S. and Canadian medical graduates and FMG's, all specialties, United States, 1946-1973. Data on numbers of vacancies and FMG's were first recorded in 1950 and 1951, respectively. There is evidence to suggest that the relative magnitude of each was not large prior to those dates.[16, 22] Source: American Medical Association: Medical education in the United States 1972-73, J. A. M. A. **226:** 938, 1973.

decrease signals a reversal of or a transient deviation from the trend toward an increase in the mean number of positions offered per year (Fig. 1).

The problem of the growth of specialization in American medicine is by no means peculiar to surgery (Table I). Since the 1940's, nonsurgical positions offered have grown by 8 percent per annum and, in the last three years, grew at a rate of 6.2 percent per annum. At this latter rate, all nonsurgical positions offered would double in 11 years. Of note, the fastest growing nonsurgical specialty is family practice,* with a 1970's growth rate in positions offered of 32 percent per annum. The recent, rapid rise of this growth rate suggests that the availability of positions in a given specialty can be made responsive to society's perceived needs. The present growth rate in family practice notwithstanding, positions offered in that specialty now equal only 6 percent of all nonsurgical positions offered and residents in that specialty account for only 5 percent of nonsurgical residents.[2] Nonsurgical positions other than family practice have grown in the seventies at a rate of 4.9 percent per annum; continuing at this rate they would double in just over 14 years.

There is much discussion at present of a possible excess of surgeons in the United States (a subject in itself requiring considerable further research). It is important, however, that the corresponding growth of nonsurgical specialization be noted, lest attempts to regulate the number of residents by specialty focus disproportionately on a possible surgical overpopulation as opposed to a nonsurgical overpopulation. It is much easier to measure a paucity of hernia equivalents in the practice of a surgical specialist (or a surgical resident) than it is to assess the degree of underutilization entailed in a highly trained internist's treating the common cold and other ailments of low morbidity.[13, 14]

There has been considerable variation in the recent growth of individual surgical specialties. Since 1966, thoracic surgical positions, which had the second highest rate of growth in the 1950's, 9 percent per year, have had the lowest rate of growth, less than 2 percent per annum. General surgery has had the next lowest rate, with obstetrics and gynecology almost equal to general surgery; both

*Includes general practice.

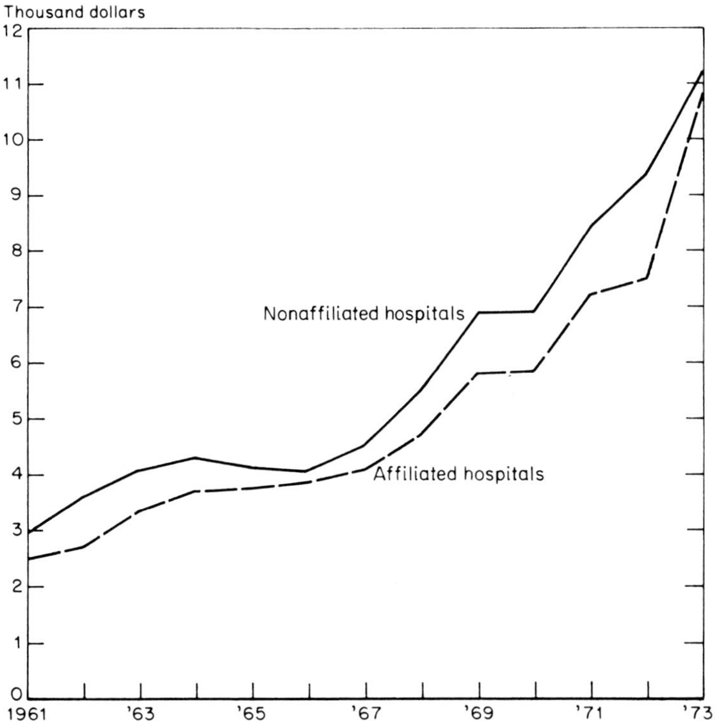

Fig. 3. Mean annual salaries offered residents in approved positions, all specialties, by hospital affiliation, 1961-1973. Source: American Medical Association: Medical education in the United States 1972-73, J. A. M. A. **226:** 930, 1973; American Medical Association: Medical education in the United States, J. A. M. A. **210:** 1505, 1969.

slightly greater than 2 percent. It would be interesting to know if the slower rates of growth of these three specialties bear any relationship to saturation (actual or surmised) in these areas. The growth of thoracic positions offered will be especially interesting to watch with regard to the ultimate determination of the efficacy of coronary bypass surgery. At the other end of the surgical spectrum lies plastic surgery, with a growth rate of 8 percent per annum since 1966 and of 11 percent in the last three years alone. Were the rate of this most recent three-year period to continue, plastic surgical positions offered would nearly double in six years. Orthopedic surgery has grown by 6 percent per annum since 1966; at this rate it would double its positions in 11 years. All other surgical specialties have grown by 3 to 4 percent since 1966 except colon and rectal surgery (which offers only 26 positions), which had a growth rate of 9 percent (not significant).

By way of contrast to this growth in the quantity of residents demanded, the population of the United States has grown, since 1940, at a rate of 1.4 percent per annum and United States medical graduates at a rate of 2.0 percent per annum.[1, 19, 20] The excess rate of growth of the quantity of all residents demanded and of all surgical residents demanded over the production of United States medical graduates has resulted in vacancy rates in all residency positions offered and in surgical positions offered that, since 1960, have averaged 17 and 10 percent per year, respectively, and are currently 12 and 8 percent, respectively (Figs. 1 and 2). This excess in demand would appear to be responsible, in large part, for the rapid growth in positions filled by foreign medical graduates (FMG's), who now occupy almost 27 percent of all residency positions filled and 29 percent of surgical residency positions filled.[2]

Evidence for the strength of this excess demand is found in the fact that, during the period 1966-1973, when positions offered in all specialties increased at 4.3 percent per

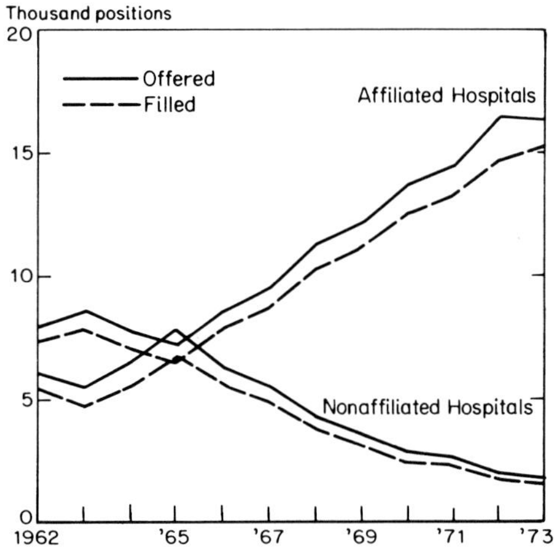

Fig. 4. Approved residency positions offered and filled by hospital affiliation, all surgical specilties, 1962-1973. Source: American Medical Association: Medical education in the United States, J. A. M. A., annually 1963-1969, 1971-1973; American Medical Association, Council on Medical Education: Unpublished 1970 data.

year, residents' mean salaries increased at 14.5 percent per year (Fig. 3).[5, 6] This increase was such that the mean salary offered residents doubled in less than five years to $10,880 in 1972-1973. This salary increase, long overdue from the perspective of residents, has three important ramifications. First, it increases the rate of return to specialization by reducing the foregone earnings that are associated with specialty training and constitute a major disincentive toward pursuing lengthy training. Second, it would appear that FMG's might be most influenced by this salary increase and their supply most sensitive to further increases. Third, this increase in salaries coincides temporally with and, in large part, would appear to be a result of federal subsidization of patient care through Medicare and Medicaid. If so, these salary increases are being financed indirectly by the Federal government. This is a point of crucial importance when it comes to the question of regulating the growth of specialization.

The subject of the demand for residents is highly complex and warrants in-depth study. A number of questions emerge at this time, however, upon which some preliminary light might be tentatively shed.

Why the growth in demand? Almost 10 years ago, Longmire,[15] in his seminal paper on graduate surgical training, noted some of the problems associated with the expansion of the supply of surgeons and the proliferation of residency positions. He stated: "One of the greatest paradoxes of our times is the overwhelming zeal of almost every surgeon to be a teacher. Practically every hospital of 200 beds or more in this country seems bent on having an approved surgical residency program. . . . Some training programs are initiated because of a sincere desire on the part of a number of staff surgeons to engage in teaching. Some programs are started for their 'prestige value' in the community, and some, unfortunately, merely to obtain the services of a group of residents to do the 'scut work'." The last of Longmire's reasons, the service contribution of residents to the care of patients of attending surgeons, not involving direct out-of-pocket expenses to these attendings, would appear in an equivocal situation to be of sufficient weight to propel the development, expansion, or, at the very least, maintenance of a surgical residency program. A potential mechanism for achieving a redistribution of residents among specialties, and still enabling the service tasks now associated with residency training to be accomplished, may lie in the utilization of paraprofessional health manpower in graduate education settings.[9, 11] To date, the utilization of paraprofessional manpower in ambulatory settings has been shown to increase physician productivity by as much as 40 to 75 percent.[17] Studies of the costs of and the quality of care implications in the use of such manpower in educational settings are warranted.

Where is the growth in the number of residency positions offered? Since 1962, the number of hospitals in the United States with approved residency programs has increased by 12.5 percent, a growth of slightly more than 1 percent per annum. In 1962, there were 1,366 such hospitals; in 1973, there were 1,562.[4, 7] In contrast to this modest growth in the number of hospitals offering approved

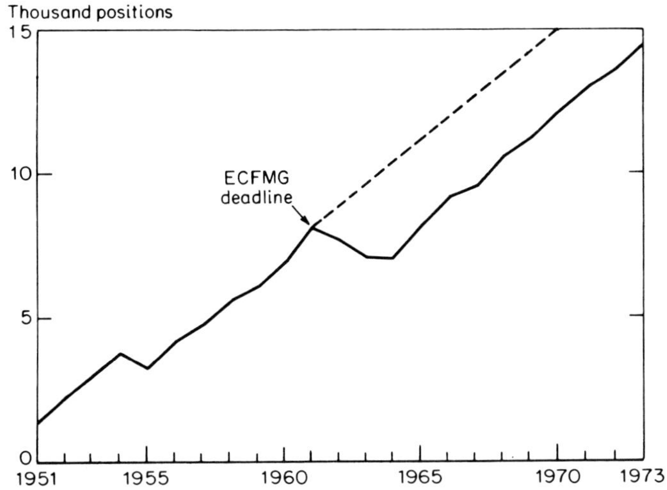

Fig. 5. FMG's in approved residency positions, all specialties, United States, 1951-1973. Source: American Medical Association: Medical education in the United States 1972-73, J. A. M. A. **226:** 938, 1973.

residency programs is a marked change in the affiliation status of these hospitals.

In 1962, 377 of the hospitals with approved programs were affiliated with academic medical centers and 989 were unaffiliated.[7] In 1973, however, the numbers were essentially reversed: 1,109 hospitals with approved programs were affiliated with academic medical centers and only 453 were unaffiliated.[4]

This trend toward academic affiliation by hospitals with approved programs is such that in 1973, 91 percent of all the 18,174 positions offered in the surgical specialties (16,487) were in affiliated hospitals and 93 percent of these were occupied (Fig. 4).[3]* Nine percent of all positions offered (1,687) were in nonaffiliated hospitals and 87 percent of these were filled. The significance of this trend toward affiliation is such that the overwhelming majority of surgical residency positions now offered are located in academic programs supervised by university surgeons. With only 9 percent of surgical residency positions in nonacademic hands, attempts to regulate positions offered will predominantly involve university personnel.

For every surgical position erased from the unaffiliated rolls since 1965, one and a half positions have appeared on the affiliated rolls.

*The same trend also exists in the nonsurgical specialties.

How has this growth occurred? Since 1965, the number of surgical affiliated programs has grown at a rate of 4.2 percent per annum and the number of positions per affiliated surgical program has grown by 6.4 percent per annum. Thus it would appear that the growth in surgical positions in affiliated hospitals is a result of: (1) the affiliation of previously unaffiliated and of new programs, (2) the creation of new programs in affiliated institutions, and (3) the expansion of existing affiliated programs.

The trend toward affiliation is complex. It has undoubtedly been hastened by policy recommendations and the behavior of accrediting agencies.[8] Cohn has also discussed the benefits, as well as the costs, entailed in an academic surgical program's affiliating with a previously unaffiliated institution.[10] The temporal coincidence of this trend with both availability of federal funds and rise in residents' salaries is worth noting (Figs. 3 and 4). This coincidence, without an obvious explanation, underscores the necessity for research in this area. It is apparent, however, that the dramatic increase in salaries for residents has given affiliated hospitals the means to wipe away the one competitive advantage unaffiliated hospitals had previously been able to use to attract residents—a substantially larger salary. In 1962, unaffiliated hospitals were offering a mean salary 30 percent in excess of affiliated hospitals. By 1973, this competitive advantage had dropped to 3.6 percent (Fig. 3).

What can be done about the demand? There is a growing consensus that the distribution of residents among specialty positions should be controlled in some fashion consistent with the long-run health interests of the American people. This consensus is developing at a time when many Americans are finding that controls do not often beget the desired results. A previous attempt at control in residency training is worthy of comment. As mentioned, foreign medical graduates comprise approximately 27 percent of all residents in the United States today. This is perceived by many as a problem for the quality of health services in the United States. (In reality, the phenomenon is a complex one deserving of considerable further evaluation of the exact costs, if any, to the United States.) This *caveat* notwithstanding, in 1958, the ECFMG examination was introduced in an attempt to improve the quality of FMG's entering graduate training in the United States and, at some level, to modulate the growth of FMG's in the United States. The year 1961 was stipulated as the deadline after which an FMG could not occupy an approved residency position without having passed this exam. In the three years following the exam deadline, there was a marked drop in the numbers of FMG's entering United States residency positions such that by 1964, 2,500 fewer FMG residents were training in the United States than would have previously been anticipated (Fig. 5). Thereafter, however, FMG's were able to adapt to the exam requirement and to begin increasing each year in the same numbers as previously. This growth now continues unabated with the one-time diminution of 2,500 still obtaining. On the basis of this experience, it would appear that regulation of specialty training would have to be directed at the demand for residents. The demand for residents is a complex problem with important economic and quality of care implications. These implications are subjects for in-depth empirical investigation. It is to be hoped that regulation would follow only upon appropriate investigation.

I am indebted to Mr. Eugene Lewit for help in the preparation of this manuscript. I am also indebted to Mr. John Wolfe and Ms. Barbara Chamberlain for research assistance and to Mr. Irving Forman for technical assistance. I would also like to thank the Council on Medical Education of the American Medical Association for supplying unpublished data.

REFERENCES

1. American Medical Association: Medical education in the United States 1972-73, J. A. M. A. **226:** 910, 1973.
2. Ibid.: p. 927.
3. Ibid.: p. 929.
4. Ibid.: p. 930.
5. Ibid.: p. 933.
6. American Medical Association: Medical education in the United States, J. A. M. A. **210:** 1505, 1969.
7. American Medical Association: Graduate medical education in the United States, J. A. M. A. **182:** 766, 1962.
8. Association of American Medical Colleges: Statement on graduate medical education, Bull. Assoc. Am. Med. Coll. **6:** 3, 1971.
9. Bergland, R. M.: We have met the enemy and he is us, SURGERY **76:** 183, 1974.
10. Cohn, I.: Surgical education and the community hospital, Am. Surg. **39:** 537, 1973.
11. Ebert, P. A.: The medical staff and the hospital, Bull. N. Y. Acad. Med. **48:** 1405, 1972.
12. Edwards, C. C.: A candid look at health manpower problems, J. Med. Educ. **49:** 19, 1974.
13. Hughes, E. F. X., Fuchs, V. R., Jacoby, J. E., et al.: Surgical work loads in a community practice, SURGERY **71:** 315, 1972.
14. Hughes, E. F. X., Lewit, E. M., and Rand, E. H.: Operative work loads in one hospital's general surgical residency program, N. Engl. J. Med. **289:** 660, 1973.
15. Longmire, W. P.: Problems in the training of surgeons and in the practice of surgery, Am. J. Surg. **110:** 10, 1965.
16. Pearse, H. E.: The effect of specialization on graduate education in surgery, J. A. M. A. **170:** 301, 1959.
17. Reinhardt, U. E.: Proposed changes in the organization of health-care delivery: An overview and critique, Health Soc. **51:** 169, 1973.
18. Rousselot, L. M.: Federal efforts to influence physician education, specialization distribution projections and options, Am. J. Med. **55:** 123, 1973.
19. Springall, A. N., Hinman, J., and Thompson,

W. V.: Graduate medical education in the U. S., J. A. M. A. 162: 1653, 1956.
20. U. S. Bureau of the Census: Statistical Abstract of the United States: 1972, ed. 93, Washington, D. C., p. 5.
21. United States Department of Health, Education and Welfare, Public Health Service, Division of Public Health Methods: Health Manpower Source Book Section 13, Hospital House Staffs, Washington, D. C., Government Printing Office, 1961, p. 17.
22. Ibid.: p. 22.

"We have met the enemy and he is us"

Richard M. Bergland, M.D., *Hershey, Pa.*

From the Department of Surgery, Division of Neurosurgery, The Milton S. Hershey Medical Center, The Pennsylvania State University, Hershey, Pa.

MY OWN SPECIALTY, neurosurgery, has problems. We already have too many neurosurgeons, yet 130 new graduates are produced each year. Many of these are poorly trained, as evidenced by the fact that one third of the graduates fail to pass their Board examinations. Most of them are eventually underemployed; Odom[6] has estimated that the average neurosurgeon handles five or six major cases a month. We have the classic problems of maldistribution as most neurosurgeons practice in and around wealthy urban areas.

Our problems came from an assembly-line approach to education that paid little heed to the market's needs. I am confident that, as we restructure our system of neurosurgical education, our problems can and will be solved. But the problems in neurosurgery are not too dissimilar from those in other specialties. Most surgical groups are producing too many of the wrong kind of surgeons who eventually practice in the wrong places. This opinion is shared by many.

Presented at the Thirty-fifth Annual Meeting of the Society of University Surgeons, St. Louis, Mo., Feb. 14-16, 1974.

Reprint address: Richard M. Bergland, M.D., Department of Surgery, The Milton S. Hershey Medical Center, The Pennsylvania State University, Hershey, Pa. 17033.

The *New York Times* wrote in an editorial,[3] "There is wide agreement that in many areas of this country there are more surgeons than are needed, with the result that a large proportion of these highly trained specialists are employed far below their capacity. If the medical profession cannot make the necessary adjustments, then the government may have to step in with all the risks of bureaucratic error and arbitrariness such a course would raise."

Dr. Harry Schwartz,[8] a sympathetic layman, in addressing the American College of Surgery in 1973, asked if we really need hundreds of general surgeons or obstetricians and gynecologists each and every year, when there is obviously a tremendous and unfilled demand for primary-care physicians. He noted the excess in production and said, bluntly, "Either you people correct these situations or they'll be corrected for you by societal action."

Dr. Paul Beeson,[1] addressing the A.A.M.C. meeting in 1973, compared our problems to those of the population explosion and advised birth control. He said, "A real campaign of education and persuasion will have to . . . aim at reversing the trend to specialty practice. I would go after it with all the passion we are giving to population control throughout the world."

Members of this group have made similar statements: Dr. Louis Rousselot[7] said, "One of the most pressing problems in the education of U. S. physicians is the residency program, the doorway to the specialties . . . there has been a continuing and explosive growth of residency programs for decades with almost no planning as to needs."

Dr. William Longmire[4] said, "We must confine the number of medical school graduates who can enter surgery or medical specialty training to the number required to meet the health needs of the country. The remaining graduates must then enter fields that will satisfy other national needs."

Dr. Francis Moore[5] said: "If American surgery and medicine do not undertake this sort of control themselves by their own voluntary efforts, government will feel constrained to move in by legislative restriction."

Yet, somehow, we cannot change. In the past three years several thousand new residency positions have been added, most of which will lead to more specialists.

Why can we not change? I am not sure I know the answer but would ask five rhetorical questions.

1. Should not the blame for this be placed squarely on the doorstep of university surgeons? If we look at the number of university-affiliated residency programs, we note that 8,000 new positions were added in the past three years. However, in nonaffiliated, nonuniversity programs, there was a loss of 600 resident positions. More specifically, if we look at the number of surgical resident positions offered in the same three years, there was an increase of 1,000 positions in university-affiliated programs, whereas in nonaffiliated programs there was a loss of 300.[2]

2. Are not we as surgical educators inconsistent? In the past three years my own institution, The Hershey Medical Center, has doubled the number of surgical interns and doubled the number of surgical trainees. Our increase is consonant with the growth of our institution but most surgical educators have good reasons for adding to the manpower excess. Very few educators have been able to slow the production of surgeons, despite their avowed belief in the need to do so.

3. Does our commitment to traditional systems of surgical residency training limit the development of perhaps better strategies of surgical education?

4. Have the boards of the various specialties, in a well-intentioned effort to maintain quality, placed surgical education in a strait jacket that makes change impossible?

5. Is not the overproduction of surgeons the natural consequence of a surgical tradition that barters service to an institution for a surgical education?

I have answered these questions for myself and concluded that I will live my life within the university but will not educate neurosurgical residents.

Traditional residency training in neurosurgery begins after one or two years of general surgery and then lasts for four or five years. Upon coming to Hershey I considered the time-honored option of having trainees complete general surgery before beginning neurosurgery; I considered a combined Ph.D./residency program; and I considered a Ph.D. program as a separate block of time between medical school and residency. Each of these hurdles would make neurosurgical education more lengthy and predictably would yield a superior product. Yet each scheme would eventually add another neurosurgeon.

I also considered an abbreviated residency. Since the practice of neurosurgery is progressively dividing into those that do minor neurosurgical procedures and those that do major neurosurgical procedures, why not train some minor neurosurgeons? But again, this would add to the existing excess.

I elected to train no residents at all and believe that this is the decision many surgical educators must eventually make.

A word about neurosurgical board requirements: After medical school the Board requirements for the neurosurgical trainee today include at least one year of internship and four years of neurosurgery, of which only 30 months must be spent on a neurosurgical service. There are now 96 training programs in America, all of which stamp out products in the same mold. The Board, in an effort to maintain quality control, does not allow many variations. Most programs are located in large urban areas which are increasingly overpopulated with neurosurgeons. As a consequence, trainees do increasingly less.

At the end of formal residency training, the Board of Neurosurgery demands that students "practice for two years." Even though the young neurosurgeon may be clinically insecure, desire subspecialty training, or wish to pursue some problem in the laboratory, the two years of practice rule usually stops either supplementary clinical education or additional scientific involvement. I believe the years immediately beyond the residency are especially critical for career development but there are few places where this can occur.

My educational effort at Hershey has been directed toward men who have completed their formal training elsewhere. Most of the

130 new graduates readily acknowledge deficiencies in their education. Because their parent training program and most other universities are committed to training residents, the young attending finds career development at this stage difficult if not impossible.

Because I do not have residents I can preserve within the boundaries of my university a place where these men have priority. The position provides a busy clinical experience, support in the laboratory, sabbatical time, travel time, and what my dean thinks is an exorbitant salary.

My program is obviously new but for my first trainee it is working well. He operates frequently; in January he did 28 cases. His laboratory investigations of the ventricular surface have earned him a high reputation among basic scientists and he participates in the teaching of the neuroanatomy course. Time will tell, but I think his career is progressing rapidly in all the right directions.

Our service has an average census of 20 beds and for eight months of this year we had no rotating interns or residents of any kind. We have hired a surgical assistant who does most of the chores usually done by the resident staff.

I do not advocate that all surgeons within the university give up training residents but so far my own individual experiment in surgical education is working well.

Historically, there appears to be a clear evolutionary trend in surgical education. The anatomy schools founded by Galen were superseded in the latter part of the eighteenth century by Hunter's development of preceptorships. Preceptorships in turn were superseded by the residencies developed by William Halsted in the later part of the nineteenth century. There seems to be little doubt that there will be further evolution in surgical education and I doubt that the current residency system of surgical education is the ultimate. Simply to alter the number of surgeons trained without devising new strategies of education could make evolutionary changes less likely.

Our surgical past belongs to those who were able to devise new forms of surgical education. Likewise, I believe that the future of surgery belongs to those institutions, specialty groups, or individuals that can build new systems.

I believe that the best changes that occur will occur as the consequence of individual responsibility which leads to individual action.

REFERENCES

1. Beeson, P. B.: Some good features of the British National Health Service, J. Med. Educ. **49:** 43, 1974.
2. Directory of Approved Internships and Residencies 1973-74, American Medical Association.
3. Editorial: Physician planning, New York Times, Nov. 8, 1972.
4. Longmire, W. P., Jr.: The surgeon, the system, and patient care: Presidential address to American College of Surgeons, San Francisco, Calif., Oct. 2, 1972, Bull. Am. Coll. Surg.
5. Moore, F. D.: Panel discussion: Annual Meeting, American Surgical Association, San Francisco, Calif., April 27, 1972, Ann. Surg.
6. Odom, G. L.: Neurological surgery in our changing times: the 1972 A.A.N.S. presidential address, J. Neurosurg. **37:** 255, 1972.
7. Rousselot, L. M.: Federal efforts to influence physician education, specialization distribution projections and options: Editorial, Am. J. Med. **55:** 123, 1973.
8. Schwartz, H.: American medicine after Watergate, Bull. Am. Col. Surg., Jan. 1974.

A model for evaluation of surgical manpower needs—Pediatric Surgery

James A. O'Neill, Jr., M.D., *Nashville, Tenn.,*
Mark M. Ravitch, M.D., *Pittsburgh, Pa., and*
Bruce Barton, M.S., *Pittsburgh, Pa.*

From the Division of Pediatric Surgery, Vanderbilt University School of Medicine, Nashville, Tenn., and the Department of Surgery, University of Pittsburgh School of Medicine, Pittsburgh, Pa.

THERE ARE now approximately 280 pediatric surgeons practicing in the United States. They are involved in surgery of the newborn,

Presented at the Thirty-fifth Annual Meeting of the Society of University Surgeons, St. Louis, Mo., Feb. 14-16, 1974.

Reprint address: James A. O'Neill, Jr., M.D., Division of Pediatric Surgery, Vanderbilt University School of Medicine, Nashville, Tenn. 37232.

abdominal and thoracic surgery of childhood, pediatric oncology, and trauma. All of these surgeons have had special training in the field ranging from 12 to 36 months (average, 24 months) in addition to full training in general surgery and, in some cases, thoracic surgery as well. All but a handful of pediatric surgeons expend 100 percent of their efforts caring for infants and children.

Since this surgical population represents a relatively small number of individuals it seemed reasonable to study the group in depth.

The Study on Surgical Services for the United States (SOSSUS) began its Manpower Evaluation activities in June, 1972. Simultaneously with this effort, the American Pediatric Surgical Association initiated its own studies of pediatric surgical manpower with the intention of contributing to SOSSUS while gathering additional data for its own use. These efforts are still in progress.

The primary aims of this study are as follows: (1) to determine the existing number and distribution of pediatric surgeons in the United States; (2) to determine, within limits, the number needed and where; (3) to determine the existing and needed number of completely equipped and staffed hospitals (centers); and (4) to determine the number of training programs and trainee output required to fulfill estimated manpower needs.

METHODS

Although pediatric surgeons perform a wide range of surgical procedures, all of them are involved in the surgical care of a number of complicated disorders in the neonate. As a first estimate of the need for pediatric surgeons, a detailed computer study was initiated in order to estimate the occurrence of nine key surgical conditions to be expected in 49 population areas of the United States having a population of 200,000 or more. The diagnoses selected were tracheoesophageal fistula, omphalocele, imperforate anus and variants, intestinal atresia and variants, diaphragmatic hernia, Hirschsprung's disease, rhabdomyosarcoma, Wilms' tumor, and neuroblastoma. From these numbers an estimate can be made of the number of surgeons required to handle this load as part of their total practice. From these data it should also be possible to identify the number of referral centers required to handle this load.

The second estimate of need involved a survey of patterns of pediatric surgical manpower distribution in other countries, especially those whose populations appear to be well served. The numbers of pediatric surgeons were divided into the population of each country in order to arrive at a ratio which could be used for comparison. Pediatric surgeons in those countries were asked to comment on the adequacy of their own numbers as well.

Finally, a questionnaire was sent to 68 pediatric surgeons, 28 of whom occupy academic positions and are involved in training and 40 of whom are in private community practice. They were selected to represent 62 of the major population areas mentioned above. These individuals were asked to estimate the need for pediatric surgeons in their own areas. It was felt that this might add information related to not only need but also demand for pediatric surgical specialists.

RESULTS

Even though results are incomplete, it has been possible to complete a projection of population estimates from 1970 through 1985 for the major population concentrations in the United States. Estimates could be made of the number of each of the nine pediatric surgical conditions which would be expected to occur in these areas and also will permit determination of how many pediatric surgical centers will be needed—and where.

Data are available from this study and the one reported by Rickham[3] on the pattern of pediatric surgical care in other parts of the world. In Great Britain the ratio of pediatric surgeons to population is 1:250,000; in Sweden, 1:800,000; in Australia, 1:500,000; and in the United States, 1:700,000.

At present there are approximately 285 surgeons who devote themselves entirely or almost so to the surgery of infancy and childhood. They are located in virtually every major population area of the United States having more than 200,000 inhabitants However, no pediatric surgeons are located in Alaska, Arkansas, Idaho, Montana, New Mexico, North Dakota, South Dakota, West Virginia, or Wyoming. Of the latter states only Arkansas, New Mexico, and West Virginia have at least one county as large as 200,000 inhabitants.

The effort is still under way to gather data relative to a local estimation of need and demand for pediatric surgeons throughout the United States. These results will subsequently be compared with the estimates obtained from the other two approaches to the question.

DISCUSSION

The American Surgical Association and The American College of Surgeons, leaders in American surgery, set a remarkable precedent when they initiated SOSSUS. The purpose of all this effort is to insure that optimum standards of surgical care are promoted. The American Pediatric Surgical Association is participating in this effort for that reason and others as well.

Pediatric surgery is a young field in the United States so there are relatively few individuals who are recognized pediatric surgeons compared with other specialty groups. This state of affairs gives pediatric surgeons an opportunity to plan the future of training in that field in a manner which is in keeping with the needs of the population it serves. A critical look is being taken at all existing and proposed training programs in order to be certain that the product is one worthy of American trust. In similar fashion, a careful look is being taken at the number of pediatric surgeons needed and how many training programs will be required for that purpose.

It is important that all surgical specialty groups take a close look at themselves at this time if they are to determine their own destinies.[2] The methods reported here may be of use to others engaged in similar efforts.

It is expected that the methods utilized in this study will provide data sufficient to give a close estimate of pediatric surgical manpower needs. We already know how many pediatric surgeons are active and that pediatric surgical expertise is available in almost every population concentration of 200,000 inhabitants or more. This has evolved from only a handful of individuals who constituted pediatric surgery in the United States less than 25 years ago.

Computer data related to the incidence of nine key diagnoses should indicate not only manpower needs but also the requirements for special facilities in various parts of the country. It should also be possible to plan transportation linkages in association with this. However, the rapidly declining birth rate must necessarily be taken into account in this regard.

A questionnaire study is presently under way on a country-wide basis to identify existing pediatric surgical care facilities which might qualify as complete centers for care. It is assumed that centralization of care of complicated problems in newborn and childhood surgery, pediatric oncology, and serious trauma is in the best interest of quality care, economy, training, and research.

At present, approximately 13 to 15 pediatric surgeons are being graduated from 13 training programs in the United States yearly. Is this enough or too many? How many cases must a surgeon perform to remain competent? What are the economic factors involved? To be sure, the problem is a broad one and control of pediatric surgical residency output is hardly the answer to manpower needs or excess. As Moore[1] has stressed, emphasis on quantity is inadequate without equal emphasis on quality of care and all its implications. It is hoped that all or at least most of these questions may be answered by the approaches described.

REFERENCES

1. Moore, F. D.: Surgical residencies: To shorten or to shrivel, SURGERY **72:** 659, 1972.
2. Moore, F. D.: Freedom and organization, Ann. Surg. **176:** 1, 1972.
3. Rickham, P. P.: An analysis of pediatric surgery in North America and Northwestern Europe, J. Pediatr. Surg. **7:** 475, 1972.

Should the total number of surgical residency training programs be regulated?

Frank Cole Spencer, M.D., *New York, N. Y.*

From the Department of Surgery, New York University School of Medicine, New York, N. Y.

SHOULD the total number of surgical residency training programs be regulated? In consideration of this question, with such far-reaching implications, the factors influencing the growth of residency programs, the question of how many residency programs are needed, and possible mechanisms of regulation are discussed.

FACTORS INFLUENCING THE GROWTH OF SURGICAL RESIDENCY PROGRAMS

In the past 30 years there has been at least a 900 percent increase in the number of residency positions in surgery[1, 2]—from 2,000 to 18,000. The present rate of growth is nearly four percent a year; if unchanged, this could double the current number of surgical residency programs in the next 17 years.

Several factors may be identified as encouraging this rapid, unprecedented growth of residency positions in different hospitals throughout the country. First, there is virtually uniform agreement that patient care is almost always significantly improved when a hospital develops a residency program. Such a program not only permits closer "around-the-clock" supervision of patient care but also enhances the entire intellectual atmosphere of the hospital with the heightened priorities on both teaching and patient care.

A second factor is undoubtedly the prestige that a hospital acquires with a training program. In general, institutions with such programs are almost always regarded as more "prestigious" or "advanced" than those without. The Board of Trustees may become more interested and helpful and voluntary financial contributions to support the hospital may be enhanced.

A third important factor is the clear fact that the availability of surgical residents, performing much of the care of individual patients, frees a significant amount of time for the individual surgeon and thus makes it possible for him either to care for more patients or to care for seriously ill patients more effectively.

Finally, a fourth factor is the widespread instinct in the medical profession to teach. This teaching instinct, a cherished and admirable characteristic of the profession, is esteemed by all and efforts to enhance any opportunity for teaching are usually enthusiastically approved.

An almost identical list of influences was briefly mentioned by Moore[5] in his Presidential Address to the American Surgical Association in 1972.

SEQUENCE OF DEVELOPMENT OF SURGICAL TRAINING PROGRAMS

The evolution of a new residency program often follows a familiar pattern. First, a physician is appointed to supervise a residency program. He is often titled "Director of Medical Education," paid a substantial salary, and, in contrast to the remaining members of the hospital staff, devotes a large percentage of his time, often 100 percent, to the teaching and training program. The development of this educational subspecialty, accelerating at a progressive rate over the past two decades, has greatly enhanced such programs, even progessing to the level of a national organization of Directors of Medical Education.

The basic question of funding of surgical residents has usually been achieved by simply adding these to the cost of patient care, in turn reimbursed to a great extent by different insurance carriers, either federal or private. This policy has been subjected to intense review and criticism in certain states, especially Pennsylvania, within the past two years.

The final step, recruitment of adequate

Presented at the Thirty-fifth Annual Meeting of the Society of University Surgeons, St. Louis, Mo., Feb. 14-16, 1974.

Reprint address: Frank C. Spencer, M.D., Department of Surgery, New York University School of Medicine, 550 First Ave., New York, N. Y. 10016.

house staff, is not unusually difficult. American medical school graduates may be in scarce supply, but to an increasing degree there has been a more than ample number of foreign medical graduates (FMG's), though quality in many instances has been minimal. This is considered in more detail shortly.

Once the basic guidelines for establishing a residency program have been followed, the program is then reviewed by the National Residency Review Committee in the specialty, usually a tripartite committee developed under the aegis of the American Medical Association. A crucial concept underlying the growth of residency programs is the fact that approval has been based solely on the quality of the program, not upon the question of whether there was actually a need for such a program to produce more surgeons, at either a local or a national level. There have been no data to suggest that such programs should be limited, with the widespread unproved assumption that so many more surgeons were needed that the question of creating too many surgical residency programs simply did not exist. Nearly a decade ago Longmire[3] cautioned that such widespread, uncontrolled proliferation of residency programs might be harmful.

THE FOREIGN MEDICAL GRADUATE

An unrelated factor, but a crucial one supporting the growth of surgical residency programs, has been the increasing number of FMG's rising at a rapid rate each year for the past 10 to 15 years. Presently, at least 10,000 such graduates enter this country each year, almost equalling the graduates from American medical schools. It is estimated that presently at least one half, perhaps two thirds, of these wish to remain permanently in this country. An excellent numerical analysis of this worldwide phenomenon was recently published by Sodeman and associates.[6] To summarize briefly, worldwide there are about 80,000 medical graduates each year. About 40,000 of these are free to emigrate. Of these, at least 50 percent take the ECFMG, the preliminary required examination before coming to the United States for residency training. Their interest in coming for training is greatly enhanced by the ready availability of residency training positions, combined with adequate salaries. About three years ago, a survey of residency positions in general surgery found that about 50 percent were filled by graduates of American schools, 25 percent by FMG's, and 25 percent were vacant. A recent survey for general surgery found 33 percent filled by FMG's, 6 percent vacant. Hence there have been readily available positions, though often varying in quality, for any qualified FMG coming to this country.

The fact that such a large percentage of medical graduates throughout the world, at least 50 percent, are interested in coming to this country indicates that this is a strong worldwide socioeconomic force that will not easily be changed. To alter this phenomenon will require an unusually decisive change in our present system of medicine.

From the foregoing paragraphs, two conclusions seem reasonable. First, residency programs have grown rapidly with little relation to the number of surgeons needed, partly because this information was not available and partly because there has been a widespread unproved assumption that there was an actual shortage of surgeons. This growth of residency programs has been greatly enhanced by the increasing immigration of FMG's whose immigration, in turn, has been enhanced by the availability of residency programs.

HOW MANY SURGEONS DOES THE UNITED STATES NEED?

From the current studies such as the SOSSUS study, initiated by the American College of Surgeons and the American Surgical Association under the chairmanship of Dr. George Zuidema, it should soon be able to calculate the approximate surgical needs of a population of 200 million. These data can be compared with experiences in England, Sweden, and other countries where a regulated system of medical care for the past two decades can provide similar data.

A second calculation can then be made about how busy a surgeon should be. In this regard, the concept of the "hernia equivalent" developed by Hughes and others[1, 2] in recent publications seems to have considerable validity, though this requires further utilization to be certain. The "hernia equivalent" has been developed from a comparison of a surgical procedure in terms of operating room time, hospitalization time, and surgical fee. A statistical analysis of different unrelated factors found a high correlation, suggesting that the concept is valid. From the concept of a "hernia equivalent," the work associated with a standard inguinal herniorrhaphy, the relative work involved in any other surgical procedure can be similarly calculated. For example, a cholecystectomy is not quite two "hernia equivalents," (1.8), an abdominal perineal resection is 2.9 "hernia equivalents," and an open-heart procedure is about 6 "hernia equivalents." This concept has been used in some states as a basis for insurance reimbursement formulas.

In a study published in SURGERY, March, 1972, an analysis of a group of surgeons, voluntarily participating in the study, found the average workload surprisingly small, little more than three "hernia equivalents" a week, necessitating a work week of about 35 hours.[1] It was considered by the group that an ideal workload would be near 10 "hernia equivalents" a week, although this was achieved only by a minority of the group. To date the concept of the ideal workload being near 10 "hernia equivalents" a week has been accepted by some group practice plans, though experience to date is limited. I imagine many surgeons, including the author, would consider even this workload far too little.

From these two designations, the surgical needs of a population of 200 million, and the ideal surgical workload, both expressed in "hernia equivalents," the theoretical number of surgeons needed for a population of 200 million can be calculated. This in turn can be compared with the output of present residency programs, and a decision readily made about whether both the present and future output is adequate, excessive, or inadequate. When the data from the SOSSUS studies are available, these calculations should be possible. Preliminary information indicates neither a surplus nor a shortage of surgeons, but the significance of the data must be interpreted with the fact that over 30 percent of operations performed nationally are *not* done by certified surgeons.[4, 5]

PATIENT CARE WITHOUT A RESIDENCY PROGRAM

An immediate implication of the consideration that many hospitals should not establish a residency program is to decide what other methods of effective patient care should be used. Dr. Bergland, a separate speaker on this program, has addressed himself to that question regarding neurosurgery. One obvious method is the greatly expanded use of physician associates in different capacities, encouraging the training, the certification, and employment of such persons, much as laboratory technicians and x-ray technicians are currently effectively used. Two members of the Society of University Surgeons, Dr. Kirklin at the University of Alabama and Dr. Sabiston at Duke University, have already had extensive experience with pilot programs of this type.

A second method is to encourage hospitals to pay junior members of their staff to perform services often performed by house staff, such as working in the emergency room, the intensive-care unit, and other areas. An adequate salary would make this position attractive to many junior surgeons seeking to supplement their income and yet represent less expense than a full residency program with current house-staff salaries.

In support of the concept that many hospitals can render excellent patient care without a residency program is the surprising fact from Hughes' studies that approximately 50 percent of operations in general surgery are less complex than one "hernia equivalent."[1] That is, their complexity is equal to or less than that required for the performance of the standard inguinal herniorrhaphy. Certainly, operations of this type do not require a residency program and, indeed, many can be performed on an ambulatory basis.

THE QUESTION: REGULATE THE NUMBER OF SURGICAL RESIDENCY PROGRAMS OR "OBSERVE?"

With the foregoing analyses it is apparent that continued growth of surgical residency programs can easily occur unless a definite decision is made that the number should be regulated. The reasons for their growth have been described, emphasizing the lack of relation to actual surgical need and their support by the increasing numbers of foreign medical graduates. One possibility of regulation is that by federal legislation. Such legislation is already being considered in Congress, in early draft form, numerically limiting the total number of positions existing. Such programs are already limited sharply in several countries, including Canada and England. For the federal government, the stimuli for limiting the number of programs are several. First, the cost of medical care, of increasing concern to everyone, can be restricted. A surplus of medical specialists tends to increase the cost of medical care, rather than decrease it. Second, the ratio between the number of specialists vs. the number of physicians in primary care may be altered. Finally, the maldistribution of physicians, with the tendency for specialists to congregate in large urban areas, may be influenced.

A more attractive possibility to the medical profession is self-regulation by the profession itself. Current mechanisms are potentially effective if strengthened. Currently regulation and certification are done through residency review committees under the auspices of the American Medical Association in liaison with the American College of Surgeons and other organizations. These are currently being regrouped with the Liaison Committee for Graduate Medical Education, to be discussed in more detail by Dr. Francis Moore on this panel.

However, for several reasons, simply defining the number of residency positions needed in surgery can be a dangerous oversimplification. First, a large number of operations are performed in the United States by persons not certified by the American Board of Surgery—perhaps as high as 30 percent of all operations performed.[5] If the number of persons doing surgery cannot be restricted to those properly certified, simply decreasing the number of residency positions does not alter the over-all quality of surgery performed.

A second consideration is the fact that simply limiting the total number of residency positions assumes that all residency programs are equal in quality. This is clearly not true, for programs vary widely in quality, depending upon resources, patient volume, faculty, and several other factors. An ideal goal should be a selective restriction of programs of limited resources and quality, little change in many programs well balanced between their resources and their responsibilities, and an actual enhancement of some programs with unusually strong resources and capacity for growth.

These objectives of estimating the total number of properly trained surgeons needed nationally, and the ideal rate of growth needed in the next decade to reach and maintain this level, should be achievable through existing organizations for regulation and certification. If these objectives cannot be reached, however, the two other alternatives seem to be either continued unchanneled growth of residency programs or federal regulation.

REFERENCES

1. Hughes, E. F. X., Fuchs, V. R., Jacoby, J. E., and Levitt, E. M.: Surgical work loads in a community practice, SURGERY **71:** 315, 1972.
2. Hughes, E. F. X., Levitt, E. M., and Rand, E. H.: Operative work loads in one hospital's general surgical residency program, N. Engl. J. Med. **289:** 660, 1973.
3. Longmire, W. P., Jr.: Problems in the training of surgeons and in the practice of surgery, Am. J. Surg. **110:** 16, 1965.
4. Moore, F. D., Boyden, C. M., Sabiston, D., et al.: The production, attrition, and biologic life-time of surgeons in relation to the population of the United States: A look into the future through the clouded computer, Ann. Surg. **176:** 457, 1972.

5. Moore, F. D.: Freedom and organization, Ann. Surg. **176:** 1, 1972.
6. Sodeman, W. A., Castenda, A. R., Moore, F. D., and Warren, R.: The foreign medical graduate's role in American medicine, Arch. Surg. **107:** 476, 1973.

Reduction in the surgical training program of the United States: Warnings for the unwary

Francis D. Moore, M.D., *Boston, Mass.*

From the Department of Surgery, Harvard Medical School, Boston, Mass.

THERE HAVE BEEN many suggestions, both on this panel and in the recent literature, that we should reduce the number of surgical residents and residency programs in this country. There is increasing evidence to suggest that any such policy must be extremely selective and accompanied by strict performance standards in surgical practice. The American Surgical Establishment must enter the "numbers game" only if we are aware of several clear warnings ahead.

It is the purpose of this presentation to review some aspects of this problem and some of the pitfalls. This is not in any sense an official report of our manpower studies, nor would I wish to represent these ideas as having any broad constituency, as many new data have only recently become available.

TWO WARNINGS

Two important warnings surface immediately.

1. Beware reduction in the number of approved surgical residency positions in the absence of strict control of surgical practice in the hospitals over the country. It should be a relatively easy matter for the American Boards and the Residency Review Committees to reduce the total number of residencies offered by cutting off the less satisfactory programs. This is a very important step, but there must be an appropriate response on the part of the hospitals of the United States if such a step is to be both safe and meaningful for society. There must be the strictest sort of limitation on continuing surgical privileges, operated either by the American Hospital Association, Joint Commission on Accreditation of Hospitals, or the American College of Surgeons, specifying a required educational level indicated by Board certification, and with evidence of continuing education. Without the establishment of such credentials as national policy, reduction in the number of qualified surgical training programs will result in a chaotic situation far worse than anything we now have. It will be an open door for all physicians who wish to carry out surgical operations to do so, while the number of well-trained surgeons (doubtless to be referred to as "elitist") shrinks both in number and authority.

2. Beware of reduction in the cohort of well-trained, dedicated surgeons who carry out surgical operations in the United States, if this leaves untouched the production of large number of persons who are carrying out surgical operations without either constraints or an educational standard of technical excellence. This merely restates the first warning, but considers it in terms of manpower production rates. It would be a tragic mistake to reduce the closely supervised surgical residencies in this country (many of them in university hospitals) while approving an increased availability of short-term residencies, family-practice programs that include major surgery, and an ever-widening scope for personal operative responsibility by unqualified persons, including allied health personnel.

With these two fundamental *caveats* clearly stated, we might now drop back and ask ourselves, in the light of the available evidence, where did we get the idea that there are too many surgeons in this country?

EVIDENCE

What is the evidence? Too many surgeons or too many people doing surgery? There are five lines of evidence.

Presented at the Thirty-fifth Annual Meeting of the Society of University Surgeons, St. Louis, Mo., Feb. 14-16, 1974.

Reprint address: Francis D. Moore, M.D., Moseley Professor of Surgery, Harvard Medical School, 721 Huntington Ave., Boston, Mass. 02115.

1. The total fraction of practicing physicians performing surgical operations is very high. Of the 345,000 people who currently have the M.D. degree in the United States, approximately 75,000 are in retirement or full-time jobs in government, administration, and research. The remainder, approximately 270,000 people, are in practice of medicine in either private, group, or University settings. Of these, 92,000 persons carry out surgical operations. This amounts to 34 percent of all licensed physicians and is a high figure by any standard. Of this total of 92,000 persons, 12,000 are residents and approximately 30,000 are persons who have completed their postgraduate education without yet passing the American Board examination. Of these, approximately 2,000 are in the Board process, not yet completed. This leaves the base number of about 52,000 Board-certified surgeons in the country or with Board-certification equivalence.

It is perfectly clear from these numbers that there are *not* too many surgeons in this country. Fifty thousand surgeons would yield a figure of a little under 20 percent for the total fraction of surgeons in this population of practicing physicians, a reasonable norm for the developed countries. The data currently at hand suggests that these 50,000 surgeons, assisted by a group of approximately 10,000 surgical residents, could easily carry the surgical load of this country given an improvement in organization, emphasizing multispecialty group practice. The 10,000 residencies would graduate approximately 2,000 men each year and this would approximately replace those leaving practice by death or retirement.

This first line of evidence therefore leaves us with the message that there are far too many people doing surgery in this country, and just about the right number of surgeons. The remedy for this difficulty has to do with standards of education and credentialing. At an early date, hospital standards should remove from the field of surgery those who are not able to show acceptable credentials, general and family practitioners who are "part-time surgeons" and who are far more effective on the front line of primary care where they are so much needed. There should be a reduction in the number of residencies whose graduates are unable to pass the various American Boards of Surgery examinations, together with the removal of major surgical experience from family and general practice residencies, yet holding the door wide open for those young people who wish to enter surgery as a full-time career. We must accept an emphasis on continuing education and recertification to maintain the fitness of this core surgical group of 50,000 surgeons for this country.

2. Comparisons with other countries. The second line of evidence to support the widespread idea that there are too many surgeons in this country lies in the comparisons to other countries, in which no correction is made for differences in the training or background of those performing surgery. In addition, some articles of this type[1] emphasize surgical comparisons with Great Britain, without mentioning other specialties and without recognizing the fact that specialization is very much a part of the American medical scene throughout all of medicine. Although there are more surgeons even of the Board-certified type, relatively speaking, than holders of the Royal College diplomas in Great Britain, there are also far more psychiatrists, pediatricians, and internal medical specialists in this country than in Britain. To isolate the surgical specialty picture from the rest of the cultural trend toward specialization in this country was to do violence to the sociologic facts of the matter.

Allowing for the tendency of many aspects of American culture to show technological specialization, and correcting the total number of persons doing surgery for that number with proper credentials, the comparison of Great Britain to the United States shows only a minor excess in the fraction of surgeons in the United States (19 percent of practitioners vs. approximately 15 percent of practitioners in Great Britain). Because the total number of physicians per 100,000 population is greater in the United States than in Great Britain (165 vs. 85) the total of surgeons per unit population is also greater. This is also true of pediatricians, psychiatrists, and internists.[2]

3. Underoccupation of surgeons. Growing statistics of a spotty or episodic nature, of underoccupation of surgeons, underemployment, and nonuniform distribution of surgical services are the third line of evidence that there are too many surgeons in this country.

One such study[3] deals with suburban New York City. The vast majority of foreign medical graduates (FMG's) in this country who are carrying out surgical operations without American type training or American Board certification are concentrated in the New York–New Jersey–Philadelphia–Baltimore megalopolis. It is not surprising to find that in certain suburban areas—always notable for an insecure relationship in tertiary care—there are some Board-certified surgeons who are feeling keenly the competition of non–Board-certified personnel. This was particularly notable in general surgery in the study mentioned above.

Our data clearly indicate that this suburban situation is neither normal nor typical of surgical activity rates for Board-certified personnel in this country. Looked at within a geographical framework, the suburban areas of large cities and some of the affluent communities appear to show underoccupation of some surgeons in severe competition with underqualified personnel. Looked at within the framework of various specialties, it appears that Neurosurgery has the largest fraction of persons carrying out an operative load that is less than ideal, with General Surgery a close second. Some of the other fields (Obstetrics-gynecology, Ophthalmology, Otolaryngology, Orthopedics, Urology) demonstrate areas of undesirable clustering of specialists but work and productivity loads are more constant. To reason from New York suburbia that Board-type surgical residency should be reduced in number because it is those very surgeons who are being outstripped by their noncertified counterparts would do a severe injustice to the public. Such operations as hysterectomy, tonsillectomy, cholecystectomy, and operations for back pain are examples of situations in which a high level of training is associated with restraint and by professional commitment to the welfare of the patient. This results in a lesser operative rate than for those whose criteria are far looser and whose approach to their surgical work load is that of an entrepreneur rather than a professional. *Blind emphasis on surgical "productivity" rates can be a severe danger to the public.*

4. The large influx of FMG's. The fourth line of evidence that there are too many surgeons comes from the general awareness that very large numbers of FMG's are entering this country[6] and that some residency programs are entirely populated by them. In addition, the enrollment, nationally, of FMG's in residency programs in some surgical specialties rises as high as 25 to 35 percent. Recent licensure data indicates some states are running as high as 65 percent FMG's in the current licensing process.[4] While it is acknowledged that this situation is undesirable because it drains expensively trained professionals away from their countries of origin and places them in substandard hospitals in this country, this matter is not in any sense confined to surgery. In addition, many hospitals have thoughtlessly extended their residency programs to help with their own work load despite minimal attention to their educational components, providing a haven for the FMG. The low pass-rate of the FMG in Board examinations is not always a matter of language because many of these men have been exploited at home, as well as in the United States, by enrollment in very large medical schools that have very low standards of educational achievement. At the present time, about 12 percent of FMG's in the United States are citizens of the U. S. A. returning to their native heath.

Although this is a severe problem that demands some sort of guideline and constraints, this influx of FMG's does not, per se, impact on the surgical problem uniquely. It contributes to the over-all capacity of advertised surgical residencies in this country, of which there are 16,000, with only 12,000 men in them. This "partial vacuum" continues to attract the FMG. The Board Committees should move rapidly and decisively on those residency programs that have not

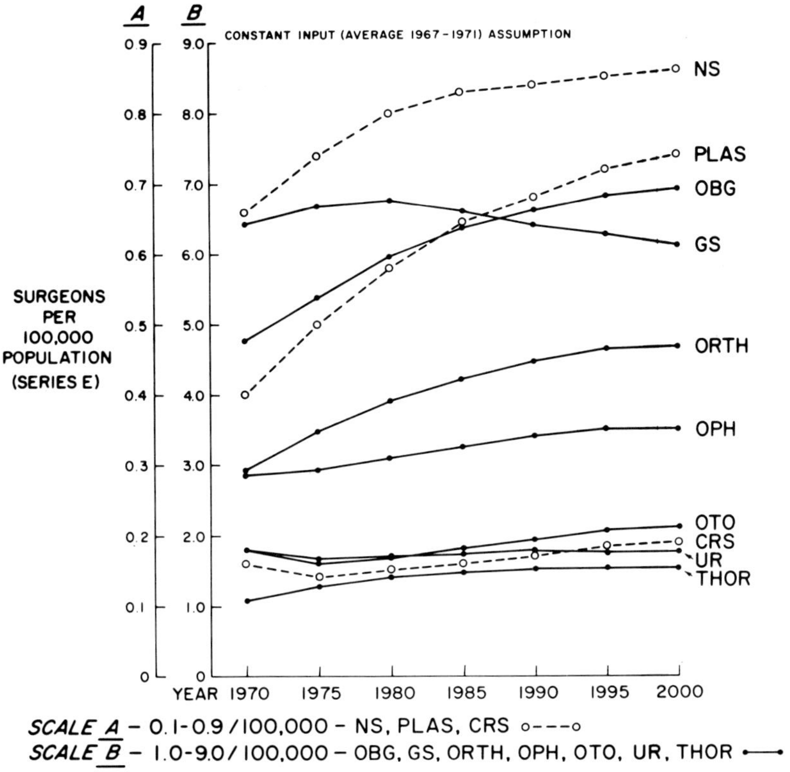

Fig. 1. Projection to 2000 A.D. for 10 specialties. Two scales are shown at the left, one to suit the less numerous specialties (dotted lines) such as neurosurgery, plastic surgery, and colo-rectal surgery. If these were all shown on the same scale as the solid lines, they would be difficult to visualize at the bottom of the chart. Most noteworthy is the continued predicted growth of the number of neurosurgeons on a population base up through the year 1985, even with constant input. This is, of course, due to the relatively young age of most neurosurgeons now in practice. The steep rise in plastic surgery is noteworthy not only for the foregoing reason, but because the plastic Board is increasing its rate of certification drastically over any previous figures. The decline in general surgery is obvious and is a trend discerned in many hospitals that have multiple residency programs. It is quite notable that urology and thoracic show an almost flat projection. (From: "Surgical manpower," Arch. Surg. **108:** 637, 1974.)

achieved any significant enrollment in the last few years.

5. Rising prediction curve for Board-certified surgeons on the population base. The fifth line of evidence was the prediction of an increased number of Board-certified surgeons over the next 30 years as presented in the panel two years ago.[5] This figure, for Board-certified surgeons alone, showed, on the basis of extremely rigid data and a closely checked computer prediction program, that even while limiting the number of surgeons to those Board certified, and making a constant input assumption at the 1967-1971 average, there would be an increase from approximately 21 per 100,000 population to approximately 27 per 100,000 population in the next 30 years. A breakdown of this overall figure for the various specialties is shown in Fig. 1. It is evident that when this gross change in number of surgeons per population in the United States is subdivided according to specialty we see a mixed picture. Quite clearly a sense of discrimination between specialties is going to be necessary if we are to balance out the training of surgeons against the needs of the country, expressing the latter in their simplest possible terms, i.e., with reference to present supply on a population base.

First are those specialties in which, assuming constant residency output at the average of 1967-1971 rates, the number of surgeons per population will remain fairly constant through the next few years. This includes Urology, Thoracic surgery, and Ootolaryngology.

Second, there is a group in which the specialists on a population base will increase strikingly even with constant input. It should be noted that all these curves are based on a "constant input assumption" (1967-1971 average) and that the Residency Review Committees for those Boards should not tolerate a gross increase in the number of residencies currently being offered.

The question is often asked as to how the number of specialists per 100,000 population can increase over a 30 year period if the input is constant. The answer is to be found in the average age group of those currently in practice. When the mean age is rather young, then constant input will swell the ranks until death and retirement begin to balance input. This appears to be the case particularly in Neurosurgery, Plastic surgery, Orthopedic surgery, and Obstetrics-Gynecology, in which all the curves show a rising trend. Interpretation of these curves is not to be taken lightly. It does appear that Neurosurgery would be wise to cut down its number of residents at this time and should make Board certification a much tighter credential. Neurosurgery is unique in having a rather large cohort of persons (estimated to be 50 percent) of excellent training and background who go on with their specialty practice without Board certification. They become so clearly identified as Neurological surgeons in their hospital staff position that they evidently do not feel a need for Board certification to the extent that those in some other fields do.

The field of Plastic surgery seems to be expanding its mandate strikingly at this time. It is still too soon to know whether this increase is in response to perceived needs, whether it represents people with Plastic surgical background increasingly taking over operations formerly carried out by others (largely General surgeons), or whether it represents expansion of Plastic surgeons carryout highly elective cosmetic surgery of the type that raises questions about the utilization of hospital space and the expensive resources of health care. Far more data are needed to answer these difficult questions. Both Orthopedics and Obstetrics-Gynecology appear to be rising in number in response to real needs. Orthopedics has taken over musculoskeletal trauma virtually entirely and even in small communities the general surgeon is less active in these fields than he used to be. In addition, Orthopedics has identified several new types of reconstructive surgery for which there is a very large need in the population. As to Obstetrics-Gynecology, there is evidence that in some parts of the country less than 60 percent of obstetrical deliveries and gynecologic operations are carried out by residency-trained personnel. It might seem wise to increase the training level in this field, which is so much concerned with the health of young women in the reproductive age group and the welfare of the newborn infant.

Third, and quite predictably, there is one field in which, with constant input, the number of specialists per population will fall in the next 30 years. This field is General surgery. It is the largest of all the surgical fields. In terms of the University, "General Surgery is general education in surgery" and it is general surgeons who have generally held together the teaching and research activities of the University departments. From a professionalistic point of view, general surgery is not the surgical equivalent of general practice* but it is a very specific field. It is surgery of the gastrointestinal tract, the breast, endocrine glands, and vascular and pediatric surgery. The latter two represent certifiable areas of interest within general surgery. With constant input the number falls because the average age of general surgeons is older than that in any of the other specialties. It is my own opinion that it would be very unwise at this time to reduce in number the well-established and highly qualified general sur-

*Sociologists on both sides of the Atlantic persist in confusing this point. General surgery, while broad in responsibility, is no longer an interdisciplinary field. The general surgeon is not a surgical "jack of all trades" but a specialist with a somewhat broader anatomical mandate than many of his colleagues.

gical residencies. A decline in numbers will occur with constant input. In this field, as in others, the marginal programs should be discontinued. The excellent programs now in existence (many of them in universities) should be strengthened with an increasing emphasis on basic biological science as well as clinical and technical excellence. To avoid the obvious accusation of favoritism, the standard constraints and inspection procedures should be especially rigorous for those programs that are to be continued.

From the above evidence it would seem clear that we should do everything in our power, both within the Society of University Surgeons and within the universities where we are employed, to increase the flow of top-flight American graduates into all fields of surgery. At the same time we must make a commitment to improved credentialing and better, more realistic tracking of young surgeons into certain specialties and into the geographical areas where they are most needed.

PLATFORM FOR ACTION

A reasonable "platform" for action in this field might appear to involve the following five steps.

1. Continued recruitment of top-flight people into surgery. This battle has already been joined as the preclinical scientist, the nonsurgical specialist, and deans who perceive their mission as related to community care all join in to discourage the brilliant young man from entering a career in specialties or in surgery. The societal responsibility of surgery in this country is very great. Surgeons are responsible for 50 to 70 percent of the patients confined to hospitals by their illness; there are 15 to 20 million surgical operations carried out per year and it is estimated that eight percent of the population have surgical care during any given year. We must learn to educate our colleagues in science, in the other fields, and in the deans' offices that this need is real and will continue to require the finest young men and women.

2. Strengthen hospital credentialing. The new staff committee guidelines of the Joint Commission on Accreditation of Hospitals represent a strong move in this direction. Unfortunately there is already a cry of "outrage" either from those who feel threatened in their work or those who sense a new level of conflict in the jurisdictional disputes within surgery. This latter point, the most distressing of any aspect of surgical manpower, can never be solved on a national level. No committee can legislate that all hands should be operated upon by orthopedists or all noses by otolaryngologists. This sort of policy decision must always be left to the local level. We would hope that the strength of the Societies as well as that of the Joint Commission would avoid the construction of "cookbook lists" of surgery to be associated with each Board Specialty certification. The equitable settlement of such questions must depend upon the strength of staff organization so that men can grow and improve their skills on the basis of continuing education.

3. Monitoring and constraint in residency program approval. This is essential. The Coordinating Committee on Medical Education, or the Liaison Committee on Graduate Medical Education, jointly sponsored by several national organizations, would seem to be the logical point of leverage here. There must be some group carrying forward with a computer program to update annually the prediction of the number of specialists present in the country, relative to the population. It is on the basis of information such as this that the total number of residency positions can be monitored and controlled, limiting some and encouraging others, always with an emphasis on quality of the total educational experience. Some sort of screening mechanism should be introduced for FMG's entering the system, such as the three parts of the National Board Examinations, an exchange visitor-student type visa, and a written commitment together with a promise of position from their professor at home. *It is simply not fair to the youth of America to exclude them from admission to medical schools, and then bring in a large flux of FMG's over their heads.* FMG's who are American citizens should have preferential treatment for obvious reasons, despite the political vulnerability of such an approach to "favorite-son" candidates for residency.

4. Appropriate geographical dissemination of trained surgeons should be encouraged. The best way to do this is to make available to all young people an annually updated printout of the population ratios for the nine surgical specialties in each of the cities, towns, and rural counties of the country. This is feasible at an estimated annual budget of $75,000. Some national agency should pick up this mission. It is my own bias that the multispecialty group, whether or not prepaid, provides the best framework for the geographical distribution of surgeons as well as specialists in other fields. Work loads are more evenly distributed in group practice and there is less evidence of nonuniformity to suggest overexploitation of certain operative procedures. A service that makes available the distributional ratios in localities as mentioned above could likewise take on the task of indicating where openings exist in such groups.

5. Evidence of continuing education by the Board-certified specialists. The surgeon cannot ask the hospital, the public, and the third-party payment mechanisms to shoulder all the burden for credentialing and residency limitation. The surgeon himself must join this action by something that may seem very distasteful. Evidence of continuing education of a solid type involving exposure to evolving clinical procedures, with examination (and possibly recertification) is an inevitable concomitant of any sort of national self-discipline in the field of surgery.

SUMMARY

The five evidences for an excessive number of full-time career surgeons in this country are not impressive, whereas there are far too many people carrying out surgical operations. Effective steps in new programs are available at this time that could help rectify this situation within the voluntary sector of our American medical establishment. It is my hope that we will move rapidly and strongly in this direction before a rigid system of inflexible government controls, derived from political pressure, loaded with coercion, and enforced by a system of penalties, becomes inevitable.

REFERENCES

1. Bunker, J. P.: Surgical manpower in the United States and in England and Wales," N. Engl. J. Med. **282:** 135, 1970.
2. Hospital Medical and Dental Staff, England and Wales: Regional tables, Department of Health and Social Security Statistics and Research Division, August, 1973.
3. Hughes, E. F. X., Lewit, E., and Rand, E.: Operative work loads in one hospital's general surgical residency program, N. Engl. J. Med. **289:** 660, 1973.
4. Massachusetts Medical Society: Applicants for fellowship, N. Engl. J. Med. **298:** 913, 1973.
5. Moore, F. D., Boyden, C., et al.: The population, attrition, and biologic life-time of surgeons in relation to the population of the United States, Ann. Surg. **174:** 457, 1973.
6. Sodeman, W. A., Casteneda, A. R., Moore, F. D., and Warren, R.: The foreign medical graduate's role in American medicine, Arch. Surg. **107:** 476, 1973.

Volume 76 Number 2

SURGERY

AUGUST, 1974

Editorials

Too many surgeons?

Claude E. Welch, M.D., *Boston, Mass.*

From the Massachusetts General Hospital and the Harvard Medical School, Boston, Mass.

SURGERY AS A CAREER choice suddenly has become unpopular with many medical students. Many reasons might be adduced including the lack of time given in many curricula to the subject, or the difficult tension-filled life that a surgeon must lead—a prospect not appealing to many students. There is a haunting fear, however, that the student may be swayed strongly by recent data that tend to indicate the career might be filled with unpleasant surprises.

Thus statements have been made that there are too many surgeons and that too many surgical operations are performed. Let us examine each of these allegations in turn.

Too many surgeons either now or in a decade? The studies of Moore and Peterson that shortly will be published in a SOSSUS report show clearly that if the present output is maintained, there will be a plethora of general surgeons and almost surely many surgical specialties such as neurosurgery, urology, and plastic surgery will be overmanned within a decade. But it should be noted also that many specialties other than surgery are filling their ranks at a rapid rate. Radiology, for example, is reaching a point of saturation. With the introduction of nurse anesthetists in many areas, anesthesiology may soon reach the same point. Assistant Secretary of HEW, Dr. Charles Edwards, stated recently that there will be no doctor shortage by the end of the decade. At the present moment it would appear that the only great vacuum that still exists is in primary care.

These projections, however, are not equivalent to the statement that we are overpopulated with surgeons at the present time; nor are they equivalent to the statement that well-trained surgeons will be too numerous in a decade. As a matter of fact, Moore's study showed that of some 86,000 U. S. A. surgeons, 15,000 are in training and only approximately 46,000 are estimated to be active Board-certified surgeons.

How many operations should a surgeon perform to maintain his skills? This is a

Accepted for publication May 13, 1974.

Reprint requests: Charles E. Welch, M.D., Suite 1104, Warren Bldg., 275 Charles St., Boston, Mass. 02114 question that is impossible to answer; but an average of perhaps five operations a week averaging one hernia equivalent each might not be an undue estimate. This would mean that approximately 250 operations should be done by a surgeon in a year. Board-certified surgeons then could perform 11 million 500 thousand operations in that period. Actually there are approximately 14 million operations done a year in this country. If all surgery had to be carried out by Board-certified surgeons, it clearly would be impossible for them to handle the load. Obviously many surgeons are extremely capable and do not have Board certifications; it could be estimated that if every one of the 86,000 doctors engaged in the practice of surgery were performing operations, an average of approximately 160 would be performed by each surgeon at the present time. Clearly in the future, however, it is to be expected that increasing percentages of surgical procedures will be done by Board-certified surgeons.

The second question is, are there too many surgical operations performed? A pioneer study by Lewis in Kansas indicated that more surgical operations were performed in the areas that had more surgeons. This would seem to be reasonable. Certainly there are more operations performed in the Mayo Clinic than in a neighboring city of like size; this does not mean that the indications for surgery are too liberal. Certainly more art works are produced where there are more artists. Some social planners, however, would interpret this fact in an entirely different light and say that surgeons acting as general practitioners generate their own practice. Echoes of this interpretation are seen in a national health plan before the Congress which states that surgeons should perform operations only when the patients are referred by primary-care physicians. It is suggested that there are too many tonsillectomies, too many hysterectomies, too many bladder neck revisions, too many operations on lumbar discs, too many vascular procedures. Actually, I believe that these statements are poorly documented and that there is still a serious problem of underutilization of surgical services that overshadows the overutilization. More rigorous peer review should weed out the occasional, often highly publicized, overenthusiastic operator.

It must be remembered that all projections of manpower and utilization must rest upon a large number of variables. Consider the extreme consequences that might follow some major development. Observe the burgeoning field of endoscopy and the possibility that malignant disease of the colon may be detected at an earlier stage than it is at present. Suppose that coronary artery surgery is established as a standard procedure. Suppose that transplantation of viscera other than the kidney becomes practical. Suppose another major war should occur. Suppose a sudden reduction of gasoline supply should render the American public far less mobile; if present services are to be maintained, decentralization and more surgical personnel would be necessary. Suppose that continuing medical education becomes a reality; there would be a corresponding reduction in the amount of time a surgeon could devote to patient care. Most likely of all, suppose that national health plans, when finally implemented, would gradually direct all surgical procedures into the hands of those surgeons who are certified and recertified by American Boards. Recommendations that would project too narrow a margin of safety could turn out to be disastrous both in the number of available surgeons or in the quality of their care.

Some future prospects seem clear. As Longmire has pointed out, the number of surgical residencies offered will become less numerous than they were in the past. They will tend to be congregated about university centers. However, practicing surgeons, as their numbers decrease and the population increases, will be expected to have a greater opportunity for service than they had in the past and be expected to perform more operations. There will be a gradual trend toward the elevation of the Board-certified surgeon.

These trends should not discourage the

young person who wants to become a first-rate surgeon. It might encourage dilettantes or those who have little desire for hard work. But there is no need for the well-motivated student who likes surgery to be troubled. Only 93 percent of the present residency openings in general surgery are filled and 34 percent of them are occupied by foreign medical school graduates; similar figures exist in the surgical specialties.

Assuming that a surgeon's average active lifetime is approximately 30 years, it could be estimated that approximately 20 percent of all medical students should enter a surgical residency in order to maintain the present level of surgical care. There may well be cause for alarm if the figure in medical schools falls below this level. Perhaps students should take another look, pay less attention to the headlines, spend more time in the operating room, and discover how many operations are necessary in our society. In many respects the opportunities have never been brighter for the well-trained surgeon.

A computer logic program in the operating room

Mark M. Ravitch, M.D., *Pittsburgh, Pa.*

From the Department of Surgery, Montefiore Hospital and the University of Pittsburgh, Pittsburgh, Pa.

C. O. KNUTSON and F. R. Watson have come up with a fascinating "surgery game" (in the sense that Pentagon planners have "war games") which allows for computer examination of alternative tactics. However, surgeons are as likely to be reluctant to refer to the computer *in medias res* as would a general in the midst of a battle. The problem is, of course, that what generals are always speaking of as "calculated risks," are really incalculable risks.

As a teaching tool for students and residents, a computer program of this type is highly attractive and a set of such programs, purchasable at a reasonable price, might be very useful.

That the present computer program had a 96 percent correlation is hardly surprising in a very strong institution with extremely competent surgeons, particularly since the surgeons who planned the program presumably planned it on the basis of their accepted practice. The value of a program such as this in "uplifting" a practice might be better assessed by a similar analysis of procedures done (1) in a neighboring community hospital, and (2) in some other major hospital. If there were any very striking differences in the computer recommendations and in the performance in those hospitals, one would then wish to compare the days of stay, the mortality, morbidity, and cure rates. There is still an enormous amount of work to be done before one could begin to say that a computer program of this kind would have a practical clinical value.

If the concern, in the opening paragraph of the paper, about the increasing proliferation of new medical information and the bulk of current pertinent literature is meant to apply to the kind of problem under discussion, i.e., carcinoma of the colon, it is open to challenge. A single publication rarely establishes the validity of a new departure in clinical surgery and there is a certain virtue in waiting to see whether a number of major investigators or major clinics are satisfied with a new departure in surgery before it is widely recommended and adopted. There is also the question of the inertia of computer programs. Who is going to change the program and how often to "maintain a working knowledge of the current pertinent literature?"

The assumption that the computer decision on clinical problems in the operating room is made in a fraction of the time required by the surgeon is incorrect. I would say that any mature surgeon goes through essentially the process involved in the logic flow diagrams and that he can do this more

Accepted for publication May 14, 1974.

Reprint requests: Mark M. Ravitch, M.D., Department of Surgery, Montefiore Hospital, 3459 Fifth Ave., Pittsburgh, Pa. 15213.

quickly than he can announce the information and have somebody type the information into a computer, although admittedly the answer would then come back from the computer almost instantaneously. As a teaching method in the operating room, I would repeat that this is superb, particularly for surgeons not gifted in logical exposition.

My own bias is that the computer is wasted on relatively simple decisions, such as those involved in the choice of operation for colon carcinoma, which have only a few variables which can be instantly seen and which do not require the analysis of trends in the patient.

Compare this with decisions to be made in the postoperative period in patients with electrolyte imbalance, with cardiac and renal inadequacy, on respirators, with gastrointestinal fistulae, diarrhea, or nasogastric suction, etc., in which there are scores of variables to be analyzed, as well as trends, and numerous bits of hard data available in terms of chemical determinations and measurements of function. The complexity of problems of this kind is infinitely greater—there are real data available. We are dealing with trends and can instantly measure and re-evaluate the effects of our change in therapy, further modifying that as required by succeeding analyses. In this sort of situation, and particularly if the computer can be fed on-line information from the patient, the computer, properly programmed, can be expected to be a vast improvement over seat-of-the-pants clinical management. The present program has weaknesses by virtue of (1) the somewhat artificial anatomical designations, (2) the failure to indicate what is entailed in a given resection (viz., in sigmoid resections take inferior mesenteric flush with the aorta? strip aorta clean? etc., in removal of attached viscera (a) always? (b) when not separable? (c) when attachment is thought to be due to malignant extension?—etc.).

These and other factors such as whether or not one uses the "no touch" technique, practices proximal and distal initial ligature of the bowel, or practices vein ligation as the first step, etc., are perhaps not as vital to the use of the computer for the "surgery game" as they would be if the computer were intended to be employed in the operating room.

The authors have presented a reasoned and well thought-out analysis of the operative problem in colorectal malignancy, on the basis of long-established and currently standard practice. If it is proposed that this will safeguard the patients of those surgeons who can operate but cannot think, the proposal is deadly.

If it is proposed that it be presented as a teaching program with the computer pointing out to the student why a given choice is fallacious, it might have real attractiveness. The program may serve to help surgeons who are technically competent and intellectually deficient, but such surgeons will be at the mercy of the individual in the operating room who is informing the computer and who may not be relied upon to discern that a surprising answer from the computer could only have come from its having received erroneous information.

Original communications

Boris Petrov, great Russian surgeon, and the Sklifosovsky Institute of Emergency Surgery

Owen H. Wangensteen, M.D., *Minneapolis, Minn.*

From the Department of Surgery, University of Minnesota, Minneapolis, Minn.

Boris Petrov (1898-1973), internationally known Russian surgeon, died of cerebrovascular thrombosis in Moscow, June 5, 1973, a few months short of his seventy-fifth birthday. His elementary education was in Moscow, where his father held a governmental position. In 1922 Petrov graduated in medicine from the University of Moscow's Medical School. His early training in surgery was under the direction of Profs. I. K. Spizparny and N. N. Burdenko.

In 1927 Petrov transferred his hospital activities to the Sklifosovsky emergency hospital,* known before 1923 as the Shernetev Hospital. There he worked initially under the direction of Professor V. A. Kransintsev and too under the guidance of that facile Master Surgeon, Sergei Yudin. Here Petrov demonstrated his engrossing love of surgery and his unfailing devotion to his patients' welfare. The fame of institutions is owing fundamentally to enduring innovations made by those who energize them. The Yudin-Petrov succession and their important contributions have placed upon the Sklifosovsky Institute of Emergency Surgery a hallmark of distinction as one of the great surgical hospitals of the world.

Through constant and inspired dedication to his work, Petrov came to be recognized as one of Russia's great surgeons. He was a general surgeon, but his primary interest concerned the alimentary canal and its appendages. His most important work involved replacement of the esophagus in children for benign corrosive stricture. Petrov had approximately 180 journal publications and an additional eight surgical monographs. For many years he was Professor of Surgery at the University of Moscow and Chief Surgeon at the Sklifosovsky Institute. He was long the Editor of *Chirurgiya* and also a member of the Editorial Committee of This Journal.

This surgeon first met Petrov, with other Russian surgical colleagues, during his visit to Minnesota in February, 1959. It was immediately apparent that he was a very knowledgeable and competent surgeon, carrying the stamp of a true gentleman, with a kindly and warm manner. The writer had the pleasure of being with Petrov at the International Cancer Congress in Tokyo in November, 1966, and subsequently at meetings in Buenos Aires (1969), at the Clinical Congress of the American College of Surgeons in October, 1970, and in his own

Accepted for publication April 18, 1974.

Reprint requests: Owen H. Wangensteen, M.D., Regents' Professor, Department of Surgery, Mayo Memorial Building, Minneapolis, Minn. 55455.

*Biographic data from the September 1973 issue of *Chirurgiya* kindly translated from the Russian by Dr. Mattew Smorstok of the Medical Faculty of the University of Minnesota.

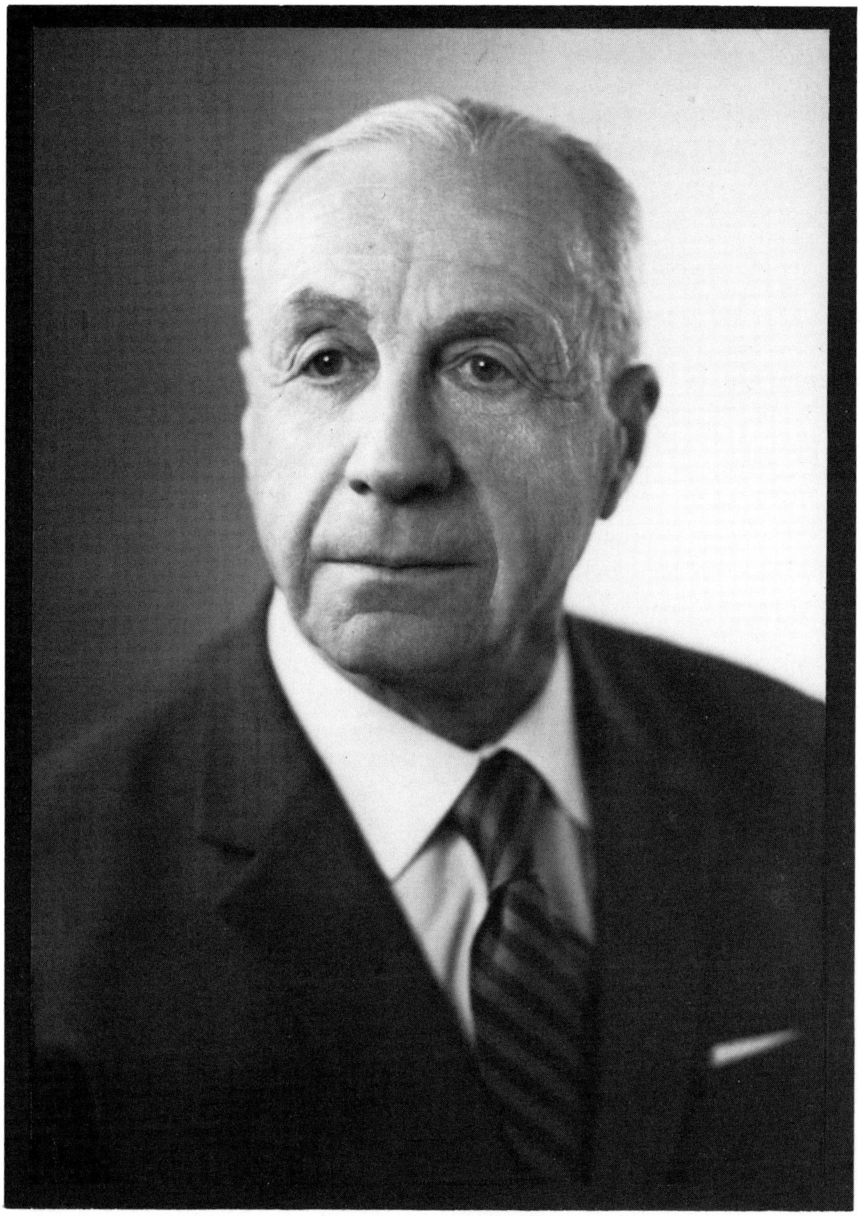

Boris Petrov, 1898-1973

Sklifosovsky hospital in August, 1971, when the Congress of the International Surgical Society convened in Moscow. There I saw several young patients for whom Petrov had re-established esophageal continuity, anxious to display their ability to swallow, revealing their unconcealed admiration, love, and adoration of their surgeon.

Prof. Petrov will be best remembered for his method of reconstruction of the esophagus for corrosive strictures. In the cold winter climate of northern Russia it is common practice to place a tumbler of sulfuric acid between the inner and outer windows, where its gradual evaporation serves to minimize frosting of the window panes. Young children who accidentally swallow such fluids suffer diffuse severe esophageal burns with virtual obliteration of the esophageal lumen. Petrov's experience with restoration of continuity for this tragic disorder was unusually large. In the beginning, like Yudin, Petrov made a presternal subcutaneous jejunal replacement, but by 1956 his preference was retrosternal positioning employing the right colon and a short length of terminal ileum, which he attached to the esophagus and/or pharynx, a procedure he initiated in 1952. Petrov's experience with cancer of the esophagus, stomach, colon, and rectum also was extensive.

Eugen Bircher of Aarau, Switzerland (1907), had made a presternal esophagocutaneous gastrostomy in several steps, an operation often complicated by leaks slow to heal. Even so, the operation proved popular, especially with German professors of surgery, many of whom retained as a hospital "diener" a successfully treated patient for purposes of demonstrating their unusual achievement to students. With the success of the Sklifosovsky surgeons with jejunal and colic replacement, the cutaneous component of the procedure disappeared completely, save for reconstruction of the cervical esophagus following removal of a high-lying cancer. Petrov stated that Yudin was continuously occupied with presternal replacement of the esophagus for benign stricture over a 20 year period, beginning in 1928. Yudin improved the Herzen-Roux operation considerably and performed the operation on more than 300 patients.

Petrov wrote two papers on retrosternal placement of a "new" esophagus in SURGERY. In his 1959 paper (SURGERY **45:** 890, 1959) Petrov indicated that Peter Herzen of Moscow first completed an esophagojejunogastric anastomosis for esophageal stricture in three stages in something less than four months on a 20-year-old girl in 1907 (Zentralbl. Chir. **8:** 219, 1908). Continued Petrov, Cesar Roux of Lausanne had done the initial stage of such an operation on an 11-year-old boy on June 12, 1906 (Sem. Med. **27:** 37, 1907). However, Roux failed to connect the upper end of the jejunum to to the esophagus until almost five years later (1911). In his 1964 paper (SURGERY **55:** 520, 1964) Petrov reported upon a succession of 88 patients operated upon between 1956 and 1962 with the remarkably low mortality for that period of 5.6 percent.

In the migration of a jejunal segment Yudin divided some of the vasa recti of the mesenteric vessels to secure adequate jejunal length for the esophageal replacement. Petrov's preference was to mobilize the entire root of the mesentery, thereby making it possible to obtain considerably greater length of the jejunal loop brought into the neck for the esophageal anastomosis.

A number of the German titans of surgery, notably Ferdinand Sauerbruch and Martin Kirschner, struggled unsuccessfully for more than a decade to excise malignancies of the thoracic esophagus with restoration of continuity. It remained for T. Ohsawa of Kyoto, Japan (1933, 1940) to succeed where they had failed. He did not employ the Meltzer-Auer technique of sustained, positive, intratracheal pressure to insure expansion of the lungs, relying solely on a tightly fitting face mask. Unlike Sauerbruch and Kirschner, Ohsawa did not believe that hurried completion of the operative procedure in an hour's time was the chief determinant of success. Many will recall that Kirschner (Arch. klin. chir. **114:** 676, 1920) said it took him 75 minutes to complete the operation; and lamented that if he could only do it in 60 minutes,* the procedure would be successful. Ohsawa made no apologies for taking approximately four hours to complete the operation. Today competent surgeons around the world are able to excise the thoracic esophagus for cancer with restitution of continuity with an acceptable operative mortality.

Another of Petrov's major interests and contributions concerns transfusion of cadaver blood. Writing in SURGERY (**46:** 651, 1959), he said that Prof. F. N. Shamov (1928, 1937), a Soviet physiologist-surgeon, showed that dogs depleted by extensive bleeding could be revived if transfused with cadaver blood from recently killed dogs. Meanwhile, Yudin (1933) had reported upon an exten-

*Repeated in a dinner conversation with this surgeon in Tübingen in March, 1928.

sive clinical experience since Shamov first apprised him of his 1928 experiments on dogs.

Petrov reported that transfusion of cadaver blood had been in use at the Sklifosovsky for 28 years; that more than 27,000 such transfusions had been given, representing 70 percent of all the blood transfused at that Institute. Petrov remarked further that cadaver blood is not only harmless with respect to infection and intoxication, but possesses some advantages over blood from living donors, in that no anticoagulant need be given because of the presence of fibrinolysins (SURGERY **46:** 651, 1959).

In the preface to Yudin's* 1933 monograph, *La transfusion du sang de cadavre à l'homme,* the Paris surgeon, Antonin Gosset, wrote that the Sklifosovsky Institute was the best organized hospital for emergency surgery in the world, a deserved distinction to which the consecutive labors and devotion successively of Yudin and Petrov have contributed greatly. The Sklifosovsky has first claim on surgical emergencies of every variety in the greater Moscow area.

Both Yudin and Petrov had large experiences with primary gastric resection for perforated peptic ulcer. v. Haberer (1919) had earlier advocated the thesis on the score that the procedure dealt more effectively with the ulcer diathesis. The success of the Sklifosovsky surgeons, Yudin and Petrov, with the procedure encouraged others to adopt it and today primary gastric resection for duodenal ulcer perforation is widely practiced and with a primary operative mortality rate not out of line with that of simple closure of the perforation.

The names of Petrov and Yudin and the Sklifosovsky Institute for Surgical Emergencies will forever be linked together for important achievements in several areas of mutual interest. Unlike Yudin, Petrov has not been a controversial figure. He has been held in the highest esteem by his Russian surgical colleagues and widely admired and honored too, as was Yudin, outside of Russia.

*Then spelled Judine.

The Sklifosovsky Institute, so named in honor of a great Russian surgeon, celebrated its 50th anniversary on Dec. 22, 1973. Prof. Petrov wrote the story of the 50 years of the Institute (Chirurgiya 1973). He had intended providing THIS JOURNAL with a history of the Institute, including the work of his eminent predecessor, Sergei Yudin. However, frail health interrupted completion of that task, generously assumed, to which the distinguished Minister of Health, Prof. Boris Petrovsky, had lent his approval and endorsement on the occasion of this writer's visit to Moscow in 1971.

Tatiana Petrova, Petrov's devoted and talented wife, shared all his interests and was of great assistance to Prof. Petrov in many of his writings, especially those of an historical nature. When this surgeon sought information concerning Carl Reyher's visit to Lister's clinic in Edinburgh, she was able to provide helpful information* from official records.

At the October, 1970, Convocation of the American College of Surgeons, Walter MacKenzie, in presenting Boris Petrov for Honorary Fellowship, speaking on behalf of the Regents of the American College of Surgeons, said: "The discipline of Surgery has an international language, and Boris Petrov speaks it, in his own tongue and ours, with sincerity and integrity. . . . Professor Petrov is one of the most outstanding surgeons of the Soviet Union . . . widely recognized and much decorated for scientific contributions to his country, . . . a member of the Academy of Medical Sciences of the U.S.S.R." Petrov had the unique "ability to develop remarkable loyalty in his own staff," an over-all assessment with which all who knew Petrov will agree.

Those who came to know Boris Petrov well will always cherish his name with great pride and warm affection, summoning recollections of a modest, kindly man with a charming, old-world courtesy, a surgeon obviously animated by the highest ideals and with a tremendous love of and complete commitment to surgery and its advance.

*SURGERY **74:** 664, 1973.

The name of Petrov (1898-1973) has now joined in memory that galaxy of celebrated Russian surgeons of the 19th century, Nikolai Pirogoff (1810-1881), Nikolai Sklifosovsky (1836-1904), and Carl Reyher (1846-1890); and the 20th century surgeon, Sergei Yudin (1891-1954)—a company of surgical luminaries whose names will endure in the history of surgery.

The world of surgery salutes this brilliant company of Russian surgeons and holds out high hopes that reciprocal respect and friendship will insure removal of the impervious veil that hampered free interchanges over recent decades. We are encouraged to hope and believe that we shall soon observe assurances and greatly heightened evidences of an improved climate of confidence, mutual trust, and cooperation, shared completely too by our respective governments, to the lasting benefits of all mankind.

The current status of vena caval replacement

J. P. Scherck, M.D., M. D. Kerstein, M.D., *and* H. C. Stansel, Jr., M.D., *New Haven, Conn.*

From the Section of Peripheral Vascular Surgery, Department of Surgery, Yale University School of Medicine, Yale–New Haven Hospital, and the West Haven Veterans Administration Hospital.

RESTORATION of vascular continuity in the venous system has been a goal of surgical research since the first experimental grafting attempts by Carrel and Guthrie[22] in the early nineteen hundreds. However, despite radical advances in the use of prostheses to replace arteries, venous grafting remains too unreliable for routine clinical application. Inconsistent or low success rates in experimental models account for this lag. The problem has not been studied as extensively as have arterial grafts, largely because venous disease is neither as dramatic in onset nor as threatening to life. Still, venous disease is a not uncommon problem which often causes significant morbidity and sometimes death. Superior vena caval syndrome, inferior vena caval syndrome, postphlebitic disease, traumatic loss of veins, and congenital absence or displacement of veins all represent potentially correctable lesions. Thus a reliable surgical treatment could be a useful adjunct to the surgeon's craft.

The lowest success rates for replacement prostheses in the venous system have consistently been obtained in the infrarenal inferior vena cava (IVC) and, like the thoracic aorta in arterial replacements, this has become the ultimate test of a vascular prosthesis for venous replacement. Most of the studies referred to herein therefore deal with attempts to maintain prosthetic patency at that level. In addition, however, IVC obstruction represents a real clinical problem for which there is as yet no treatment. Consistently successful bypass grafting of this vein area would not only satisfy the most stringent theoretical requirements for venous grafting but also could benefit patients suffering from a particular clinical syndrome.

INFERIOR VENA CAVAL SYNDROME

In a 20 year survey done at the Johns Hopkins Hospital,[114] IVC obstruction represented 18 of 400,000 cases treated and 16 of 3,000 which came to autopsy. The earliest medical reference to the disease was by Schenck[142] in 1644; he described autopsies of two cases, one occurring secondary to "peripneumonia," the other secondary to caries of the lumbar vertebrae. The first thorough study was done by Pleasants[114] in 1911 and remains a classic in the field. A thorough study of 18 cases and review of 296 others from the literature was presented (see Table I). Etiologies, symptoms, morbid anatomy, and studies of the collateral vessels which develop were discussed in detail.

Accepted for publication March 20, 1974.

Reprint requests: Dr. H. C. Stansel, Jr., Department of Surgery, Yale University School of Medicine, 333 Cedar St., New Haven, Conn. 06510.

Table I. *Causes of inferior vena caval obstruction as reported by Pleasants*[114]

			No. of cases
I.	Obstruction due to thrombosis		171
II.	Obstruction due to new growth of the IVC wall		2
III.	Obstruction due to nonmalignant diseases of the abdomen		42
	Liver	31	
	Other	11	
IV.	Obstruction due to new growths		88
	By invasion	48	
	By pressure	21	
	By thrombosis	19	
	Kidney	29	
	Peritoneum	11	
	Liver	9	
	Testicle	9	
	Uterus	6	
	Other	26	
V.	Obstruction due to "kinking"		2
VI.	Obstruction due to congenital obliteration		9
VII.	Obstruction of both venae cavae		6
VIII.	Obstruction due to ligation		8
	Total		328

A more recent review was presented by Boruchow and Johnson[15] in 1972.

Obstruction usually occurs caudal to the renal veins; it is often asymptomatic; sometimes it causes edema of both lower extremities and dilatation of the superficial collateral vessels; chronic venous stasis disease is the usual result, though gangrene of the extremities has been reported.[24, 56, 60, 104] Sometimes the renal veins are involved, giving the characteristics of the nephrotic syndrome; mild renal impairment or death[39, 85, 87, 108] may occur, depending on the rapidity of occlusion and time for development of collaterals. Sometimes the upper segment of the IVC occludes and thrombosis of the hepatic veins is the result, leading to the Budd-Chiari syndrome with ascites, hepatomegaly, and liver failure.

Obstruction of the IVC may result from diverse causes and the course and prognosis are largely dependent on the cause. Thrombosis is the most common primary inciting factor, representing 68 percent of Pleasants' series, and usually reaches the IVC by extension from distal phlebitis. Thrombosis, of course, may also be a secondary consequence of any of the other causes for IVC obstruction. Neoplasms, especially renal-cell carcinomas, are next most common, causing obstruction by invasion more often than by pressure. Liver disease may also give IVC occlusion, due to either pressure from hepatic enlargement[55] or ascites.[115]

Rarer causes of IVC syndrome have also been reported. Leiomyosarcomas[25, 159] and other tumors[114] of the vein wall, retroperitoneal fibrosis,[145] congenital membranes,[10, 17, 167] congenital agenesis,[14] hypercoagulable states, and even physical exertion[94] have been among reported etiologies. The syndrome may occur in association with cyanotic heart disease.[80] Despite the fact that infrarenal IVC ligation is used to prevent pulmonary emboli, the procedure has been shown to produce hemodynamic disturbances,[111, 171] continual pulmonary emboli,[113, 130] disability,[149] and even death.[59]

Therapy is limited. If thrombosis is acute, thrombectomy has been successful[41, 89] and is especially recommended if the renal veins are involved. Treatment of the liver disease or removal of the ascites could theoretically open the constricted IVC. Surgical removal of IVC coarctation[167] and of a constricting tumor mass[89] has been reported. Radiation or chemotherapy directed at lymphomas or other malignancies may palliate IVC obstruction.

Despite generally unsuccessful experimental results, bypass grafting has been tried clinically when no other therapy was possible. Many of these attempts have been successful; more have not. The need for further experimentation to determine why some are successful and how these successes can be reproduced is obvious.

The only real successes in experimental work have been accomplished when the infrarenal IVC graft was inserted in conjunction with a distal arteriovenous fistula (originally tried by Stansel[158]), which increases the flow through the vascular prosthesis.

Other experimental techniques have been sometimes encouraging, but mostly inconsistent; these include newer graft materials, rigid rings to support the anastomoses, and anticoagulants. Results have been particularly independent of the type of graft material chosen.

Rosenberg and associates[120] have reported extensive experience with vascular grafting using bovine carotid arteries which are digested to collagen tubes by a process developed in their laboratory. These grafts are extremely easy to handle, cause no immunologic stimulation, and have given good long-term success rates in arterial replacement. Use in the venous system[19, 153] has shown this to be as good as any other prosthetic material.

HISTORICAL DATA: IVC GRAFTING

Experimental work. The first attempt at vena caval grafting was reported by Jeger and Israel with experimental replacement of the IVC at the level of the renal veins, giving equivocal results.[81] Further experimentation awaited the surge of successful results with grafts in the arterial system; in 1951 Klassen and associates[79] reported a clinical five-month success for a femoral vein autograft used to relieve SVC obstruction. In the subsequent years a wealth of experimental and clinical data has been reported (Tables II, III, and IV). In general, variable success has resulted from SVC grafts but the IVC has consistently resisted attempts at bypass. The remainder of this discussion will relate to these IVC grafting attempts.

The fate of fresh venous autografts, venous homografts, aortic homografts, and Orlon tubes in the thoracic IVC of growing pigs was studied by Sauvage and Wesolowski.[135] All eight venous autografts remained patent for 209 days, as did the one venous homograft. The two aortic homografts had strictures and the two Orlon tubes occluded and remained so for 60 and 116 days. The animals were killed after a sixfold weight gain, at which time the venous grafts had doubled in length and diameter. Silk sutures were found to restrict growth; catgut did not.

Ohara and Sakai[109] had some success with SVC replacement by aortic heterografts and homografts, but infrarenal vena cava grafts in 29 dogs all obstructed. Alcohol-preserved heterografts, Amylan, and silicone rubber tubes were tried.

Bryant and associates[20] did control studies on suture technique in the IVC and decided on No. 5-0 silk in a continuous over-and-over stitch interrupted at four quadrants for end-to-end anastomoses. They were able to maintain patency in eight of 10 dogs for six weeks using 3 cm. fresh venous autografts in the infrarenal cava, but were uniformly unsuccessful with fresh and freeze-dried venous homografts, freeze-dried arterial homografts, Orlon, nylon, and Teflon.

Thoracic vena cava grafts were studied by MacLean and his colleagues.[86] They reported two of 11 dogs patent at 16 months with aortic homografts. They also discovered that by adding Lucite support rings they could improve the patency of Ivalon grafts from none of 25 to nine of 13 at 10 months. Davalos and associates[32] reported 13 patent grafts from the diaphragm to the right atrium in evaluating that material for the Baffes operation used to treat transposition of the great vessels.

The superiority of venous autografts was further confirmed in 1960 by Bower and associates[18] and Earl and associates.[44] Bower had 10 of 11 autografts patent up to eight months in the infrarenal vena cava with only four of 22 using other materials; Earl had five of six patent autografts, but none of six patent homografts and four of eight patent grafts compiled by suturing panels of smaller veins together.

Though Collins, Burrus, and De Bakey[23] did not mention where in the IVC their grafting was done, they had some short-term successes, all of which occluded by four months. Materials included reanastomosis of the vena cava, autogenous aorta, peritone-

Table II. *Inferior vena cava bypass: Experimental work*

Ref. No.	*Date*	*Patency*	*Percent*	*Follow-up*	*Comment*
INFRARENAL IVC:					
Autogenous vein:					
20	1958	8/10	80	6 wk.-9 mo.	
44	1960	4/8	50	?	
18	1960	10/11	90	to 8 mo.	
34	1961	6/7	85	10 wk.	
175	1962	1/19	5	188 d.	Common iliac to IVC
161	1964	8/9	88	3 wk.	Patch graft
151	1964	5/10	50	6/18 wk.	Jugular vein
Total		43/93	46		
Homologous vessels:					
20	1958	0/4	0	3 wk.	Vein
20	1958	0/2	0	2 wk.	Freeze-dried veins
20	1958	0/8	0	5 wk.	Freeze-dried arteries
135	1960	1/8	12	5 mo.	
166	1963	1/11	9	4 mo.	Veins
Total		2/33	6		
Other biological materials:					
109	1957	0/1	0	6 mo.	Heterograft
166	1963	1/7	14	5 mo.	Tracheal homograft
151	1964	1/10	10	8 wk.	Compilation autograft
19	1965	1/10	10	30 d.	Bovine collagen tube
153	1965	1/5	20	1 yr.	Bovine collagen tube
116	1972	0/15	0	—	Small bowel
Total		3/48	6		
Dacron:					
166	1963	0/7	0	—	Crimped
166	1963	0/2	0	—	Noncrimped
166	1963	1/7	14	3 mo.	Woven, carbonized, with acrylic spiral
166	1963	2/4	50	3 mo.	Teflon thread reinforced
173	1968	—	—	—	See text
Total		3/10	15		
Teflon:					
20	1958	0/2	0	3 wk.	
18	1960	1/8	12	5 d.	Crimped
63	1962	0/8	0	1 wk.	
161	1964	2/15	13	3 wk.	Patch graft
42	1964	0/8	0	1-7 mo.	Crimped
105	1967	0/10	0	2-4 wk.	Isodiametric
173	1968	—		—	See text
96	1968	1/8	12	3 mo.	Control group
157	1972	1/3	33	2 mo.	"Gore-Tex"
Total		5/54	9		
Other synthetic materials:					
109	1957	0/2	0	60 d.	Amylan
109	1957	0/2	0	—	Silicone rubber
20	1958	0/4	0	3 wk.	Orlon
20	1958	0/4	0	3 wk.	Nylon
18	1960	2/6	33	125 d., 8 mo.	Seamless nylon
34	1961	0/5	0	—	Dacron, Vinyon, Teflon
166	1963	0/3	0	—	Polypropylene
107	1971	1/5	20	3-6 mo.	Elastor Td 24/2
Total		1/31	3		

Table II—*Cont'd*

Ref. No.	Date	Patency	Percent	Follow-up	Comment
Using rigid support:					
166	1963	0/3	0	—	Dacron, rubber rings
151	1964	7/10	70	7-19 wk.	Jug. vein, Teflon rings
49	1968	2/3	60	117, 142 d.	Tetoron, steel coil
6	1969	5/9	55	7 d-2 yr.	Rigid silicone rubber helix
92	1969	0/12	0	up to 3 wk.	Dacron, silastic reinforced
107	1971	2/5	40	3-6 mo.	Elastor Td 24/2, steel rings
Total		16/42	38		
Using anticoagulants:					
34	1961	8/9	88	10 wk.	Autogenous IVC
34	1961	0/5	0		Dacron, Vinyon, Teflon
175	1962	4/9	44	9 d.	Autogenous vein
61	1964	4/11	36	4 mo.	Autogenous vein
Totals		16/34	47		
		0/5	0 synthetics		
Using arteriovenous fistula:					
158	1964	2/5	40	8-24 mo.	Dacron, isodiametric
158	1964	3/3	100	8-24 mo.	Dacron, larger than IVC
158	1964	1/2	50	8-24 mo.	Teflon, isodiametric
158	1964	6/6	100	8-24 mo.	Teflon, larger than IVC
160	1966	7/8	87	72-219 d.	Teflon
160	1966	5/6	83	22-222 d.	Dacron
160	1966	5/5	100	10-154 d.	Autogenous vein
96	1968	3/5	60	3 mo.	Teflon
8	1972	5/5	100	1 mo.	Peritoneum
116	1972	10/30	30	to 3 mo.	Small bowel
Total		47/75	62		
Other experiments:					
72	1966	16/35	45	0-500 d.	Tetoron with pseudointima*
72	1966	1/27	3	5 wk.	As above into cats
96	1968	12/15	80	3 mo.	Teflon with fistula and support
150	1970	4/9	44	23-36 wk.	Teflon with fistula and support
8	1972	10/10	100	1 mo.	Peritoneum with fistula and rigid polyethylene support
SUPRARENAL IVC:					
Synthetics:					
105	1967	7/11	63	1-1½ yr.	Teflon, isodiametric
6	1969	2/2	100	—	Silicone rubber helix
107	1971	2/5	40	3 mo.	Elastor Td 24/2
107	1971	2/5	40	6 mo.	As above with support rings
157	1972	3/3	100	1 d.-2 mo.	Teflon ("Gore-Tex")
Total		16/26	61		
THORACIC IVC:					
Autologous vein:					
135	1955	8/8	100	209 d.	In pigs
136	1960	3/3	100	21, 2,700, 2,741 d.	
		11/11	100		
Homologous vessels:					
135	1955	1/1	100	200 d.	Pigs, vein
135	1955	2/2	100	62, 244 d.	Pigs, aorta
86	1959	2/11	18	10 mo.	Dogs, aorta
136	1960	0/5	0	—	Dogs, aorta
Total		5/19	26		

*See text.

Table II—*Cont'd*

Ref. No.	*Date*	*Patency*	*Percent*	*Follow-up*	*Comment*
Other biological materials:					
136	1960	3/3	100	—	Pericardial autograft
82	1971	19/19	100	6-18 mo.	Intestinal submucosa
Synthetics:					
135	1955	0/2	0	116 d.	Orlon
86	1959	0/25	0	—	Ivalon
32	1960	13/13	100	30 wk.	Teflon
63	1962	13/15	86	1 wk.	Teflon
49	1968	2/6	33	30, 451 d.	Tetoron
157	1972	3/3	100	2-6 mo.	Teflon ("Gore-Tex")
Totals		29/31	93 Teflon		
		2/33	6 all others		
Other experiments with synthetics:					
86	1959	9/13	69	10 mo.	Ivalon, Lucite support rings
170	1965	9/10	90	2 mo.	Teflon, end support rings, graphite-Benzalkonium-heparin bonded surface
106	1970	10/10	100	2 mo.	Dacron, wall bonded heparin
Total		28/33	84		
OTHER OR NOT SPECIFIED LOCATION:					
Autogenous vein:					
23	1960	0/?	0	4 mo.	Location unspecified
30	1963	3/7	43	100-150 d.	Location unspecified
152	1964	7/9	78	3-6 wk.	Suprarenal to thoracic
Other biological materials:					
23	1960	0/?	0	4 mo.	Autogenous peritoneum, location unspecified
23	1960	0/?	0	4 mo.	Autogenous aorta, location unspecified
152	1964	1/5	20	3-6 wk.	Bovine heterograft suprarenal to thoracic
91	1966	40/40	100	to 14 mo.	Inverted jejunum, SVC and IVC locations unspecified
82	1971	0/12	0	3 wk.	Jejunal mucosa, "abdominal IVC"
Dacron:					
23	1960	0/?	0	4 mo.	Location unspecified
30	1963	0/5	0	"few days"	Location unspecified
152	1964	1/10	10	3-6 wk.	Suprarenal to thoracic
49	1968	6/9	66	2-421 d.	Tetoron, "thoracoabdominal"
92	1969	0/12	0	3 wk.	Silicone reinforced
Other materials or experiments:					
152	1964	4/6	60	3-6 wk.	Nylon, suprarenal to thoracic
152	1964	0/2	0	3-6 wk.	Teflon, suprarenal to thoracic
49	1968	3/3	100	16-250 d.	Tetoron, "thoracoabdominal," with steel support coil
147	1969	8/8	100	100 d.	Electrolour, location unspecified

um, and Dacron. They noted both fibrous constriction of the anastomotic sites and thrombus throughout the graft and attributed failures to low flow and pressure rather than graft material.

Sauvage and Gross[136] replaced segments of both SVC and thoracic IVC with 100 percent patency in both sites with autogenous vein and complete occlusion with aortic homografts. Three pericardial autografts remained patent in the IVC. A later report[139] showed continued patency of the composite

Table III. *Superior vena cava bypass: Experimental work*

Ref. No.	*Date*	*Patency*	*Percent*	*Follow-up*	*Comment*
Autogenous veins:					
38	1955	0/4	0	1 mo.	—
136	1960	3/3	100	21-243 d.	—
30	1963	0/7	0	1-150 d.	Azygous patent
30	1963	3/6	50	10-250 d.	Azygous ligated
30	1963	4/4	100	60-130 d.	IVC
174	1964	5/5	100	11 d.-9 mo.	Infrarenal IVC
174	1964	7/10	70	4-6 mo.	Panelled IVC
174	1964	3/4	75	8-28 d.	SVC
141	1964	2/5	40	—	—
137	1967	2/2	100	1700, 2941 d.	Composite vein
Total		29/50	58		
Autogenous aorta:					
97	1958	30/33	90	1 d.-12 mo.	—
102	1964	33/33	100	—	—
Total		63/66	96		
Homologous aorta:					
38	1955	"good"	—	—	—
5	1956	0/6	0	1-5 mo.	Freeze-dried
53	1957	5/10	50	—	—
53	1957	9/9	100	to 1 yr.	Azygous ligated
109	1957	4/12	33	5 d.	Alcohol-preserved
136	1960	0/5	0	21-243 d.	—
137	1967	0/2	0	2-2889 d.	—
Total		18/44	40		
Other biological materials:					
118	1958	0/12	0	3 hr.-3 mo.	Autogenous pericardium
117	1958	23/24	96	3 hr.-6 mo.	Pedicle tube from right atrial appendage
136	1960	0/3	0	21-243 d.	Autogenous pericardium
100	1961	25/35	71	2-467 d.	Fresh SVC homografts
102	1964	0/12	0	—	Autogenous pericardium
153	1965	2/3	67	10, 13 mo.	Bovine collagen tube
Totals		59/100	59		
		0/27	0 autogenous pericardium		
Teflon:					
38	1959	0/8	0	1 wk.	—
45	1960	6/7	85	2-24 wk.	—
99	1960	19/20	90	2-413 d.	⅝" + ¾" crimped
99	1960	21/32	68	2-413 d.	5/16" + ⅜" crimped
112	1960	17/30	56	1 wk.-10 mo.	—
16	1960	12/16	75	1-6 mo.	Sponge
164	1962	3/7	42	1 wk.-14 mo.	Fabric
164	1962	2/10	20	"long term"	Rigid fabric
30	1963	1/8	12	250 d.	⅜"
30	1963	6/6	100	50-250 d.	⅜", azygous ligated
30	1963	2/6	30	250 d.	½"
30	1963	5/6	83	80-250 d.	½", azygous ligated
102	1964	8/12	27	—	Gelatin impregnated
102	1964	43/50	86	—	Crimped
42	1964	6/7	85	1-7 mo.	Crimped
141	1964	3/5	60	—	—
69	1965	6/14	44	1-56 wk.	—
95	1966	6/10	60	6 mo.	3 cm. long
95	1966	0/5	0	6 mo.	8 cm. long
Totals		165/259	63		
		11/12	91 azygous ligated		

Table III—*Cont'd*

Ref. No.	*Date*	*Patency*	*Percent*	*Follow-up*	*Comment*
Dacron:					
164	1962	0/4	0	1 d.-6 wk.	Fluflon
164	1962	0/3	0	3-6 mo.	Acylamide impregnated
101	1963	15/18	83	5 d.-9.5 mo.	Knitted
101	1963	9/14	64	8 d.-9 mo.	Woven
30	1963	4/6	66	180-250 d.	½", knit, azygous ligated
30	1963	4/6	66	10-180 d.	15 mm., Ehhigraft, ligated
141	1964	0/5	0	—	—
102	1964	9/14	64	—	Woven
102	1964	15/18	83	—	Knitted
Total		56/88	63		
Other synthetic materials:					
38	1955	0/4	0	—	Ivalon sponge
38	1955	1/3	33	—	Dacron, nylon taffeta
38	1955	0/1	0	—	Nylon tubing
109	1957	0/5	0	26 d.	Silicone rubber tubing
75	1958	0/6	0	2-20 wk.	Ivalon
45	1960	6/7	85	1-34 wk.	Nylon
164	1962	1/7	14	6 wk.	Rigid nylon
Total		8/33	24		
Using arteriovenous fistula:					
141	1964	5/5	100	—	Teflon
141	1964	4/6	67	—	Dacron
141	1964	5/5	100	—	Autogenous vein
69	1965	17/18	95	9 d.-14 mo.	Teflon
95	1966	10/10	100	6 mo.	Teflon, 3 cm.
95	1966	8/10	80	—	Teflon, 8 cm.
52	1967	15/15	100	4 mo.	Teflon, 2-4 cm.
Total		64/69	93		
With anastomotic support rings:					
74	1962	18/18	100		Aortic homograft, nylon support rings

venous autografts in two dogs living at 2,700 and 2,941 days.

DeMeetz and associates[34] had 100 percent thrombosis of infrarenal plastic prostheses despite the operative and postoperative use of fibrinolysin.

Hambraeus and Anderson[63] compared thoracic and abdominal IVC grafts using a crimped, knitted Teflon prosthesis. Of 11 dogs with thoracic IVC grafts surviving 7 to 11 months, all were patent; all eight infrarenal grafts thrombosed in less than a week.

Todd and co-workers[166] studied tracheal homografts, venous homografts, peritoneal autografts, and numerous plastic prostheses. The highest patency (14 percent) was with the tracheal homografts. Low-molecular-weight dextran was tried without effect. Six dogs were given warfarin for 1 week postoperatively and, though they all died of bleeding complications, all grafts were thrombosed at autopsy.

Sive and associates[155] reported a 90 percent patency using autogenous veins and 20 percent with homogenous veins.

Haimovici and colleagues[61] and Zinicola and associates[175] studied the effects of anticoagulants on the fate of autogenous iliac vein bypass of the infrarenal cava. With pre- or postoperative anticoagulation they maintained patency in eight of 20 dogs for up to 120 days, compared with one of 19 without anticoagulants. Similar grafts to the jugular vein remained patent in all cases; the authors accounted for these differences by the differences between isogravitational flow and antigravitational flow.

Dale and Scott[30] presented a succinct re-

Table IV. *Vena cava grafts: Clinical reports*

Ref. No.	*Date*	*Indication*	*Results*	*Follow-up*
SUPERIOR VENA CAVA:				
Autogenous vein:				
79	1951	"Calcified node"	Patent	5 mo. by venogram
139	1954	Fibrosis	Patent	8 d. by autopsy
139	1954	Fibrosis	Patent	1 yr.
132	1954	Fibrosis	Occluded	5 mo.
76	1954	Fibrosis	Patent	5 yr. at death
1	1958	Benign obstruction	Patent	1 yr. clinically
1	1958	Fibrous mediastinitis	Postoperative	death
1	1958	Fibrous mediastinitis	Occluded	5 yr.
1	1958	Mediastinitis	—	—
1	1958	Radiation fibrosis	Patent	8 d. by autopsy
1	1958	Organized hematoma	Patent	1 yr. clinically
Aortic Homografts:				
13	1954	TB nodes	Patent	5 yr.
67	1954	Fibrous mediastinitis	Patent	10 mo. clinically
64	1954	Tumor	Patent	4 mo. at death
116	1955	Tumor, fibrosis	Patent	3 mo. clinically
38	1955	TB node	Patent	18 mo.
66	1956	Granuloma	Patent	11 mo. by venogram
66	1956	Tumor	Patent	4.5 mo. at autopsy
66	1956	Tumor	Patent	6 wk. at autopsy
1	1958	Metastatic sarcoma	Patent	6 wk. at death
1	1958	Malignant obstruction	Asymptomatic	6 wk. at death
1	1958	Benign obstruction	Patent	4 mo. at death
1	1958	Benign obstruction	Occluded	1 mo.
1	1958	Radiation fibrosis	Patent	5 mo. clinically
1	1958	Fibrous mediastinitis	Patent	10 mo. clinically
1	1958	Lung carcinoma	Patent	5 mo. clinically
1	1958	Granuloma	—	—
30	1963	Nonspecific fibrosis	Occluded	Postoperatively
Venous homografts:				
165	1972	Lung carcinoma	Patent	1 yr.
Aortic heterografts:				
5	1956	Lung carcinoma	Patent	7 mo. clinically
1	1958	Tumor	Patent	7 mo. clinically
Synthetic materials:				
1	1958	Fibrous mediastinitis (nylon)	Patent	4 mo. clinically
2	1962	Fibrous mediastinitis (Teflon support rings)	Patent	7 wk.
30	1963	Lung carcinoma (Teflon, 6 by 1 cm.)	Occluded	Postoperatively
57	1964	Lung carcinoma (Teflon)	Occluded	By venogram
36	1964	Lung carcinoma (Dacron)	Patent	9 mo. by venogram
INFERIOR VENA CAVA:				
Aortic homografts:				
14	1956	Agenesis infrarenal IVC (heparin used)	Patent	11 mo. by venogram
3	1956	Retroperitoneal tumor	Occluded	4 mo. by venogram
7	1957	Transposition (thoracic IVC to atrium, 23 of 38 cases patent)	Patent	26 mo.
93	1961	Retroperitoneal sarcoma (iliacs to suprarenal, heparin used)	Occluded	10 d. by venogram
30	1963	Nonchromaffin paraganglioma (infrarenal)	Patent	42 mo. by venogram
Inverted small bowel:				
91	1966	Carcinoma (infrarenal)	Patent	13 d. at autopsy
Synthetics:				
110	1963	Budd-Chiari syndrome (suprarenal to right auricle: Dacron, 2.5 by 22 cm.)	Patent	4 mo. by venogram

Table IV—*Cont'd*

Ref. No.	*Date*	*Indication*	*Results*	*Follow-up*
36	1964	Trauma (suprarenal to thoracic: Dacron)	Patent	30 d. by venogram
36	1964	Squamous-cell carcinoma (left renal vein to IVC: Dacron)	Patent	9 mo. by venogram
48	1966	Budd-Chiari syndrome (infrarenal to thoracic: (Teflon)	Patent	7 mo. by venogram
133	1970	Wilms' tumor (complete IVC replacement: Teflon)	Patent	2 yr.

view of the literature on venous grafting to 1963 and their results with autogenous jugular vein and knitted Dacron in the IVC. Three of seven autogenous venous grafts remained patent for up to 150 days; all of the Dacron occluded. They also reported successful SVC grafts and first noted the importance of ligating tributaries (i.e., the azygous vein) to maintain patency.

Silver and associates[152] attempted grafts from the suprarenal vena cava to the intrathoracic level and later successfully applied this method for decompression of suprahepatic vena caval obstruction. Of Dacron, Teflon, and bovine grafts, few remained patent, where seven of nine autogenous vein and four of six nylon were open at six weeks.

Anastomotic support by Teflon rings was first attempted by Shore and associates[151] using jugular vein autografts. Seven of 10 were patent compared to five of 10 without the rings. Larger grafts created by suturing panels of jugular vein had the lowest patency (one of 10); the suture lines presumably predisposed to thrombosis.

Patch grafting in the infrarenal vena cava was suggested by Stickel and Moorman[161] but, though eight of nine dogs with autologous vein patches maintained patent venae cavae for 3 weeks, only two of 15 did so with Teflon.

D'Silva and colleagues[42] were able to increase patency rates in SVC Teflon grafts by consistently using right-angle end-to-end anastomoses, but none of their IVC grafts were patent.

Whiffen and Gott[170] had nine of 10 thoracic IVC grafts remain patent for 2 months by the use of a Teflon graft with end-support rings and a GBH (graphite-benzalkonium-heparin) -coated inner surface. Later (1970), Najjar and Gott[106] reported 100 percent 2 month patency using heparin bonded by a cationic detergent to either woven or knitted Dacron.

A unique approach to the problem was developed by Inokuchi and Ono,[72] who placed Tetoron (Dacron) grafts in the abdominal aortas of dogs for several weeks, allowing a pseudointima to develop. They then transplanted the grafts to infrarenal venae cavae in dogs and cats. Sixteen of the 35 remained patent in dogs up to 500 days and 11 of 27 in cats up to 5 weeks. No immunosuppressive drugs were used. Histologic studies showed that the implanted pseudointima became necrotic and was replaced by pseudointima from the host animal.

A comparison of infrarenal and suprarenal grafting was done by Najafi and associates.[105] They placed 6 cm. Teflon grafts in the venae cavae of 21 dogs. All grafts below the kidneys thrombosed; seven of 11 above the kidneys were patent up to 18 months. They concluded that the patency rate was solely dependent on flow.

Egusa[49] reported on the effects of stainless steel support coils on the patency of Tetoron grafts. All of his thoracoabdominal IVC grafts with the coil remained patent from 16 to 250 days, compared with two thirds without the coil. Two of three infrarenal grafts with the coil remained patent 117 and 142 days.

Sharp and associates[147] placed negatively charged Dacron velour (Electrolour) grafts somewhere in the IVC of eight dogs; all were patent at 100 days. McCaughan[92] placed silicone rubber reinforced Dacron grafts in the infrarenal IVC of 12 dogs; all thrombosed in less than 3 weeks.

Ashton and associates[6] used a rigid prosthesis to theoretically counteract the force of constriction from fibrosis. A multilayer helix of silicone rubber was placed in the infrarenal IVC of nine dogs, four of which were patent up to 26 months. Two successes were also reported with the material in the suprarenal IVC.

Beilin and co-workers[9] used a temporary femoral-to-jugular bypass with GBH-coated polyvinyl to relieve acute experimental suprarenal IVC ligation in five dogs. Survival was maintained, but all shunts were noted to be closed in 48 hours.

Matsumoto[91] and his colleagues evaluated free segments of small bowel in the infrarenal vena cava. All 19 dogs thrombosed at less than 72 hours. However, of 40 grafts using inverted bowel, either as such or with removal of mucosa or of mucosa and serosa, all remained patent with follow-up to 14 months. Lawler and associates[82] used canine intestinal submucosa as a substitute in the thoracic IVC of 19 dogs; all were functional at 6 to 18 months with minimal inflammatory response. However, of 12 grafts of preserved jejunal mucosa placed in the abdominal IVC, all thrombosed in less than 3 weeks.

A recent study of the effects of anastomotic support rings was reported by Noszczyk.[107] That author used a Polish fiber Elastor Td24/2 and metal rings at the anastomosis in 10 dogs. Two of five dogs each had patent grafts in the infra- and suprarenal locations.

Soyer and associates[157] evaluated tubes of a porous Teflon product (Gore Tex) in growing piglets. All of their thoracic and suprarenal IVC grafts remained patent, with follow-up of 1 day to 6 months. Only one of the three infrarenal grafts did not occlude.

Clinical trials. The greater frequency and greater morbidity of SVC obstruction, over that of the IVC, prompted earlier clinical trials of bypass grafting, beginning with the patent femoral vein autograft reported by Klassen and associates[79] in 1951. The need to bypass IVC obstructed by tumors, however, also led to early clinical trials despite lack of overwhelming success in experimental models.

Thus in 1956 Crawford and De Bakey[26] presented the results obtained in a patient who had undergone wide excision of a retroperitoneal tumor involving aorta, IVC, and their bifurcations, followed by replacement of both with aortic bifurcation homografts. The symptoms of IVC obstruction were relieved postoperatively, but venogram at 4 months showed obstruction of the venous graft.

In the same year Blum and associates[14] reported a 29-year-old woman who had presented with symptoms of IVC occlusion and at operation was shown to have agenesis of the infrarenal IVC. She was treated with an aortic bifurcation homograft and given a heparin drip in both saphenous veins for 72 hours postoperatively. Cavagrams at 11 months showed patency.

Baffes and co-workers[7] reported the use of aortic homografts in the operation they devised for repair of transposition of the great vessels. The operation consisted of shifting the right pulmonary vein to the right atrium, inserting an end-to-side aortic homograft from the thoracic IVC to the left atrium, and then ligating the IVC between the anastomosis and the right atrium. The operation was reported as successful in 23 of 38 patients for periods of up to 26 months.

Schramel and Olinde[146] reported bypassing a vena cava obstructed by malignancy by connecting the left saphenous vein to the external jugular vein through a subcutaneous tunnel. Symptoms were relieved for the 1 month duration of the patient's life.

McPeak[93] replaced a 13.5 cm. segment of abdominal vena cava with freeze-dried aortic homograft to which he anastomosed the left renal vein. The retroperitoneal sarcoma necessitated removal of the IVC and right kidney. Heparin was used. Though the iliac veins were shown to be obstructed at 10 days, the patient did well clinically.

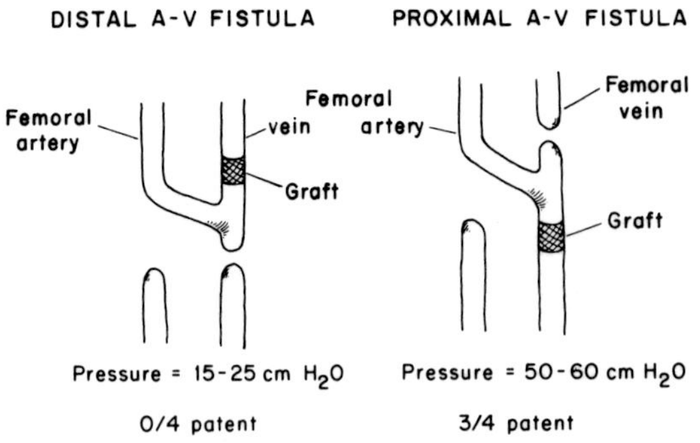

Fig. 1. Diagram of experiments of Bryant and associates.[20]

Dale and Scott[30] reported a 17-year-old boy with a large retroperitoneal nonchromaffin paraganglionoma involving the wall of the aorta, vena cava, and right renal vessels. Treatment was with en bloc resection and replacement of aorta and IVC with 12 cm. segments of freeze-dried aortic homografts. The patient had no clinical evidence of venous thrombosis and cavagram at 42 months postoperatively showed patency.

A Dacron graft 22 cm. long placed from below the renal veins to the right auricle was used by Ohara and co-workers[110] to bypass hepatic IVC occlusion. The patient improved clinically and patency was confirmed by venogram at four months.

Two successful grafts were reported by DeLaurentis and Tyson.[36] A traumatic injury to the IVC was bypassed with a knitted Dacron graft from the supra-renal to the thoracic IVC, and was patent by venogram at 30 days. A technical error during right nephrectomy necessitated the placement of a segment of aortic homograft from the left renal vein to the IVC in the second patient. She remained clinically well for at least 5 years.

Eguchi and associates[48] used a 20 cm. Teflon graft from the infrarenal IVC to the thoracic IVC to bypass the obstruction of Budd-Chiari syndrome. It was patent by cavagram at seven months.

After successfully experimenting with inverted small bowel in dogs (see above), Matsumoto[91] used a segment of inverted jejunum placed from below the renal vein to the iliac bifurcation. Autopsy at 13 days showed neither occlusion nor infection.

Sarti[133] totally replaced the IVC with a Teflon graft in a child with Wilms' tumor. The remaining renal vein was anastomosed to the graft. The graft was patent at 2 years.

HISTORICAL DATA: THE USE OF A-V FISTULAS IN VENOUS GRAFTING

Because the early thrombosis of vena caval grafts was attributed to low pressure and low flow in the venous system, several investigators designed experiments to overcome these hemodynamic factors. In 1949, Gerbode and associates[54] studied operations to relieve SVC obstruction in dogs and proposed that increased venous pressure might help hold the lumen open. So in 1953, Kunlin[81] first attempted an arteriovenous (A-V) fistula to increase venous pressure and prevent stenosis and occlusion of a peripheral venous graft; both reported cases failed.

In 1958, however, Bryant and associates[20] (see Fig. 1) used the adjunct of a proximal A-V fistula to maintain patency of 3 cm. segments of nylon graft inserted end-to-end in the femoral vein. This arrangement elevated the pressure within the grafts to 50 to 60 cm. H_2O and provided patency in three of four grafts for 3 months. A distal A-V fistula only elevated the intraluminal pressure to 15 to 25 cm. H_2O and all four grafts occluded in 3 weeks. The authors concluded that a pressure of 50 to 60 cm. H_2O was necessary to maintain patency of venous grafts.

Schauble and associates[140] elevated venous pressure in autogenous femoral veins grafted to femoral veins by ligating the infrarenal IVC. Pressures were 25 to 35 cm. H_2O. Of 12 grafts with normal femoral vein pressures, 58 percent were patent; of the seven with elevated pressures, 71 percent were patent. Nylon grafts occluded in every instance, however.

Smith and Schisgall[156] succinctly noted that since venous grafts do not fail in arterial systems, there must be nothing inherently thrombogenic about them, and related the high failure rate to three factors: (1) low flow rate, (2) low blood pressure, and (3) low oxygen tension. They noted that an A-V fistula alters all three factors. Of 11 dogs with A-V femoral fistulas, eight (72 percent) had patent autogenous femoral vein grafts proximal to the fistula, and two of two remained patent for one year after repair of the fistula. However, in the control group with no fistula, 13 of 18 (72 percent) also remained patent. They concluded that A-V fistulas were of no benefit. No measurements were reported.

Increased patency in iliac artery grafts was obtained by Dean and Read[33] by the insertion of a femoral A-V fistula on the same side, but not by distant fistulas which did not directly increase flow through the graft.

Application of the A-V shunt technique to the difficult problem of IVC grafts was first reported by Stansel,[158] who reported a patency of 11 of 15 end-to-end infrarenal IVC grafts of Dacron and Teflon with a femoral fistula. Venous pressures in the IVC distal to the graft were measured later to be from 7.6 to 17 cm. of saline in those grafts which remained patent. The author noted that significantly elevated venous pressure was not necessary to insure patency of IVC grafts, and attributed the success to increased flow.

Increased patency rates were also obtained by using common carotid artery–external jugular vein fistulas in SVC grafting. Thus Scheinin and Jude[141] used Dacron, Teflon, and autogenous vein with over-all patency of 88 percent (14 of 16), compared with 33 percent (five of 15) with no fistula. Fistulas were repaired at 1 month; grafts were followed for 4 to 8 months. Holt and Lewis[69] used woven Teflon with a 95 percent patency in 18 dogs. Shunts were repaired in 7 to 12 days; follow-up was 88 weeks. Various other parameters were measured as increased by the 1 L. per minute fistula, including cardiac output, by 25 to 40 percent, and SVC pressure, by 2 to 4 cm.

Table V. *Results of experiments of Steinman and associates[160]: Infrarenal IVC grafts combined with A-V fistulas*

Material	*No. patent/total*	*Average follow-up (days)*	*Average diameter change (%)*
Teflon	7/8	159	−71
Dacron	5/6	129	−74
Vein	3/3	127	+217
Total	15/17 (88%)		

H_2O. Mitsuoka and associates[95] reported a 100 percent patency (10 of 10) with 3 cm. Teflon grafts and 80 percent (eight of 10) with 8 cm. lengths. The fistulas were closed at 3 weeks, followed for 6 months. All three studies with fistulas showed significant improvement over control groups without fistulas.

The internal mammary artery was anastomosed to the SVC by Ellis and Del Rosaria[52] to enhance patency of 2 to 4 cm. Teflon SVC prostheses. Fistulas were repaired at 30 days. Patency was shown in all 15 dogs at 4 months.

Steinman and associates[160] used Teflon, Dacron, and autogenous vein grafts in an end-to-side anastomosis, bypassing ligatures in the infrarenal vena cava. A 2 to 2½ cm. A-V femoral fistula was created prior to the grafting and ligated at three weeks. The grafts were 12 mm. in diameter and varied in length from 8 to 10 cm. Results were as shown in Table V.

A thorough study of the effect of A-V fistulas on Teflon and Dacron grafts was presented by Yamaguchi and associates[173] in 1968 (see Fig. 2). Various places for the fistulas were studied, flow measurements were done, and the effect of late ligation of the fistula was noted. In the group (V) with distal aortocaval fistulas closed "later than 20 days postoperatively," 10 Teflon grafts and one Dacron graft were all patent at 1 month to 4 years. The authors noted a much thinner pseudointima in those grafts which were given increased flow than was found in those few grafts which stayed pat-

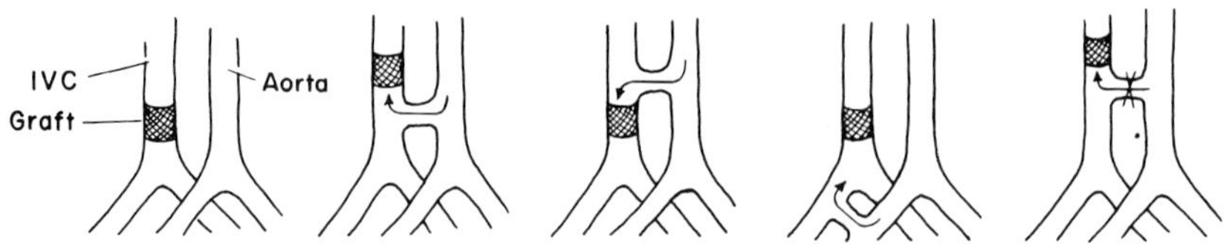

GROUP	I	II	III	IV	V
Patency[a]	6/16	20/24	17/20	5/7	11/11
Per Cent	33 %	83 %	85 %	71 %	100 %
Flow[b]	5-10.3	58.3	12.2	23.4	—
Pressure[c]	59	152	257	65	—

Fig. 2. Results of experiments of Yamaguchi and associates.[173] *(a)* Flow and pressure measurements were done in separate groups of dogs from those with the reported patency rates. *(b)* Blood flow in milliliters per minute per kilogram. *(c)* Pressure in millimeters of saline.

ent with normal flow. Patency was attributed solely to increased flow.

Mitsuoka and Howard[96] used 3 cm. Teflon grafts and 5 cm. Teflon grafts supported by five Teflon rings in conjunction with a 5 mm. femoral A-V fistula to replace resected infrarenal IVC. The fistulas were closed at 3 weeks. Of five grafts with only the fistula, three (60 percent) were patent; of 15 grafts also having support rings, the first three thrombosed due to technical difficulties and the last 12 remained patent for from 3 to 9 months.

Johnson and Eiseman[74] reported on jugular vein grafts bypassing the femoral veins using distal A-V fistulas. All five remained patent, and four had fistulas closed at 6 weeks and continued to be patent. They also discussed a 51-year-old woman who had presented with pain and swelling after inadvertant femoral vein ligation. The occlusion was bypassed with an 8 cm. segment of jugular vein autograft; a distal A-V fistula was constructed. Leg swelling diminished when the fistula was ligated at 3 weeks. The graft was patent by venogram at 7 months and clinically for at least 1½ years.

The neointima of Teflon prostheses placed in the infrarenal IVC and subject to a distal A-V fistula was studied by Shimamura and associates.[150] Stainless steel rings were used to insure patency, though only four of nine remained patent. The neointima on the patent grafts at 34 and 36 weeks was compared with the IVC intima distally. Minor morphologic differences in the endothelial cells were noted on electron microscopy (i.e., less invagination of basal cytoplasmic membrane into underlying connective tissue and less endoplasmic reticulum) but the differences were considered insignificant.

Baumann[8] applied the A-V fistula technique to peritoneal grafts in the infrarenal vena cava. The 7 mm. fistula was occluded at 1 month. In those grafts with polyethylene supports, all were patent; in those without the support, all were patent with hour-glass strictures.

Aureggi[3] studied the effect of an A-V fistula on the patency of inverted segments of free intestine with mucosa removed and inserted into the infrarenal IVC. A 1.5 cm. iliac fistula was used. Thrombosis was prevented in 33 percent of 30 dogs followed up to 3 months.

In the continuing search for better prostheses to replace arteries or veins, one which has proved especially promising is the ficin-digested bovine carotid artery preparation originally described by Rosenberg and associates.[121] Heterografts had been tried as arterial replacement since the pioneering—but unsuccessful—attempts by Hopfner[70] in 1903, and later successes of dog vessels transplanted into cat aortas by Carrel.[21] However, results were unpredictable and the heterografts more often than not were subject to thrombosis or aneurysm formation with rupture. Microscopic examination[27] showed that untreated heterografts brought forth an intense reaction by the host which uniformly led to severe inflammatory and degenerative changes within the graft.

In 1956, Rosenberg and colleagues[121] reported the results of enzyme-modified bovine carotid arteries used as aortic replacements in dogs. The elastic and muscle fibers were digested by the proteolytic enzyme ficin, and the resultant nonantigenic collagen tube was then tanned with formaldehyde. Seventy percent patency was obtained at 3 months to 1 year. Detailed histologic studies revealed the following: (1) There was minimal cellular reaction at 14 days and thereafter, limited to the suture lines (silk was used). (2) The grafts were immediately coated by a thin mural thrombus, which was infiltrated by fibroblasts by 90 days. (3) At 90 days, indeed, the original prosthesis could often no longer be identified. Later, DeFalco[35] performed detailed immunologic studies with the graft preparation and found no immunologic reactions whatsoever. Rosenberg and associates[122] also showed that the essential component of arterial wall for resistance to stress was indeed collagen and found[123] that the tensile strength of the grafts even increased after implantation.

However, 5 year follow-up of Rosenberg's original grafts[124] showed a success of 50 percent, due to aneurysm, dilatation, wall irregularities, and mural thrombi. Inserted into the thoracic aorta by deTakats and associates,[37] the grafts also had a high rate of aneurysm formation. It was determined that the enzyme had not been adequately deactivated and later grafts were prepared with a more controlled digestion period, deactivation of the enzyme, and more permanent tanning using dialdehyde starch.

Results of the newer graft preparation in arterial replacement have been encouraging.[126, 127] Seven-year follow-up of seven thoracic or thoracoabdominal grafts in dogs[129] revealed (1) no dilatation or aneurysm formation, (2) complete intimization except for small areas of erosion or thin mural thrombus, (3) limited and rare suture line pannus (Mersilene was used), and (4) no cellular reaction on microscopic examination. Interestingly, in one dog, the implant was disorganized by foci of chondrification and osteoid formation. Seventeen human arterial replacements were first reported by the same authors[128] with seven femoropopliteal, iliofemoral, and popliteal grafts still patent at 1 year. More recently[120] they reported results of 90 arterial implants followed from 2 to 6 years. Fifty had received femoropopliteal bypass, with a 60 percent patency at two years. Of grafts used in iliofemoral (7), femorofemoral (3), axillary-branchial (1), and aortorenal (2) bypass, all were patent. Other authors[31, 77, 78, 172] have reported similar results.

Results of the bovine heterograft in the venous system have been variable, and closely parallel results with other graft materials. Thus, Ohara and Sakai[109] had four of 12 grafts patent in the SVC, but the infrarenal IVC graft thrombosed. Moore and coworkers[98, 102] and Riberi and Moore[119] reported an 82 percent patency in 11 dogs with SVC grafts followed up to 26 months. Ashburn and associates[5] presented a patient who had been relieved of malignant SVC obstruction for 7 months by an aortic heterograft. These early experiments were done with freeze-dried or alcohol-preserved arteries.

Use of the ficin-digested bovine carotid artery in the venous system was first reported by Todd and associates,[166] who reinforced the collagen tube with Dacron rings. They reported three grafts patent at 3 months. Silver and Anlyan[154] put five grafts in dogs from the suprarenal to the thoracic IVC; one was patent at 6 weeks. A later report[153] studied the collagen tube in various venous settings, including pulmonary artery, IVC, and SVC. Continuous over-and-over No. 5-0 silk sutures interrupted at the angles were used in both end-to-end and end-to-side anastomoses. Segments of 1 cm. in the left pulmonary artery were all patent at 6 months, but three of six occluded by 13 months. All but one of the seven 3 to 4 cm. segments were patent up to 16 months. SVC

Table VI. *Results of five IVC grafts by Silver[153] with bovine collagen tube*

Duration of patency	*Necropsy findings*
Occluded at 1 wk.	Thrombosis of entire graft, adherent to proximal anastomosis
Occluded at 3 wk.	Graft completely filled with adherent, organized thrombus
Occluded at 3 wk.	Similar to above dog
Occluded at 8 mo.	Fibrotic stricture of both anastomoses causing occlusion; marked degeneration of graft
Patent at 12 mo.	Well endothelialized; longitudinal thickened folds in graft; as compared to other grafts, (1) less adventitial fibrosis and inflammation, (2) greatest degree of fibrous ingrowth into implanted graft material, (3) more residual elastic tissue in implanted graft material

Table VII. *Results of 10 IVC grafts by Breslau and associates[19] with bovine collagen tube*

Four graft thrombosed at less than one week:
One dog had severe polymorphonuclear cell infiltration throughout the graft and adjacent tissues
Three dogs had a lumbar tributary vein which had escaped ligation

Five grafts thrombosed at more than one week:
Five had external fibrotic encirclement of both anastomotic lines by dense fibrous tissue producing marked stenosis; four of these were distended with firm, adherent, laminated thrombus

One graft was still patent at 61 days:
One had (a) longitudinal wrinkling of the graft intima, (b) fibrous thickening of neointima, especially present in the midportion of the graft, (c) fragmentation of outer one third of graft wall by invading host fibrous tissue

grafts were complicated by a high rate of infection; two of three dogs without infection remain patent up to 13 months. The results of 2.5 cm. segments in the infrarenal IVC are outlined in Table VI.

Histologic studies were also done by Silver. Fibrous invasion did not occur diffusely throughout the graft and only a sparse infiltration was noted near the anastomosis. However, the most successful grafts were noted to have the most fibrous ingrowth. An ingrowth of endothelialized connective tissue was noted from the anastomotic sites along the luminal surface. The tissue consisted of apparently multipotential mesenchymal cells which sometimes differentiated into chondroblasts or osteoblasts. Intense proliferation of this fibrous subendothelial layer was found in all grafts with late occlusions.

Breslau and associates[19] also studied the heterograft preparation in the infrarenal vena cava. The 4.5 to 7.5 cm. grafts were sutured end-to-end to the vein using a single everting layer of No. 5-0 silk. Of 10 dogs, six were patent at 1 week, but only one was patent at 1 month. This sole patent graft was uniformly narrowed but remained patent until sacrifice at 61 days. Histologically, the grafts were said to be much as described for those in the arterial system.[121] Thrombosed grafts were followed for up to 22 weeks and no recanalization was noted. Results are summarized in Table VII.

DISCUSSION

Despite extensive study, numerous published reports, and a thorough background of experimental and clinical work in vascular surgery of arteries, replacement of venous segments has still not been nearly successful enough to be realistically applied to any but the most desperate of clinical situations.

Collected reports have indicated a fair number of successes by some investigators in specific situations, and this may indicate the feasibility of venous replacement and certainly shows that the problem warrants further investigation. However, for each success by one worker, there are a number of failures by others; comparison is difficult largely because the personal technical aspects are so significant in venous surgery and also because methods and timing of measurements, specifics for surgical procedures, criteria for patency, and follow-up periods vary widely.

A cursory review of the literature reveals some results which are difficult to reconcile with others. Some authors[23] state that prosthetic material type is of no importance;

others[30] do not agree. Theoretical considerations and studies by some authors[42] would stress the importance of suture methods (i.e., the everting stitch), others[134, 154] find it unimportant. Some[140] stress failures found in veins with antigravitational flow; others[64] find no difference from isogravitational flow. Some[53, 107, 151] find anastomotic support by rigid rings to be of great benefit; others[69, 166] find them useless. Some[61] find significant benefit from anticoagulation; most[34, 40, 43] report occluded grafts in dogs dying from hemorrhage. Many authors[30, 46, 99, 100, 141, 162] assert that grafts patent for short periods (i.e., 1 week) will remain so; others[72, 102] report more significant problems with late (i.e., 1 month) occlusions. Many[20, 140, 162] conclude from their studies that increased pressure is what keeps a venous graft patent; an equal number[33, 105, 141, 158] assert that it is purely a matter of flow. At least one author[1] condemned ligating of collateral channels as risky when a graft might thrombose; others[19, 30] noted patency only after the collaterals had been ligated.

But despite a certain element of ambiguity in the above reports, enough pertinent data have accumulated that some generalizations can be made about venous grafting in general and IVC grafting in particular. Some of these are presented below. A cogent analysis of venous surgery was presented by Dale and Scott[30] in 1960; a more recent analysis was done by Haimovici and associates.[62]

1. The particular vein being replaced is significant. For whatever reasons, grafts in the SVC are more likely to remain patent than those in the IVC. Various authors[30, 62] have explained this on the basis of negative thoracic pressure holding a graft open whereas positive abdominal pressure obliterates it. This is supported by the increased patency of thoracic over abdominal IVC grafts,[157] and a similar patency of SVC and thoracic grafts.[136] However, differences in flow tend to better explain why suprarenal grafts are more successful than infrarenal,[105] and one might wonder how graft lumina obliterated by high abdominal pressure consistently come to be distended with thrombi at autopsy. That SVC collateral vessels (i.e., the azygous vein) can be ligated whereas those of the IVC cannot has also been offered as an explanation, but is equally conjectural.

Grafts in the portal vein or jugular vein are also likely to remain patent.

2. Most grafts fail in the first week due to thrombosis. This is evident from examination of early occluded grafts distended with thrombus.[18, 166] How to prevent thrombosis is a more difficult question to answer, but it is generally assumed that this is a matter of surgical technique—as it is in arterial surgery. However, venous surgery is more difficult: veins are thin walled and collapse and retract; tearing of the vein wall occurs easily; twisting, buckling, and ridging all predispose to thrombosis.[20] Prosthetic material and suture and anastomotic technique also relate to this problem but have not been adequately studied.

3. Late occlusion of venous grafts is due to sclerosis. Histologic examination of nearly all authors[61] has demonstrated obliteration of the anastomotic diameter by scar tissue in those few grafts which occlude late (i.e., after 1 week and usually before 5 weeks) and even narrowing in those which remain patent. In general, the use of steel rings to support the anastomoses has been successful, but is a technically difficult procedure.

4. Highest patency rates are obtained when the graft lumen is isodiametric with the vein. Eiken[51] and Malan and associates[88] have shown that the greatest flow and least turbulence are obtained with isodiametric grafts. It should be noted that for a synthetic graft's lumen to remain isodiametric the diameter of the inserted graft must be greater[158, 160] to allow for the thickness of the pseudointima which develops on the inside luminal wall and is especially thick in venous implants. Autogenous vein grafts, however, are more likely to dilate after insertion.[28]

5. The type of prosthetic material is important; autogenous veins remain patent; synthetics do not. Every conceivable prosthetic material has been tried in venous surgery, from rubber tubes[109] to small bowel.[116] It is clear that autogenous vein is the best substitute, but this may be because it is the only material shown to recanalize following thrombosis.[29, 30, 40, 43, 160] With the exception of pericardial tubes, small bowel, and some unusual synthetics, all other materials are usually unsuccessful in the abdomen, but have been reported as highly successful by at least one investigator. Other differences may be noted (Tables II, III, and IV) but may relate more to the technical factors in the graft or investigator than in the material itself.

Various theories have been used to explain why one prosthesis might have a higher patency rate than another; this subject has been extensively studied in arterial grafts. Certainly short-term failure is related to thrombosis and some grafts appear less likely to thrombose. Negative charge on the inner luminal surface (negative zeta potential) tends to repel clot formation,[131] which may explain the high patency reported[147] with negatively charged Dacron velour. Heparin-coated materials also tend to prevent thrombosis.[106, 170]

Factors such as biologic reactivity and porosity, which are important to the success of arterial grafts,[61, 65, 168, 169] are also important in the venous system. Of particular significance is the thickness and viability of the pseudointima which develops by organization of the mural thrombus which forms along the inner luminal surface immediately after insertion of the graft. Various authors[158, 173] have noted that the pseudointima developing in venous grafts is thicker (by about 200 microns) than in arteries; Eiken[50] and Sharp and associates[147] have shown this thickness to be related to lower flow. Stansel[158] accounted for the decreased success rate of Dacron over Teflon as due to the thicker, less adherent pseudointima. Wesolowski[169] noted that graft failure in arteries is often related to necrosis of areas of pseudointima which become too thick for their limited blood supply.

6. A distal arteriovenous fistula increases patency. From Table II it is obvious that the only consistently successful graft attempts have been obtained by using this experimental technique. The one reported failure of the A-V fistula to benefit results[156] was when the 3 cm. fistula was within 1 cm. of the femoral vein graft, and turbulence cannot be ruled out as the factor inciting thrombosis.

There are at least four effects from creating an A-V fistula: (1) increased pressure, (2) increased flow, (3) pulsatile flow, and (4) arterialization of venous blood with increased oxygen saturation and possible changes in the acidity and solute content. There have been no studies evaluating the third and fourth factors, and few good studies evaluating the first two, so it is impossible to state which factor or combination of factors may be necessary to maintain patency of venous grafts.

That flow is the main factor is supported by differences between infrarenal and suprarenal graft successes,[6, 105, 157] by the finding of Stansel[158] and Yamaguchi and associates[173] that vena caval pressure did not increase significantly with the fistula, and by the studies of Schenk and associates[143, 144] showing that in a femoral side-to-side fistula the proximal femoral vein pressure does not increase while the flow does. However, Yamaguchi's studies were not done in the same dogs which later had patent grafts, Stansel's measurements were taken some time after the operation, and Schenk's fistula studies did not deal with the obstruction resulting from a graft anastomosis.

There are various reasons why increased flow could logically be thought to prevent occlusion. It could provide better mechanical cleansing of fibrin, formed elements, and the thromboplastin which Huggins[71] considers important in small artery thrombosis. It has been shown[83, 103] to affect the initiation, structure, and propagation of thrombi, and has been suggested[158] to affect the electrostatic charge on the luminal surface.

That pressure is the important factor is supported by the difference between SVC and IVC graft patency, by the increased patency obtained by Schauble and associates[140] where pressure was increased and flow decreased by IVC ligations, and by the findings obtained by Bryant and associates[20] that only in the setting where peripheral resistance was high (hence, low flow)* did internal pressure rise enough for the grafts to remain patent. However, in none of these cases can other factors be excluded completely.

Pressure could logically be thought to prevent occlusion simply by opposing those forces (e.g., abdominal pressure, fibrosis, the negative pressure of increased flow by Bernouille's law)† which tend to obliterate the lumen or anastomosis. The elevation necessary appears to be near 50 to 60 cm. H_2O.

The other changes from an A-V fistula have not been investigated. One would guess from Eiken's[51] studies that pulsatile flow would increase the chances for thrombosis. Arterialization of venous blood could, however, decrease failure by promoting nourishment of the pseudointima.

The duration of the A-V fistula necessary to maintain patency has been empirically determined to be about 3 weeks,[96, 160, 173] though no studies have been reported with attempts at fistulas of shorter duration. Steinman and associates[160] theorized that the 3 week fistula might allow for the development of a pseudointima, but Yamaguchi and associates[173] have shown that neither organization nor endotheliazation is achieved in this period, and that these processes consistently take 2 months whether or not a fistula is present. Those authors simply speculate that the fistula promotes a perfectly smooth fibrin layer over the suture lines and graft lumen. It may thus remove the excessive fibrin at the anastomoses which, when organized, would lead to fibrous constriction.

7. There are some other less certain facets of venous system grafting which should be mentioned. The effect of graft length on patency has not been adequately studied and, indeed, most experimental work has been done with grafts much too short for clinical applicability. Mitsuoka and associates[95] did find a lower patency (i.e., eight of 15, or 53 percent) with 8 cm. grafts than with 3 cm. one (i.e., 16 of 20, or 80 percent).

The studies by Dale and Scott[30] and by Emerson and Galente[53] give fairly convincing evidence that, at least in the SVC, the collateral system (i.e., the azygous vein) should be ligated. Dale and Scott had only 19 percent (four of 21) patency without ligation, compared with 74 percent (26 of 35) with ligation. On the other hand, pointing out untied collaterals on venograms as the cause for occlusion[19] may be faulty reasoning, since untied collaterals might not be visible without occlusion and it is thus impossible to determine whether they represent the cause or the effect.

Finally, from the examination of Table IV it is readily apparent that clinical success rates are far better than experimental ones. This may be a real phenomenon, possibly related to the fact that thrombi form more readily in dogs; it is more likely due to hesitancy on the part of investigators to report clinical failures.

*I.e., with the proximal A-V fistula; with the distal fistula pressure rose only slightly and grafts occluded.

†I.e., within a tube pressure is inversely related to flow.

REFERENCES

1. Allansmith, R., and Richards, K.: SVC obstruction, Am. J. Surg. **96:** 353, 1958.
2. Allansmith, R.: Surgical treatment of SVC obstruction due to malignant tumor, J. Thorac. Cardiovasc. Surg. **44:** 258, 1962.
3. Aureggi, A.: Plastic substitutions of the IVC, Policlinico (Chir.) **79:** 49, 1972 (English abst.).
4. Aschberg, S., and Hindmarsh, T.: Distal A-V shunts in autotransplantation of canine venous valves, Acta Chir. Scand. **137:** 503, 1971.
5. Ashburn, F. S., Seuell, W. H., and Huggins, C. E.: Experimental replacement of the SVC with homologous arteries and report of a case with malignant obstruction replaced with a heterologous artery, J. Thorac. Surg. **31:** 618, 1956.
6. Ashton, F., Geddes, R., and Fejfar, J.: Woven silicone rubber as a venous prosthesis, Br. Med. J. **3:** 409, 1969.
7. Baffes, T. G., Riker, W. L., DeBoer, A., and Potts, W. J.: Surgical correction of transposition of the aorta and pulmonary artery, J. Thorac. Surg. **34:** 469, 1957.

8. Baumann, G.: Segment replacement of the IVC in dogs with peritoneum. Dtsch. Med. Wochenschr. **97:** 957, 1972 (German).
9. Beilin, L., Campbell, R. N., and Bassaniga, A. B.: Ligation of the supra-renal IVC: Application of a graphite-benzalkonium-heparin coated femoral to jugular vein shunt, Ann. Surg. **174:** 837, 1971.
10. Bennett, I. L.: A unique case of obstruction of the IVC, Bull. Johns Hopkins Hosp. **87:** 290, 1940.
11. Benvenuto, R., and Lewis, R. J.: Anastomosis between the SVC and the right atrium, SURGERY **45:** 173, 1959.
12. Benvenuto, R., Rodman, F. S. B., Gilmour, J., Phillips, A. F., and Callagham, J. C.: Composite venous graft for replacement of the SVC, Arch. Surg. **84:** 570, 1962.
13. Bhonslay, S.: A discussion of Earl et al., Arch. Surg. **80:** 124, 1960.
14. Blum, L., Medl, W. J., and Keefer, E. B. C.: Aortic homograft substitution for the post-renal IVC, Arch. Surg. **72:** 567, 1956.
15. Boruchow, I., and Johnson, J.: Obstructions of the vena cava, Surg. Gynecol. Obstet. **134:** 115, 1972.
16. Botham, R. J., Dracopoulos, T. T., and Gale, J. W.: SVC replacement with sponge Teflon prosthesis: A preliminary report, J. Thorac. Cardiovasc. Surg. **39:** 202, 1960.
17. Boutelier, P., and Couinand, C.: Primitive anomalies of the IVC, J. Chir. **83:** 199, 1962 (French).
18. Bower, R., Fredericci, V., and Howard, J. M.: Continuing studies of replacement of segments of the venous system, SURGERY **47:** 132, 1960.
19. Breslau, R. C., Schwartz, S. I., Smith, D. W., and Rob, C. G.: IVC replacement with bovine heterografts, N. Y. State J. Med. **65:** 1967, 1965.
20. Bryant, M. F., Lazenby, W. D., and Howard, J. M.: Experimental replacement of short segments of veins, Arch. Surg. **76:** 289, 1958.
21. Carrel, A.: Heterotransplantation of blood vessels in cold storage, J. Exp. Med. **9:** 226, 1907.
22. Carrel, A., and Guthrie, C. C.: Uniterminal and biterminal venous transplantation, Surg. Gynecol. Obstet. **2:** 266, 1906.
23. Collins, H. A., Burrus, G., and De Bakey, M. E.: Experimental evaluation of grafts of the canaine IVC, Am. J. Surg. **99:** 40, 1960.
24. Contescu, N.: Gangrene of the extremities from phlebitis of the IVC, Presse Med. **69:** 2209, 1961 (French).
25. Cope, J. S., and Hunt, C. J.: Leiomyosarcoma of the IVC, Arch. Surg. **68:** 753, 1954.
26. Crawford, E. S., and De Bakey, M. E.: Wide excision including involved aorta and vena cava and replacement with aortic homograft for retroperitoneal malignant tumors: Report of two cases, Cancer **9:** 1085, 1956.
27. Creech, O., De Bakey, M. E., Self, M., and Halpert, B.: The fate of heterologous arterial grafts: An experimental study, SURGERY **36:** 431, 1954.
28. Creech, O., Deterling, R. A., Edwards, S., Julian, O., Linton, R., and Shumacker, H.: Vascular prostheses: Report of the Committee for Study of Vascular Prostheses, of The Society for Vascular Surgery, SURGERY **41:** 62, 1957.
29. Dale, W. A.: Thrombosis and recanalization of veins used as venous grafts, Angiology **12:** 603, 1961.
30. Dale, W. A., and Scott, H. W.: Grafts of the venous system, SURGERY **53:** 52, 1963.
31. Dale, W. A., and Lewis, M. R.: Modified bovine heterografts for arterial replacement, Ann. Surg. **169:** 927, 1969.
32. Davalos, C. A., Sewell, S. H., and Harrison, J. H.: Experimental use of a Teflon prosthesis for elongation of IVC in the Baffes operation, Surg. Forum. **10:** 657, 1960.
33. Dean, R. E., and Read, R. C.: The influence of increased blood flow in thrombosis of prosthetic grafts, SURGERY **55:** 581, 1964.
34. DeMeetz, A., Phillips, U., Habif, D. V., and Jacobson, J. H.: Use of fibrinolysin in IVC replacement, Arch. Surg. **83:** 883, 1961.
35. DeFalco, R. J.: Immunologic studies of untreated and chemically modified bovine carotid arteries, J. Surg. Res. **10:** 95, 1970.
36. DeLaurentis, D. A., and Tyson, R. R.: Surgical reconstruction of major veins, Circulation **29:** 176 (Suppl. 1), 1964.
37. deTakats, G., Thompson, I. D., and Dolowy, W. C.: Bovine arterial grafts: An experimental study, Ann. Surg. **150:** 1017, 1959.
38. Deterling, R. A., and Bhonslay, S. B.: Use of vessel grafts and plastic prostheses for relief of SVC obstruction, SURGERY **38:** 1008, 1955.
39. Devon, H. W., Schlesinger, M. J., Savitz, H.: Chronic progressive occlusion of the IVC and the renal and portal veins, Arch. Int. Med. **63:** 626, 1939.
40. DeWeese, J. A., and Niguidula, F.: The replacement of short segments of veins, Surg. Gynecol. Obstet. **110:** 303, 1960.
41. Dillard, R. A., Lyons, C., and Salter, P. P.: Thrombosis of the vena cava to the level of renal veins with recovery, Am. Surg. **23:** 539, 1957.
42. D'Silva, J., Crampton, A. R., and Hohf, R. P.: SVC prosthesis: A comparison of

types and sites of anastomosis, J. Thorac. Cardiovasc. Surg. **48:** 276, 1964.
43. Ducharme, J. C.: End to end venous anastomosis in small puppies: Techniques, results, growth, and some factors influencing thrombosis, Ohio Med. J. **57:** 777, 1961.
44. Earl, A. S., Horsley, J. S., Villavicencio, J. L., and Warren, R.: Replacement of venous defects by venous autografts, Arch. Surg. **80:** 119, 1960.
45. East, W. M., and Muller, W. H.: Experimental study of resection and replacement of the SVC, Am. J. Surg. **99:** 6, 1960.
46. Edwards, W. S., Dalton, D., and Quattlebaum, R.: Anastomoses between synthetic graft and artery, Arch. Surg. **86:** 477, 1963.
47. Egdahl, R. H., Hume, D. M., and Schlag, H. A.: Plastic venous prostheses, Surg. Forum **5:** 235, 1955.
48. Eguchi, S., Endo, S., Yamaguchi, A., and Asano, K.: IVC occlusion associated with the Budd-Chiari syndrome: Treatment with bypass operation, J. Cardiovasc. Surg. **7:** 490, 1966.
49. Egusa, S.: Experimental study on vascular grafts. I. Replacement of IVC with crimped woven Tetoron (polyester) grafts and those reinforced with stainless steel coil, Acta Med. Okayama **22:** 65, 1968.
50. Eiken, O.: Combined Teflon-autologous vein grafts for small artery replacement in dogs, Acta Chir. Scand. **121:** 200, 1961.
51. Eiken, O.: Pressure-flow relationships and thrombotic occlusion of experimental grafts, Acta Chir. Scand. **121:** 398, 1961.
52. Ellis, P. R., and Del Rosaria, V. C.: Internal mammary artery–SVC fistula: An adjunct to SVC replacement, Ann. Thorac. Surg. **4:** 74, 1967.
53. Emerson, D. M., and Galente, W.: The use of externally supported aortic homografts in the SVC, Surg. Forum **8:** 450, 1957.
54. Gerbode, F., Yee, J., and Rundle, F. F.: Experimental anastomoses of vessels to the heart: Possible application to SVC obstruction, SURGERY **25:** 556, 1949.
55. Gliedman, M., Girandet, R., Ryzoff, R., and Karlson, R. E.: Hepatic swelling and IVC constriction, Ann. Surg. **161:** 344, 1965.
56. Gonzales, E. G.: Thrombosis of the IVC with gangrene of both legs, Br. J. Surg. **51:** 235, 1964.
57. Gothman, B., and Anderson, T.: SVC replacement with woven Teflon tube, J. Cardiovasc. Surg. **5:** 29, 1964.
58. Hatch, W.: Collateral circulation in IVC occlusion, Med. Klin. **66:** 1574, 1971 (German).
59. Haimov, M., Kirchner, D., and Kark, A. E.: Fatal complications following IVC interruption, Vasc. Surg. **5:** 228, 1971.
60. Haimovici, H.: Gangrene of the extremities of venous origin, Circulation **1:** 225, 1950.
61. Haimovici, H., Zinicola, N., Noovani, M., and Hoffert, P. W.: Vein grafts in the venous system, Arch. Surg. **87:** 542, 1963.
62. Haimovici, H., Hoffert, P. W., Zinicola, N., and Steinman, C.: An experimental and clinical evaluation of grafts in the venous system, Surg. Gynecol. Obstet. **131:** 1173, 1970.
63. Hambraeus, B., and Anderson, M.: Experimental vena cava replacement with Teflon prosthesis, Arch. Surg. **85:** 220, 1962.
64. Hanlon, C. R.: Discussion of Scannel and Shaw, J. Thorac. Surg. **28:** 172, 1954.
65. Harrison, J. H., and Davalos, P. A.: Influence of porosity on synthetic grafts, Arch. Surg. **82:** 8, 1961.
66. Higginson, J. F.: Aortic homograft substitution and bypass in SVC obstruction, J. Thorac. Cardiovasc. Surg. **32:** 684, 1956.
67. Holman, C. W., and Steinberg, I.: Treatment of SVC occlusion by arterial graft, J. A. M. A. **155:** 1403, 1954.
68. Holman, E., and Taylor, G.: Problems in the dynamics of blood flow. II. Pressure relations at the site of an A-V fistula, Angiology **3:** 415, 1952.
69. Holt, M. H., and Lewis, F. J.: Experimental grafts of the SVC with temporary A-V shunts, J. Thorac. Cardiovasc. Surg. **49:** 818, 1965.
70. Hopfner, E.: On vascular suture, vascular transplant, and replantation of amputated extremities, Arch. Klin. Chir. **70:** 417, 1903 (German).
71. Huggins, C. E.: Blood vessel thromboplastins and early thrombosis after vascular operations, SURGERY **48:** 724, 1960.
72. Inokuchi, K., and Ono, K.: Experimental venous replacement by transplanted synthetic grafts, SURGERY **60:** 862, 1966.
73. Johns, T. N. P.: A comparison of suture and non-suture methods for the anastomosis of veins, Surg. Gynecol. Obstet. **84:** 939, 1947.
74. Johnson, V., and Eiseman, B.: Evaluation of A-V shunt to maintain patency of venous autograft, Am. J. Surg. **118:** 915, 1969.
75. Jones, T. W., Stevenson, J. K., Jesseph, J. E., and Harkins, H. N.: A critical evaluation of polyvinyl sponge (Ivalon) as a vascular and tissue substitute, Ann. Surg. **24:** 401, 1958.
76. Kay, E. B.: Discussion of Scannell and Shaw, J. Thorac. Surg. **28:** 171, 1954.
77. Keshishian, J. M., Smyth, N. P. D., Adkins,

P. C., Camp, F., and Yahr, W. Z.: Clinical experience with the modified bovine arterial heterograft Ann. Surg. **172:** 690, 1970.
78. Keshishian, J. M., Smythe, N. P. D., Adkins, P. C., Camp, F., Yahr, W. Z., and Hill, L.: Clinical experience with the modified bovine arterial heterograft, J. Cardiovasc. Surg. **12:** 433, 1971.
79. Klassen, K. P., Andrews, N. C., and Curtis, G. M.: Diagnosis and treatment of SVC obstruction, Arch. Surg. **63:** 311, 1951.
80. Kuehl, K. S., Perry, L. W., and Scott, L. P.: Thrombosis of IVC in patients with cyanotic congenital heart disease, J. Pediatr. **79:** 430, 1971.
81. Kunlin, J.: The reestablishment of venous circulation with grafts in cases of obliteration from trauma or thrombophlebitis, Mem. Acad. Clin. **79:** 109, 1953 (French).
82. Lawler, M. R., Foster, S., and Scott, H. W.: Evaluation of canine intestinal submucosa as vascular substitute, Am. J. Surg. **122:** 517, 1971.
83. Leonard, E. F.: The role of flow in thrombogenesis, Bull. N. Y. Acad. Med. **48:** 273, 1972.
84. Lillehei, C. W., Bobb, J. R. R., and Visscher, M. B.: Occurrence of endocarditis with valvular deformities in dogs with A-V fistulas, Ann. Surg. **132:** 577, 1950.
85. Lutembacher, D.: Thrombophlebitis of the IVC and renal and portal veins, Presse Med. **43:** 1175, 1935 (French).
86. MacLean, L., Phibbs, C. M., Flom, R. S., and Brainard, J. B.: Replacement of vital veins: A comparative experimental study, Ann. Surg. **149:** 549, 1959.
87. Madden, J. L.: Ligation of the IVC, Ann. Surg. **140:** 200, 1954.
88. Malan, E., Noseda, G., and Longo, T.: Approach to fluid dynamic problems in reconstructive vascular surgery, Surgery **66:** 994, 1969.
89. Martinek, J. B.: Surgical treatment of renal tumors penetrating into the great veins, Int. Surg. **55:** 417, 1971.
90. Mason, R. G.: Personal communication, September 2, 1969, noted in description of product: Arterial graft (bovine origin), Johnson and Johnson, New Brunswick, N. J.
91. Matsumoto, T.: Replacement of large veins with free inverted segments of small bowel, Ann. Surg. **164:** 845, 1966.
92. McCaughan, J.: Evaluation of silastic-reinforced Dacron for replacement of the IVC, Surgery **66:** 375, 1969.
93. McPeak, C. J.: Resection of IVC and graft replacement for retroperitoneal sarcoma, Surgery **50:** 778, 1961.
94. Missal, M. E., Robinson, J. A., and Tatum, R. W.: IVC obstruction: Clinical manifestations, diagnostic methods, and related problems, Ann. Intern. Med. **62:** 133, 1965.
95. Mitsuoka, H., Vega, R. E., and Howard, J. M.: Experimental venous replacement utilizing the adjunct of a temporary A-V fistula, Arch. Surg. **93:** 382, 1966.
96. Mitsuoka, H., and Howard, J. M.: Experimental grafting of the IVC, J. Cardiovasc. Surg. **9:** 190, 1968.
97. Moore, T. C., and Riberi, A.: SVC replacement. III. Successful use of fresh autogenous aorta, Surgery **44:** 898, 1958.
98. Moore, T. C., Heimburger, I. L., and Teramoto, S.: Experimental replacement of SVC, Bull. Soc. Int. Surg. **19:** 340, 1960.
99. Moore, T. C., Teramoto, S., and Heimburger, I.: Successful use of Teflon grafts for SVC replacement, Surg. Gynecol. Obstet. **111:** 475, 1960.
100. Moore, T. C., Teramoto, S., Heimburger, I., and Hershum, J. D.: SVC replacement. V. Use of fresh homografts of SVC, J. Thorac. Surg. **43:** 379, 1961.
101. Moore, T. C., and Mandelbaum, I.: SVC replacement. VII. Experimental use of toluene di-isocyanite treated Dacron, Surgery **54:** 340, 1963.
102. Moore, T. C., and Yong, N. K.: Experimental replacement and bypass of large veins, Bull. Soc. Int. Surg. **23:** 274, 1964.
103. Mustard, J. F., Murphy, E. A., Rowsell, H. C., and Downie, H. G.: Factors influencing thrombus formation in vivo, Am. J. Med. **33:** 621, 1962.
104. Myhre, J., and Ylvisaker, R. S.: Venous gangrene with thrombosis of the IVC, Arch. Surg. **69:** 732, 1954.
105. Najafi, H., Battung, V., Sarfatis, D., Hirose, M., and DeWall, R. A.: Experimental IVC replacement, J. Thorac. Cardiovasc. Surg. **53:** 243, 1967.
106. Najjar, F. B., and Gott, V. L.: Small diameter Dacron grafts with wall bonded heparin for venous and arterial replacement, Surgery **68:** 1053, 1970.
107. Noszcyk, W.: Experimental prosthesis of the abdominal segment of the IVC, Pol. Med. J. **10:** 140, 1971.
108. Oakes, W. W., and Hawthorne, H. R.: Pseudoembolic phlebitis with ligation of the IVC, Ann. Surg. **127:** 1247, 1948.
109. Ohara, I., and Sakai, J.: Transplant of large venous system with blood vessel substitutes, Surgery **42:** 928, 1957.
110. Ohara, I., Ouchi, H., and Takahashi, K.: A bypass operation for occlusion of the

hepatic IVC, Surg. Gynecol. Obstet. **117:** 151, 1963.
111. Olivier, C., Fontaine, J. L., Devien, W., and Levy: Early dynamic effects of ligation of IVC, Chirurgie **97:** 506, 1971 (French).
112. Peter, M. Y., Hering, A. C., and Watkins, E.: Experimental Teflon replacement of the SVC and atriocaval junction, J. Thorac. Surg. **40:** 224, 1960.
113. Piccone, V. A., Vidal, E., Yarnoz, M., Glass, P., and LeVeen, H. H.: Late results of caval ligation, Surgery **68:** 980, 1970.
114. Pleasants, J. H.: Obstruction of the IVC with a report of eighteen cases, Johns Hopkins Hosp. Rep. **16:** 363, 1911.
115. Ranninger, K., and Smetz, D. M.: Local obstruction of the IVC by massive ascites, Am. J. Roentgenol. **93:** 935, 1965.
116. Reveno, W. S., Reynolds, L., and Dodrell, F. S.: Occlusion of both innominate veins: Restoration of blood flow by arterial grafts, J. A. M. A. **159:** 1192, 1955.
117. Riberi, A., and Moore, T. C.: SVC replacement. II. Successful use of a pedicle tube, Surgery **43:** 355, 1958.
118. Riberi, A., and Moore, T. C.: SVC replacement, Arch. Surg. **76:** 384, 1958.
119. Riberi, A., and Moore, T. C.: SVC replacement. IV. Experimental use of alcohol-preserved bovine heterograft aortas, J. Thorac. Cardiovasc. Surg. **38:** 172, 1959.
120. Rosenberg, D. M., Glass, B. A., Rosenberg, N., Lewis, M. R., and Dale, W. A.: Experience with modified bovine heterografts in arterial surgery, Surgery **68:** 1064, 1970.
121. Rosenberg, D. M., Gaughran, E. R. L., Henderson, J., Lord, G. H., and Douglas, J. R.: The use of segmental arterial implants prepared by enzymatic modification of heterologous blood vessels, Surg. Forum **6:** 242, 1956.
122. Rosenberg, N., Henderson, J., Douglas, J. F., Lord, G. H., and Gaughran, E. R. L.: Use of arterial implants prepared by enzymatic modification of arterial heterografts, Arch. Surg. **74:** 89, 1957.
123. Rosenberg, N., Henderson, J., Lord, G. H., Gaughran, E. R. L., and Douglas, J. F.: Use of enzyme digested heterografts as segmental arterial substitutes. III. Follow-up observations on two year old implants, Arch. Surg. **76:** 275, 1958.
124. Rosenberg, N., Henderson, J., Lord, G. H., Bothwell, J. W., and Gaughran, E. R. L.: The use of enzyme treated heterografts as segmental arterial substitutes. IV. Follow-up observations on five year old implants, Arch. Surg. **83:** 950, 1961.
125. Rosenberg, N., Henderson, J., Lord, G. H., Bothwell, J. W., and Gaughran, E. R. L.: Use of enzyme treated heterografts as segmental arterial substitutes, Arch. Surg. **85:** 192, 1962.
126. Rosenberg, N., Henderson, J., Lord, G. H., Bothwell, J. W., and Gaughran, E. R. L.: Biologic arterial prostheses of heterologous vascular origin: A progress report, Bull. Soc. Int. Surg. **21:** 13, 1962.
127. Rosenberg, N., Henderson, J., Lord, G. H., and Bothwell, J. W.: An arterial prosthesis of heterologous vascular origin, J. A. M. A. **187:** 741, 1964.
128. Rosenberg, N., Martinez, A., Sawyer, P. N., Wesolowski, S. A., Postlethwait, R. W., and Dillon, M. L.: Tanned collagen arterial prostheses of bovine carotid origin in man, Ann. Surg. **164:** 247, 1966.
129. Rosenberg, N., Lord, G. H., Henderson, J., Bothwell, J. W., and Gaughran, E. R. L.: Collagen arterial graft of bovine origin: Seven-year observations in the dog, Surgery **67:** 951, 1970.
130. Rosseau, J., Dupuy, J. P., Lebloys, Y., Buy, B., and Comte, B.: The long-term outcome of ligature of the IVC, J. Radiol. **51:** 821, 1970 (French).
131. Sadd, J. R., Koepke, D. E., Daggett, R. C., Zarnstorff, W. C., Yount, W. P., and Gott, V. C.: Relative ability of different conductive surfaces to repel clot formation on intravascular prostheses, Surg. Forum **12:** 252, 1961.
132. Samson, P. C.: Discussion of Scannel and Shaw, J. Thorac. Surg. **28:** 170, 1954.
133. Sarti, L.: Total prosthetic transplantation of the IVC with venous drainage restoration of the one remaining kidney on the graft, successfully performed on a child with Wilms' tumor, Surgery **67:** 851, 1970.
134. Sauvage, L. R., and Wesolowski, S. A.: The influence of suture method upon the incidence of thrombosis in artery-artery, vein-vein, and artery-vein-artery anastomoses, Surgery **36:** 227, 1954.
135. Sauvage, L. R., and Wesolowski, S. A.: Anastomoses and grafts in the venous system with special reference to growth changes, Surgery **37:** 714, 1955.
136. Sauvage, L. R., and Gross, R. E.: Observations of experimental grafts in intra-thoracic vena cavae, Surg. Gynecol. Obstet. **110:** 509, 1960.
137. Sauvage, L. R., and Gross, R. E.: Evaluation of venous autografts and aortic homografts in canine thoracic vena cavae for periods up to eight years, J. Thorac. Cardiovasc. Surg. **53:** 549, 1967.

138. Sawyer, P. N., editor: Biophysical mechanisms in vascular homeostasis and intravascular thrombosis, New York, 1965, Appleton-Century-Crofts, pp. 306-313.
139. Scannel, J. G., and Shaw, R. S.: Surgical reconstruction of the SVC, J. Thorac. Surg. **28:** 163, 1954.
140. Schauble, J. R., Anlyan, W. G., and Postlethwait, R. W.: A study of grafts in the venous system, Arch. Surg. **78:** 288, 1959.
141. Scheinin, T. M., and Jude, J. R.: Experimental replacement of the SVC: Effect of temporary increase in blood flow, J. Thorac. Cardiovasc. Surg. **48:** 781, 1964.
142. Schenck: Observationum medicarum variorum. Lugduni: 1644, Lib III, p. 339, noted in Pleasants, J. H.: Johns Hopkins Hosp. Rep. **16:** 363, 1911.
143. Schenk, W. G., Martin, J. W., Leslie, M. B., and Portin, B. A.: Regional hemodynamics of experimental acute A-V fistulas, Surg. Gynecol. Obstet. **105:** 733, 1957.
144. Schenk, W. G., Martin, J. W., Leslie, M. B., and Portin, B. A.: Regional hemodynamics of chronic experimental A-V fistulas, Surg. Gynecol. Obstet. **110:** 44, 1960.
145. Schneider, C. F.: Idiopathic retroperitoneal fibrosis producing vena caval, biliary, and duodenal obstruction, Ann. Surg. **159:** 316, 1964.
146. Schramel, R., and Olinde, H. D. H.: A new method of bypassing the obstructed vena cava, J. Thorac. Cardiovasc. Surg. **41:** 375, 1961.
147. Sharp, W., McVay, W. P., Flaksman, R. J., and Wright, J.: Electrolour: Achievement of long term vascular tolerance, Surg. Forum **20:** 141, 1969.
148. Sharp, W. V., Wright, J., Flaksman, R. J., and McVay, W. P.: Promotion of a viable neo-intima, Vasc. Surg. **3:** 243, 1969.
149. Shea, P. C., and Robertson, R. L.: Late sequelae of IVC ligation, Surg. Gynecol. Obstet. **93:** 153, 1951.
150. Shimamura, T., Gyorkey, F., Kanakami, T., Beall, A. C., and De Bakey, M. E.: The ultrastructure of neointima of canine infrarenal vena caval Teflon prostheses, Exp. Molec. Pathol. **13:** 190, 1970.
151. Shore, J. M., Greenstone, S. M., Mussel, T. B., Heringman, E. C., and Wagner, K.: A comparative study of canine venous autografts (The influence of graft diameter and external anastomotic support), J. Cardiovasc. Surg. **5:** 67, 1964.
152. Silver, C. E., Azuilizan, A. A., and Hurwitt, E. S.: Experimental ascites, Arch. Surg. **89:** 428, 1964.
153. Silver, C. E.: Fate of enzyme digested bovine arterial heterografts in low pressure systems, Am. J. Surg. **110:** 918, 1965.
154. Silver, D., and Anlyan, W. G.: Peripheral vein grafts in dogs, Surg. Forum **12:** 259, 1961.
155. Sive, E. B., Danese, C., and Howard, J. M.: Exhibit A. M. A., New York, June 26 to 30, 1961, noted in Haimovici, H., et al.: Surg. Gynecol. Obstet. **131:** 1173, 1970. p. 1176.
156. Smith, C. A., and Schisgall, R. M.: The effects of a distal A-V fistula upon an autogenous vein graft in the venous system, J. Surg. Res. **3:** 412, 1963.
157. Soyer, T., Lempinen, M., Cooper, P., Norton, L., and Eiseman, B.: A new venous prosthesis, SURGERY **72:** 864, 1972.
158. Stansel, H. C., Jr.: Synthetic IVC grafts, Arch. Surg. **89:** 1096, 1964.
159. Staley, C. J., Valaitis, J., Trippel, O. H., and Franzblau, S.: Leiomyosarcoma of the IVC, Am. J. Surg. **113:** 211, 1967.
160. Steinman, C., Alpert, J., and Haimovici, H.: IVC bypass grafts, Arch. Surg. **93:** 747, 1966.
161. Stickel, D. L., and Moorman, C. T.: Experimental patch grafts of the canine IVC, J. Surg. Res. **5:** 465, 1964.
162. Symbas, P. W., Foster, J. H., and Scott, H. W.: Experimental vein grafting in the portal venous system, SURGERY **50:** 97, 1961.
163. Szilagyi, D. E., Whitcomb, J. G., Schenker, W., and Waibel, P.: The laws of fluid flow and arterial grafting, SURGERY **47:** 55, 1960.
164. Takaro, T., Smith, D. E., Peasley, E. D., and Kim, J. S.: Experimental vena caval anastomosis and grafts, Surg. Gynecol. Obstet. **115:** 49, 1962.
165. Tice, D. A., and Zerbino, V.: Clinical experience with preserved human allografts for vascular reconstruction, SURGERY **72:** 260, 1972.
166. Todd, R. S., Sive, E. B., Devore, L. R., Damese, C., and Howard, J. M.: Replacement of segments of the venous system, Arch. Surg. **87:** 998, 1963.
167. Watkins, E., Jr., and Fortin, C. L.: Surgical correction of a congenital coarctation of the IVC, Ann. Surg. **159:** 536, 1964.
168. Wesolowski, S. A., Fries, C. C., Karlson, K. E., De Bakey, M. E., and Sawyer, P.: Porosity: Primary determinant of ultimate fate of synthetic vascular grafts, SURGERY **50:** 91, 1961.
169. Wesolowski, S. A.: Performance of materials as prosthetic blood vessels, Bull. N. Y. Acad. Med. **48:** 331, 1972.

170. Whiffen, J. D., and Gott, V. L.: Prosthetic thoracic vena cava grafts, J. Thorac. Cardiovasc. Surg. **50:** 31, 1965.
171. Williams, B. T., Roding, B., and Schenk, W. G.: Experimental evaluation of hemodynamic effects of IVC ligation, J. Cardiovasc. Surg. **11:** 454, 1970.
172. Wimberly, J. E., Lewis, M. R., and Dale, W. A.: Modified bovine heterografts for arterial patches, SURGERY **64:** 433, 1968.
173. Yamaguchi, A., Eguchi, S., Iwasaki, T., and Asano, K.: Influence of A-V fistula on patency of synthetic IVC grafts, J. Cardiovasc. Surg. **9:** 99, 1968.
174. Yong, N. K., Klein, N., and Moore, T. C.: SVC replacement (experimental use of fresh autogenous vein grafts), Br. J. Surg. **51:** 374, 1964.
175. Zinicola, N., Hoffert, P. W., and Haimovici, H.: Autogenous vein bypass grafts in the venous system, an experimental evaluation, Bull. Soc. Int. Surg. **21:** 265, 1962.
176. Description of product, package insert, Arterial graft (bovine origin), Johnson & Johnson, New Brunswick, N. J.

Long-term results of hepatic portoenterostomy for biliary atresia: Special reference to postoperative portal hypertension

Masahiko Miyata, M.D., Minoru Satani, M.D., Takashi Ueda, M.D., *and* **Eizo Okamoto, M.D.,**
Osaka, Japan

A long-term clinical analysis of congenital biliary atresia was made in 51 patients who had undergone hepatic portoenterostomy. Jaundice disappeared completely in 15, who were all under 4 months of age at the time of initial surgery. Seven of these patients demonstrated critical signs of portal hypertension postoperatively and four died. Thus the widely accepted "surgical cure" for congenital biliary atresia should be re-evaluated. Transient episodes of definitive retrograde cholangitis were evident in 71 percent of postoperative patients in whom jaundice had disappeared. It is strongly suggested that retrograde cholangitis plays an active role in producing postoperative portal hypertension.

From the First Department of Surgery, Osaka University Medical School, and the Children's Medical Center of Osaka, Osaka, Japan.

ABOUT five years has passed since Roux-Y–fashioned hepatic portojejunostomy[1] was adopted as a routine surgical procedure for congenital biliary atresia in Japan. Although this procedure has already been utilized in more than 60 instances in our clinics, a retrospective evaluation appears necessary. Such being the case, the following analysis was carried out.

MATERIALS AND METHODS

Included are 44 patients with hepatic portojejunostomy, six patients on whom exploratory laparotomy had been done prior to hepatic portojejunostomy, and one hepatic portoduodenostomized patient who had a Billroth II gastrectomy as a second operation. These 51 patients with noncorrectable types of congenital biliary atresia underwent Roux-Y–fashioned portoenterostomy at the First Department of Surgery, Osaka University Medical School, and Children's Medical Center of Osaka City, from January, 1969, to March, 1973. Hepatic portoenterostomy was

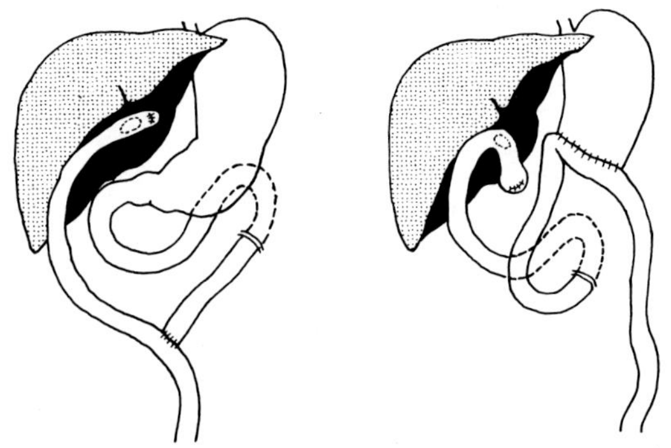

Fig. 1. Surgical procedures applied to 51 cases of noncorrectable types of congenital biliary atresia (see text).

Accepted for publication, May 14, 1974.

Reprint requests: Masahiko Miyata, M.D., First Department of Surgery, Osaka University, Medical School, Fukushima-ku, Osaka, Japan.

Table I. *Rate of disappearance of jaundice and age at time of surgery*

	Age (mo.)					
	1	2	3	4	5	Total
Jaundice disappeared	1	9	5	0	0	15
Number of operations*	1	22	12	2	4	41
Rate (percent)	100	40.9	41.7	0	0	36.6

*Ten patients who died within one month postoperatively are not included.

done according to the procedure of Kasai and associates,[1] in which, following amputation of a dense fibrous mass of the porta hepatis and the whole hypogenetic extrahepatic bile duct system *en bloc,* an end-to-side anastomosis was carried out between the cut edge of the mass and an opening of the alimentary tract (Fig. 1).

Diagnosis of portal hypertension was limited to those with ascites and/or ruptured esophageal varices. Hepatosplenomegaly and venous dilatation over the abdomen were not considered positive indications of portal hypertension in this study. A diagnosis of retrograde cholangitis was made when leukocytosis, transient elevation of serum bilirubin concentration, and lightened color of the stool were present during a febrile period.

RESULTS

Disappearance of jaundice. Bilirubin was detected in the stool postoperatively in 31 out of the 51 patients; however, jaundice disappeared completely in only 15, all of whom were under 4 months of age at the time of operation (Table I).

Mortality and survival rates. Ten patients died within 1 month postoperatively due to complications. Four in whom jaundice had disappeared died within 18 to 41 months postoperatively. The other 11 patients in whom jaundice had disappeared are still alive 12 to 71 months postoperatively. Twenty-two jaundiced patients died within 2 to 18 months postoperatively and the other three are alive 4 to 39 months postoperatively (Table II). The cause of death in all but six patients (76.9 percent) was portal hypertension (Table III).

Postoperative portal hypertension. Portal hypertension was evident in seven out of 15 patients in whom jaundice had disappeared (Table IV). Its first appearance was 6 to 36 (mean, 16.1) months postoperatively (Table V). On the other hand, preoperatively to 18 (mean, 4.1) months postoperatively, portal hypertension was clearly evident in those patients in whom the jaundice had not disappeared.

Postoperative retrograde cholangitis. Portal hypertension was also demonstrated in five out of eight (62.5 percent) with an episode of cholangitis and two out of seven (28.6 percent) without such an episode in those patients in whom jaundice had disappeared (Table VI). Among patients in whom jaundice disappeared after hepatic portoenterostomy, five out of seven (71.4 percent) with portal hypertension and three out of eight (42.9 percent) without portal hypertension developed retrograde cholangitis.

Table II. *Mortality rate and survival*

	Jaundice disappeared	Jaundice remaining
No. of survivals	11	3
Survival period (mo.)	12-71	4-39
Mean (mo.)	46.5	16.7
No. of deaths	4	22
Survival period (mo.)	18-41	2-18
Mean (mo.)	35.3	7.8

Table III. *Cause of death*

	Jaundice disappeared	Jaundice remaining
Portal hypertension	4	16
Postoperative infection	0	3
Measles	0	1
Infantile diarrhea	0	1
Intestinal obstruction	0	1
Total	4	22

Table IV. *Postoperative portal hypertension and age at time of surgery*

	Age (mo.)					
	1	2	3	4	5	Total
Jaundice disappeared:						
Number of patients	1	9	5	0	0	15
Portal hypertension	0	5	2	0	0	7
Incidence (percent)	0	55.6	40.0	—	—	46.7
Jaundice remaining:						
Number of patients	0	13	7	2	4	26
Portal hypertension	0	9	5	2	4	20
Incidence (percent)	—	69.2	71.1	100	100	76.9

Table V. *Appearance of portal hypertension*

	No. of cases	Range (mo.)	Mean (mo.)
Jaundice disappeared	7	6-36	16.1
Jaundice remaining	20	0-18	4.1

DISCUSSION

Hepatic portoenterostomy is recognized as the most effective surgical procedure for the cure of jaundice in noncorrectable types of congenital biliary atresia.[1-6] Apparently there is no difference regarding results when this procedure is applied to noncorrectable types of congenital biliary atresia and when choledochoenterostomy is done in correctable types of the disease.[2, 4, 5]

It is generally been accepted that patients in whom jaundice had disappeared and those who had no clinical abnormalities one year postoperatively are cured.[1, 4, 5] There are instances, however, where these "cured" patients have been readmitted with complaints of esophageal bleeding and/or ascites. Critical signs of portal hypertension were indeed evident in postoperative patients, in whom jaundice disappeared (46.7 percent), in their early childhood (Table V). Four out of seven died as a result of this complication. In three patients in whom jaundice had disappeared, surgical procedures for decompression of portal venous pressure were required and one patient died in the early postoperative period due to hepatic coma. Thus, a number of patients whose jaundice disappeared following hepatic portoenterostomy for congenital biliary atresia cannot be classified as cured.

It can be argued that in patients in whom jaundice had not disappeared, a biliary cirrhosis developed and demonstrated itself as portal hypertension; however, there is no feasible explanation of why portal hypertension occurred postoperatively in congenital biliary atresia patients in whom jaundice had disappeared completely. Histological findings in the liver at the time of the initial operation for congenital biliary atresia revealed very slight hepatic fibrosis in those cases where jaundice had disappeared completely postoperatively.[2-5] Such was also the case in the present study; however, in all patients in this series in whom jaundice had disappeared, a definite hepatosphlenomegaly was present. Typical cirrhosis of the liver was also demonstrated histologically in all three patients in whom jaundice had disappeared and who had a second operation to remedy portal hypertension. In addition, many patients had neither ascites nor esophageal varix yet had considerable venous dilatation over the abdomen.[3] In these cases, portal hypertension of some degree is usually suspected, but such suspects were not among those in the present series. It is thus hypothesized that hepatic fibrosis developed and, in many cases, cirrhosis of the liver did actually occur even though the jaundice disappeared following hepatic portoenterostomy.

It was observed that in many cases retrograde cholangitis occurred, after which portal hypertension developed during the postoperative course. In those patients in whom jaundice had disappeared, 53.3 percent had

Table VI. *Postoperative retrograde cholangitis and portal hypertension in patients in whom jaundice disappeared*

	Portal hypertension	No portal hypertension	Total
Cholangitis	5 (62.5%) 71.4%	3 (37.5%) 42.9%	8 (100%)
No cholangitis	2 (28.6%) 28.6%	5 (71.4%) 57.1%	7 (100%)
Total	7 100%	8 100%	15

episodes of evident retrograde cholangitis. This postoperative disorder was also evident among 71.4 percent of the patients in whom jaundice had disappeared and portal hypertension had developed. On the other hand, 62.5 percent of patients in whom jaundice had disappeared and had episodes of retrograde cholangitis showed critical signs of portal hypertension (Table VI). Thus postoperative portal hypertension appears to be closely related to retrograde cholangitis.

In these patients, laboratory tests revealed without exception a high concentration of serum alkaline phosophatase. Such evidence suggests that some mechanical obstruction of the bile flow remains even though jaundice has indeed disappeared.

One factor contributing to the development of postoperative portal hypertension in patients in whom jaundice has disappeared may be the irreversibility of hepatic fibrosis; another may be the presence of a heretofore unknown fibrogenetic factor of the liver specific to congenital biliary atresia. In view of the present results, however, postoperative retrograde cholangitis is the most probable contributing factor to portal hypertension in cases of congenital biliary atresia after hepatic portoenterostomy where jaundice disappears.

Although this operation has been widely acclaimed for eliminating jaundice,[1-6] nevertheless in many cases the so-called "cures" are incomplete.

Gratitude is due to Professor H. Manabe, First Department of Surgery, Osaka University Medical School, for his promotion of this study; to Drs. Y. Kujiraoka, T. Fugino, Y. Ohkuma, and N. Nagahara for their kind support; to Dr. Y. Iida, Assistant Professor of Pediatrics, Osaka University Medical School, for advice and suggestions; and to Miss M. Ohara, Kyoto University, for assistance with manuscript.

REFERENCES

1. Kasai, M., Kimura, S., Asakura, Y., Suzuki, H., Taira, Y., and Ohhashi, E.: Surgical treatment of biliary atresia, J. Pediatr. Surg. **3:** 665, 1968.
2. Kasai, M., Watanabe, I., Asakura, Y., and Ohi, R.: Follow-up study of long-term survivors after surgical correction of biliary atresia, J. Jap. Soc. Pediatr. Surg. **9:** 231, 1973 (in Japanese).
3. Miyata, M., Okada, A., Takao, T., Kuwata, K., Ohkuma, Y., Satani, M., Okamoto, E., Manabe, H., Nagahara, N., Fugino, T., and Ueda, T.: A long-term analysis of hepatic portoenterostomy in congenital biliary atresia (abst.), J. Jap. Soc. Surg. **74:** 68, 1973 (suppl. in Japanese).
4. Ohkuma, Y.: Histopathological study on intrahepatic bile ducts of congenital biliary atresia: with special reference to results of surgical treatment, J. Jap. Soc. Pediatr. Surg. **8:** 189, 1972 (in Japanese).
5. Okamoto, E., and Ohkuma, Y.: Hepatic fibrosis of congenital biliary atresia. Unpublished data.
6. Suruga, K., Nagashima, K., Hokno, S., Miyano, T., Kitahara, T., and Inui, M.: A clinical and pathological study of congenital biliary atresia, J. Pediatr. Surg. **6:** 655, 1972.

Attitudes of British graduates on surgical research fellowships in the United States

Michael J. Knight, F.R.C.S., *London, England, and* **Ceri M. Griffiths, F.R.C.S.(C)**
Galveston, Texas

Forty-one British graduates who had completed surgical research fellowships in the United States during the five-year period 1968 through 1972 were surveyed by questionnaire. The average fellow was aged 33, was married, had two children, and had had six years of clinical experience and considerable research experience before leaving the United Kingdom. The main reasons for coming to America were to improve the curriculum vitae and to learn research techniques. During their fellowship term graduates received an annual salary of about $9,000; one third considered this inadequate. All graduates consider their fellowship term well worthwhile and stated that they would at a future date recommend a similar fellowship to their juniors. One third of all graduates did not have an appointment arranged to follow their fellowship year, and during their stay in America 22 percent considered that they were bypassed for an appointment in Great Britain because of their nonavailability.

From the Department of Surgery, St. George's Hospital, London, England, and the Department of Otorhinolaryngology, University of Texas, Galveston, Texas

IN THE LAST DECADE it has been the custom for British medical graduates to include a research year in their specialty training program. Many of these graduates, particularly those in the surgical sciences, have by personal preference or at the request of their directors of study spent this research year in academic centers in the United States. Although reliable statistics are not available there appears at the present time to be a general impression among British academics and surgical trainees that fewer graduates are inclined to spend such a fellowship year in America and at least one recent study has shown that the flow of medical graduates from Europe to the United States is on the decline.[3] A number of factors could be responsible for this apparent fall-off in numbers, perhaps the main one being the fact that less money is now available for research posts generally in the United States. However, to determine whether or not a personal factor is involved, a questionnaire was sent to British graduates who were on, or who had completed, a surgical research fellowship in the United States during the 5 year period 1968 through 1972.

Supported by grants to M. J. K. from St. George's Hospital, London, and the Wellcome Foundation. Presented at the 1973 Congress of the American College of Surgeons.

Accepted for publication April 18, 1974.

Reprint requests: Michael Knight, F.R.C.S., St. George's Hospital, Hyde Park Corner, London SW 1X 7EZ, England.

METHODS

The names and present addresses of graduates were supplied by heads of surgical departments at 14 university medical centers distributed throughout the United States. Fifty-eight of these graduates were contacted and 41 returned completed questionnaires suitable for inclusion in the survey. Graduates on pure clinical fellowships were not included in the study. To encourage frankness in replies the graduate's name and medical center did not appear on the questionnaire.

RESULTS

Each of the five years covered by the study was well represented (Table I), there being approximately eight graduates from each year who returned questionnaires.

Personal status. The average age on taking up the fellowship appointment was 33 years. Forty of the 41 were male and 75 percent of all graduates were married, with an average of two children. The wives of all married graduates accompanied their husbands during the fellowship. Fifty-four percent of graduates had passed the E.C.F.M.G. examination before arriving in the United States and three percent acquired the qualification during the fellowship term. In fact, only 23 percent of all graduates were involved with clinical work in addition to their research activities at the American center.

Inquiries as to the previous experience of all graduates in the survey showed that the average number of clinical years spent in their specialty prior to starting the fellowship had been six and 64 percent had had previous research experience (mean, 3 years) in the United Kingdom.

Fellowship appointment. The duration of the fellowship term in the United States had in the majority of instances (80 percent) been one year. Twelve percent of graduates spent two years and 5 percent three years completing their projects. Only one graduate came for less than a year.

The fellowship appointment itself had been arranged between heads of departments at the home and American centers in 63 percent of cases, by application in 27 percent, and by invitation in 10 percent. Sixty-six percent of the graduates had appointments

Table I. *Number of graduates in each of the five years studied*

Fellowship year	*No. of graduates*
1968	8
1969	5
1970	8
1971	8
1972	12

Table II. *Objectives in spending fellowship year in the United States*

	Points
Curriculum vitae	28
Research techniques	19
Publications	13
Overseas travel	12
Project participation	12
Association with U. S. surgeon	11
Emigration reconnaissance	2
Clinical experience	2
Salary	1
Total	100

in Britain arranged to follow their fellowships; 34 percent had not.

Motivation. In the questionnaire graduates were asked to indicate in order of importance their objectives in taking their fellowship in America and the results were assessed according to a points system (Table II). By far the most important reasons for coming to the United States would appear to be improvement in curriculum vitae with a view to advancing career prospects in Great Britain and to learn research techniques. Other factors such as publications, overseas travel, interest in program project, and the wish to be associated with the name of a particular American specialist play a relatively minor role in their motivation. It would also appear from this study that hardly anyone came for the remuneration offered or with a view to permanent residence in the United States.

Having then decided to come to the United States for his fellowship term, what attracts the British graduate to a particular medical center? Again priorities were assessed according to a points system (Table III) and showed that the most important factor in-

Table III. *Factors influencing choice of program*

	Points
Reputation of U. S. head	34
Advice from U. K. head	33
Interest in program project	13
Reputation of U. S. center	7
Established exchanges	7
Geographical location of U. S. center	6
Salary	0
Total	100

Table IV. *Fellowship salaries*

Year	*Salary*
1968	$6,300
1969	$8,600
1970	$8,100
1971	$9,200
1972	$9,100

volved was the reputation of the departmental head in the United States. Of almost equal importance was advice from the British chief of the prospective fellow. Other minor reasons were interest in the program project, reputation of the American medical center, established exchange programs, and geographical location. None chose a particular medical school for the salary which it offered.

Remuneration. The average salary for each of the five years studied is shown in Table IV. Thirty-four percent of graduates considered that their remuneration was more than their British salary, while 64 percent regarded it as equal, less, or less in buying power than their pay in Great Britain. Twelve percent of all graduates supplemented their American stipend with a private income from home. The source of the American salary was difficult to determine as many graduates were paid from composite research funds but it would appear at an approximate estimate that 50 percent received their remuneration from the United States government, 7 percent from the British government, and 43 percent from private and commercial organizations through research grants to the American medical center.

Long-term plans. Inquiries were made into the long-term plans of these graduates before and after their fellowship term. Ninety-three percent intended to return to the United Kingdom, the majority (39 percent) into teaching hospital staff appointments; 25 percent planned to continue in academic surgery in Great Britain; another 24 percent intended to apply for nonteaching hospital staff posts on their return. Five percent had arranged full-time research posts in England and 7 percent of all graduates proposed to stay in the United States after completion of their year's research.

The effect of the fellowship term on these plans was minimal; only two graduates changed their minds and stayed in the United States rather than return to the United Kingdom.

General attitudes. All graduates considered their fellowship term as time well spent and all stated that they would at a future date recommend a similar fellowship term to their juniors. Ninety-three percent of graduates considered that all their objectives in coming to the United States had been achieved; the other 7 percent thought that their objectives had been partly achieved. The average fellow published five articles based on his research work in the United States.

On the negative side, 22 percent considered that they were bypassed for an appointment in Great Britain because they were not available at the time the post was advertised or vacant.

Finally, these graduates were asked for their opinions on how the fellowship term could have been of more value. Twenty percent could think of no improvement. Thirty percent considered that an increase in salary would have allayed some of the anxieties and restrictions they felt in coming to America. The point was made several times that because of family safety considerations a substantial proportion of their salary was taken up in paying for accommodation in a nonviolent area and that in these areas house rents were invariably higher. Twenty percent thought that the fellowship term would have been more productive had they been advised of the details of the research project a few months before their arrival in the United States. This period could have been used for preparatory reading, accumulation of references, and planning of protocols which would have allowed more time for practical laboratory work while actually in the United States. Fifteen percent suggested that tighter control of the research program and more constructive criticism from the departmental head would have been welcome, while another 10 percent would have liked to have visited other surgical centers during their year's stay in America.

DISCUSSION

Of the 63,000 foreign medical graduates at present in the United States,[2] approximately 500 are engaged in surgical research.[1] As 4.6 percent of all doctors on exchange visitor visas in the United States come from Great Britain we can estimate that approximately 23 British graduates arrive in America every year to start such a surgical research fellowship. Thus the 41 graduates who returned questionnaires represent about one third of the total number who have been on these fellowships in the 5 year period ending in 1972. Although the numbers are small and the study restricted to one nationality, it was felt worthwhile to present these data to illustrate some of the aspirations, achievements, difficulties, and general attitudes of the foreign medical graduate on such fellowships in the United States.

It is commonly assumed that British graduates come to the United States to develop an investigative background to their clinical work and this study would tend to support this impression. However, it would also appear that the majority of these doctors already have considerable knowledge of research techniques before leaving Great Britain, indicating that other factors must be involved in their motivation. From this study the most important reason for crossing the Atlantic seems to be improvement in curriculum vitae with a view to advancing career prospects in Great Britain. The fellowship year then practically assumes qualification status and indicates that the authorities in Britain still regard a year spent in the United States as a valuable experience for prospective surgical consultants.

The fellowships themselves are usually arranged between departmental heads and the reputation of the American surgeon is a major factor in the choice of center rather than the actual project in progress at his institution. On completion of their research terms the unanimous verdict of these graduates is that their fellowships were well worthwhile and that they would at a future date recommend a similar fellowship term to their juniors. Practically all these graduates return to Great Britain after completing their projects, the majority with plans to apply for teaching-hospital staff posts. A quarter intend to remain in academic surgery and an equal number plan to spend their professional life on the staff of nonteaching hospitals.

During their stay in America these graduates are paid about $9,000 a year and a third consider this to be inadequate. If consideration is given to the higher cost of living in the United States and the fact that the average fellow at the present time is aged 33 and married with two children, this salary level may well cause some hardship and have a deterring influence on prospective fellows. The answer to this problem could well come from the home country in the form of subsidies from the British government, Royal Colleges, or similar institutions with an interest in international education.

A disturbing feature of this survey is that nearly one quarter of all graduates consider that they were bypassed for an appointment at home because they were not available at the time the post was advertised or vacant. This, together with the fact that one third of the graduates surveyed did not have any appointment arranged to follow their research year, indicates that these fellowships should be part of a properly organized surgical rotation scheme based in the graduate's country of origin.

The authors express their thanks to Professor Walter F. Ballinger of Washington University, St. Louis, Mo., for his encouragement and help in this project. We also thank the surgical research fellows for completing the questionnaire and the heads of surgical departments who kindly supplied the names and addresses of these graduates.

REFERENCES

1. Balte, B. E., Lorant, J. H., and Todd, C., editors: The profile of medical practice, American Medical Association, U. S. A., 1971, p. 23.
2. Dublin, T. D.: N. Engl. J. Med. **286:** 870, 1972.
3. Editorial: Med. World News **14:** 20, 1973.

Changes and trends in graduate medical education and credentialling

J. W. Humphreys, Jr., M.D., *Philadelphia, Pa.*

THE WINDS of change are today blowing with typhoon force over the landscape of medical education. For the second time in the century there is occurring a great upheaval in all of its foundations and structures. Many forces are at work; among them are the population increase, the growing public demand for medical care, the rising cost of medical education and of medical care, the striving by various components of the profession and in fact the entire health-care team for individual places in the sun, the increasing interest of organized groups other than medicine in the systems of medical education and health-care delivery, the ever mounting involvement of the federal and other governments in health care with the inevitable burgeoning bureaucracy and burdening regulations, the influences of third-party payers, the impatience of students flayed by their desire to complete their education in the shortest possible span of time, and the reactions of the profession to the attacks being made upon its current structure and goals. All these forces and others are driving medical education in many directions, with movement first one way and then another, some of it appearing to be almost truly "Brownian" in nature. Although the compass is still searching, it may be possible by carefully looking at the vectors to plot the general direction being taken but not, at this time, at least, to prepare a detailed flight plan or even to designate a final destination or an estimated time of arrival.

The first great cataclysym in medical education in the United States occurred following the issuance, in 1910, of the now classic and famous report by Abraham Flexner.[4] This report stressed the need for a scientific basis for medical practice, the need for medical education to be vested in accredited schools and universities where scholarly pursuits would advance applicable knowledge, and the need for a supervised clinical education in a hospital environment prior to entering practice. It produced a chain reaction affecting every facet of medicine and health care over the ensuing fifty years. The effects of the report reached their peak in the 1950's and 1960's, when federal funding became available in large amounts to support research and education and even to a large part the salaries of the faculties. The result, as we all know, was that medicine and its allied disciplines became heavy on the side of science with a (perhaps unfortunate) loss of some of the mass of the art. The literal explosion in the volume and complexity of knowledge and the almost incomprehensible technological developments made it impossible for men to truly store and use all the available knowledge and thus forced medicine to assume its present shape of increasing specialization. No longer was it possible to become expert in medicine through undergraduate education alone and more and more students of medicine sought and

Presented as the Robert E. Lee Memorial Lecture, Society of Air Force Clinical Surgeons, Las Vegas, Nev., April 9, 1974.

Accepted for publication May 13, 1974.

Reprint requests: J. W. Humphreys, Jr., M.D., Secretary and Executive Director, American Board of Surgery, Inc., 1617 John F. Kennedy Blvd., Philadelphia, Pa. 19103.

entered courses of graduate education of the appropriate length and content to suit their career goals.

In the mid 1960's the clamor for social changes requiring funding by the federal government could no longer be ignored, students became agitated activists for almost any cause, and it became obvious that the honeymoon between federal funding and medical education was approaching an end and that a new interest—primary health care—was already in ascendancy.

Several reports of vital importance were published between 1965 and 1971. They are admirably summarized in the Introduction to The Report of the Goals and Priorities Committee of the National Board of Medical Examiners[5] published in 1973. The Coggeshall[2] Report in 1965 suggested reorganization of the relationships of the multitude of educational institutions and focused on the Association of American Medical Colleges. The now famous Millis[6] Report in 1966 defined primary care, dealt with the problems of hospital-based graduate education, and made recommendations concerning graduate medical education. In 1966 the Willard[8] Report further defined primary care by creating a description of family practice and offered proposals for the education and role of primary-care physicians. These reports led to the establishment of the Specialty Board in Family Practice. Then, in 1970, came the Carnegie Commission[1] Report proposing that "University Health Science Centers" be established and that they assume a patient care/service function in addition to their educational responsibilities. This latter proposal creates an entirely new role for universities, one in which they have little or no experience and which appears to be in conflict with their traditional purposes and goals.

All these reports have led to the initiation of fundamental changes in the process of medical education which bid fair to have a profound effect upon it and the processes of evaluation, certification, and licensure. They are briefly as follows.

1. The concept of the *continuum* of medical education from entrance into medical school throughout a medical career is evolving. This will create new responsibilities for the academic centers and will require a significant accommodation on the part of the agencies now responsible for accreditation of medical education and evaluation of professional competence.

2. The formalized and similarly structured curricula of the many medical schools are becoming more flexible and more personalized with a resultant loss of understanding exactly what the M.D. degree really means. This will require more precise evaluation of individuals and can only lead to the conclusion that an M.D. degree connotes that the student is now ready to commence his second phase—graduate education—which upon completion will equip him for independent practice of the type he chooses.

3. The acceptance or partial acceptance of the AAMC concept of "Corporate, Institutional, or Organizational Responsibility" as enunciated in its position statement of 1971,[7] will change the educational environment of medical schools and teaching hospitals and will certainly affect the authorities and operations of the evaluating and accrediting agencies related to graduate education. By the way, the "position of AAMC" (briefly, all education should be vested in the Academic Centers) has not been accepted as yet and is still being discussed and defined.

4. Accountability to the public will continue to become more important and will most likely place new demands upon those agencies responsible for evaluating clinical competence, such as the Boards.

The changes enumerated are in process, having moved forward to greater or lesser degrees; they are still under debate, and will probably come to pass, but in a somewhat different form from that envisioned by the groups that first proposed the changes and even those involved today.

Of all the studies and reports, the most important to the future of graduate medical education is the Millis[6] Report and, although it sets forth many recommendations, it may be well to summarize for consideration a few of the more pertinent ones:

1. That each teaching hospital or institution organize its staff so as to make its programs of graduate medical education a *corporate responsibility* rather than the individual responsibilities of particular services or heads of services.
2. That the internship, as a separate portion of medical education, be abandoned, and that there be a single period of graduate education called a residency and planned as a unified whole. (Note that this requires amendment of certain State Licensure acts and other statements of requirements.)
3. That graduation from medical school be recognized as the end of general medical education and that specialized education then begin to prepare the student for independent practice.
4. That institutions experiment with various forms of graduate medical education and that Specialty Boards and Residency Review Committees encourage such experimentation.
5. That Specialty Boards not increase the length of their required periods of training to compensate for the loss of the internship year.
6. That programs of graduate education not be approved unless they cover the entire span from graduation from medical school through completion of the residency.
7. That formal approval of programs in graduate medical education be given to the institution rather than the particular department or service concerned.
8. Although not recommended, it is implied that the University or Academic Medical Center should become the keystone of a network which brings together many institutions and disciplines. (If taken too literally this could mean that free-standing residencies in community and/or governmental hospitals would be forced to join the University or Academic complexes.)
9. That there be *created* a Commission on Graduate Medical Education specifically for the purpose of planning, coordinating, and periodically reviewing standards and for reviewing and approving the institutions in which that education is offered. It was further suggested that membership on this commission consist of appointees from the American Medical Association, The Association of American Medical Colleges, and The National Academy of Sciences, who could then consider individuals who might be suggested by other interested bodies. It is of great importance to note that such a composition of the Government Body for Graduate Medical Education provides for the exclusion of those groups most intimately concerned with, currently involved in, and most knowledgeable about the subject, i.e., the learned Specialty Societies and Colleges, the Specialty Boards, and the Program Directors. How intriguing this concept is.

Having looked very briefly and superficially at recent history and a few of the proposed changes, it then follows that a summary description of the situation as it exists today may be pertinent.

The concept of a Continuum of Medical Education has been quite universally accepted by the profession and the approved free-standing "internship" will be abandoned, starting in July, 1975. The first postgraduate year will become known as a "categorical" or "flexible" year. While these terms are not yet finally understood, it appears that they apply more to the intentions of the student than to fixed content. One entering a "categorical" first year declares his intent to pursue a course of graduate education in a designated specialty, such as Surgery. Those entering a "flexible" first year are keeping the option open of continuing in one of two or more specialties. It is therefore possible that in certain instances the content of both a categorical and a flexible year could be exactly the same; for example, a first year of surgical graduate education may include up to six months of clinical experience on a service other than Surgery, and therefore both categorical and flexible could have six months of surgery and six months of medicine, but the student who enters "flexible" could have entry into a second year in either medicine or surgery while the "categorical" must continue in Surgery. A "flexible" year must be approved as a first year by the appropriate Residency Review Committees of the applicable specialties. Admittedly there are many questions to be answered and it is expected that there will be a certain amount of confusion initially, but time should solve most of the problems.

Experimentation and innovation in the structure of graduate programs is being accepted by the Boards and Residency Review Committees. The American Board of Surgery and the Conference Committee on Graduate Education in Surgery have established a mechanism for joint review of such proposals and, as some of you may know, Thoracic Surgery has several "special programs" which do not equip the graduate for certification by the American Board of Surgery as is generally required. There is another program approved by the American Boards of Surgery and of Otolaryngology which provides for entry into the certification process of both Boards.

None of the surgical specialty Boards has increased the minimal educational requirements for entry into their certification examinations. Certain modifications in required program content have been made in those programs using only the minimal time; for example, the minimal requirements of the American Board of Surgery are for four years of clinical experience after medical school, three and one half of which must be in clinical surgery. Other full-time nonclinical experience, such as research laboratory, basic sciences, radiology, etc., must be in addition to the four clinical years. The surgical Boards in general feel that there is an irreducible minimum of time required for the student to obtain an adequate exposure to a wide variety of clinical entities and adequate operative experience. We do not plan to compromise quality regardless of administrative or other pressures.

The organization of the American Board of Family Practice, the approval of the Essentials for Graduate Education, and the establishment of approved residencies in this field brought the entire spectrum of clinical medicine into the same focal plane. Now there is no basic sphere of medical expertise that does not have recognized graduate educational requirements. Most of the profession has already recognized and accepted the fact that graduation from medical school does not equip one for the practice of medicine and that a single graduate year is inadequate preparation for independent practice. This fact has not yet been accepted by all members of the profession nor by most of the State Licensing Authorities and it may well be years before the political exigencies will allow definitive action by them. All states now license broadly in Medicine and Surgery, 39 require only one graduate year, and the remaining ones have no such requirement for licensure. This situation can be expected to change, but very slowly.

Since 1933 there has been in existence a loose federation of the specialties known as the Advisory Board of Medical Specialties. Recognizing that the various forces playing upon graduate education and upon the process of credentialling would not treat with the multitude of agencies such as each specialty Board and each Residency Review Committee, it was mutually agreed between the Boards to form a more cohesive body. Thus came into being, in 1970, the American Board of Medical Specialties, which is a chartered and incorporated nonprofit organization, the purposes of which are: (1) to improve the standards of medical care; (2) to act as spokesman for all approved specialty Boards, as a group; (3) to deal with the applications for approval of proposed new specialty Boards, subsidiary Boards, new types of certification, modification of existing types of certification, and related matters; (4) to endeavor to avoid duplication of effort by specialty Boards; and (5) to

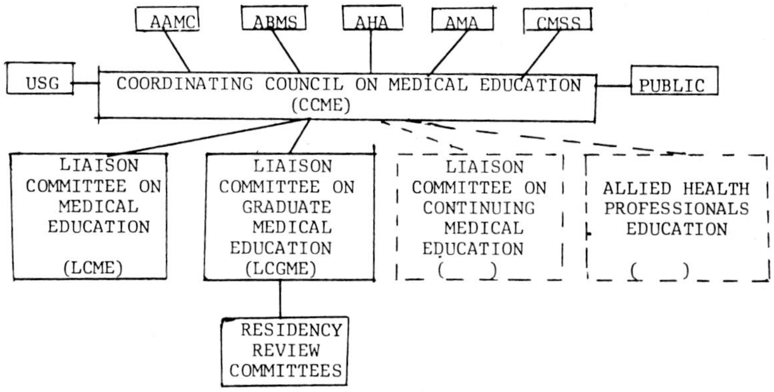

Fig. 1. Accreditation structure—medical education. Solid lines, existing; broken lines, proposed. USG, U. S. Government; AAMC, Association of American Medical Colleges; ABMS, American Board of Medical Specialties; AHA, American Hospital Association; AMA, American Medical Association; CMSS, Council of Medical Specialty Societies.

establish and maintain minimal standards of organization and operation of specialty Boards.

The regular members of the ABMS are the 20 primary specialty Boards and two conjoint Boards. There are certain associate members, also, but the power to determine policies, procedures, and actions lies within the voting strength of the regular members. The ABMS is still finding its way, but is proving its worth as a spokesman, as a forum for all the Boards, and as a body to resolve differences between the various member Boards.

It was hoped by many that the ABMS could become the formal accrediting agency for programs of graduate education, but this was not to be the case.

Perhaps (and there would be some to quarrel) the greatest contribution of the ABMS, to date, has been to bring to a halt the proliferation of independent specialty Boards with a very limited interest. This is not to say that subspecialties are not being recognized. They are being recognized by the granting of special certifications by the primary Boards, each of which requires review and approval by the member Boards that form the body of ABMS. Its greatest potential lies in the fact that by virtue of its membership on several bodies in the developing hierarchy concerned with medical education it represents all the approved specialties and therefore the mass of those practicing medicine.

The process of review and the authority for approval of programs of graduate medical education has undergone drastic change within the past few months. Previously the process and authority had been vested primarily in the specialty Board alone or in conjunction with its primary specialty society. For example, the Residency Review Committee for Orthopedic Surgery has been composed of members from the Board and the American Academy of Orthopedics. Others have been purely an extension of the Board. In Surgery the function has long been vested in a tripartite committee with members from the Board, the College, and the Council on Medical Education of the AMA. The Residency Review Committees have taken their guidance from their parent bodies and until recently have been the final authority as to a program's status.

For reasons too numerous and complex to discuss at this time, and under a threat that the Commissioner of Education of the HEW would not deal with a group, but only with a single accrediting agency, a new hierarchy concerned with all of medical education, "from the cradle to the grave," has been recently established. By reference to Fig. 1 it may be seen that the structure now consists of a Coordinating Council on Medical Education (CCME) whose chief functions are coordination of all aspects of medical education, approval and/or promulgation of broad policies related thereto, and review of the actions of subordinate elements. Under the guidance of the CCME are the Liaison Committees, Medical Education, and Graduate Medical Education, which now are functioning, and two additional ones being discussed—Continuing Medical Education and Allied Health Education. When the Liaison Committee on Continuing Medical Education is formed the educational process of a physician from entry into medical school throughout his career will be under the surveillance and control of a formal system of accreditation.

The Liaison Committee on Medical Education has been in existence for a number of years and is responsible for the accreditation of schools of medicine in the undergraduate phase.

The Liaison Committee on Graduate Medical Education (LCGME) has as its purpose the accreditation of programs in graduate medical education. The functions of this new organization as quoted from the latest version of its by-laws are to:

(1) develop standards and criteria common to all programs in graduate medical education for approval by the CCME;
(2) approve specific guidelines provided by the individual Residency Review Committees (Essentials and Guidelines);
(3) establish general standards and criteria for evaluation of programs in graduate medical education;
(4) recommend and initiate studies pertinent to improving the organization and conduct of programs in graduate medical education;
(5) receive and consider proposals for new types of programs in graduate medical education for which accreditation is being sought;
(6) review periodically the criteria by which programs of graduate medical education are evaluated;
(7) provide a means whereby programs in graduate medical education may appeal adverse decisions;
(8) receive from and provide information to the public and the government concerning the evaluation and accreditation of programs in graduate medical education; and
(9) initiate studies and recommend policy to keep programs in graduate medical education responsive to public and social needs.

It is obvious from the functions that the LCGME has assumed control of the process of graduate medical education and it is most probable that it will increase its power over all aspects once it receives approval from the federal government on its application to be recognized as the single accrediting agency in the United States.

The Residency Review Committees which had previously been the accrediting authorities, and creatures of the Specialty concerned, now are subordinated to the LCGME and all their functions and actions subject to review by the LCGME. The Residency Review Committees will continue to carry out the mechanics of development of criteria for programs and inspection of the programs, but all their actions must be approved by the LCGME. As a matter of fact the letters going out to programs and/or institutions informing them of their status will be on LCGME letterheads and not that of the Residency Review Committee, a small matter, but indicative of the trend.

We are being assured that the LCGME will not be dictatorial, but it is obvious that the Boards and Major Specialties Societies no longer occupy the front rank in the system. Their influences must now be exerted through the representatives to CCME and LCGME from the ABMS, the Council of Medical Specialty Societies, and the AMA, since the representatives from the AHA, the AAMC, the public, and the government will certainly not be speaking for them.

Thus the much-debated recommendation of the Millis Report, that there be created a

National Commission on Medical Education, has now been implemented, though in a somewhat different form.

What will be the long-range effect of the changes in the governing structure of graduate medical education is not foreseeable, but I believe we are going to experience more standardization and more regimentation, which all too often leads not to excellence but to mediocrity. Even though the product may eventually be better, the process will be painful until we accommodate to it.

The proposition that approval should be awarded to institutions rather than to individual programs or to program directors is still being pushed by certain factions, but is meeting resistance from the Boards and program directors. While we are generally in favor of "corporate or organizational responsibility" we do not believe that blanket approval should be given to institutions for all graduate education. We know that the quality of programs varies within each institution and we do not wish to see approval withheld from a good surgical program because of poor quality in others and vice versa. This problem remains to be brought to solution and the specific responsibilities and authorities of all concerned must be clearly defined.

These are the high days of the consumer advocate and accountability to the public is on an ever-rising spiral in all walks of life. It is probably a good thing and, although it is disturbing to the status quo, the profession recognizes that it must cope. Certification has traditionally been a one-time action and due to the dedication of most physicians it has been adequate as a measure of competence. However, we must all agree that it is related only to one point in time and that many of us in a busy practice do fall behind. It is an obligation of all who follow Aesculapius to strive for continuing improvement of their services to their patients and continuing education is a very necessary part thereof. No longer will it be acceptable to leave this to the good intentions of the individual and we believe that periodic measurement of competence both is desirable and will be forced upon us by pressures originating outside the profession, if we do not act in time. Is it not better for the profession to take the lead and devise the system rather than have it dictated from the lay community? We think yes!

Recertification on a periodic basis is upon us. When formed, the American Board of Family Practice announced that recertification would be required every seven years. Most of the Boards have developed a policy in support of recertification. All of the surgical Boards have announced that they will recertify, with the sole exception of Neurological Surgery.

The American Board of Surgery recently announced that all diplomates certified on or after Sept. 1, 1975, would be required to be recertified at 10 year intervals and their certificates will bear a date showing the termination of validity. All diplomates certified before Sept. 1, 1975, will be offered voluntary recertification with the process beginning in 1980. The exact mechanism is not yet settled upon, but the process will be highly clinically oriented and may well involve other factors than examination.

It appears certain that in the near future the credentials of all specialists and probably generalists are going to be re-examined periodically. This may become a factor in reducing the unwarranted claims to being a specialist and could result in steady improvement of quality of care given to the public.

There are three sides to the triangle encompassing the life of a medical professional. They may be termed *accreditation* of the educational process; *credentialling,* or the recognition of competence; and *licensure,* or the legal entitlement to practice. These three sides have all been of different length, so to speak, in the past, but with the changes occurring in accreditation and credentialling the triangle is becoming an isosceles. All of medical education is being brought into a continuum and into a structured accreditation system and credentialling is following the same three-phase pattern. The third side,

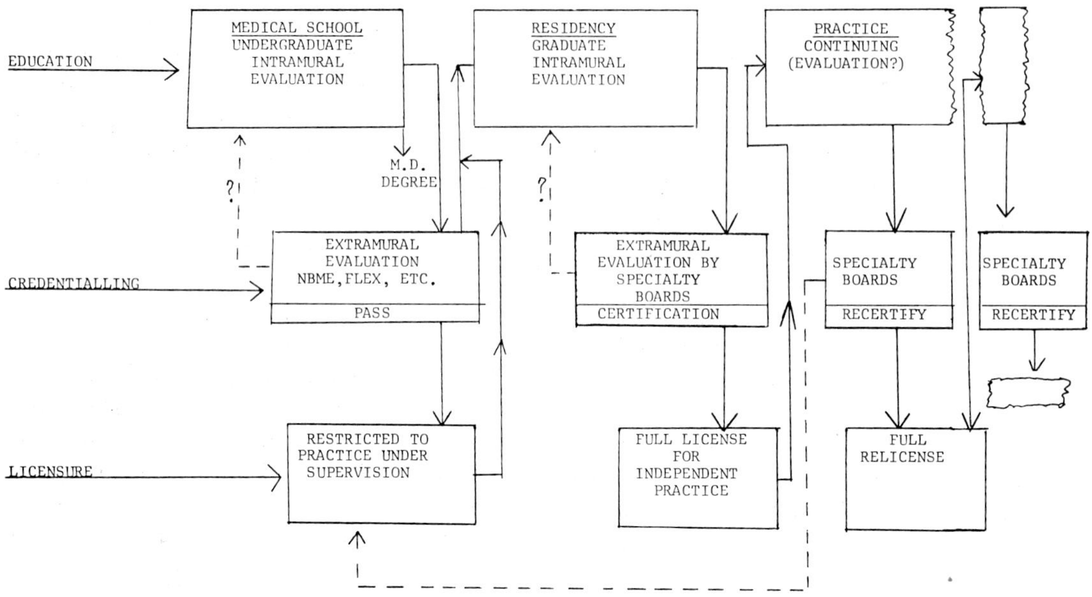

Fig. 2. Education, credentials, licensure—future relationships? Solid lines, currently proposed; broken lines, presumption only.

licensure, which is a function of state legislative acts, does not bear a relationship to the entire process, but in some states is related only to Phase I (undergraduate) and in others to that plus a portion of Phase II (graduate). Licensure bears almost no relationship to the credentialling occurring at the completion of graduate education and, except in two or three states, none to continuing education and credentialling. This is an anomalous situation, to say the least, if the purpose of licensure is to protect the public weal.

In June, 1973, very interesting developments occurred in both the United States and Canada which may reshape the triangle to an equilateral configuration, although the reshaping will probably be very slow in the United States. The Goals and Priorities Report of the National Board of Medical Examiners and the Proceedings of the General Council of the Canadian Medical Association[3] of June, 1973, contain somewhat similar recommendations relating licensure to education and competence. For the sake of brevity only an outline is presented at this time. (Fig. 2) presents the essentials with certain added presumptive indications of my own.

The proposals are that the institution offering undergraduate education be accredited and that it provide an intramural assessment of the knowledge of its graduate. Upon receipt of the M.D. degree the graduate would then be subject to an assessment by an extramural agency and mechanism, such as the National Board Examinations or the FLEX, which would, if passed, entitle him to *license to practice under supervision only* or, as the Canadians put it, a *restricted license.* This may be considered Phase I.

Most, if not all, M.D.'s enter into graduate education programs of variable lengths, depending upon their interests and goals. Those who successfully complete the requirements of an accredited program and who then pass a second milestone, certification by the appropriate Board in the United States, would be granted an *unrestricted license* or a *licensure for independent practice.* The Canadian proposal goes further than the U. S. in that it proposes to delineate the field in which he had been judged competent (Phase II).

Each individual who completes Phase II will be expected to engage in continuing education, preferably in approved programs, courses, or institutions, and will periodically be reassessed, or recertified, at which time he will either be fully relicensed or presumably revert to a restricted status of being licensed to practice under supervision until he attains certified status. No one has openly addressed the question of what happens in the event of failure at any milestone, but the answer is implied in Fig. 2.

The proposals mentioned express a philosophy with which it is extremely difficult to disagree on logical grounds. The idea seems relatively simple, but upon reflection, it becomes obvious that the pathway is strewn with many unknowns and that each step is fraught with extremely serious implications, each of which must be illuminated and fully understood if wise choices and decisions are to be made. The great danger lies in the fact that the profession may be panicked into implementation of such a system by political and/or social demands before the problems have been fully thought through.

It is clear, to me at least, that we will in time come to a more structured formal linking of education, credentialling, and licensure, and it most probably will be an improvement over the variegated "no system" in effect today. Whatever is the final structure, I predict that the trip thereto will be bumpy and pass through enormous volumes of "hot air."

It is a basic biologic law that an organism or species must adapt to the changing environment or it must perish. Medicine may struggle, but as we move into a new age we must endeavor, each of us, to insure that the genetic code we are building will result in a profession which is properly equipped and dedicated to provide an adequate supply of the highest possible quality medical care to those whom we serve.

The "old order changeth." Let us wisely shape the future.

REFERENCES

1. Carnegie Commission on Higher Education: Special report and recommendations on higher education and the nation's health, New York, 1970, McGraw-Hill Book Company, Inc.
2. Coggeshall, L. T.: Planning for medical progress through education; report to the Executive Council of the Association of American Medical Colleges, Evanston, Ill., 1965.
3. Council on Medical Education: Recommendations approved by the General Council of the Canadian Medical Association, Vancouver, June 1973.
4. Flexner, A.: Medical education in the United States and Canada; report to the Carnegie Foundation for the Advancement of Teaching, Bull. No. 4, Boston, 1910, The Merry Mount Press.
5. Mayer, W. D., Chairman: Report of the Committee on Goals and Priorities, National Board of Medical Examiners; evaluation in the continuum of medical education, Philadelphia, June 1973.
6. Millis, J. S., Chairman: Report of the Citizens' Commission on Graduate Medical Education; the graduate education of physicians, Chicago, 1966, American Medical Association.
7. Statement on Graduate Medical Education: Bull. Assoc. Am. Med. Coll. **6:** 3, 1971.
8. Willard, W. R., Chairman: Report of the Ad Hoc Committee on Education for Family Practice of the Council on Medical Education of the American Medical Association; meeting the challenge of family practice, Chicago, 1966.

The fate of kidney transplants from donors with minor renal abnormalities

Panayiotis K. Spanos, M.D., Richard L. Simmons, M.D., Luca C. Rattazzi, M.D., Marvin E. Goldberg, M.D., *and* John S. Najarian, M.D., *Minneapolis, Minn.*

A total of 142 living related donors gave kidneys at the University of Minnesota between August, 1967, and June, 1971. All recipients have been followed for a minimum of 2½ years. Out of 142 donors, 35 had minimal abnormalities of the urinary tract, including abnormalities of the IVP, renogram, and renal arteriogram, a strong history of recurrent urinary tract infections, and some donors on initial evaluation were found to have positive urine cultures containing more than 100,000 colonies on repeated specimens. None of the donors had evidence of upper tract infection. Of the 35 patients who received abnormal kidneys, 27 (77 percent) currently have good kidney function with a follow-up 2½ to 6½ years. No kidney loss or patient death appeared related to the abnormality of the donor kidney. With careful evaluation of donor urinary tract, the use of related kidneys demonstrating minor abnormalities is safe for both donor and recipient.

From the Departments of Surgery and Radiology, University of Minnesota Hospitals, Minneapolis, Minn.

LIVING RELATED DONORS continue to provide about half of the kidneys to patients reqiring renal transplantation because related kidneys continue to function better than do cadaver kidneys.[1] The general criteria for the selection of living donors have long been established[5] and strict adherence to certain principles of donor selection is essential since we have found that 20 to 25 per cent of apparently healthy relatives of patients with renal failure will also have evidence of renal disease.[6] Some of these abnormalities are apparently minor, however, and it is important to determine how well kidneys with such abnormalities function in the new host. In this report we present the long-term results of 35 kidneys which were known to possess minor abnormalities prior to transplantation to related recipients.

This work was supported by United States Public Health Service Grant No. AM 13083.

Accepted for publication April 4, 1974.

Reprint requests: Richard L. Simmons, M.D., Box 185, University of Minnesota Hospitals, Minneapolis, Minn. 55455.

MATERIAL

Living related donors gave kidneys to 142 recipients at the University of Minnesota between August, 1967, and June, 1971. All recipients have been followed a minimum of 2½ years. Of 142 living related donors 35 had minimal abnormalities of the urinary tract: These included abnormalities of the intravenous pyelogram (IVP), the renogram, and renal arteriogram, a strong history of recurrent urinary tract infections, and some of the donors on initial evaluation were found to have positive urine cultures containing more than 100,000 of colonies in two different clean-catch urine cultures. The group of

Table I. *Fate of kidneys from living related donors with history of recurrent urinary tract infections*

Pt. No.	*Age (yr.)*	*Donor relation**	*Current serum creatinine (mg./ 100 ml.)*	*Current blood pressure (mm. Hg)*	*Comment*
1	40	S	1.5	110/70	Well, 54 mo.
2	20	P	2.7	132/102	Chronic rejection; fair function, 65 mo.
3	28	P	1.4	90/56	Well, 54 mo.
4	19	P	1.7	132/92	Well, 30 mo.
5	37	S	—	—	Died, 10 mo., cytomegalovirus, hepatitis; normal kidney function

*S = Sibling; P = parent.

donors with bacteriuria on initial evaluation were treated with appropriate antibiotics for 10 days and the nephrectomy was undertaken only after repeated urine cultures became negative and there was no evidence of concurrent upper tract disease.

The 35 donors were grouped into four major categories according to the abnormality found in the donor. A fifth group consists of donor organs with a combination of abnormalities.

All kidneys regardless of abnormality were transplanted by standard techniques[5] and treated with standardized immunosuppressive regimens.[5]

RESULTS

Group 1. Kidneys from living related donors with history of recurrent urinary tract infections. Five recipients received kidneys from relatives who had a history of recurrent urinary tract infections (Table I) but no evidence of renal functional impairment or evidence of active urinary tract infection. These patients have been followed from 2½ to 5 years and four of the five are well. One patient (No. 5), who had juvenile diabetes, died 10 months after the transplant of cytomegalovirus hepatitis despite normal kidney function. Patient No. 2 has moderate impairment of renal function 5 years post transplant. Apparently kidneys from donors with a history but no current evidence of urinary tract infections function as well as normal kidneys for prolonged periods.

Group II. Kidneys from living related donors with bacteriuria at initial evaluation. Eight kidneys from living related donors with bacteriuria (>100,000 colonies of the same organism in two different clean-catch urine cultures) were used for eight recipients. The donors underwent antibiotic treatment until the cultures were negative, and there was no anatomic evidence of upper tract infection.

The results of these eight kidneys are seen in Table II. Patient No. 11 died 1½ years after the operation from a cerebral thrombosis and other complications following kidney rejection. Patient No. 13 died of pneumonia 2½ years post transplant with normal renal function. The remaining six kidney grafts (75 percent) are functioning satisfactorily 3 to 6 years after transplantation, though patient No. 12 has some impairment of renal function due to recurrent Goodpasture's disease six years post transplant. No patient has shown evidence of persistent or recurrent urinary tract infections.

Group III. Kidneys from living related donors with evidence of minimal stasis of the excretory system. Table III shows the results of 17 transplants performed using the abnormal kidney from a donor with a unilateral abnormal kidney on IVP or renography. Five patients demonstrated delayed emptying of the renal pelvis on IVP, seven showed evidence of delayed emptying of portions of the excretory system on the renogram, and another five had evidence of up-

Table II. *Kidneys from living related donors with bacteriuria at initial evaluation*

Pt. No.	*Age (yr.)*	*Donor relation**	*Current serum creatinine (mg./ 100 ml.)*	*Current blood pressure (mm. Hg)*	*Comment*
6	3	P	1.2	140/70	Well, 38 mo.
7	15	P	1.9	118/84	Well, 48 mo.
8	4	P	0.7	90/56	Well, 56 mo.
9	22	S	0.8	110/60	Well, 67 mo.
10	20	S	1.5	122/90	Well, 62 mo.
11	48	O	—	—	Died, 18 mo.; rejection
12	13	P	2.4	140/98	Goodpasture's disease recurrence; fair function, 77 mo.
13	27	P	—	—	Died, 2.5 yr.; bacterial pneumonia with normal function

*S = Sibling; P = parent; O = other relative (cousin, uncle, aunt, etc.).

Table III. *Kidneys from living related donors with evidence of minimal stasis of the excretory system on IVP and/or renogram*

Pt. No.	*Age (yr.)*	*Donor relation**	*Current serum creatinine (mg./ 100 ml.)*	*Current blood pressure (mm. Hg)*	*Comment*
6†	3	P	1.2	140/70	Well, 38 mo.
7†	15	P	1.9	118/84	Well, 48 mo.
8†	4	P	0.7	90/56	Well, 56 mo.
14	20	S	1.1	130/90	Well, 33 mo.
15	58	O	1.2	112/80	Well, 30 mo.
16	52	O	—	—	Died, 1 yr.; septicemia
17	19	S	5.9	110/70	Goodpasture's recurrence at 38 mo.
18	34	S	1.1	100/64	Well, 37 mo.
19	36	P	1.7	120/88	Well, 44 mo.
20	23	P	1.1	124/82	Well, 33 mo.
21	8	P	0.8	120/78	Well, 57 mo.
22	48	S	1.3	130/70	Well, 34 mo.
23	45	S	1.1	96/58	Died, 25 mo.; pancreatitis; normal function
24	50	O	0.9	120/70	Well, 30 mo.
25	36	S	—	—	Renal artery thrombosis
26	36	O	—	—	Died, 1.5 mo.; myocardial infarction
27	12	P	1.1	128/86	Well, 84 mo.

*S = Sibling; P = parent; O = other relative (cousin, uncle, aunt, etc.).
†These patients are also listed in Table II.

per tract stasis on both IVP and renogram. Typical IVP's and retrograde pyelograms of this type are shown in Fig. 1. One diabetic patient (Nos. 25 and 26) received two such transplants; the first kidney was lost 1½ months after transplant secondary to acute thrombosis of the renal artery and she died of a myocardial infarction about 1½ months after the second graft. The remaining 15 kidneys (87 percent) functioned for at least one year. At one year, another kidney was lost when Patient 16 died from septicemia. At two years, 14 (82 percent) kidneys were functioning and currently 13

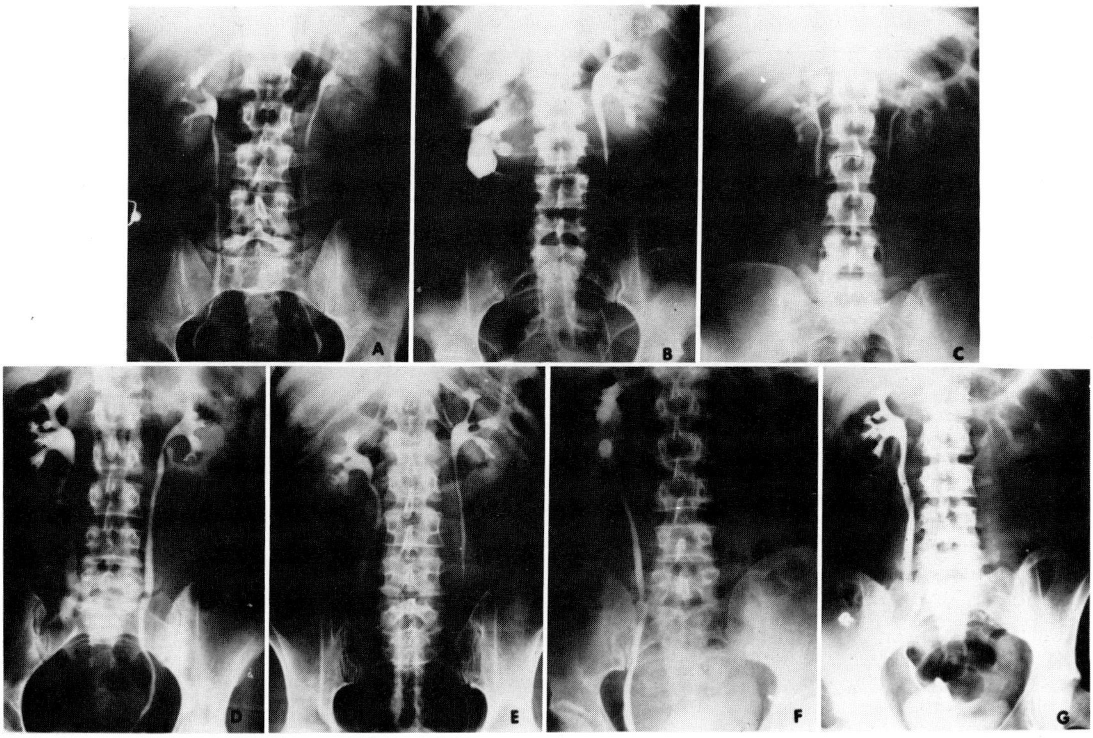

Fig. 1. Ureteropelvic abnormalities in living kidney donors. *A,* calyectasis of the right upper pole is present. *B,* malrotation of the right kidney. *C,* a large upper polar diverticulum can be recognized. *D* and *G* show compression of the right ureter at the level of the right ovarian vein (right ovarian vein syndrome) on intravenous and retrograde pyelograms. *E* illustrates scarring of the infundibulum of the left middle calyx. *F,* pyelocaliectasis and pressure of the U-P junction is present. All abnormal kidneys were utilized and continue to function well at least two years later. The normal kidney was left in the donor in each case.

(77 percent) of the recipients of kidneys from living related donors with minimal stasis of the excretory system have excellent renal function at 30 to 84 months after transplantation. Patient 17 however, has borderline function at 38 months, because of recurrence of Goodpasture's disease. Only one recipient (No. 12) lost his kidney secondary to sepsis which might have originated within the urinary tract. None of the patients has any evidence of partial urinary obstruction or recurrent urinary tract infections.

Group IV. Kidneys from living related donors with miscellaneous anomalies. The fates of kidneys from living related donors with miscellaneous abnormalities are listed in Table IV. Three of these kidneys had double excretory systems, two patients had small kidneys ($<$ 11 cm. long or $>$ 2 cm. smaller than that on the other side), two had kidneys with cysts diagnosed prior to operation, and two had minor vascular anomalies (fibromuscular dysplasia and a small aneurysm of the renal artery with minimal atherosclerosis).

The results with the three recipients of kidneys with double excretory systems are not very encouraging even though failure does not seem related to the double excretory system. One of these kidneys is functioning 53 months postoperatively but the other two kidneys have been lost (Table IV). Patient 29 rejected the kidney 3½ months post transplantation and is currently well with a second transplant. Patient 31 hyperacutely rejected her son's kidney, underwent a second transplant, which was promptly rejected, and died while on dialysis.

Table IV. *Kidneys from living related donors with miscellaneous anomalies*

Pt. No.	*Age (yr.)*	*Donor relation**	*Current serum creatinine (mg./ 100 ml.)*	*Current blood pressure (mm. Hg)*	*Comment*
Double excretory system:					
29	42	S	—	—	Rejected, 3.5 mo.; well with second transplant
30	10	P	0.8	122/70	Well, 59 mo.
31	39	O	—	—	Hyperacute rejection
Small kidney < 11 cm. or 2 cm. smaller than other side:					
28	4	O	—	—	Rejected, 2 mo.; well with second transplant
32	10	P	0.7	98/68	Well, 39 mo.
Kidneys with cysts:					
33	12	S	—	—	Rejected, 1 mo.; well with second transplant
34	57	S	0.8	112/70	Well, 30 mo.; cyst proved to be cortical adenoma
Minor vascular anomalies:					
23†	45	S	1.1	96/58	Died, 25 mo.; pancreatitis
35	57	S	1.0	132/78	Well, 30 mo.

*S = Sibling; P = parent; O = other relative (cousin, uncle, aunt, etc.).
†This patient was listed in Table III.

Two patients received small but apparently normal kidneys, i.e., kidneys less than 11 cm. long or a kidney at least 2 cm. smaller than the contralateral one. One of them (No. 28) was from a grandmother to her 4-year-old grandson. Although her kidneys were small (11.1 and 11.0 cm.), both IVP and renogram were normal and the creatinine clearance was 110 ml. per minute. The transplanted kidney never functioned well and at 2 months it was rejected and removed. The recipient currently is well with a second kidney. Patient 32 received the right kidney of his mother. This kidney was 11.6 cm. and her left kidney measured 13.6 cm. This patient is doing well 39 months post transplant.

Two kidneys from living related donors were thought to contain single renal cysts. Patient 33 received a kidney with a 6 cm. diameter cyst that was unroofed before transplantation; the kidney was rejected and removed after one month. Patient 34 received a kidney in which a small cyst had been diagnosed near the renal hilum but during nephrectomy a cortical adenoma was found. The adenoma was enucleated and the kidney transplanted with excellent results.

In the last subgroup of miscellaneous anomalies (Table IV) we included two kidneys with minor vascular abnormalities. Patient 35 received a kidney with the diagnosis of minor fibromuscular dysplasia on the arteriogram. During evaluation no hypertension was encountered and the rest of the studies were also normal. The recipient of this kidney (No. 35) has excellent renal function 30 months after transplantation. The second transplant (No. 23) was from a living related donor with a small aneurysm of the right renal artery and evidence of delayed emptying of the right renal pelvis (also included in Tables III and V). During nephrectomy the small aneurysm was excised prior to anastomosis. The recipient was well for 21 months. She died of pancreatitis with good renal function 25 months post transplant.

Group V. Patients receiving kidneys from living related donors with multiple minimal abnormalities, history of urinary tract infection or bacteriuria, and abnormal IVP, renogram, and/or arteriogram. Ten kidneys were classified in this group, which is a

Table V. *Kidneys from living related donors with multiple minimal abnormalities, history of urinary tract infection or bacteriuria, and abnormal IVP, renogram, and/or arteriogram*

Pt. No.	*Age (yr.)*	*Donor relation**	*Current serum creatinine (mg./100 ml.)*	*Current blood pressure (mm. Hg)*	*Comment*
1	40	S	1.5	110/70	Well, 54 mo.
2	20	P	2.7	132/102	Well, 65 mo.
6	3	P	1.2	140/70	Well, 38 mo.
7	15	P	1.9	118/84	Well, 48 mo.
8	4	P	0.7	90/56	Well, 56 mo.
17	19	S	5.9	110/70	Goodpasture's recurrence at 38 mo.
19	36	P	1.7	120/88	Well, 44 mo.
21	8	P	0.8	120/78	Well, 57 mo.
22	48	S	1.3	150/90	Well, 34 mo.
23	45	S	1.1	96/58	Died, 25 mo. pancreatitis

*S = Sibling; P = parent.

combination of Groups I to IV. All ten kidneys functioned for at least 2 years (Table V). Patient 23 died 25 months post transplant from complications of pancreatitis. All the remaining patients have functioning grafts 35 to 65 months after transplantation, and seven of these have ideal function. One patient (No. 30) has compromised function secondary to chronic rejection, and one (No. 17) has recurrent Goodpasture's syndrome. None of the patients have lost their kidneys of causes attributable to the donor abnormalities.

DISCUSSION

No one can doubt that kidneys from living related donors survive better than those from cadaver donors.[1] However, as more living related kidney donors are investigated, major and minor abnormalities of the donor kidney will be found more frequently. We refuse to utilize 20 to 25 percent of potential volunteer related donors because of major abnormalities found during evaluation.[6] A dilemma arises, however, when the abnormality is minimal, its significance is unknown, and there is no other volunteer donor available. The dilemma is compounded if the prospective recipient cannot tolerate hemodialysis. We have chosen to use the kidney with the minor abnormality for transplantation, relieving the donor of the abnormal kidney and leaving the normal kidney in place. If both kidneys have minor abnormalities the volunteer is not allowed to donate.

Analysis of Tables I and II shows that a history of urinary tract infection or bacteriuria in the donor in the absence of structural changes does not affect the outcome or the long-term function of the grafted kidney. In these groups there was no kidney or patient loss that could be attributed to transplanted kidneys. In fact, only one of these recipients has been treated for bacteriuria. Though the number of recipients is small and a definite conclusion cannot be made, it would seem reasonable to utilize living related donors with history of past urinary tract infection or bacteriuria if upper tract abnormalities are not found.

Stasis on IVP or renogram accounted for almost half of the kidneys with minor abnormalities that we transplanted (Table III). The stasis most often localized to the level of a calyx or the ureteropelvic junction, and was usually caused by vessels crossing across calyceal necks or at the ureteropelvic junction.[2, 3] This pressure can most often be relieved during dissection at nephrectomy and if there is doubt about the caliber of the narrow point, a rubber catheter of known diameter can be passed up the ureter to calibrate it. Analysis of this group of patients also showed no kidney loss secondary to the physiological anomaly present. This was an excellent group of transplants and their outcome can be compared to the results of any group of transplants from normal living related kidneys. The same statement can be made for the group of combined anomalies (Table V). Actually, the results in this group were better than any other.

The worst results occurred in the fourth group of kidneys—those with miscellaneous anomalies (Table IV).

Recipients of kidneys from living related donors with double excretory system had poor results. Only one of the three is currently functioning although both losses were from rejection. That technical problems should not predispose to post-transplant problems has been shown by our use of double pediatric cadaver kidneys which also require double ureteral implantations into the bladder.[4] Thus, we must conclude that double collecting systems are no contraindications to donor use.

On the other hand, we believe that small kidneys should not be routinely used for donation. Their smaller size may be secondary to early atherosclerosis of the renal artery or from scarring of the renal cortex from an old infectious process. In the two patients mentioned here we found no such evidence during the donor evaluation. Nevertheless, had another relative been available we would have preferred not to use the smaller kidneys.

Renal cysts should not cause any post-transplant problem. The only reservation is the difficulty in their diagnosis; our second "cyst" was in reality an adenoma. Exploration of the kidney may even be necessary to assure that the potential donor does not have a malignant tumor. We have encountered a potential donor with a 2.0 cm. "cyst" which on exploration proved to be an invasive renal cell carcinoma. Minor vascular problems should be faced with a positive view. If the rest of the evaluation is normal, related kidneys with minor vascular anomalies should be preferred over cadaver donor kidneys.

REFERENCES

1. Advisory Committee to the Renal Transplant Registry: The 11th report of the Human Renal Transplant Registry, J. A. M. A. **226:** 1197, 1973.
2. Fraley, E. E.: Vascular obstruction of superior infundibulum causing nephralgia, N. Engl. J. Med. **275:** 1402, 1966.
3. Harbert, J. C., and Fraley, E. E.: Scintillation camera renography in superior infundibular obstruction, J. A. M. A. **207:** 2433, 1969.
4. Kinne, D. W., Spanos, P. K., DeShazo, M. T. M., Simmons, R. L., and Najarian, J. S.: Double renal transplants from pediatric donors into adult patients, Am. J. Surg. **127:** 292, 1974.
5. Simmons, R. L., Kjellstrand, C. M., and Najarian, J. S.: Kidney: Techniques, complications and results, *in* Najarian, J. S., and Simmons, R. L., editors: Transplantation, Philadelphia, 1972, Lea & Febiger, Publishers, pp. 445-495.
6. Spanos, P. K., Simmons, R. L., Kjellstrand, C. M., Buselmeier, T. J., and Najarian, J. S.: Screening for renal disease. Renal abnormalities of potential related transplant donors. Lancet **1:** 645, 1974.

Adjuncts to the abdominal wall reconstruction following extensive cancer surgery

Tomoo Tajima, M.D., *and* **John C. McDonald, M.D.,** *New Orleans, La.*

This paper reports the use of Marlex mesh, porcine xenografts, and human autografts to reconstruct a large full-thickness defect of the abdominal wall produced by extensive cancer surgery. This combined method was found useful and resulted in rapid recovery and rehabilitation.

From the Department of Surgery, Tulane University School of Medicine, New Orleans, La.

RATHER favorable survival and significant tumor control have been obtained in patients with colonic cancer involving the abdominal wall,[4, 5] yet there is a general tendency to avoid resection in such patients. Marlex mesh has been successfully utilized to reconstruct the defects of the abdominal wall following extensive cancer surgery.[7] Porcine xenografts have been widely used as biological dressings for open soft-tissue wounds. We are unaware of any report in which a combination of Marlex mesh and porcine xenografts was used to repair an abdominal wall defect. This paper records a case in which Marlex mesh, porcine xenografts, and split-thickness autografts were used to reconstruct a large abdominal wall defect which resulted from extensive cancer surgery.

CASE REPORT

A 49-year-old woman was admitted to H. P. Long Charity Hospital of Louisiana complaining of a large mass in her right lower abdomen and a 27 kilogram weight loss in the previous five-month period. The mass measured 13 by 10 cm. and was firmly attached to the anterior abdominal wall. It was slightly fluctuant and tender. A diagnosis of appendiceal abscess was entertained. The patient was operated upon. An abscess was encountered which was drained. These drain sites persisted. Mixed coliform organisms were cultured from the drainage on several occasions. Subsequently a large filling defect was demonstrated in the cecum by barium enema. Fistulograms demonstrated colocutaneous fistulas. An intravenous pyelogram was normal. Fig. 1, *a,* shows local physical findings.

The patient was prepared for operation and underwent an extended right colectomy with en bloc excision of the anterior abdominal wall on July 25, 1972. This included the distal two feet of the ileum, the right colon, two thirds of the transverse colon, a wide area of the mesentery, the omentum, and approximately 40 percent of the surface area of the anterior abdominal wall. An end-to-end ileotransverse colostomy was performed (Fig. 1, *e*). The skin was included in the specimen because of the presence of two infected fistulous tracts and direct tumor involvement of abdominal wall musculature. The specimen is shown in Fig. 2. Microscopic examination of the specimen revealed a well-differentiated adenocarcinoma of the cecum with rectus muscle involvement. No metastatic disease was found in the mesenteric lymph nodes. The full-thickness defect of the anterior abdominal wall measured 25 by 15 cm. and could not be closed primarily (Fig. 1, *b*). Because of the presence of multiple infected colocutaneous fistulas

Accepted for publication April 4, 1974.

Reprint requests: John C. McDonald, M.D., Department of Surgery, Tulane University School of Medicine, 1430 Tulane Ave., New Orleans, La. 70112.

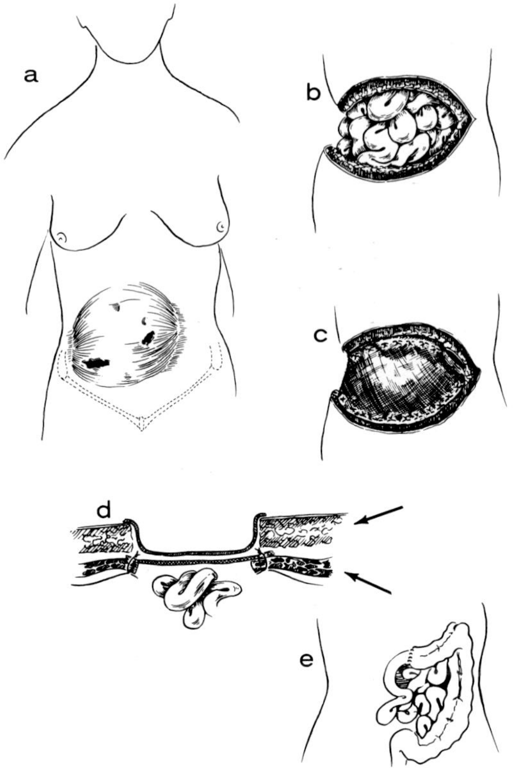

Fig. 1. *a,* Large abdominal mass firmly attached to abdominal wall with multiple colocutaneous fistulas. *b,* Abdominal wall defect. *c,* One layer of Marlex mesh covering the defect. *d,* Porcine xenografts directly placed over the Marlex mesh overlying loops of intestine. *e,* Reconstruction with ileotransverse colostomy.

it was thought unwise to close the defect with large pedicle flaps; therefore, one sheet of Marlex mesh was sutured to the fascial defect directly overlying loops of intestines (Fig. 1, *c*). The mesh was covered with a bulky dressing. The patient lost a large amount of peritoneal fluid through the mesh during her first two postoperative days. We elected to apply porcine xenografts directly on the Marlex mesh as a biological dressing (Fig. 1, *d*). After the first xenograft was applied on the third postoperative day, no further loss of peritoneal fluid occurred. The biological dressing made the care of the patient much simpler. The grafts were changed every three or four days in the operating room with strict aseptic technique. Granulation tissue was allowed to grow through the interstices of the mesh, and completely covered it by the twenty-first postoperative day. Autogenous split-thickness skin grafts were then applied and the patient was discharged from the hospital on the sixth day following autograft application. She now weighs 82 kilograms and has no evidence of disease 19 months after resection.

DISCUSSION

It is generally accepted that multiorgan involvement by colonic cancer carries a poor prognosis, and that extension of tumor into the abdominal wall often precludes its resectability; however, the seemingly advanced colorectal cancer which has invaded another organ often bears favorable biological characteristics and multiple organ resection in judiciously selected patients will control the tumor in a substantial number of patients.[9] Tumor size is not a determinant of regional metastases in colonic cancer[12] and direct neoplastic extension to an adjacent organ is not a statistically more adverse prognostic sign than metastases to one to five regional lymph nodes.[13] Indeed, rather favorable survival, significant tumor control, and significant palliation have been obtained among the patients whose colonic cancer involved the abdominal wall.[4, 5]

One of the major problems following these extensive operations is the large defect of the abdominal wall. Similar problems are often seen in extensive trauma, surgical infections, and abdominal wall hernias.

Prosthetic mesh has been widely used for reconstruction of abdominal wall defects[6-8, 10] although some believe that permanent use of prosthetic meshes is undesirable.[8]

Porcine xenografts have been clinically satisfactory[1-3] as temporary biological dressings and are felt to be adequate substitutes for fresh human allografts in the preparation of open granulating wounds for autografts or secondary closure.[11] Many advantages of biological dressings have been listed[1] and the porcine xenografts for the present case indeed prevented the loss of peritoneal fluid. Pain was decreased, the patient was more mobile, infection was prevented, and the wound was ready for autografting in a short period of time. The use of prosthetic mesh frequently causes excessive delay in grafting.[8] This delay may have been pre-

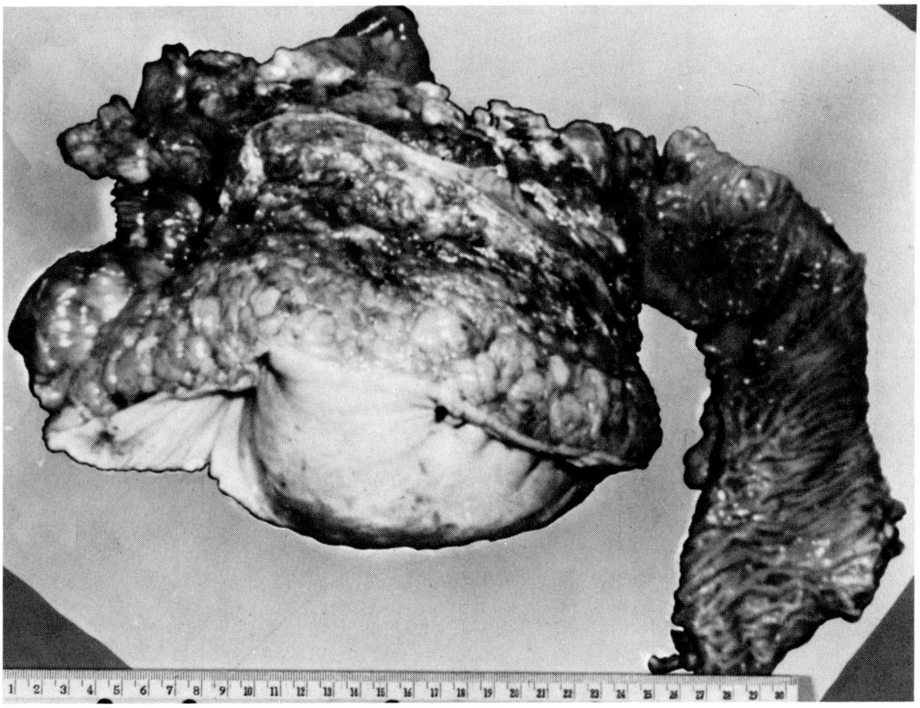

Fig. 2. Gross appearance of the specimen.

vented by the xenografts,[11] although this is difficult to prove.

Subcutaneous fluid frequently collects in the space between prosthetic mesh and skin if the mesh is covered directly with full-thickness skin[7] and as in this case potential contamination often prohibits primary closure by rotating a pedicle flap. The temporary use of heterografts until the wound becomes optimal for autografts may prove a beneficial innovation.

REFERENCES

1. Artz, C. P., Rittenbury, M. S., and Yarbrough, D. R., III: An appraisal of allografts and xenografts as biological dressings for wounds and burns, Ann. Surg. **175:** 934, 1972.
2. Baxter, C. R.: Homografts and heterografts as a biologic dressing in the treatment of thermal injury. Presented at the First Annual Congress of the Society of German Plastic Surgeons in Munich, Sept. 28, 1970.
3. Bromberg, B. E., Song, I. C., and Mohn, M. P.: The use of pig skin as a temporary biological dressing, Plast. Reconstruct. Surg. **36:** 80, 1965.
4. El-Domeiri, A., and Whitely, H. W., Jr.: Prognostic significance of abdominal wall involvement in carcinoma of cecum, Cancer **26:** 552, 1970.
5. Jenson, H. E., Balslev, I., and Nielsen, J.: Extensive surgery in treatment of carcinoma of the colon, Acta Chir. Scand. **136:** 431, 1970.
6. Kus, H., Wozniewski, A., and Szypillo, S.: Large tumor of the abdominal wall. Resection and reconstruction using knitted polyester net, Int. Surg. **49:** 436, 1968.
7. Mays, E. T., and Weakley, S.: Alloplasty of the abdominal wall after extensive cancer surgery, Am. J. Surg. **122:** 781, 1971.
8. Morgan, A., Morain, W., and Eranklis, A.: Gas gangrene of the abdominal wall: Management after extensive debridement, Ann. Surg. **173:** 617, 1971.
9. Polk, H. C., Jr.: Extended resection for selected adenocarcinomas of the large bowel, Ann. Surg. **175:** 892, 1972.
10. Schmitt, H. J., Jr., and Grinnan, G. L. B.: Use of Marlex mesh in infected abdominal war wound, Am. J. Surg. **113:** 825, 1967.
11. Silverstein, P., Curreri, P. W., and Munster,

A. M.: Evaluation of fresh, viable porcine cutaneous xenograft as a temporary burn wound cover, Annual Progress Report (Project No. 3A061101A91C-00) U. S. Army Institute of Surgical Research, Brooke Army Medical Center, June 30, 1971.

12. Spratt, J. S., Jr., and Ackerman, L. V.: Relationship of the size of colonic tumors to their cellular composition and biological behavior, Surg. Forum **10:** 56, 1959.

13. Spratt, J. S., Jr., and Spjut, H. J.: Prevalence and prognosis of individual clinical and pathologic variables associated with colorectal carcinoma, Cancer **20:** 1976, 1967.

Proteolysis of preformed protein in wound nutrition

H. Paul Ehrlich, Ph.D., Harold Tarver, Ph.D., *and* **Thomas K. Hunt, M.D.,**
San Francisco, Calif.

Plant protein with its amino and imino acids uniformly labeled with ^{14}C was diluted with unlabeled albumin and dusted into polyvinyl sponges which were implanted subcutaneously in rats. At 7 days, 12 percent of the implanted radioactivity was recovered from TCA extracts of the wound. Only traces of ^{14}C were found in other wounds from the same animal not loaded with labeled protein. Though no labeled hydroxyproline was implanted, 1.3 percent of the radioactivity recovered was found specifically in collagen hydroxyproline, and it is estimated that a minimum of 10 percent of the label was incorporated into collagen. The results indicate that cells in healing wounds are able to degrade preformed protein through proteolysis and can reuse the liberated amino acids for collagen synthesis. A hypothesis for the pathway of this form of wound nutrition is presented.

From the Department of Surgery, School of Medicine, University of California, San Francisco, Calif.

ALTHOUGH it is well established that nutrition and wound healing are intimately related, how the wound receives its nutrition is still incompletely understood.

Apparently, carbohydrate is presented to the wound by glucose in the circulation. Amino acids from blood plasma diffuse into the wound where they are used for protein synthesis. However, the normally low serum amino acid levels, the relationship of hypoalbuminemia to poor healing, the proteolytic aspects of the inflammatory response, and the sensitivity of wound healing to corticosteroids in the first few days after healing suggest that protein nutrition may be derived at least in part from the products of lysis of macromolecules within the wound itself. Furthermore, it would seem to be biologically advantageous for the wound to use breakdown products of damaged tissue to build new tissue.

This work was supported by United States Public Health Service Grant No. GM-12829.

Accepted for publication April 10, 1974.

Reprint requests: Thomas K. Hunt, M.D., Department of Surgery, School of Medicine, University of California, 3rd and Parnassus, San Francisco, Calif. 94143.

This study was designed to determine whether wound cells can digest macromolecules and reuse the amino acids locally for protein synthesis.

METHODS

Eighteen polyvinyl sponge disks, 1.0 cm. in diameter and 0.2 cm. thick, were dried to constant weight and heat sterilized. Six of the disks were placed into a vial with lyophilized and powdered bovine serum albumin. The vial was shaken for several minutes in a test tube mixer and each sponge was removed and reweighed.

By this means, 6 to 10 mg. of the albumin powder were deposited into each disk. Similarly, six more sponges were dusted with a mixture of 100 parts of bovine serum albumin to 1 part of radioactive Chlorella plant protein* with its amino acids uniformly labeled with ^{14}C (Amersham/Searle). The final specific activity was 233,000 disintegrations per minute (d.p.m.) per milligram of protein. Six more disks remained empty of protein. One of each type of disk was implanted under the abdominal skin of each of six adult male Sprague-Dawley rats.

In preliminary testing of acid hydrolysates, no hydroxyproline was detected in either the albumin or the labeled Chlorella protein. However, the Chlorella protein contained 5.0 percent proline and the serum albumin contained 4.5 percent proline by weight.

Seven days after implantation, the sponges and their contents were removed and were dried to constant weight for 24 hours at 68° C. The collagen was extracted from each dried sponge with 2 ml. of hot 5 percent trichloracetic acid (TCA), according to the method of Fitch and associates.[4] A Teflon-lined screw cap was secured on each test tube and the tubes were heated for 30 minutes at 90° C. After the tubes had been centrifuged at 1,700 G for 5 minutes at room temperature, the supernatant was removed. This procedure was repeated once and the two supernatants from each sponge were pooled.

Then 1 ml. of the pooled supernatant fluid of the TCA extraction was placed in a counting vial with 0.5 ml. of Soluene solubilizer (Packard Instrument Company) and 15 ml. of Toluene PPO-POPO liquid scintillation fluid and the mixture was counted. Duplicate determinations were not done, but each of the six samples in each group was counted until the 2 percent confidence range was reached.

Two milliliters of the pooled TCA supernatant and all of the TCA precipitate were taken up separately in concentrated hydrochloric acid to make a 6N solution which was hydrolyzed at 110° C. for 24 hours. After hydrolysis, the contents of each tube were filtered through a glass filter paper; the entire filtrate was dried over sodium hydroxide pellets in a vacuum desiccator.

*Chlorella protein has a mixture of molecules of varying molecular weights.

The dried TCA supernatant and precipitate hydrolysates were dissolved in 200 μl of water and 200 μg of hydroxyproline were added; 100 μl of this mixture were spotted on a silica gel thin-layer chromatography plate, 20 by 20 cm. in diameter. The plate was developed in 9:1 phenol:water solution and dried at room temperature.[7] The dried plate was sprayed with a solution of 0.2 percent isatin with 4 percent acetic acid in acetone. The plate was dried and sprayed again with 1 percent dimethylaminobenzaldehyde in acetone and concentrated hydrochloric acid in the proportions of 9:1.[1] The red spot, hydroxyproline, was scraped from the plate and placed in a counting vial with 1 ml. of NCS solubilizer (Nuclear-Chicago Corporation) and 15 ml. of toluene PPO-POPOP and counted. There was no appreciable loss of counting efficiency with this method.

The total hydroxyproline contents of the remaining 100 μl of TCA solution and precipitate hydrolysates were then determined by the automated method of Grant.[5]

The remaining 1 ml. of the 6 percent TCA solution was used to determine total protein by the method of Lowry and associates.[6]

In a second experiment two sponges containing bovine serum albumin conjugated with a fluorescent label, rhodamine RB200 (Cal-Biochem), were implanted into each of two rats. On the second day, the sponges were removed, fixed in 10 percent formalin, and sectioned for microscopic examination. The sections were then viewed in a fluorescent microscope.

RESULTS

The mean wet and dry weights of the sponge and the tissue within were identical in all three types of sponges (mean of the albumin sponges 60 ± 3.2 mg. [±1 S.E.], mean of the labeled protein sponges 59 ± 2.3 mg., and mean of the "empty sponges" 56 ± 4.4 mg.).

The total collagen—that is, the hydroxyproline content of the sponges—was also the same in all three groups. The sponges implanted with albumin alone contained a mean of 570 ± 60 μg (±1 S.E.) of hydroxyproline, the labeled protein group contained 609 ± 28 μg, and the average content in the "empty" group was 596 ± 25 μg. The groups are not statistically distinguishable from each other.

At the time of harvesting the sponges, seven days after implantation, 10 percent of the isotope originally placed in the Chlorella protein remained in the sponge in which it was implanted. In the same animals, less than 0.1 percent of the total radioactivity implanted. In the same animals, less than 0.1 percent of the total radioactivity implanted was found in the sponges originally implanted with albumin alone and less than 0.5 percent was found in the "empty" sponge. Samples of liver and plasma contained negligible amounts of radioactive isotope.

A mean of 172,000 ± 32,700 (±1 S.E.) d.p.m. (approximately 10 percent of the total implanted label) was recovered in the sponges implanted containing labeled protein. The 5 percent TCA fraction, which is mostly collagen (mixed with some small polypeptides and free amino acids), contained 20,600 ± 503 d.p.m. or 12 percent of the label found in the sponges. A mean total of 1,970 ± 641 d.p.m., approximately 1 percent of the label found in the sponges, was found in the hydroxyproline fraction isolated by thin-layer chromatography.

The sponges loaded with albumin labeled with fluorescent rhodamine contained extracellular fluorescent material. In the 2-day-old wounds, however, fluorescent label was detected in "granules" in the cytoplasm of phagocytic cells.

DISCUSSION

Histochemical and biochemical investigations of wounds have revealed a variety of proteolytic enzymes. These studies, together with microscopic evidence that protein debris disappears in the inflammatory reaction, can leave no doubt that proteolysis is an active and prominent process in repair after injury. The present study indicates that the products of proteolysis are to some extent reutilized for collagen synthesis. Reutilization of products of proteolysis would seem particularly useful in early repair when injured tissue and inflammatory exudate are plentiful.

Ninety percent of the labeled protein implanted with sponges was not recoverable in these wounds at seven days. Yet the amount which was recovered in each of these implants exceeded that found in the other wounds in the same animal by 20 to 100 times. Obviously, amino acids freed by proteolysis are reused locally within the wound.

In all, 1.3 percent of total counts found in the harvested sponges was from new hydroxyproline. This seems a small fraction, but this figure is deceptive. Hydroxyproline radioactivity was measured because significant amounts of hydroxyproline are found only in collagen. It is not present in albumin, or Chlorella protein, or other noncollagenous protein found in wounds. Hydroxyproline accounts for only 10 percent of the amino acids found in collagen. If one assumes that the diffuse Chlorella label contributed as much ^{14}C to all the amino acids in collagen as it did to hydroxyproline, the collagen would then contain 10 times as much label as found in hydroxyproline alone. The TCA extract, in fact, contained 12 times as much. It seems reasonable to conclude, therefore, that approximately 1 percent of the labeled amino acids in preformed protein placed in the wound on day 0 was found in new collagen on day 7. The collagen label must be somewhat less than the 12 percent found in the TCA fraction since this fraction contains small amounts of peptides and free amino acids in addition to collagen.

Unfortunately, any attempt at quantitative estimation of the portion of collagen synthesis dependent upon preformed protein as an amino acid resource is severely hampered by the rapid turnover of collagen normally occurring in the wound. Since wound collagen turns over fairly rapidly, we would estimate that more than 1 percent of the label was incorporated into collagen at some time during the seven-day experiment. In tissue culture, some collagen is lysed before it is even secreted from the cell.[8] Therefore, the amount of ^{14}C label found in the TCA extract represents that amount of label which *remains* in collagen after a long sequence of metabolic steps including collagen synthesis, lysis, and resynthesis. Furthermore, collagen represents only a fraction of the total protein synthesis in a wound. New cells and mucopolysaccharides, and new vessels, must be synthesized as well.

The seventh day was chosen for removal of the sponges because collagen synthesis is active at this time, and to avoid the possibility that excessive amounts of radioactivity would be lost due to collagen turnover.

The finding of rhodamine fluorescent label in the cytoplasm of the phagocytic cells in the model wound suggests that the nutritional pathway from preformed protein to collagen has an intermediate intracellular phase. It is theoretically possible, of course, that the rhodamine alone was phagocytized, but this is unlikely since rhodamine is covalently bound to albumin. It seems that preformed protein, or fragments thereof from extracellular proteolysis, are ingested by phagocytes and lysed to smaller peptides or amino acids, presumably in digestive vacuoles. Possibly, some digestion could also take place extracellularly. The resulting amino acids would seem to be available for use by fibroblasts for collagen synthesis. Analogous processes have been demonstrated for hemoglobin phagocytosed by macrophages.[2, 3]

This hypothesis has several interesting aspects. First, it proposes a nutritional role for the inflammatory process with phagocytic cells deriving useful amino acids from the injured tissue. We realize that specific depletion of polymorphonuclear leukocytes or lymphocytes does not retard primary repair. However, primary repair requires minimal nutrition as compared to the synthesis of new tissue to fill the sponge dead space. Furthermore, no one has yet succeeded in excluding macrophages from the wound, and preliminary evidence suggests that they are important to repair. In fact, where fibroblasts are seen, macrophages almost always occur as well. Furthermore, fibroblasts are capable of phagocytosis and this may play an important role in the reutilization of amino acids from ingested protein. Second, the findings support our previous hypothesis that the inhibitory effect of cortisone on repair may occur partly because cortisone interferes with the normal digestive activities of phagocytes. This implies that among its other actions, cortisone blocks a significant nutritional pathway in early wound-healing nutrition. In support of this thesis, Rudolph and Klein[10] have shown that cortisone diminishes lysis of tritium-labeled collagen as well as synthesis of new collagen.

There is no evidence that collagen synthesis is enhanced or inhibited by the addition of protein to the sponges. The total hydroxyproline content was the same in all sponges, including those containing added protein.

REFERENCES

1. Dawson, R. M. C., Elliott, D. C., Elliot, W. H., and Jones, K. M.: Data for biochemical research, ed. 2, New York, 1969, Oxford University Press, pp. 529-532.
2. Ehrenreich, B. A., and Cohn, Z. A.: The fate of hemoglobin pinocytosed by macrophages in vitro, J. Cell. Biol. **38:** 244, 1968.
3. Ehrenreich, B. A., and Cohn, Z. A.: The fate of peptides pinocytosed by macrophages in vitro, J. Exp. Med. **129:** 227, 1969.
4. Fitch, S. M., Harkness, M. L. R., and Harkness, R. H.: Extraction of collagen from tissues, Nature **176:** 163, 1955.
5. Grant, R. A.: Estimation of hydroxyproline by the Auto-Analyzer, J. Clin. Pathol. **17:** 685, 1964.
6. Lowry, O. H., Rosenbrough, N. J., Farr, A. Z., and Randal, R. J.: Protein measurement with the Folin phenol reagent, J. Biol. Chem. **193:** 265, 1951.
7. Pataki, G.: *In* Techniques of thin-layer chromatography in amino acid and peptide chemistry, ed. 2, Ann Arbor, Mich., 1969, Humphrey Science Publication, Inc., p. 53.
8. Priest, R. E.: Collagen synthesis by cultured cells: The appearance of free hydroxyproline, Fed. Proc. **31:** 2440, 1972 (abst.).
9. Ross, R.: Personal communication. To be published in the report of the International Symposium on Wound Healing, Rotterdam, April 8-12, 1974.
10. Rudolph, R., and Klein, L.: Inhibition of ^{3}H-collagen destruction by triamcinolone, J. Surg. Res. **14:** 435, 1973.

Rabbit anti–rat lymphocyte serum-induced lymphopenia in thoracic duct lymph and peripheral blood

Roland Girardet, Eli A. Friedman, *and* **Karl E. Karlson,** *Brooklyn, N. Y.*

The simultaneous effect of a single intraperitoneal injection of rabbit anti–rat lymphocyte serum (ALS) on thoracic duct (TDL) and blood lymphocytes (BL) was studied in Sprague-Dawley rats by means of a thoracic duct side fistula. ALS produced an immediate lymphopenia of equal magnitude in thoracic duct lymph and blood suggesting activity against all lymphocytes in circulation at the moment of injection. The lymphopenia remained sustained for eight days in the thoracic duct lymph but was only transient in the blood. This differential response suggests that thoracic duct lymph may be the medium of choice for in vivo assay of ALS.

From the Departments of Surgery and Medicine, State University of New York, Downstate Medical Center, Brooklyn, N. Y.

PARTICIPATION of thymus-dependent lymphocytes (T-lymphocytes) in allograft rejection is well established.[3, 9, 16] T-lymphocytes are a main target for ALS[5, 13, 14, 19, 22] which either destroys lymphocytes, through lysis by cytotoxic antibody and complement or opsonization, or impairs their function by blindfolding or sterile activation, or possibly accomplishes both. The ALS-induced decrease in the pool of T-lymphocytes may also be responsible for blood lymphopenia because 75 percent of small lymphocytes in the blood are long-lived.[4, 10, 15, 21, 23]

Thoracic duct lymph carries an almost pure population of ALS-susceptible lymphocytes.[1, 18, 20] The present experiment was designed to study and compare simultaneously the action of ALS on thoracic duct lymph and peripheral blood in the rat.

METHOD

TDL's from male Sprague-Dawley rats were used as antigen to develop ALS in two male New Zealand rabbits. Lymphocytes collected during the first 24 hours of drainage via a thoracic duct fistula[7] were utilized. The schedule for preparation of the ALS was as follows: on day 0, each rabbit received a total of 100 × 10[6] lymphocytes injected into the footpads with complete Freund's adjuvant. On days 21, 22, and 23, each rabbit received a single intravenous injection of 100 × 10[6] lymphocytes. The antiserum was collected under sterile conditions on day 30, pooled, heated for 30 minutes at 56° C., and stored at –20° C. The lymphagglutination titer of the antiserum was 1:1536 and the cytotoxic titer was 1:256. Normal rabbit serum (NRS), used as control serum, was obtained from the same rabbits one week before the first injection of lymphocytes and processed in a similar fashion as the antiserum.

The ALS was tested in five male Sprague-Dawley rats weighing 400 to 600 grams (experimental group). A T-tube thoracic duct fistula was constructed in each animal according to a technique reported previously.[8] For two days after establishment of the fistula,

Accepted for publication April 4, 1974.

Reprint requests: Roland E. Girardet, M.D., Department of Surgery, University of Louisville School of Medicine, Health Sciences Center, Louisville, Ky. 40201.

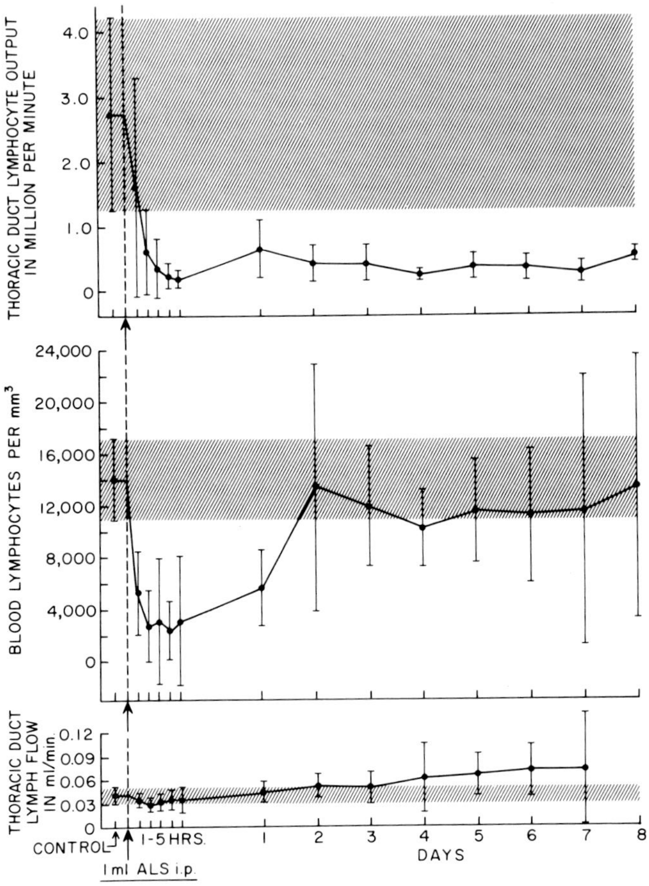

Fig. 1. Effect of one injection of ALS on thoracic duct lymphocyte output, blood lymphocyte concentration, and thoracic duct lymph flow in five experimental rats. Mean values and S.D. are indicated. The shaded area corresponds to the S.D. of the control (preinjection) values.

control mean values were obtained for thoracic duct lymph flow, TDL output, and tail blood lymphocyte concentration. On the second postoperative day, each rat received 1 ml. of ALS intraperitoneally. The thoracic duct lymph flow, TDL output, and BL concentration were then measured hourly for five hours and subsequently two to four times daily for an additional eight days.

A control group of five additional rats had T-tube thoracic duct fistulas created. Normal rabbit serum was administered to this group and the animals followed according to the same protocol as ALS recipients.

RESULTS

Control values for the experimental group were as follows: thoracic duct lymph flow, 0.046 ml. per minute (±0.011); TDL output, 2.73×10^6 per minute (±1.51); and blood lymphocyte concentration, 14,000 per cubic millimeter (±3,145) (Fig. 1). For the control group, the respective values were: 0.036 ml. per minute (±0.008), 1.91×10^6 cells per minute (±0.78), and 12,557 cells per cubic millimeter (±4,384) (Fig. 2).

The responses of each of the ALS-treated rats were superimposable. As compared with pre-ALS injection values, thoracic duct lymph flow remained unchanged while TDL output decreased rapidly and remained below control values after the second postinjection hour. BL concentration was significantly decreased only during the first two days after injection of ALS, with return to preinjection level on day three. The mean values for five ALS-

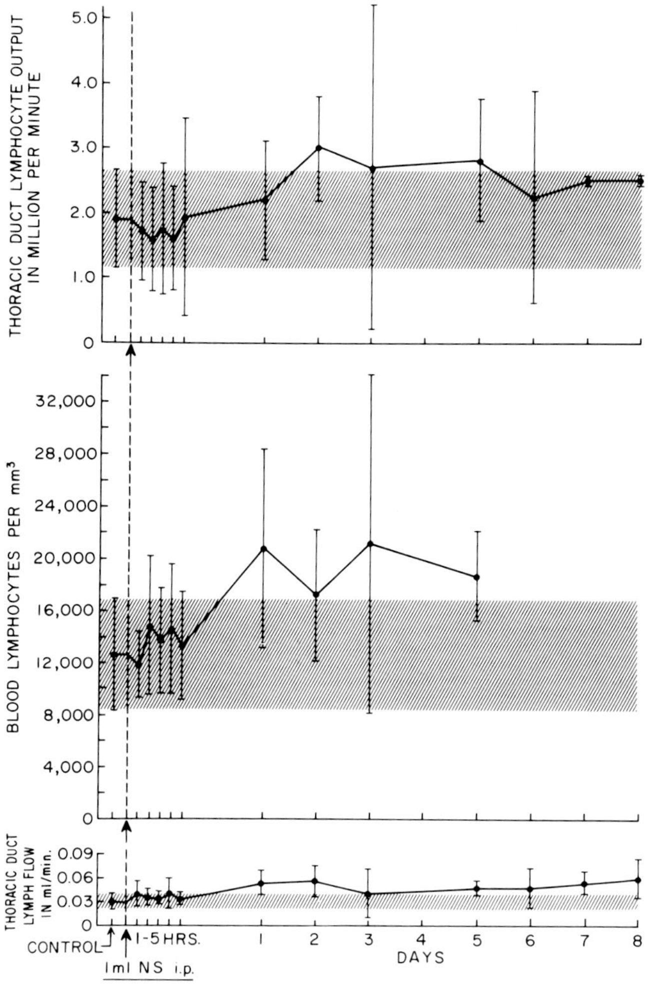

Fig. 2. Effect of one injection of normal serum on thoracic duct lymphocyte output, blood lymphocyte concentration, and thoracic duct lymph flow in five control rats. Mean values and S.D. are indicated. The shaded area corresponds to the S.D. of the control (preinjection) value.

treated experimental rats (mean fistula function of seven days, with a range of five to eight days) are presented in Fig. 1.

Comparable function of thoracic duct fistulas was noted in the NRS-treated rats (mean fistula function of five days, with a range of four to eight days). Neither TDL output nor lymph flow changed significantly following NRS injection. Peripheral BL concentration also remained unchanged in this group (Fig. 2).

DISCUSSION

Intraperitoneal or intravenous injection of ALS produces peripheral blood lymphopenia which may be transient, even in the face of continuing ALS administration.[11] Denman and Denman[6] and Tyler and associates[20] explain this "escape" by a modification of the small lymphocyte population in blood such that the long-lived fraction remains reduced while the short-lived fraction increases to restore a normal total small lymphocyte count. Because short-lived and long-lived small lymphocytes are morphologically indistinguishable, the compositional change is not detectable in blood smears. Thus, attempts to use blood lymphopenia as an in vivo index of ALS activity have met with inconsistent results.[11, 17]

Table I. *Mean concentrations of lymphocytes in TDL and in BL, and their ratio, before and after intraperitoneal injections of 1 ml. of ALS in five rats*

Time (related to ALS injection)	*TDL (concentration/ mm.³)*	*BL (concentration/ mm.³)*	*Ratio: TDL/BL*
Before injection (control)	72,000	14,000	50/10
After injection:			
4-5 hours	10,500	2,500	40/10
1 day	15,600	5,500	28/10
2 days	8,600	13,500	6/10
3 days	10,200	12,000	8/10
4 days	5,800	10,300	5/10
5 days	6,600	11,600	5/10
6 days	6,100	11,100	5/10
7 days	9,200	11,500	8/10
8 days	4,700	13,300	3/10

Examination of thoracic duct lymph permits detection of selective T-cell lymphopenia in the absence of potentially confusing short-lived lymphocyte repletion, as short-lived lymphocytes do not enter lymph. Long-lasting thoracic duct lymphopenia has been previously documented following ALS injection.[1, 20] These studies, however, required the use of inbred rats, serially examined by continuous thoracic duct drainage, which itself resulted in pronounced and nonspecific lymphopenia, rapidly obliterating the specific changes attributable to the action of ALS alone. Prior attempts to study the simultaneous effect of ALS on thoracic duct lymph and in blood of the same animal by Bollman fistulas[2] have had only limited success.[7] The present experiment, with an intermittent sampling technique,[8] obviates the limitations of the Bollman fistula and facilitates study and comparison of thoracic duct and blood lymphocytes under stable conditions in the same animal. A single injection of ALS produced marked and persistent lymphopenia in thoracic duct lymph with only transient blood lymphopenia.

Calculation of the ratio of thoracic duct lymphocytes to peripheral blood lymphocytes (per cubic millimeter) provides an estimate of the relative proportion of long-lived to short-lived lymphocyte pools (Table I). This ratio before ALS injection (50/10) remained unchanged four to five hours after ALS injection (40/10) at a time of maximal lymphopenic effect and marked reduction in the total number of lymphocytes. The unchanging ratio supports the hypothesis that ALS is effective on all lymphocytes, with little regard to their function as either long-lived or short-lived variety, as long as the cells are in circulation at the moment of ALS administration.[12] The reversal of the concentration ratio, from the second postinjection day on, probably reflects a relative increase in the short-lived lymphocyte pool in the blood.

The different responses of thoracic duct and blood lymphocytes to ALS administration under the conditions of these experiments point to the unreliability of blood lymphopenia in assessing ALS activity. This suggests that thoracic duct lymphopenia might be a sensitive in vivo system to assay the lymphopenic potency of ALS and to correlate this action with the immunosuppressive properties of ALS.

We thank Kathy Grice and Linda Stackhouse for their technical assistance.

REFERENCES

1. Agnew, H. D.: The effect of heterologous anti-lymphocytic serum on the small lymphocyte population of rats, J. Exp. Med. **128:** 111, 1968.
2. Bollman, J. L., Cain, J. C., and Grindlay, J. H.: Techniques for the collection of lymph from the liver, small intestine, or thoracic duct of the rat, J. Lab. Clin. Med. **33:** 1349, 1948.
3. Chanana, A. D., Cronkite, E. P., Joel, D. D., Schiffer, L. M., and Schnappauf, H.: Studies on lymphocytes. XII. The role of immunologically committed lymphocytes in rejecting skin allografts, Transplantation **7:** 459, 1969.
4. Chew, W. B., and Lawrence, J. S.: Antilymphocytic serum, J. Immunol. **96:** 217, 1937.
5. DeMeester, T. R.: Mode of action of antilymphocyte serum, Surg. Gynecol. Obstet. **129:** 717, 1969.
6. Denman, A. M., and Denman, E. J.: Changes in the life span of circulating small lymphocytes in mice after treatment with antilymphocyte globulin, Lancet **1:** 321, 1968.
7. Gelfand, M. C., Girardet, R., and Friedman, E. A.: Thoracic duct lymphopenia: An effect

of antilymphocyte serum, Transplant. Proc. **1:** 439, 1969.
8. Girardet, R. E., and Karlson, K. E.: T-tube side-fistula in thoracic duct: A surgical technique for the study of lymph and lymphocytes in the rat under normal conditions of thoracic duct circulation, J. Lab. Clin. Med. **79:** 157, 1972.
9. Gowans, J. L.: The effect of the continuous re-infusion of lymph and lymphocytes on the output of lymphocytes from the thoracic duct of unanesthetized rats, Br. M. Bull. **21:** 106, 1965.
10. Gray, J. G., Monaco, A. P., Wood, J. R., and Russel, P. S.: Studies on heterologous anti-lymphocyte serum in mice, J. Immunol. **96:** 217, 1966.
11. Jeejeebhoy, H. F., and Vela-Martinez, J. M.: Studies on the mode of action of heterologous anti-lymphocyte plasma. 2. The effect of anti-lymphocyte plasma on lymphocyte counts, Transplantation **6:** 149, 1968.
12. Levey, R. H., and Medawar, P. B.: Further experiments on the action of anti-lymphocytic serum, Proc. Natl. Acad. Sci. **58:** 470, 1967.
13. Martin, W. J., and Miller, J. F. A. P.: Cell to cell interaction in the immune response. IV. Site of action of antilymphocyte serum, J. Exp. Med. **128:** 855, 1968.
14. Medawar, P. B.: Antilymphocyte serum: Its properties and potential, Hosp. Pract. **4:** 26, 1969.
15. Medawar, P. B.: Biological effects of heterologous antilymphocyte sera, *in* Rapaport, F. T., and Dausset, J., editors: Human transplantation, New York, 1968, Grune & Stratton, Inc., p. 501.
16. Moller, G.: Immunocompetent cells in graft rejection, Transplant. Proc. **3:** 15, 1971.
17. Rule, A. H., and Judd, K. P.: Rabbit anti-rat lymphocyte serum: Relationship between dosages, circulating lymphocytes, and the primary immune response, Transplantation **6:** 970, 1968.
18. Schwarz, M. R., Tyler, R. W., and Everett, N. B.: Mixed lymphocyte reaction: An in vitro test for anti-lymphocyte serum activity, Science **160:** 1014, 1968.
19. Seifert, J., and Brendel, W.: The effect of antilymphocytic serum on homologous ^{51}Cr-labelled lymphocytes in rats, Transplantation **8:** 806, 1969.
20. Tyler, R. W., Everett, N. B., and Schwarz, M. R.: Effect of antilymphocytic serum on rat lymphocytes, J. Immunol. **102:** 179, 1969.
21. Waksman, B. H., Arbouys, S., and Arnason, B. G.: The use of specific "lymphocyte" antisera to inhibit hypersensitive reactions of the "delayed" type, J. Exp. Med. **114:** 997, 1961.
22. Woodruff, M. F. A.: Antilymphocytic serum and its mode of action, Transplant. Proc. **3:** 34, 1971.
23. Woodruff, M. F. A., and Anderson, N.: The effect of lymphocyte depletion by thoracic duct fistula and the administration of anti-lymphocyte serum on the survival of skin homografts in rats, Ann. N. Y. Acad. Sci. **120:** 119, 1964.

Effect of single dose irradiation on isolated perfused canine kidney

G. H. Malek, M.D., M. J. S. Richards, M.D., P. M. Burkholder, M.D., *and*
W. L. Caldwell, M.D., *Madison, Wis.*

Passenger leukocytes may be a primary stimulus for renal allograft rejection. Massive single dose in vitro irradiation in a cold, hypoxic environment has been suggested as a method of eradicating such leukocytes. This study was undertaken to evaluate the tolerance of isolated, cooled, hypoxic canine kidneys to massive in vitro irradiation before autotransplantation, a critical factor if such a method would be useful in delaying rejection. Sixteen dogs were divided into eight groups, with two dogs serving as controls. After perfusion for 4 to 5 minutes, doses of irradiation ranging from 2,000 to 10,000 rads were delivered to each isolated test kidney in a cold, hypoxic environment prior to autotransplantation. Single doses of less than 3,000 rads were tolerated, with acceptable renal function remaining for up to eight months. However, this dose of irradiation is not sufficient to delay significantly allograft rejection. It seems unlikely that renal tissues can be sufficiently protected by a cold, hypoxic environment at the time of irradiation to allow preferential killing of passenger leukocytes to the extent to make this approach clinically feasible.

From the Departments of Surgery (G. H. M.), Pathology (P. M. B.), and Radiology (M. J. S. R. and W. L. C.), The University of Wisconsin Medical School, The University of Wisconsin Medical School, Madison, Wis.

It has been suggested that passenger leukocytes may be a primary stimulus for renal allograft rejection.[2, 5-7] Therefore, in vivo and in vitro irradiation of the donor kidney has been utilized in experimental animals as a method for eliminating these cells in order to prevent and delay acute rejection of renal allografts. Steinmuller and Hart[6] observed that rejection of rat heart allografts was delayed significantly by irradiating the cold, anoxic, donor heart in vitro to 2,000 rads. Stuart and associates[8] similarly found that rat kidneys massively irradiated to a dose of 10,000 rads in vitro prior to transplantation into a histocompatible animal delayed the onset of uremia significantly, but follow-up on these animals was brief and the degree of renal irradiation damage could not be assessed adequately. They[7, 8] hypothesized that such high single doses of irradiation were necessary to eradicate passenger leukocytes not removed by previous perfusion since such a delay was not seen in animals receiving 5,000 rads. However, they[7, 8] did express concern that such massive doses might be potentially injurious to renal parenchyma. There is no published information indicating the tolerance of an isolated, cooled, perfused kidney to single-dose irradiation,[8] a critical factor if such a method would be useful. The

Accepted for publication May 13, 1974.

This work was supported in part by a National Cancer Institute funded University of Wisconsin Training Program in Radiotherapy, Physics, and Biology (5-TO1-CA-05104).

Reprint requests: Marcia J. S. Richards, M.D., Radiotherapy Center, 1300 University Ave., Madison, Wis. 53706.

Table I. *Radiation dose and maximum values of creatinine and BUN before being put to death*

Radiation dose (rads)	Dog No.	Status	Creatinine	BUN	Time after transplant (mo.)
0 (controls)	1	Alive	1.5	21	10
	2	Alive	1.8	29	10
2,000	3	Alive	2.5	46	8
	4	Alive	3.5	50	8
3,000	5	Alive	2.1	45	8
	6	Alive	2.7	56	8

Table II. *Radiation dose and maximum values of creatinine and BUN before death*

Radiation dose (rads)	Dog No.	Status	Creatinine	BUN	Time after transplant (wk.)
4,000	7	Dead	12.0	209	4
	8	Dead	7.0	185	6
5,000	9	Dead	2.4	30	3*
	10	Dead	6.2	94	5
6,000	11	Dead	13.9	211	8
	12	Dead	12.7	220	4
8,000	13	Dead	5.0	99	5
	14	Dead	4.0	65	5
10,000	15	Dead	16.6	302	5
	16	Dead	7.0	98	4

*Pneumonia.

present study was undertaken to evaluate the tolerance of resected, cooled, canine kidneys to a single dose of irradiation. Functional and pathological changes in irradiated, reimplanted kidneys were evaluated.

MATERIAL AND METHODS

Sixteen mongrel dogs, with normal baseline serum creatinine and blood urea nitrogen (BUN), weighing between 18 and 22 kilograms, were dewormed and immunized against distemper. All dogs underwent unilateral nephrectomy two weeks prior to the experiment. After the dog had been anesthetized with sodium Pentothal and inhalation anesthesia maintained with methoxyflurane,* the remaining kidney of the dog was removed and perfused with 4° C. Ringer's lactate solution which contained 10,000 U. of heparin and 60 mg. of papaverine. Perfusion was carried out for 4 to 5 minutes to allow the kidney to cool to 6 to 9° C. Subsequently, the kidney was placed in cold slosh of Ringer's lactate in a sterile container, which was put in crushed ice. The temperature was maintained at 6 to 9° C. and the kidneys were irradiated in the cold slosh container with 4 MvP x-rays produced by a Varian linear accelerator with a 6 by 6 cm. field at a target-to-kidney distance of 60 cm. The dose rate was approximately 350 rads per minute at the point of maximal dose.

The dogs were divided into eight groups: two dogs served as controls and the remaining 14 were test animals. Control kidneys were brought to the radiation therapy department in the cold slosh container and allowed to remain in the treatment room for the same length of time as required for the average irradiation (approximately 18 minutes). The test kidneys also were irradiated in the cold slosh container; doses of irradiation to the midplane of the kidney for each pair ranged from 2,000 to 10,000 rads. Subsequently, the kidneys were autotransplanted to the iliac fossa; the renal artery was anastomosed to

*Penthrane: Abbott Laboratories, Chicago, Ill.

Table III. *Histologic findings after being put to death*

Animal No.	*Radiation dose (rads)*	*Survival of graft (days)*	*Glomeruli*	*Tubules*	*Interstitium*	*Other*
1	0	300 living	Segmental slight mesangiol cellularity, segmental capillary dilation	Rare vacuolization PT*	Normal, single calicific focus in medulla	—
2	0	300 living	Slight mesangiol cellularity, segmental capillary dilation	Vacuolization, PT, DT	Normal, single calicific focus in medulla	—
3	2,000	240 living	Prominent juxtaglomerular apparatus (2/30 glomeruli); moderate mesangiol thickening; capsular fibrosis and adhesions (1/30 glomeruli)	Normal	Normal	—
4	2,000	240 living	Endothelial vacuolization, slight thickening of Bowman's capsular basement membrane; isolated capsular synechiae	Vacuolization, PT; thickening basement membrane DT	Moderate fibrosis; focus of chronic inflammation with tubular atrophy	—
5	3,000	240 living	Segmental mesangiol thickening (1/10 glomeruli); prominent juxtaglomerular apparatus (1/10 glomeruli); capillary dilation (1/10 glomeruli)	Vacuolization PT, normal DT	Normal	—
6	3,000	240 living	Normal	Vacuolization PT, DT	Normal	—

*PT = proximal tubules; DT = distal tubules; CD = collecting ducts.

the iliac artery, end-to-end, and the renal vein end-to-side to the iliac vein with 6-0 prolene. Ureteroneocystotomy was accomplished by the Leadbetter-Politano technique, creating a 1.5 to 2 cm. submucosal tunnel. All dogs received sodium ampicillin (500 mg. per day) for the first five postoperative days.

Serum creatinine and BUN were checked every day for the first seven days, then biweekly until the animals were killed at 8 months or died. The kidneys were biopsied if serum creatinine rose above 2.5 mg. per 100 ml.

Irradiation dose, maximum values of serum creatinine and BUN before sacrifice or death, and survival data are tabulated in Tables I and II. Specimens of kidney obtained by needle biopsy or autopsy were fixed in buffered 10 percent formalin and processed routinely for staining of sections with hematoxylin and eosin.

RESULTS

All kidneys produced urine within 4 to 6 minutes after completion of the vascular anastomosis. Dogs 1 and 2 (controls) were alive and well 10 months after autotransplantation; their renal function was normal. Dogs 3 and 4 and dogs 5 and 6, which received 2,000 and 3,000 rads, respectively, were alive and well eight months after autotransplantation, but there was some deterioration in renal function when compared with the control dogs, as seen by examination of levels of maximal creatinine and BUN before sacrifice listed in Table I. Whether renal dysfunction would have eventually led to renal failure had the animals not been sacrificed at 8 months is unknown. All dogs which received 4,000 rads or over died or had to be killed because of severe deterioration of renal function within 4 to 8 weeks after autotransplantation (Table II).

Fifteen kidneys were studied for patho-

Table IV. *Histologic findings after death*

Animal No.	*Radiation dose (rads)*	*Survival of graft (days)*	*Glomeruli*	*Tubules*	*Interstitium*	*Other*
7	4,000	25	Protein in Bowman's space; prominent juxtaglomerular apparatus	Focal necrosis, PT*; vacuolization, PT; occasional crystals and calcium, DT; granular debris and necrotic cells, CD	Occasional focal chronic inflammation; edema	—
8	4,000	44	Normal	Extensive necrosis, PT; prominent yellow in pigment, PT; extensive necrosis, DT; debris and necrotic cells, CD	Edema	Thick capsule
10	5,000	41	Normal	Vacuolization, mild PT; vacuolization, DT; dilation, DT; rare focal necrosis, PT	—	Thick capsule
11	6,000	60	Normal; occasional prominent juxtaglomerular apparatus	Hyaline casts, DT; vacuolization, PT; vacuolization focal, DT; dilation, DT	Edema; rare focal inflammation (plasma cells)	Thick capsule; squamous metaplasia calyx
12	6,000	8	Cortical necrosis			
13	8,000	30	Normal; rare enlarged juxtaglomerular apparatus	Dilation, DT; vacuolization mild, PT; rare necrosis, PT, DT; rare cast, hyaline or granular, DT; rare regeneration in necrotic tubules	—	Thick capsule
14	8,000	39	Normal; rare enlarged juxtaglomerular apparatus	Dilation, mild, DT; vacuolization, PT, DT; rare hyaline casts, DT; one site of squamous metaplasia	Focal chronic inflammation (plasma cells), focal necrosis	Vacuolization of calyceal mucosa; thick capsule
15	10,000	36	Normal; protein in Bowman's space	Vacuolization, PT; dilation, DT; necrotic cellular debris casts, DT	Edema slight	Thick capsule
16	10,000	30+	Normal; protein in Bowman's space; mild prominence of juxtaglomerular apparatus	Vacuolization, PT, DT; cellular debris, DT; hyaline, granular casts, DT, CD; mild dilation, DT; iron pigment mitoses (rare)	Normal	—

*PT = proximal tubules; DT = distal tubules; CD = collecting ducts.

logical changes. The essential histologic alterations observed are described in Tables III and IV. Glomeruli, arterioles, and arteries were remarkably normal. No intimal thickening, hypertrophy, or hyperplasia of endothelial cells or mural necrosis (except very rarely in dog 10) was observed in intrarenal arteries or arterioles. There also was no significant increased cellularity, atrophy, endothelial swelling, or sclerosis of glomeruli.

Among the most striking alterations were those observed in various tubular segments of the nephrons. Nearly all animals had some vacuolar cytoplasmic swelling of mild, moderate, or occasionally severe degree in proximal and/or distal tubules. In dogs 7, 10, and 13 there was limited focal necrosis and in dog 8 extensive necrosis of proximal tubules. In one instance there was complete generalized necrosis of the entire kidney (dog 12), presumably the result of a mechanical vascular problem. Dog 4 had prominent thickening of basement membrane of distal convoluted tubules. Most of these autografted kidneys had tubular casts, either of the hyaline variety (dogs 11, 13, 14, and 16) and/or of a granular variety including debris from necrotic tubular cells (dogs 7, 8, 13, 15, and 16). The frequency and severity of such findings correlated poorly with dose of irradiation except these changes were not seen in the control kidneys or those irradiated to 2,000 or 3,000 rads; dog 16, whose kidney received the highest radiation dose, had rather severe tubular vacuolar changes and cast formation. About one third of the kidneys (dogs 10, 11, 13, 15, and 16) also had mild to moderate dilation of distal tubules, which seemed to correlate somewhat with the extent of accumulation of debris and casts in tubules.

In most cases of animals receiving irradiation dose of 4,000 rads or more, all of whom were ill or moribund when specimens of kidney were obtained, had congestion of interstitial capillaries and in addition dogs 7, 8, 11, and 15 had some degree of interstitial edema. The capsular surface of most kidneys was covered by moderately to markedly increased amounts of fibrocellular—often well-vascularized—connective tissue.

DISCUSSION

Irradiation of an isolated kidney prior to transplantation with doses of up to 10,000 rads has been used to destroy passenger leukocytes in experimental animals.[7, 8] But obviously this is only a futile exercise if the renal tissues also are significantly injured in the process. Apparently tolerable doses (approximately 2,000 rads in a single dose) may not be adequate to eradicate all of the leukocytes, since allograft rejection is not delayed by this dose in dogs, whereas higher doses do delay rejection.[8] This is not to say that other factors are not involved in the allograft rejection.

Hypoxic tissues show less postirradiation effect than well-oxygenated tissues when irradiated to the same dose of x- or gamma radiation. The ratio of the irradiation dose to produce a specific effect under extreme hypoxia and the dose required to produce the same effect under full oxygenation (oxygen enhancement ratio) may reach values as high as three in mammalian systems.[1, 9] Different tissues show varying degrees of alteration of radiosensitivity in response to various oxygen tensions.

Alteration of the irradiation response with tempertaure change has been less well studied by radiobiologists, but it is generally accepted that cooler tissues are less radiosensitive than normothermic ones. Again, there is considerable variability of different tissues in response to the same irradiation doses.[3, 4] It was hoped that the cold, hypoxic environment used during the in vitro renal irradiation would accentuate the difference in radiosensitivity between passenger leukocytes and renal parenchymal cells to a degree that would allow the delivery of radiation doses that could feasibly destroy leukocytes without causing serious renal injury. Unfortunately, our results do not support such a hypothesis.

Functional changes in the kidneys, at the doses of irradiation used, were more pronounced than the histologic abnormalities. At doses of 2,000 and 3,000 rads, minimal increases in serum creatinine and BUN were found and histologic examination revealed only nonspecific changes. At 4,000 rads or above, renal failure or death was seen within eight weeks with limited histologic changes. Values for BUN and serum creatinine, and the time of death secondary to renal failure, did not vary significantly with dose in this range. Perhaps this reflects a steep dose-response curve for the development of postirradiation nephritis between 3,000 and 4,000 rads in a single dose for the dog kidney irradiated in vitro in a cold, hypoxic environment. As additional irradiation above 4,000 rads did not contribute to the rate of onset or degree of severity of the functional changes during life, and at the time of death resulted in no apparent increase in the histologic abnormalities, perhaps it can be assumed that postirradiation effects had revealed an asymptomatic plateau with a dose of 4,000 rads.

We must conclude that in vitro renal tolerance for the previously described environment is approximately 2,000 rads in a single dose, since functional abnormalities were demonstrated at this dose even though no histologic abnormalities were demonstrated at sacrifice at 8 months after irradiation. None of the findings typical of subacute or chronic irradiation nephritis were seen in animals with renal transplants that received less than 4,000 rads, and which survived at least 8 months, despite the increased serum creatinine and BUN. Focal necrosis, vacuolization, cast formation, and regeneration of tubules were seen most conspicuously at dose levels in excess of 4,000 rads. Probably in the other animals, whose renal grafts received 4,000 or more rads, the time course before death was too short for the typical histologic manifestations of postirradiation nephritis to develop.

Without further studies, it seems clear that in the dog under the conditions suitable for irradiation of isolated kidneys, any differential response to irradiation of leukocytes and renal tissues is not sufficient to utilize this approach to forestall rejection. Since at least a twofold increase of dose is required for even delaying allograft rejection,[8] there is little likelihood that irradiation under different conditions will be successful in destroying passenger leukocytes without functional injury of renal tissue.

CONCLUSIONS

This study has attempted to evaluate the tolerance of isolated, cooled, hypoxic canine kidneys to massive in vitro irradiation. It is apparent that single doses less than 3,000 rads are tolerated by autotransplanted kidneys with acceptable function remaining for up to eight months. However, this dose of irradiation, which is tolerated by the renal parenchyma, is not sufficient to delay significantly allograft rejection. It seems unlikely that renal tissues can be sufficiently protected by a cold, hypoxic environment at the time of irradiation to allow preferential killing of passenger leukocytes to the extent to make this approach clinically feasible.

REFERENCES

1. Grey, L. H., Conger, A. D., Ebert, M., Horsey, S., and Scott, O. C. A.: The concentration of oxygen dissolved in tissues at the time of irradiation as a factor in radiotherapy, Br. J. Radiol. **26:** 638, 1953.
2. Guttmann, R., and Lindquist, R.: Hematopoietic origin of immunological target in enhancement of renal allografts, Transplant. Proc. **3:** 717, 1971.
3. Leibner, E. J., Moos, W. S., Hochhauser, M., and Harvey, R. A.: Lowering the skin temperature of the irradiated field, Am. J. Roentgenol. **88:** 976, 1962.
4. Selawry, O. S., Carlsen, J. D., and Moore, G. E.: Tumor response to ionizing rays at elevated temperatures, Am. J. Roentgenol. **80:** 833, 1958.
5. Snell, G. D.: The homograft reaction, Ann. Rev. Microbiol. **11:** 439, 1957.
6. Steinmuller, D., and Hart, E.: Passenger leukocytes and induction of allograft immunity, Transplant. Proc. **3:** 673, 1971.
7. Stuart, F. P., Bastien, E., Holter, A., Fitch, F. W., and Elkins, W. L.: The role of passenger leukocytes in the rejection of renal allograft, Transplant. Proc. **3:** 461, 1971.
8. Stuart, F. P., Garrick, T., Holter, A., Lynch, A., and Bastien, E.: Delayed rejection of renal allografts in the rat and dog by reduction of passenger leukocytes, SURGERY **70:** 128, 1971.
9. Tomlinson, R. H.: The oxygen effect in mammals, *in* Fundamental aspects of radiosensitivity, Brookhaven Symposium in Biology, No. 14, Technical Services, Department of Commerce, 1961, pp. 204-219.

Effect of complete parenteral nutrition including fat emulsion on plasma lipid

Yoshiko Koga, M.D., Keiichi Ikeda, M.D., *and* **Kiyoshi Inokuchi, M.D., D.Sc.,** *Fukuoka, Japan*

Four to 8 week complete parenteral nutrition including fat emulsion, 10 percent Intralipid, from 2 to 4 Gm. per kilogram per day, was carried out on immature dogs. The following conclusions were reached: In the first 2 weeks of complete parenteral nutrition using the infusion of fat emulsion, α- and β-lipoproteins and plasma lipid levels, particularly phospholipids and cholesterol, increased remarkably. Thereafter, throughout the entire experiment using fat emulsion, they remained at nearly the same high level, returning to the approximate normal level in a short period after the interruption of the infusion of the fat emulsion. This enhancement in lipid metabolism was considered to be caused by an accelerated metabolic process for the fat emulsion and would seem to indicate that the daily infusion of the fat emulsion from 2 to 4 Gm. could be performed safely for an extended period.

From the Second Department of Surgery, Kyushu University School of Medicine, Fukuoka, Japan.

HYPERALIMENTATION and complete parenteral nutrition are often used in pediatric surgery. For many reasons, fat emulsion is necessary in order to obtain the required intravenous supply of energy in such cases. This study was designed to determine the levels of lipid components of the serum in immature dogs which were maintained on a complete parenteral nutrition, including Intralipid,* for 4 to 8 weeks.

MATERIALS AND METHODS

Seven litters of immature dogs each containing two or three members, or a total of 17 animals, 8 to 10 weeks old, were used. A silicone rubber catheter was inserted into an external jugular vein and threaded into the superior vena cava of one or two animals of each litter.[4] The animals were sustained exclusively by vein, receiving 140 Cal. per kilogram of body weight per day. The solution, infused over a 21 to 23 hour period daily, consisted of 4 Gm. of amino acid mixtures per kilogram of body weight, carbohydrate, fat, and all the vitamins and minerals recommended for growth in dogs[4] (Table I). The provision of carbohydrate varied according to the fat intake. The experimental animals were divided into three groups. In Group 1, two animals (4 week experiment) received 2 Gm. of fat per kilogram per day. In Group 2, three animals (4 week experiment) received 3 Gm. of fat per kilogram per day. In Group 3, three animals (4 week experiment) and two (8 week experiment) received 4 Gm. of fat per kilogram per day. Ten percent Intralipid was used as the fat emulsion (Table II). It was infused over an 8 to 10-hour period in each 24 hours with

Accepted for publication April 10, 1974.

Reprint requests: Yoshiko Koga, M.D., The Second Department of Surgery, Kyushu University School of Medicine, Fukuoka City, Fukuoka Prefecture, Japan.

*Blood Plasma Co. of Japan, Ohsaka, Japan.

8 U. of heparin per kilogram of body weight per hour. Complete parenteral nutrition, with 31 Gm. of carbohydrate and 4 Gm. of amino acid mixtures per kilogram of body weight, was continued after the 4 week experiment for 5 days in one animal (dog 36, Group 2) and for 10 days in a second animal (dog 44, Group 3). The littermate controls (seven animals) were fed Clea dog food (commercial food with an adequate content of calories, minerals, and vitamins) at the same caloric levels as the experimental animals. The average daily fat intake was 3.5 Gm. per kilogram of body weight. During the first 4 weeks in both the 4 week and 8 week experimental groups, blood samples were taken at 2 week intervals, 3 hours after the completion of the fat emulsion. This pattern was continued throughout the experiment in the 8 week experimental group. On the last day of the fourth week, following the administration of the last fat emulsion, in the 4 week experimental group, blood samples were drawn at intervals of 3, 6, and 12 hours. In dogs 36 and 44, the blood was drawn immediately after the completion of the last carbohydrate solution. In the control animals, blood samples were obtained after an overnight fast. The concentrations of plasma lipids were determined by the following methods: lipid phosphorus, method of Bauman[2]; total cholesterol, method of Zurkowski[11]; triglycerides, method of Fletcher[7]; nonesterified fatty acids (NEFA), method of Duncombe.[5] The fatty acid composition of the plasma lipids was determined by gas-lipid chromatography. Electrophoretic analysis of plasma was carried out by the method of Noble[9] and the quantitative determinations were performed by the densitometric scan. In addition, blood sugar, blood ketones, venous blood pH, and other various determinations were carried out.

RESULTS

Plasma lipid phosphorus (Fig. 1). The three experimental groups averaged twofold increases in the plasma lipid phosphorus levels in 2 weeks. After that, the plasma lipid phosphorus levels increased only slightly. At

Table I. *Composition of the intravenous diet*

Nutrients (per kilogram per day):
Protein, 4.0 Gm.
Carbohydrate, 22-31 Gm.
Fat, 2-4 Gm.
Calories, 140
Water, 140-190 ml.
Vitamins (per kilogram per day):
A, 1,000 I.U.
D, 100 I.U.
E, 0.5 I.U.
Choline, 2 5mg.
B_{12}, 0.003 mg.
Folic acid, 0.015 mg.
Thiamine, 5.0 mg.
Riboflavin, 1.0 mg.
Pyridoxine, 1.5 mg.
Pantothenic acid, 2.5 mg.
Niacin, 1.0 mg.
K, 0.1 mg.
Biotin, 0.007 mg.
PABA, 2.0 mg.
Minerals (mg. per kilogram per day):
Calcium, 72
Phosphorus, 96
Sodium, 120
Potassium, 170
Chloride, 315
Magnesium, 20
Copper, 0.1
Cobalt, 0.05
Manganese, 0.2
Zinc, 0.2
Iodine, 0.06
Iron, 1.0

Table IIA. *Lipid composition of Intralipid and Clea dog food*

	Intralipid (Gm./100 ml.)	Clea dog food (Gm./100 Gm.)
Triglycerides	9.79	3.35
NEFA	0.11	0.53
Lipid phosphorus	0.04	0.01
Cholesterol	0.06	0.02

Table IIB. *Fatty acid composition (weight percent) of Intralipid and of triglycerides of Intralipid and Clea dog food*

Fatty acid	Intralipid	Triglycerides of Intralipid	Triglycerides of Clea dog food
C16=0	11.6	11.2	20.4
C16=1	0.4	1.1	2.5
C18=0	3.8	3.2	11.1
C18=1	26.6	27.6	36.3
C18=2	50.0	49.4	25.2
Others	7.6	7.5	4.2

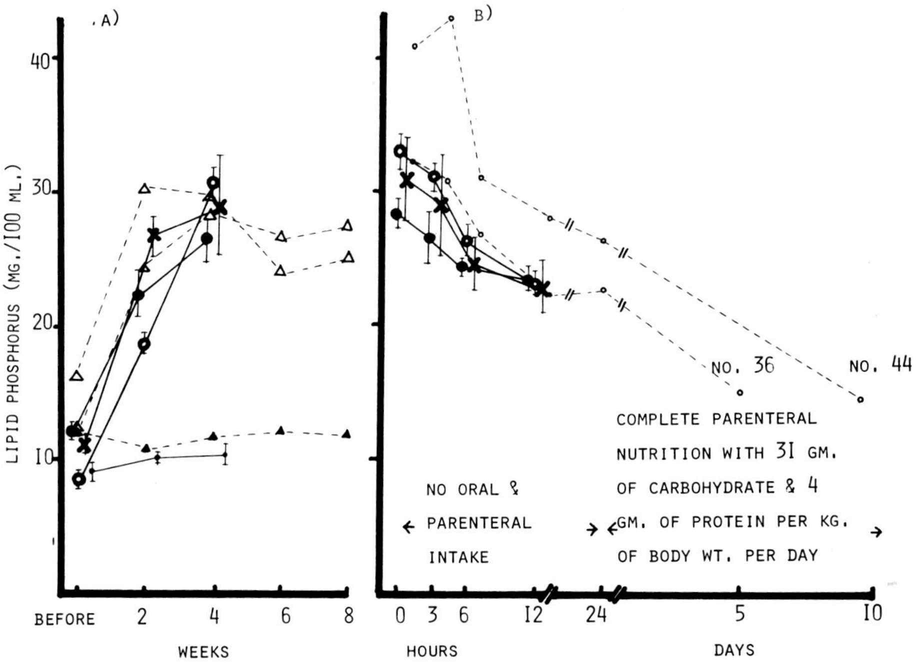

Fig. 1. Effect of complete parenteral nutrition including fat emulsion on the plasma lipid phosphorus level. *A,* Changes in the lipid phosphorus level in the 4 and 8 weeks experiments. *B,* Disappearance of plasma lipid phosphorus following the administration of the last fat emulsion on the last day of the 4 week experiment. ●, Group 1 (4 week experiment); ○, Group 2 (4 week experiment); **X**, Group 3 (4 week experiment); •, control group (4 week experiment); △, Group 3 (8 week experiment); ▲, control group (8 week experiment). Dogs 36 and 44 are single animals (see text). Vertical lines indicate mean ± S.E. of the mean.

2 and 4 weeks, there was a significant difference between the three 4 week experimental groups and the control group, but no significant difference among the three experimental groups. After 5 and 10 days on a fat-free solution, the levels of dogs 36 and 44 returned to approximately their initial values.

Plasma cholesterol (Fig. 2). Almost threefold increases in the plasma cholesterol levels were detected at the second week in the three experimental groups, which were significantly higher than that of the control. At successive week intervals, all the plasma cholesterol levels in the experimental groups were elevated only slightly. At the fourth week, they were significantly elevated. No significant difference was found among the three experimental groups. After 5 and 10 days on a fat-free solution, the levels of dogs 36 and 44 decreased to approximately the initial value.

Plasma triglycerides (Fig. 3). The three experimental groups averaged threefold increases in the plasma triglyceride levels in 2 weeks. After that, the plasma triglyceride levels increased only slightly. At the fourth week, they were significantly higher than that of the control. No significant difference was found among the three experimental groups. At the end of the last fat emulsion, in the 4 week experiment, the levels were high. Thereafter, they fell rapidly.

Plasma NEFA (Fig. 4). The plasma NEFA levels remained at approximately the initial values in the experimental animals during the 4 and 8 weeks of the infusion of the fat emulsion. At the end of the last fat emulsion, in the 4 week experiment, the levels were high. Then they fell at 3 hours. The levels of dogs 36 and 44 were at a low value after 5 or 10 days on a fat-free solution.

The fatty acid composition of plasma lipid fractions (Fig. 5).

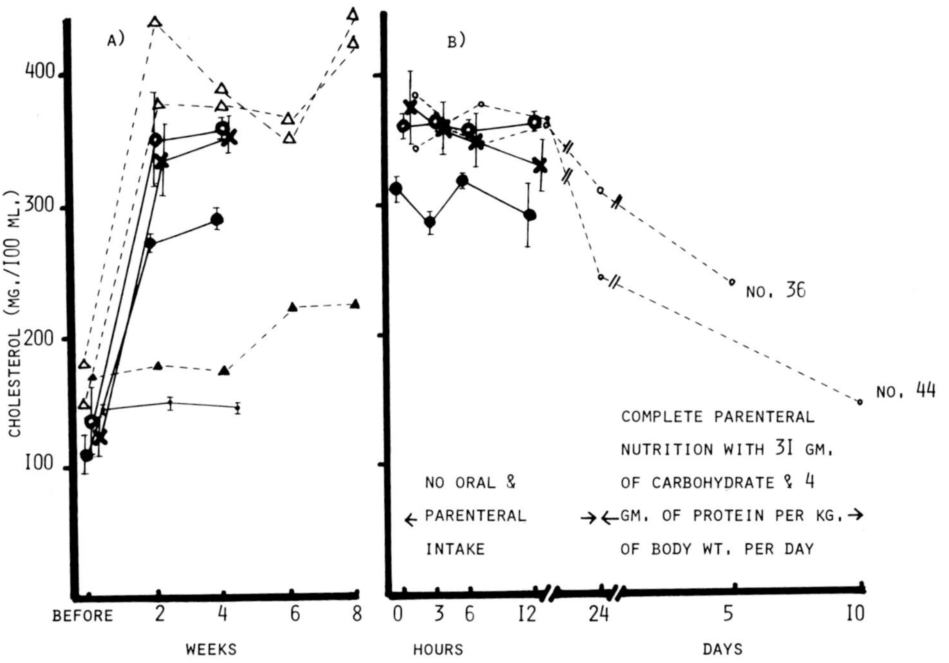

Fig. 2. Effect of complete parenteral nutrition including fat emulsion on the plasma cholesterol level. *A,* Changes in the plasma cholesterol level in the 4 and 8 week experiments. *B,* Disappearance of plasma cholesterol following the administration of the last fat emulsion on the last day of the 4 week experiment. ●, Group 1 (4 week experiment); ○, Group 2 (4 week experiment); **X**, Group 3 (4 week experiment); •, control group (4 week experiment); △, Group 3 (8 week experiment); ▲, control group (8 week experiment). Dogs 36 and 44 are single animals (see text). Vertical lines indicate mean ± S.E. of the mean.

Phospholipids. In the experimental animals, the fatty acid composition of plasma phospholipids differed from that of the fat emulsion and of its phospholipid component.

Cholesterol esters. In the 4 and 8 week experimental animals, the fatty acid composition of the cholesterol esters differed from that of the fat emulsion and of dogs 36 and 44 obtained after 5 or 10 days on a fat-free solution. However, it had considerable similarity to the fatty acid composition of the fat emulsion as a whole.

Triglycerides. There was a remarkable similarity in the fatty acid composition of the plasma triglyceride fraction of the 4 and 8 week experimental animals, that of the triglyceride component of the fat emulsion, and that of the fat emulsion as a whole. Dogs 36 and 44, after 5 or 10 days on a fat-free solution, differed in their patterns of acids from other experimental animals.

Lipoprotein electrophoresis on agarose gel. The fat emulsion remained at the point of its origination. In the 4 and 8 week experimental animals whose blood samples were drawn 3 hours after the interruption of the fat emulsion, the percentages of α- and β-lipoproteins were 64-78, and 22-35, respectively. There was no clear evidence of pre-β-lipoproteins. At the point of origination, lipoproteins were not detectable. Though the percentage of lipoproteins remained at about the same value, circulating lipoproteins were considered to be increased due to the elevation of the plasma lipid levels. Trails of lipid were usually observed extending from α- and β-lipoprotein regions to the origin. At the end of the last fat emulsion, in the 4 week experiment, 0 to 10 percent of lipoprotein concentrations were seen at the origin and were surmised to be the fat emulsion in the circulation. After 5 and 10 days on a fat-free

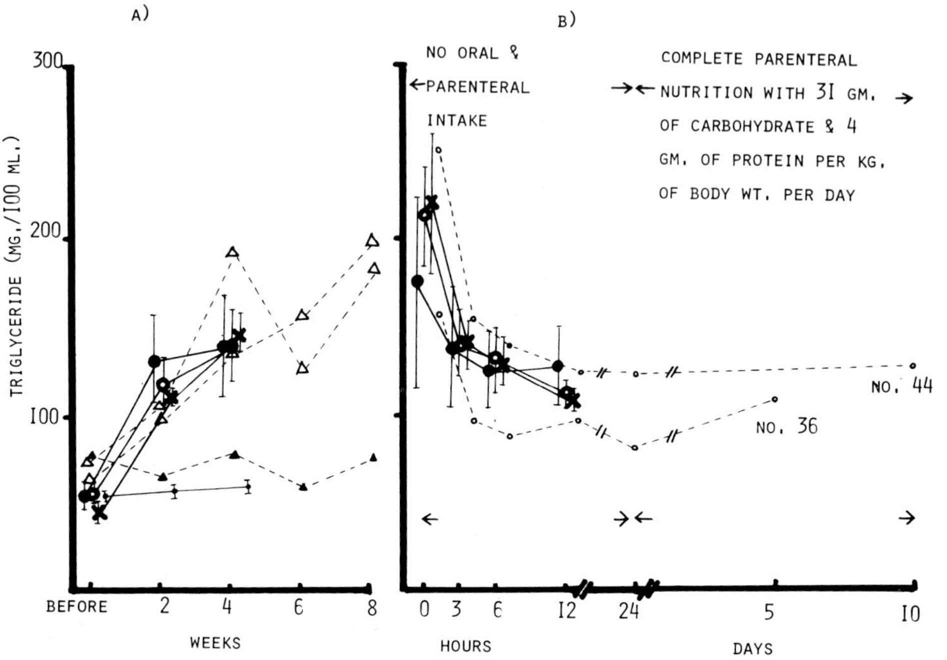

Fig. 3. Effect of complete parenteral nutrition including fat emulsion on the plasma triglyceride level. *A,* Changes in the plasma triglyceride level in the 4 and 8 week experiments. *B,* Disappearance of plasma triglycerides following the administration of the last fat emulsion on the last day of the 4 week experiment. ●, Group 1 (4 week experiment); ○, Group 2 (4 week experiment); **X**, Group 3 (4 week experiment); •, control group (4 week experiment); △, Group 3 (8 week experiment); ▲, control group (8 week experiment). Dogs 36 and 44 are single animals (see text). Vertical lines indicate mean ± S.E. of the mean.

solution, the percentage of the α-lipoprotein decreased to 54-55 and that of the β-lipoprotein increased to 43-46.

Slight ketonemias were observed during the 4 and 8 weeks of the infusion of the fat emulsion. There were no remarkable changes in blood sugar, venous blood pH, or other various determinations. The animals were in good condition and, in both the experimental and the control animals, growth, development, and weight gains were observed to be approximately normal.

DISCUSSION

Because Intralipid consists of triglycerides, phospholipids, cholesterol, and NEFA, it would seem important to investigate whether the increased plasma lipid fractions were of exogenous origin, i.e., whether they were the accumulation of the fat emulsion in the circulating blood or were of endogenous origin. To determine this, the fatty acid composition of the plasma lipid fractions and the electrophoretic analysis of plasma by the agarose method were examined. Because of the extremely short half-life of NEFA,[10] the NEFA of the infused fat emulsion might be metabolized rapidly and those in the plasma were assumed to be endogenous. Lipoprotein electrophoresis on agarose gel exhibited that the fat emulsion remained at the origin and, in the case of the blood samples obtained, there was nothing at the origin when observations were made 3 hours after the interruption of the fat emulsion. This made it clear that the plasma lipids were mostly endogenous. Moreover, it was found that the fatty acid compositions of phospholipid component of the fat emulsion and the plasma lipids were dissimilar, as were those of cholesterol esters in the fat emulsion and the plasma lipids. The fatty acid profile of the plasma triglycerides had striking similarity to that of the fat emulsion as a whole. There is experi-

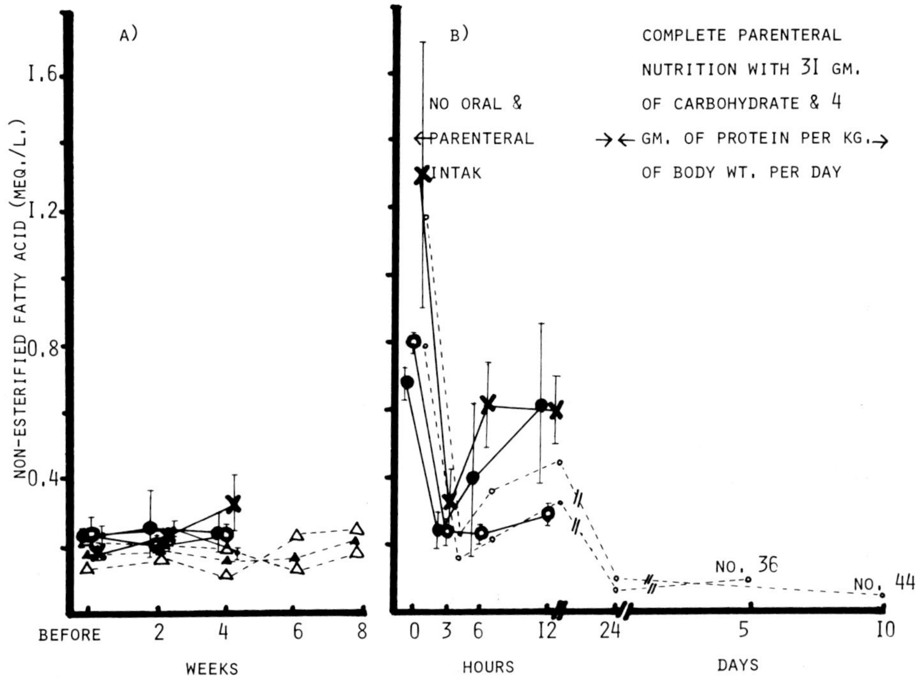

Fig. 4. Effect of complete parenteral nutrition including fat emulsion on the plasma NEFA level. *A,* Changes in the plasma NEFA level in the 4 and 8 week experiments. *B,* Disappearance of plasma NEFA following the administration of the last fat emulsion on the last day of the 4 week experiment. ●, Group 1 (4 week experiment); ○, Group 2 (4 week experiment); X, Group 3 (4 week experiment); •, control group (4 week experiment); △, Group 3 (8 week. experiment); ▲, control group (8 week experiment). Dogs 36 and 44 are single animals (see text). Vertical lines indicate mean ± S.E. of the mean.

mental evidence that the acid mixtures of the triglycerides are altered by the dietary fats.[1] Therefore, in the case of the intravenous fat administration, the same phenomenon might apply to the plasma triglycerides. Thus, the evidence has been obtained that the increased plasma lipid fractions might come from endogenous synthesis.

In this experiment, in the three experimental groups, the plasma lipid fractions and α- and β-lipoproteins increased rapidly within the first 2 weeks. Thereafter, regardless of the daily volume of the fat emulsion administered and the length of the total infusion period, they remained at approximately the same high levels. Those changes in the plasma lipids, however, diminished and returned to nearly the initial values shortly after the interruption of the fat emulsion as noted in dogs 36 and 44.

It is worthy of note that the long-term daily fat emulsion, largely composed of triglycerides, led to marked rises in the plasma phospholipid and cholesterol levels as well as in triglyceride levels; the increases in the former were more prominent. Either at the capillary surface or immediately upon entering cells, particularly in the liver, the fat emulsion glycerides might be hydrolyzed.[6] The elevated plasma NEFA level in the experimental animals at the end of the last fat emulsion, in the 4 week experiment, and the decrease, concomitant with the removal of the fat emulsion from the circulation, represented the hydrolysis of the fat emulsion at the capillary surface–intravascular lipolysis. This caused slight ketonemias observed during the experimental period. On the other hand, the constituent of the fat emulsion might be reformed into other esters within the liver[3] and re-enter the blood stream as lipoproteins. In this experiment, α- and β-

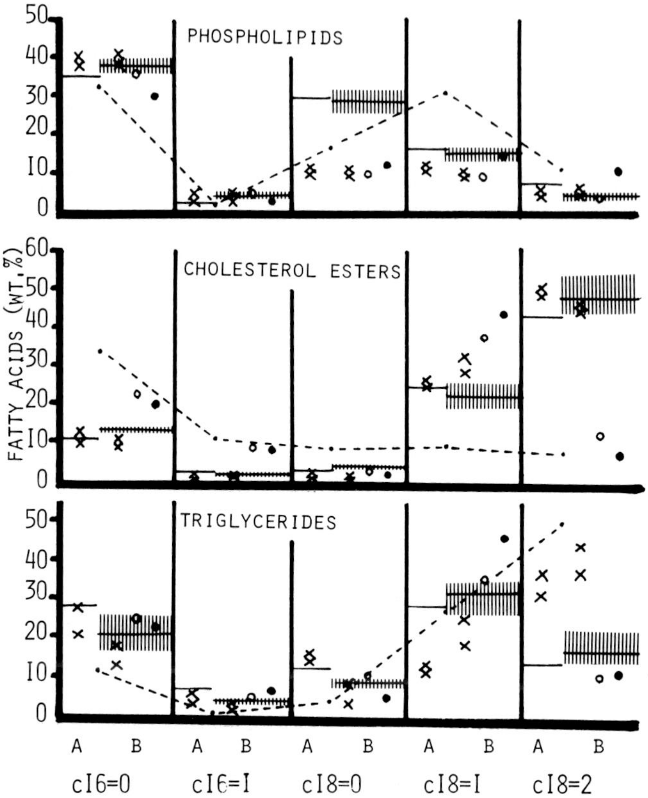

Fig. 5. Changes in the fatty acid composition (weight percent) of plasma phospholipids, cholesterol esters, and triglycerides in the 4 to 8 week complete parenteral nutrition. *A* represents the result of the 8 weeks experiment. *B* represents the result of the 4 weeks experiment and of dogs 36 and 44 after 5 and 10 days, respectively, on a fat-free solution after 4 weeks of complete parenteral nutrition including fat emulsion. ×, Group 3; ○, dog 36; ●, dog 44. Rows of vertical lines indicate the control group (the mean value and the range of the value). Broken lines, Intralipid.

lipoproteins, reportedly rich in cholesterol and phospholipids,[8] seemed to perform the major lipid transport tasks in the experimental animals. What is actually responsible for the increase in the plasma lipid, particularly with phospholipids and cholesterol, is not completely understood; however, enhanced endogenous synthesis of α- and β-lipoproteins in the liver appears to have an important role. The infused fat emulsion might lead to the enhancement in lipid transport tasks for final uptake by the utilizing tissues. The α- and β-lipoproteins seemed to be produced vigorously for this purpose and the cholesterol and phospholipids might be demanded as structural components of lipoproteins. It is thus quite reasonable to presume that the enhancement in lipid metabolism was caused as a proper metabolic process of the fat emulsion.

Although, in this experiment, the experimental and the control animals received approximately the same amount of fat, the plasma lipid was markedly increased when the experimental animals were compared with the control animals. This might be due to the difference in the metabolic pathway between the fat given orally and that given intravenously.[3] After the completion of the last fat emulsion, however, agarose lipoprotein electrophoresis of plasma and the fatty acid composition of the plasma cholesterol esters and triglycerides showed different results from those obtained during the 4 and

8 weeks of the infusion of the fat emulsion. The phospholipids appeared to be influenced little in their fatty acid composition by the fat emulsion, as in the case of dietary fat.[1] These phenomena were presumed to indicate that the enhanced lipid metabolism, because of the fat emulsion, returned approximately to its initial level in 5 to 10 days after its interruption, exerting no residual ill effect. Furthermore, it was ascertained that the animals remained in good condition, and their growth, development, and weight gain were observed to be approximately normal. Thus, daily infusion of fat emulsion, from 2 to 4 Gm. per kilogram of body weight, could be performed safely for an extended period of time.

REFERENCES

1. Ahrens, E. H., Jr., Insull, W., Jr., Hirsh, J., Stoffel, W., Peterson, M. L., Farquhar, J. W., Miller, T., and Thomasson, H. J.: The effect on human lipids of a dietary fat, highly unsaturated, but poor in essential fatty acids, Lancet **1:** 115, 1959.
2. Bauman, E. J.: On the estimation of organic phosphorus, J. Biol. Chem. **59:** 667, 1924.
3. Cornell, R. P., and Saba, T. M.: Vascular clearance and metabolism of lipid by the reticuloendothelial system in dogs, Am. J. Physiol. **221:** 1511, 1971.
4. Dudrick, S. J., Wilmore, D. S., Vars, H. M., and Rhoads, J. E.: Long-term total parenteral nutrition with growth, development and positive nitrogen balance, SURGERY **64:** 134, 1968.
5. Duncombe, W. G.: The colorimetric microdetermination of long-chain fatty acids, Biochem. J. **88:** 7, 1963.
6. Edgren, B.: The lipolytic activity in dog plasma after intravenous fat emulsion, Arch. Int. Pharmacodyn. Ther. **126:** 255, 1960.
7. Fletcher, M. J.: A colorimetric method for estimating serum triglycerides, Clin. Chim. Acta **22:** 393, 1968.
8. Hillyard, L. A., Entenman, C. C., and Reinhardt, W. O.: Composition and concentration of lymph and serum lipoproteins during fat and cholesterol absorption in the dog, J. Biol. Chem. **233:** 838, 1968.
9. Noble, R. P.: Electrophoretic separation of plasma lipoprotein in agarose gel, J. Lipid Res. **9:** 693, 1968.
10. Yoshitoshi, Y., Naito, C., Okaniwa, H., Usui, M., Mogami, T., and Tomono, T.: Kinetic studies on metabolism of lipoprotein lipase, J. Clin. Invest. **42:** 707, 1963.
11. Zurkowski, O.: A rapid method for cholesterol determination, Clin. Chem. **10:** 451, 1964.

Thrombosis in the superior mesenteric and portal veins: Report of a case treated with thrombectomy

Sven-Erik Bergentz, M.D., Björn Ericsson, M.D., Ulla Hedner, M.D., Lennart Leandoer, M.D., *and* **Inga Marie Nilsson, M.D.,** *Malmö, Sweden*

A case of acute, spontaneously appearing thrombosis in the superior mesenteric and portal veins was reported. A laparotomy catheterization of the superior mesenteric vein was done, followed by a phlebography, pressure measurement, and removal of fresh and old thrombi. The patient, who had a history of repeated episodes of deep-vein thrombosis, was found to have a marked decrease in the content of fibrinolytic activators in the vein walls.

From the Department of Surgery and the Coagulation Laboratory, Malmö General Hospital, University of Lund, Malmö, Sweden.

Superior mesenteric vein thrombosis may occur following abdominal surgery, sepsis, or shock in congestive heart failure,[9, 10] as a complication to cancer or to liver cirrhosis, and occasionally after a blunt trauma to the abdomen.[11] A number of cases with "idiopathic" superior mesenteric vein thrombosis have been described, sometimes associated with recurrent deep-vein thrombosis in the legs, or during treatment with contraceptive pills.[1, 3, 4, 5, 13, 17]

It is the purpose of this communication to report a case of spontaneously appearing superior mesenteric vein thrombosis, with thrombotic masses also in the portal and splenic veins. The patient had a history of recurrent deep-vein thrombosis in the legs, and was found to have a pronounced lack of fibrinolytic activators in the vein wall, which was probably responsible for his thrombotic disease. He was treated with venous thrombectomy, combined with a relatively minor intestinal resection.

Supported by grants from the Swedish Medical Research Council (B74-19X-87-10, B74-40X-759-09C) and Riksbankens Jubileumsfond.

Accepted for publication April 11, 1974.

Reprint requests: Sven-Erik Bergentz, Department of Surgery, Malmö General Hospital, 214 01 Malmö, Sweden.

METHODS

The following laboratory studies on coagulation factors, platelets, and components of the fibrinolytic systems were made on three occasions between December, 1972, and April, 1973: platelet count, platelet adhesiveness, one-stage prothrombin time, recalcification time of plasma, prothrombin + factor VII + factor X (Owren's P & P test), factor V, factor VIII, fibrinogen, antithrombin III, fibrinolytic activity of plasma and resuspended euglobulin precipitate on fibrin plates, plasminogen (immunochemical method), inhibitors of the plasminogen activation, alpha-2 macroglobulin and fibrin degradation products (FDP). The methods described earlier[2, 6, 7, 14] were used. The local blood fibrinolytic activity after venous occlusion of the arms was determined according to Nilsson and Robertson.[14]

The fibrinolytic activator level of the vein wall. A segment from a hand vein was excised under local anesthesia (0.5 percent Carbocain). The veins were examined by Pandolfi's[18] modification of Todd's[20] fibrinolysis autography technique. The activity was expressed in arbitrary units according to Pandolfi. The mean value in healthy volunteers is 7.5 arbitrary units (range 6 to 11 units in 60 healthy volunteers).

CASE REPORT

The patient was a 47-year-old man with a 25 year history of recurrent deep-vein thrombosis in both legs. Phlebography had shown complete occlusions of his deep veins in the lower leg. He had severe post-thrombotic symptoms with swelling of his legs, and he had previously had recurrent leg ulcers.

The patient's symptoms started on Oct. 16, 1972, with diffuse, slowly progressing abdominal pain, vomiting, and diarrhea. He did not have bloody stools. He was hospitalized elsewhere on the twentieth of October. Because of progressing pain, vomiting, and abdominal distension, laparotomy was carried out on Oct. 23. He was found to have gangrene of about 40 cm. of jejunum. This part of the intestinal tract was resected. The resection line in the mesentery showed multiple thrombotic venous occlusions.

Following the laparotomy the patient was transferred to Malmö General Hospital for further treatment. He was well hydrated by intravenous infusions and had a good diuresis. Because of progressing abdominal distension and signs of peritonitis he was operated on again on Oct. 26. Another 20 cm. of the small intestine, immediately proximal to the anastomosis, was gangrenous. The liver appeared normal. The remaining part of the small intestine was heavy, edematous, and cyanotic. The limit between the gangrenous and nongangrenous small bowel was diffuse, and about 35 cm. of the jejunum, including the previous anastomosis, was resected. Thrombotic occlusions were found in the transected mesenteric veins. Because of the borderline viability of the remaining part of the small intestine, with risk for impaired healing of the anastomosis and further gangrene, it was decided to do a thrombectomy.

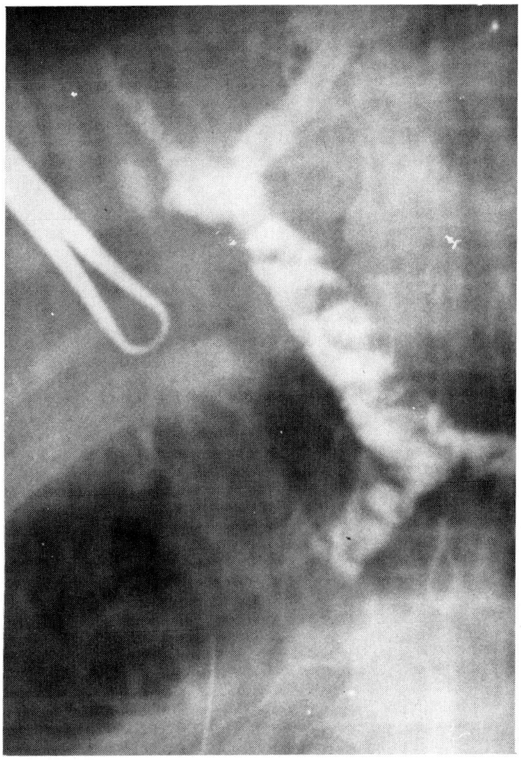

Fig. 1. Portography on the operating table. Note the filling defects in the portal vein and the occlusions of the peripheral branches. The splenic vein is not filled.

A baby-feeding tube was introduced into a peripheral mesenteric vein and passed into the portal vein. The pressure there exceeded 50 cm. of water, indicating a pronounced portal hypertension. Contrast was injected through the catheter. A phlebogram showed wide-spread filling defects in the superior mesenteric veins and portal vein, indicating thrombotic masses. The splenic vein did not fill with contrast (Fig. 1). The superior mesenteric vein was explored and opened as it passed in front of the pancreas, and just below the entrance of the splenic vein. Using a Fogarty catheter, thrombotic material was extracted from the portal vein and its intrahepatic branches, as well as from the splenic vein and superior mesenteric vein. Some of the thrombi could be felt to be adhering to the vessel wall and could not be removed. Following closure of the opening in the mesenteric vein, there was a marked im-

Table I. *Data on coagulation and fibrinolysis obtained from the patient and corresponding normal values*

	Patient's range 12/72 to 4/73	*Normal range*
Platelet number (per mm.³)	180,000-320,000	150,000-400,000
Platelet adhesiveness (%)	29-33	17-33
Recalcification time (sec.)	120-160	112-195
One-stage prothrombin time (sec.)	14-16	14-16
P & P (%)	70-90	80-120
Factor V (%)	94-100	80-120
Factor VIII (%)	180	60-160
Fibrinogen (Gm./100 ml.)	0.22-0.24	0.20-0.40
Antithrombin III	62-97	60-140
Spontaneous fibrinolytic activity (lysed area in mm.²)		
Plasma	0	0-50
Resusp. euglob. prec.	10-20	0-70
FDP (μg/ml.)	6-12	0-10
Plasminogen (%)	70-90	60-140
Urokinase inhibitors of plasminogen activation	80-132	60-140
Alpha-2 macroglobulin (%)	119	80-120
Fibrinolytic response to venous stasis of arms (lysed area in mm.²)		
Right arm	**160**	
Left arm	**108**	160-500
Fibrinolytic activity of venous biopsy (arbitrary units)		
Arm vein	**0-1**	6-11

provement in the color and the motility of the small intestine. The portal pressure dropped to 25 cm. of water. The baby-feeding tube was left in the peripheral mesenteric vein when the wound was closed. The patient was given a continuous drip through this tube for 5 days, containing 100 mg. of heparin the first day, increasing to up to 400 mg. a day. He was also given 500 ml. of dextran-40 a day, as a prophylaxis against recurrence of the thrombosis.

During the postoperative period, the patient developed an intestinal fistula which healed spontaneously after a few weeks. He also developed a thrombosis of the subclavian vein as a complication to a subclavian catheter. Phlebographic studies were carried out by injection of contrast medium into the superior mesenteric vein through the baby-feeding tube during the 6 days it was kept in the patient. These studies showed a good passage of contrast into the intrahepatic branches of the portal vein but there were still filling defects, obviously due to remaining wall-adherent thrombotic material. The liver function studies were normal with the exception of a temporary, moderate rise in serum bilirubin. The catheter in the superior mesenteric vein was removed without complications 6 days postoperatively. At that time the portal pressure was 20 cm. of water.

The patient was discharged on Dec. 12. He was in good condition and had no diarrhea. Arteriography was done in January, 1973, by contrast injection through the superior mesenteric and coeliac arteries. No visualization of the portal vein was found. The vascularization of the liver through the hepatic artery appeared to be increased, suggesting portal vein occlusion.

Results of coagulation and fibrinolytic studies. The results 2 to 6 months postoperatively are given in Table I. The patient had a normal platelet count and normal platelet adhesiveness. The levels of the various coagulation factors were essentially normal, as was the antithrombin III level. The various components of the fibrinolytic system were normal and the patient had a normal level of inhibitors of plasminogen activation. The fibrinolytic activator content of the walls of superficial arm veins, measured on biopsy specimens on two different occasions, was markedly decreased. The biopsies were taken from the arm *not* affected by subclavian vein thrombosis. The response of the fibrinolytic activity to venous stasis of the arms was also abnormally low.

Pathology. The resected part of the small intestine showed edema and hyperemia as well as venous stasis and incipient gangrene. The veins in the resection line were filled with thrombotic material. Some of these thrombi showed signs of organization. Histological study of the thrombi showed both fresh and older thrombotic material.

DISCUSSION

The usual therapy in superior mesenteric vein thrombosis is intestinal resection. The mortality rate is high, partly because of delayed operation due to diagnostic difficulties, partly due to the fact that the thrombosis usually is very wide-spread, causing generalized circulatory disturbances in the intestinal tract. In only one case reported in the literature was a thrombectomy done[12] on a patient in whom the thrombosis occurred during the performance of a pancreatectomy for carcinoma of the pancreas. A marked cyanosis, edema, and hemorrhagic mottling appeared in the small intestine as the thrombosis developed, and disappeared after thrombectomy.

There are many similarities between the circulatory disturbances appearing in the intestine in the course of a superior mesenteric vein thrombosis and phlegmasia cerulea dolens in the lower extremities. Both conditions are due to wide-spread occlusions, not only of the large veins, but also of the small branches, combined with marked edema and severe arterial spasm. Such a spasm, markedly impairing the arterial circulation, has been demonstrated experimentally in mesenteric vein occlusion.[19]

Thrombectomy following deep-vein thrombosis in the lower leg has been found to give relatively unsatisfactory late results due to rethrombosis. The initial results, particularly with regard to restoration of blood flow in phlegmasia cerulea dolens, are, however, quite impressive. It seems, therefore, to be a logical approach to remove as much of the thrombotic material as possible in the superior mesenteric and portal veins to improve intestinal circulation. It was quite obvious in our patient that both the portal pressure decreased and the color and motility of the small intestine improved markedly as soon as thrombotic material had been extracted from the veins. Some of the thrombotic material was probably almost 10 days old at that time and a definite success could not be expected. Even a temporary effect on the blood flow may, however, be of importance in making it possible to decrease the extent of intestinal resection and in helping the patient through the critical period of the impaired intestinal circulation.

As to the etiology of the mesenteric vein thrombosis in this patient, the almost complete absence of fibrinolytic activators of the arm vein walls is of interest.

In recent years abnormalities in the fibrinolytic system have been reported to cause recurrent deep-vein thrombosis in the lower leg. (For review, see Nilsson and Isacson.[15]) Such abnormalities are characterized by a deficiency in the fibrinolytic activators normally occurring in the vessel wall.[8] This can be demonstrated as an abnormally low release of such activators during stasis[14] and/or as a lack of fibrinolytic activators, using a histochemical technique on superficial arm or leg biopsies.[18] Patients with spontaneous, recurrent, deep-vein thrombosis have been found to have an abnormally low activity, as demonstrated with one of these techniques, in not less than 73 percent of the cases.[8] The fibrinolytic activity in the arm veins is three to four times greater than that *in* the leg veins, but a deficiency in the arm veins *always* parallels a deficiency in the leg veins. For practical reasons it is impossible to obtain biopsies from the deep veins in the leg or viscera. Most of the patients reported have, however, thrombosis in the *deep* leg veins, though the abnormality was demonstrated in biopsies from superficial arm and/or leg vein biopsies. It is, therefore, reasonable to assume that this abnormality is generalized. The case presented here represents, to our knowledge, the first patient with spontaneous thrombosis in superior mesenteric vein in whom such an abnormality has been demonstrated.

REFERENCES

1. Berry, F. B., and Bougas, J. A.: Agnogenic venous mesenteric thrombosis, Ann. Surg. **132:** 450, 1950.
2. Cronberg, S., Nilsson, I. M., and Silwer, J.: Studies on the platelet adhesiveness in von Willebrand's disease, Acta Med. Scand. **180:** 43, 1966.
3. Cruickshank, A. H.: Venous thrombosis in internal organs associated with thrombosis of leg veins, J. Pathol. **71:** 383, 1956.
4. Cuschieri, A., Brearley, R., Bradley, J., and Moossa, A. R.: Recurrent venous thrombosis and portal hypertension, N. Engl. J. Med. **287:** 1083, 1972.
5. Gerber, I. E., and Mendlowitz, M.: Visceral thrombophlebitis migrans, Ann. Intern. Med. **30:** 560, 1949.
6. Hedner, U., and Nilsson, I. M.: Clinical experience with determination of fibrinogen degradation products, Acta Med. Scand. **189:** 471, 1971.
7. Hedner, U., Nilsson, I. M., and Jacobsen, C. D.: Demonstration of low content of fibrinolytic inhibitors in individuals with high fibrinolytic capacity, Scand. J. Clin. Lab. Invest. **25:** 329, 1970.
8. Isacson, S., and Nilsson, I. M.: Defective fibrinolysis in blood and vein walls in recurrent "idiopathic" venous thrombosis, Acta Chir. Scand. **138:** 313, 1972.
9. Johnson, C. C., and Baggerstoss, A. M.: Mesenteric vascular occlusion. I. Study of 99 cases of occlusion of veins. II. Study of 60 cases of occlusion of arteries and of 12 cases of occlusion of both arteries and veins, Proc. Staff Meet. Mayo Clin. **24:** 629, 649, 1949.
10. Laufman, H. S., Nora, P. F., and Mittelpunkt, A. I.: Mesenteric blood vessels: Advances in surgery and physiology, Arch. Surg. **88:** 1021, 1964.
11. McCune, W. S., Keshishian, J. M., and Blades, B. B.: Mesenteric thrombosis following blunt abdominal trauma, Ann. Surg. **135:** 606, 1952.
12. Mergenthaler, F. W., and Harris, M. N.: Superior mesenteric vein thrombosis complicating pancreatoduodenectomy: Successful treatment by thrombectomy, Ann. Surg. **167:** 106, 1968.
13. Naitove, A., and Weismann, R. E.: Primary mesenteric venous thrombosis, Ann. Surg. **161:** 516, 1965.
14. Nilsson, I. M., and Robertson, B.: Effect of venous occlusion on coagulation and fibrinolytic components in normal subjects, Thromb. Diath. Haemorrh. **20:** 397, 1968.
15. Nilsson, I. M., and Isacson, S.: New aspects of the pathogenesis of thrombo-embolism, Prog. Surg. **11:** 46, 1973.
16. Nilsson, I. M., Krook, H., Sternby, N.-H., Söderström, E., and Söderberg, N.: Severe thrombotic disease in a young man with bone marrow and skeletal changes and with a high content of an inhibitor in the fibrinolytic system, Acta Med. Scand. **169:** 323, 1961.
17. North, J. P., and Wollenman, O. J., Jr.: Venous mesenteric occlusion in the course of migrating thrombophlebitis, Surg. Gynecol. Obstet. **95:** 665, 1952.
18. Pandolfi, M.: Histochemistry and assay of plasminogen activator(s), Rev. Eur. Etud. Clin. Biol. **17:** 254, 1972.
19. Polk, H. C.: Experimental mesenteric venous occlusion. III. Diagnosis and treatment of induced mesenteric venous thrombosis, Ann. Surg. **163:** 432, 1966.
20. Todd, A. S.: Histological localization of fibrinolysin activator, J. Pathol. **78:** 281, 1959.

Control of capillary bleeding by topical application of microcrystalline collagen

Lars M. Vistnes, M.D., David A. Goodwin, M.D., *Palo Alto, Calif.,* **John H. Tenery, M.D.,** *Fort Worth, Texas,* **George A. Ksander, M.S.,** *and* **Ronald P. Gruber, M.D.,** *Palo Alto, Calif.*

In 15 patients, each serving as his own control, 90 comparisons were made between the hemostatic effect of disks composed of microcrystalline bovine collagen and control disks composed of cellulose fiber. Split-thickness skin graft donor sites provided a reproducible homogeneously bleeding wound model. Measurements of blood loss were made by radioisotope and photometric techniques in a double-blind procedure that was used to evaluate various methods of application of the test material. Microcrystalline bovine collagen, when applied to the wound for 30 seconds without pressure, reduced blood loss by 40 to 50 percent over untreated controls.

From the Departments of Surgery and Nuclear Medicine, the Veterans Administration Hospital and Stanford University Medical Center, Palo Alto, Calif., and from Alcon Laboratories, Fort Worth, Texas

MOST, if not all, surgeons will agree that bleeding from identifiable vessels should be permanently controlled by mechanical occlusion (tying) or by some form of electrocoagulation. Brisk capillary bleeding, however, precludes the use of these methods for two reasons: the vessels are too small and too numerous. Accordingly, every surgeon has his own favorite method of dealing with this aggravating problem, such as pressure on cold packs, hot packs, dry packs, or wet packs. When these measures fail, other agents are resorted to as local surgical hemostatic agents. Principal among these are gelatin sponge, oxidized cellulose as a fabric or as a cotton-like fluffy material, thrombin, and epinephrine. Orthopedic surgeons have an agent to themselves in the form of bone wax.

The variety of methods, and the search for new ones, suggest that these present methods and agents leave room for improvement.

Microcrystalline bovine collagen (MBC) was initially described in 1969 as a novel child of polymer chemistry.[1] It is a dry, tangled, fibrous substance that is easily compressible. It is a water-insoluble acid salt of bovine collagen prepared by a process which conserves the normal helical configuration of the tropocollagen molecule and most of the lateral bonding forces between these molecules. Because of its potential multiplicity of form, it was thought that it would be ideal as a vascular prosthesis. It was only when intense thrombogenic activity in these grafts was noted[4] that its potential use as a hemostatic agent was considered.[4, 5]

Since that time, other reports indicate that MBC is probably effective as a local hemostatic agent.[6, 9] These reports, however, evaluate the effect of the agent either by comparing its efficiency to another similar agent or by attempting to measure the difference in

Accepted for publication April 22, 1974.

Reprint requests: Dr. Lars M. Vistnes, Department of Surgery (Plastic and Reconstructive), Stanford University Medical Center, Stanford, Calif. 94305.

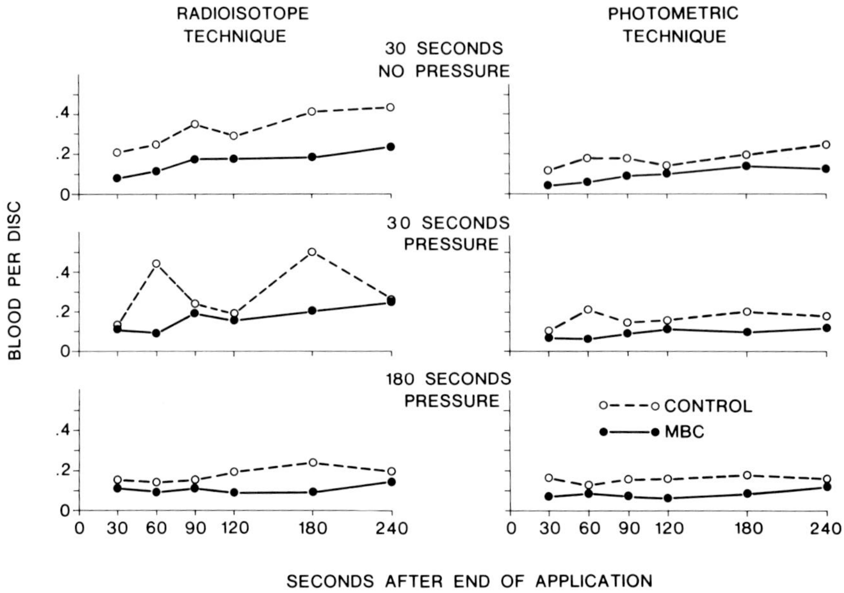

Fig. 1. The course of bleeding following each method of application of the test materials. Each point measures the total blood loss up to removal time of that disk.

bleeding between a treated and nontreated area.

Valid evaluation of any of these agents is difficult for two main reasons: it is difficult to find an easily duplicated homogeneously bleeding surface and it is difficult to measure the minute quantities of blood lost on such a surface in a controlled double-blind experiment. We believe that the idea of Wilkinson and associates[9] of using the skin graft donor site as a model solves the first one of these two problems and our approach, as described below, solves the second one.

METHODS

A uniformly bleeding wound model was obtained by utilizing 15 split-thickness skin graft donor sites (0.012 to 0.015 inch) from 10 patients in 15 separate procedures for a variety of surgical problems. Routine screening failed to detect any coagulation or bleeding problems.

Test materials were applied with an apparatus consisting of a plastic holder (17.5 by 8 cm.) and 12 cups fitted with plungers used to provide pressure during application. Six cups were filled with MBC tamped manually into a loose disk (0.14 Gm.) while the remaining six cups were filled with control disks of cellulose fiber (0.10 Gm.). The area of all disks was 3.14 $cm.^2$ In vitro tests showed that the absorbancy of both disks was much greater than any experimentally measured values. The assembly was covered with a rectangle of x-ray film, inverted, and placed on the bleeding site immediately following removal of the skin graft. Application began when the film was slid from between the disks and the wound surface.

The position of each experimental and control disk on the bleeding site was randomly determined for each patient to eliminate any systematic effects due to application technique. In addition, disks were coded throughout application and measurement to eliminate experimenter bias.

In one group of five patients, the disks were allowed to rest on the wound for 30 seconds. No pressure was applied. In a second group of five patients, uniform pressure was applied manually for 30 seconds. In a third group of five patients, the same pressure was applied for 180 seconds. After delays of 30, 60, 90, 120, 180, and 240 seconds, one MBC disk and one control disk were removed from the wound and placed in coded test tubes.

Data were thus gathered on *total bleeding* at six intervals following application under

Table I. *Means and standard errors of all MBC and control disks for each method of application*

	Blood absorbed (ml.)					
	30 seconds, no pressure		30 seconds, pressure		180 seconds, pressure	
	$\bar{X}$	S.E.	$\bar{X}$	S.E.	$\bar{X}$	S.E.
Radioisotope technique:						
Control	0.33	0.04	0.29	0.06	0.18	0.02
MBC	0.16	0.02	0.17	0.02	0.11	0.01
t	4.58		2.48		4.41	
P	< 0.001		< 0.02		< 0.001	
Photometric technique:						
Control	0.18	0.03	0.19	0.03	0.16	0.01
MBC	0.09	0.01	0.10	0.01	0.08	0.01
t	3.63		3.53		5.78	
P	< 0.005		< 0.005		< 0.001	

three conditions of application. With each patient serving as his own control, 90 separate comparisons of MBC and control disks were made.

Blood absorbed by each disk was measured by both a radioisotope and photometric technique, first by counting the level of radioactivity of ^{113m}In-labeled serum[8] and second by assaying hemoglobin content with the cyanmethemoglobin technique, which this laboratory has previously used to measure small amounts of bleeding.[7]

Prior to application of the test materials, 4 to 8 ml. (8 to 14 millicuries) of radioactive ^{113m}Indium were injected intravenously and allowed to circulate for a minimum of 10 minutes. Immediately prior to and immediately following application, 5 ml. venous blood samples were drawn. ^{113m}In binds almost instantaneously to the beta-1-globulin fraction of plasma.[3] It has the advantage of a short half-life of 100 minutes and can, therefore, be used in high dosage to obtain significant counts in small amounts of blood. It is the same material used in liver and brain scans.[8]

After completion of the entire application procedure, the coded test tubes were placed in a Picker Autowell II counter and the radioactivity of each disk counted for one minute. The amount of blood absorbed by each disk was calculated from the mean activity of the venous samples.

Next, each disk was eluted in 15 ml. of Drabkin's cyanmethemoglobin reagent. Disks from the 180 second pressure group were eluted for one minute with vigorous agitation. Later groups were eluted for 90 minutes with periodic vigorous agitation to maximize extraction of blood. Following elution, the contents of each tube were filtered through No. 4 paper and the optical density was measured against a Drabkin's reagent blank in a Coleman Jr. 6D Spectrophotometer, diluting with reagent where necessary.

Optical density measurements were transformed to milliliter volume measurements by reference to linear calibration curves based on 0.0, 0.5, 1.5, and 2.5 ml. samples of pooled blood added to MBC and control disks and eluted as above.

RESULTS

The time course of bleeding following each method of application is shown in Fig. 1. Each point on these curves is the mean of five patients. Straight lines fitted to these data are close to horizontal and parallel (all slopes between 0.000 and 0.001 ml. per second).

The absence of a large difference in rate of blood loss between MBC and control curves was felt to justify the pooling of all data within each application method to obtain estimates of the effect of each treatment that are more reliable than those based on only five observations at each disk removal time. For each application method, the difference between the means of all MBC and control disks was tested for statistical significance by the t test for paired comparisons with 29 degrees of freedom based on the 30 comparisons between disks. (The 30 second no-pressure radioisotope test is based on 27 degrees of freedom due to the loss of data from two control disks.) These results are shown in Table I.

The means in Table I indicate a reduction of blood loss with increasing amounts of pressure. Analysis of variance[2] shows that this is a significant trend ($P < 0.05$) for the radioisotope data but not for the photometric data.

DISCUSSION

These data strongly support the hypothesis that MBC is an effective hemostatic agent. In every comparison, there is significantly less blood loss from sites treated with MBC.

Both measurement techniques agree in confirming the effect of MBC. Throughout the data, however, the radioisotope technique yields larger values than does the photometric technique. This can plausibly be attributed to the sensitivity of this technique to the seepage of greater amounts of labeled serum relative to red cells as clotting proceeds. The same explanation can also be applied to the differing effects of the application methods as measured by the two techniques. With this in mind, there does not appear to be much difference between the three application methods, a significant reduction in blood loss occurring simply with application of MBC without pressure for 30 seconds.

These measurements do not begin until 30 seconds after the end of application. This is the minimum time necessary to remove the applicator, and it was not possible to measure blood loss before this time. The absence of a difference in time trends between MBC and control data indicates that the reduction in blood loss attributable to the difference in effect of the MBC and control treatments has, therefore, largely occurred before the first measurements were made. Since there was a significant reduction in bleeding in the 30 second groups, it can be concluded that the hemostatic effect of MBC occurs during the first 30 seconds of application, and does not greatly increase after this time.

Although the data show strong statistical significance, evaluation of the clinical significance of the measured effect is of more interest. The mean difference between the MBC and control disks ranges from 0.07 to 0.17 ml., a reduction in blood loss of 40 to 50 percent over the control disks. The reduction over totally uncontrolled bleeding must be much greater, but because of the need to absorb blood with some material in order to measure blood loss, thereby controlling bleeding to some degree, uncontrolled bleeding could not be evaluated with the present techniques.

Under clinical conditions where bleeding is critical, as in neurosurgery, or occurs over large areas, as in multiple skin graft procedures in the management of burns, a bleeding reduction of 40 to 50 percent can be of considerable value.

REFERENCES

1. Battista, O. A., Erdi, N. Z., Ferraro, C. F., and Karasinsky, F. J.: Novel microcrystals of polymers, Part II, J. Appl. Polymer Sci. **11:** 481, 1967.
2. Croxton, F. E.: Elementary statistics with application in medicine, New York, 1953, Prentice-Hall, Inc., pp. 295-310.
3. Goodwin, D. A., et al.: In^{113m} colloid: a new radiopharmaceutical for liver scanning, Nucleonics **24:** 65, 1966.
4. Hait, M. R., Battista, O. A., Stark, R. B., and McCord, C. W.: Microcrystalline collagen as a biologic dressing, vascular prosthesis, and hemostatic agent, Surg. Forum **20:** 51, 1969.
5. Hait, M. R.: Microcrystalline collagen: a new hemostatic agent, Am. J. Surg. **120:** 330, 1970.
6. Hait, M. R., et al.: Comparative evaluation of Avitene microcrystalline collagen hemostat in experimental animal wounds, Am. J. Surg. **125:** 284, 1973.
7. Siegel, R. J., Vistnes, L. M., and Iverson, R. E.: Effective hemostasis with less epinephrine, Plast. Reconstruct. Surg. **51:** 129, 1973.
8. Stern, D. A., Goodwin, D. A., Scheffel, U., Wagner, H. N., and Kramer, H. H.: In^{113m} for blood-pool and brain scanning, Nucleonics **25:** 62, 1967.
9. Wilkinson, T. S., Tenery, J. H., and Zufi, D.: The skin graft donor site as a model for evaluation of hemostatic agents, Plast. Reconstruct. Surg. **51:** 541, 1973.

Effect of aspirin on microaggregate formation in banked blood

Paul J. Arrington, M.S., *and* **J. Judson McNamara, M.D.,** *Honolulu, Hawaii*

Banked blood in CPD solution from donors who have ingested aspirin or with exogenously added aspirin develops microaggregate debris at a slower rate than blood collected from donors who have not ingested aspirin. This is apparently a consequence of the effect of aspirin on platelet aggregation.

From the Department of Surgery, Queen's Medical Center and the University of Hawaii School of Medicine, Honolulu, Hawaii

BLOOD STORED at 4° C. in ACD solution develops microaggregates composed primarily of platelets and fibrin.[1, 10, 14] This debris in transfused blood has been shown to produce changes in pulmonary hemodynamics in animals[3, 8] and has been implicated in the pathogenesis of post-traumatic pulmonary insufficiency in man.[5, 9, 12]

The present studies were undertaken to more clearly define the mechanism by which microaggregates are formed, to evaluate the effect of aspirin (ASA) in microaggregate formation, and to compare the formation of debris in CPD-anticoagulated blood with the formation of debris in ACD-anticoagulated blood.

MATERIALS AND METHODS

All blood was drawn in the customary fashion and stored in plastic bags at 4° C. Ten units were drawn in ACD from healthy young men (ages 20 to 30) with no history of ASA ingestion for 10 days prior to donation (Group 1), 10 U. were drawn in CPD from healthy young men with no history of ASA ingestion for 10 days prior to donation (Group 2), 10 U. were drawn in CPD from healthy young men who had ingested 20 gr. of ASA per day for three days prior to donation (Group 3), and 5 U. were drawn in CPD from healthy young men with no history of ASA ingestion for 10 days prior to donation (Group 4). To Group 4 on the day of collection, 1 ml. of aqueous sodium acetylsalicylate (10 mg. per milliliter) was added to each of the units.

Blood in Groups 1, 2, and 3 was studied on the day of collection, on each subsequent day for three days, and at three-day intervals thereafter. These studies included the following: (1) Hematocrit—microhematocrit method; (2) screen filtration pressure (debris weights)—determined quantitatively by measuring dried debris deposited on a 20 micropore tared screen after 5 c.c. of whole blood had been passed through the screen at a constant rate.[8]

Blood in Group 4 was studied on the day of collection and on day 21. These studies included hematocrit and screen filtration pressure. Since exogenous material was added to these samples, further studies were not

Supported by USARDC Contract DADA17-71-C-1023.
Accepted for publication May 11, 1974.

Reprint requests: J. Judson McNamara, M.D., Director of Surgical Education, The Queen's Medical Center, P.O. Box 861, Honolulu, Hawaii 96808.

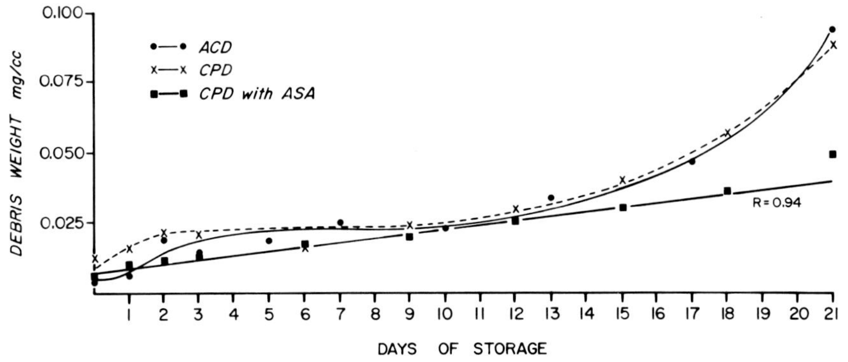

Fig. 1. Mean debris formation.

performed in an attempt to prevent bacterial growth.

RESULTS

The mean hematocrit in all three groups was 42 percent and remained constant throughout the 21 days of storage.

Fig. 1 shows mean debris formation in all three groups. The rate of debris formation in CPD blood without ASA was nearly identical with that in ACD blood. Day 0 debris weights were slightly higher for CPD without ASA than for ACD blood. Debris accumulation in CPD leveled off on day 2, remained constant through day 10, and rapidly increased during the next 11 days of storage. In ACD blood, debris accumulation began on day 2 but continued to increase through day 5, to reach a level identical with that of CPD at day 5, remained constant through day 10, and then increased in a fashion identical with CPD blood without ASA during the next 11 days of storage.

The SFP increased in a fashion nearly identical with increases in debris weight except in the period before day 2 and after day 17 at which point the pressures leveled off.

Mean debris accumulation in CPD blood with ASA samples was linear during the entire 21 days of storage (Fig. 1). Statistical evaluation revealed a Cor Mat = 0.94. The debris accumulated in CPD blood with ASA was at all times less than debris in CPD blood without ASA or ACD blood. Blood in CPD with exogenous ASA (Group 4) had identical day 0 and day 21 debris weights as Group 3 (CPD with ingested ASA).

DISCUSSION

The present study demonstrates that debris formation in CPD and ACD is almost identical. It also demonstrates that the rate of debris formation and total debris from ASA-ingesting donors is less than the debris from non–ASA-ingesting donors. The initial increase in debris weight at day 2 in the non-ASA samples is absent in the ASA samples. This initial increase has been attributed to platelet microaggregate formation. The debris weight of the non-ASA samples is constant from day 2 through day 10 and then increases rapidly during the next 11 days of storage while the debris weight of the ASA samples increases in a linear fashion throughout the 21 day storage period. This tends to support our postulation that debris formation is at least in part a result of platelet aggregation followed by fibrin deposition.

Aspirin has been shown to suppress prothrombin synthesis.[6] Furthermore, it is known that thrombin plays an important role in platelet aggregation.[2, 4] It is possible that the observed decrease in debris weight in blood from ASA-ingesting donors may have resulted from limitation of fibrinogen conversion to fibrin through a reduction in available thrombin. Prothrombin is not manufactured in the blood, however; therefore, the observed reduction in debris formation resulting from addition of aspirin to the blood can result only from a direct effect on the blood constituents.

This is consistent with our previous postulate that debris formation is initiated by platelet aggregation and that aspirin inhibits debris formation by preventing the secondary release phase of platelet aggregation. This is consistent with the known effect of aspirin on platelet release reaction and the consequent decrease in platelet aggregation both in vivo and in vitro.[11, 13]

REFERENCES

1. Arrington, P. J., and McNamara, J. J.: Mechanism of microaggregate formation in stored blood, Ann. Surg. **179:** 146, 1974.
2. Bettex-Gallond, M., and Luscher, E. F.: Extraction of an actomyosin-like protein from human thrombocytes, Nature **184** (Suppl. 5): 276, 1959.
3. Hissen, W., and Swank, R. L.: Screen filtration pressure and pulmonary hypertension, Am. J. Physiol. **209:** 715, 1965.
4. Hovig, T., Rowsell, H. C., Dodds, W. J., Jorgensen, L., and Mustard, J. F.: Experimental hemostasis in normal dogs and dogs with congenital disorders of blood coagulation, Blood **30:** 636, 1967.
5. Jenevein, E. P., and Weiss, D. L.: Platelet microemboli associated with massive blood transfusion, Am. J. Pathol. **45:** 313, 1964.
6. Link, K. P., Overman, R. S., Sullivan, W. R., Huebner, C. F., and Scheel, L. D.: Studies on the hemorrhagic sweet clover disease, J. Biol. Chem. **147:** 463, 1943.
7. McNamara, J. J.: Effective filtration of banked blood, SURGERY **71:** 394, 1972.
8. McNamara, J. J., Burran, E. L., Larson, E. J., et al.: Effect of debris in stored blood on pulmonary microvasculature, Ann. Thorac. Surg. **14:** 133, 1972.
9. McNamara, J. J., Molot, M. D., and Stremple, J. F.: Screen filtration pressure in combat casualties, Ann. Surg. **172:** 334, 1970.
10. McNamara, J. J., Molot, M. D., and Stremple, J. F.: Changes in some physical properties of stored blood, Ann. Surg. **174:** 58, 1971.
11. Mielke, C. H., Kaneshiro, M. M., Mather, J. A., et al.: The standardized normal Ivy bleeding time and its prolongation by aspirin, Blood **34:** 204, 1969.
12. Moore, F. D., et al.: Post-traumatic pulmonary insufficiency, Philadelphia, 1969, W. B. Saunders Company.
13. Schwartz, A. D.: Platelet aggregation in blood donors, Blood **38:** 815, 1971.
14. Swank, R. L.: Alterations of blood on storage: Measurement of aging platelets and leukocytes and their removal by filtration, N. Engl. J. Med. **265:** 728, 1961.

Preliminary results of a computer logic program for the operative management of colon cancer

Carl O. Knutson, M.D., *Louisville, Ky.*, *and* **Francis R. Watson, Ph.D.**, *Columbia, Mo.*

Surgical judgment decisions can be expressed in sequential statements of explicit logic which are consistent, highly reliable, and computer-adaptable. A sequential logic on-line program which evolves the intraoperative management decisions for the surgical treatment of colorectal neoplasms has been developed and tested with 304 cases of operable colorectal neoplasms. In 291 cases (96 percent) the ultimate programmed management decisions demonstrated a perfect correlation with the clinical management decisions independently expressed by the experienced operating surgeon. In three cases (one percent) the surgeon's decision to transect extensive neoplasm was challenged by the programmed logic, resulting in different ultimate management decisions. The remaining four percent were composed of ten situations in which the surgeon's judgment decisions to temporize the ideal ultimate management due to the patient's precarious preoperative status resulted in conflicting ultimate management decisions. The system promises to minimize intraoperative errors in judgment and provide a mechanism for the prospective collection of pertinent data and an objective basis for quality control.

From the Department of Surgery, University of Louisville School of Medicine, Health Sciences Center, Louisville, Ky., and the Department of Biomathematics, Ellis Fischel State Cancer Hospital–Cancer Research Center, Columbia, Mo.

THE APPLICATION of computers to clinical medicine, as opposed to laboratory medicine, has not earned acceptance in the minds of most physicians. However, the increasing proliferation of new medical information may require further consideration of such techniques if physicians are to keep abreast of current concepts. The best organized clinician can no longer maintain a working knowledge of the current pertinent literature. If the present rate of proliferation of information continues, the frustration of keeping abreast in the future will likely be increased further, even for physicians limited to very circumscribed fields.

Accepted for publication March 15, 1974.

Reprint addresses: C. O. Knutson, M.D., Department of Surgery, University of Louisville School of Medicine, Health Sciences Center, Louisville, Ky. 40201; and F. R. Watson, Ph.D., Department of Biomathematics, Ellis Fischel State Cancer Hospital–Cancer Research Center, Columbia, Mo. 65201.

The modern computer can assist the medical profession in this matter. Although computer hardware is highly advanced, the explicit medical logic software essential to developing an effective clinical system has not been successfully developed.

The development of explicit medical logic programs by necessity must be problem oriented. Medicine is far too vast and complex to attempt the development and integration of the entire explicit medical logic in one step. The disillusionment stemming from the current failure of computer techniques to be of any real assistance to the practicing physician in the past is largely attributable to too much attempted too rapidly. Explicit logic programs for indi-

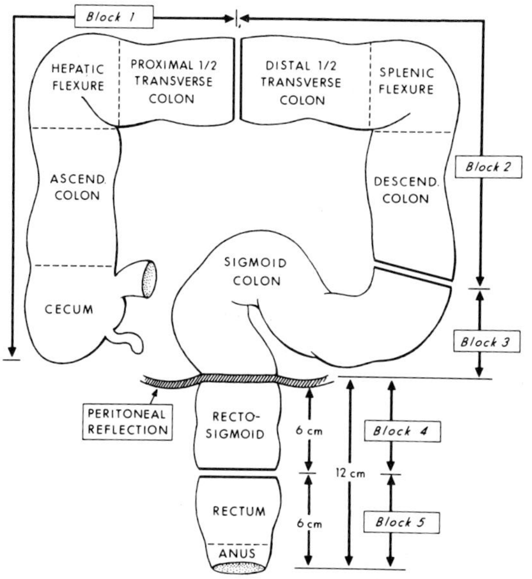

Fig. 1. Schematic diagram of regional divisions of the colon.

vidual problem areas must be developed. When they have been developed and tested for reliability, the programs may become a part of a multiple problem-solving system.

This report describes the first phase of an explicit logic program for the operative treatment of colon cancer. Although the program is not yet ready for general use, the authors present the current status of the program in terms of the explicit logic utilized and in terms of the results of pilot tests in order to stimulate interest and constructive comments pertaining to the feasibility of this approach as well as refinement of the incorporated logic.

DESCRIPTION OF THE COLON CANCER MANAGEMENT PROGRAM

Certain assumptions must be made at the present time which will necessarily require revision and refinement in the future. (1) The patient is an acceptable risk for operation and can tolerate any procedure deemed necessary to remove the cancer once the intraoperative findings are known. (2) The surgeon is qualified to perform any procedure deemed necessary at the time of surgery. (3) There are no synchronous tumors.

Table I. *Ten questions which must be answered at the time of surgery prior to making a management decision*

1. Tumor location
2. Distant metastasis
3. Contiguous spread
    4. Involves 1 kidney and contralateral kidney abn/abs?*
    5. Involves 1 ureter and contralateral ureter abn/abs?*
    6. Involves both ureters in pelvis?
    7. Involves nonremovable vital organ?
    8. Attachment to pelvic wall prevents resection?
9. Perforation
10. Obstruction

*Abnormal or absent.

Table II. *The elements of the operative procedure: Options*

I. Primary procedure (conventional or en bloc):
- A. Right hemicolectomy
- B. Right hemi- and partial left colectomy
- C. Left hemicolectomy
- D. Left hemi- and partial right colectomy
- E. Anterior sigmoid resection
- F. Abdominal perineal resection
- G. Segmental (sleeve, wedge) resection
- H. Internal intestinal bypass
    - A. Ileotransverse
    - B. Ileosigmoid
- I. Pelvic exenteration
- J. Delayed colectomy
- K. Nothing

II. Anastomosis:
- A. Direct
    - 1. End to end
    - 2. End to side
    - 3. Side to side
- B. None
    - 1. Proximal colostomy
        - A. Temporary
            - 1. Diverting
            - 2. Decompressing
        - B. Permanent-end
    - 2. Distal mucous fistula
    - 3. Close distal rectal stump

III. Other considerations:
- A. Drain
- B. Delay primary skin closure
- C. Close perforation

Given the above limitations and a carcinoma at any location within the colon or rectum which is associated with any combination of intraoperative findings, a series of simple sequential questions and answers will lead the surgeon through the entire

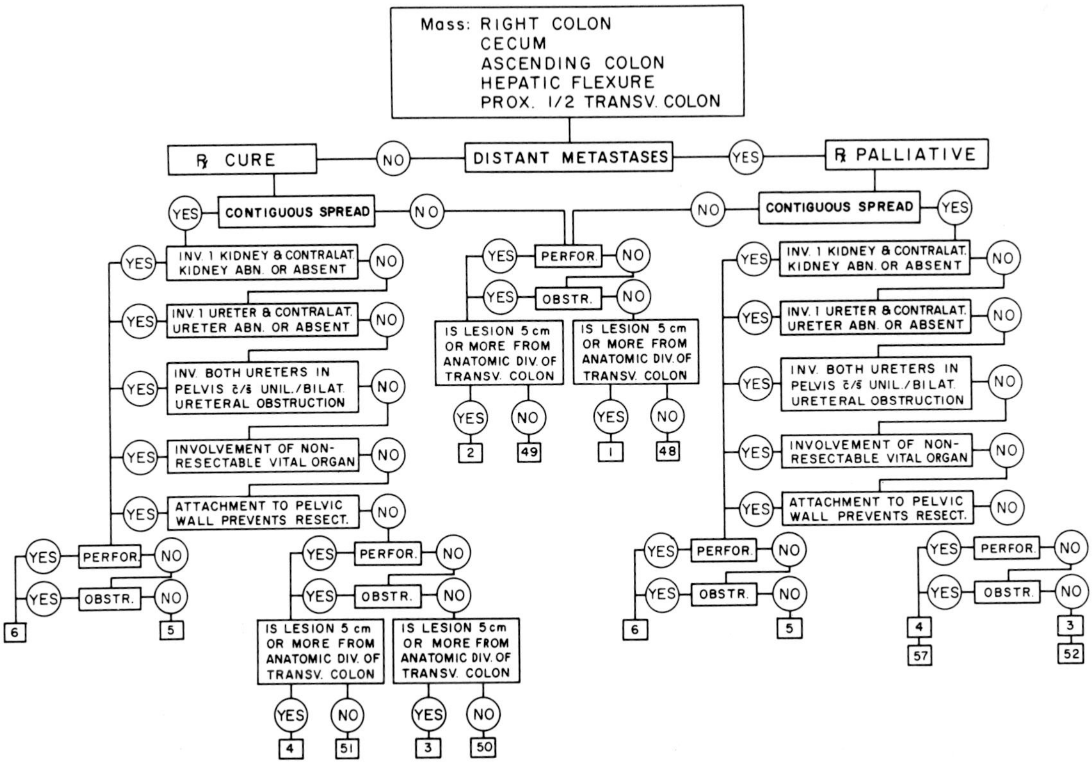

Fig. 2. Logic flow diagram for lesions of the right colon.

thought process necessary to decide the best management method. Following the completion of analysis of all pertinent considerations, the program will display a suggested list of acceptable procedures in order of preference, based on the operative findings as interpreted by the surgeon and on the most currently available medical knowledge. No attempt has been made to "limit" the surgeon in his choice of procedures. However, procedures which are not generally accepted in the specific operative setting in question are not listed. This obviously confines the operator to those options best suited to the operative setting. For any given combination of intraoperative findings, all acceptable management procedures are illustrated by the computer with only two exceptions: (1) the patient with a cancer of the right colon should not be left with an ileostomy and (2) if at all possible, any perforated cancer should be removed at the initial procedure.

Beyond these two considerations, any currently acceptable operation is considered in the list of treatments. In addition, other considerations are displayed, such as potential curability, initial colostomy with delayed resection vs. primary resection, primary or delayed anastomosis, abdominal drainage, and delayed vs. primary skin closure.

DESCRIPTION OF THE MANAGEMENT LOGIC FOR COLON CANCER

The colon is divided into five segments determined by the colonic blood supply (Fig. 1). Any neoplasms arising within the same anatomical segment are treated in a similar fashion. For example, a cecal lesion will be approached with the same set of programmed questions and treatment options as a lesion of the hepatic flexure, providing the intraoperative findings are similar.

Analysis of the surgical decision-making process on an element-by-element basis raises 10 basic questions which must be

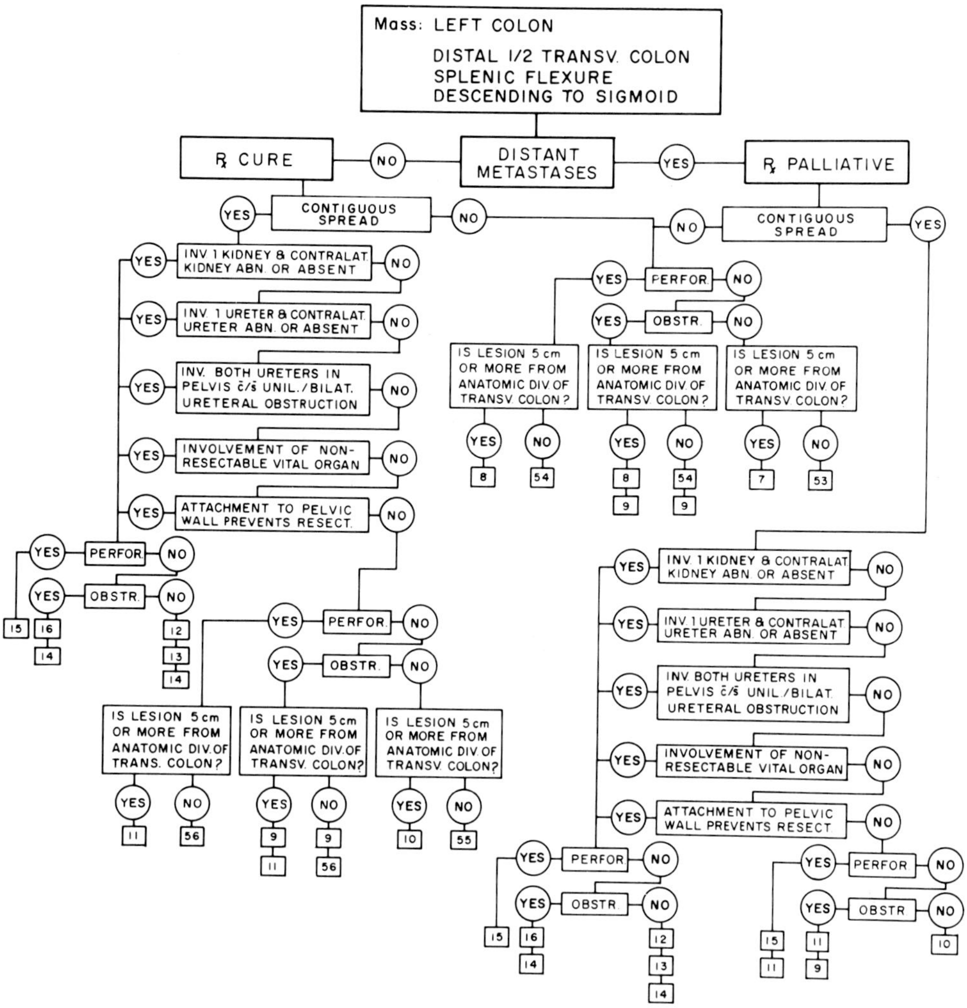

Fig. 3. Logic flow diagram for lesions of the left colon.

answered before a valid management decision can be made (Table I). Various combinations of yes/no answers to the basic questions encompass nearly all conditions which may be encountered intraoperatively. The same basic questions apply to neoplasms arising in any segment of the colon, but the surgical options differ, depending on which colon segment is involved.

The basic elements of the surgical procedures combined in various orders formulate the exact operation to be used (Table II). In essence, there are 12 basic operative procedures commonly used for colon cancer: three types of direct anastomosis, five methods of handling the transected ends of the bowel if direct anastomosis is not desirable, and three additional considerations pertaining to the skin closure, perforated bowel, and abdominal drainage.

Although there are 288 possible combinations of the elements listed in Table II, only 57 of the combinations contribute to acceptable treatments for the operative management of colon neoplasms.

Therefore, based on the location of the neoplasm and accurate documentation of any combination of 10 operative considerations, the program not only displays the options of surgical procedures and optional methods of management of the transected bowel but it also lists the optional procedures

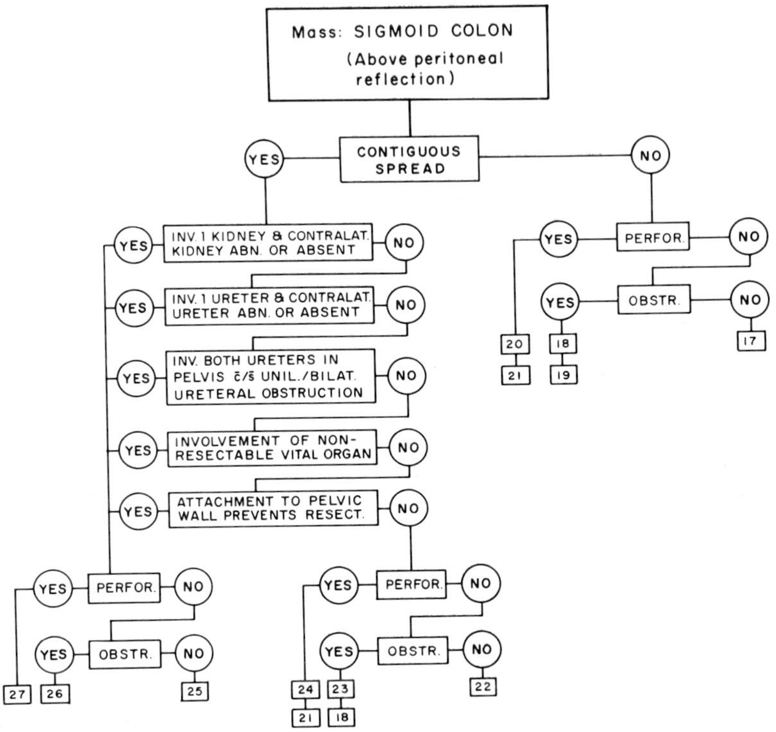

Fig. 4. Logic flow diagram for lesions of the sigmoid colon (above the peritoneal reflection).

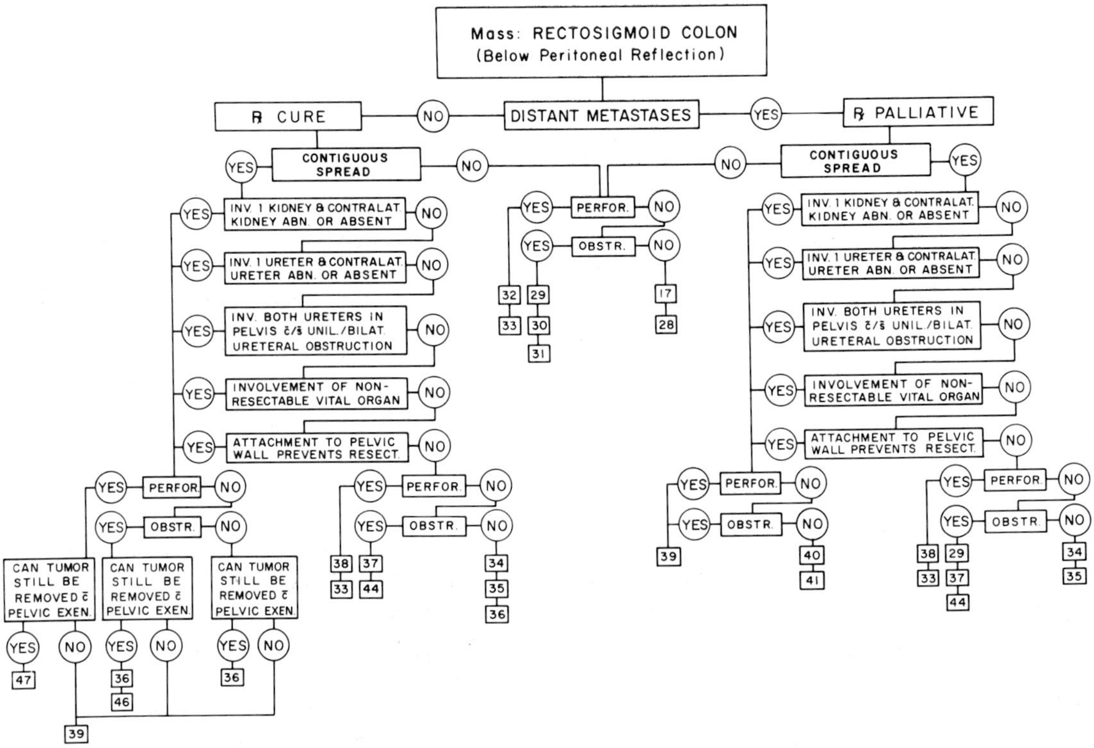

Fig. 5. Logic flow diagram for lesions of the rectosigmoid colon (below the peritoneal reflection).

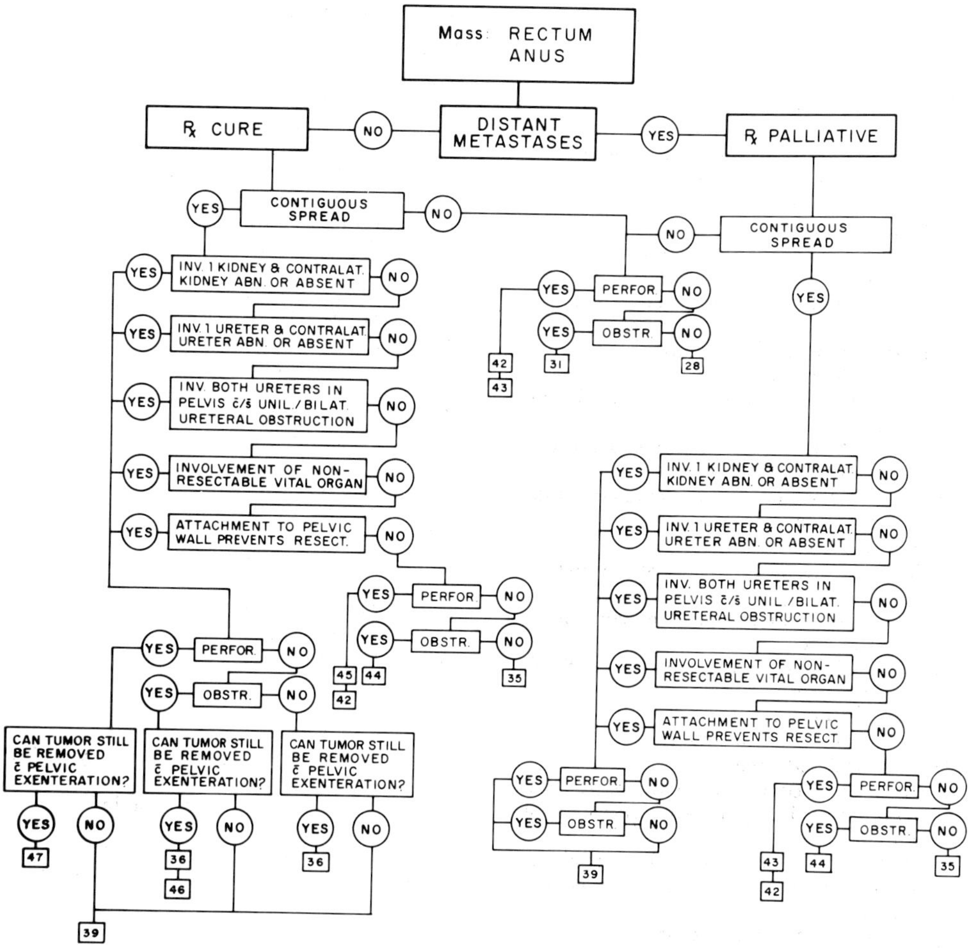

Fig. 6. Logic flow diagram for lesions of the rectum and anus.

in order of preference based on the most current knowledge available.

The logic flow diagrams for each colon segment are illustrated in Figs. 2 to 6.

The corresponding management options are illustrated in Tables III through VII. The numbers in the squares at the bottom or at the end of each logic diagram correspond to the treatment numbers for the respective neoplasm location which are tabulated in Tables III through VII.

Example. Let us assume that the surgeon is confronted with a carcinoma of the descending colon. Referring to Fig. 3, which is the logic flow diaram for lesions of the left colon, the following questions are asked:

1. Are distant metastases present? No
2. Is there contiguous spread? No
3. Is there a perforation? No
4. Is there obstruction? No
5. Is the lesion 5 cm. or more from the anatomical division of the transverse colon? Yes

Given the above responses to the questions, only one treatment option would be suggested by the computer program: treatment 7. Referring to Table IV, which includes all treatment options for left colon lesions, treatment 7 is a left hemicolectomy with an end-to-end colocolostomy.

By defining the different intraoperative settings in the above manner one can follow the logic flow diagrams to the suggested therapy options for any lesion of the colon or rectum.

RESULTS

To establish the validity and practical applicability of this logic model, 304 cases of colon cancers treated at the Ellis Fischel

Table III. *Treatment options for right colon lesions*

T1	(A)	Right hemicolectomy with end-to-end ileotransverse colostomy
T2	(A)	Right hemicolectomy with end-to-end ileotransverse colostomy
	(B)	Delay primary skin closure
	(C)	Drain (if indicated)
T3	(A)	En bloc right colon resection with end-to-end ileotransverse colostomy
T4	(A)	En bloc right colon resection with end-to-end ileotransverse colostomy
	(B)	Delay primary skin closure
	(C)	Drain (if indicated)
T5	(A)	Interval ileotransverse colostomy bypass either: (1) end-to-end with two mucous fistula exclusion or: (2) end-to-side with one mucous fistula exclusion or: (3) side-to-side
T6	(A)	Internal ileotransverse colostomy bypass either: (1) end-to-end with two mucous fistula exclusion or: (2) end-to-side with one mucous fistula exclusion or: (3) side-to-side
	(B)	Delay primary skin closure
	(C)	Drain (if indicated)
T48	(A)	Right hemicolectomy with partial left colectomy with end-to-end ileocoloanastomosis
T49	(A)	Right hemicolectomy with partial left colectomy with end-to-end ileocoloanastomosis
	(B)	Delay primary skin closure
	(C)	Drain (if indicated)
T50	(A)	En bloc right colon and partial left colon resection with ileocoloanastomosis
T51	(A)	En bloc right colon and partial left colon resection with ileocoloanastomosis
	(B)	Delay primary skin closure
	(C)	Drain (if indicated)
T52	(A)	Segmental resection of tumor with end-to-end ilecolo- or colocolostomy
T57	(A)	Segmental resection of tumor with end-to-end ilecolo- or colocolostomy
	(B)	Drain (if indicated)
	(C)	Delay primary skin closure

Table IV. *Treatment options for left colon lesions*

T7	(A)	Left hemicolectomy with end-to-end anastomosis
T8	(A)	Left hemicolectomy with end colostomy
	(B)	Distal mucous fistula (if possible)
	(C)	Drain pelvis (if indicated)
	(D)	Delay primary skin closure
T9	(A)	Temporary proximal diverting colostomy
	(B)	Delay primary skin closure
	(C)	Definitive colectomy at later date
T10	(A)	En bloc resection with left colectomy and end-to-end anastomosis
	(B)	Proximal colostomy (temporary)
T11	(A)	En bloc resection with left colectomy and end colostomy
	(B)	Distal mucous fistula (if possible)
	(C)	Drain pelvis (if indicated)
	(D)	Delay primary skin closure
T12	(A)	Proximal end colostomy with distal mucous fistula
T13	(A)	Do nothing at this time
	(B)	When symptomatic—do proximal end colostomy
T14	(A)	Ileosigmoid colostomy bypass (end to side)
	(B)	Exteriorize proximal colon as mucous fistula
T15	(A)	Proximal end colostomy with distal mucous fistula
	(B)	Close perforation (if indicated)
	(C)	Drain pelvis (if indicated)
	(D)	Delay primary skin closure
T16	(A)	Proximal end colostomy and distal mucous fistula
	(B)	Delay primary skin closure
T53	(A)	Left hemicoletomy and partial right colectomy with end-to-end colocolostomy
T54	(A)	Left hemicolectomy and partial right colectomy with end-to-end colocolostomy
T55	(A)	En bloc resection of left hemi- and partial right colectomy with end-to-end anastomosis
T56	(A)	En bloc resection of left hemi- and partial right colectomy with end colostomy
	(B)	Distal mucous fistula
	(C)	Drain pelvis (if indicated)
	(D)	Delay primary skin closure

State Cancer Hospital–Cancer Research Center (EFSCH–CRC) were retrospectively reviewed with no attempt to preselect cases other than to gain specific numbers of patients representing each possible location of neoplasm. This institution has been the site of continuing clinical research referable to large bowel cancer for many years. The results of this review are shown in Table VIII.

The 10 intraoperative questions used in the logic program were answered from recorded intraoperative findings. The coder was instructed not to use the pathologist's report to answer the 10 questions.

The options displayed on the computer were then compared to the procedures actually performed by placing them into one of four categories (Table VIII).

In 291 instances (96 percent) the programmed treatment recommendations correlated well with what was actually done. In three cases (one percent) the tumor was transected to remove some of the neoplasm. These three procedures, performed in the 1950's, were considered inadequate based on current philosophy; in each case, given the operative findings, the program suggested currently more appropriate procedures. In no case was the program's suggested approach inadequate. There were 10 situations (three percent) which arose that the computer program was not able to handle in the preliminary stage of logic development because of previously conceded assumptions (see Description of program). Because of the limited sophistication of development, the current program cannot yet preoperatively evaluate the risk to the patient and, in all 10 patients, the actual procedure performed was of a lesser magnitude than that suggested by the computer program. In addition, had those patients been better operative risks, the procedures suggested by the program would have been more acceptable.

Even in its infancy, this computer program has attained a clinical accuracy of 97 percent. Further refinement of the logic and the integration of preoperative evaluation will likely significantly reduce, if not eliminate altogether, the remaining three percent.

DISCUSSION

This colon cancer management logic program was initiated at the Ellis Fischel State Cancer Hospital–Cancer Research Center in September, 1970. It represents one of two specific cancer sites which have been developed according to explicit logic principles which are computer adaptable. The other site developed is a system for the management of breast cancer.

Distinct advantages and tremendous potential exist in a system of this nature. It represents a uniform, complete, and systematic method for collecting and analyzing data essential to the evaluation of currently used surgical procedures. Not only will physicians have ready access to the most current medical knowledge in terms of the most acceptable modes of therapy for any given set of operative circumstances, but the various options can be presented in order of priority based on the continuing accumulation of new data. In addition, each option can be footnoted and referenced for the convenience of the viewer to minimize the amount of time and effort required to obtain the same data. This approach affords the

Table V. *Treatment options for sigmoid colon lesions (above peritoneal reflection)*

T17	(A)	Anterior resection with colorectal anastomosis
	(B)	Temporary proximal colostomy (if indicated)
T18	(A)	Temporary proximal decompression colostomy
	(B)	Delay primary skin closure
	(C)	Definitive sigmoid resection at later date
T19	(A)	Anterior resection with proximal end colostomy (Hartman)
	(B)	Distal mucous fistula (if possible)
	(C)	Delay primary skin closure
T20	(A)	Anterior resection with proximal end colostomy
	(B)	Distal mucous fistula (if possible)
	(C)	Drain pelvis (if indicated)
	(D)	Delay primary skin closure
T21	(A)	Temporary proximal decompression colostomy
	(B)	Close perforation (if possible)
	(C)	Drain pelvis
	(D)	Delay primary skin closure
T22	(A)	En bloc resection with sigmoid colectomy and colorectal anastomosis
	(B)	Temporary proximal colostomy (if indicated)
T23	(A)	En bloc resection of sigmoid colon and proximal end colostomy
	(B)	Distal mucous fistula (if possible)
	(C)	Delay primary skin closure
T24	(A)	En bloc resection of sigmoid colon and end colostomy
	(B)	Distal mucous fistula (if possible)
	(C)	Drain pelvis (if indicated)
	(D)	Delay primary skin closure
T25	(A)	Permanent proximal end colostomy with distal mucous fistula
T26	(A)	Permanent proximal end colostomy with distal mucous fistula
	(B)	Delay primary skin closure
T27	(A)	Permanent proximal end colostomy with distal mucous fistula
	(B)	Close perforation (if possible)
	(C)	Drain pelvis (if indicated)
	(D)	Delay primary skin closure

Table VI. *Treatment options for rectosigmoid colon lesions (below peritoneal reflection)*

T17	(A)	Anterior resection with colorectal anastomosis
	(B)	Temporary proximal colostomy (if indicated)
T28	(A)	Abdominal perineal resection
T29	(A)	Proximal end colostomy with distal mucous fistula
	(B)	Delay primary skin closure
	(C)	Definitive colectomy at later date (anterior resection or abdominal perineal resection)
T30	(A)	Anterior resection, oversew rectal stump (Hartman)
	(B)	Proximal end colostomy
	(C)	Delay primary skin closure
T31	(A)	Abdominal perineal resection
	(B)	Delay primary skin closure
T32	(A)	Anterior resection, oversew rectal stump (Hartman)
	(B)	Proximal end colostomy
	(C)	Drain pelvis (if indicated)
	(D)	Delay primary skin closure
T33	(A)	Proximal end colostomy
	(B)	Drain pelvis (if indicated)
	(C)	Close perforation (if possible)
	(D)	Delay primary skin closure
	(E)	Definitive colectomy at later date (anterior resection or abdominal perineal resection)
T34	(A)	En bloc anterior resection with colorectal anastomosis
	(B)	Temporary proximal colostomy (if indicated)
T35	(A)	En bloc abdominal perineal resection
T36	(A)	Pelvic exenteration
T37	(A)	En bloc anterior resection, oversew rectal stump (Hartman)
	(B)	Proximal end colostomy
	(C)	Delay primary skin closure
T38	(A)	En bloc anterior resection, oversew rectal stump (Hartman)
	(B)	Proximal end colostomy
	(C)	Drain pelvis (if indicated)
	(D)	Delay primary skin closure
T39	(A)	Permanent proximal end colostomy with distal mucous fistula
	(B)	Close perforation (if present and if possible)
	(C)	Drain pelvis (if indicated)
	(D)	Delay primary skin closure
T40	(A)	Nothing at this time
	(B)	Permanent proximal end colostomy when signs of obstruction appear
T41	(A)	Permanent proximal end colostomy
	(B)	Distal mucous fistula
T46	(A)	Permanent end colostomy
	(B)	Distal mucous fistula
	(C)	Delay primary skin closure
	(D)	Definitive pelvic exenteration at later date
T47	(A)	Permanent end colostomy
	(B)	Distal mucous fistula
	(C)	Treat perforation
	(D)	Drain pelvis (if indicated)
	(E)	Delay primary skin closure
	(F)	Definitive pelvic exenteration at later date

surgeon a reliable checklist for avoiding errors of omission and commission in addition to forming a basis for uniform operative notes and a peer review system.

Another advantage of this program is in the training of house officers and students. Traditionally, every generation of new physicians have initially devoted their time to learning the medical knowledge accumulated from preceding generations before they could acquire new knowledge. There is an obvious voluminous and accumulative effect of this type of educational system, the efficiency of which leaves much to be desired. The repercussions of past teaching methods are reflected in the current, widespread revisions being made in the medical educational system. At present surgeons have no truly objective method for teaching surgical house officers "good" surgical judgment. The sample program presented, which incorporates "good" surgical judgment in explicit statements in a logical sequential flow diagram, has significant potential as a method of teaching. It demonstrates the often nebulous components of that judgment decision; not only will it save time for the student of surgery but in addition the answers are consistent and reproducible. The fact that logic flow diagrams can be periodically reviewed by recognized authorities in a particular field enables the program to reflect the most current accepted views, as opposed to reading many textbooks which are often outdated shortly after they have been published.

We have relegated certain functions to the clinical laboratories, to paramedical personnel, and to physician's assistants. Once a set medical management decision has be-

Table VII. *Treatment options for rectal or anal lesions*

T28	(A)	Abdominal perineal resection
T31	(A)	Abdominal perineal resection
	(B)	Delay primary skin closure
T35	(A)	En bloc abdominal perineal resection
T36	(A)	Pelvic exenteration
T39	(A)	Permanent proximal end colostomy with distal mucous fistula
	(B)	Close perforation (if present and if possible)
	(C)	Drain pelvis (if indicated)
	(D)	Delay primary skin closure
T42	(A)	Proximal end colostomy with distal mucous fistula
	(B)	Drain pelvis (if indicated)
	(C)	Close perforation (if indicated)
	(D)	Delay primary skin closure
	(E)	Definitive abdominal perineal resection at later date
T43	(A)	Abdominal perineal resection
	(B)	Drain pelvis
	(C)	Delay primary skin closure
T44	(A)	En bloc abdominal perineal resection
	(B)	Delay primary skin closure
T45	(A)	En bloc abdominal perineal resection
	(B)	Drain pelvis
	(C)	Delay primary skin closure
T46	(A)	Permanent end colostomy
	(B)	Distal mucous fistula
	(C)	Delay primary skin closure
	(D)	Definitive pelvic exenteration at later date
T47	(A)	Permanent end colostomy
	(B)	Distal mucous fistula
	(C)	Treat perforation
	(D)	Drain pelvis (if indicated)
	(E)	Delay primary skin closure
	(F)	Definitive pelvic exenteration at later date

Table VIII. *Summary of the results of a review of 304 cases of colon cancer comparing the procedures suggested by the computer program with the actual procedures performed*

Cameo: Colon cancer logic (Phase 1)	*No.*	*%*
Total charts reviewed	304	—
1. Actual and Cameo treatments correlate	291	96.0
2. Actual treatment inadequate (probable)	3	1.0
3. Cameo treatment inadequate	0	0.0
4. Cameo could not evaluate (at present development)	10	3.3

Colon site	*Result of chart review* 1	2	3	4
Cecum	32	0	0	0
Ascending colon	27	0	0	1
Hepatic flexure	29	1	0	0
Proximal one-half transverse colon	18	0	0	0
Distal one-half transverse colon	13	0	0	2
Splenic flexure	24	0	0	0
Descending colon	29	0	0	1
Sigmoid colon	49	1	0	3
Rectosigmoid colon	24	1	0	0
Rectum or anus	46	0	0	3
	291	3	0	10

come widely accepted by the profession, does it seem unreasonable to convert this "art" to explicit medical logic and commit it to the memory of a computer which permits rapid retrieval in a fraction of the time required for a physician to store and appropriately recall the same amount of information?

Concern has been expressed for the surgeon's role, if such computer programs are instituted. Will programs of this nature reduce the surgeon to the status of a surgical technician? To answer this question, reiteration of several inevitable limitations of the computer are in order. The computer cannot think, it cannot create, and it does not have a sensitivity and ability to draw unprogrammed conclusions. Indeed, it requires a skilled surgeon to make the observations requisite for the program's decisions; in the operating room it functions only as a very reliable, rapid recall memory for the surgeon. It may serve as a checklist to help the surgeon to be thorough in his evaluation, to consider all essential variables, and to keep him current with new trends and consensus opinions of the profession. It might be considered a highly skilled secretary, totally trained by the surgeon and totally subservient to him. It offers the surgeon a quality control mechanism which gives him added assurance that his endeavors are in keeping with modern surgical knowledge. Therapeutic decision-making logic programs will not lower the status of the surgeon to the level of a technician. Rather, the surgeon will be taking another assistant to the operating table.

The rationale for the need and desirability of computer systems in clinical medicine has been thoroughly discussed elsewhere.[1, 2]

CONCLUSIONS

1. The preliminary results of a computer-adaptable logic program for the operative management of colon cancer are discussed.

2. The feasibility and validity of this computer logic program were tested by comparing its results with the actual surgical procedures performed on 304 patients with colon cancer. The computer program suggested appropriate operative management decisions in 97 percent of the intraoperative situations reviewed.

3. Advantages and potential of this method are briefly discussed.

4. The program's potential as an objective method of teaching "good" surgical judgment is stressed. The logic flow diagrams are displayed herein for professional scrutiny and comments.

5. Although the program is still under development, this publication is intended to stimulate interest in this area and promote constructive comments and discussion with the end result being a refinement of the program's decision-making logic.

The authors wish to thank Hiram C. Polk, Jr., M.D., for critical review and constructive suggestions during the preparation of the manscript.

REFERENCES

1. Watson, F. R.: Will the art of medicine be destroyed by the automation of medical logic? Mo. Med., 936, Dec. 1971.
2. Watson, F. R., and Glass, R. L.: Cameo: Cancer management and education optimization, Mo. Med., 875, Dec. 1971.

Teratomas in infancy and childhood: Experience with 81 cases

G. Hossein Mahour, M.D., M.Sc.(Surgery), Morton M. Woolley, M.D., Sulochana N. Trivedi, M.D., *and* Benjamin H. Landing, M.D., *Los Angeles, Calif.*

Teratomas in 81 patients seen at the Childrens Hospital of Los Angeles during the years 1941 through June, 1970 were studied. Thirty-six teratomas (44.5 percent) were from the sacrococcygeal area and 30 (37 percent) were ovarian. Teratomas occurred in the testis in 5 patients (6.2 percent), in the retroperitoneum in 4 (5 percent), in the mediastinum in 3 (3.7 percent), and there was one each (1.2 percent) in brain, soft palate, and base of the umbilical cord. In 61 patients, the teratomas contained benign (mature) tissue only. Mature as well as embryonic tissues were found in 10 tumors, and 10 patients had malignant teratomas, with frankly malignant tissue in addition to mature and/or embryonic tissue. Types of malignant component included germinoma (seminoma or dysgerminoma), embryonal carcinoma, yolk sac carcinoma, and choriocarcinoma. Tumors which contained one or more of these malignant elements, but no mature or embryonic tissues, were not included in this series. In patients with teratoma containing frankly malignant tissues, the occurrence of local recurrence and/or metastasis was lethal regardless of therapy. In our series, there has been no survivor among these patients.

From the Departments of Surgery and Pathology, Childrens Hospital of Los Angeles and the University of Southern California School of Medicine, 4650 Sunset Blvd., Los Angeles, Calif. 90027.

TERATOMAS ARE TUMORS which contain elements "derived" from more than one of the embryonic germ layers, so that the tissue components are often foreign to the anatomic site of the tumor.[10] Theories of their origin thus have included: (1) parthenogenetic development of germ cells within the gonads or in extragonadal sites; (2) nonparthenogenetic origin from "wandering" germ cells left behind during the migration of embryonic germ cells from yolk sac to gonad; (3) origin from other totipotent embryonic cells which escaped organizer influence during development. Teratomas are distinguished from mixed tumors like those of the salivary glands, from embryomas and similar tumors (e.g., nephroblastoma, hepatoblastoma), and from other "tumors" grouped as "hamartomas," composed of a mixture of elements normally found in the site. In contrast to incomplete conjoined twins, which may superficially mimic a teratoma, a true teratoma has a high degree of disorganization and may be inherently malignant or have the potential of malignant degeneration.

Supported in part by the Los Angeles County Chapter of the National Foundation–March of Dimes.

Accepted for publication Feb. 19, 1974.

Reprint requests: G. Hossein Mahour, M.D., Childrens Hospital of Los Angeles, 4650 Sunset Blvd., Los Angeles, Calif. 90027.

MATERIALS AND METHODS

Seventy-nine patients had their initial surgical treatment at the Childrens Hospital of

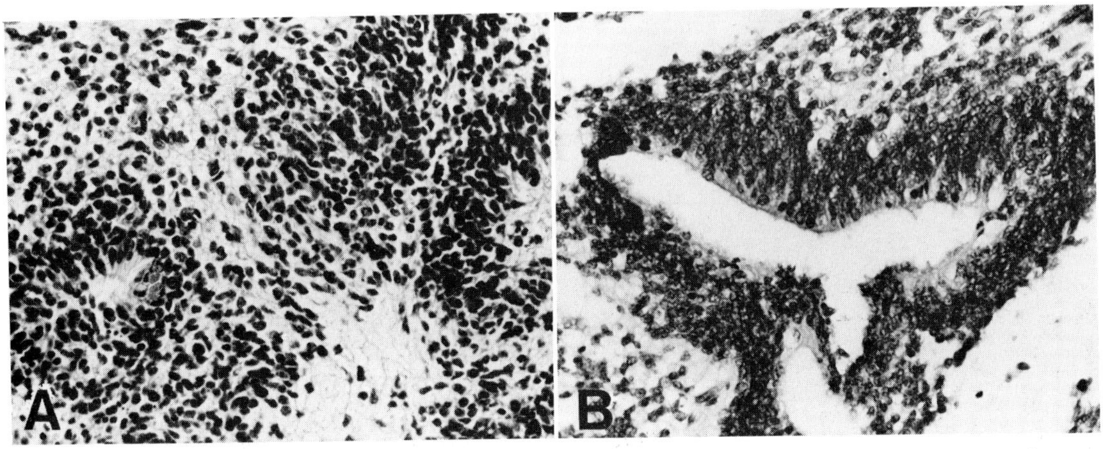

Fig. 1. Embryonic tissues in *A,* ovarian and *B,* sacrococcygeal teratomas (Hematoxylin and eosin; ×400).

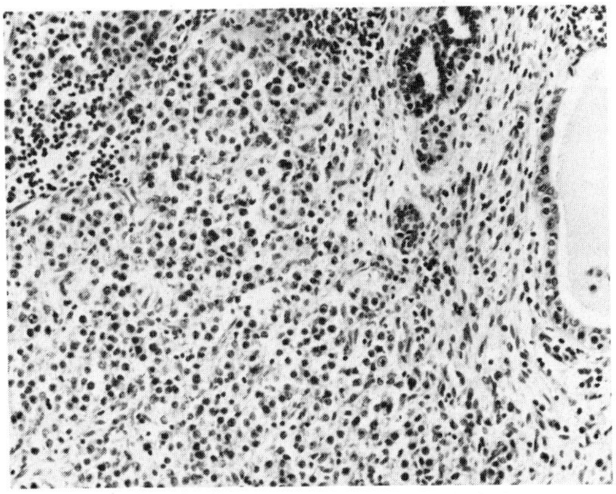

Fig. 2. Ovarian teratoma with embryonal carcinoma and dysgerminoma elements, plus a small area showing mature tissue (Hematoxylin eosin; ×225).

Los Angeles. Two patients with ovarian teratomas were operated upon elsewhere, and were referred to the Childrens Hospital for evaluation of recurrence. Clinical records and autopsy protocols of the patients were reviewed, and follow-up data on all but seven were obtained. Microscopic sections of the tumors were available for review in all cases, and in many instances tissue was available for more detailed study.

The teratomas of the various anatomic locations are classified in three pathologic categories, based on histologic findings: (1) benign teratomas, containing mature tissue only; (2) teratomas with mature and immature (embryonic) tissues which were not frankly malignant; and (3) malignant teratomas, with frankly malignant tissue in addition to mature and/or embryonic tissues. This last group is further divided according to the type of malignant component, whether germinoma (seminoma or dysgerminoma), embryonal carcinoma, yolk sac carcinoma, or choriocarcinoma (Figs. 1 through 4). Teratoid tumors which contained one or more of these malignant components, but no mature or embryonic tissues, were not included in this series. Therefore, four patients with this type of tumor included in a previous review of teratomas from this institution[11] were excluded from the series.

GENERAL OBSERVATIONS

Of the 81 patients, 57 were female, and 24 were male (Table I). Excluding ovarian and testicular tumors, the female preponderance fell to 27 to 19 since ovarian teratomas are more common than testicular teratomas.

Thirty-six teratomas were from the sacrococcygeal area. The ovary was the next most common site, accounting for 30 patients. Teratomas occurred in the testis in five patients, in the retroperitoneum in four, in the mediastinum in three, and one each in the brain, soft palate, and base of the umbilical cord (Fig. 5 and Table I).

In 61 patients, the teratoma contained

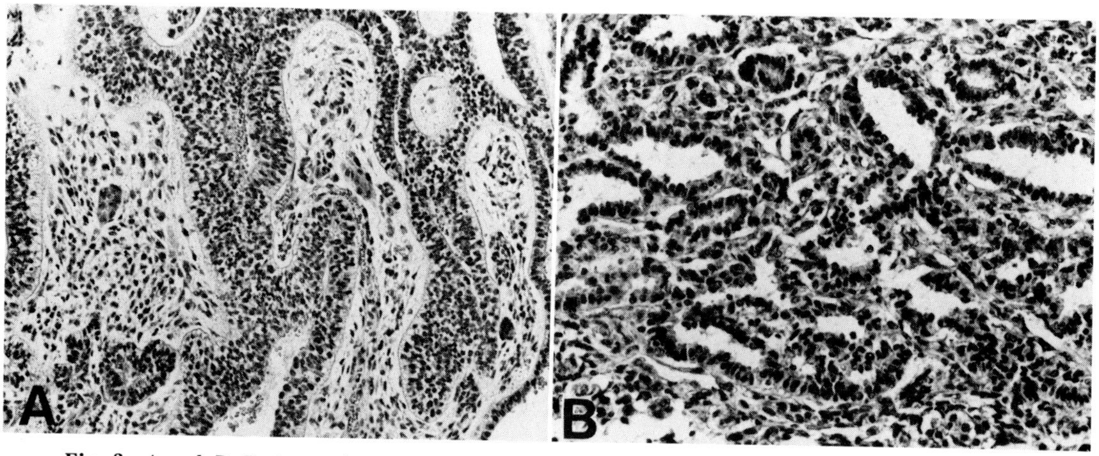

Fig. 3. *A* and *B,* Embryonal carcinoma in ovarian teratoma (Hematoxylin and eosin; ×175 and 400).

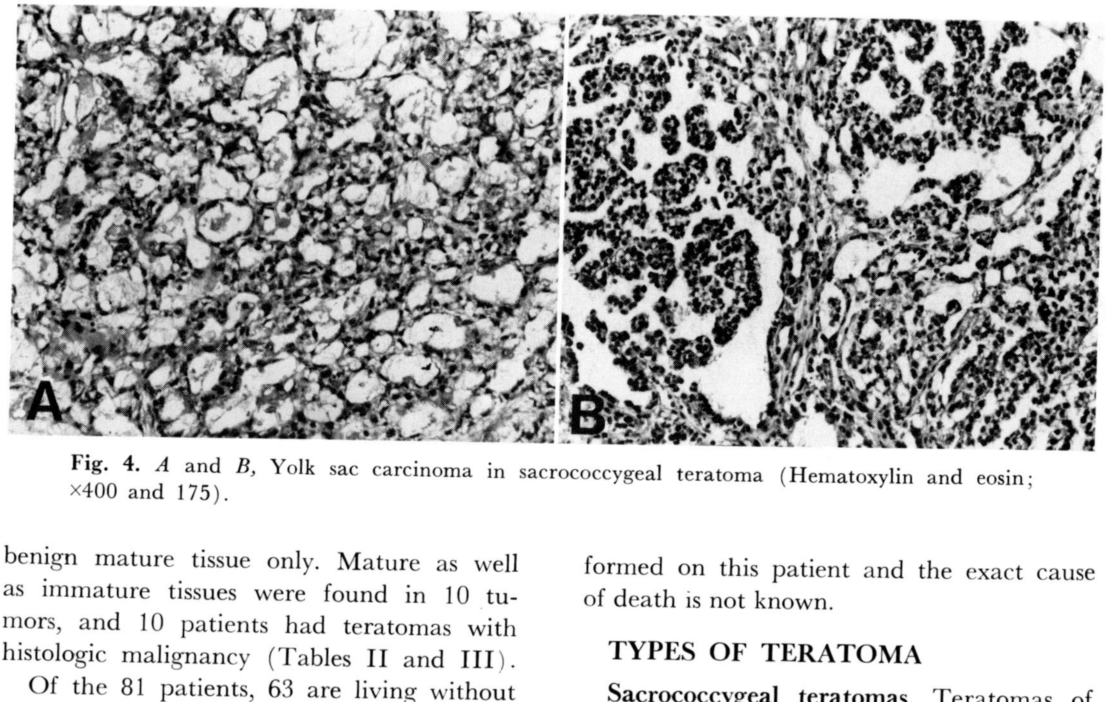

Fig. 4. *A* and *B,* Yolk sac carcinoma in sacrococcygeal teratoma (Hematoxylin and eosin; ×400 and 175).

benign mature tissue only. Mature as well as immature tissues were found in 10 tumors, and 10 patients had teratomas with histologic malignancy (Tables II and III).

Of the 81 patients, 63 are living without known residual tumor, seven patients have been lost to follow-up, eight are dead as a result of malignant teratoma, and three patients have died of causes other than malignancy. Of this last group, one patient with retroperitoneal teratoma died of hydrocephalus, one death was due to postoperative peritonitis in a patient with sacrococcygeal teratoma, and one patient with intracranial teratoma died at home 10 months after the operation. No autopsy was performed on this patient and the exact cause of death is not known.

TYPES OF TERATOMA

Sacrococcygeal teratomas. Teratomas of the sacrococcygeal region occurred in 36 patients (Table I). Twenty-two (61.1 percent) were female, and 14 (38.9 percent) were male, a marked female preponderance which has been observed in many other series.

Twenty-five patients had a mass visible at birth over the sacrococcygeal area. In five patients, an external sacrococcygeal mass was recognized later at the age of 5 months to 2½ years, and six patients had

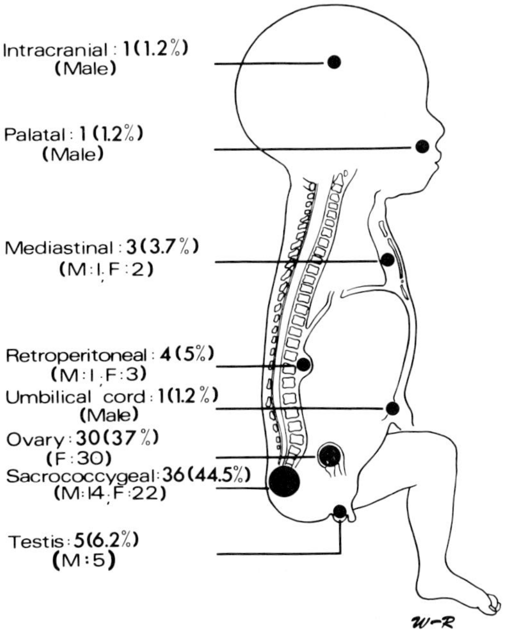

Fig. 5. Diagram to indicate the location of teratomas in 81 patients.

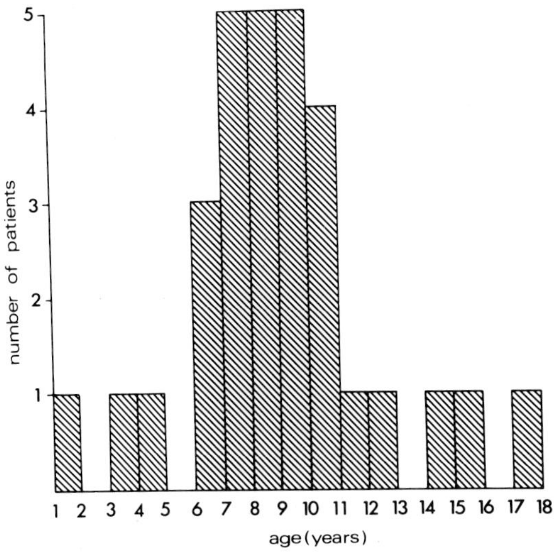

Fig. 6. Age distribution of 30 patients with ovarian teratoma. Note that the majority are between the ages of 6 and 11 years.

a tumor located anterior to the sacrum (Table IV). Of these last six patients, the mass was discovered at the age of 5 to 6 months in three patients, at 21 months in two, and at 9 years of age in one patient. Radiographic examination of the sacrococcygeal area demonstrated calcification within the tumor in 19 patients, including three of the five with frankly malignant teratoma.

Three patients had paralysis, pain, or weakness of a leg due to pressure of benign tumor. Constipation alone, or alternating with frequent stools, in three patients was indicative of colon obstruction. Two patients had urinary tract infection and/or distended bladder because of bladder neck obstruction. In the patients with presacral tumor, intravenous pyelogram and barium enema were helpful in demonstrating dysfunction or displacement of the urinary tract or colon.

Of the 36 patients with sacrococcygeal teratoma, one patient died due to postoperative enterocolitis and peritonitis 2 weeks after excision of the teratoma, 32 have been followed (Table V), and 3 have been lost to follow-up.

Of the 32 patients who have been followed (Table V), 19 were operated on at age one month or less. Of these, 16 are living without known residual tumor, five patients for 1½ to 5 years and 11 for more than 5 years, and three patients are dead due to recurrence and/or metastases of the teratoma. The three deaths occurred between 12 and 27 months after excision of the primary tumor with the initial diagnosis of malignant teratoma in two and teratoma with mature and immature tissue only in one. Eight patients were operated on from 2 to 7 months of age. Four of these patients had had a visible mass which, for 2 to 6 months prior to the operation, had been "growing with the child," and three patients had tumor anterior to the sacrum. All eight patients of this group are living and well, three for 2½ to 3 years and five for 5 years or more since the initial operation. Four patients were operated on between 20 and 30 months of age. Of these, two are dead and two have remained well for 3 and 19 years after the operation. The two deaths occurred in children with malignant teratoma; one child died one month after biopsy of the sacrococcygeal mass and the other died 5 months after excision of the mass. One ad-

Table I. *Anatomic locations of 81 teratomas (1941 through June, 1970)*

Location	No. of Cases			
	Male	Female	Total No.	Total %
Sacrococcygeal	14	22	36	44.5
Ovary		30	30	37
Testis	5		5	6.2
Retroperitoneal	1	3	4	5
Mediastinal	1	2	3	3.7
Intracranial	1	0	1	1.2
Palate	1	0	1	1.2
Umbilical cord	1	0	1	1.2
Total	24 (29.6%)	57 (70.4%)	81	100

Table II. *Histologic classification of 81 teratomas (1941 through June, 1970)*

Location	Benign "adult"		Embryonic tissue present		Malignant component present		Total
	No.	%	No.	%	No.	%	
Sacrococcygeal	24	66.7	7	19.4	5	13.9	36
Ovary	25	84	1	3	4	13	30
Testis	3	60	2	40	0		5
Retroperitoneal	4	100	0		0		4
Mediastinal	2	67	0		1	33	3
Intracranial	1		0		0		1
Palate	1		0		0		1
Umbilical cord	1		0		0		1
Total	61	75.3	10	12.35	10	12.35	81

Table III. *Location and histological classification of 10 malignant teratomas*

Location	No. of cases	Germinoma	Embryonal carcinoma	Yolk sac carcinoma	Chorio-carcinoma
Sacrococcygeal	5	0	5	2	0
Ovarian	4	2	4	2	1
Mediastinal	1	0	0	0	1
Total	10	2	9	4	2

ditional patient, a 9 year-old girl, presented with persistent pain in the sacral area for one month. She was found to have a benign teratoma anterior to the sacrum. This patient is living and well 2 years after excision of the tumor and coccyx.

Of the 36 sacrococcygeal teratomas, 24 were histologically benign (mature tissues only), seven had embryonic tissues in addition to mature components, and five had admixture of malignant with benign tissues (Tables II and III). Although a significant number of the tumors contained pancreatic tissue, in addition to squamous and respiratory epithelium, none of the patients demonstrated preoperative clinical manifestations of hypo- or hyperglycemia.

The patient who died due to postoperative peritonitis had teratoma with mature and immature tissues. In the three patients who are lost to follow-up, teratoma contained mature and embryonic tissues in two and only mature tissues in one.

Of the 32 patients with long term follow-

Table IV. *Presenting symptoms and signs in 36 patients with sacrococcygeal teratoma*

Symptoms or signs	*No. of cases* Male	Female	*Total*
Mass:	14	22	36
Visible, discovered at birth	8	17	25
Visible, discovered later	1	4	5
Intrapelvic (presacral)	5	1	6
Calcification on plain film	10	9	19
Paralysis, pain, or weakness of a leg	2	1	3
Constipation and/or frequent stools	3	0	3
Distended bladder	2	0	2

Table V. *Cases of sacrococcygeal teratoma with long-term follow-up*

Survival	*Age at operation (mo.)* ≤ 1	2 to 7	≥ 20	*Total*
Alive	16	8	3	27
Dead	3	0	2	5
Total	19	8	5	32

ups, 23 patients had teratoma containing mature tissues only. All these patients are living for 2½ years or more after diagnosis (Table VI). Four patients had tumor with mature and embryonic tissues but without frankly malignant element. Of these, three are living and well for three or more years after the initial operation, while one died with local recurrence and pulmonary and liver metastases one year after excision of the mass and coccyx at the first day of age. The metastatic lesions in this patient contained embryonal carcinoma. Five patients, three male and two female, all 2 years of age or younger, had malignant tumor. Four of these patients died of tumor within the first 27 months after the diagnosis. In two patients, in whom the diagnosis was made during the first 3 days of life, survival was 20 and 27 months respectively; while in the other two patients, in whom the diagnosis was made at 21 months and 2 years of age, survival was only 1 month and 5 months respectively. The only long-term survivor among the patients with malignant tumor was an infant with teratoma containing admixture of embryonal carcinoma and mature tissues. In this child, the tumor was resected on the first day of life; she received no further therapy and has remained well without known residual tumor for 11½ years.

Among the patients with teratoma without frankly malignant tissue, five are known to have had local recurrences; four of these patients are among the survivors. Two patients had primary tumor containing mature tissues only. In both, the recurrences occurred within the first year after the initial operation; and in one, the coccyx had not been removed at the primary operation. The other 3 patients had teratoma containing mature as well as embryonic tissues without frankly malignant element. In one, local recurrence occurred 4½ years after the primary operation. The second patient had had multiple operations for "sacral abscess" and "pilonidal sinus" before the coccyx was finally removed and definite diagnosis of teratoma was made with no further recurrence thereafter. The third patient is the one who died with local recurrence and distant metastases one year after excision of the mass and coccyx. The metastatic lesions in this last patient contained embryonal carcinoma.

Of the six patients with purely presacral tumor, one was female and five were male. Five patients had benign tumor. Of these, one has been lost to follow-up and four have remained well for 2 to 8 years. The sixth patient, a 21-month-old boy with malignant tumor (embryonal and yolk sac carcinomas), died one month after diagnosis.

Ovarian teratomas. In this series, there were 30 patients with ovarian teratoma (Tables I, II, and III). Patients with "dermoid" tumor are also included in this series. The most common complaint was that of abdominal pain, found in 24 patients (80 percent). Of these, eight patients had abdominal pain acute at onset, with nausea and/or vomiting, and were found to have torsion of the tube and tumor. Three to 4 month histories of abdominal pain and enlarge-

Table VI. *Cases of sacrococcygeal teratoma with long-term follow-up*

Survival	Benign "adult" No.	Benign "adult" %	Embryonic tissue present No.	Embryonic tissue present %	Malignant component present No.	Malignant component present %	Total No.	Total %
Alive	23	100	3	75	1	20	27	84.3
Dead	0		1	25	4	80	5	15.7
Total	23	100	4	100	5	100	32	100

Table VII. *Presenting symptoms and signs in 30 patients with ovarian teratoma*

Symptoms and signs	No. of cases
Abdominal pain	24
Acute torsion of tube and ovary	8
Urinary tract infection or obstruction	4
Constipation	2
Abdominal mass	15
Calcium within the mass	18

Table VIII. *Ovarian teratomas (1941 through June, 1970)*

Site	Benign "adult"	Embryonic tissue present	Malignant component present	Total
Right	12	1	1	14
Left	11	0	3	14
Bilateral	2	0	0	2
Total	25	1	4	30

ment were common among the others, and one patient had had abdominal pain and vomiting for 7 years. Other presenting symptoms were constipation (in two) and urinary tract infection and/or radiologic evidence of urinary tract obstruction (in four), (Table VII).

The most common physical finding was palpable lower abdominal mass, detected in 15 (50 percent). Eighteen patients (60 percent) had calcium visible within the tumor on plain film. Of two with bilateral ovarian teratomas, one had areas of calcification visible in both tumors, while the other had an apparently unilateral mass with no calcification.

Only one patient was under 2 years of age at the time of diagnosis, the majority being between 6 and 11 years of age (Fig. 6). Fourteen patients had teratoma in the right ovary, 14 in the left, and two in both ovaries (Table VIII). Of the 28 patients with unilateral teratoma, 17 patients were treated by ipsilateral salpingo-oophorectomy, seven had excision of the affected ovary, and four had excision of tumor only, with ovarian tissue left in place. Of the two patients with bilateral teratoma, one had excision of tumor from both ovaries, with ovarian tissue being left bilaterally. The other patient had salpingo-oophorectomy for a large cystic left ovarian teratoma. The right ovary appeared to be normal, but when it was bivalved, two teratomas were found and excised.

Twenty-five patients, including the two with bilateral tumor, had ovarian teratoma with mature tissues only. One patient had teratoma of the right ovary containing embryonic and mature tissues, and four patients (13.3 percent) had teratomas with frankly malignant components in addition to mature tissues (Tables II, III, and VIII). These last four patients were all between 8 and 10 years of age at the time of diagnosis; three had teratoma in the left, and one in the right ovary.

Twenty-six patients, including one of the two with bilateral tumors, have remained well, without sequelae, for 5 months to 23½ years after the operation. Twenty patients have been followed for 2 or more years, and three are known to have had one or more children. Two patients, both with malignant teratomas, have died and two, including one with bilateral teratoma, have been lost to follow-up.

A 10 year-old girl underwent right oophorectomy and partial omentectomy elsewhere for teratoma with mature tissue, embryonal carcinoma, and choriocarcinoma. At that time, there had been no demonstrable intra-abdominal metastasis except for a small peritoneal implant over the bladder which had been excised. Four months later, she was referred to the Childrens Hospital for evaluation of abdominal mass. Abdominal exploration revealed widespread intra-abdominal metastases of embryonal carcinoma and choriocarcinoma with involvement of the liver, right diaphragm, bowel wall, and pelvic organs. She died 12 days after the operation, with massive intra-abdominal bleeding from necrotic tumors, despite postoperative chemotherapy (methotrexate). Postmortem examination confirmed the operative findings in addition to the pulmonary metastases.

Another death occurred in an 11 year-old girl 2 years after salpingo-oophorectomy, performed elsewhere, for teratoma containing mature tissue, embryonal carcinoma, dysgerminoma, and yolk sac carcinoma. She was referred to the Childrens Hospital 3 months after the initial operation for evaluation of recurrence. At that time, abdominal exploration revealed pelvic tumor, containing embryonal carcinoma, which was partially resected, with no other demonstrable metastasis. She received postoperative radiotherapy as well as chemotherapy (methotrexate, Cytoxan, and actinomycin D). At autopsy, she had widespread intra-abdominal metastases with liver involvement.

Of the other two patients with malignant teratomas, one is living, without known residual tumor, 9 years after left salpingo-oophorectomy and omentectomy for teratoma with mature tissue, embryonal carcinoma and dysgerminoma. She has had no further treatment. The other patient has remained well for 3½ years, without residual tumor, following left salpingo-oophorectomy plus partial cystectomy and omentectomy for teratoma with mature tissue and embryonal and yolk sac carcinomas. She received postoperative actinomycin D, Cytoxan, and methotrexate, plus radiotherapy.

Testicular teratoma. Five patients had testicular teratomas, two on the right and three on the left (Table I). The youngest patient was 6 months of age and the oldest 2 years at the time of diagnosis. All were seen because of enlarged testis, none of which were painful or appeared inflammatory. None of these patients had diagnostic x-rays of the testicular area, but the pathological specimens of each contained calcium.

Four patients had resection of the affected testis and accompanying cord structures up to the internal inguinal ring, and one patient had resection of the teratoma with the testis left in situ. Three of the five teratomas had benign tissue only and two, both of the left testis, contained embryonic in addition to mature tissues without frankly malignant elements (Table II).

Four of these patients have been followed. Two, with benign tumors, are alive and well for 16 years and 22 months, respectively. The other two patients, both with teratomas containing embryonic tissues, have remained well, without known residual tumor, for 18 and 3 years respectively after the operation.

Retroperitoneal teratoma. There were four patients, three girls and one boy, with retroperitoneal teratomas (Tables I and II). In one patient, an 8 month-old boy, the tumor was discovered at autopsy after the patient had died of hydrocephalus. An asymptomatic abdominal mass was found on routine physical examination of two female patients at 2 and 6½ months of age, respectively. The fourth patient was a 15 year-old girl who had complained of weight loss for one year, and who was found to have an abdominal mass on physical examination. All of the retroperitoneal teratomas contained mature tissues only.

Surgical excision of the teratoma was performed in three patients and the spleen was resected in one of them because of its contiguity with the tumor. These patients have been followed for 21 months and 4 years after the operation. They all have remained well and asymptomatic.

Teratoma of the mediastinum. Three patients had teratoma of the mediastinum. A 15 month-old female infant presented with wheezing and fever. Radiographic examination of the chest demonstrated a calcified tumor in the anterior mediastinum. The tumor was excised and found to be teratoma containing benign tissues only. Her postoperative course was uneventful, but no long term follow-up is available.

A 14 year-old boy presented with progressive dyspnea, chest pain, and fever, for one month. Radiologic examination of the chest revealed an anterior mediastinal mass, without calcification, plus bilateral extensive pulmonary infiltrates. Examination of the urine showed markedly elevated chorionic gonadotropin level, and biopsy of the pulmonary lesions revealed choriocarcinoma. The patient died 3 days after the operation; at autopsy the mediastinal mass contained small areas of mature tissues, in addition to choriocarcinoma.

In an 11 year-old girl with recurrent epigastric pain, an anterior mediastinal mass, with calcification, was demonstrated by x-ray. The tumor was excised and found to contain benign tissues only. This patient has remained well and asymptomatic for 13 months after the operation.

Miscellaneous teratomas. One patient with intracranial teratoma was admitted to the hospital at 9 months of age with increased intracranial pressure. Skull x-ray revealed suprasellar calcification. The patient had excision of a histologically benign teratoma from the anterior and middle cranial fossae. Postoperatively, she had gastrointestinal bleeding and transient diabetes insipidus. She died 10 months later at home; no autopsy was performed.

A female neonate was noted to have a tumor of the palate at birth (epignathus). At age 6 weeks, the tumor was resected. Excess bleeding was controlled by ligation of the right external carotid artery. The tumor contained benign tissues only. This patient is alive and well, 22 years of age, and the mother of a 4 year-old child.

The remaining patient in this series was born with an intact omphalocele, associated with a small teratoma at the base of the umbilical cord. The teratoma, containing benign tissues only, was resected during the course of the omphalocele repair. She has remained well for 12 years.

COMMENTS

The cause of teratomas remains obscure.[4, 8, 10] The most frequent site of these tumors in children is the sacrococcygeal region, [1, 2, 5, 7, 11] but they may occur almost anywhere in the body; [7, 11] they are more common in females.[1, 2, 3, 9, 11]

Most teratomas contain both solid and cystic areas,[4, 5] although completely solid teratomas do occur. Benign teratomas are usually well encapsulated and the presence of areas of necrosis or hemorrhage is strongly suggestive of malignant tumor.

Microscopic examination of teratomas usually reveals a variety of tissues from more than one germ layer. Benign and malignant, mature and immature elements may be found side by side in the same tumor and it is entirely possible that malignant areas would escape being sectioned. Thus, very extensive sectioning of the tumor is necessary to eliminate the presence of cancer.[2, 4, 11] In some tumors, the histologic distinction between neoplastic and poorly differentiated embryonic tissues is difficult.[11] In the series reported here, one patient died with local recurrence and metastatic lesions containing embroyonal carcinoma one year after excision of a sacrococcygeal teratoma containing embryonic tissues without frankly malignant element.

The treatment of teratomas is primarily surgical, regardless of the size of the mass, or the young age, even prematurity, of the patient. The operation should be instituted as soon as possible.[4, 5, 9]

It appears that in teratomas with frankly malignant tissues, the occurrence of local recurrence and/or metastasis is lethal, regardless of the site of origin of the tumor or modalities of the treatment. In our series, 10 patients had malignant teratoma. Of these, seven died of tumor at various intervals within 27 months after the diagnosis; and three are living for 3½, 9, and 11½ years respectively after the initial operation. None of the survivors has as yet demonstrated evidence of local recurrence or metastasis.

Sacrococcygeal teratomas are usually detected during infancy, if not at the time of birth. The most common finding is a mass in the sacral-buttock area. Occasionally, especially in older children, no external mass is present. In these cases, rectum or bladder obstruction is common[6, 11] and the principal differential diagnostic considerations are meningocele, chordoma, duplication of the rectum, neurogenic tumors, lipoma, and hemangioma.[2, 3, 4, 5, 6] In some children, a mistaken diagnosis of pilonidal cyst or sinus, or perirectal abscess, has been made.

The surgical technique for removal of sacrococcygeal teratoma has been well described.[2, 3, 4, 5, 11] In excision of these tumors, failure to resect the entire coccyx has been associated with a high incidence of recurrence. In our series, a 20-month-old girl had multiple procedures for "sacral abscess" and "pilonidal sinus" at various intervals. At age 3½ years, she had excision of the coccyx and "total removal of the mass with draining sacrococcygeal sinus." At this operation the diagnosis of sacrococcygeal teratoma was finally made; she has had no further recurrence for 3 years.

At operation for unilalteral ovarian teratoma, the "normal" opposite ovary should be bivalved and inspected for the presence of teratoma. In our series, one patient had a large cystic left ovarian teratoma. At operation, the right ovary appeared to be normal, but when it was bivalved, two small separate teratomas were found buried in the ovarian tissue.

REFERENCES

1. Carney, J. A., Thompson, D. P., Johnson, C. L., and Lynn, H. B.: Teratomas in children: Clinical and pathological aspects, J. Pediatr. Surg. **7:** 271, 1972.
2. Dillard, B. M., Mayer, J. H., McAlister, W. H., McGavrin, M., and Strominger, D. B.: Sacrococcygeal teratoma in children, J. Pediatr. Surg. **5:** 53, 1970.
3. Donnellan, W. A., and Swenson, O.: Benign and malignant sacrococcygeal teratomas, SURGERY **64:** 834, 1968.
4. Exelby, P. R.: Sacrococcygeal teratomas in children, CA **22:** 202, 1972.
5. Gross, R. E., Clatworthy, H. W., and Meeker, I. A.: Sacrococcygeal teratomas in infants and children. A report of 40 cases, Surg. Gynecol. Obstet. **92:** 341, 1951.
6. Gwinn, J. L., Dockerty, M. B., and Kennedy, R. L. J.: Presacral teratomas in infancy and childhood, Pediatrics **16:** 239, 1955.
7. Lynn, H. B.: Teratomas in children, Postgrad. Med. **25:** 427, 1959.
8. McCune, W. S.: Management of sacrococcygeal tumors, Ann. Surg. **159:** 911, 1964.
9. Waldhausen, J. A., Kilman, J. W., Vellios, F., and Battersby, J. S.: Sacrococcygeal teratoma, SURGERY **54:** 933, 1963.
10. Willis, R. A.: Pathology of tumours, ed. 4, London, 1967, Appleton-Century-Crofts.
11. Woolley, M. M., Ginsburg, S., DiCenso, S., Snyder, W. H., Mirabal, V. Q., and Landing, B. H.: Teratomas in infancy and childhood, Kinderchir. **4:** 289, 1967.

Choledochoduodenostomy: An 18 year study of 175 consecutive cases

George A. Degenshein, M.D., *Brooklyn, N. Y.*

Lateral choledochoduodenostomy is slowly gaining favor with American surgeons. The theoretical objections to this procedure have not been borne out in practice. Although used originally for ampullary stenosis, the indications have extended to include multiple small stones in the common duct, retained stones, hepatic stones, strictures, and benign tumors. There is also a place for this operation in malignancies of the head of the pancreas. Two absolute requisites are evident. The common duct must be dilated and the anastomosis must be made no less than 2.5 cm. in its longest diameter. This series of 175 consecutive cases was carried out over an 18 year period with low mortality and morbidity rates in an aged population. The two cases of subsequent cholangitis are well documented and confirm the need for an adequate size for the anastomosis. Lateral choledochoduodenostomy is a safe, effective procedure which should receive wider application for proper indication.

From the Departments of Surgery, Maimonides Medical Center and Coney Island Hospital affiliate and Downstate Medical Center, State University of New York, Brooklyn, N. Y.

DESPITE the increase in volume of favorable literature in the United States on the value of lateral choledochoduodenostomy, there is still considerable resistance to the utilization of this procedure for proper indication. It is also noteworthy that there has been almost no adverse literature. We thought it important to report the results of a series of 175 consecutive cases followed over an 18 year period from 1955 to 1973. This report includes the 48 cases reported by us previously.[5]

In 1891, Sprengel[12] reported the first lateral or side-to-side choledochoduodenostomy. The next year Riedel[9] reported that he had done one two years before Sprengel. A review of that case revealed that he used a complementary cholecystostomy. Following the turn of the century, the operation gained popularity on the continent and Sasse[10] in 1913 reported a significant number of cases. In 1928 at the meeting in Freiburg, Germany, Flörcken[3, 4] reported 100 cases with excellent results. There were vigorous objections from other surgeons who claimed that this procedure would cause cholangitis because of reflux of duodenal content into the biliary tree and they brought reports of barium swallows which showed flooding of the biliary tree.

In response to these objections, Flörcken and another surgeon named Göetze set the guideline for this procedure, which is still valid today.[3] They stressed the need for a large anastomosis and agreed that "the more barium the better." The danger of cholangitis was purely theoretical and the objections came only from those who never did the procedure, or those who made a small anas-

Accepted for publication May 13, 1974.

Reprint requests: George A. Degenshein, M.D., Department of Surgery, Maimonides Medical Center, 4802 Tenth Ave., Brooklyn, N. Y. 11219.

Table I. *Data*

	No. of cases
Jaundice	112
Dilated common duct	173
Previous cholecystectomy	50
Previous cholecystostomy	3
Cholecystojejunostomy	1
Cholecystocolic fistula	1
Two-layer anastomosis	148
One-layer anastomosis	27
Average hospital stay	15.23 days

Table II. *Indications*

	No. of cases	Percentage
1. Multiple small stones	78	44.6
2. Ampullary stenosis	25	14.3
3. Retained or recurrent common duct stones	24	13.7
4. Malignant obstructions	22	12.7
5. Sludge	18	10.3
6. Cholangitis	8	4.7
7. Impacted ampullary stone	8	4.7
8. Hepatic stones	7	4.0
9. Stricture of common duct	5	2.8
10. Pancreatitis	4	2.3
11. Benign tumors of common duct	2	1.2
12. Not indicated	2	1.2

tomosis. They also made clear the necessity for a dilated common duct as a requisite for this operation.

In 1955, stimulated by the work of Nansen and Saunders,[11] Dr. Alfred Hurwitz, former Director of Surgery at this institution, became interested in this procedure almost exclusively for ampullary stenosis. At that time, the methods of treatment for ampullary stenosis were not particularly satisfactory, with dilatation resulting in re-stenosis and accompanied by the danger of instrument perforation of the lower end of the duct. Sphincterotomy gained in popularity, but the results of this procedure were not entirely satisfactory. The introduction of the sphincteroplasty was a marked improvement and the report of Jones and associates[6] of 132 cases showed excellent results, but there were three deaths associated with pancreatitis. The sphincteroplasty is, in effect, a transduodenal choledochoduodenostomy. It seemed logical, therefore, to do a choledochoduodenostomy at a more convenient level. In the early series, we reserved this procedure primarily for ampullary stenosis. As we gained experience, it became a safety operation for us each time we were in a dilemma with the problem of adequately cleansing the common duct. At the present time our indications for doing this procedure have extended widely.

AGE AND SEX

There were 107 women and 68 men. Their ages ranged from 19 to 95; but 21 were over the age of 80 and three over the age of 90.

SIGNIFICANT DATA

There were 112 patients with jaundice and every common duct, (except two) was dilated. It was a primary procedure in 120 cases and secondary in 55. The average hospital stay was 15.23 days (Table I) Table II lists our indications today, and each is worthy of discussion.

INDICATIONS

Multiple stones. Whenever a large number of small stones is removed from a common duct, it is almost impossible to be certain, despite cholangiography, that there is not a stone or the nidus for a stone left behind. It is most protective to carry out a choledochoduodenostomy where the slightest suspicion exists that there may be a residual small stone. Cleansing this "uncommon" duct has defied the ingenuity and talent of surgeons for almost a century, despite the use of fiberoptic scopes, Fogarty catheters, special metal instruments, and table cholangiograms. There is not a surgeon of experience who has not cleansed a common duct, done a table cholangiogram, and been completely satisfied that he had left no stones behind. Then some 10 or 12 days later, with another cholangiogram prior to T-tube removal, a residual stone is found. I think our average would be even worse than it is if not for a generally unpublicized physiological fact that following cholecystectomy the sphincter of Oddi usually remains patent for a few months and there is reason to believe that many small stones that we leave behind are passed through this open sphincter. All of us have had patients tell us that, in the immediate postoperative period or within a month or two afterward, they felt as though they had their gallbladder back in again because they had an attack which mimicked the original reason for the cholecystectomy. This probably reflects the passage of some small residual stones through the patent ampulla.

Ampullary stenosis. This indication is clear-cut. Soft stasis stones tend to recur in the presence of stenosis and may actually form a cast of the common duct. Flörcken[3] reported a patient whose ducts were explored seven times before choledochoduodenostomy provided the cure. Dennis[2] had a patient who was cleansed of stasis stones adequately four times by excellent surgeons, but only choledochoduodenostomy resolved the problem.

Retained or recurrent stones. There were 24 cases of retained or recurrent stones and, although many of them were from other institutions, we are certain that some of our cases were reoperated elsewhere. Choledochoduodenostomy is ideally suited for any repeat operation on the common duct provided that the duct is dilated. It is a definitive procedure and overcomes the possibility of further re-explorations.

Malignant obstructions. Although there are some basic objections to doing an anastomosis adjacent to a pancreatic or lower bile duct malignancy, it is often the least traumatic and the most effective procedure available. It functions more reliably than a cholecystojejunostomy and, with a markedly dilated duct, is a much lesser procedure than a Longmire operation.

Sludge. Sludge is rarely a primary indication. We have become distrustful of the muddy, murky bile with soft lumps and bumps, despite the fact that they are not true calculi. They imply stasis or a metabolic aberration and, if there are several small stones in the duct, the presence of sludge is a secondary factor which may lead to the decision to do choledochoduodenostomy.

Cholangitis. Cholangitis is also a relative indication and is more often an indication to explore the common duct than to specifically indicate the procedure.

Impacted ampullary stone. Impacted ampullary stone is a controversial indication. We have had the experience of opening the duodenum and searching for the impacted stone, which is not rarely tucked in a side pocket or outpouching of the lower end of the duct and requires a great deal of trauma in the region of the pancreatic duct. If it cannot be gently disimpacted from above, one may consider a lateral choledochoduodenostomy and leave the stone behind. We have done this in eight cases without subsequent difficulty, but the series is not large enough to state firmly that this type of stone may be left behind. One thing is certain, if the duodenum is already opened and there is difficulty in dislocating the stone, a sphincteroplasty is more logical than a lateral choledochoduodenostomy, since the duodenal incision would be improperly placed for a lateral anastomosis. The leaving of a blind segment below the anastomosis has come under criticism, but in our 175 cases we have not had one instance of accumulation of sufficient debris to obstruct the anastomotic site. It is our feeling that a large enough anastomosis prevents the accumulation of debris sufficient to cause obstruction or cholangitis.

Hepatic stones. Hepatic stones represent an excellent indication. It may be difficult to flush out such a stone and one has to regard the future possibility of its passing. Providing a large vent guarantees that it will not subsequently cause obstruction (see Fig. 2).

Stricture of the common duct. Stricture of the common duct is a self-evident indication if the proximal duct is dilated.

Pancreatitis. Pancreatitis is a relative indication depending upon associated common duct stones and the desire to avoid instrumentation in the region of the pancreatic ducts.

Benign tumors. Benign tumors of the common duct also represent an excellent indication if biopsy proof of benignity is available.

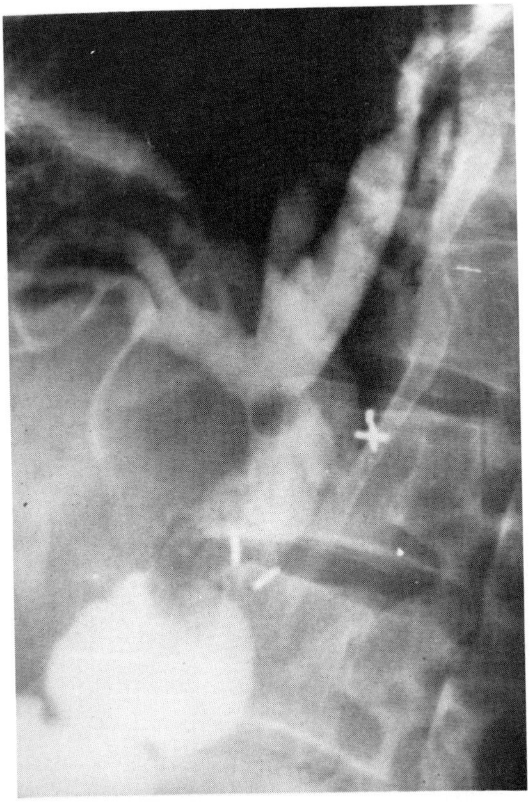

Fig. 1A. Close-up view of retained common hepatic duct stone cholangitis.

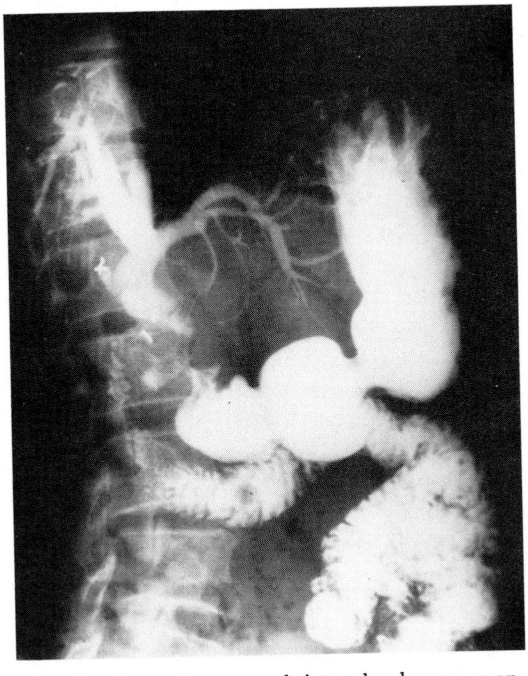

Fig. 1B. Stone has passed into duodenum spontaneously with relief of cholangitis.

Not indicated. There were two cases with nondilated ducts which were done without proper indication. One was a small duct and the anastomosis leaked postoperatively and drainage was instituted. This patient was ultimately reoperated upon at another institution where the choledochoduodenostomy was taken down and the appropriate procedure carried out directly on the duct with a successful outcome. The second case was one with a relatively small duct and suspicion of a sclerosing cholangitis for which we feel there is no indication for this procedure.

Complications. We had a 5.1 percent wound infection rate reflecting a group of acute cases and a generally aged population, many of whom had associated diseases not conducive to wound healing. There were four leaks with bile peritonitis, three of which will be discussed under mortality rate. The fourth is classified as "not indicated" (Table III).

There were two cases of cholangitis in the entire series and they are worthy of discussion. The first occurred in a 61-year-old woman who developed cholangitis six months postoperatively. She was found to have a small stoma which was revised to a 3 cm. stoma and, during a 10 year follow-up, was completely asymptomatic. The second case was a most fascinating one in one of our attending physicians. He had a choledochoduodenostomy for an extremely large number of stones and the suspicion that there was a hepatic duct stone that could not be retrieved. Less than one year postoperatively, he was admitted for cholangitis. A gastrointestinal swallow revealed a large stone in the common hepatic duct (Fig. 1*A*). While in hospital on antibiotics, he had a sudden dramatic relief of pain and fever and a subsequent gastrointestinal swallow fortuitously showed the passing of the stone into the duodenum (Fig. 1*B*). He has been asymptomatic for more than a year since that time.

MORTALITY RATE

Of the 153 cases of benign disease, there were five deaths—an incidence of 3.2 percent. There were two deaths in the malignant

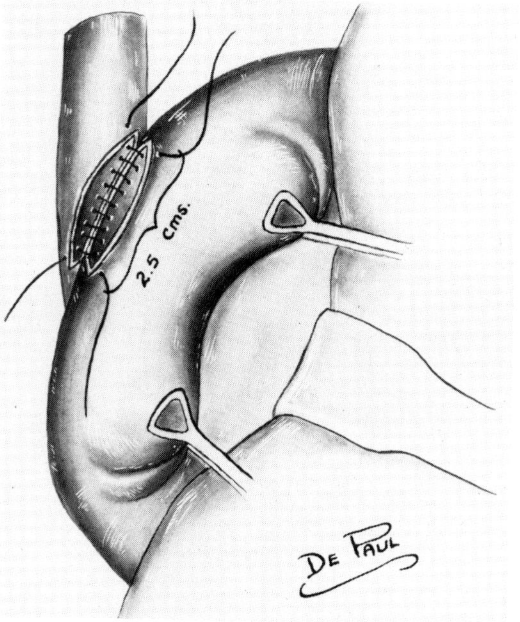

Fig. 2A. Oblique or vertical incision in common duct with duodenum rolled away. Note suture above and below anastomosis.

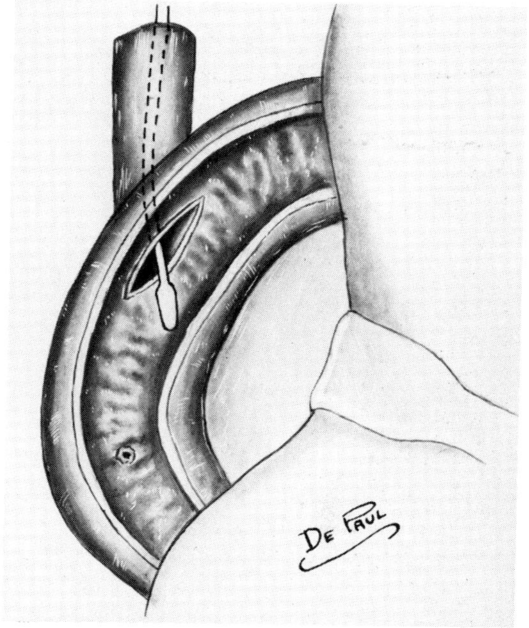

Fig. 2B. Completed anastomosis. Note relationship to papilla.

Table III. *Complications*

	No. of cases
Wound infection	9
Significant atelectases	5
Leak with bile peritonitis	4
Thrombophlebitis	3
Cholangitis	2
Renal failure	2
Peritonitis	2
Gastrointestinal bleeding	2
Pancreatitis	1
Wound dehiscence	1
Myocardial infarction	1
Atrial fibrillation	1
Psychosis	1

Table IV. *Deaths*

1. Man, 84 years old, died on postoperative day 8: renal failure
2. Woman, 68 years old, died on postoperative day 9: bile peritonitis, cancer of common bile duct, tension
3. Man, 77 years old, died on postoperative day 21: adenocarcinoma of bile duct, nephrosis, ascites, metastases
4. Women, 75 years old, died on postoperative day 14: bile peritonitis, ulcerative colitis
5. Woman, 74 years old, died on postoperative day 7: multiple myeloma, meningitis, arteriosclerotic heart disease
6. Woman, 71 years old, died on postoperative day 7: basilar artery occlusion, myocardial infarction
7. Woman, 70 years old, with bile peritonitis

group—an incidence of 9.1 percent. There was an over-all mortality rate of seven cases out of 175—an incidence of 4 percent. Causes of death are noted in Table IV.

TECHNIQUE

This has been covered in a previous publication,[1] but some comments are warranted. The terms lateral or side-to-side are really misnomers. The duodenum is in a more superficial plane than the common duct and when it is Kocherized and rolled over, the duodenal incision is made somewhat posteriorly. When allowed to roll back, it comes to sit on the common duct like a hen sits on an egg and in this way is most protective.

Tension on the anastomosis is completely unacceptable and is avoided by placing the incisions correctly and a suture above and below the anastomosis (Fig. 2*A*). The duct must always be dilated and the longest diameter of the anastomosis must never be less than 2.5 cm. (Fig. 2*B*). The suture material does not seem to be important; Madden used 5/0 silk typing knots on the inside[7] and Pi-Figueras[8] used No. 2 chromic. The number of layers is not critical; some use two layers, others one layer, and still others two layers posteriorly and one anteriorly or one layer posteriorly and two anteriorly. It is important for the surgeon to make an anastomosis technically satisfactory to himself. Despite the above comments, the most critical factor in carrying out this procedure is premeditation. The decision to do this operation must be made before the duodenum is opened. If one explores the common duct, finds problems that lead to a duodenotomy and exposure of the papilla, is still dissatisfied, and now considers a lateral choledochoduodenostomy, he will now find himself with an improperly placed duodenal incision and with an elderly patient who has been on the operating table for a long period of time, especially if multiple cholangiographs have been taken. It is probably wise to settle for sphincteroplasty under those circumstances. On the other hand, if, upon exploration of the duct, the need for the procedure becomes evident, one may proceed with a choledochoduodenostomy in many instances without even doing a cholangiogram. The technique is rarely difficult.

One caution! There is always a danger of overlooking an ampullary carcinoma, so that part of the operative procedure is to slip a finger into the duodenotomy and palpate the papilla.

CONCLUSIONS

1. Results of a consecutive series of 175 cases of choledochoduodenostomy have been reported.

2. The traditional objections to this procedure are not valid.

3. The requisites of proper indications, dilated duct, and large anastomosis are stressed.

4. This is a safe, simple, effective procedure for a high-risk population.

This represents a cooperative study involving almost all of our general surgeons and the house staff, who have given considerable time to the documentation and follow-up of the cases reported.

REFERENCES

1. Degenshein, G. A., and Hurwitz, A.: The techniques of side-to-side choledochoduodenostomy, SURGERY **61:** 974, 1967.
2. Dennis, C.: Personal communication.
3. Flörcken, H.: Freie Vereinigung Frankfurter Chirurgen. 22. Sitzung vom 24 November 1927 in der chir. Abt. des Diakonissen hauses, Zentralbl. Chir. No. 3, 1928.
4. Flörcken, H.: Die "Ruckfalle" nach Gallensteinoperationen und die Bedeutung des Verbindung Zwischen Gallengang und Zwolffingerdarm, Munch. Med. Wochenschr. **70:** 498-499, 1923.
5. Hurwitz, A., and Degenshein, G. A.: The role of choledochoduodenostomy in common duct surgery: Reappraisal, SURGERY **56:** 1147, 1965.
6. Jones, S. A., Smith, L. I., Keller, T. B., and Joergenson, E. J.: Choledochoduodenostomy to prevent residual stones, Arch. Surg. **86:** 1014, 1963.
7. Madden, J. L., Gruqez, J. A., and Tan, P. Y.: Obstructive (surgical) Jaundice: an analysis of 140 consecutive cases and a consideration of choledochoduodenostomy in its treatment, Am. J. Surg. **109:** 89, 1965.
8. Pi-Figueras, J.: Technique de panastomose choledochoduodenale pour la lithiase de la voie biliare principale, Iconogr. Chir. **31:** 17, 1958.
9. Riedel, B. M. C. L.: Erfahrungen uber die Gallensteinkrankheit mit und ohne Icterus, Berlin, 1892, Hirschwald, pp. 116-119.
10. Sasse, Fr.: Choledochoduodenostomie, Arch. Klin Cherierg. **100:** 313, 1913.
11. Saunders, R. L.: Indications and value of choledochoduodenostomy, Ann. Surg. **123:** 847, 1946.
12. Sprengel, L.: Exstirpatiore der Gallenblase mit Anbegung Eiver Kommuni Kation Zwischen Duodenum und Ductus Choledochus, Dtsch. Med. Zeitung, **12:** 354, 1891.

Trace elements in normal and malignant human breast tissue

Arthur E. Schwartz, M.D., *New York, N. Y.,* **George W. Leddicotte, Sc.D., Richard W. Fink, Ph.D.,** *Atlanta, Ga., and* **Eugene W. Friedman, M. D., New York, N. Y.**

Normal and malignant breast tissue from nine patients undergoing radical mastectomy was analyzed for concentrations of trace metals by neutron activation analysis. The levels of potassium, phosphorus, copper, magnesium, and zinc were substantially higher in the malignant tissue. The significance of these differences requires further study.

From the Mount Sinai School of Medicine, City University of New York, New York, N. Y. (Drs. Schwartz and Friedman), The Nuclear and Biological Sciences Division, Georgia Institute of Technology, Atlanta, Ga. (Dr. Leddicotte), and the School of Chemistry, Georgia Institute of Technology, Atlanta, Ga. (Dr. Fink)

THE ROLE of trace elements in malignant disease evokes increasing interest with the advent of accurate methods of detecting their presence in human tissue. The observation that substantial differences exist in the concentration of such metals as potassium, zinc, copper, phosphorus, and magnesium in malignant and normal tissue suggests that these elements may play a role in the etiology or metabolic alterations of cancer and excites interest in their possible use in diagnostic tests.

In this study, the concentration of trace elements in malignant breast tissue from a series of nine patients is compared to that of normal breast tissue from the same patients.

METHODS AND MATERIALS

Tissue was obtained at operation from nine patients who had undergone radical mastectomy for cancer of the breast. In each patient, two specimens were removed for study: (1) 1 c.c. of cancerous breast tissue and (2) 1 c.c. of normal breast tissue from a remote area of the same breast. In every case, microscopic sections of the malignant tissue was reported "infiltrating duct carcinoma" and the grossly normal tissue was histologically confirmed. Thus, 18 specimens of tissue were available for study representing normal and malignant breast tissue from each of nine patients. Samples were preserved in formalin and transported in polyethylene vials.

Concentrations of trace elements in tissues were determined by neutron activation analysis.[6] Tissue samples were irradiated in a thermal neutron flux of 1.5×10^{13} n./cm.^{2} sec. for specific time periods. This neutron bombardment produces radioactive isotopes in the chemical elements of the sample material. Each radioisotope has a specific half-life and characteristic gamma ray energy level; these are identified and measured by a lithium-drifted germanium detector. The

Accepted for publication April 4, 1974.

Reprint requests: Arthur E. Schwartz, M.D., Mount Sinai School of Medicine, City University of New York, New York, N. Y. 10028.

Table I. *Concentration (in μg% wet weight) of trace elements in normal and malignant breast tissue*

Element	Patient 1		Patient 2		Patient 3		Patient 4	
	*N**	*M*	*N*	*M*	*N*	*M*	*N*	*M*
Sb								
Br	540	41	210	250	50	91	69	43
Cl	71,000	64,000	110,000	73,000	20,000	47,000	39,000	68,000
Cr								
Cu								
Au								
I	<25	280	<22	<34	<11	26	120	<70
Fe	760	1,700	<450	2,100	490	1,300	730	
Mg	<1,000	13,000	<1,000	5,600	<1,000	2,000	<1,000	12,000
Mn	<2.2	10	<2.2	6.9	<2.2	7.3	9	18
Hg								
P								
K	12,000	160,000	24,000	64,000			5,600	68,000
Rb								
Se	180	110	31	96	12	32	77	
Na	52,000	38,000	80,000	57,000	17,000	36,000	24,000	49,000
Zn	250	1,200	180	220	88	580	210	

*N = Normal tissue; M = malignant tissue.

total system is interfaced with a computer. This nondestructive method of analysis offers a precision and sensitivity which exceeds that of conventional chemical and physical methods.

The analysis of the 95 hour irradiated samples revealed considerable activity in the low-energy range (<300 keV.) which was determined to be due to Bremstrahlung radiation or beta particle decay. Malignant tissue showed a consistently higher level of this activity. The entire source of this beta radiation was identified as ^{32}P (14.3 day half-life) and, therefore, phosphorus concentration in the samples from the fifth to the ninth patient were studied in greater detail with a beta detector.

RESULTS

Table I is a complete tabulation of the results obtained from gamma ray data as well as phosphorus concentrations based on beta decay data in samples of benign and malignant breast tissue from nine patients.

Fig. 1 presents the weight ratios for specific elements in malignant and benign breast tissue. These ratios were obtained by dividing the concentration of each element in malignant tissue by the corresponding concentration in benign tissue.

An analysis of the pure formaldehyde drained off from the benign and malignant tissue samples of patient nine showed that most—if not all—of the chromium, gold, and antimony in the samples arose from the formaldehyde (Table II). It also appears that a certain amount of copper and zinc in the samples was due to formaldehyde. On the other hand, there is a loss of certain elements from the tissue due to their solubility in formaldehyde: mercury, manganese, rubidium, sodium, potassium, and chlorine. Although the results of this study were not significantly affected by the preservation and transporting of specimens in formalin, we feel that freeze-drying offers greater accuracy and plan to use this method in the future.[7]

DISCUSSION

Potassium. The concentration of potassium was found to be eight times greater in malignant breast tissue than in normal breast tissue. Increased potassium content of malignant tissue has been noted by others[2] and may simply be a reflection of the largely intracellular location of potassium in normal tissues and the highly cellular nature of malignancy. Whether there is a real difference in the potassium concentration of malignant cells per se is not known at this time.

Phosphorus. The phosphorus concentration in malignant breast tissue was found to *from nine patients treated by radical mastectomy*

Patient 5 N	Patient 5 M	Patient 6 N	Patient 6 M	Patient 7 N	Patient 7 M	Patient 8 N	Patient 8 M	Patient 9 N	Patient 9 M
<0.3	<0.3	0.3	0.4	0.4	0.6	1	0.4	1	2
3,100	990	840	140	1,500	730	1,300	1,100	1,300	360
46,000	98,000	13,000	130,000	75,000	46,000	86,000	55,000	22,000	26,000
10	12	72	5	10	<5	<1	<1	11	5
<30	50	<30	250	100	80	<30	230	170	460
<0.01	<0.01	0.04	0.05	0.08	0.02	0.05	<0.01	0.03	<0.01
<10	<10	370	30	23	29	30	20	<10	88
1,500	6,300	1,800	1,700	2,300	2,300	670	2,100	980	3,300
1,100	16,000	920	6,400	850	10,000	1,700	9,400	3,000	13,000
14	21	8	20	12	30	24	32	11	55
31	18	10	28	92	29	38	47	14	77
3,500	71,000	2,800	54,000	2,400	26,000	15,000	32,000	4,000	86,000
8,100	180,000	7,800	95,000	5,000	40,000	21,000	42,000	6,400	54,000
<4	38	<4	25	<4	15	10	20	5	25
25	91	10	78	15	60	37	59	21	97
40,000	88,000	9,300	110,000	4,700	49,000	78,000	71,000	20,000	30,000
340	2,600	170	1,800	94	1,500	700	1,900	280	2,200

be 11.4 times greater than that in normal breast tissue. DeJeorge and associates[3] noted a significant increase in the phosphorus concentration of malignant breast tissue, as did Mulay and associates.[8]

Copper. This element was found to be 2.3 times greater in concentration in malignant than in benign breast tissue. Mulay et al.[8] reported similar results. DeJeorge and associates[3] felt that one of the first tissue disorders in breast cancer is the accumulation of copper in malignant tissue, and also noted an increase in blood serum copper in these patients. Danielson and Steinnes[2] reported no increase in copper concentrations in malignant tissues from other organs, but did not study breast tissue. DeJeorge and associates[4] noted increased blood levels of copper in patients with cancer of the larynx correlated with increased levels in the malignant tissue.

Magnesium. The mean concentration of magnesium was eight times greater in malignant breast tissue than in normal mammary tissue. Seltzer and associates[9] reported a twofold increase in the magnesium concentration of human breast cancer with high significance ($p < 0.002$). Mulay and associates[8] reported similar results in breast cancer, but the serum concentration of this element in their study was not abnormal. DeJorge and associates,[3] however, found normal levels of tissue magnesium in mammary cancer.

Zinc. Mammary cancer was found to have a mean concentration of zinc 5.7 times that of normal breast tissue. Mulay and associates[8] reported increased zinc concentration in breast cancer compared to normal breast tissue. Danielson and Steinnes[2] cited a de-

Table II. *Trace elements in formalin preservative**

Element	Raw formalin	Formalin used for Patient 9 samples N†	Formalin used for Patient 9 samples M
Sb	14	4	6
Br	7	170	42
Cl	1,300	76,000	35,000
Cr	21	5	6
Cu	36	60	40
Au	<0.06	0.04	0.03
I	<7	<20	60
Fe	350	430	230
Mg	160	1,300	250
Mn	9	13	6
Hg	<1.0	16	11
P	240	3,000	7,500
K	6,000	25,000	53,000
Rb	4	24	52
Se	<3	<3.0	<3.0
Na	1,800	55,000	26,000
Zn	620	240	170

*Concentration: μg% wet weight.
†N = Normal breast tissue; M = malignant breast tissue.

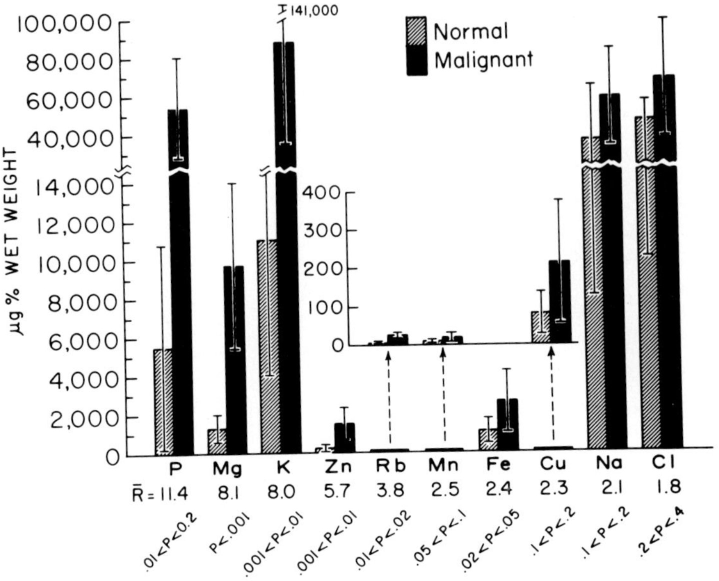

Fig. 1. Weight ratios of trace elements in malignant and normal breast tissue (nine patients). $\bar{R}$ is a mean of ratios: malignant/normal. Its limits represent 99 per cent confidence interval for this mean.

crease in zinc levels of various malignant tissues but did not study breast. Tupper and associates[10] demonstrated a small but statistically significant uptake of zinc in mammary tumors in mice.

Concentrations of this element in the blood, serum, and tissues of other malignancies are variably reported. Valberg and associates[11] reported an increased zinc content of erythrocytes in acute leukemia, chronic lymphatic leukemia, chronic myeloid leukemia, Hodgkin's disease, and metastatic carcinoma. Addink and Frank[1] concluded "unless neoplasms develop in tissues rich in zinc, the zinc level of both serum and whole blood in carcinoma cases is subnormal." They found increased blood levels of zinc in leukemia and carcinoma of the lungs (leukocytes and lung tissue being rich in zinc) and reduced levels in other cancers.

Iron. We found cancerous breast tissue to have a concentration of iron 2.4 times greater than its normal counterpart. Mulay and associates[8] found increased iron concentration in malignant breast tissue but also noted that in bronchiogenic carcinoma of the lung, the iron content of the cancerous tissue was significantly lower than normal bronchial tissue.

CONCLUSIONS

There appears to be a substantial difference in the concentration of certain trace elements in malignant and normal breast tissue, as well as in other cancers. The significance of these variations remains a matter of speculation.

Reduced adhesiveness of malignant cells was noted by Heinmets,[5] who cited evidence that some tissues can be dissociated into individual viable cells by treatment with reagents that remove positive ions. Others have suggested that differences in trace metal concentrations may reflect the known role of metaloenzymes in the anaerobic metabolism of malignancy. Trace metals are known to be essential ingredients of many metabolic activities: copper is present in enzyme systems concerned with oxidation; zinc and iron are vital to cell metabolism; manganese, magnesium, and cobalt are known to be active parts of important enzyme systems. These same elements and others, such as tin, lead, and cadmium, are also known to inhibit enzyme activity, whereas metals such as chromium, molybdenum, arsenic, asbestos, nickel, and others have been implicated as carcinogens.

Tissue levels of trace metals appear to vary not only with age, sex, and other factors, but particularly with the organ of origin.[1, 8] Differences in concentration must, therefore, be evaluated in terms of normal values for a particular organ rather than in absolute terms.

An understanding of the role of trace elements in malignancy awaits more information on normal values in specific tissues and the pattern of change in each cancer. Neutron activation analysis offers an accurate and effective method of assembling these data.

The advice and technical support of Milton E. McLain, Jr., and the laboratory work of John H. Jackson, both of the Nuclear and Biological Sciences Division, Georgia Institute of Technology, are gratefully acknowledged.

REFERENCES

1. Addink, N. W. H., and Frank, L. J. P.: Remarks appropos of analysis of trace elements in human tissue, Cancer **12:** 544, 1959.
2. Danielson, A., and Steinnes, E.: A study of some selected trace elements in normal and cancerous tissue by neutron activation analysis, J. Nucl. Med. **11:** 260, 1970.
3. DeJeorge, F. B., Sampaio Goes, J., Jr., Guedes, J. L., and DeUlhoa Cintra, A. B.: Biochemical studies on copper, copper oxidase, magnesium, sulfur, calcium and phosphorus in cancer of the breast, Clin. Chim. Acta **12:** 403, 1965.
4. DeJeorge, F. B., Paiva, L., Mion, D., and DaNova, R.: Biochemical studies on copper, copper oxidase, magnesium, sulfur, calcium and phosphorus in cancer of the larynx, Acta Otolaryngol. **61:** 454, 1966.
5. Heinmets, F.: Analysis of normal and abnormal cell growth; model-system formulation and analog computer studies, New York, 1966, Plenum Press.
6. Leddicotte, G. W.: Activation analysis of the biological trace elements. Meth. Biochem. Anal. **19:** 345, 1971.
7. Maletskos, C. J., and Tang, C. W.: Multielement trace analysis of human tissues by neutron activation after removal of 24 Na and 42K, Phys. Med. Biol. **15:** 155, 1970.
8. Mulay, I. L., Roy, R., Knox, B. E., Suhr, N. H., and Delaney, W. E.: Trace-metal analysis of cancerous and noncancerous human tissues, J. Natl. Cancer Inst. **47:** 1, 1971.
9. Seltzer, M. H., Rosato, F. E., and Fletcher, M. J.: Serum and tissue magnesium levels in human breast carcinoma, J. Surg. Res. **10:** 159, 1970.
10. Tupper, R., Watts, R. W. E., and Wormall, A.: The incorporation of Zn^{65} in mammary tumors and some other tissues of mice after injection of the isotope, Biochem. J. **59:** 264, 1955.
11. Valberg, L. S., Holt, J. M., and Card, R. T.: Erythrocyte magnesium, copper and zinc in malignant diseases affecting the hemopoietic system, Cancer **19:** 1833, 1966.

Brief clinical reports

Duodenal duplication cysts: Diagnosis and operative management

Norman B. Ackerman, M.D., Ph.D., *Kansas City, Mo.*

Duplication cysts of the duodenum, although uncommon, are important because of the difficulties in diagnosis and surgical treatment. A case report is presented in which the preoperative diagnosis was made accurately and the symptoms of nausea and upper gastrointestinal vomiting were readily controlled by a simple surgical procedure. Awareness of the condition, with x-ray and endoscopic techniques, should increase the accuracy of preoperative diagnosis. Because of the proximity of many of these cysts to the ampulla of Vater, segmental resection of the diaphragm between the cyst and duodenal lumen or a cystojejunostomy should be performed.

From the Department of Surgery, Menorah Medical Center, and The School of Medicine, University of Missouri–Kansas City, Mo.

DUPLICATION CYSTS of the duodenum are uncommon lesions, representing only 4 to 12 percent of all duplications in the alimentary tract. Patients with this condition are of particular interest because of the difficulty in establishing a preoperative diagnosis and because of the variety of operative procedures proposed for treatment. An accurate preoperative diagnosis of this condition was first reported only in 1965 by Inouye and associates.[5] Their patient, a 4-year-old child, had a large cyst, 10 cm. in diameter, which was easily palpable on physical examination. In the present report, a preoperative diagnosis was made in an adult with a lesion measuring only 3 cm. in diameter. The combination of a greater awareness of this condition with newer diagnostic techniques, including fiberoptic endoscopy, has made it possible to improve diagnostic accuracy. Surgical management of this lesion is often complicated by its location adjacent to the biliary and pancreatic drainage systems and also, in some situations, by the size of the cyst. The patient in this report was treated by a simple, safe procedure, which has been effective for this type of lesion.

Accepted for publication April 4, 1974.

Reprint requests: Norman B. Ackerman, M.D., SUNY, Upstate Medical Center, Syracuse, N. Y. 13210.

CASE REPORT

The patient, a 51-year-old woman, had a 2 week history of nausea, vomiting, and mild epigastric pain. The vomiting was unrelated to eating and dark green. An upper gastrointestinal x-ray study demonstrated a filling defect within the descending limb of the duodenal sweep (Fig. 1). The patient was then admitted to the hospital for further work-up and treatment. Her past medical history included a cholecystectomy, 19 years previous to admission, and an appendectomy, 35 years ago. The physical examination at time of admission was essentially negative. The abdomen was soft, nontender, not distended, and no masses or hypertrophied organs were palpated. Pelvic and rectal examinations were negative. Admitting laboratory studies were also unremarkable. The hemoglobin, hematocrit, and white blood counts were normal,

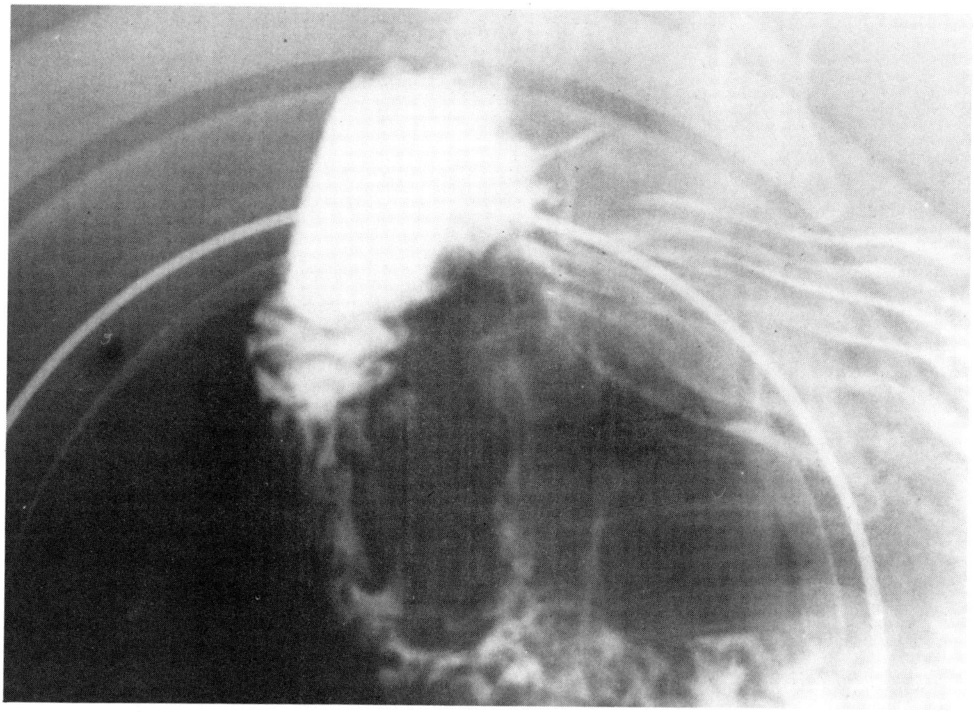

Fig. 1. Intraluminal defect seen in descending portion of duodenum on upper gastrointestinal x-rays.

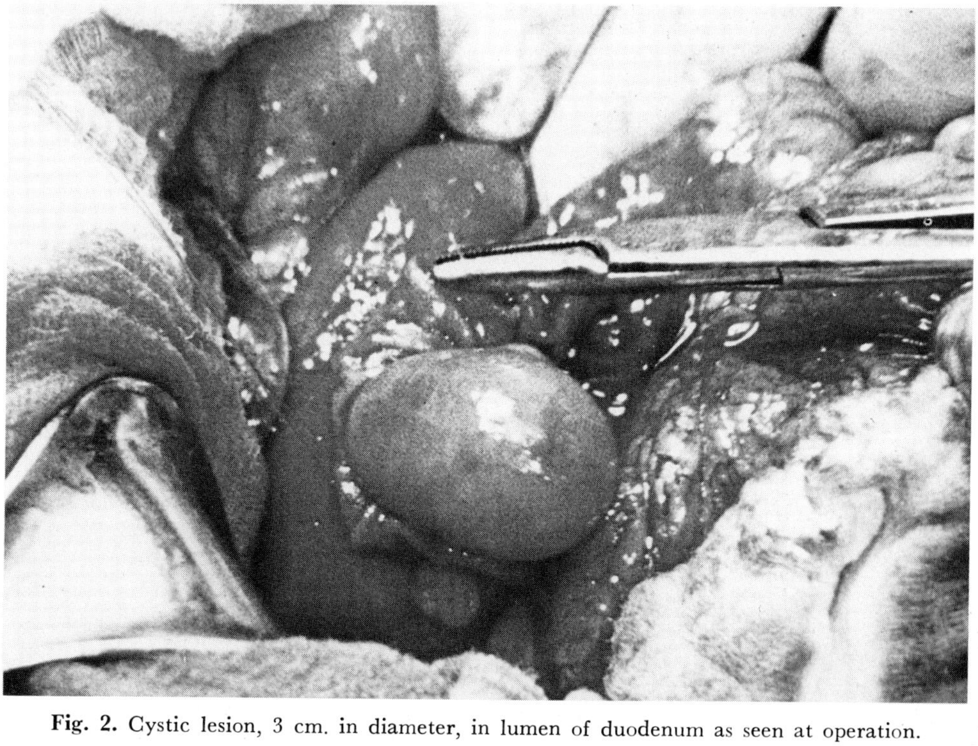

Fig. 2. Cystic lesion, 3 cm. in diameter, in lumen of duodenum as seen at operation.

as were serum electrolytes and the SMA-12. An ECG was also read as normal. Fiberoptic endoscopy was performed and revealed a 1 by 3 cm. cystic lesion of the descending duodenum. A biopsy was taken of this tissue and revealed normal duodenal mucosa. A repeat upper gastrointestinal x-ray series again revealed the filling defect in this area. This lesion appeared to move about, changing in position and outline. Barium did not enter into this mass. A diagnosis of duplication cyst of the duodenum was made, but intraluminal diverticulum and choledochal cyst were also considered. While in the hospital, the patient continued to have nausea and frequent vomiting.

An exploratory abdominal operation was then performed through a right paramedian incision. After freeing adhesions in the area of the previous cholecystectomy, a Kocher maneuver was carried out to permit full access to the descending portion of the duodenum. A cystic lesion was felt in the duodenum, corresponding to that described in the diagnostic studies. A longitudinal duodenotomy, approximately 2 inches long, was performed and a smooth-surfaced cystic lesion about 3 cm. in diameter revealed itself in the lumen (Fig. 2). The ampulla of Vater was identified proximal to the cyst, just above the superior surface. A decision was made to excise the portion of the cyst which was projecting into the lumen of the duodenum. As this tissue was being excised, the milky mucous fluid within the cyst was aspirated. The cut edges of the cyst were then oversewn with 3-0 chromic catgut for hemostasis and the back wall of the cyst, which blended with the posteriomedial surface of the duodenum, was left intact. After this operation, any further drainage from this tissue would be able to flow into the intestinal lumen. The ampulla was not disturbed and bile was seen draining from this at the conclusion of the procedure. The duodenotomy was then closed transversely with 3-0 silk.

On pathological study, the excised tissue was reported to be lined with columnar epithelium, and Paneth cells were seen in the depths of the glands. A lamina of smooth muscle was noted, which ultimately joined with the smooth muscle of the muscularis mucosa of the bowel. The patient made an uneventful postoperative recovery. A postoperative upper gastrointestinal x-ray no longer showed the duodenal lesion.

DISCUSSION

Most duodenal duplication cysts are found in infants and young children, but they also can be discovered in adults of fairly advanced years. Although these are congenital, it is not known why these cysts become symptomatic, in some patients, only after many years. They appear to be equally distributed between male and female patients. The cysts have been reported as ranging in size from 2 to 12 cm. in diameter and can be single or multiple. They usually occur in the first or second part of the duodenum and share a common wall and blood supply with the duodenum. They can be either spheroid or elongated and have been described as either submucosal or intramuscular. Essentially, they can present themselves as an inwardly projecting mass within the lumen, not obviously apparent on observation of the outer surfaces of the duodenum, or they can appear to project outward, beyond the serosal surface of the normal duodenum. The duplication can communicate with the intestinal lumen or with the biliary tract, although most duplication cysts are completely intact. Related to these lesions is the so-called intraluminal diverticulum, which is believed by some to represent a partial duplication of the duodenum.[3]

Histologically, the mucosal lining of duplication cysts resembles that of the duodenum or other gastrointestinal structures, including stomach, small bowel, and pancreas. In some cysts evidence of necrosis, due to high pressures within the cyst, is apparent. The cystic fluid varies from clear to reddish-brown in color and is often milky or mucous.

The symptoms relating to these cysts are caused by partial obstruction, as the cyst projects into the duodenal lumen. Nausea and high intestinal vomiting are most commonly seen. Gastrointestinal bleeding has also been described. In some patients, where the cyst is large, a palpable mass can be identified on physical examination. Since some of the cysts have gastric mucosal linings, peptic ulceration and, rarely, perforation have been described.[1] In establishing a diagnosis, one must be aware of the possibility of duplication cysts as an explanation for the symptoms. The use of upper gastrointestinal x-rays plus gastroduodenoscopy should increase the accuracy of preoperative diagnosis. Fiberendoscopy should be especially helpful in these patients.

The treatment of choice would be a segmental resection of the bowel containing the duplication cyst.[2] However, this should not be performed when the cyst is adjacent to the biliary and pancreatic drainage systems. In these situations, if the lesion is small enough, excision of the diaphragm or roof between the cyst and intestinal lumen should be carried out. This technique is described by Harkins and Nyhus,[4] who attributed it first to Gardner and Hart in 1935. This technique offers the surgeon a simple, safe, effective means of eliminating the clinical symptoms. If the duplication is relatively large, internal drainage by cystojejunostomy, with the use of a loop of jejunum, appears to be the treatment of choice. Aspiration alone, external drainage, and marsupialization have no place in the treatment of this condition.

REFERENCES

1. Dickinson, W. E., Weinberg, S. M., and Vellios, F.: Perforating ulcer in a duodenal duplication, Am. J. Surg. **122:** 418, 1971.
2. Grosfeld, J. L., O'Neill, J. A., Jr., and Clatworthy, H. W., Jr.: Enteric duplications in infancy and childhood: An 18 year review, Ann. Surg. **172:** 83, 1970.
3. Guerrier, H. P., and Turner, M. J.: A case of intraluminal diverticulum of the duodenum, Br. J. Surg. **59:** 324, 1972.
4. Harkins, H. P., and Nyhus, L. M.: Surgery of the stomach and duodenum, ed. 2, Boston, 1969, Little, Brown & Company, p. 358.
5. Inouye, W. Y., Farrell, C., Fitts, W. T., Jr., and Tristan, T. A.: Duodenal duplication: Case report and literature review, Ann. Surg. **162:** 910, 1965.

Hepatic and splenic lymphangiomatosis with skeletal involvement: Report of a case and review of the literature

Morris J. Asch, M.D., Arthur H. Cohen, M.D., *and* **Thomas C. Moore, M.D.,**
Torrance, Calif.

A 10-year-old girl with massive hepatomegaly, splenomegaly, and lytic lesions of the second and fourth ribs due to cystic lymphangiomatosis is reported. This syndrome is discussed and 11 other cases with hepatic or splenic lymphangiomatosis are reviewed. Prognosis of this lesion is poor if significant pulmonary or hepatic involvement occurs. The differential diagnosis of cystic lesions of the liver and spleen is discussed.

From the Division of Pediatric Surgery and Renal Transplantation, Departments of Surgery, Pediatrics, and Pathology, Harbor General Hospital Campus, UCLA School of Medicine, Torrance, Calif.

Lymphangiomas are well-recognized benign tumors, frequently seen in infancy and childhood, which generally affect the somatic soft tissue. Involvement of the abdominal viscera is an extremely rare and more serious form of this process. A 10-year-old girl with diffuse hepatic and splenic lymphangiomatosis and lytic rib lesions was treated recently at the UCLA–Harbor General Hospital. The diagnostic and therapeutic problems posed by this patient prompted the following report and review of the literature.

CASE REPORT

A 10-year-old Mexican-American girl was hospitalized because of a 7 pound weight loss, decreased appetite, and occasional abdominal pain of several months' duration. Physical examination revealed massive hepatosplenomegaly (Fig. 1). No cutaneous lesions were seen. Laboratory evaluation

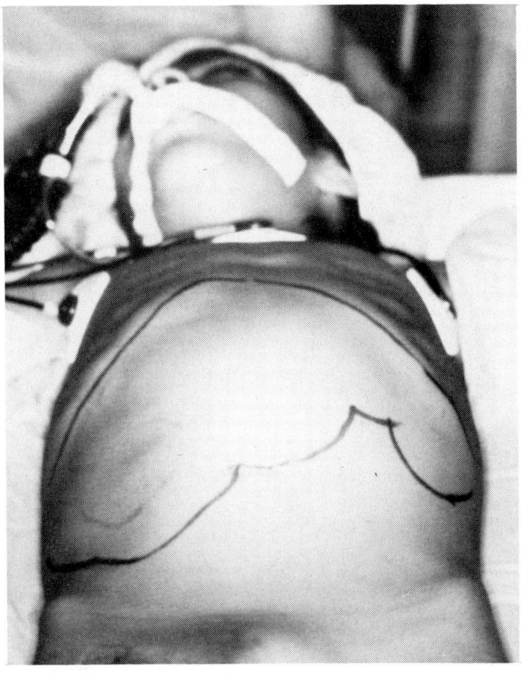

Fig. 1. Confines of massive hepatosplenomegaly outlined on abdomen.

Accepted for publication April 25, 1974.

Reprint requests: Morris J. Asch, M.D., Department of Surgery, Harbor General Hospital, 1000 W. Carson St., Torrance, Calif. 90509.

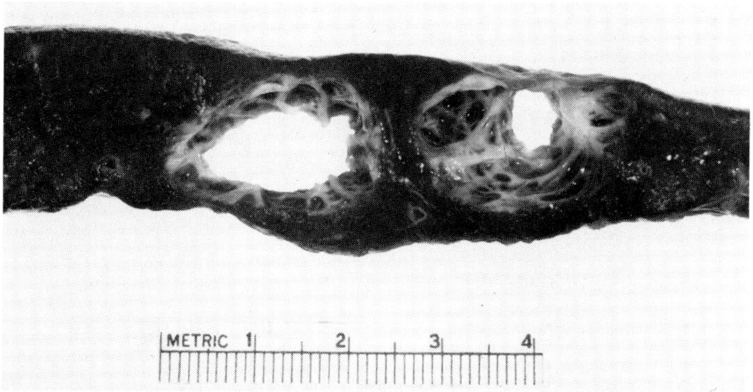

Fig. 2A. Cut surface of enlarged spleen showing multiloculated thick-walled cystic spaces.

was normal, including a negative alpha-fetoprotein and normal liver function and clotting studies. Radiological evaluation showed hepatic and splenic calcifications and lytic lesions of the second and fourth ribs. Liver scan and ultrasound studies revealed diffuse involvement of the liver and spleen with cystic lesions. Selective hepatic and splenic angiography indicated a benign appearance of these lesions. Calcified cystic lesions of the spleen raised the possibility of parasitic disease and a positive Casoni skin test led to a presumptive diagnosis of echinococcosis. At laparotomy an enlarged spleen with multiple cysts was removed. The spleen weighed 75 grams and was the site of numerous uni- and multilocular cystic spaces (Fig. 2A), containing clear serous or bloody fluid. Solid well-circumscribed nodules of firm white or yellow necrotic material were also seen (Fig. 2B).

Microscopic examination revealed many vascular channels filled with pink fluid and lined by flattened endothelial cells (Fig. 3). The largest cysts had thick fibrous walls and foci of calcification. Those cysts with a solid gross appearance were filled with amorphous eosinophilic debris, cholesterol crystals, calcium, and hemosiderin.

The massively enlarged, diffusely cystic liver (Fig. 4) was biopsied. Histological features of the liver biopsy were those of multiple small and medium-sized, endothelial-lined, vascular channels filled with eosinophilic fluid and occasionally with erythrocytes (Fig. 5). This process occupied approximately 60 percent of the hepatic parenchyma studied. Calcification was present in fibrous walls of the larger cysts. The intervening liver tissue displayed no abnormalities.

The postoperative course was uncomplicated. A hemagglutination titer obtained preoperatively was reported in the postoperative period as negative for echinococcosis. The patient has been followed for one year and remains active and well. She was the all-star catcher in her softball league. Liver size is unchanged by physical examination and scan and liver chemistries remain normal. The skeletal lesions are unchanged.

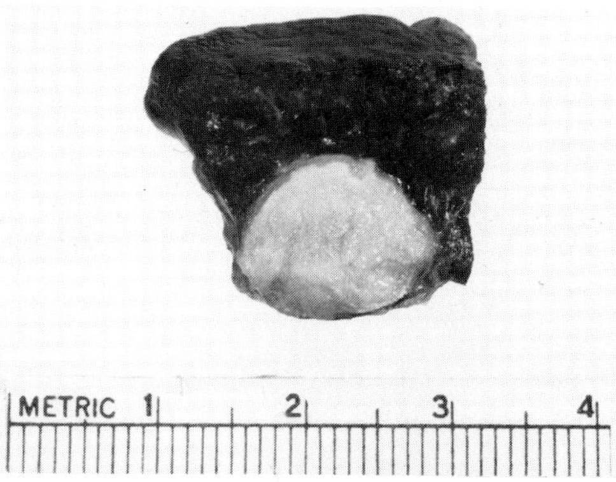

Fig. 2B. Portion of spleen containing well-circumscribed nodule, representing cyst filled with cholesterol, calcium, debris, and hemosiderin, the result of degeneration of the cyst wall and surrounding tissue.

DISCUSSION

Lymphangiomas are congenital malformations of the lymphatic system composed of lymph containing endothelial-lined spaces. Landing and Farber[10] classified lymphangiomas into three categories: (1) simple, composed of capillary-sized thin-walled lymphatic channels; (2) cavernous, made up of dilated lymphatic channels, often with fibrous adventitial coats; (3) cystic. In a recent review of 61 cases of lymphangioma, Bill and Sumner[1] described only six cases classified as "internal," five in the mediastinum and one in the mesentery. Lymphangiomas have, how-

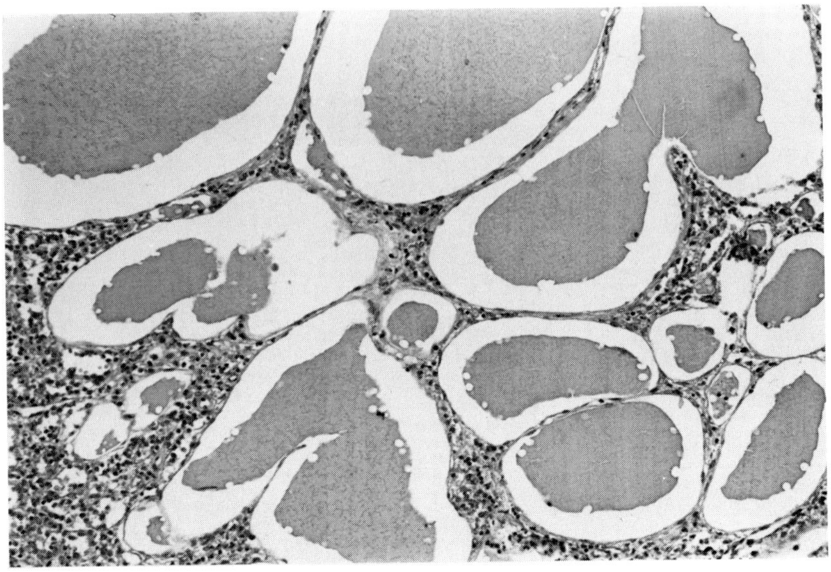

Fig. 3. Splenic parenchyma with dilated lymphatic channels filled with eosinophilic fluid and lined by flattened endothelium. (Hematoxylin and eosin; ×250.)

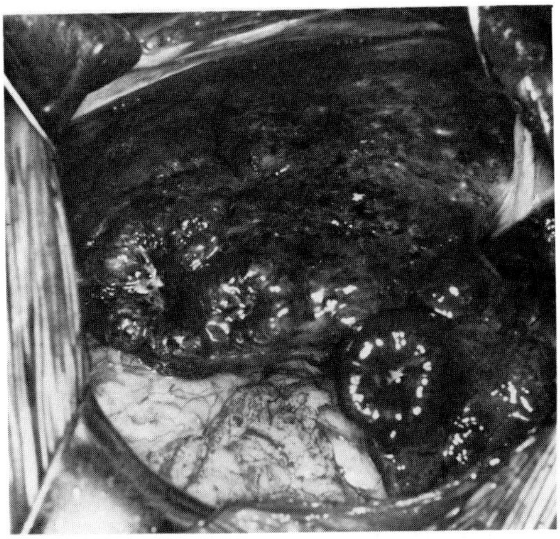

Fig. 4. Variable-sized cysts occupying most of both lobes of the liver.

ever, been described in a variety of organs, including the colon, kidney, and penis.[11, 13, 18]

When lymphangiomas involve the skeletal system this is frequently part of a generalized disorder with cystic involvement of many organs and tissues. Seckler and associates[19] first pointed this out while reviewing 12 cases and used the term "systemic cystic angiomatosis." Eight of these patients had extraosseous involvement: four had lesions of the liver, spleen, kidneys, or mediastinum and four had cystic hygromas of the neck or axilla without internal lesions. Patients with cystic angiomatosis may present with bone pain or fractures, respiratory distress, or massive hepatomegaly depending on which organ system is most involved. Gutierrez and Spjut[6] reviewed 36 cases of skeletal angiomatosis. In this report there was only one death in the 11 patients in whom the disease was confined to bone whereas 11 of the 22 patients with extraskeletal involvement died from their disease one to 12 years after diagnosis. The poor prognosis of skeletal angiomatosis with extraosseous involvement is readily apparent when one reviews the 12 cases with liver and/or spleen involvement[3-5, 7-9, 15-17, 20, 21] which have been reported (Table I). Death occurred one to 12 years after diagnosis in seven of the nine patients available for follow-up. One patient was alive and well 8 years after diagnosis and the present case has been followed for only one year; in three of the cases no follow-up is given. Diffuse pulmonary involvement was the cause of death in three patients and diffuse hepatic involvement was the cause of death in two patients.

The present case brought up the differ-

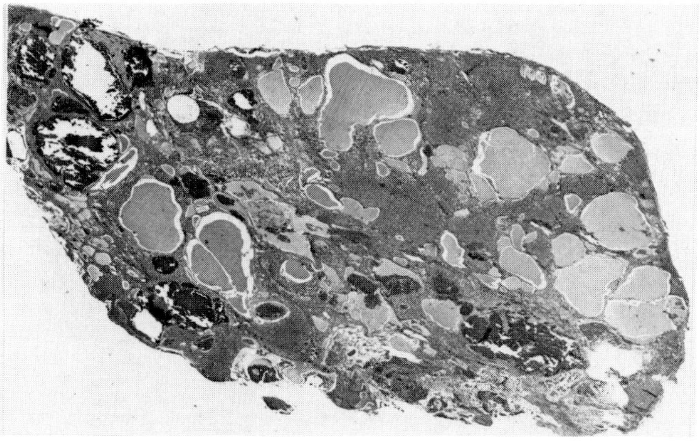

Fig. 5. Liver biopsy showing dilated lymphatics filled with lymph or blood and occupying much of the hepatic parenchyma. (Hematoxylin and eosin; ×12.)

Table I. *Review of reported cases of cystic angiomatosis of the liver and spleen*

Case No.	*Reference No.*	*Age, sex*	*Liver involved*	*Spleen involved*	*Other structures involved*	*Clinical course*
1	3	1, F	No	Yes	Vertebrae, humerus, femur, clavicle, ribs, scapula, pelvis, soft tissue of neck and shoulder	Multiple problems secondary to severe bone involvement and cervical cord compression; died age 9 of respiratory problems
2	9	1½, F	No	Yes	Skull, vertebrae, long bones, clavicle, ribs, scapula, lungs, pleura, skin	Recurrent pleural effusions; died age 5 of respiratory problems
3	17	2, M	No	Yes	Skull, vertebrae, long bones, ribs, pelvis, scapula	Multiple fractures; doing well at age 10
4	Present case	10, F	Yes	Yes	Ribs	Doing well 1 yr. follow-up
5	16	14, F	Yes	Yes	Skull, long bones, sternum, clavicle, mandible, skin, thymus, kidney, pericardium, pleura, lungs	Respiratory death age 14
6	20	15, F	Yes	Yes	Vertebrae, sternum, clavicles, thymus, kidneys, lungs	Hemoptysis, bloody ascites, pleural effusion; death age 23
7	8	21, F	Yes	Yes	Anterior mediastinum	Well after splenectomy (? length of follow-up)
8	8	26, F	No	Yes	No	Well after splenectomy (? length of follow-up)
9	7	22, F	Yes	Yes	Femur, pelvis omentum, pleura, lungs	Bloody ascites, cachexia; death age 23
10	15	27, M	Yes	Yes	Skull, sacrum	No follow-up reported
11	5	37, F	Yes	No	Skull, vertebrae, ribs, larynx, brain	Rapid development of new tumors, age 49; hemiparesis and death age 49
12	21	72, M	No	Yes	Vertebrae, femur, ribs, scapula, pelvis	Progressive sciatic pain, cachexia; death age 75

Table II. *Cystic disease of the liver**

I. True cysts:
A. Epithelial
1. Bile duct
a. Polycystic
b. Solitary
2. Squamous
a. Dermoid
3. Endothelial
a. Lymphangiomatous
b. Hemangiomatous
II. False cysts:
A. Traumatic
B. Inflammatory
1. Parasitic
2. Second to cholangitis
C. Degenerative
1. Malignant tumors

*Modified from DeBakey and Jordan.[4]

ential diagnosis of cystic lesions of the spleen and liver. McClure and Altemeier[14] divided splenic cysts into true and false categories. True splenic cysts are either epithelial (dermoid or epidermoid) or endothelial (lymphangioma, hemangioma, or serous). Epidermoid cysts are the most common true cysts of the spleen and, as pointed out by Blank and Campbell,[2] may calcify. False splenic cysts are hemorrhagic, inflammatory, or degenerative.

Hepatic cysts can also be divided into the true and false varieties (Table II). The most common cystic lesion of the liver, by far, is that which occurs as part of generalized polycystic disease.[12]

Current diagnostic measures in evaluating enlargement of the liver and spleen usually include scan and ultrasound techniques. If cystic lesions are seen the differential diagnosis described above should be considered. Skeletal x-rays should be obtained, in search of lytic lesions as part of the cystic angiomatosis syndrome. Diagnostic laparotomy usually is necessary.

If cystic lymphangiomatous disease involves only a portion of the liver, surgical removal should be considered because progression of the disease is likely. With diffuse involvement, as seen in the present case, one has little to offer in the way of therapy except, perhaps, liver transplantation. Prognosis is poor in this patient and in most patients with cystic lymphangiomatosis involving noninteg-umental extraskeletal structures.

REFERENCES

1. Bill, A. H., Jr., and Sumner, D. S.: Unified concept of lymphangioma and cystic hygroma, Surg. Gynecol. Obstet. **120:** 79, 1965.
2. Blank, E., and Campbell, J. R.: Epidermoid cysts of the spleen, Pediatrics **51:** 75, 1973.
3. Cohen, J., and Craig, J. M.: Multiple lymphangiectasis of bone, J. Bone Joint Surg. **37A:** 585, 1955.
4. De Bakey, M. E., and Jordon, G. L., Jr.: Surgery of the liver, *in* Schiff, L., editor: Diseases of the liver, Philadelphia, 1972, J. B. Lippincott Company, pp. 864-923.
5. Fischer, C., and Roeckl, H.: A case of systematized hemangiomatosis, Hautarzt **12:** 79, 1961.
6. Gutierrez, R. M., and Spjut, H. J.: Skeletal angiomatosis: Report of three cases and review of the literature, Clin. Orthop. **85:** 82, 1972.
7. Hambach, R., and Hendrich, F.: Ein Fall von generalisierter Haemangiomatose, Zentralbl. Allg. Pathol. **100:** 236, 1959.
8. Harshman, J. A., Smith, E. B., and Evans, P. V.: Cystic lymphangiectasis of the spleen, Arch. Pathol. **71:** 344, 1961.
9. Koblenzer, P. J., and Bukouski, M. J.: Angiomatosis (hamartomatous hem-lymphangiomatosis), Pediatrics **28:** 65, 1965.
10. Landing, B. H., and Farber, S.: Tumors of the cardiovascular system, *in* Atlas of tumor pathology, Washington, D. C., 1956, Armed Forces Institute of Pathology.
11. Laughlin, J. C., and Islam, M.: Lymphangiectasis of the penis: First reported case in the literature, J. Urol. **102:** 515, 1969.
12. Lieberman, E., Salinas-Madrigal, L., Gwinn, J. L., Brennan, L. P., Fine, R. N., and Landing, B. H.: Infantile polycystic disease of the kidneys and liver, Medicine **50:** 277, 1971.
13. Lindsey, J. R.: Lymphangiectasia simulating polycystic disease, J. Urol. **104:** 658, 1970.
14. McClure, R. D., and Altemeier, W. A.: Cysts of the spleen, Ann. Surg. **116:** 98, 1942.
15. Paden, P. A., and Mantz, F. A.: Benign systemic hemangiomatosis without cutaneous involvement, Radiology **64:** 252, 1955.
16. Parson, L. S., and Ebbs, J. H.: Generalized angiomatosis presenting the clinical characteristics of storage reticulosis with some observations on the reticuloendotheliosis, Arch. Dis. Child. **15:** 129, 1940.
17. Ritchie, G., and Zeier, F. G.: Hemangioma-

tosis of the skeleton and the spleen, J. Bone Joint Surg. **38A:** 115, 1956.

18. Schaeffer, J. W., Griffen, W. O., and Dubilier, L. D.: Colonic lymphangiectasis associated with a potassium depletion syndrome, Gastroenterology **55:** 515, 1968.
19. Seckler, S. G., Rubin, H., and Rabinowitz, J. G.: Systemic cystic angiomatosis, Am. J. Med. **37:** 976, 1964.
20. Shennan, T.: Histologically non-malignant angioma with numerous metastases, J. Pathol. Bacteriol. **19:** 139, 1915.
21. Zdansky, E.: Zei seltene Falle von Knochënhamangiom, Fortschr. Geb. Roentgenstr. Nuklearmed. **54:** 263, 1936.

Ischemic colitis following rectal prolapse

Y. Kawarada, M.D., S. Satinsky, M.D., *and* T. Matsumoto, M.D., Ph.D., F.A.C.S.,
Philadelphia, Pa.

A case of ischemic colitis due to prolapse of the rectum is presented. The clinical manifestation and management of ischemic colitis were reviewed and discussed.

From the Department of Surgery, Hahnemann Medical Hospital and College, Philadelphia, Pa.

ISCHEMIC COLITIS may produce several clinical syndromes due to insufficiency of the blood supply to the intestine. This disease was known by many different names until Marston and associates[13] described "ischemic colitis" due to vascular insufficiency. They divided it into three groups: gangrenous, stricturing, and transient.

Recently we had a patient who suffered from a rectal prolapse for 4 hours and reduced it by himself with difficulty. Three days prior to admission, he developed moderate rectal bleeding and lower abdominal pain and was brought to the Hahnemann Hospital emergency room.

CASE REPORT

W. W. was a 55-year-old black man who had felt well until 4 days prior to admission. He presented with a 3 day history of diarrhea, with moderate amounts of bright red rectal bleeding. He denied any previous history of bleeding, abdominal pain, constipation, and indigestion except a rectal prolapse for 2 years. He had had an episode of prolapse of the rectum 4 days previously and reduced it himself, with difficulty, after 4 hours.

Physical examination revealed a healthy black male who looked older than his stated age and was in no acute distress. The pulse was 120 per minute and regular; temperature, 99.4° F.; respirations, 18 per minute; blood pressure, 140/100 mm. Hg. The chest had an increased A-P diameter and expiratory wheezing and rhonchi were evident. The abdomen was soft, with normal bowel sounds and without tenderness. Liver was palpable at 2 cm. below the right costal margin. Rectal examination revealed engorged internal hemorrhoids, hard irregular masses at the end of the examining finger, and fresh blood stains.

On admission, laboratory studies showed normal results except slightly elevated glucose; chest x-ray was normal; the ECG was abnormal with ST changes; hematocrit, 32; hemoglobin, 9.8; white blood cells, 13,000, with normal differential; urinalysis, normal.

Sigmoidoscopy revealed multiple, nodular, circumferential, darkish brown masses, up to 20 cm., with small amounts of brightish blood. Colonoscopy revealed extensive ischemic changes up to 30 cm. from the anus. Barium enema performed on the same day showed irregular surface and thumbprinting marks on the rectum and the lower portion of the sigmoid (Figs. 1 and 2). Ischemic proctitis was diagnosed at this time. Three days later a selective superior and inferior mesenteric arteriogram was performed. There was no evidence of stenosis or occlusion at the origin or main branches of either the inferior or superior mesenteric arteries but the findings in the terminal branches of these arteries were unclear due to the previous barium enema. Both veins were patent. The patient was treated conservatively but, on the fourth day after admission, he developed rectal

Accepted for publication April 4, 1974.

Reprint requests: Teruo Matsumoto, M.D., Department of Surgery, Hahnemann Medical College and Hospital, 230 N. Broad St., Philadelphia, Pa. 19102.

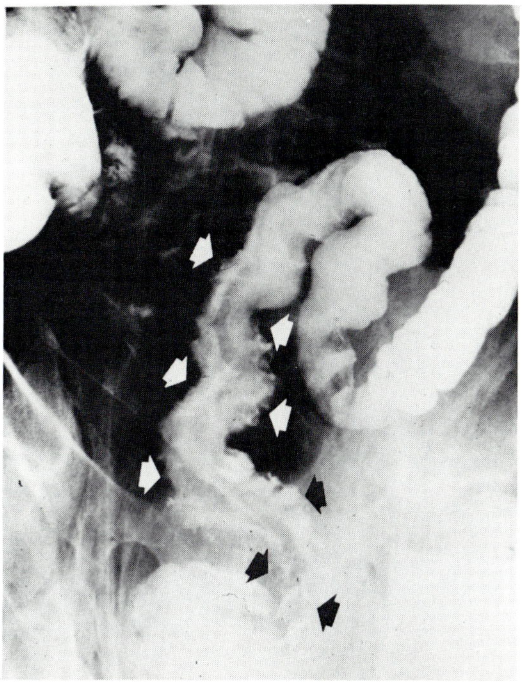

Fig. 1. Barium enema on admission. White and black arrows show irregular surface of rectum and middle portion of sigmoid with slightly narrowed lumen.

bleeding (approximately 500 ml.) and underwent an operation on the same day. Sigmoidoscopic examination again revealed hyperemic and edematous sigmoid and rectum but there was no evidence of gangrene on the surface of the colon or of active bleeding. Transverse colostomy was performed. The patient had an uneventful recovery and was discharged in satisfactory condition on the seventh postoperative day with a carefully scheduled follow-up program. On the six-month follow-up examination the patient was doing well and no further rectal bleeding had been noted. Barium enema at that time revealed severe stricture of the rectum and the middle portion of the sigmoid (Fig. 3). A sigmoidoscope could not be passed beyond 6 cm. from the anus.

ETIOLOGY

This disorder is often caused by reduction in blood flow to the involved segment of bowel with resultant infarction dependent on the site of occlusion and collateral circulation. Those occlusions can be of the middle colic or inferior mesenteric vessels, but can also be localized to the marginal arteries, rectal vessels, or intramural arteries. The most frequent site is the splenic flexure because of its vascular vulnerability. Less frequently it is the descending and transverse colon. Rarely the ascending colon, sigmoid, and rectum are involved.

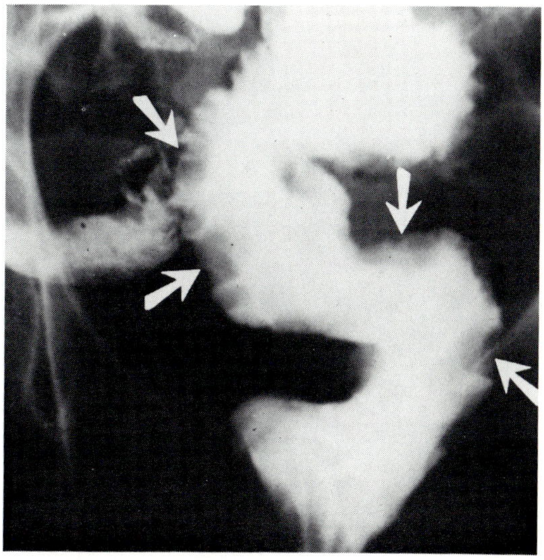

Fig. 2. Barium enema on admission. White arrows show "fingerprints or thumbprints."

Artherosclerotic plaques are common at the origins of the three main visceral arteries in the old-age group and blood pressure fluctuations may result in shut-down of peripheral vessels.[10] Reduced cardiac output and hypertension in congenital heart failure and shock may be implicated. An embolism may occur in a patient with mitral valve disease or a myocardial infarction.

Among other causes Boley and associates[4] listed local compression of the intramural vessels in ileus of the colon or in severe fecal impaction, diabetes, allergy, volvulus,[1] and parasitic infections. Trauma,[6] ruptured extrauterine pregnancy[7] with hypotension and local vascular compression, oral contraceptive agents,[11] rheumatoid vasculitis,[13] and amyloidosis[5] have also been described. Acute nonspecific colitis may infrequently occur proximal to a partially obstructing neoplasm[8, 9] but a case has been reported of the ischemic features of the disease with the presence of a nonobstructing carcinoma.[14] Patients are definitely at risk from ischemic colitis if the inferior mesenteric artery has been previously ligated surgically.[3, 13]

No case report of ischemic colitis following

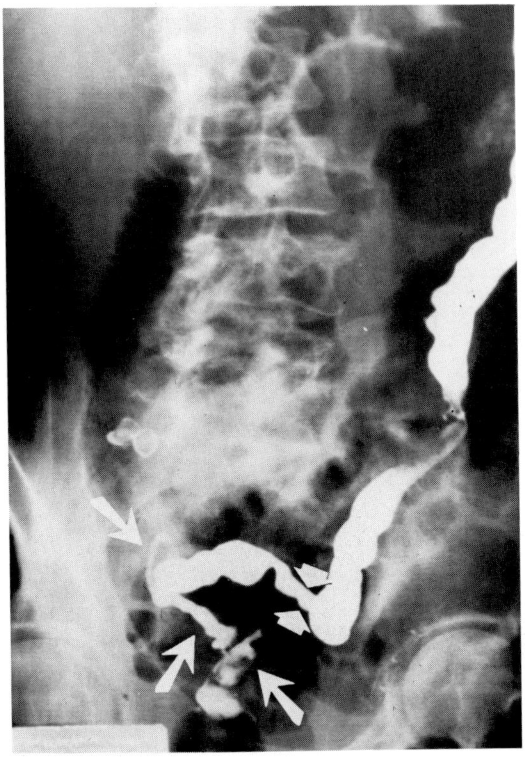

Fig. 3. Barium enema 6 months after transverse colostomy. White arrows show stricture of rectum and sigmoid.

a rectal prolapse has been published. This report presents the unusual case of a patient with the typical findings of ischemic colitis after the prolapse.

PATHOLOGICAL FINDINGS

The pathological changes of ischemic colitis are characteristic. Varying amounts of stricture formation and thickening of the intestinal wall and narrowing of the lumen and mucosal ulceration are seen. There are necrosis, ulceration, and hemorrhage. The mucosa has lost its full thickness in the ulcerated areas and epithelial regeneration is present at the edges. If the submucosa is involved it is most conspicuously changed by being widened and filled with granulation tissue. The cellular infiltrate includes many hemosiderin-filled microphages similar to those seen in resolving ischemic myocarditis.[13]

DIAGNOSIS

Ischemic colitis appears in patients usually above the age of 50 with the majority in the sixth and seventh decades. Usually their bowel habits have been regular and have not previously suggested ulcerative colitis or regional enteritis. Sometimes patients have had one episode similar to their presenting one. Rarely, abdominal angina is in the history. Presenting symptoms are lower abdominal pain, usually in the lower left quadrant, and the passage of bright red blood and clots per rectum. Occasionally patients are febrile and have some vomiting. Leukocytosis may be present. If gangrene followed by perforation occurs, it develops within the first 24 hours.[2] If stricture formation follows later in the patients' course, anorexia, increasing constipation, distension, and pain may be evident.

Physical findings are tenderness and spasm in the left lower quadrant. Sigmoidoscopy may be suggestive of proctocolitis, but most usually reveals only bloody material from above. In a rare case of rectal involvement, findings ranging from flat, superficial mucosal ulcers to an irregular, nodular type of necrosis are seen, as in our case.

X-ray. On plain film of the abdomen, dilatation of the colon may be seen. Barium enema demonstrates the stricture formation characteristically involving the splenic flexure. Four types of abnormalities have been noted in the examination of the stricture: "thumbprinting" representing a polypoid change in bowel mucosa, ragged "saw-tooth" irregularity of mucosa, tubular narrowing, and sacculation. Results of a repeat barium enema in patients with transient ischemic colitis can return to normal.

Differential diagnosis. This disease must be differentiated mainly from Crohn's disease, ulcerative colitis, and carcinoma. Differentiation is by site of involvement. Sacculation is not found on x-ray in any of the abovementioned diseases. Stricturing is seen in carcinoma, but usually an extension of the neoplasm into the lumen and a short segment of stricture can be ruled out.

TREATMENT

Marston and associates[13] divided ischemic colitis into three types, corresponding to the degrees of ischemia. The first type includes the progression to gangrene with clostridial superinfection requiring immediate operation, resection, and exteriozation. The second group, which includes the majority of cases, consists of patients with rapidly developing ischemic strictures. These patients are also treated surgically, but on an elective basis. The third group of patients have transient ischemic colitis with abdominal pain, rectal bleeding, and thumb-printing on x-ray. The disease in this group subsides with antispasmodic drugs and mild mechanical laxatives.

The treatment of ischemic colitis is dependent upon the stage. There is no special treatment for transient ischemia[12] but careful observation must be applied. Ischemic stricture without clinical indications of gangrene may usually be treated by elective resection and anastomosis if the upper rectum is not involved; if the bowel seems to be viable, then a temporary colostomy may be considered for further evaluation. Gangrene of the colon should be treated by replacement of blood volume, antiboitics, and excision of the necrotic bowel.

REFERENCES

1. Avnet, N. L., and Elkin, M.: Unusual appearance of the colon following sigmoid volvulus, Radiology **77:** 836, 1961.
2. Balsleu, Jensen, H. E., Norgaard, F., and Poll, P.: Ischemic colitis, Acta Chir. Scand. **136:** 235, 1970.
3. Bentlif, P. S., and Chir, M. B.: Ischemic disease of the colon, South. Med. J. **62:** 1452, 1969.
4. Boley, S. J., Schwartz, S., Krieger, H., Schultz, L., Sieu, F., and Allen, A. C.: 1965.
5. Brom, B., Bank, S., Marks, I. N., et al.: Ischemic colitis, gastric ulceration, and malabsorption in a case of primary amyloidosis: Gastroenterology **57:** 319, 1969.
6. Corbett, R.: Stenosed segment of descending colon associated with trauma, Pro. R. Soc. Med. **50:** 271, 1957.
7. Curr, J. F.: Rectal stricture due to ischemia following ruptured ectopic gestation, Gut **8:** 178, 1967.
8. Glotzer, D. J., Roth, S. I., and Welch, C. E.: Colonic ulceration proximal to obstructing carcinoma, Surgery **56:** 950, 1964.
9. Hurwitz, A., and Khafif, R. A.: Acute necrotizing colitis proximal to obstructing carcinoma, Surg. Gynecol. Obstet. **111:** 749, 1960.
10. Jordan, P. H., Boulafendis, D., and Guinn, G. A.: Factors other than major vascular occlusion that contribute to intestinal infarction, Ann. Surg. **171:** 189, 1970.
11. Kilpatrick, Z. M., Silverman, J. F., Betancourt, E., Farman, J., and Lawson, J. P.: Vascular occlusion of the colon and oral contraceptives, N. Engl. J. Med. **278:**.438, 1968.
12. Lewis, M. I.: Reversible ischemic colitis, Dis. Colon Rectum **16:** 121, 1973.
13. Marston, A., Pheils, M. T., Thomas, M. L., and Morson, B. C.: Ischemic colitis, Gut **7:** 1, 1966.
14. Petigrow, N., and Ludwig, W.: Ischemic colitis associated with carcinoma of the sigmoid colon, Am. J. Gastroenterol. **56:** 559, 1971.

Letters to the editors

Is the author the writer? Who cares?

To the Editors:

As a writer, I cheered Lois DeBakey on as I read her article entitled "Rewriting and the by-line: Is the author the writer?" in the January, 1974, issue of SURGERY. After all, what writer wants the nicotine-stained fingers of some ruthless editor striking out one's best prose and penciling in gross inaccuracies?

As an editor, however, I found her article extremely naive. I even bit down very hard on my pipe stem when I read her conclusion that, because a scientist has worthwhile information to communicate, "it is reasonable to expect such an informed person to know how to convey that information intelligibly." Would that it were always so! It is as reasonable to expect all architects to be fine carpenters and all football players to be great sports writers. The two skills do not necessarily co-exist in the same person.

Ideally, the author of a scientific article is attempting to present important information to a specific audience for that audience's benefit. If the scientist is not an accomplished communicator, then the job of helping him convey that important information falls to the editor. If the author shows writing ability, the editor may return the manuscript with an outline for specific revision. If the author doesn't, then the editor must recognize that his primary responsibility is to the reader. The editor will reorganize articles, rewrite turgid prose, repair poor construction, delete superfluous material, challenge unsupported statements, and request additional information from the author. Most importantly, the editor will then present a prepublication copy of the revised manuscript to the author for suggestions and corrections. Through all of this, the editor will also attempt to preserve the author's distinctive style and language as much as possible—not so much for the author's ego but to give variety to the journal for the reader's sake.

If a scientist truly wants to be a writer, or to be a better writer, surely it is reasonable to expect such an informed person to seek out one of the many courses of instruction in expository writing offered by universities and even by some high school adult education programs. Probably he doesn't; he wants to be a scientist.

That does not excuse him from attempting to make his paper clear, well-organized, and complete or from attempting to improve with each new paper. But it means the scientist should not be reluctant to allow a good editor (and there are many) to help him communicate better to those in his field. To communicate knowledge—not to boost the egos of editors or authors—is the reason articles and journals are published. The degree of communication determines how well they are read.

John H. Lavin
RN Magazine
Medical Economics Co.
Oradell, N. J. 07649

Reply: Authorship in scholarly journals

To the Editors:

Mr. Lavin's letter regarding "Rewriting and the by-line: Is the author the writer?" is best answered by suggesting that he reread my article.

Mr. Lavin's argument resorts to logical fallacies. His description of my article as "naive" amounts to an *argumentum ad hominem*. I continued to read beyond that characterization in expectation of an explanation, but found no factual evidence—only an emotional reaction: "I even bit down very hard on my pipe stem." My statement, "Presumably the author is writing because he has worthwhile information to communicate, and it is reasonable to expect

Vol. 76, No. 2, pp. 344-358

such an informed person to know how to convey that information intelligibly," in no way contradicts the fact that some such informed persons may not be able to do so; yet that is what Mr. Lavin implies. Those who cannot convey the information intelligibly, I urged to acquire the skill to do so.

Nor did I state that ability to do research and ability to write well always coexist. The point I made was that anyone who has information that is worthy of publication in a scholarly journal should learn how to write it himself instead of relying on someone else's words.

The analogies Mr. Lavin offers, I cannot accept. The architect is to the carpenter not as the scientist is to the writer, but as the scientist is to the technician or as the writer is to the typist or printer. In the one case (architect, scientist, writer), the activity is primarily cerebral, and in the other (carpenter, technician, typist), it is primarily mechanical. The tired analogy of football players–sports writers is too far-fetched for me to comment on.

Mr. Lavin suggests that there is something contradictory about being a scientist and a writer at the same time, as though the two activities were antithetical. Does he imagine that da Vinci, Vesalius, Galileo, Harvey, Newton, Darwin, Pasteur, Bernard, Huxley, and Einstein all had ghostwriters? I doubt it. I happen to know a number of physicians and a number of scientists who write entirely competently—far better than any copy-editor or ghostwriter I know. And these physicians and scientists would not allow their names to be placed in the by-line of an article written or totally recast by someone else.

I challenge Mr. Lavin or anyone else to perform the miracle he describes: He will "reorganize articles, rewrite turgid prose, repair poor construction, [and] delete superfluous material" without—mind you—notably changing "the author's distinctive style and language."

A word about Mr. Lavin's closing statement: "The degree of communication determines how well they [journals] are read." Perhaps how *widely* journals are read depends, at least partly, on how well they are written, but how *well* one reads depends on his educational background and the development of his critical faculties.

Mr. Lavin asks: "Is the author the writer? Who cares?" My reply: History, the integrity of science, and the scholar care. In addition and in particular, I hope that the person named in the by-line cares.

Lois DeBakey, Ph.D.
Professor of Scientific Communication
Baylor College of Medicine
Houston, Texas 77025

A splendid statement on a taboo subject

To the Editors:

Permit me to commend you and any others on the editorial staff of SURGERY responsible for having accepted and published Dr. Lois DeBakey's recent courageous paper in which she raises certain pertinent and timely, if to some embarrassing, questions as to the righteousness of factitious authorship. The acceptance of "ghost writing" as a necessary expedient to certain contemporary surgeons because of uncommon demands on their time absurdly implies that the great titans of world surgery in the past were less pressured, less busy, a reasoning which is of course unacceptable in the light of well-recorded history.

It is more likely that the current practice on the part of too many who willingly turn over their "material" to professional writers springs from faulty capabilities on the part of him to whom the finished paper is accredited, or perhaps in addition from his desire to produce a bibliography more notable for the quantity, not quality, of its papers.

Be these things as they may, the true scholar should be as capable as he is ardently desirous of personally expressing the results of his own studies and observations. I could not agree more with Dr. DeBakey's conclusion that those without the fundamental talent of acurate expression represent a dubious species of scholarship which assuredly must be considered suspect.

In closing, I would like to say it's always a stimulating and delightful experience to read and relish communications by Dr. Lois DeBakey, whose limitless dynamic vocabulary coupled with facile rhetorical perfection yields prose of the very highest order. And beyond all this, I've never known her precise language ever to have been mobilized except when she has had something important to say.

Again, my appreciation for SURGERY having published a splendid statement on a heretofore neglected and seemingly taboo subject.

R. Gordon Holcombe, Jr., M.D.
1607 Foster St.
Lake Charles, La. 70601

Myocardial glycogen

To the Editors:

I have read the interesting article by Hewitt and his associates in the January issue of SURGERY and I would like to suggest an additional study for their model which would be to perfuse the saline Group II with intralipid which together with the heparin in the system should provide fatty acids to meet the energy requirements during the aerobic period and build up glycogen for the anaerobic period. Another group would be to perfuse the system with isotonic three percent amino acids which would also provide a fuel source and save glycogen. Thus during the anaerobic period glycolysis or glycogenolysis is available for the fuel source.

In the intact animal the high rate of gluconeogenesis in the liver produces an excess of glucose even without exogenous infusion of energy substrate to meet the energy requirements of brain and heart and other tissues dependent upon anaerobic glycolysis. It is our opinion that in the intact animal the exogenous administration of dextrose and water makes it necessary for the substrate for gluconeogenesis in the liver to come from the viscera amino acid by protein catabolism and inhibit the rate of skeletal muscle protein breakdown by overriding the insulin resistance. This occurs both by the mass action of the infused glucose raising the circulating glucose level and the endogenous stimulation of insulin which overrides the skeletal muscle insulin resistance and blocks mobilization of amino acids from the source.

Regarding the mechanism of "GKI" I would like to suggest that it is due to the inotrophic effect of insulin rather than the provision of additional glucose or potassium. Insulin, besides regulating fuel utilization, has a direct hyperplastic effect on cellular membranes and activates ATPase, protein kinase and other important components of membrane contractility and ion exchange that are necessary for the electrical activity of heart and other contracting cells.

A means of differentiating the effect of insulin vs. that of glucose would be to look at the affluent/effluent PO_2 in these various group studies, a measure of free fatty acids, glucose and insulin.

George L. Blackburn, M.D., Ph.D.
Assistant Professor of Surgery
Senior Research Associate,
Massachusetts Institute of Technology
Cambridge, Mass. 02139

Reply

To the Editors:

Dr. Blackburn has contributed significantly to our understanding of the importance of mobilization and use of endogenous fat and to use of isotonic amino acid infusates for protein sparing in patients. He has suggested use of intravenous fat and isotonic amino acids as possible methods of increasing or conserving cardiac glycogen content during aerobic metabolism. Both of these approaches deserve investigation.

We would agree with the general concept that in the intact animal with adequate circulation a high rate of gluconeogenesis produces adequate glucose to meet energy requirements of the heart under anaerobic conditions. Our studies relate only to the anoxic heart as produced by ischemic arrest.

Certainly, the possible direct effects of insulin upon contractility, must be considered as important in the experiments utilizing perfusion of the isolated heart with glucose, potassium, and insulin during ischemic arrest although our studies did not evaluate the effects of insulin without glucose. The best evidence for the direct effect of glucose was observed in the group perfused with glucose but not insulin. Work in progress suggests additional evidence for a direct effect of potassium.

Robert L. Hewitt, M.D.
Theodore Drapanas, M.D.
Department of Surgery
Tulane University School of Medicine
New Orleans, La. 70112

Debridement

To the Editors:

May I add a footnote to the article on debridement by Owen H. Wangensteen and Sarah A. Wangensteen (SURGERY 74: 641, 1973) to point out the role of linguistics in the development of the concept particularly during and in the years following the First World War. The primary meaning of the French verb "débrider" is "to unbridle" (bride [Fr.] = bridle), and this was extended by French surgeons to express the release of tension in wounds by incision of potentially or actually constricting fascial layers. For their English-speaking colleagues the term was, not unnaturally but wrongly, assumed to come from the anglicized French word "débris," and it was used to express the removal of necrotic tissue and other debris from wounds.

Linguistic xenophobia after the war led several English surgeons to propose the abandonment of the term and the substitution of the term "excision," which they presumably thought of as a pure English word in spite of its derivation from the Latin. This had an unfortunate effect on the development of the concept in two ways. First, by stressing the act of cutting away rather than what should be cut away, it often led to the unnecessary sacrifice of healthy tissue, particularly skin. Second, the idea gradually crept in that the object was the excision not just of dead but of potentially infected tissue, and from this was developed a variable but fallacious series of rules limiting the procedure to certain time intervals after the receipt of the wound.

The marriage of the French and English interpretations of the term so clearly expresses the principle of the surgical procedure that its survival and present general acceptance are fortunate, purists of English perhaps being satisfied by the dropping of the acute accent on the first "e."

David Patey
2, Cannongate Close
Hythe, Kent CT21 4AG
England

The role of débridement—Reply to Mr. Patey's Interrogatory

To the Editors:

Mr. David Patey, well-known London surgeon and teacher at the Middlesex Hospital, very properly proposes a critical interrogatory concerning what surgeons strive to achieve in performing débridement and/or revision of contaminated wounds. The choice of terms, I would agree, is a secondary consideration. Unfortunately, Mr. Patey's query is not susceptible of a simple and satisfying answer without a look at the history of the procedure.

First, an explanation perhaps is in order how it happened that this paper appeared in SURGERY, when it had been presented at a session of the Société Internationale de Chirurgie in August, 1971. When this writer noted that the Editor of the Society's Journal had published the authors' paper on Carl Reyher in a few lines in four languages, he appreciated the Journal's Editor and the Society's Secretary-General had no intention of publishing the paper as submitted. An office copy was sent to the Editors of SURGERY, who kindly assented to its publication.

In his great book, *That Knight Errant of Surgery,* Ambroise Paré (1579) (Thomas Johnson's translation, 1634, pp. 408-425) sketched the need for immediate dilatation of gunshot wounds, accompanied by extraction of all lodged foreign bodies including wood, clothing, armor, bone splinters, bullets, and bruised or lacerated muscle and blood clots, together with provision for drainage, an instruction that he had previously made in his initial publication on wound management on the abandonment of boiling oil (1545).

Larrey, Napoleon's celebrated military surgeon (1812, v. 1, p. 50), a keen advocate of preventive débridement, credited his teacher, Desault, with reviving interest in the procedure. Even so, most military surgeons of several nations including the British and the French disaffected any suggestion of serious interest in débridement or wound revision over many decades in the 19th century. A notable exception was Begin, who, in debates at the French National Academy lasting many months in 1848, defended débridement on the basis of personal experience in military action.

The authors felt the significant work of Reyher needed to be better known. Whereas the names of Paré, Larrey, and Friedrich (1898) have stood out prominently in the history of wound revision, actually it was Carl Reyher who, in the Russo-Turkish Wars of 1876-1878, established in carefully projected prospective studies that a combination of wound antisepsis with early débridement succeeded in lowering considerably the mortality of gunshot injuries of the extremities. It is to be remembered too that Reyher had spent considerable time with Lister in Edinburgh and reported upon his observations on Listerian wound management at the German Surgical Congress in April, 1874. It may well be that the corroborative evidence, provided later by Richard Volkmann (Dec. 1874) and by Johann Nussbaum (1875) and brought to the support of Lister's work, stemmed in part from the earlier favorable report of Reyher. He was the first to perform débridement under reasonably well-controlled antiseptic conditions.

It was actually World War I which served to focus attention upon revision of wounds attending military action. The English surgeon, Colonel H. M. Gray, wrote in the Aug. 28, 1915, issue of the *British Medical Journal* that he had employed wound revision with primary suture since November, 1914, and had been greatly impressed by the results. The Inter-Allied Surgical Council held conferences and debates in Paris (1917) upon the matter of revision of contaminated wounds. It was agreed that primary wound closure was justifiable only when less than eight hours had elapsed since infliction of the wound. The French surgeon, Lemaitre, disagreed, making an emotional appeal for primary suture after revision, much as it had been done by Gray (Lyon Chir. **15:** 107, 1918). The advices of Theodore Tuffier, who strongly favored delayed closure, carried the day. In World War II the Surgeon General of the American Army, Norman Kirk, placed in the hands of all military surgical personnel an instruction that read, "Primary suture of all wounds of extremities under war conditions is never to be done." This directive has continued to be carried out in all subsequent American military conflicts, which experience has confirmed the virtue and important role of early débridement for contaminated wounds, confirming the opinion of Reyher (1881) and of Friedrich (1898).

In writing of the management of war wounds (Lancet **2:** 521, 1848), the British military surgeon, G. J. Guthrie, wrote of "débridement" of gunshot wounds, perhaps the first use of the word débridement in British literature to characterize wound revision, antedating its use by the lexicographer, Mayne (1854), by several years. Said Guthrie in this discussion, "France and England are much too proud to take the slightest advantages of each other in matters of science," a very appropriate instruction.

Since the days of the Hippocratic writings, the cautery had often been used as a last resort to control wound infection and hospital gangrene by pre-Listerian surgeons, notably Nussbaum (1875), a practice that adoption of Listerian principles brought to a halt, save for a very few enthusiastic worshippers of the curative powers of the cautery, represented by Mitchell Banks (1892).

Reyher (1881) brought a new dimension to débridement with the simultaneous use of Listerian practices. Prior thereto, in performing wound revision, surgeons had brought unclean hands and instruments to the task. Reyher deserves the major credit for terminating primary amputation for gunshot injury of an extremity in military action. The great military surgeons of the early 19th century including Percy (1811), Larrey (1812), Guthrie (1815), Thomson (1816), and Hennen (1818) all advocated early amputation for gunshot injuries of warfare, of which practice Larrey was the chief exponent. From the Napoleonic Wars (1792-1815) up through the Franco-Prussian War of 1870-71, including the Crimean (1854-56) and the American Civil War (1861-65), amputation continued to be the favored remedy of military surgeons for gunshot wounds of the extremities; in fact such too had been the practice for compound fracture by many prominent 18th and 19th century surgeons up to the time of Lister (1867).

Whereas Paré (1579) did excise contused and damaged tissue, his primary emphasis was upon removal of foreign bodies and wound drainage (Johnson's translation, 1634, pp. 408-25). Reyher's emphasis was upon early excision of traumatized and necrotic tissue, employing Listerian antiseptic wound practices to combat infection. In World War I, the military surgeons of the Allied Command in performing débridement had substituted irrigation with Dakin's hypochlorite for phenol for contaminated wounds, with a view to overcoming infection. Fleming (1919), an experienced microbiologist of wounds in World War I, very courageously advised surgeons to abandon placement of antiseptics into gunshot wounds, noting that more damage was done the tissues than the bacteria thereby.

That cellulitic infections can be neither drained nor excised every wound surgeon came to know in the era prior to the availability of sulfanilamide (1935) and antibiotics (1942-45). This surgeon has cited such an instance (Surg. Gynecol. Obstet. **137:** 694, 1973). In fact, there was no treatment for any of the cellulitic infections such as erysipelas, puerperal fever, or scarlet fever, prior to sulfanilamide and penicillin, a statement that the vital statistics of all countries will substantiate. Prior thereto the role of the surgeon in dealing with wound infection was essentially that of a pus excavator.

Fasciotomy in American surgical literature has come to replace one of the early meanings of débridement, decompression by incision of overlying fascia, a procedure especially applicable to situations in which an obstructed venous outflow from an extremity threatens tissue viability. Some surgeons have mistranslated the French word *refraîcher* as freshening the edges of the contaminated wound ("primäre anfrischung"). To Desault and Larrey, this writer believes débridement meant primary pruning or paring of the contaminated wound. I am convinced that most students of wound management today, whether they speak of débridement or wound excision or revision, are in general agreement over what is to be done in carrying out the procedure though they may provide somewhat differing explanations of why it is done.

Domagk, the Trefouëls, Fleming, Florey, and Chain brought again a new dimension to débridement with the first definitive suggestion of control of bacterial infection in wounds by chemotherapeutic means.

Bhaskar and his associates (1971) at the Walter Reed Hospital Research Center have injected still another dimension into the problem of débridement, viz., the role of energized jet irrigation with penicillin at 60 psi in the hope of lessening the need and the extent of excision of damaged and devitalized tissue. Whether such a device will relegate conventional débridement to a secondary role in the management of contaminated wounds, resulting from military action or civil trauma, would appear to be highly speculative. In the absence of crushed or devitalized tissue, this writer's experience with wounds of rabbits and guinea pigs, contaminated with 10^8 staphylococcus, suggests that such jet irrigations with penicillin do compare favorably in early hours with débridement. Only clinical trials and experience, however, can definitely settle the issue. Certainly the experience of both World Wars and the observations of American military surgeons in the Korean and Vietnam conflicts serve to stress the need of continued emphasis upon excision of dead tissue, a point made by Reyher (1881) and strongly reaffirmed by Friedrich (1898) in his experimental studies upon the guinea pig.

In the closing years of his brilliant career as Surgeon General of our Army, Leonard Heaton (1966), in writing of military surgical practices in Vietnam, said, "Proper and adequate débridement is the foundation of success in handling combat wounds. It may be defined as a procedure for the removal of all devitalized tissue, blood clots, and foreign bodies and for the control of hemorrhage"—an interpretation not dissimilar from that of Ambroise Paré in his discourse on wound care "which King Charles the Ninth, . . . enquired of me concerning wounds made by gunshot" (p. 411, et seq.).

Foreign words do not come readily into use in any language. The 1971 edition of the *Oxford Dictionary* fails to include the word débridement, though it can be found in a 1933 supplement. In citing Henry Gray's (1915) significant contribution on revision of gunshot wounds, the well-known bibliographer, Leslie Morton of London's National Institute of Medical Research wrote, in both the second (1965) and third editions of Garrison and Morton's *Medical Bibliography* (1970), "Gray revised débridement of wounds, with primary suture, a procedure with which Desault and Larrey were familiar."

Jet irrigation of contaminated wounds with penicillin and other antibiotics may lessen the need for débridement when severely contused or necrotic muscle is not present. Certainly chemotherapeutic agents have been a tremendous boon in overcoming infection in contaminated wounds, whether administered systemically or used as a local penicillin irrigant. Until biochemical and microbiologic research devise new ways of getting rid quickly of necrotic tissue by lesser means than excision, débridement must continue to occupy a prominent place in the armamentarium of the surgeon who deals with contaminated wounds of trauma.

Finally, and briefly, in reply to Mr. Patey's very appropriate and penetrating query of what today's surgeon may expect to achieve by débridement in management of the contaminated wound, this surgeon is persuaded that its main thrust is to be directed at excision of devitalized tissue; its value in the control of infection is probably minimal, for which antibiotics have supplied a much-needed extension. How much wound irrigation with penicillin contributes beyond provision for adequate wound drainage and irrigation with saline solution, accompanied by systemic administration of antibiotics, we must look to future experiments and clinical trials for a satisfying and convincing answer. Energized jet wound irrigation does facilitate removal of wound debris; though it lessens the bacterial count in contaminated wounds, it cannot sterilize them; for that achievement we must depend upon chemotherapeutic agents.

Owen H. Wangensteen, M.D.
Regents' Professor
Department of Surgery
Mayo Memorial Building
Minneapolis, Minn. 55455

Anatomic approach to vagotomy

To the Editors:

In their paper entitled "Identification of vagal structures at the esophageal hiatus" (SURGERY **75:** 233, 1974) Drs. Skandalakis, Rowe, Gray, and Androulakis quoted me quite frequently and disagreed with some of my anatomic descriptions (Griffith, C. A.: A new anatomic approach to the problem of incomplete vagotomy, Surg. Clin. North Am. **44:** 1239, 1964). In view of the fact that surgeons reading these disagreements may become more confused than enlightened, I want to clarify matters.

First, the authors agreed with me that the positions of the vagal trunks at the hiatus are quite variable (their Fig. 2 agrees with my Fig. 2), but disagreed that the trunks always assume right posterior and right anterior positions. This disagreement lies in both semantics and failure to define the exact anatomic region in question. The authors described the vagal system at the hiatus. I described the vagal system at the hiatus and also at the lower level of the distal abdominal esophagus and gastric cardia. With this in mind, the facts are these: Although the positions of the vagal trunks at the hiatus vary relative to the left and right aspects of the esophagus, the anterior gastric division from the anterior trunk and the posterior gastric division from the posterior trunk always assume constant anterior and posterior positions below the hiatus when they reach the lesser curve at the gastric cardia. Some small gastric fibers to the fundus arising above the level of the cardia may lie to the patient's left of the lesser curve at the cardia, but not the main gastric divisions (nerves of Lataret). It is this constant position of the main gastric vagal divisions along the lesser curve that permits the technique of parietal cell (or highly selective) vagotomy.

Second, the authors stated, "Griffith found cases in which the posterior trunk was closer to the aorta. In our material it was always closer to the aorta." Rather than replying to this discrepancy, I will point out its surgical significance. In encircling the vagal fibers with the esophagus by digital dissection at the higher level of the hiatus or at the lower level of the cardia, or in between these levels, the finger often does not readily feel a large "trunk" posteriorly. By palpating more dorsally (i.e., away from the esophagus and toward the aorta), a large "trunk" will always be felt. This "trunk" may be either the actual posterior vagal trunk or its large celiac division. If the latter, and if the posterior gastric division is not identified, the result conceivably could be a selective celiac vagotomy and an incomplete posterior gastric vagotomy. However, as shown in my Fig. 3, at the level of the most distal esophagus and cardia the posterior gastric division from the posterior trunk always lies well away from the aorta adjacent to the cardia. (In unusual cases the posterior gastric division runs to the lesser curve with the left gastric artery.)

Third, "We cannot agree with Griffith's view that it is the level of the diaphragm that varies with respect to the esophageal plexus." What I actually stated was, "The trap is the diaphragm, a structure that has nothing whatsoever to do with the embryology or anatomy of the vagus nerves. At the esophageal hiatus the vagal system may occur in the form of any one of three components . . . the esophageal plexus or the trunks or the truncal divisions." The authors illustrated these variations in their Figs. 1 and 3, which are the same as in my Fig. 4.

To sum up, I shall once again attempt to clarify pertinent surgical anatomic points that the late Henry Harkins and I felt we never really succeeded in getting across. The surgeon performing vagotomy within the confines of the hiatus does not know either how many vagal fibers there are or where they are in the individual patient. Failure to recognize the exact component of the vagal system at hand (the two trunks or multiple fibers of either the esophageal plexus or the truncal divisions) has been and continues to be the basic cause of incomplete vagotomy. In contrast, at the most distal esophagus and cardia, which is the one and only place where all gastric vagi always gather to innervate the stomach, the surgeon has a much better anatomic opportunity to accomplish a complete vagotomy—be it selective or total. In this regard, I would answer John Alexander-Williams' question, "How to be an adequate vagotomist" (SURGERY **75:** 308, 1974) by first sending the inadequate vagotomist to the morgue so that he could demonstrate to himself the anatomic basis for accomplishing complete or adequate vagotomy. Then, and only then, would I follow Alexander-Williams' advice concerning the various tests for completeness of vagotomy (Burge, Lee, Grassi and Hollander). Dr. Harkins and I proved the validity of this approach to our own satisfaction during a two-year evaluation several years ago. When we deemed vagotomy complete on the basis of an accurate anatomic dissection, the Burge and Hollander tests were consistently negative. At that time we were in the midst of the controversy concerning selective vagotomy. Although we repeatedly emphasized that the cardinal advantage of the selective technique was anatomic assurance of accomplishing a complete gastric vagotomy, this advantage was overshadowed by the great debate about diarrhea and, judging from what appears in the current literature, is now largely lost and not appreciated by the majority of surgeons. Only a minority (e.g., Sawyers, J. L., Scott, H. W., Edwards, W. H., Shull, H. J., and Lay, D. H.: Comparative studies of the clinical effects of truncal and selective vagotomy, Am. J. Surg. **115:** 165, 1968) recognizes the advantage of consistently successful results of adequate vagotomy by dissecting at the gastric cardia and avoiding the anatomic pitfalls at the hiatus.

Charles A. Griffith, M.D.
1041 116th Ave., N. E.
Bellevue, Wash. 98004

Reply: The vagaries of the vagus

To the Editors:

Thank you for the opportunity to reply to Dr. Griffith's discussion of our paper, "Identification of vagal structures at the esophageal hiatus."

First, we reported what we actually found. The discrepancy is not entirely a matter of "semantics and failure to define the exact anatomic region in question." At the hiatus, in our material, 91 percent of anterior vagal trunks and 86 percent of posterior vagal trunks were to the right of the esophageal midline (Fig. 2). An abdominal esophagus of variable length was always present; this was taken into consideration.

We made no attempt to discuss the topographic anatomy of the vagi distal to the hiatus. Since selective vagotomy is currently so important, the authors will discuss identification of vagal structures distal to the hiatus in a future paper.

Second, we do not understand Dr. Griffith. We can only repeat that the posterior trunk, at the hiatus, was always closer to the aorta than to the esophagus.

Third, we are in error here. We cited Dr. Griffith's 1964 paper and we read, but unfortunately failed to refer to his chapter in Maingot's *Abdominal operations,* ed. 2, chap. 16. In Fig. 2, p. 240, "various levels of esophageal hiatus" are shown. Perhaps we misunderstood this figure. If so, we sincerely apologize for both the misunderstanding and the failure to refer to it. We believe we have no disagreement.

To sum up, we agree with Dr. Griffith without quarreling with Dr. Alexander-Williams. The vagaries of the vagus are many and we do not wish to muddy the waters.

John E. Skandalakis, M.D., Ph.D., F.A.C.S.
Professor of Anatomy
Division of Basic Health Sciences
Department of Anatomy
Emory University
Atlanta, Ga. 30322

Phagocytosis

To the Editors:

The inference made by Olcay and associates' that depression of phagocytosis is "due exclusively to Kupffer cell dysfunction"[1] is tenuous. It would seem that further information on hepatic blood flow is necessary to draw this conclusion. Clearance rates and total organ uptake of materials eliminated from the blood by phagocytosis are dependent upon the function of the phagocyte, on the rate of blood flow, and on the dose of the material used.

The Kupffer cell population constitutes an estimated 70 to 90 percent of the blood-clearing phagocytic population of cells,[2] hence even small changes in blood flow through the liver may be reflected in altered clearance rates. Clearance studies under controlled conditions of blood flow can be performed, however, by applying the isolated perfused rat liver technique.[3-6]

In the reported experiments, considerable manipulation of hepatic bloodflow took place six hours preceeding the actual clearance study.[1] Hence, the conclusion that the observed changes are exclusively due to Kupffer cell dysfunction is misleading in the absence of information concerning hepatic blood flow. What evidence is there to indicate that the period of Kupffer cell dysfunction would exceed that of altered hepatic blood flow? As a consequence, some of the conclusions drawn by the authors may not be valid.

Also, the Limulus lysate test is not what it once was thought to be; it has serious limitations that deserve emphasis here,[7, 8] in view of its current popularity. It is less specific for endotoxin, since it has been found to react also with thromboplastin, nucleoproteins, and thrombin.[8]

Evidence for the enteric origin of clotting and fibrinolytic agents has previously been provided.[9, 10, 11] In addition we noted, while doing portacaval shunts in rats that the mortality rate is considerably reduced if the animals are heparinized prior to cross-clamping the portal vein, also suggesting that a thrombinlike material escapes from the intestine into the portal blood to exert its deleterious effect.[12] Whether the authors measured endotoxin activity or thrombinlike activity remains to be established, although its absence in germ-free rats would suggest that both activities may well be identical.

H. Gans, M.D., Ph.D.
Department of Surgery
New York Hospital–Cornell Medical College
New York, N. Y. 10021

REFERENCES

1. Olcay, I., Kitahama, A., Miller, R. H., Drapanas, T., Trejo, R. A., and Di Luzio, N. R.: SURGERY **75:** 64, 1974.
2. Gans, H., Stern, R., and Tan, B. H.: Thromb. Diath. Haem. **22:** 1, 1969.
3. Gans, H., and Lowman, J. T.: Blood **29:** 517, 1961.
4. Gans, H., Lowman, J., and Fahr, G.: Fed. Proc. **25:** 2900, 1966.
5. Gans, H., Subramanian, V., and Tan, B. H.: Science **159:** 107, 1968.
6. Subramanian, V., McLeod, J. and Gans, H.: SURGERY **64:** 775, 1968.
7. Stumacher, R. J., Kovnat, M. J., and McCabe, W. R.: N. Engl. J. Med. **288:** 1261, 1973.
8. Elin, R. J., and Wolff, S. M.: J. Inf. Dis. **128:** 349, 1973.
9. Gans, H.: SURGERY **55:** 544, 1964.
10. Rutherford, R. B., and Hardaway, R. M.: Ann. Surg. **163:** 51, 1966.
11. Gans, H., Mori, K., Quinlan, R., Richter, D., and Tan, B. H.: Proc. Soc. Exp. Biol. Med. **136:** 627, 1971.
12. Gans, H., and Matsumoto, K.: In preparation.

Reply

To the Editors:

Dr. Gans is obviously correct in that vascular clearance of particulate materials can be influenced by hepatic blood flow, and indeed, under certain conditions, small changes in blood flow are reflected in altered clearance rates. This statement is, however, correct only when a relatively minute particulate load is employed and hepatic extraction of the colloid is 100 per cent. Under these conditions liver blood flow becomes the rate-limiting factor in colloidal clearance and the fractional clearance rate × blood volume is, therefore, a measure of sinusoidal liver blood flow.

The studies of the influence of transient portal vein occlusion on reticuloendothelial (RE) function in the rat[6] followed an extensive series of studies on the effect of total normothermic hepatic ischemia on hepatic parenchymal and RE function in the baboon. In these studies, liver blood flow was measured and correlated with changes in vascular clearance of the RE test lipid emulsion.[4] By employing differential doses of the colloid in which the dose for measuring liver blood flow was below the "critical colloid dose," it was observed that sinusoidal blood flow was decreased 50 to 60 per cent at the three-hour postocclusion interval. When phagocytic function was ascertained by employment of a particulate load which was above the "critical colloidal dose," it was noted that despite the pronounced alteration in liver blood flow, vascular clearance of the lipid emulsion was normal. Indeed, at the 24 hour postocclusion interval when phagocytic dysfunction, as reflected by an approximate sevenfold impairment in vascular clearance of the emulsion, occurred in the group which ultimately succumbed to the insult, liver blood flow was normal. These studies clearly indicate that liver blood flow alterations in this liver ischemic model played no role in the impaired clearance rates seen following the ischemic insult.

The observed reduction in the mortality rate which Dr. Gans has noted to result following the administration of heparin prior to cross-clamping the portal vein when performing portacaval shunts in rats may or may not be due to the influence of heparin on coagulation mechanisms. Previous studies in our laboratory have demonstrated that heparin has a profound ability to reduce lethality associated with endotoxin shock. Heparin administration prior to endotoxin-maintained normal leukocyte levels. Additionally, heparin was found to prevent endotoxin-induced enhancement of colloidal carbon clearance. Anticoagulation with Dicumarol was inffective in modifying endotoxin-induced alteration in colloidal carbon clearances, suggesting that the prevention of coagulation per se was not the mechanism of heparin action. Indeed, suggestions were made at this time that heparin interaction with endotoxin might act to alter the fate of the injected endotoxin. Heparin has also been shown to modify phagocytic events in vitro[3] and in vivo.[2] In view of the diverse actions of heparin, the postulate of Dr. Gans of a single mode of action of heparin in modifying lethality following temporary portal vein occlusion may be somewhat restrictive.

Relative to the specificity of the Limulus lysate technique, it is quite obvious that caution should be employed in the lysate procedure as Elin and Wolff[1] have indeed raised questions regarding the specificity of this test.

We have conducted extensive studies employing the Limulus lysate technique on various biologicals and fluids and have also attempted to modify the lysate procedure test to increase its quantitation. In view of the widespread environmental presence of endotoxin, and indeed, its presence on occasion in "deionized" and "distilled water," there is clearly no evidence that certain materials which produce positive endotoxin reactions are indeed free of endotoxin. While this point is extremely difficult to ascertain, the possibility exists that traces of endotoxin might be present in certain isolated natural products or introduced in these preparations. Additionally, clinical and experimental studies in this laboratory conducted during periods of marked alterations in coagulation mechanisms and following injury have not been associated with a positive Limulus lysate test. Indeed, in situations of liver failure where Dr. Gans has observed changes in plasminogen activity, we have, to date, never observed a positive Limulus lysate test.

Our finding that germ-free animals which underwent identical periods of portal vein occlusion did not display at any time interval the presence of positive Limulus lysate test supports the observations that the factor producing a positive lysate test is of intestinal bacterial origin. The alternate concept according to the postulate which Dr. Gans puts forth would be that "thrombin-like material" would not escape from the intestine to portal blood from germ-free animals, an assumption which would have to be evaluated.

It would appear that, based upon our composite data, the nonspecific factors, which as Elin and Wolff denoted, consisted of not only certain coagulation factors but also polynucleotides, are not of importance in the hepatic ischemia model. This may be due either to their absence or to their presence at concentrations which do not interfere with the lysate test. Clearly, the definitive nature of this conclusion can only be resolved when newer and more specific methods are available for the assessment of gram-negative bacterial endotoxins.

Nicholas R. Di Luzio, Ph.D.
Isik Olcay, M.D.
Theodore Drapanas, M.D.
Departments of Physiology and Surgery
Tulane University School of Medicine
New Orleans, La. 70112

REFERENCES

1. Elin, R. J., and Wolff, S. M.: Nonspecificity of the Limulus amebocyte lysate test: positive reactions with polynucleotides and proteins, J. Infect. Dis. **128:** 349, 1973.

2. Filkins, J. P., and Di Luzio, N. R.: Effects of gelatin and heparin on intravascular phagocytosis, J. Reticuloendothel. Soc. **3:** 471, 1966.
3. Filkins, J. P., and Di Luzio, N. R.: Effect of heparin and sulfated polysaccharides on in vitro hepatic phagocytosis, Proc. Soc. Exp. Biol. Med. **122:** 548, 1966.
4. Holper, K., Olcay, I., Kitahama, A., Miller, R. H., Brettschneider, L., Drapanas, T., Trejo, R. A., and Di Luzio, N. R.: Effect of ischemia on hepatic parenchymal and reticuloendothelial function in baboon, SURGERY. In press.
5. Olcay, I., Holper, K., Kitahama, A., Miller, R. H., Drapanas, T., Trejo R. A. and Di Luzio, N. R.: Reticuloendothelial function: determinant for survival following hepatic ischemia in the baboon, SURGERY. In press.
6. Olcay, I., Kitahama, A., Miller, R. H., Drapanas, T., Trejo, R. A., and Di Luzio, N. R.: Reticuloendothelial dysfunction and endotoxemia following portal vein occlusion, SURGERY **75:** 64, 1974.

Subclavian steal syndrome

To the Editors:

In the February, 1974, issue of SURGERY, LeVeen and his co-workers[3] have proposed what we believe is a most ingenious solution to the problem of the subclavian steal syndrome. In January of 1973, two papers were published in the *Archives of Surgery*,[2, 4] which described in detail our experiences with four patients undergoing axillary-axillary bypass. In one case the procedure was identical to that suggested by Dr. LeVeen and his colleagues. In the other three, the bypass was performed with the use of the first portion of the axillary artery, an approach which I believe to be easier and less hazardous. Dr. LeVeen has suggested that this operation is capable of restoring normal hemodynamic relationships. We have investigated this thoroughly and reported our findings in December of 1972.[5] It is interesting to note that no mention of these papers or the pioneering work of Ehrenfeld and colleagues,[1] who reported the first subclavian-subclavian bypass, is made in Dr. LeVeen's rather extensive bibliography. At the present time, all grafts which we initially reported are patent with the exception of one patient who died of a nonrelated cause. The longest survivor[5] is now three years postoperative and has no recurrence of symptoms. An additional four cases have been added to my personal experience and in every instance the grafts have been performed with ease and without complications. No graft has failed. The subsequent experience with this procedure and the verbal communications of others that have performed the operation since our original description have confirmed the usefulness of axillary-axillary bypass in subclavian steal syndrome.

David J. Mozersky, Lt. Col., USAF, MC
Assistant Chief, Vascular Surgery
General Surgery Service
Wilford Hall USAF Medical Center (AFSC)
Lackland Air Force Base, Texas 78236

REFERENCES

1. Ehrenfeld, W. K., Levin, S. M., and Wylie, E. J.: Venous crossover bypass grafts for arterial insufficiency, Ann. Surg. **167:** 287, 1968.
2. Jacobson, J. H., Mozersky, D. J., Mitte, H. A., and Brothers, M. J.: Axillary-axillary bypass for the subclavian steal syndrome, Arch. Surg. **106:** 24, 1972.
3. LeVeen, H. H., Piccone, V. A., Sr., Diaz, C., Christoudias, G., Slade, W., and Norshand, I.: A simplified correction of subclavian steal syndrome, SURGERY **75:** 299, 1974.
4. Mozersky, D. J., Sumner, D. S., Barnes, R. W., and Strandness, D. E., Jr.: Subclavian revascularization by means of a subcutaneous axillary-axillary graft, Arch. Surg. **106:** 20, 1972.
5. Mozersky, D. J., Sumner, D. S., Barnes, R. W., Calloway, G. P., and Strandness, D. E., Jr.: The Hemodynamics of the axillary-axillary bypass, Surg. Gynecol. Obstet. **135:** 925, 1972.

Reply

To the Editors:

Obviously, Dr. Mozersky would not be piqued if axillary-to-axillary bypass were not such an important procedure. Axillary-to-axillary bypass avoids difficult intrathoracic surgery by substituting an equally satisfactory subcutaneous procedure.

The idea of a venous crossover graft for subclavian steal syndrome was becoming obvious to many skilled in the art at about the same time. Although our case may have preceded Dr. Mozersky's, Dr. Piccone and I make no claim to originality. Finkelstein and associates[1] described a six-year experience with 15 cases treated by subclavian-to-subclavian bypass before the reports of Mozersky or our own. Once one is aware of the principle of crossover grafts, one can scarcely call a move down the vessel from the subclavian to the axillary artery ingenious. The procedure became obvious to us after reviewing the literature in 1970.[2] Unfortunately, the case reported by Ehrenfeld and associates[3] did not come to light at that time, else it would have been included in the literature review.

Our first candidate for a vein crossover was encountered in 1971 about the same time as Dr. Mozersky was independently doing his work.

As to Dr. Mozersky's point about prefering the first part of the axillary artery, his article gives no hint of the technical details. He seems to have done two cases to the first part and one case to the third part. We must bow to his greater experience, and can only leave up to the readers whether they would prefer: the first part of the axillary artery, which is short (2.5 cm.) and deep under the costocorticoid membrane lying in a hole between the pectoralis minor and the first rib; the second part of the artery surrounded by the cords and under the pectoralis minor; or the third part, which is 6.5 cm. long and, although surrounded by nerves, is accessible without difficulty and offers unobstructed superficial exposure.

Although Dr. Mozersky is enthusiastic about the content of our article, his comments are directed toward the Editors of SURGERY as much as toward ourselves. His letter cries out "Wake up, SURGERY. I published that article a year ago." Dr. Mozersky finds our solution to the problem of subclavian steal most ingenious and novel because after all it is his idea he is praising. Dr. Mozersky's letter turns out to be a poultice for his own bruised ego. If he really believes we secretly plagiarized without credit, his only solace is that "imitation is the sincerest flattery."

Perhaps the editors of SURGERY are saying, "Here is another successful application of a crossover graft for the subclavian steal syndrome. The method seems to have merit enough to bring it to the attention of our readers."

Harry H. LeVeen, M.D.
Department of Surgery
State University of New York
Downstate Medical Center
Brooklyn, N. Y. 11203

REFERENCES

1. Finkelstein, N. M., Byer, A., and Rush, B. F., Jr.: Subclavian-to-subclavian bypass for the subclavian steal syndrome, SURGERY **71:** 142, 1972.
2. Piccone, V. A., and LeVeen, H. H.: The subclavian steal syndrome (collective review), Ann. Thorac. Surg. **9:** 51, 1970.
3. Ehrenfeld, W. K., Lewin, S. M., and Wylie, E. J.: Venous crossover bypass grafts for arterial insufficiency, Ann. Surg. **167:** 288, 1968.

Painless removal of sutures

To the Editors:

According to most patients, the removal of skin sutures is a painful and unpleasant experience; consequently, many patients, especially female patients, who have to undergo elective surgery, are afraid to have it done because they have heard of or have already experienced the pain when sutures are removed.

The pain is caused when a suture is cut and removed immediately since there is no time for the tissues (skin and subcutaneous tissue) either to accommodate or to relax; furthermore, the sutures are still adherent to one or both sides of the surgical incision.

Skin sutures are painlessly removed only if cut one by one and, once they are all cut, a few seconds or minutes should be allowed before starting to remove them gently, in the same order as they were cut, until the last one is removed. In very sensitive patients, the sutures may be cut one day and removed the next.

This is the best procedure for the removal

of sutures with the added advantage that your patients will always be happy and grateful.

"The art of surgery" is to arrive at a correct diagnosis followed by the right surgical procedure; this will cure your patients, keep them alive, satisfied, and grateful. All this can be done from beginning to end with little or no pain.

It really works. Try it.

Leon Bialostozky, M.D.
Cardiovascular Surgery C. H.
"20 de Noviembre" (ISSSTE)
Mexico 5, D. F.

Value of intraoperative tests in vagotomy

To the Editors:

I would like to make a brief comment on two contributions to the February, 1974, issue of SURGERY.[1, 3] Both the article by Grassi and Orecchia and the editorial by Alexander-Williams were concerned with the continued efforts to develop a satisfactory intraoperative test for determining the completeness of a vagal section.

In 1949, we did experimental and clinical studies on the gastric excretion of neutral red.[4] These studies included the use of the dye as an intraoperative test, as well as a postoperative test. We also combined the use of neutral red and Hollander's insulin test, with the drugs given both simultaneously and separately. We were well satisfied with the tests as employed for a late postoperative check on the completeness of the vagal section. There were some failures in its use as an intraoperative test because no intraoperative test can distinguish a temporary physiologic interruption of small numbers of remaining intact nerve fibers due to operative trauma from a complete or nearly complete anatomic interruption of all vagal nerve fibers. If the test is positive, however, additional fibers should be searched for.

We did not investigate the simultaneous use of a vagal stimulant and parenteral neutral red during the operation as suggested by Cole.[2] While this might be expected to increase the incidence of the positive results, false negatives could again occur due to physiologic interruption of the nerve fibers.

The great advantage of the use of neutral red is the simplicity of the procedure. Simple gastric lavage through a Levine tube already in the stomach, using normal saline, will indicate the presence of neutral red excreted by the parietal cells after intravenous injection.

To assist in becoming an adequate vagotomist, the employment of some intraoperative test during a surgeon's training would be of definite value.

Miles J. Gullickson, M.D.
Clinical Professor of Surgery
Rockford School of Medicine
Rockford, Ill. 61108

REFERENCES

1. Alexander-Williams, J.: How to be an adequate vagotomist (editorial), SURGERY **75:** 308, 1974.
2. Cole, R. E.: An intra-operative test for completeness of vagotomy, Am. J. Surg. **123:** 543, 1972.
3. Grassi, G., and Orecchia, C.: A comparison of intraoperative tests of completeness of vagal section, SURGERY **75:** 155, 1974.
4. Gullickson, M. J., and Campbell, D. A.: Gastric secretion of neutral red as influenced by vagotomy, Gastroenterology **12:** 454, 1949.

Central venous catheter maintenance

To the Editor:

The long-term maintenance of a central venous catheter inserted in the subclavian or internal jugular vein for monitoring a seriously ill patient or for administration of parenteral alimentation is clearly needed. However, accidental dislocation of the catheter and the danger of infection are troublesome. Infection usually starts at the puncture wound of the catheter where chronic irritation by the catheter produces a serous accumulation and subsequent infection. For the past three years we have utilized the following technique and were able to eliminate most of the complications.

A tight suture encompassing the soft tissue around the catheter prevents serous accumulation in the space between the catheter and tissue. As a result, the puncture wound stays dry and clean, rendering itself resistant to external contamination. Also, the catheter is securely anchored to the skin using ends of the same suture in order to protect it from accidental dislocation.

Dong K. Kim
Joseph G. Fortner
Gastric and Mixed Tumor Service
Memorial Sloane-Kettering Cancer Center
1275 York Ave.
New York, N. Y. 10021

Bifurcation of canine abdominal aorta

To the Editors:

The article entitled "Systemic and renal responses to a graded reduction in cardiac output," by L. L. Michaelis and associates (SURGERY **74:** 853, 1973), contains a small anatomical error. Fig. 1 on p. 854 shows the bifurcation of the abdominal aorta in a humanoid fashion when in fact the dog's anatomy varies somewhat from this arrangement, with a common internal iliac artery.

R. Adar, M.D.
Department of Surgery
Beth Israel Hospital
330 Brookline Ave.
Boston, Mass. 02215

Volume 76 Number 3 SURGERY

SEPTEMBER, 1974

Editorials

The Carrel-Guthrie letters revisited

L. G. Walker, Jr., M.D., *Charlotte, N. C.*

From the Department of Surgery, Nalle Clinic, Charlotte, N. C.

Recent publications have offered a revisionist stance in the history of vascular surgery regarding the individual contributions of Carrel *vis à vis* Guthrie. Hershey and Calman, in their *Atlas of Vascular Surgery,* third edition, state: "Of these pioneers, Garrison mentioned only Eck and Carrel. Much of the early work was quite ignored, and the commanding position of Guthrie seems to be completely overlooked."[5] Saunders in his chapter entitled, "A Conceptual History of Transplantation," makes even stronger claims for Guthrie.[6] Since an excellent article by Harbison,[4] entitled "Origins of Vascular Surgery: The Carrel-Guthrie Letters," published in Surgery in August, 1962, seems to have served as the source for some of these opinions, it seems timely to review the evidence albeit 12 years after publication of Harbison's paper and to add new information, namely the other side of the correspondence—the Guthrie to Carrel letters obtained from the Carrel Archives, Georgetown University, Washington, D. C.

Accepted for publication Apr. 25, 1974.

Reprint requests: L. G. Walker, Jr., M.D., 1350 S. Kings Dr., Charlotte, N. C. 28207.

Let it be noted that the "Carrel-Guthrie Letters" of Harbison's article are all letters from Carrel to Guthrie. Every man is entitled to his opinion, but needless to say, the more information available, the more apt one is to make a fair judgment. Thus some of the letters that Guthrie wrote to Carrel may shed light and will be quoted.

Carrel had begun work in Lyon in 1901 on blood vessel anastomosis. He published his classic paper, "The operative technique of vascular anastomoses and the transplantation of organs," in *Lyon Medical* in 1902[1] and had spoken to an international medical and surgical meeting in Montreal in 1904 on blood vessel anastomosis and transplantation. He had had two articles on the subject published in Canadian journals before he was invited in 1905 by Dr. G. N. Stewart of the University of Chicago to work with Guthrie who, up until this time, had been doing "some gastrointestinal experimentation." As Harbison relates, the two worked together from June through August, 1905, and from January through March, 1906. The originator of the concept of vascular surgery and transplantation is clearly Carrel, as attested by his earliest publications. Harbison acknowledges that this was "brilliant original work." I personally know of no original contribution to the field of vascular surgery solely by Guthrie that can match Carrel's early achievements.

That there was later ill will by Guthrie toward Carrel cannot be denied. Guthrie wrote a stinging two page letter in the January 1, 1909, issue of *Science* in which he stated: "As to priority, it gives me great pleasure to express my high regard for Dr. Carrel's persistence in the face of a long series of unsuccessful operations and I desire to in no way endeavor to attach any of the credit he deserves for this devotions." He is referring to Carrel's results prior to their collaboration at Chicago. Guthrie concludes the letter piously, "The dubious distinction of priority which it would appear is the goal sought by some of our contemporaries, presents slight attraction to the sincere investigator whose reward largely is the consciousness that his labors may in the end add a line to the encyclopedia of science."[3] This statement is not at all in the spirit of his communications to Carrel in the fall of 1905.

What then are some of the claims made the Carrel to Guthrie letters) and later by about Carrel by Harbison (on the basis of Saunders in his article?

First Harbison says, "The work of Guthrie and Carrel was not unknown to the popular press. Guthrie felt deeply about the inadvisability of this, and *even Carrel at times* (my emphasis) was outraged, although he was very sensitive to priority and publishing immediately." Saunders refers to Carrel's publishing articles with "precipitate alacrity which was to become characteristic" of him.

Now note Guthrie's interest in publishing immediately, although neither Harbison nor Saunders relate this. Columbia, Mo., Sept. 11, 1905 (Guthrie to Carrel):

". . . I think *Science* would issue the earliest publication of any American journal and if you desire to send it there, the write up should be short as possible. I regret that the work is so widely known at this time as our experiments are. I think, in the preliminary stage as yet—comparatively speaking of course.

"If such men as Cushing take it up now it means that we will be 'beat out' in making human applications as their facilities for such work are at present vastly superior to ours—you understand I mean opportunities to get and operate suitable patients. Still I cannot believe that anyone, or set of surgeons can equal our results before they have worked much longer on the techniques that you and I have together. I think it might be a good plan to keep the *important details* of the actual technique to ourselves for a time—not many of them will take the time to look up your first paper and besides, I believe certain details are somewhat improved since then, are they not? A few blood clots would serve to cool their ardor."

On Sept. 16, 1905, from Columbia, Mo. (Guthrie to Carrel):

". . . The newspaper notoriety is deplorable but it cannot be helped. We should, I suppose, show our animals to absolutely no one in the future. If we could maintain secrecy for say a year and write all our results in book form, it would be the ideal way, I think but that is not possible, I suppose, now. I myself do not care to go on acknowledging assistance (?) from any third party for it is not fair to ourselves. Still our circumstances place us in rather a dependent attitude as regards this point. I am not surprised that all of the animals are doing well. At first I lacked complete confidence in the permanency of the results but now we have overwhelming data to my mind, to assure us on the results."

And on Oct. 4, 1905, Guthrie wrote Carrel:

"The note for *Science* is very good. The statements are clear and concise. I hope it will be published immediately. . . . We certainly have a lot of interesting work ahead of us. I wrote Dr. Stewart about the 'sacredness' of the rooms and advised the special lock and new animals quarters immediately. Also that we attributed our uniform success mainly to the fact that we got the place clean and were able to keep it so."

Second, referring to some of Carrel's difficulty with an inept assistant about whom he had written to Guthrie, Harbison concludes: "Apparently Guthrie planned carefully, was successful in training people. It was not so happy a situation with Carrel." However, in Guthrie's letter on Oct. 31, 1905, he told Carrel about some of his own trouble with assistants:

". . . Your results with Mr. Wilson emphasize the importance of coordination between the operators. I have been anastomosing some cat vessels. . . . The results were good considering my assistant has so much astigmatism that he cannot distinguish the vessels without looking through a tube. I have him hold the vessels by the first ligature while I sew the sides of the triangle. Dr. Miller is the pathologist and has just returned from spending the summer in England and Germany. He says we have great international reputation on having successfully transplanted the heart! Is it not ridiculous? Newspaper fame again. It is a pity for so much advertising to go to waste. It would be worth thousands to anyone of dozens of 'surgeons' I could name. I have no doubt at all but that at this moment the work is being assayed in a dozen different laboratories. Our main protection is the difficulty of the technique. . . . The medical men here are just beginning to evidence an interest in the work. The Dean spent an afternoon with me not long ago and he tried to persuade me to operate for them. I refused as I have nothing to operate with and it is doubtful if I get anything."

Third, Saunders goes so far as to suggest that Carrel was mistaken about the newspaper publicity that ensued and that Guthrie was not and speculates, "One wonders whether Guthrie's magnificent statement in his book on the necessity of exercising care, consideration, and humanitarianism in animal experimentation was not a rebuttal to all this publicity." Carrel never solicited newspaper publicity and fully understood its perils, especially in a age of yellow journalism.

Fourth, Saunders also states, "Although the leading American surgeons of the period (Halsted, Murphy, Matas, Cushing, Bloodgood, Crile) were familiar with Guthrie's work, they passed it by almost in silence." The most that can be said was that they overlooked the joint work of Carrel and Guthrie, although Guthrie's letter of Sept. 11, 1905, implies that he was hoping to be overlooked at the time. Saunders' statement is most effectively countered by Cushing's own account of the visit of the members of the Society of Clinical Surgery to Carrel's laboratory in Chicago in October, 1905. "While the remaining few of us were at lunch, Matas passed the word around that in the physiological laboratory at the University of Chicago a young Frenchman named Alexis Carrel was doing some interesting work on anastomosing blood vessels and transplanting vessels and were we interested, he would be glad to give us a demonstration." (Cushing had written to Carrel earlier asking if the group might visit.) "We certainly were interested, and though the anastomosis had to be made on a dog no longer alive for reasons that need not be gone into, it was the only original work that had been shown to us for some time. In retrospect, it now proves to have been an historic milestone in the checkered history of blood transfusion."[2]

Harbison concludes his article in SURGERY with the opinion, "It is difficult fifty years later to assess priorities and value of contributions, but certainly to Charles Claude Guthrie the modern surgeon owes a very sizeable debt, probably greater than to Alexis Carrel." I disagree.

REFERENCES

1. Carrel, A.: La technique opératoire des anastomoses vasculaires et la transplantation des visceres, Lyon Med. **98:** 859, 1902.
2. Cushing, H.: The Society of Clinical Surgery in retrospect, Ann. Surg. **169:** 1, 1969.
3. Guthrie, C. C.: On misleading statements, Science **29:** 29, 1909.
4. Harbison, S. P.: Origins of vascular surgery: The Carrel-Guthrie letters SURGERY **52:** 406, 1962.
5. Hershey, F. B., and Calman, C. H.: Atlas of vascular surgery, ed. 3, St. Louis, 1973, The C. V. Mosby Co., p. 4.
6. Saunders, J. B. D. M.: A conceptual history of transplantation, *in* Najarian, J. S., and Simmons, R. L., editors: Transplantation, Philadelphia, 1972, Lea & Febiger, p. 17.

Ischemia and the gastric mucosal barrier: A note of caution

W. P. Ritchie, Jr., M.D., Ph.D., *Charlottesville, Va.*

From the Department of Surgery, University of Virginia School of Medicine, Charlottesville, Va.

THE BELIEF that acute post-traumatic hemorrhagic gastritis is a consequence of an incompetent gastric mucosal barrier is widely held. The "back diffusion" hypothesis postulates that the common initial underlying pathophysiologic event in the development of this disease entity is ischemia of the gastric mucosa which renders it more permeable to secreted acid. This circumstance, in turn, permits excessive enterosorption of H^+ and pepsin with resulting autodigestion of the gastric mucosa, manifested by erosion formation and bleeding into the gastric lumen.[23] Experimentally, this thesis is based principally upon the observations of Skillman and his co-workers[24] who studied the properties of the gastric mucosal barrier in the intact innervated stomach of the rabbit (1) during a one-hour baseline period, (2) during a 15 minute period of hypotension produced by hemorrhage, and (3) 3 hours following the reinfusion of the shed blood. In those animals in which acid was instilled into the stomach during each phase of the experiment, a net gain of H^+ was noted during the baseline period. During the period of blood pressure manipulation, a small net loss of H^+ was observed. By the third hour after shock, net loss of H^+ was markedly accentuated and was associated with the development of multiple linear gastric ulcers in nine of the 10 animals studied. The results of this study have prompted the suggestion that, in man, gastric mucosal ischemia per se leads to a generalized increase in gastric mucosal permeability.[9, 22, 23] Because of the therapeutic implications of this thesis, it would seem prudent to examine its component parts in some detail.

Although no direct evidence exists to link an incompetent gastric mucosal barrier to the subsequent development of acute post-traumatic hemorrhagic gastritis clinically, a considerable body of circumstantial data tends to support this relationship. The responsible lesions occur early following injury; they are multiple and are confined in large part to the proximal acid-pepsin secreting area of the stomach,[12, 14] all of which suggests that autodigestion has occurred. If patients with central nervous system injury are excluded, there is no evidence of "hypersecretion" of gastric acid following injury in patients who ultimately develop clinically apparent upper gastrointestinal hemorrhage. Rather, the gastric juice of these individuals is usually characterized by relatively high volume, a high concentration of Na^+, and a low concentration of recoverable acid. In addition, it has been reported that, follow-

This study was supported by contract No. DAMD 17-74-C-4014.

Accepted for publication May 13, 1974.

Reprint requests: W. P. Ritchie, Jr., M.D., Ph.D., Department of Surgery, University of Virginia School of Medicine, Charlottesville, Va. 22901.

ing trauma, protein unassociated with the glycoprotein of mucus appears in the gastric content, a finding particularly prominent just prior to the development of hemorrhage.[25] The most direct evidence to support the hypothesis is contained in the report of Skillman and associates,[24] who studied the barrier properties of 26 critically ill patients. All of these were of the type most susceptible to the development of stress ulcer disease. When compared to healthy nonhospitalized volunteer controls, 12 demonstrated significantly greater disappearance of H^+ following instillation of a 160 mM. HCl solution into the stomach. In general, a rough correlation could be developed between the magnitude of the patient's illness and the degree of "back diffusion" observed. In assessing these data, it should be noted that several critical and, in some instances, largely unproven assumptions exist with respect to the requisite calculations. These assumptions relate primarily to the rate of flow and composition of nonparietal secretion, to the $[Cl^-]$ in parietal secretion, and to the use of ΔPEG as a measure of pyloric loss. Recently, this same group has studied the ability of the gastric mucosa to maintain a high intraluminal $[Li^+]$ in a similar patient population and has demonstrated in some an apparent increase in mucosal permeability to this ion, an increase which correlates well both with the severity of the patient's illness and with the later development of upper gastrointestinal hemorrhage.[9] That change in the magnitude of unidirectional Li^+ movement is a valid measure of alterations in gastric mucosal permeability to other intraluminal cations is likely but remains to be convincingly demonstrated.[3]

Considerable clinical and experimental evidence exists to suggest (but not to prove) that gastric mucosal ischemia may also play a role in the development of acute hemorrhagic gastritis. Sequential gastroscopy in susceptible patients indicates that the earliest observable lesion in the proximal stomach consists of small areas of mucosal pallor surrounded by a zone of hyperemia. These areas appear to progress to the formation of punctate erosions and, ultimately, in a few cases, to confluent ulcers.[14] The pathologic anatomy of resected specimens also indicates that, in some instances, the responsible lesions are microscopically consistent with a coagulation type of ischemic necrosis.[12] Using a variety of experimental designs, lesions which resemble those found in man have been produced in the dog,[16] pig,[8] rat,[15, 21] and rabbit[11, 24] by bleeding animals to a mean arterial pressure of 40 to 80 mm. Hg for variable periods of time (15 minutes to 4 hours). Hemorrhage of the magnitude usually employed is associated with a significant reduction in superior mesenteric arterial blood flow (and presumably in celiac axis flow as well) in every species in which it has been studied.[1, 13] E. coli endotoxemia has also been reported to reduce markedly gastric mucosal blood flow in the piglet associated with the development of typical ulcers in the areas of ischemia.[18] Finally, both single and multiple intravenous injections of vasopressin, an α-adrenergic agonist which does not demonstrate a marked degree of autoregulatory escape, have been reported to result in typical erosion formation in the dog stomach.[17]

With the demonstration in the rabbit that a brief episode of hemorrhagic shock followed by reinfusion of shed blood resulted in an apparent increase in mucosal permeability to H^+ associated with lesion formation and intraluminal bleeding, these disparate sets of data appeared to fit the unifying hypothesis described earlier. Unfortunately, attempts to reproduce the basic experimental data in other species or by other techniques in the same species have been uniformly unsuccessful. Using chambered segments of fundic mucosa exposed to 0.15N HCl, Moody and Aldrete[16] could demonstrate no evidence of an impaired gastric mucosal barrier in dogs subjected to 30 to 90 minutes of hemorrhagic shock despite the development of punctate erosions and a marked reduction in aminopyrine clearance. Nevertheless, acid was an important factor in lesion formation in this study, since no erosions were observed during shock when the mucosa was in contact with a neutral solution. Ritchie and Fischer[20] could also find no evidence of increased mucosal permeability in the denervated fundic pouch of the dog exposed to an acid solution during a 3½ hour period of hemorrhagic shock, even though the ability of the mucosa to maintain an electrical gradient was markedly impaired. Similar changes in electrical parameters, unassociated with changes in mucosal permeability, have been noted during endotoxemia in the dog.[4] DenBesten and Hamza[6] studied the fluxes of H^+, Na^+, and Cl^- in normotensive animals and in animals shocked to a mean arterial blood pressure of 40 to 50 mm. Hg for one hour, with and without concomitant topical sodium taurocholate application. They found that movement of these ions, although increased several fold by the presence of bile salts, was not significantly different between the normotensive or shocked states. Recently, Davenport and Barr,[5] using the aminopyrine clearance technique, have demonstrated in the dog that mucosal ischemia caused by subcutaneous vasopressin, by intravenous vasopressin, by intravenous norepinephrine, or by a single venous hemorrhage of 30 percent of the calculated blood volume had no detectable effect on the gastric mucosal barrier for up to 6 hours. This circumstance was also true when administration of the vasoconstrictor drugs was combined with the infusion of a variety of secretagogues. Dorricott and associates[7] have shown that large doses of vasopressin infused directly into the arterial supply of canine denervated fundic pouches markedly reduced aminopyrine clearance but did not alter in a significant way the net fluxes of H^+ and Na^+. The end organ effect of one deleterious consequence of prolonged ischemia, tissue anoxia, was recently studied by Birkett and Silen.[2] Using in vivo rabbit gastric mucosa, these investigators were unable to demonstrate any significant increase in H^+ loss during a 30 minute period of total anoxia, either alone or in combination with bile salts. Finally, recent studies from our laboratory demonstrate that, in a species phylogenetically more akin to man than either dog or rabbit, the rhesus monkey, neither a 2.5 hour period of hypotension induced by hemorrhage nor subsequent reinfusion of the shed blood significantly affected the ability of the innervated isolated intact stomach to maintain electrical or pH gradients.[19] These data clearly indicate that the alterations observed in mucosal permeability to H^+ in the rabbit after a brief period of hemorrhagic shock do not occur in the dog during pharmacologically induced ischemia of the gastric mucosa or in the anoxic mucosa of the rabbit in vitro. Nor do they occur in the dog or subhuman primate subjected to relatively prolonged periods of hemorrhagic shock and subsequent reinfusion of shed blood, a circumstance in which the animal is subjected to rheological and humoral insult over and above mucosal ischemia alone. It is possible that longer periods of either ischemia or hypovolemic hypotension may be required to unmask flux changes of the sort observed during classical disruption of the barrier (e.g., during topical bile salt application), but until such a demonstration is available, the thesis that gastric mucosal ischemia per se increases gastric mucosal permeability must be regarded as completely unproven.

This conclusion does not, of course, invalidate the "back diffusion" hypothesis. The clinical studies noted above remain relevant, subject to the limitations of the assumptions employed. Also germane is the observation that topically applied bile salts enhance ulcer formation in the intact stomach of the dog subjected to hemorrhage, even though increased "back diffusion" of H^+ is not observed during the shock period.[10] In addition, ulcerogenesis induced in this way can be prevented by the concomitant administration of cholestyramine, an exchange resin which binds bile acids, renders them unabsorbable, and prevents "back diffusion" of H^+ of any magnitude in this experimental preparation.[26] A synergistic relationship may therefore exist between impaired gastric mucosal blood flow and "back diffusion" of intraluminal acid, even though the mucosal barrier is "normal" under these circumstances. The precise nature of this relationship remains to be defined. It is likely that the development of more suitable experimental models and additional relevant patient data will do much to resolve the ambiquities inherent in this challenging clinical problem.

REFERENCES

1. Barton, R. W., Reynolds, D. G., Swan, K. G.: Mesenteric circulatory responses to hemorrhagic shock in the baboon, Ann. Surg. **175:** 204, 1972.
2. Birkett, D., and Silen, W.: Effect of severe anoxia and sodium taurocholate on H+ loss from luminal surface of in vivo gastric mucosa, Surg. Forum **24:** 421, 1973.
3. Chung, R. S. K., Field, M., and Silen, W.: Permeability of gastric mucosa to hydrogen and lithium, Gastroenterology **64:** 593, 1973.
4. Chou, A. C., Miller, J., Jacobson, E. D., et al.: Effects of endotoxin on gastric mucosal active transport processes, Gastroenterology **64:** 710, 1973.
5. Davenport, H. W., and Barr, L. L.: Failure of ischemia to break the dog's gastric mucosal barrier, Gastroenterology **65:** 619, 1973.
6. DenBesten, L., and Hamza, K. N.: Effect of bile salts on ionic permeability of canine gastric mucosa during experimental shock, Gastroenterology **62:** 417, 1972.
7. Dorricott, N. J., Isenberg, H., and Silen, W.: Effect of intraarterial vasopressin on canine gastric mucosal permeability, Gastroenterology **65:** 625, 1973.
8. Goodman, A., and Osburn, M.: An experimental model and clinical definition of stress ulceration, Surg. Gynecol. Obstet. **134:** 563, 1972.
9. Gordon, M. J., Skillman, J. J., Zervas, N. T., et al.: Divergent nature of gastric mucosal permeability and gastric acid secretion in sick patients with general surgical and neurosurgical disease, Ann. Surg. **178:** 285, 1973.
10. Hamza, K. N., and DenBesten, L.: Bile salts producing stress ulcers during experimental shock, Clin. Res. **19:** 393, 1971.
11. Harjola, P., and Sivula, A.: Gastric ulceration following experimentally induced hypoxia and hemorrhagic shock: In vivo study of pathogenesis in rabbits, Ann. Surg. **163:** 21, 1966.
12. Lev, R., Molot, M. D., McNamara, J. J., et al.: "Stress" ulcers following war wounds in Viet Nam: A morphological and histochemical study, Lab. Invest. **25:** 491, 1971.
13. Lillehi, R. C., Longerbeam, J. K., and Rosenberg, J. C.: The nature of irreversible shock: Its relationship to intestinal changes, *in* Bach, K. D., editor: Shock: pathogenesis and therapy, Berlin, 1962, Springer-Verlag, p. 106.
14. Lucas, C. E., Sugawa, C., Riddle, J., et al.: Natural history and surgical dilemma of "stress" gastric bleeding, Arch. Surg. **102:** 266, 1971.
15. Mersereau, W. A., and Hinchey, E. F.: Effect of gastric acidity on gastric ulceration induced by hemorrhage in the rat utilizing a gastric chamber technique, Gastroenterology **64:** 1130, 1973.
16. Moody, F. G., and Aldrete, J. S.: Hydrogen permeability of canine gastric secretory epithelium during formation of acute superficial erosions, SURGERY **70:** 154, 1971.
17. Nedzel, A. J.: Experimental production of gastric ulcers in dogs by inducing vascular spasm with pitressin, Am. J. Dig. Dis. **10:** 283, 1943.
18. Richardson, R. S., Norton, L. W., Sales, J. E. L., et al.: Gastric blood flow in endotoxin induced stress ulcer, Arch. Surg. **106:** 191, 1973.
19. Ritchie, W. P., Jr.: Effect of hemorrhage on gastric mucosal permeability in the subhuman primate, Gastroenterology. In press.
20. Ritchie, W. P., Jr., and Fischer, R. P.: Studies on the pathogenesis of "stress ulcer": Electrical potential difference and ionic fluxes across canine gastric mucosa during hemorrhagic shock, J. Surg. Res. **3:** 173, 1972.
21. Ritchie, W. P., Jr., Roth, R., and Fischer, R. P.: Studies on the pathogenesis of "stress ulcer": Effect of hemorrhage, transfusion, and vagotomy in the restrained rat, SURGERY **71:** 445, 1972.
22. Skillman, J. J., and Silen, W.: Acute gastroduodenal "stress" ulceration: Barrier disruption of varied pathogenesis? Gastroenterology **59:** 478, 1970.
23. Skillman, J. J., and Silen, W.: Stress ulcers, Lancet **2:** 1303, 1972.
24. Skillman, J. J., Gould, S. A., Chung, R. S. K., et al.: The gastric mucosal barrier: Clinical and experimental studies in critically ill and normal man and in the rabbit, Ann. Surg. **172:** 564, 1970.
25. Stremple, J. F., Molot, M. D., McNamara, J. J., et al.: Post-traumatic gastric bleeding: Prospective gastric secretion composition, Arch. Surg. **105:** 177, 1972.
26. Zike, W. L., Safaie-Shirazi, S., Paluska, G., et al.: The role of cholestyramine in the prevention of stress ulcers, Gastroenterology **64:** 826, 1973.

The academic surgical body count

B. Eiseman, M.D., *Denver, Colo.*

From the Department of Surgery, Denver General Hospital, and the University of Colorado Medical Center, Denver, Colo.

THERE WERE 18 empty chairs of surgery in the one hundred–odd medical schools in the United States during 1973. In addition, three to seven other surgical department heads, though not officially listed as KIA (killed in administration), were certainly WIA (wounded in administration) to an extent that several inevitably will be invalided out of Academia.

When 20 percent of top management positions in an industry fall vacant in one year and the mean survival time approximates that of cancer, it seems reasonable to seek the cause and to perform an epidemiologic study of the disease.

Two factors characteristically presage an epidemic: (1) a new pathogen emerges or (2) a large group of virginal hosts are caught with their immune defenses down. Both probably apply to the current mortality and morbidity among surgical chairmen.

THE PATHOGEN

Chairmen in the '70's are exposed to administrative, economic, and academic viruses unknown to their predecessors. Governmental regulation, insurance carrier demands, and organized administrative militants are among the new slings of their administrative misfortune. Endless unstructured committee meetings sap their energies and are typical of the archaic corporate structure and operative methods of most medical schools. Business and managerial techniques suitable for trading in an Oriental bazaar are being forced to serve the conglomerates that now constitute a modern department of surgery. The strain on those caught in the system is predictable. Surgeons are at double risk because of the time and energy demands of the operating room. They do not have the leisure of their clinical colleagues who can devote long hours to administration. Both are at the mercy of the basic science faculty, whose teaching requirements are at best episodic. Seasonally some glandular curricular stimulus sponsors their emergence, grumbling and disheveled from their cavernous laboratories, briefly to perform their academic rites. The function completed within a few weeks, they retire exhausted and still grumbling whence they came.

Their lack of involvement in hospital matters and the brief duration of their teaching duties keep them primarily immune from attack in the current epidemic.

RESISTANCE

Debilitating administrative influences on surgical chairmen have been analyzed else-

Accepted for publication June 24, 1974.

Reprint requests: B. Eiseman, M.D., Director, Department of Surgery, City and County of Denver, W. 8th Ave. & Cherokee St., Denver, Colo. 80204.

where but not so their lack of administrative resistance or immunity.

It seems incongruous to depict bright, highly organized, and occasionally aggressive young staff surgeons after 35 years of intense training as being virginal—even in an administrative, immunologic sense. Although their training prepares them superbly for clinical care, research, and teaching, it is almost totally lacking in exposure to the antigenic stimuli necessary to provoke a second-set immunologic memory when they are challenged as new department chairmen. No wonder they fall easy prey to predatory deans or fellow chairmen trained essentially from academic puberty for the administrative lists. Some of their adversaries even have served the ultimate academic indignity as assistant deans! Such unfortunates may be hyperimmunized to administrative challenge to the border of anergy.

The lack of managerial training in new surgical chairmen is the fault of those of us responsible for training young surgeons for academic responsibility. In our zeal to prepare our preceptors as clinicians, teachers, and investigators, we have neglected to train them as managers. When named to a chair they suddenly assume the chilling responsibility of leading a big business. The first step in solving this problem is to appreciate that an academic surgical department is big business. Economically the department of surgery characteristically generates 30 to 60 percent of patient income to run a multimillion dollar university hospital. Their responsibilities for complex research grants, contracts, equipment, buildings, and personnel all parallel the duties of the chief executive officer (CEO) of any similar multimillion dollar industry. Yet where else is an industry so naive in training and choosing its CEO's? Our CEO candidates are trained only in their primary craft (clinical surgery, teaching, and research)—not as managers. No sane owner of a multimillion dollar professional football franchise would place a wide receiver as its combined business manager and coach simply because he had good hands and clever, classy moves. Yet this is the analogous pattern for surgical chairman training and selection. Other industries require previous and progressive managerial experience prior to CEO selection.

Since World War II America has become the surgical center of the world. Simultaneously there has been a revolution in the science of management in this country. The phenomenal growth of business schools and the success of their M.B.A. graduates in industry and government reflect the effectiveness of this new science. Alas, those swept along and occasionally leading the surgical pack have not profited by the advances in managerial sciences—and for this oversight we are now paying a fearful price in disgruntled, discarded, and depressed exchairmen. Their poor prognosis was as predictable as the Christian vs. lion encounters in the Roman arena.

A few examples where surgical chairmen have come to grief by ignoring established managerial principles are in order. Names are withheld but the *cognoscenti* can identify where the violated principles caused grief in their own institution.

1. Span of control. One person can efficiently supervise only four to eight immediate subordinates. This is the recognized maximum span of control. To exceed such a table of organization inevitably results in poor upward and downward communication and administrative chaos. Yet everyone knowledgeable of medical school affairs can identify dozens of deans and surgical chairmen in trouble because they have violated this simple organizational rule.

2. Communication. A lot of lip service is given to "lack of communication" as responsible for administrative confusion and personal antagonism—yet few enough surgical chairmen (or deans) have bothered to study techniques by which vertical and horizontal communications can be performed with optimal efficiency. Committee meetings, the bane of a chairman's existence, characteristically are little more than unstructured sensitivity sessions in medical schools. Few surgical chairmen know the maximum number of participants that can be included in a managerial committee that is expected to perform effectively. Without agenda categorized (a) for information only, (b) for discussion, and (c) for decision, committee meetings degenerate into unproductive anecdotal gripe sessions wherein policy and operational problems become hopelessly confused. Items requiring decision must be presented with appropriate staff work, prior warning, and suggested options for solution.

There are good models for the frequency and form of manager–middle management meetings. It matters not whether these people are called surgical chairman and specialty division chiefs or the equivalent titles in the automobile, soap, or fertilizer business!

3. Relation of line, staff, and service departments. There are several acceptable relations between those whose duties provide the primary function of an organization and those whose existence solely rests on providing an environment that will simplify and make the line more effective. Confusion in the role and relative priority of line, staff, and service continually causes chaos in a medical school. Those in-service organizations, such as personnel, auditing, business office, grants management, or even housekeeping, become arrogant and ultimately power mad simply because their self-image becomes blurred and they forget that they exist solely to serve their line masters. In a medical school those who teach, take care of patients, and do research are the masters. Where this obvious principle is overlooked simply because it may offend a few administrators or service department personnel, the resulting antagonisms, wasted energies, poor morale, and administrative chaos are predictable. Just because a hospital will be in trouble if the garbage collectors strike, this does not equate these vital "sanitary engineers" with professors of surgery. This is an unpleasant, undemocratic realism.

4. Budgeting. Preparing the department of surgery budget, with a cash flow of one to ten million dollars a year, is at least as complex as the preparation of an equivalent document of an equally large hardware or grocery store. The manager and budget officer in the real world outside Academia prepare such budgets in relation to a long-range plan, use systems and cost-effective analysis, and often employ so-called planning programming budget techniques. The neophyte surgical chairman characteristically does not even know the meaning of these managerial terms, much less their implications for him as the CEO of a sizable organization. No wonder he is putty in the hands of a predatory medical center comptroller or vice president in charge of health affairs, scarred by years of administrative karate!

5. Conflict resolution. Of all the managerial techniques that are violated by surgical chairmen, perhaps the most vital of these is conflict resolution—a science extensively analyzed by experts in labor-management relations, international diplomacy, psychology, behavioral science, and even by experts in winning at poker! Surgical academicians as a rule have studied only the latter.

A single fundamental fact may serve in illustration. When resolution of a conflict is desired, the participant should identify both his own and his adversary's primary and subsidiary goals. He must act so as to give his antagonist room to maneuver with dignity. The resolution compromise must allow his antagonist to save face. The alternative is total Clausewitzian obliteration of the antagonist, a luxury granted a manager only once or twice in a lifetime. Austerlitz and Wagram, Trafalgar and Waterloo—those were the last of the great routs. Even the winner can only occasionally afford such victories.

Cornered with no room to maneuver, even the timid antagonist has no alternative but to bare his teeth and go for the jugulars. Such is seldom a productive environment for mutually acceptable conflict resolution, be it with a bow-tied, superficially mild pediatric colleague seeking additional hospital beds or with an economy-minded dean committed in print to emphasis on community medicine or experiments in health care.

Newspaper publicity inevitably solidifies

the bargaining position of an antagonist and destroys his ability or desire to find a solution to an odious academic-administrative confrontation. This unproductive scenario seems to have a fatal fascination for untutored chairmen.

These five examples will serve to illustrate the need for training surgical chairmen as scientific managers. The mere listing of other techniques by title brings to mind their applicability in an academic department of surgery. They include: criteria for departmentalization, functional organization, unity of authority and responsibility, use of project managers to solve unexpected problems, long-range planning, scalar principles (supervisor-subordinate relationships), authority responsibility, dissatisfiers (hygienic factors), built-in role conflicts, decision making (pay-off matrix, decision trees, zero-sum gaming, minorant game vs. majorant) (study of alliances), linear programming, motivation models, identifying, and use of administrative power.

SOLUTIONS

"By nature surgeons are more interested in finding solutions than merely defining problems," thus recently spoke a very successful chairman of our close personal acquaintance. And so it should be as we have defined the lack of managerial training among surgical chairman aspirants. How can this be achieved in the busy life of an academically oriented surgical resident, or as he progresses into the ranks of the junior faculty? Those of us dedicated to training surgical chairmen must recognize our responsibility by giving them managerial experience.

1. Managerial job rotation. Managerial training has received careful analysis by large corporations such as General Electric, Sears, and General Motors, where a constant flow of top management candidates is vital for continued corporate success. One technique employs rotation of administrative assignments to those with managerial potential. Surgical chairmen can annually rotate the administrative assignments of the aspirants on their subordinate staff. Assignments can include administration of the O.R., interfacing with the emergency department, supervising the intensive-care unit, budgeting, or junior student curriculum and grading. By the time such a man has come up through the ranks he is administratively ready to be CEO on his own. He need not neglect his devotion to clinical surgery, teaching, or research while thus growing up administratively. The chairman must be willing to delegate not only responsibility but equivalent authority to his subordinate in such a role—a demand that the insecure or selfish chairman may be unwilling to meet. If he wisely so delegates his responsibilities, he reaps double benefit. He has time for his own curricular and extracurricular interests and simultaneously is hailed as a wise and generous statesman. Rarely does laziness pay off so handsomely.

2. Technical administrative assistants. Regardless of what other techniques are employed, the surgical chairman requires an administrative assistant. He must equate his staff needs to those of a bank, store, or department manager in industry who deals in equal sums of money, equal numbers and complexity of outside grants and contracts, and equal numbers of people. When the dean begins to balk at the expense of such an assistant, the surgical chairman should invite him to compare the size and annual cash flow of the surgical department with those of other preclinical and clinical chairmen. As one whose department generates millions of dollars of hospital and medical school income the surgeon can be in a favorable position to resolve this conflict if he but uses his bargaining potential.

3. Seminars and workshops in managerial techniques. Progressive corporations intermittently collect their middle management personnel with advancement potential into management instruction seminars and workshops. Sometimes these conventions are simply didactic expositions of proved principles. More experienced personnel enter the learning process on case-study techniques popularized by the Harvard Business School.

Such techniques could easily be included in the meetings of organizations such as the Society of University Surgeons or they could be made the theme of an entire meeting of the Whipple Society. Experienced chairmen could translate the theoretic exposition of managerial principles to the real problems facing surgical department chairmen. Some of the surgical casualties might even perform their own administrative postmortem!

4. Sequestered full-time training in managerial techniques. Although block study time in managerial technique would probably be most productive in making junior-grade M.B.A.'s of surgical academicians, the professional surgical demands and interests of academic surgeons probably exclude devotion of very many days solely to such training. Many business schools hold short "cram" courses for executives. Rather than become involved with our industrial-managerial counterparts, where such items as merchandising and advertising techniques are of importance, we would be better served by having our own two- to three-week "cram" course, perhaps in a suitable resort environment.

5. Surgical war college. Both the Departments of State and Defense have long recognized the necessity for training potential managers. Junior and senior command and staff schools are a vital part of the Army, Navy, Air Force, and National War Colleges. Their mission is both to teach managerial principles and to provide experience in solving anticipated tactical and strategic problems that the student will face when he assumes a position of managerial responsibility within the profession. The technique and even the environment is applicable to the training of surgical chairmen. We could activate a surgical war college!

Realistic administrative surgical problems could be computer programmed. Aspiring chairmen could play their game on the computer against an adamant dean, a recalcitrant neurosurgeon demanding departmental status, a self-appointed group of dissident residents protesting about food or parking, or a drastic budget cut resulting in cessation of a training grant. Misplays in such computer play have the advantage of not resulting in real casualities. By the time the student faces the real problem as a chairman he would have worked out analogous solutions against a machine.

The programmer for such a surgical academic war college will have an easy assignment. His scenarios have all been written in blood and acted out in tragedy or triumph throughout the land. Conflicts with the dean's office, solved theoretically at the computer console without the emotional charge of real-life confrontation that occasionally overshadows the true issue, will prepare our chairman aspirant for future campaigns. When they occur, he can, with the cold efficiency of *dejà vu,* plot his moves objectively while his adversaries, faced with the problem for the first time, waste their emotional energy inefficiently trying to reach a planned course of action.

The American College of Surgeons could (with a grant) become the headquarters for our academic surgical command center. For security reasons it probably should be located in its Chicago headquarters' sub-basement.

The problem for academic surgery is real. Too many capable academic surgeons have been sacrificed and the appeal of an academic career has, without question, been lessened in the eyes of those who should be candidates for chairs. The first step in solution involves admitting the fundamental nature of our problem. As an academic specialty we are untrained in managerial techniques. It is time to restore sanity, dignity, and some degree of tranquility to the life style of a surgical chairman. The techniques are well known in industry. We simply must apply them and stop the wastage among the best and brightest of surgical academicians.

Physician supply, residency programs, and the foreign medical graduate

Lucian L. Leape, M.D., *Boston, Mass.*

From the Division of Pediatric Surgery, Tufts University School of Medicine, Boston, Mass.

In recent years there has been a significant increase in the number of foreign medical graduates (FMG) entering residency programs in the United States. In 1971, 11,000 FMG's entered the United States, 5,000 of them on exchange visas and 6,000 on immigrant visas.[1] The influx of FMG's has steadily increased in the past 2 decades. In 1951, 2,072 interns and residents were FMG's (10 percent). By 1960 this figure had increased to 20 percent. In 1972, 18,395 of the 56,244 filled intern and residency positions were taken by FMG's, 33 percent of the total.[5] There is no reason to think that this steady influx of FMG's will significantly abate in the near future. Although many FMG's assert their intent to return to their home country at the completion of training, in practice only 10 to 20 percent actually do so on a permanent basis.[3] This significant augmentation of the physician supply poses serious ethical and practical problems which so far have been addressed inadequately in both the professional and lay press.

THE NEEDS OF ALL CONCERNED

In an attempt to clarify the issues, and hopefully to stimulate a solution, the following analysis is presented. The problem is considered from four points of view: (1) the needs the individual FMG himself, (2) the needs of the countries of origin, (3) the needs of the residency programs involved, and (4) the needs of this nation.

1. The needs of the individual. The FMG may not be able to realize his professional ambitions in his home country. The classic example is the physician who comes to the United States, obtains training in cardiac surgery, and returns to his homeland to find that not only is he unable to carry on such a practice (absence of supporting equipment and personnel), but that there really is no need for his services. There may well be people who have cardiac disease, but their medical care is not a top priority item. As in the United States, distribution is a problem. In Iran, for example, there is a surplus of specialists in the cities. The individual has little choice but to emigrate if he is to pursue his professional ambition. Emigration represents "overflow" rather than "drain."[4]

Most Americans admire and support the ambition of an individual to improve himself. In practice, the FMG may be shortchanged. Rather than acquiring a good educational experience, he may find himself in a "work" residency where he is hired to help take care of patients, but in actuality is given very little training. American graduates select the residencies which they think give the best educational experience. Since program

Accepted for publication June 27, 1974.

Reprint requests: Lucian L. Leape, M.D., Boston Floating Hospital, 171 Harrison Ave., Boston, Mass. 02111.

directors tend to favor American graduates, the best programs fill with U. S. graduates. Less desirable programs and those in specialties with less appeal must select FMG's if they are to fill their positions. Thus, although one may support the concept of American training for FMG's, in practice it may not be carried out very well.

2. Needs of the country of origin. Although the home country may well not need cardiac surgeons, it most certainly does need physicians. Major recent suppliers of FMG's to the U. S. (India, Philippines, Korea, Iran, and Thailand) desperately need more physicians in general practice and in public health and can ill afford to lose the national resource represented by each emigrating physician. Unfortunately, inducements to practice in rural areas are often meager,[4] so an increased number of physicians alone is not the solution to their problems, any more than it is in the U. S.

A strong argument can be developed for an American aid program of training foreign physicians to return to help with their nations' problems. The Fulbright program sought to accomplish this goal. Its objectives were lost, however, as American residency programs sought FMG's to fill their positions irrespective of educational value. An effective program requires certain safeguards: (1) The residency programs have to be training programs, not work programs. They must be educationally valid. (2) They have to be appropriate for the needs of the recipient nation. Family practice, public health, and tropical medicine programs are likely to be most useful. (3) The return of the physician to his homeland must be assured. One way to accomplish this would be by an absolute denial of immigration privileges for 10 years. This type of program would give tremendous benefit at little cost. It would provide a type of foreign assistance that is needed, and which we are eminently qualified to carry out.

3. Needs of residency programs in the United States. The total number of residency positions available in 1972 was 51,658. Only 30,610 of these were filled by U. S. medical school graduates. Even though FMG's filled an additional 14,471, there were 6,577 unfilled positions. From a numbers standpoint, we clearly need the FMG in our residency program.

The number of residency positions available results from a myriad of factors, many of little educational significance: increasing complexity of patient care requires constant availability of skilled physicians; a residency program lightens the load on the staff and enhances the prestige of the institution; patient care is improved; many doctors like to teach; etc. Because of the confusion of educational objectives with local service needs, the number of positions available is not a valid indicator of educational need, in terms of either total number of physicians or individual specialties. Approval of a residency program is not difficult to achieve, and the number of positions available in a given program is even more loosely regulated. To date, there have been few attempts to tailor the number of residency programs to national need, either generally or in specific specialties.

4. Needs of the United States. Do we need the FMG? The question has two parts: First, do we need trained FMG's to supplement the practicing physicians in the United States, and second, do we need the number of residency positions we currently have?

At the present time our ratio of physicians to population is 163:100,000. This is higher than in any other country. There is increasing evidence that our physician-availability problems have to do more with geographic distribution and the specialty "mix" than with numbers per se. We clearly need more primary physicians. Similarly we probably have too many general surgeons. Many cities have a surplus of physicians, while rural communities go without.

Interestingly, the FMG tends to aggravate these problems, rather than relieve them. Although in 1970, 17 percent of U. S. physicians were FMG's, they represented only 14 percent of primary care specialists (GP's, internists, pediatricians, and obstetricians).

However, 30 percent of physicians in anesthesiology, pathology, and pediatric cardiology were FMG's.[1] FMG's also shun the rural areas. Eighteen percent of U. S. graduates practice in towns of less than 50,000, but only 11 percent of FMG's do.[2]

Do we need the number of residency positions we currently have? Until decisions are made as to the number of physicians needed, and more particularly the numbers in each of the individual specialties, a rational appraisal of residency numbers is impossible. There is reason to think that there are too many residency positions available in certain specialties, but too few in primary care. Alteration in the number of residency positions available is the surest way to redress that imbalance.

At present the FMG occupies an important role in both residency programs and the practice of medicine, especially in urban areas. Certainly this is not something which we can ethically defend. Even if we do need FMG's, we need them less than their countries of origin whose physician-patient ratios may be only one tenth of ours. It is truly a national disgrace for this affluent nation to deplete other nations of this precious resource simply because we are not willing to do what it takes to produce enough physicians from our own population. It is particularly ironic when so many qualified Americans are denied the opportunity to study medicine. This is not, of course, an overt or endorsed policy, but it is the current practice, and one which we are responsible for by inattention, if not by direction.

Our physician supply/distribution problems urgently need redress. Decisions need to be made about the numbers of physicians who must enter practice each year. If we need more, then clearly we need more medical schools, or larger classes. If our problem is distribution, then answers must be found. For example, a period of required national service might be an acceptable alternative. Exploitation of underdeveloped nations is not the answer to either of these problems.

With these considerations in mind, the following proposal is presented in the hope of stimulating a national debate which will lead to resolution of this serious problem.

1. Responsible parties, in particular the Coordinating Council on Medical Education, representing the A. M. A., A. A. M. C., and the American Board of Medical Specialties, must make hard decisions as to the number of new physicians needed to enter each specialty each year. These decisions must, of course, be based on the best available data and scientific predictions of population changes and needs. (The SOSSUS study should go a long way toward definition of these parameters for surgery and the surgical specialties.) Periodic review must bring about alterations in these numbers as needs change in the future, but a decision must be made, and made soon. From information already available it seems clear that the number of openings in family practice must be markedly increased while those in some other specialties, such as general surgery, must be decreased.

2. Once these numbers are determined the number of first-year postgraduate positions (internship or first-year residency) approved for each specialty must be altered to match. For most specialties, this will require a reduction in the number of positions offered. Regulation should take place at the *input* side, so that we do not have oversupply or wasted individual investment of time and money in unnecessary training.

3. If the total number of first-year residency positions, exceeds the projected annual number of graduates from U. S. medical schools, then the number of medical school graduates must be increased. Although substantial federal financial assistance will be necessary, there are many ways of doing this. But it must be done, and it must be done rapidly. Even with an immediate expansion it will be 3 to 4 years before graduates are available for residency, so an early decision is urgently needed. In the unlikely event that the calculated number of first-year residency positions is less than the predicted number of graduates, then medical schools should reduce their numbers accordingly.

4. "Work" residencies must be eliminated.

Residency programs should be educational programs, most under university administration (though not necessarily *in* university hospitals). If "extra hands" are needed in hospitals, persons should be hired for that purpose: trained physicians who are hired as assistants, or physician's assistants, or nurses. *There is no justification for a residency program that is not a bona fide, effective, worthwhile, educational experience.* Alternatives must be sought to the use of residents largely to help out with the work. Senior academic physicians will have to adjust to the concept of not having their own resident just because of their rank or local prestige.

Assessment of the needs and distribution of physicians and the relative numbers in various specialties is a difficult and inexact exercise. It will never be completed, and it must, of necessity, constantly change as the nature of medical practice changes. However, it is not impossible, and a reasonable decision, based on data that are already available, is certainly far better than no decision, which is the current situation. Clearly the potential benefits are enormous: better fulfillment of our national medical needs, better realization of the undeveloped countries' medical needs, better training for the FMG himself, and the possibility of increased opportunities for qualified Americans who want to study medicine but cannot currently find openings in U. S. medical schools.

REFERENCES

1. Contributions to a Comprehensive Health Manpower Strategy, Center for Health Services Research and Development, Chicago, 1973, American Medical Association.
2. Dublin, Thomas D.: The migration of physicians to the United States, N. Engl. J. Med. **286:** 870, 1972.
3. Haug, J., and Stevens, R.: Foreign medical graduates in the United States in 1963 and 1971: A cohort study, Inquiry **10:** 26, March 1973.
4. Joorabchi, B.: Physician migration: Brain drain or overflow? With special reference to the situation in Iran, Br. J. Med. Educ. **7:** 44, 1973.
5. Status of internship and residency programs in the United States, J. A. M. A. **226:** 938, 1973.

Original communications

Adrenalectomy with chemotherapy in the treatment of advanced breast cancer: Objective and subjective response rates; duration and quality of life

Francis D. Moore, M.D., Susan Bland VanDevanter, M.D., Caryl Magnus Boyden, M.S., Jacob Lokich, M.D., *and* **Richard E. Wilson, M.D.,** *Boston, Mass.*

It is appropriate to examine the results achieved with adrenalectomy and chemotherapy employing 5-fluorouracil, after a decade of standard usage in the treatment of advanced breast cancer. This report covers a consecutive series of 238 adrenalectomized patients, in 158 of whom a prolonged course of 5-fluorouracil was commenced shortly after operation. The objective response rate for adrenalectomy within chemotherapy was 40 percent. With chemotherapy, the objective response rate was increased to 58 percent. In 64 percent of the patients, the subjective palliation involved a return to essentially normal living during the period of improvement. The operative mortality rate was 1.8 percent; chemotherapy did not complicate replacement hormone therapy. Those patients showing an objective response had a significantly longer survival by life-table analysis; when the responders only are considered, it is apparent that those without chemotherapy had a better life-table curve after 30 months. It is concluded that this combination represents a significant improvement in the treatment patterns now available; evidence suggests that the program of chemotherapy should be changed after 24 months.

From the Department of Surgery, Harvard Medical School at the Peter Bent Brigham Hospital, and the Children's Cancer Research Foundation, Boston, Mass.

IN THE evaluation of any treatment for malignancy in which cure is beyond reach, the response rate should be determined both by objective changes and by subjective response, the latter being based on the patient's own evaluation of her feelings and of the meaning of the treatment to her. There are two important time intervals to be measured and one subjective judgment to be made. These two intervals are the duration of remission and the duration of life after treatment, while the subjective judgment concerns the quality of the patient's life during those two intervals. It is the latter that determines the value of the treatment to the patient and her family and helps to answer the question: does the achievement of a remission actually mean a longer and better life for the patient, or is it merely a transient medical improvement, of little actual worth, in an otherwise downhill course?

This study was supported in part by the Breast Cancer Research Fund, The Charlotte Rudnick Fund, and the Virginia Gibson Fund of the Peter Bent Brigham Hospital.

Accepted for publication April 8, 1974.

Reprint requests: Francis D. Moore, M.D., 721 Huntington Ave., Boston, Mass. 02115.

We are reporting here the results of treatment in 238 consecutive patients subjected to adrenalectomy as the principal modality in the treatment of advanced breast cancer. About one half of the patients had undergone oophorectomy previously; the remainder had oophorectomy at this time. After treating the initial group without chemotherapy, chemotherapy was then added to the treatment program. The 5-fluorouracil was commenced soon after operation and continued for a prolonged period thereafter. The present report, therefore, does not cover a randomly selected or concomitant series specifically designed to examine the effects of chemotherapy. Instead, it reports an evolving treatment program from which observations can be made on the results of endocrine ablation as well as on the early and late effects of additional chemotherapy. Some of these patients have been included in prior preliminary studies or reports.[12, 21, 22]

METHODS

Case selection. After many fruitless attempts to improve case selection by endocrine, biochemical, or cytologic means,[2, 8, 19] case selection has been based primarily on clinical criteria. Advanced liver disease with jaundice, extensive brain involvement with focal signs or seizures, and pulmonary lymphangitic spread with respiratory insufficiency have been consistent contraindications. Such patients were treated instead by a course of corticosteroids with chemotherapy, and in all cases died within 90 days.

Table I shows the composition of the treated population. The study series, 238 patients, represents the total of all those appropriate for follow-up study, out of a total of 268 patients with advanced breast cancer subjected to adrenalectomy between January, 1952, and February, 1972. The 30 patients excluded as being inappropriate for this follow-up study were as follows. A total of 16 were operated upon too recently (less than 6 months prior to the beginning of follow-up study in April, 1971), 9 patients were not at risk for a late-treatment result because they died of other diseases, while 5 patients who died immediately after operation were included for calculation of the mortality rate, but were excluded because they were likewise not at risk for a late result.

Of the 238 patients under consideration, 80 (34 percent) underwent adrenalectomy without chemotherapy. This group is termed *adrenalectomy alone*. Of these, 54 had under-

Table I. *Composition of treated population*

Age at onset of primary disease:	
Under 40	24
41 to 50	63
51 to 60	100
61 to 70	51
	238
Primary treatment:	
Simple mastectomy	6
Same plus radiotherapy	10
Modified radical mastectomy	3
Same plus radiotherapy	4
Radical mastectomy	88
Same plus radiotherapy	89
Inoperable; radiotherapy	38
	238
Duration of free interval:	
Less than 1 year	104
1 to 2 years	40
2 to 3 years	20
3 to 5 years	35
Over 5 years	39
	238
Events during free interval:	
(Zero free interval)	(47)
No treatment events	135
Prophylactic oophorectomy	46
Prophylactic hormones	5
Prophylactic oophorectomy plus chemotherapy	5
	238
Pattern of metastatic disease predominating:	
Skin and soft tissue	24
Bone	95
Pleura, lung	47
Viscera and others	72
	238
Prior treatment of secondary disease	
None	104
Oophorectomy with chemotherapy	54
Radiotherapy alone	35
Radiation with hormones	25
Hormones with chemotherapy	14
Oophorectomy alone	6
	238

gone a prior oophorectomy or prior radiation castration, and in 26 patients the ovaries were removed at the same operation as were the adrenal glands.

In 158 patients (66 percent of the total series of 238) adrenalectomy was followed by early and continuous chemotherapy with 5-fluorouracil. This group is referred to as *adrenalectomy with chemotherapy.* Of these, 77 had undergone prior oophorectomy or radiation castration, and in 81 patients the ovaries were removed at the same operation as were the adrenal glands.

Local radiotherapy was used liberally for local painful bone metastases. In the group of *adrenalectomy alone* patients, 8 of the 80 (10 percent) had radiotherapy to local symptomatic areas whereas in the group with *adrenalectomy with chemotherapy,* 13 of the 158 patients (8.2 percent) had such local radiotherapy. There is no significant difference in these rates for the employment of local radiotherapy, a response to which was not counted as evidence of an objective remission to the systemic treatment.

All but five of the patients were treated in the decade 1962-1972. The use of chemotherapy was commenced in 1963 and was applied to all patients operated on after 1966.

TREATMENT PROGRAM

Operative procedure. Adrenalectomy was combined with oophorectomy in those patients with ovaries still in place. Oophorectomy by pelvic laparotomy was performed first, permitting evaluation of the state of the liver and peritoneal cavity. The ovaries were removed without the Fallopian tubes or uterus. The patient was then turned under anesthesia, care being taken to avoid inadvertent pathologic fractures, and likewise to position the patient ideally for lighting and exposure. Both adrenal glands were then removed by the bilateral simultaneous twelfth rib lumbar approach.

Hormone management. Cortisone replacement was commenced during adrenalectomy at a dose of 300 mg. per day. This was reduced over the next few days and the patients were carried thereafter at a dose of 75 mg. of cortisone per day by mouth with 0.1 mg. of α-fluorohydrocortisone twice a week. Minor changes in hormone dosage were made from time to time to suit minor symptomatic alterations; cortisone dosage was increased for intercurrent injury or illness.

Chemotherapy. The 5-fluorouracil was commenced between the third and fifth postoperative day. The drug was administered by a slow intravenous infusion daily for 6 days at a dose of 15 mg. per kilogram and continued thereafter by weekly injections or by mouth, with periodic checks of hematologic response. The patient's home physician frequently joined in the supervision of this prolonged chemotherapy, employing the index of "35" as a signal for a hiatus in drug administration lasting 2 to 3 weeks. By this it was meant that an hematocrit was below 35 percent, the white count was below 3,500 per cubic millilimeter or the platelet count was below 35,000 per cubic millimeter. The simultaneous administration of chemotherapy did not render cortisone maintenance any more difficult or hazardous than had been observed in those without chemotherapy.[11, 17]

FOLLOW-UP AND EVALUATION

No patients were lost to follow-up. The patient's hospital record was reviewed as well as the notes of her home physician, including follow-up visits, x-rays, laboratory studies, and enzyme tests. Evaluation of the quality of the patient's life during remission was based on personal interviews, and letters from the patient or from members of her family.

The term *objective response* was used when there was a reduction in measurable size of lesions on the skin by x-ray, lasting for a period of 6 months or more, or significant changes, such as those from an osteolytic to an osteoblastic bone lesion, similarly persisting for a period of 6 months or more with no evidence of disease advancing elsewhere. A patient showing an objective response is referred to as a "responder."

The term *subjective response* was used to denote symptomatic improvement for 6 months or more, or the maintenance of an asymptomatic state in the presence of stationary or advancing metastases for 6 months or more. In both instances the patient's own evaluation or that of her family was used. Patients demonstrating this sort of subjective response are referred to as "palliated."

The *quality of life* during the interval of palliation was judged from the patient's statement as to what activities she could undertake, as reported either by her or her family. These activity gradations ranged through six stages, three of which were considered arbitrarily as indicating a satisfactory quality of life, and three indicating an unsatisfactory quality of life or poor palliation despite the patient's own statement that she felt better. In the tabulations, the notation of a "satisfactory quality of life" indicates that the patient's activity was in the three more favorable grades. The gradations were as follows:

Satisfactory quality of life during palliation.

Grade 1. Full return to activity with a full normal life.

Grade 2. Slight reduction in strength but with normal activity.

Grade 3. Activity 50 percent of normal, asymptomatic.

Unsatisfactory quality of life during palliation.

Grade 4. Very slight activity but without pain.

Grade 5. Ambulatory and comfortable but with very limited activity, without pain.

Grade 6. Comfortable but not ambulatory, without pain.

STATISTICAL METHODS

All data were entered on a standard data computer retrieval system. This was programmed by the UCLA Biomedical Fortran Program (BMDOIS) for data reduction to life-table and survival-rate configurations.[7] The life-table method used is that described by Cutler.[4] The percentages of response rate were compared among groups within this series and with the literature, using the chi-square test with Yates' correction. The entire life-table curve can be analyzed and compared with other curves at intervals, using a combined test of significance as described by Cochran.[3]* In certain instances the cumulative survival rates were also transformed to semilog plots and the resulting lines were analyzed by covariance analysis.

RESULTS

Mortality and morbidity rates, hormone replacement, and drug toxicity. Of the 238 patients under consideration, 195 (82 percent) were dead at the time of the close of the study (March 1, 1972).

The 5 surgical deaths should be applied against the 268 total adrenalectomy group for a postoperative mortality rate of 1.9 percent, but are not included in the later evaluation. Five additional patients died within 30 days of operation from rapid progession of their disease; they are included as treatment failures. When these are combined, the hospital mortality rate of 10 patients within thirty days becomes 3.8 percent.

Surgical complications of serious note occurred in six instances (2.3 percent). Of these six patients, five suffered pulmonary embolism and one a postoperative hemorrhage. In one of the patients suffering embolism, a vena cava ligation was carried out. In addition, there were 12 patients who had minor complications such as suture abscesses or transient urinary tract infections that did not prolong their hospital stay alter their degree of palliation. Most patients were up and about the day following operation and were ready for discharge 5 to 9 days later.

The addition of chemotherapy did not appear to complicate hormone management; hormone dosage was unchanged and detailed management was not altered in contrasting the two groups. Facial appearances or bodily configurations analogous to those seen in

*We are indebted to Kathryn Erat for assistance in statistical methods and to Linda Desmond at the Health Sciences Computing Facility at the Harvard School of Public Health for additional collaboration in statistical evaluation, data storage, and retrieval.

Table II. *Objective response rates*

Line	Group	Total No.	Objective response No.	Objective response %	No response No.	No response %	Indeterminate response No.	Indeterminate response %	Comparisons in response rate: Line vs. line	Significance† (P)
1	Entire series	238	123	52	102	43	13	5		
2	Adrenalectomy with chemotherapy	158	91	58	59	37	8	5	1 vs. 2	NS
3	Adrenalectomy alone	80	32	40	43	54	5	6	2 vs. 3	< 0.02
4	Free interval less than 1 year	104*	43	41	53	51	8	8		
5	Free interval more than 1 year	134	80	60	49	37	5	3	4 vs. 5	< 0.01
6	Free interval less than 2 years	144	63	44	72	50	9	6		
7	Free interval more than 2 years	94	60	64	30	32	4	4	6 vs. 7	< 0.005
8	Premenopausal	20	12	60	7	39	1	1	8 vs. 9	NS
9	Less than 1 year after menopause	42	16	38	24	57	2	5		
10	1 to 5 years after menopause	63	24	38	36	57	3	5		
11	5 to 10 years after menopause	32	20	62	11	34	1	4	10 vs. 11	< 0.05
12	Age under 40	24	8	33	14	59	2	8		
13	Age over 40	214	115	54	88	41	11	5	12 vs. 13	NS
14	Age under 50	87	38	44	45	51	4	5		
15	Age over 50	151	85	56	57	38	9	6	14 vs. 15	NS

*All figures from line 4 downwards refer to the entire series.
†In this and the subsequent tables "P" values over 0.05 are considered to indicate nonsignificant differences (NS).

Cushing's syndrome were rare in this group of patients, although weight gain was sometimes troublesome. In no instance did such changes alone alter the patient's evaluation of her subjective response. In several patients there was considerable skin pigmentation, made much more marked by exposure to the sun.

The occurrence of clinically dangerous toxic reactions to this program of 5-fluorouracil administration was exceptionally rare.[11, 17] There were no severe hematologic, cutaneous, or gastrointestinal manifestations, although one patient, subsequent to the close of this study, has developed upper-gastrointestinal hemorrhage requiring cessation of chemotherapy. Hair loss was never bothersome in patients on 5-fluorouracil alone. In about one third of the patients the drug had to be stopped for a few weeks to permit the hematologic indices to return to normal, but the patients were asymptomatic and did not develop septic complications during this time. In many patients the occurrence of nausea and malaise after intravenous injection abated when the drug was administered orally.

Objective response rates. An objective response was achieved in 123 patients (52 percent), identified as "responders." There were 102 patients (43 percent) who achieved no objective response ("nonresponders"). There were an additional 13 patients (5 percent) who were indeterminate as to response. That is, their condition remained stable; objectively their lesions were the same while subjectively they felt better. Of these 13 patients, three showed a response only to local radiotherapy and therefore could not be deemed as "responders" to systemic therapy (Table II).

Adrenalectomy alone yielded a lower response rate (40 percent) than adrenalectomy with chemotherapy (58 percent). This difference is strongly significant. Those patients with the longer free intervals and those who were farther past the menopause showed a significantly higher response rate. Age differ-

Table III. *Effect of chemotherapy on objective response rates in various categories*

Line	Category	With chemotherapy		Without chemotherapy		Comparison significance (P)
		No.	Objective response (%)	No.	Objective response (%)	
1	Adrenalectomy	158	58	80	40	< 0.02
2	Zero free interval	35	63	12	0	< 0.001
3	Free interval less than 1 year	73	52	31	16	< 0.002
4	Free interval less than 2 years	101	52	43	23	< 0.003
5	Age under 40	18	44	6	0	NS
6	Age over 40	140	59	74	43	< 0.05
7	Less than 1 year after menopause	32	47	10	10	NS
8	Bone metastases predominate	60	67	35	34	< 0.005
9	Skin and soft tissue metastases	12	58	12	50	NS
10	Pleura and lung metastases	36	53	11	55	NS
11	Visceral metastases	50	50	22	36	NS

ences were not clear cut considering the series as a whole.

As shown in Table III, the addition of chemotherapy showed a marked effect in patients with very short free intervals or in whom primary and secondary disease was first diagnosed simultaneously (so-called "zero free interval"); in these groups chemotherapy yielded much higher response rates than did adrenalectomy without chemotherapy. Patients around the age of 40 and close to the time of the menopause did not show clear-cut differences in response, with or without chemotherapy, when judged by these criteria alone. When the criterion of metastatic pattern was considered, chemotherapy showed a most marked beneficial effect on bone metastases, with the other patterns showing a less clear improvement with the addition of chemotherapy. When bone metastases predominated, chemotherapy provided a strongly significant increase in objective response rate (67 percent as opposed to 34 percent for adrenalectomy alone).

Examination of the objective response rates to treatment of the advanced disease, according to certain details of the primary disease, included study of the effect of the original location of the tumor, size of the tumor, spread of tumor, and prior oophorectomy. In these areas* there was only one finding relative to the nature of the primary tumor or its treatment that appeared to have a strong bearing on subsequent response to treatment of the advanced disease. This one factor was the performance of oophorectomy prior to the development of the primary tumor. This group of 19 patients, who by chance had undergone oophorectomy at a younger age for other unrelated reasons, showed the highest response rate of any subcategory in the study (79 percent), with no statistically significant difference according to whether or not they received chemotherapy. The next most advantageous setting for oophorectomy was its performance at the same time as adrenalectomy (64 percent objective response) to be contrasted to various other patterns of oophorectomy showing objective response rates in the range of 42 to 49 percent.

*Tabulations of these and many other variables are available from the authors upon request.

Subjective response. A subjective response, as judged by the patient herself or her family, was experienced for periods of 6 months or more in 160 (67 percent) of the 238 patients (Table IV). Of these a total of 154 patients (64 percent of the series) could return to living conditions arbitrarily established as "satisfactory quality of life" (i.e., Grades 1, 2, or 3). Of this same total of 160 patients who had experienced satisfactory palliative response for 6 months or more, 28 patients were those who were asymptomatic but with widespread metastatic disease, and remained so.

Table IV. *Subjective response rates*

Line	Nature of palliation	Total series subjective responses No.	%	With subjective response (%)	With chemotherapy No.	%	Without chemotherapy No.	%	Comparisons by chemotherapy (P)
1	Subjective improvement	132	55	82	93	59	39	49	NS
2	Remained asymptomatic	28	12	18	22	14	6	8	NS
3	Total subjective responses (lines 1 + 2)	160	67	100	115	73	45	56	< 0.02
4	No improvement	62	26	—	32	20	30	38	< 0.005
5	Brief improvement	16	7	—	11	7	5	6	NS
6	Total no subjective response (lines 4 + 5)	78	33	—	43	27	35	44	< 0.02
7	Grade 1:* "Normal life"	111	47	69	83	53	28	35	< 0.02
8	Grade 2: "Decreased strength"	38	16	24	27	17	11	14	NS
9	Grade 3: "50 percent activity"	5	2	3	3	2	2	2	NS
10	Grade 4: "Marked reduction in activity"	0	0	0	0	0	0	0	—
11	Grade 5: "Ambulatory and comfortable"	6	3	4	2	1	4	5	NS
12	Grade 6: "In bed, comfortable"	0	0	0	0	0	0	0	—

*See text for grading of subjective responses.

Table V. *Objective response rates—comparisons with literature*

Line	Series	No. in series	Objective response rate (%)	Comparisons: Line vs. line	Significance (P)
1	This, entire series	238	52	1 vs. 2	NS
2	This, adrenalectomy alone	80	40	2 vs. 3	< 0.02
3	This, adrenalectomy with chemotherapy	158	58	2 vs. 4	NS
4	Fracchia et al.,[9] adrenalectomy	500	32	3 vs. 4	< 0.001
5	Fracchia et al.,[10] hypophysectomy	203	23	2 vs. 5	< 0.007
6	Dao et al.,[5] adrenalectomy	573	34	3 vs. 6	< 0.001
7	Macdonald,[15] adrenalectomy	690	28	3 vs. 7	< 0.001
8	Macdonald,[14] hypophysectomy	340	33	3 vs. 8	< 0.001
9	Yonemoto et al.,[23] adrenalectomy	280	39	3 vs. 9	< 0.001
10	Ansfield et al.,[1] 5-fluorouracil	676	23	3 vs. 10	< 0.001
11	Drug Council,[6] androgens	580	21	3 vs. 11	< 0.001
12	Drug Council,[6] estrogens	364	36	3 vs. 12	< 0.001

Of the 154 patients who achieved a "satisfactory quality of life," 111 returned to an essentially normal life (47 percent of those treated).

There was a total of 78 patients (33 percent of the series) in whom no subjective response was achieved or, if noted at all, was very transient. The effect of chemotherapy on subjective response rate was clear cut: a significantly higher subjective response rate and a higher incidence of "satisfactory quality of life" was achieved in those patients receiving chemotherapy (73 percent) than in those without chemotherapy (56 percent).

Contrast of objective response rates with comparable series in the literature. In Table V are data evaluating these results by comparison with other series reported in the literature for a variety of modalities of therapy. The series included in the table are those of Fracchia and associates[9] for adrenalectomy alone, of Fracchia and associates[10] for hypophysectomy, of Dao and associates[5] for adrenalectomy alone, of Macdonald[15] for adrenalectomy alone, of Macdonald[14] for hypophysectomy, of Yonemoto and associ-

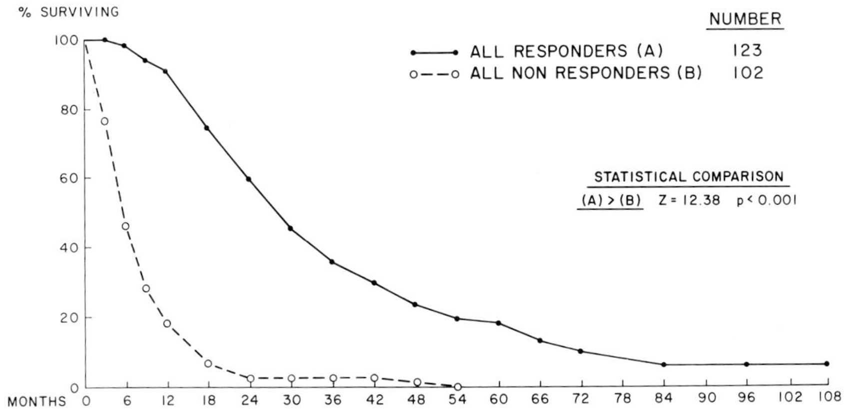

Fig. 1. Life-table analysis: survival, all categories, by objective remission. Responders have a longer survival than nonresponders. In this and subsequent charts the value "Z" is the cumulative normal deviate criterion of Cochran.[3] The appropriate corrected p value is shown.

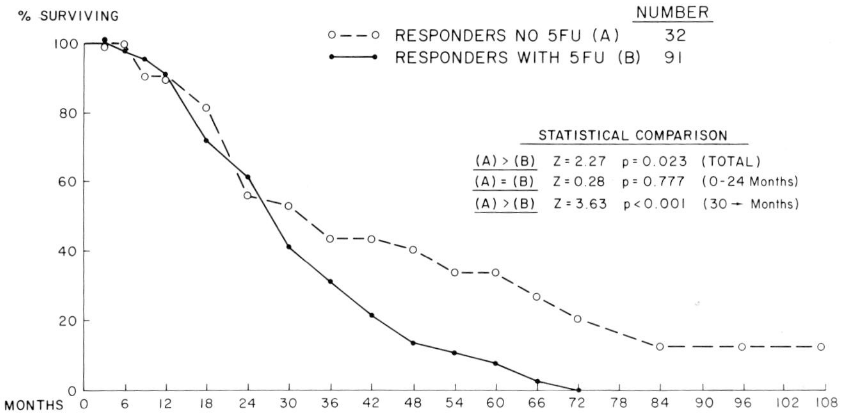

Fig. 2. Life-table analysis: survival, responders only, contrasting by chemotherapy. There is no significant difference in the life-table curve configuration for the first 24 months; thereafter, responders without initial chemotherapy show a significantly longer survival. Both groups received secondary or tertiary chemotherapy when the inital modalities failed.

ates[23] for adrenalectomy alone, of Ansfield and associates[1] for 5-fluorouracil alone, and of the Drug Council Report for androgens and estrogens.[6]

The objective response rate in this series for adrenalectomy alone is essentially the same as that previously reported for adrenalectomy alone by other workers. This suggests that the subset of patients undergoing adrenalectomy alone does not present any bias in selection, viewed retrospectively. In none of the other series reported was an endocrine manipulation combined with a chemotherapeutic modality. Those patients of the present series who received chemotherapy after adrenalectomy showed a higher response rate than did patients of any other series reported in the literature. The response rates for adrenalectomy alone and adrenalectomy plus chemotherapy were both notably higher than those reported for chemotherapy alone using 5-fluorouracil, as described by Ansfield and associates[1] and likewise significantly higher than those reported for either androgens or estrogens alone.[6] Although there is always an uncertainty in comparing data from one hospital with those obtained by an alternative treatment in another hospital, the similarity of our results for adrenalectomy alone (40 percent objective response rate) when compared with the results of Dao (34 percent), Macdonald (28 percent),

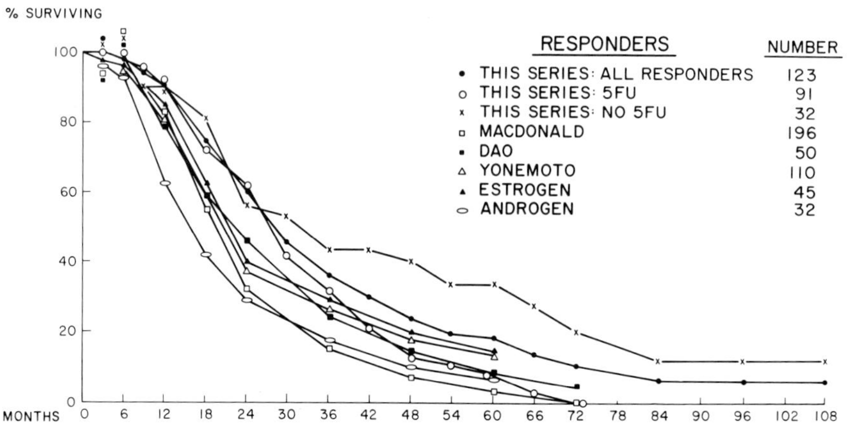

Fig. 3. Life-table analysis: comparison with the literature, responders only. Differences in slope are noted only after 30 months. Prior to that the slopes are essentially the same for all modalities. Early slopes for androgen therapy are less promising than those for the other modalities shown.

and Yonomoto (39 percent) suggests that there are no gross differences in case selection. This factor renders even more significant the much higher response rate (58 percent) when chemotherapy was added to adrenalectomy.

Life-table analysis. Life-table curves for this and other series are shown graphically in Figs. 1 through 5. In all cases the initial 2 to 3 year part of the curve is linear on semilog paper. This signifies that the early slope can be described as a single exponential decay and embodies a constant fractional survival decrement per unit time. Therefore the curve may be described by its half-time. This is the meaning of the term "$T_{1/2}$" in Tables VI and VII. This value for half-time describes the number of months required for the cohort to show a 50 percent decrease in numbers surviving. The whole life-table curves are compared by the method of Cochran[3] in Table VI.

It is notable that in those patients showing an objective response ("all responders") there was a statistically significant longer survival rate (28 months half-time) than in those who did not respond (5.6 months half-time).

In this group of responders, we find that the subset of 32 patients who achieved an objective response without chemotherapy had a longer life-table curve (half-time 32 months) than those responders who were given chemotherapy (half-time 27 months). This difference in survival (by comparison of whole life-table curves) was significant at a P value of 0.023.

There was no difference in the survival curves (half-times of 5.4 and 5.8 months) between those nonresponders without chemotherapy and those with chemotherapy.

Comparison of life-table curves with literature. In Table VI are also shown selected life-table curves contrasted with the literature.* Responders in the chemotherapy subgroup of this series (adrenalectomy plus chemotherapy responders) show a longer half-time than did those in any other series reported in the literature for whom life-table curves can be constructed by this technique. Again it is noteworthy that the chemotherapy-treated nonresponders lived about the same length of time (half-time 5.6 months) as did those reported in the literature without chemotherapy, indicating again the absence of an adverse effect of chemotherapy in nonresponders.

Comparison of this series with patients who received 5-fluorouracil alone. The series reports by Ansfield and associates[1] for the

*In constructing life-table curves from the literature we have taken the reported numbers of cases and the sequential survival rates and entered them in the standard life-table method as described by Cutler and Ederer.[4]

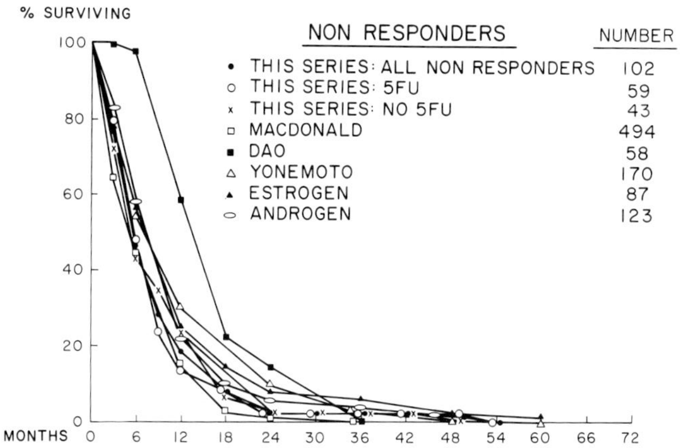

Fig. 4. Life-table analysis: comparison with the literature, nonresponders only. Nonresponders show no essential differences, suggesting that the addition of chemotherapy does not shorten survival.

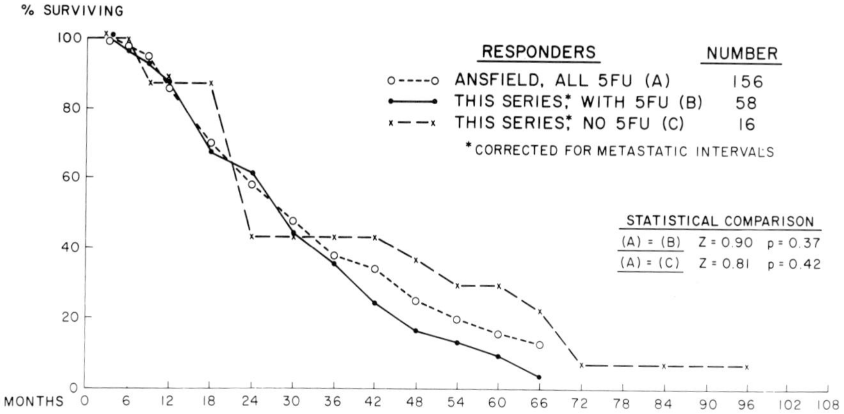

Fig. 5. Life-table analysis: responders only, comparisons with the studies of Ansfield[1] (5-fluorouracil alone). The data from the present series are modified as described in the text to include only those patients operated upon within 6 months of the appearance of metastases, to make a consistent comparison with Ansfield's data. Although the group undergoing adrenalectomy and chemotherapy have a much higher response rate (58 percent) than Ansfield's patients (23 percent) there is no statistical difference between the life-table survivorship slopes of the responders treated by the two methods. After 30 months there is a more prolonged survivorship among those treated by adrenalectomy without chemotherapy.

response to 5-fluorouracil alone is important in interpretation of findings in this group of patients receiving both adrenalectomy and 5-fluorouracil. Although the response rate reported here for the combination treatment is 58 percent, and significantly higher than the response rate of 23 percent reported by Ansfield and associates[1] in 676 patients having 5-fluorouracil alone, the life-table slope of declining survivorship of responders is identical (Fig. 5). To avoid bias in this comparison, resulting from the time interval that often elapsed after metastases were noted but before therapy was begun, we have modified our data as shown in Fig. 5 to include only those patients treated by adrenalectomy and chemotherapy within 6 months of onset of metastases. This renders them directly comparable with Ansfield's data, based on patients in whom chemotherapy was begun immediately when metastases were observed. This comparison indicates that

Table VI. *Life table curves—this series and comparisons with the literature*

Line	Series	No.	$T_{1/2}$ (Mos. ± S.D.)	Two-year survival (%)	Comparisons: Line vs. line	Comparisons: Whole curve (P)	Comparisons: 2 Year survey (P)
1	This, entire series	238	16 ± 1.4	35			
2	This, adrenalectomy with chemotherapy	158	17 ± 1.7	40			
3	This, adernalectomy alone	80	13 ± 1.9	26	2 vs. 3	< 0.93	< 0.05
4	This, all responders	123	28 ± 2.0	60	4 vs. 7	< 0.018	< 0.001
5	This, responders to adrenalectomy with chemotherapy	91	27 ± 1.6	62			
6	This, responders to adrenalectomy alone	32	32 ± 5.7	56	5 vs. 6	< 0.023	NS
7	Yonemoto et al.,[23] responders	110	21 ± 1.3	37	5 vs. 7	< 0.163	< 0.001
8	Dao et al.,[5] responders	50	22 ± 2.5	46	4 vs. 8	< 0.024	NS
9	Macdonald,[15] responders	196	20 ± 0.8	32	4 vs. 9	< 0.001	< 0.001
10	Drug Council,[6] estrogens (all)	132	11 ± 1.0	19	1 vs. 10	< 0.006	< 0.002
11	Drug Council,[6] androgens (all)	155	9 ± 0.6	10	1 vs. 11	< 0.001	< 0.001
12	Drug Council,[6] estrogen responders	45	21 ± 1.9	40	4 vs. 12	< 0.135	< 0.04
13	Drug Council,[6] androgen responders	32	16 ± 2.0	29	5 vs. 13	< 0.005	< 0.003
14	This, nonresponders entire series	102	5.6 ± 0.4	2			
15	This, nonresponders to adrenalectomy with chemotherapy	59	5.8 ± 0.6	2			
16	This, nonresponders to adrenalectomy alone	43	5.4 ± 0.8	2	15 vs. 16	< 0.85	NS
17	Yonemoto et al.,[23] nonresponders	170	7.3 ± 0.9	8	14 vs. 17	< 0.034	< 0.08
18	Macdonald,[15] nonresponders	494	5.2 ± 0.3	1	14 vs. 18	< 0.097	NS

Table VII. *Early and late life-table curves of responders only: Comparisons according to chemotherapy covariance analysis of log plots*

Line	Period	Chemotherapy: With	Chemotherapy: Without	Comparison (P)
0 to 24 months:				
1	Number of cases	91	32	
2	Slope ($\bar{S}_6$)*	0.864	0.857	NS
3	Slope ($T_{1/2}$) (mo.)	28.4	27.0	NS
4	Correlation coefficient (r)	0.97	0.93	
5	Variance			NS
6	Adjusted means			NS
30 to 96 months:				
7	Number of cases	36	18	
8	Slope ($\bar{S}_6$)*	0.657	0.865	< 0.001
9	Slope ($T_{1/2}$) (mo.)	9.9	28.7	< 0.001
10	Correlation coefficient (r)	0.97	0.97	
11	Variance			NS
12	Adjusted means			< 0.001

*$\bar{S}_6$ = six-monthly decremental fraction of linear decay survivorship.

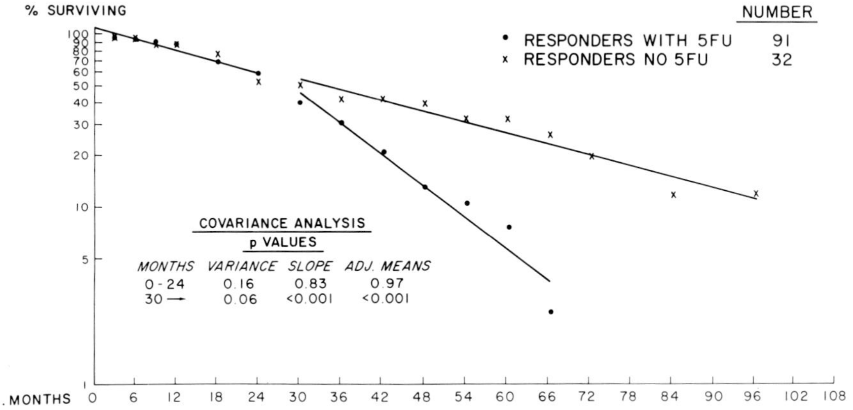

Fig. 6. Life-table analysis: responders only, contrasting patients with and without chemotherapy. Here semilog plots are shown for the life-table curves, demonstrating their linear behavior as a constant decremental-decay fraction. These responders with and without chemotherapy are identical up to 24 months. Thereafter the slopes depart sharply from each other with a strongly significant difference between the slopes after 30 months, those with chemotherapy departing downwards.

although the response rate for the present series is significantly higher than in those patients reported by Ansfield, the survival-slope characteristic of those who responded to therapy is strictly comparable between the two series.

Late effects of added chemotherapy. It is evident from Fig. 2 that patients who received chemotherapy with adrenalectomy showed an interesting deviation in survival curves when considered for the period after 30 months. When adrenalectomy and chemotherapy were used together, there was a clear increase in response rate, as previously mentioned. Prior to 30 months, the life-table curves of the two groups of responders are identical. After the interval of approximately 30 months, the responders appeared to show a somewhat better survival curve if they had not received chemotherapy. It must be noted that this comparison is between *responders only* in both groups; there is no significant difference in survival at the 2 year level, but, comparing the whole curve, there is a small difference (half-time 32 months vs. 27 months).

Because of this unexpected finding of improved late survival curves of those responders who did not receive chemotherapy, a variety of additional comparisons were made. These are shown in Fig. 6 and Table VII. When the late curves for responders are dealt with either by standard (linear) life-table techniques or by covariance analysis on the logarithms of the data, the group without chemotherapy shows a clearly longer survival and a lesser slope after 30 months. Prior to that time there was no difference. For example, during the period of 30 to 96 months, the group without chemotherapy showed a slope described by a half-time of 28.7 months, while those with chemotherapy showed a slope described by half-time of 9.9 months. This difference in the late slope configuration is significantly different with a P value of 0.001. It is evident from Fig. 6 that the group on prolonged chemotherapy show a downward departure from their prior life-table slope after 30 months.

DISCUSSION

The modalities combined here (adrenalectomy, oophorectomy, if not previously performed, and chemotherapy with 5-fluorouracil) were standardized about 10 years ago in this department. Although it had been anticipated that early chemotherapy might improve response rates, more toxicity was expected than was experienced, and the improvement in response rates exceeded expectations. The improvement in response rate, palliation, and the fine quality of life experienced, together with the prolonged survivorship, appeared to set this combination therapy apart from our previous experience and that of others reported in the literature.

As based on our experience with these 238 patients, it is evident that if the patient achieves an objective remission from adrenalectomy either with or without chemotherapy she then has a significant likelihood of having a much longer life (half-time 27 months) than her sister patient who underwent the same treatment but did not achieve an objective remission (half-time 5.6 months). The addition of chemotherapy adds to the likelihood of her favorable response (58 vs. 40 percent) and, if she fails to respond, does not shorten her life. She has a somewhat better chance of experiencing a return to essentially normal living if she is given chemotherapy at the time of adrenalectomy and is maintained on the drug thereafter. These data, therefore, provide a baseline against which further improvements in the treatment of late metastatic breast cancer can be compared.

The stimulus to employ chemotherapy with 5-fluorouracil very early after adrenalectomy and to continue it thereafter for an indefinite period was an outgrowth of the immediate pain relief often observed after adrenalectomy alone. This phenomenon suggested that the endocrine ablation produced some acute alteration in the tumor cell membrane itself, its water content, its metabolism, or its cell-cycle kinetics that might well provide an ideal opportunity for exposure to a cytotoxic chemotherapeutic agent. Based on this highly theoretical consideration, combined therapy was commenced in a patient suffering from extensive pulmonary metastases. A remarkably favorable result encouraged continuance of the program. Thereafter, in an increasing fraction of patients, chemotherapy with 5-fluorouracil was commenced early in the postoperative period. This evolution of the treatment program has been associated with the high and maintained objective response rate indicated above. This naturally raises questions as to whether case selection was especially favorable in the more recent group or especially unfavorable earlier. Although the two groups were not contemporaneous nor randomly selected, we have reviewed the age groups, metastatic patterns, symptomatology, free intervals, late drug treatment, and other clinical indices.* Only minor differences were revealed for the group of patients subjected to adrenalectomy with chemotherapy as compared to those without; there was a slightly longer free interval and a slightly lower incidence of premenopausal patients in the group without chemotherapy. The fact that the patients who underwent adrenalectomy alone show a response rate that is virtually identical with other case series reported in the literature suggests that they were not adversely selected. That the group undergoing adrenalectomy alone was not adversely selected is also suggested by the fact that it is in this category (adrenalectomy alone) that late survival appeared to be improved when responders were contrasted with those responders in the chemotherapy group.

Although the objective response rate to adrenalectomy is higher with chemotherapy than without, the explanation of this late difference in survival time of responders is not clear. Several alternative explanations offer themselves, including an immunosuppressive effect of chemotherapy, prior withholding of chemotherapy and its subsequent administration, or alterations in case selection unknown to us. We have examined all three of these possibilities and again have no conclusive evidence to favor any one explanation. In most patients in the series there was some late alteration in drug treatment when final relapse began and if drugs had not been given they were then added. Review of this tertiary chemotherapy in both groups shows that they were entirely comparable.

Recent evidence concerning the growth of tumors under immunosuppression raises the

*The changeover from no chemotherapy to universal use of chemotherapy in these patients was rather abrupt. There were 34 patients operated upon in 1964 and 1965; fourteen received chemotherapy. Thereafter, all patients received chemotherapy with adrenalectomy.

possibility that any drug used for cancer chemotherapy might have unfavorable side effects on the patient's immune resistance to the tumor, ultimately coming to dominate any favorable effect on tumor cell mitosis or protein synthesis.[16, 20] Although this potentially adverse effect of cancer chemotherapy has long been suspect, we have previously found no evidence for it in our prior studies nor in reports from the literature. We now report this unexpected finding: after 2 years responders in the group without chemotherapy appear to survive longer than responders in the group with chemotherapy. A variety of statistical methods have been applied to examine this small difference in two groups of cases. By all criteria used it holds up as statistically significant. This suggests that after 24 to 30 months chemotherapy should be changed or stopped. Again it must be noted that this difference is exhibited among two groups of *responders* in whom the *response rates* are quite different.

Using adrenalectomy one occasionally encounters patients who are made clinically worse.[18] We have not experienced this phenomenon in patients treated by adrenalectomy plus chemotherapy. Estrogen and androgen therapy, either separately or together, are capable of producing severe exacerbation with hypercalcemia after only a few days or weeks of treatment.[13] We have not seen this response in adrenalectomy with or without chemotherapy. Some of the more toxic chemotherapeutic drugs are also capable of making the patient very ill and of destroying a palliative result. The use of 5-fluorouracil has been singularly free of this unfavorable issue. In discussing treatment with the patient and her family, these simple considerations often rise to the top of the conversation. A patient suffering from late cancer must consider not only the likelihood of success of palliative treatment, but also the potential price of failure.

This paper should close by re-emphasizing the fact that these patients still die of breast cancer and that our best results still yield only a few extra years of life for the patient.

The authors acknowledge with gratitude the collaboration and assistance throughout this study received from members of the hospital staffs in Surgery, Medicine, Chemotherapy, and Radiotherapy at the Peter Bent Brigham Hospital and the Children's Cancer Research Foundation.

REFERENCES

1. Ansfield, F. J., Ramirez, G., Mackman, S., Bryan, G. T., and Curreri, A. R.: A ten year study of 5-fluorouracil in disseminated breast cancer with clinical results and survival times, Cancer Res. **29:** 1062, 1969.
2. Castellanos, H., Fairgrieve, J., O'Morchoe, P. J., and Moore, F. D.: Corticotropin stimulation of urethral cornification. A measure of adrenal estrogen capacity in carcinoma of the breast, J. A. M. A. **184:** 123, 1963.
3. Cochran, W. G.: Some methods for strengthening the common χ^2 tests, Biometrics **10:** 417, 1954.
4. Cutler, S. J., and Ederer, F.: Maximum utilization of the life-table method in analyzing survival, J. Chron. Dis. **8:** 699, 1958.
5. Dao, T. L., Nemoto, T., and Bross, I.: A continuing randomized comparative study of early and late adrenalectomy in women with advanced breast cancer, *in* Forrest, A. P. M., and Kunkler, P. B., editors: Prognostic factors in breast cancer, First Tenovus Symposium, Cardiff, Wales, 1967, Edinburgh, E. & S. Livingstone, Ltd., 1968.
6. DeNoseguo, N. (secretary): Report of council on drugs—androgens and estrogens in the treatment of disseminated mammary carcinoma, J. A. M. A. **172:** 1271, 1960.
7. Dixon, W. J., editor: UCLA biomedical fortran program (BMDOIS) for data-reduction to life-table and survival-rate configuration, *in* Biomedical computer programs—Health Sciences Computing Facility, Department of Preventive Medicine and Public Health of the School of Medicine, University of California at Los Angeles (privately printed).
8. Fairgrieve, J.: Selected criteria for surgical removal of the endocrine glands in advanced breast cancer, Surg. Gynecol. Obstet. **122:** 371, 1965.
9. Fracchia, A. A., Randall, H. T., and Farrow, J. H.: The results of adrenalectomy in advanced breast cancer in 500 consecutive patients, Surg. Gynecol. Obstet. **125:** 747, 1967.
10. Fracchia, A. A., Farrow, J. H., Miller, T. R., Tollefsen, R. H., Greenberg, E. J., and Knapper, W. H.: Hypophysectomy as compared with adrenalectomy in the treatment of advanced carcinoma of the breast, Surg. Gynecol. Obstet. **133:** 241, 1971.
11. Hall, T. C., and Wilson, R. E.: A safe and

effective method of administering 5-fluorouracil to adrenalectomized patients, Surg. Gynecol. Obstet. **121:** 978, 1966.

12. Jantet, G., Crocker, D. W., Shiraki, M., and Moore, F. D.: Adrenal suppression in disseminated carcinoma of the breast. I. The effect on adrenal morphology of hypophysectomy and corticosteroid treatment, N. Engl. J. Med. **269:** 1, 1963.
13. Jessiman, A. G., Emerson, K., Shah, R. C., and Moore, F. D.: Hypercalcemia in carcinoma of the breast, Ann. Surg. **157:** 377, 1963.
14. Macdonald, I.: Adrenalectomy and hypophysectomy in disseminated mammary carcinoma; Preliminary statement by the Joint Committee on Endocrine Ablative Procedure in Disseminated Mammary Carcinoma, J. A. M. A. **175:** 787, 1961.
15. Macdonald, I.: Endocrine ablation in disseminated mammary carcinoma, Surg. Gynecol. Obstet. **115:** 215, 1962.
16. Penn, I., Hammond, W., Brettschneider, L., and Starzl, T. E.: Malignant lymphomas in transplantation patients, Transplant. Proc. **1:** 106, 1969.
17. Piro, A. J., Wilson, R. E., Hall, T. C., Aliapoulios, M. A., Nevinny, H. B., and Moore, F. D.: Toxicity studies of fluorouracil used with adrenalectomy in breast cancer, Arch. Surg. **105:** 95, 1972.
18. Wilson, R. E., Jessiman, A. G., and Moore, F. D.: Severe exacerbation of cancer of the breast after oophorectomy and adrenalectomy. Report of four cases, N. Engl. J. Med. **258:** 312, 1958.
19. Wilson, R. E., Crocker, D. W., Fairgrieve, J., Bartholomay, A. F., Emerson, K., and Moore, F. D.: Adrenal structure and function in advanced carcinoma of the breast. II. The relation of steroid excretion to adrenal morphology and the outcome of adrenalectomy, with description of a new discriminant function, J. A. M. A. **199:** 134, 1967.
20. Wilson, R. E., Hager, E. B., Hampers, C. L., Corson, J. M., Merrill, J. P., and Murray, J. E.: Immunologic rejection of human cancer transplanted with renal allograft, N. Engl. J. Med. **278:** 479, 1968.
21. Wilson, R. E., Piro, A. J., Aliapoulios, M. A., and Moore, F. D.: Evaluation of adrenalectomy and hypophysectomy in the treatment of metastatic cancer of the breast, Cancer **24:** 1322, 1969.
22. Wilson, R. E., Piro, A. J., Aliapoulios, M. A., and Moore, F. D.: Treatment of metastatic breast cancer with a combination of adrenalectomy and 5-fluorouracil, Progr. Rep. Cancer **28:** 962, 1971.
23. Yonemoto, R. H., Byron, R. L., Jr., and Keating, J. L.: Long term survival following adrenalectomy for advanced breast cancer, Cancer **20:** 254, 1967.

Safe limits of hemodilution in cardiopulmonary bypass

Yasunaru Kawashima, M.D., Zengo Yamamoto, M.D., *and* **Hisao Manabe, M.D.,** *Osaka, Japan*

Eleven adult mongrel dogs were subjected to cardiopulmonary bypass at normal temperature with a constant perfusion flow rate. The hematocrit value was reduced stepwise to investigate the blood-gas exchange during hemodilution perfusion. The arterial O_2 saturation was maintained at the physiological level whereas the venous O_2 saturation decreased progressively. The arterial and venous O_2 contents declined with the fall of hematocrit value, the decrease in venous O_2 content being rather slow at hematocrit values below 20 percent. The systemic O_2 consumption, consequently, was maintained within the range of that under whole blood perfusion when the hematocrit value was above 20 percent, whereas it fell drastically with a decrease in hematocrit below 20 percent. Neither the CO_2 tension nor the CO_2 content of arterial blood showed any significant relationship with the hematocrit value. The A-V difference in CO_2 tension increased progressively with the fall in hematocrit values, whereas there was no correlation between the A-V difference in CO_2 content and hematocrit. The results of the present study indicate the safe limits of hemodilution in the practice of cardiopulmonary bypass at normal temperature with the flow rate of 80 ml. per kilogram per minute to be not lower than a hematocrit value of 20 percent.

From the First Department of Surgery, Osaka University Medical School, Osaka, Japan

CARDIOPULMONARY bypass with hemodilution is currently used as a common adjunctive measure in open-heart surgery. With recent technological improvements in the design of the pump oxygenator and in the technique of perfusion, the extracorporeal circulation requiring no blood for priming is now also in clinical use. However, reports of basic studies designed to determine how far the circulating blood can be diluted with safety or without serious complications are surprisingly few, although a considerable number of communications[9, 14-17] have appeared in an effort to assess these factors clinically.

Accepted for publication Jan. 29, 1974.

Reprint requests: Yasunaru Kawashima, M.D., First Department of Surgery, Osaka University Medical School, Fukushima-Ku, Osaka, Japan.

The present report deals with an experimental study which the authors conducted from a viewpoint of blood-gas exchange; it is an attempt to determine the safe limits of hemodilution in cardiopulmonary bypass.

MATERIALS AND METHODS

Eleven adult mongrel dogs ranging in weight from 6.0 to 13.5 kilograms were used. The animals were intubated, and respiration was controlled with a volume respirator using room air. Cardiopulmonary bypass was performed by means of a disc oxygenator pump whereby the blood was drawn through catheters inserted into venae cavae and returned into the right femoral artery. Flow rate during bypass was maintained at a constant rate of 80 ml. per minute per kilogram of body weight. Blood temperature was maintained at

Table I. *Data from arterial and venous blood experimental animals undergoing cardiopulmonar*

	Pv_{O_2} (mm. Hg)	Sa_{O_2} (%)	Sv_{O_2} (%)
-10	45.3 ± 3.4	99.3 ± 0.3	48.3 ± 3.7
11-20	35.4 ± 2.0	98.0 ± 0.5	44.4 ± 3.2
21-30	39.3 ± 2.6	97.1 ± 0.9	52.1 ± 3.9
31-40	44.7 ± 1.9	96.9 ± 0.8	64.4 ± 3.4
41-	45.6 ± 2.0	94.3 ± 1.6	66.9 ± 2.2

	Pa_{CO_2} (mm. Hg)	Pv_{CO_2} (mm. Hg)	ΔP_{CO_2}(mm.Hg)	Ca_{CO_2} (ml./100 ml.)
-10	36.6 ± 3.3	62.8 ± 5.3	26.2 ± 2.8	28.5 ± 5.4
11-20	43.9 ± 2.1	63.5 ± 2.7	19.6 ± 1.5	32.2 ± 2.9
21-30	41.5 ± 2.2	56.1 ± 2.9	14.5 ± 1.6	28.9 ± 2.1
31-40	34.2 ± 3.3	43.1 ± 4.0	8.9 ± 1.5	27.7 ± 2.6
41-	33.6 ± 4.2	40.1 ± 4.6	7.1 ± 0.9	24.5 ± 3.1

*All values are mean ± standard error of the mean.
Pv_{O_2}, venous O_2 tension
Sa_{O_2}, arterial O_2 saturation
Sv_{O_2}, venous O_2 saturation
Pa_{CO_2}, arterial CO_2 tension
Pv_{CO_2}, venous CO_2 tension
ΔP_{CO_2}, A-V difference in CO_2 tension
Ca_{CO_2}, arterial CO_2 content

37° C. by way of a Gabauer heat exchanger. The rate of oxygen supply to the disc oxygenator was constantly 1.4 times that of blood flow.

The cardiopulmonary bypass was begun with whole donor blood, and aliquots of circulating blood were taken out while equal amounts of buffered Ringer's lactate solution were infused to replace it in the pump oxygenator at 30 minute intervals in order to reduce the hematocrit value of the circulating blood stepwise by about ten percent each time.

Arterial and venous blood samples were obtained after initiation of the cardiopulmonary bypass before dilution and between 15 and 30 minutes following each blood dilution. Hematocrit and hemoglobin values, partial pressures of O_2 and CO_2, and pH were measured, and the O_2 and CO_2 content, O_2 consumption, and CO_2 elimination were calculated. These data were classified into five groups according to hematocrit values, less than 10, 11 to 20, 21 to 30, 31 to 40, and more than 41. The relationship between the hematocrit value and the various blood gas data was investigated.

RESULTS

The results are summarized in Table I. The venous O_2 tension remained within a range between 22 and 74 mm. Hg. It demonstrated a tendency to decline in accord with a decrease in hematocrit value within the range between 10 and 50 percent, whereas beyond the lower limits of this range and downward, the venous O_2 tension failed to show any fall but, conversely, rose in some instances (Fig. 1).

The arterial O_2 saturation was maintained at levels more than 90 percent irrespective of the hematocrit value. The venous O_2 saturation varied between 28 and 84 percent and was noted to diminish progressively with the decrease in hematocrit value. It, however, did not decline with a fall in hematocrit value below 20 percent.

The arterial O_2 content declined progressively in proportion to the fall of hematocrit value, with a positive correlation between them (Fig. 2). The venous O_2 content as well proved to decline with the decrease in hematocrit value; again there was a positive correlation between them although the trend of diminution of venous O_2 content became progressively less pronounced as the fall in hematocrit progressed. Insomuch as the arterial O_2 content decreased linearly with a fall of hematocrit, the arteriovenous difference in O_2 content eventually diminished with the decrease in hematocrit value.

In the study reported, the arteriovenous difference in O_2 content was directly proportionate to the oxygen consumption as the *ypass with various hematocrits**

Ca_{O_2} (ml./100 ml.)	Cv_{O_2} (ml./100 ml.)	$\dot{V}_{O_2}$ (ml./Kg./min.)
4.33 ± 0.45	1.79 ± 0.24	2.01 ± 0.19
8.43 ± 0.48	3.54 ± 0.44	3.76 ± 0.21
12.14 ± 0.63	6.48 ± 0.70	4.53 ± 0.35
17.21 ± 0.65	11.29 ± 0.86	4.74 ± 0.40
20.14 ± 1.15	14.07 ± 1.15	4.86 ± 0.35

Cv_{CO_2} (ml./100 ml.)	$\dot{V}_{CO_2}$ (ml./Kg./min.)	RQ	ΔpH
32.5 ± 5.7	3.20 ± 0.60	1.63 ± 0.41	0.188 ± 0.018
37.1 ± 2.8	3.92 ± 0.42	1.23 ± 0.17	0.098 ± 0.013
34.6 ± 2.3	4.56 ± 0.64	0.98 ± 0.17	0.084 ± 0.014
31.7 ± 2.4	3.20 ± 0.44	0.78 ± 0.11	0.045 ± 0.008
28.1 ± 3.0	2.88 ± 0.55	0.59 ± 0.12	0.035 ± 0.004

Ca_{O_2}, arterial O_2 content
Cv_{O_2}, venous O_2 content
$\dot{V}_{O_2}$, O_2 consumption
Cv_{CO_2}, venous CO_2 content
$\dot{V}_{CO_2}$, CO_2 elimination
RQ, respiratory quotient
ΔpH, A-V difference in pH

blood flow rate was kept constant throughout the experiment. Oxygen consumption remained roughly constant irrespective of any variation in hematocrit value, provided that the hematocrit was over 20 percent, whereas with a hematocrit below 20 per cent, it fell drastically with a decrease in the hematocrit value (Fig. 3). That is, there was no significant difference in mean O_2 consumption among the three groups showing hematocrit values from 21 to 30 percent, from 31 to 40 percent, and more than 41 percent. The mean O_2 consumption of these groups was 4.69 ± 0.37 ml. per kilogram per minute. By contrast, blood samples with hematocrit values from 11 to 20 percent displayed a mean O_2 consumption of 3.76 ± 0.21 ml. per kilogram per minute, and this value differed significantly from the foregoing value ($P < 0.01$). The remaining group with hematocrit values of less than ten percent showed a further significant decrease in mean O_2 consumption, being 2.01 ± 0.19 ml. per kilogram per minute ($P < 0.01$).

Arterial blood samples exhibited a rather broad range of CO_2 tension and of CO_2 content, from 14 to 54 mm. Hg and from 8.2 to 58.0 vol. percent, respectively. There was no relationship between these values and the hematocrit value. Both venous CO_2 tension and content were noted to vary in parallel with variation in the arterial CO_2 tension and content, respectively, with positive correlations between them ($r = +0.80$; $r = +0.97$). The arteriovenous difference in CO_2 tension increased with the fall of hematocrit value (Fig. 4). There was no correlation between the arteriovenous difference in CO_2 content and the hematocrit value, as shown in Fig. 5. It follows that there was no significant relationship between the hematocrit value and CO_2 elimination.

The results heretofore described indicate that the blood CO_2 transport and elimination is minimally influenced by hemodilution. Since the O_2 consumption fell drastically at hematocrit values below 20 percent as described above, there was a tendency for the respiratory quotient to rise with the fall of hematocrit value (Fig. 6).

The pH of arterial blood and that of venous blood fell with the decrease in hematocrit value, and this tendency was particularly prominent in the venous blood. Consequently, the difference in pH between arterial and venous blood tended to increase as the hematocrit value decreased (Fig. 7).

DISCUSSION

Hemodilution perfusion was initially designed to avoid homologous blood syndrome[1, 5, 8] or to meet the necessity of saving blood. Many reports emphasizing its clinical safety[2, 3, 6, 7, 10] have appeared to date while

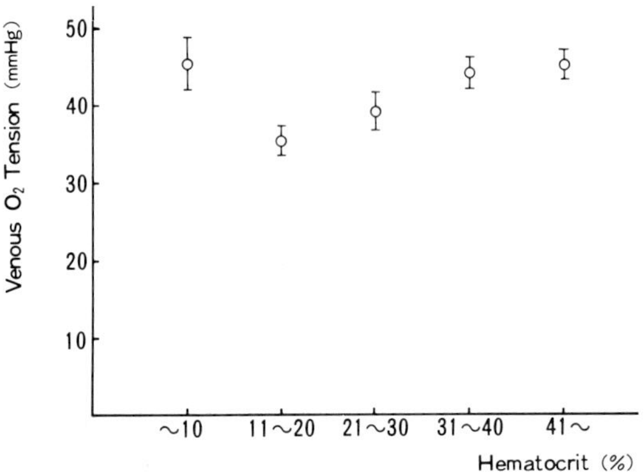

Fig. 1. Relationship between venous O_2 tension and hematocrit. Points are mean ± S.E. for given intervals of hematocrit.

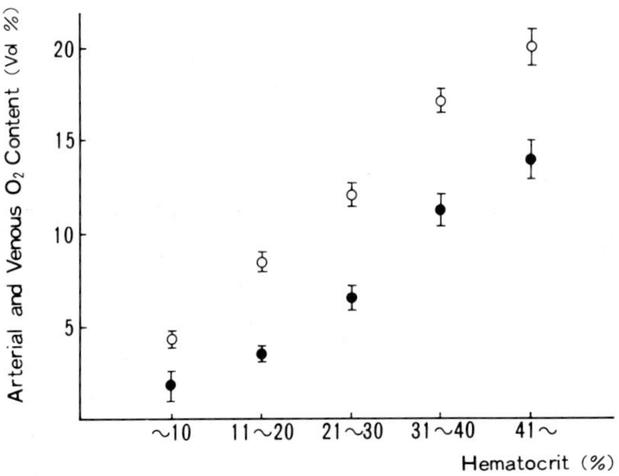

Fig. 2. Arterial and venous O_2 content with various hematocrits. Open circles: arterial O_2 content. Closed circles: venous O_2 content.

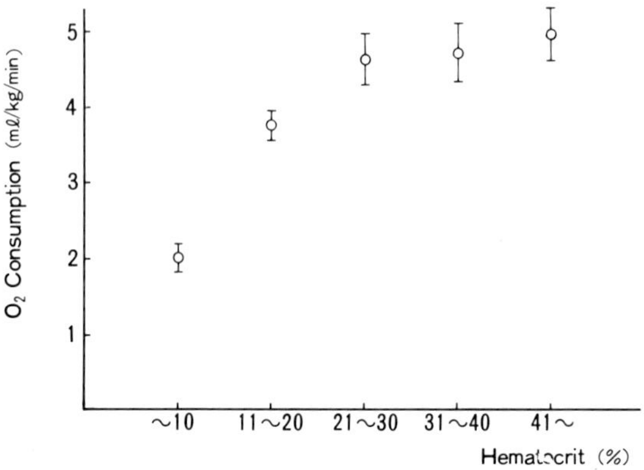

Fig. 3. Relationship between O_2 consumption and hematocrit.

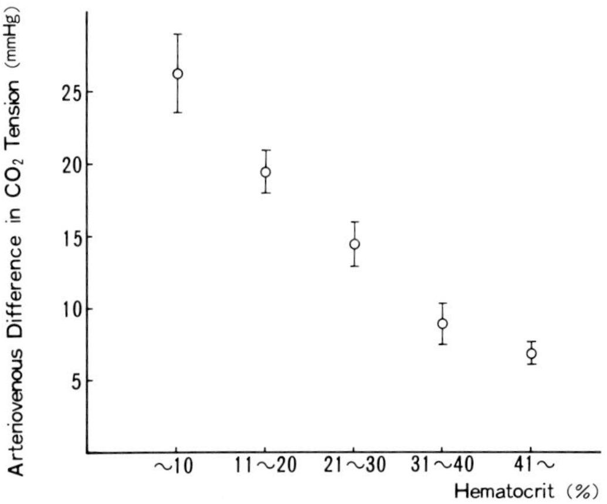

Fig. 4. Relationship between arteriovenous difference in CO_2 tension and hematocrit.

there is surprisingly a dearth of published information on the basic pathophysiologic study of this procedure.

Acid-base imbalance has been discussed as a major complication of hemodilution,[15] whereupon assessments of various diluents and the importance of proper adjustment of pH have been urged from a practical point of view.[9, 16] The underlying cause, however, is no doubt a disturbance in the O_2-carrying capacities of the blood which is precipitated by a decrease in hemoglobin value resulting from hemodilution. Cardiac output has been shown to increase in induced normovolemic anemia.[12, 13] It is also possible, under cardiopulmonary bypass, to compensate for the hemodilution by increasing the perfusion flow rate and with the concomitant use of hypothermia. However, there do exist certain limitations both for the increase in flow rate and in the degree of hypothermia. In view of this, the authors made an initial attempt in the study described to determine the safe limits of hemodilution by investigating the influence of hematocrit diminution on the O_2- and CO_2-carrying capacities under the normothermic condition with a constant perfusion flow rate.

With a stepwise reduction in hematocrit value, when the arterial O_2 content was diminished progressively, there was a proportionate decline in the venous O_2 content, resulting in a constant arteriovenous difference in O_2 content to a level of 20 percent

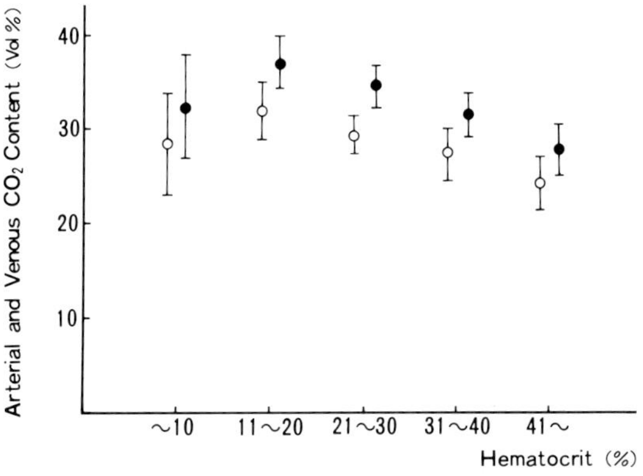

Fig. 5. Arterial and venous CO_2 content with various hematocrits. Open circles: arterial CO_2 content. Closed circles: venous CO_2 content.

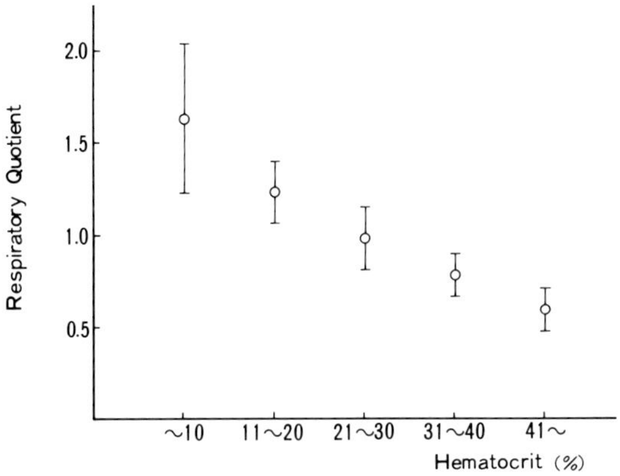

Fig. 6. Relationship between respiratory quotient and hematocrit.

hematocrit. That is, the arteriovenous difference in O_2 content was maintained at a constant by the reduction of venous O_2 saturation, although the O_2-carrying capacity of blood diminished with a decrease in the hematocrit value. However, a certain range of O_2 tension is necessary for the diffusion of O_2 into the tissues,[18] and the possible decline in the venous O_2 saturation is limited. Therefore, it is necessary for the O_2 dissociation curve to shift to the right so as to ensure an adequate arteriovenous difference in O_2 content. The factors that operate to shift the O_2 dissociation curve to the right are a diminution of pH and an elevation of CO_2 tension.[11] As shown in Fig. 7, the arteriovenous difference in blood pH increased with the fall of

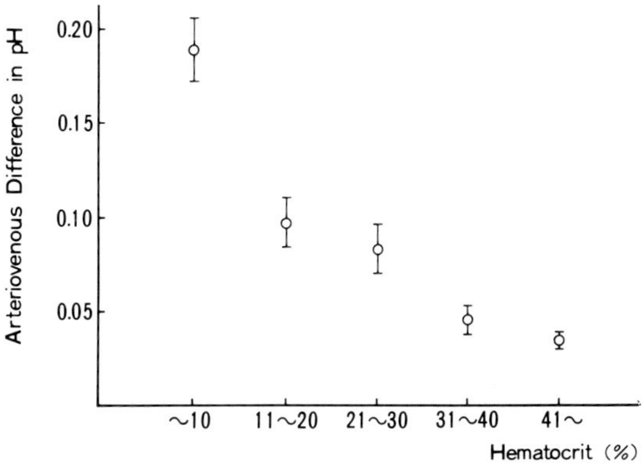

Fig. 7. Relationship between arteriovenous difference in pH and hematocrit.

hematocrit value, and as shown in Fig. 4, the arteriovenous difference in CO_2 tension also increased with the fall of hematocrit value. Thus, the arteriovenous difference in O_2 content is maintained at a constant by the reduction of venous O_2 saturation.

Once the hematocrit value has fallen below 20 percent, however, the body is no longer capable of compensating for the decline in O_2 supply (even by the abovementioned compensatory mechanisms), and as a result, a drastic decrease in O_2 consumption follows (Fig. 3). Salient increase in the arteriovenous difference in blood pH and CO_2 tension can no longer obviate this tendency. The fact that some venous blood samples show elevations of O_2 tension despite a marked fall in hematocrit value seems to indicate that the tissues were already incapable of taking up the O_2 supplied.

Meanwhile, the arterial CO_2 content was noted to be independent of the hematocrit value, and the venous CO_2 content was found to be intimately correlated with the arterial CO_2 content, again unrelated to the hematocrit value (Fig. 5). Consequently, no correlation was found between the hematocrit value and the arteriovenous difference in CO_2 content nor between the hematocrit value and the systemic CO_2 elimination. This finding suggests that the hemodilution scarcely interferes with CO_2 transport and elimination.

The fact that an elevation in the venous CO_2 tension occurred with a fall in hematocrit appears to be due to probable inhibition of HCO_3^- formation that might arise from an impairment of buffering capacity of the hemoglobin with the decrease in hematocrit value. The absence of any significant rise in venous blood CO_2 content therefore was probably derived from a flattening of the CO_2 dissociation curve. Thus, the increase in the venous CO_2 tension and a fall of pH are suggested to be the compensatory homeostatic mechanisms of the body whereby the CO_2 elimination is maintained at a certain level. Furthermore, the shift of the O_2 dissociation curve to the right renders possible further diminution of O_2 saturation. As the reduced hemoglobin is superior to oxyhemoglobin with respect to its buffering capacity, the decrease in venous O_2 saturation associated with the fall of hematocrit value eventually compensates for the loss of buffering activity of the hemoglobin, with the subsequent compensation for the disturbance in HCO_3^- production.

As described above, the systemic O_2 consumption decreases drastically when the hematocrit value has fallen below 20 percent, and the respiratory quotient tends to rise with the decline in hematocrit value. The phenomenon appears to demonstrate that there was no obvious tendency for the CO_2 elimination to diminish despite a significant decrease in O_2 consumption at hematocrit below 20 percent under the given experimental conditions. It seems to suggest that the anaerobic metabolic process is taking place. The authors' observation that the pH fell and the base excess diminished progressively with the lapse of time in animals undergoing prolonged cardiopulmonary bypass with extreme hemodilution may provide evidence in support of the latter view.

The experimental study herein reported was performed with the donor blood drawn immediately prior to perfusion. In the clinical cases, however, heparinized blood taken the day before operation and/or acid-citrate-dextrose (ACD) blood drawn more than 24 hours before operation were utilized. The inadequate level of 2,3-DPG in such blood[1] necessitates further consideration in relation to this study.

REFERENCES

1. Beutler, E., Meul, A., and Wood, L. A.: Depletion and regeneration of 2,3-diphosphoglyceric acid in stored red blood cells, Transfusion **9:** 109, 1969.
2. Cooley, D. A., Beall, A. C., and Grondin, P.: Open-heart operations with disposable oxygenators, five percent dextrose prime, and normothermia, SURGERY **52:** 713, 1962.
3. DeWall, R. A., Lillehei, R. C., and Sellers, R. D.: Hemodilution perfusion for open-heart surgery, N. Engl. J. Med. **266:** 1087, 1962.
4. Gadboys, H. L., Slonim, R., and Litwak, R. S.: Homologous blood syndrome. I. Preliminary observations on its relationship to clinical cardiopulmonary bypass, Ann. Surg. **156:** 793, 1962.
5. Gadboys, H. L., Jones, A. R., Slonim, R., Wisoff, B. G., and Litwak, R. S.: The homologous blood syndrome. III. Influence of plasma, buffy coat and red cells in provoking its manifestations, Am. J. Cardiol. **12:** 194, 1963.
6. Greer, A. E., Carey, J. M., and Zuhdi, N.: Hemodilution principle of hypothermic perfusion, J. Thorac. Cardiovasc. Surg. **43:** 642, 1962.
7. Hellström, G., and Björk, V. O.: Hemodilution with Rheomacrodex during total body perfusion, J. Thorac. Cardiovasc. Surg. **45:** 395, 1963.
8. Litwak, R. S., Slonim, R., Wisoff, B. G., and Gadboys, H. L.: Homologous blood syndrome during extracorporeal circulation in man. II. Phenomena of sequestration and desequestration, N. Engl. J. Med. **268:** 1377, 1963.
9. Litwak, R. S., Gadboys, H. L., Kahn, M., and Wisoff, B. G.: High flow total body perfusion utilizing diluted perfusate in a large prime system, J. Thorac. Cardiovasc. Surg. **49:** 74, 1965.
10. Long, D. M., Sanchez, I., Varco, R. I., and Lillehei, C. W.: The use of low molecular weight dextran and serum albumin as plasma expanders in extracorporeal circulation, SURGERY **50:** 12, 1961.
11. Mitchell, J. H., Sproule, B. J., and Chapman, C. B.: The physiological meaning of the maximal oxygen intake test, J. Clin. Invest. **37:** 538, 1958.
12. Murray, J. F., Gold, P., and Johnson, B. L.: Systemic oxygen transport in induced normovolemic anemia and polycythemia, Am. J. Physiol. **203:** 720, 1961.
13. Murray, J. F., Gold, P., and Johnson, B. L.: The circulatory effects of hematocrit variations in normovolemic and hypervolemic dogs, J. Clin. Invest. **42:** 1150, 1963.
14. Neville, W. E., Spinazzola, A., Banuchi, F.,

Scicchitano, L. P., and Peacock, H.: Clinical experience with buffered Ringer's lactate solution for total prime of the disc oxygenator during cardiopulmonary bypass, J. Thorac. Cardiovasc. Surg. **48:** 101, 1964.

15. Neville, W. E., Faber, C. P., and Peacock, H.: Total prime of the disc oxygenator with Ringer's and Ringer's lactate solution for cardiopulmonary bypass: Clinical and experimental observations, Dis. Chest **45:** 320, 1964.
16. Neville, W. E., Scicchitano, L., Maben, M., Banuchi, F., and Peacock, H.: Cardiopulmonary bypass with large volume nonblood perfusate, Circulation **31** (Suppl. 1): 130, 1965.
17. Roe, B. B., Hutchinson, J. C., and Swenson, E. E.: High-flow body perfusion with calculated hemodilution, Ann. Thorac. Surg. **1:** 581, 1965.

Positive-contrast peritoneography for accurate delineation of diaphragmatic abnormalities

John J. White, M.D., C.M., Kook Sang Oh, M.D., *and* **J. Alex Haller, Jr., M.D.,**
Baltimore, Md.

Positive-contrast peritoneography, a technique for accurately delineating abdominal abnormalities by coating or filling them with contrast medium, was used to investigate three children with apparent diaphragmatic abnormalities. Eventration was accurately confirmed in two, and the presence or absence of contained abdominal viscera was established. The anatomic extent of the sac of a foramen of Morgagni hernia was outlined exactly preoperatively in the third case. The ease and simplicity of positive-contrast peritoneography, its relative safety, the opportunity to obtain concomitant studies, and, most importantly, the accuracy and direct delineation of abnormalities recommend the procedure. Our preliminary experience suggests that positive-contrast peritoneography can provide an accurate, simple, and safe method for the direct diagnosis of diaphragmatic abnormalities.

From The Division of Pediatric Surgery and Pediatric Radiology, The Johns Hopkins University School of Medicine, Baltimore, Md.

STRUCTURAL abnormalities of the diaphragm may be suspected clinically or from chest roentgenograms, but an accurate diagnosis without operation is often difficult to obtain. Moreover, the functional significance of an abnormality and differentiation among diaphragmatic hernia, tumor, and eventration may be uncertain. Various diagnostic techniques have been advocated which may provide indirect information, such as abnormal organ position on radioisotope scanning or angiography. Indirect techniques provide evidence that is only suggestive, and they fail to delineate accurately the diaphragmatic defect itself. Direct visualization of the diaphragmatic structural abnormalities has been attempted with the use of negative-contrast peritoneography with air or other gaseous insufflation into the abdomen. These techniques have suffered from imperfect resolution and delineation. Positive-contrast peritoneography has been reported to provide better definition than negative-contrast studies do.[1]

We have previously reported our experience with positive-contrast peritoneography for the accurate diagnosis of congenital inguinal hernias.[2, 3] We have performed more than 600 of these examinations with few complications. During this period, we have utilized positive-contrast peritoneography as well for the investigation of three children with lesions of the upper peritoneal cavity, and we have obtained clear definition of the diaphragmatic structural abnormalities involved. Appropriate therapy was confidently selected. Our early experience with positive-contrast peritoneography for diaphragmatic

Accepted for publication April 4, 1974.

Reprint requests: John J. White, M.D., Department of Surgery, Division of Pediatric Surgery, The Johns Hopkins Hospital, Baltimore, Md. 21205.

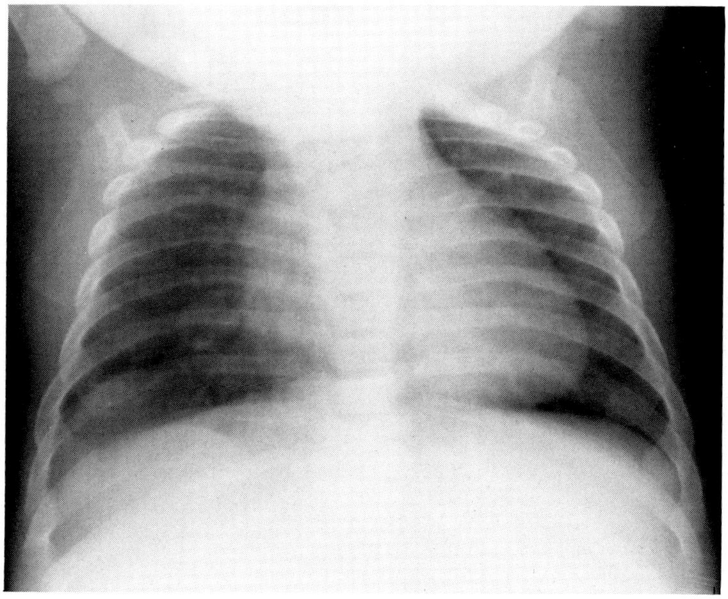

Fig. 1. A-P chest roentgenogram (case 1). There is a scoliosis of the midthoracic spine with abnormal segmentation at the level of the fifth and sixth vertebrae. Cephalad bulging of a dome-shaped soft tissue mass in the lateral portion of the right hemidiaphragm is present.

abnormalities suggests that it is a simple, uncomplicated, and highly accurate technique for the delineation of structural diaphragmatic abnormalities.

TECHNIQUE

Our technique is a modification of that previously described for the investigation of inguinal hernias.[2] With the patient supine, the skin of the abdomen in the midline about 2 to 3 cm. below the umbilicus is prepared with one percent iodine, which is allowed to dry and then removed with alcohol. Meglumine diatrizoate, in a volume depending on weight (Table I), is injected into the peritoneal cavity through the prepared site with the use of a suitably sized syringe and a 19G, 1½ inch needle. A longer needle should be used for obese or larger children. Before injecting, the syringe is aspirated for air or urine to rule out inadvertent bowel or bladder penetration. After injection, a Band-Aid is applied.

The patient is immediately placed prone or supine on the radiographic table, depending on whether the lesion is in the anterior or posterior portion of the diaphragm, respectively, and the head of the table is depressed 15 to 20 degrees. Gentle rocking from side to side is carried out to ensure adequate intraperitoneal distribution of the contrast medium. A single posteroanterior roentgenogram is obtained 5 minutes following injection and checked to ensure that complete delineation of the diaphragmatic abnormality has been accomplished. If the delineation is incomplete, further positioning and rocking are carried out, and a repeat view is obtained as soon as possible. Once delineation is complete, lateral and oblique films can be obtained as necessary.

Table I. *Dose of 30 percent meglumine diatrizoate employed in inguinal herniography**

Weight (Kg.)	*ml./Kg.*
<7	3
8–10	25
11–15	30
16–20	40
21–30	50
>30	60

*Mix one half Hypaque meglumine 60 percent and one half sterile distilled water.

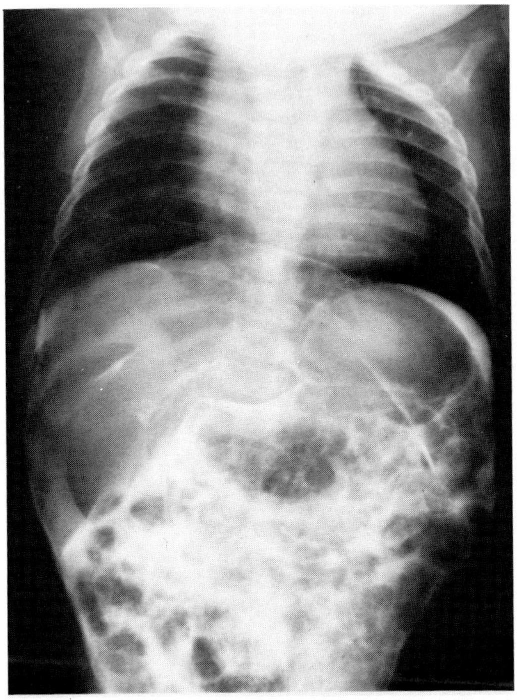

Fig. 2A. Positive-contrast peritoneogram (case 1). A well-delineated eventration is demonstrated in the right lateral diaphragm, located posterolaterally (see Fig. 2*B*). The abnormality is localized and does not contain any herniated viscera.

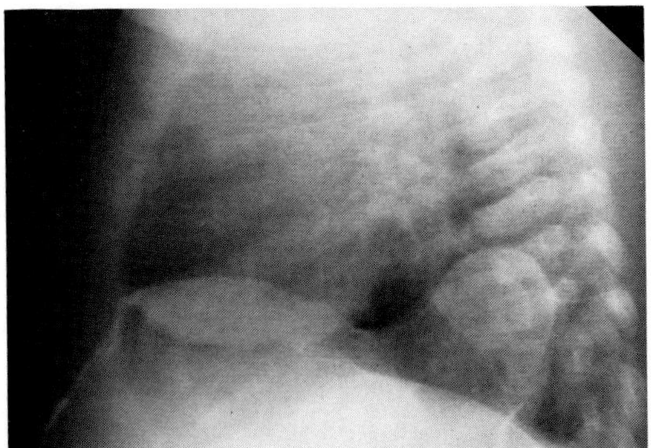

Fig. 2B. Side view of lesion shown in Fig. 2*A*.

Following completion of the diaphragmatic study, the patient is allowed to relax in the waiting area. About 60 minutes after injection of the contrast material, an anteroposterior roentgenogram of the abdomen is obtained; the gonads are shielded in the case of a male patient. Absorption of contrast material from the peritoneum usually is sufficient by this time to provide an excretory urogram adequate to screen most patients for urinary tract pathology. This "bonus" study has proved valuable in children who may have urinary tract pathology in association with other congenital anomalies.[4]

CLINICAL MATERIAL

Case 1. A 3-week-old boy was seen in the Harriet Lane Home Clinic with cough and coryza. Chest roentgenograms failed to confirm pneumonitis but did show scoliosis of the upper and midthoracic spine with abnormal segmentation at the level of the fifth and sixth thoracic vertebrae, as well as a soft tissue density bulging cephalad in the posterolateral portion of the right hemidiaphragm (Fig. 1). This was thought to represent an eventration but, in view of the thoracic vertebral anomalies, a split notochord syndrome or neuroenteric cyst, as well as pulmonary sequestration, bronchogenic cyst, Bochdalek hernia, and soft tissue tumor were also considered. Because his mother had noticed intermittent groin bulging, an inguinal herniogram was obtained. When satisfactory visualization of the inguinal areas had been obtained, he was positioned as described so that the suspected diaphragmatic abnormality could be outlined. Eventration was confirmed, well outlined with contrast material (Figs. 2*A* and 2*B*); there was no evidence of liver, kidney, or bowel herniated into the eventration defect. The excretory urogram was normal.

Case 2. A 6-month-old girl was seen at the Harriet Lane Home Clinic with cough and high fever. A posteroanterior chest roentgenogram demonstrated a dome-shaped soft tissue density bulging cephalad in the posteromedial portion of the left hemidiaphragm (Fig. 3). She had undergone a 9 day hospital investigation elsewhere at 2 months of age which included fluoroscopy, intravenous pyelogram, and pneumoperitoneum. The latter was suggestive of eventration with a soft tissue mass, probably spleen, contained within. Since we could not rule out a posterolateral diaphragmatic hernia on review of these films, positive-contrast peritoneography was obtained. Eventration was confirmed and noted to contain both bowel and a

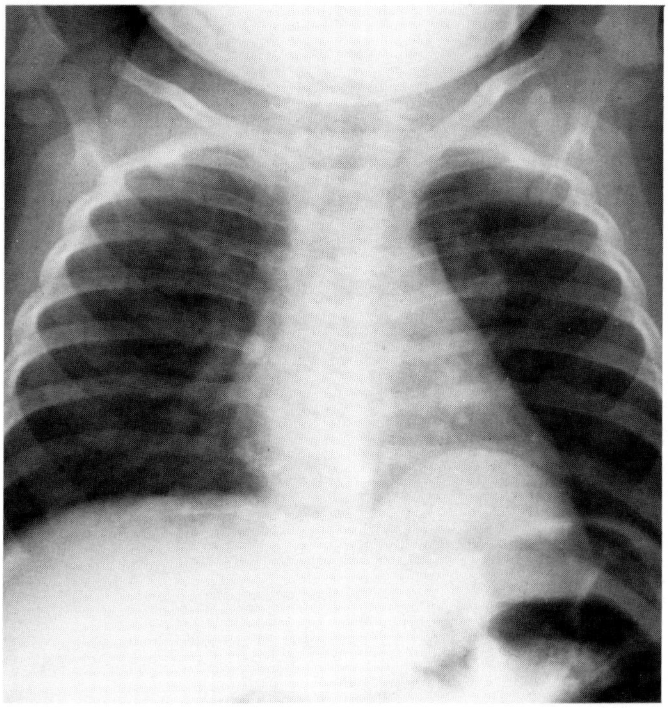

Fig. 3. A-P chest roentgenogram (case 2). Cephalad bulging of a dome-shaped soft tissue density is evident behind the heart in the medial portion of the left hemidiaphragm.

solid viscus, probably speen (Figs. 4*A* and 4*B*). The excretory urogram showed the left kidney to be positioned somewhat more cephalad, but it was not in the eventration. The child was positioned so that the contrast material outlined the inguinal areas as well. The concomitant inguinal herniogram demonstrated bilateral small peritoneal sacs; clinical hernias were not present. In view of her lack of abdominal symptoms, it was elected to follow clinically both the eventration and the patent vaginal processes, and operative therapy was deferred. She has remained asymptomatic.

Case 3. An 11-month-old boy was admitted to the Children's Medical and Surgical Center of The Johns Hopkins Hospital for investigation of a cyanotic "spell" 3 weeks prior to admission and of failure to thrive. Born prematurely, he was less than the third percentile in height, weight, and head circumference, and he was the twelfth and youngest child in a socially poor family environment. A loud precordial systolic murmur was present with split pulmonic heart sounds. There was also congenital ptosis of the left eyelid. An electrocardiogram showed right cardiac hypertrophy, and chest fluoroscopy demonstrated an apparently normal heart shifted to the left by a nonpulsatile anterior mass (Fig. 5). Cineangiocardiography showed an anterior mass pressing on the right heart, with peripheral pulmonic stenosis; right ventricular and pulmonary artery pressures were 40 mm. Hg. An upper gastrointestinal series demonstrated a transverse stomach with normal position of the ligament of Treitz and cecum. On liver scan, the anterior thoracic mass consisted mainly of the liver (Fig. 6). Negative contrast peritoneography, performed with the use of CO_2, was obtained with indistinct visualization of the diaphragmatic abnormality. Positive contrast peritoneography (Figs. 7*A* and 7*B*) demonstrated a large anteromedial diaphragmatic defect (foramen of Morgagni) with a hernia sac extending into the thorax to the level of the fourth thoracic vertebra. A successful repair of the foramen of Morgagni hernia was carried out.

DISCUSSION

Hitherto, diagnosis of diaphragmatic abnormalities has been possible either through indirect assumption based on chest roentgenography and radioisotope studies or directly with the use of negative-contrast (gas) peritoneography. Neither group of techniques has provided definitive delineation and reliably accurate diagnosis. The advent of posi-

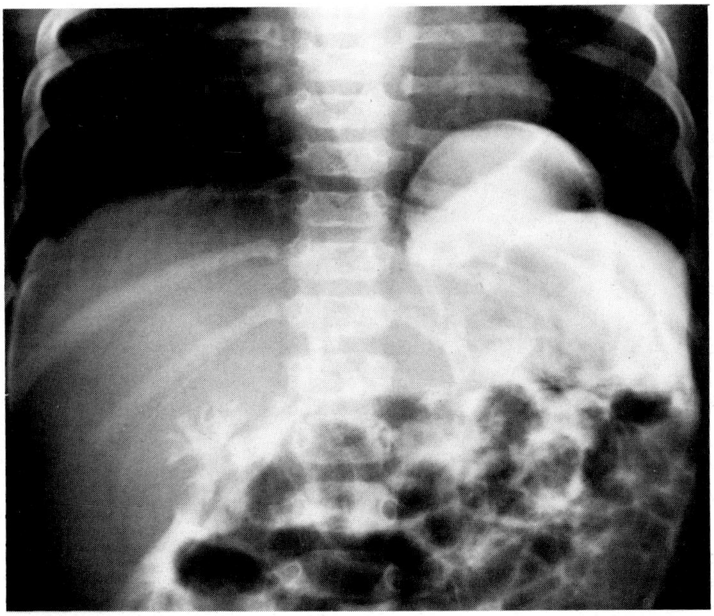

Fig. 4A. Positive-contrast peritoneogram (case 2). The eventration is well outlined in the posteromedial portion of the right hemidiaphragm. The excretory urogram shows a normal right calyceal system and a somewhat more cephalad positioned but normal left kidney.

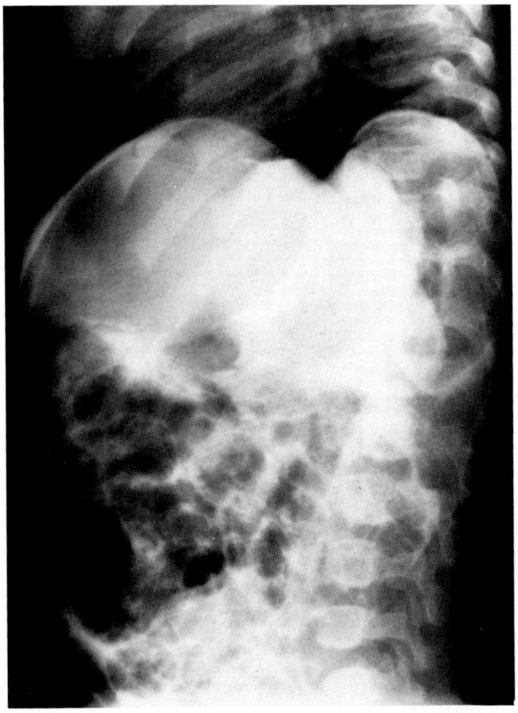

Fig. 4B. Side view of lesion shown in Fig. 4*A*. Spleen and bowel are present within and below the abnormality.

tive-contrast peritoneography promises to correct these deficiencies.

Positive-contrast peritoneography is a rapid and relatively safe procedure. More than 600 studies for inguinal herniography have been carried out in The Johns Hopkins Hospital without any deaths and with only one mild urticarial reaction to the contrast medium.[2] Clinically insignificant peritoneal contamination has occurred in three patients from inadequate skin preparation but otherwise there has been no morbidity despite occasional injections of contrast medium into the abdominal wall, or inadvertent bladder or bowel puncture. The procedure is as simple to perform as intravenous pyelography and can be carried out by any of the radiology staff.

Positive-contrast peritoneography can clearly delineate diaphragmatic abnormalities and provide an accurate preoperative assessment of the extent and anatomy of a hernia (Case 3; Fig. 7). Likewise, this technique can provide accurate definition of the size and location of diaphragmatic eventrations and

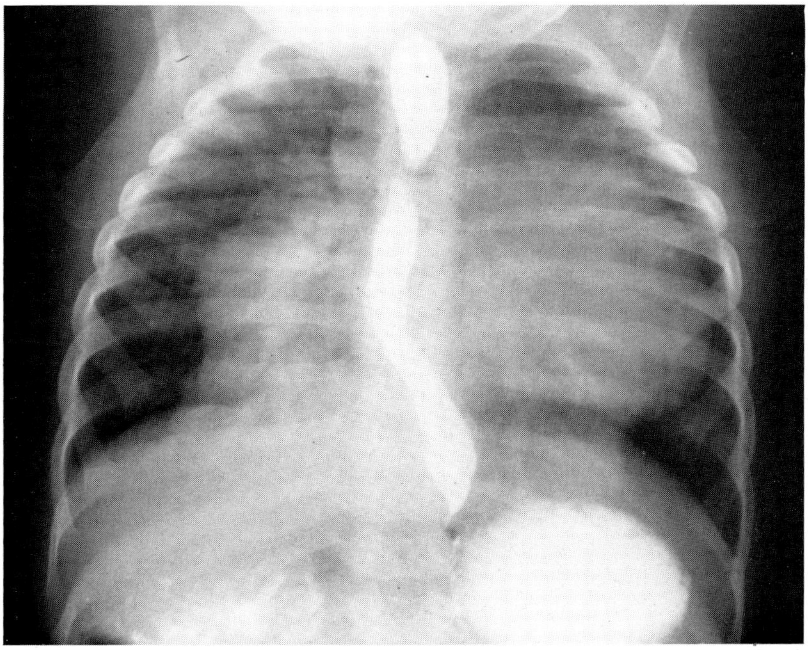

Fig. 5. Cardiac series (case 3) demonstrates shift of the heart to the left with a sharp deviation of the lower esophagus also to the left, both apparently the result of a large lobulated mass in the lower right anterior mediastinum.

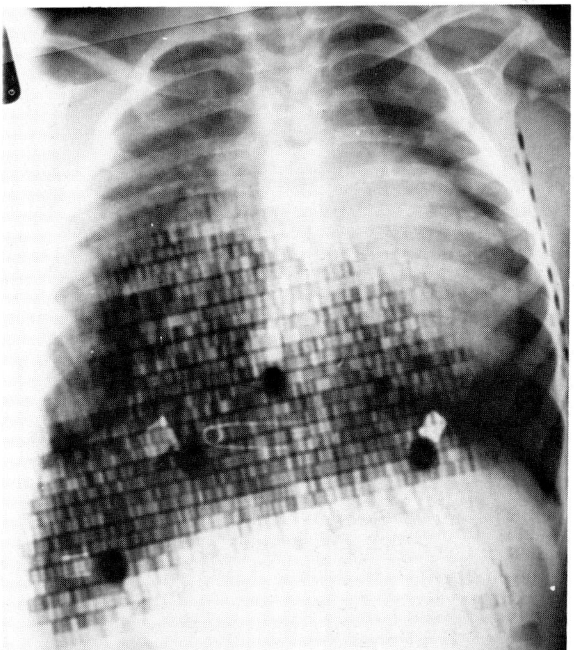

Fig. 6. Liver scan (case 3) shows the liver to lie partially above the diaphragm, particularly in its right medial aspect.

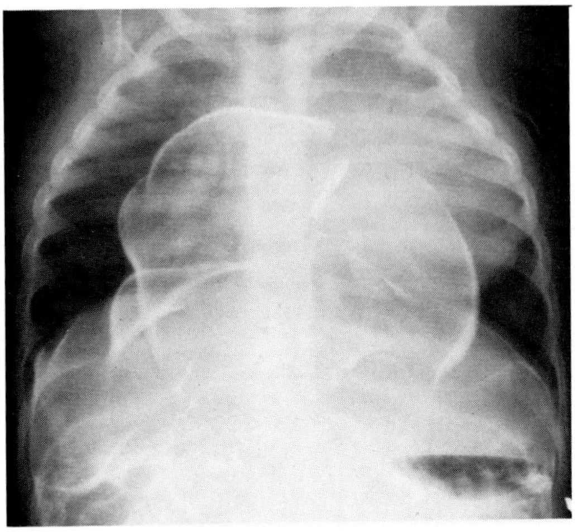

Fig. 7A. Positive-contrast peritoneogram (case 3). A large hernia sac in the anteromedial portion of the diaphragm, containing a solid organ and extending cephalad to the level of the fourth thoracic vertebra, is present.

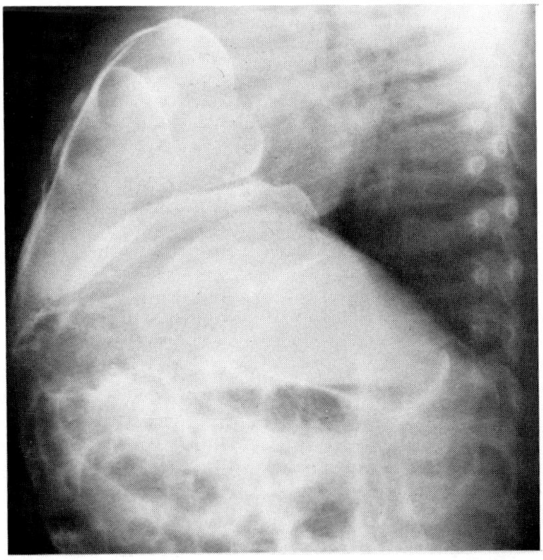

Fig. 7B. Side view of lesion shown in Fig. 7*A*. Its anterior position confirms the diagnosis of hernia of the foramen of Morgagni.

demonstrate whether they contain abdominal viscera (Fig. 4). Cineradiography of the contrast-coated diaphragmatic abnormality can be obtained to investigate explicitly whether the abnormal portion of the diaphragm undergoes paradoxical motion or moves synchronously with the rest of the diaphragm.

Diagnostically, free spillage of the contrast medium from the peritoneum into the thoracic cavity, with a sharp angle between the diaphragm proper and the abnormality, suggests a ruptured diaphragm or a posterolateral diaphragmatic hernia (Bochdalek hernia) without a peritoneal sac. A blunt angle between the diaphragm proper and the lesion, with a laggard movement on fluoroscopy of the intact and contrast-coated abnormal portion of the diaphragm suggests eventration. A foramen of Morgagni hernia can be diagnosed by its typical anteromedial location. An abnormal distance between the undersurface of a normal diaphragm and the lower border of aerated lung suggests a tumor, sequestration, or congenital cyst.

Positive-contrast peritoneography provides, as well, an opportunity to investigate other possible intra-abdominal pathology with the same procedure. Inguinal herniography can be concomitantly obtained by semierect positioning and may demonstrate unsuspected open peritoneal sacs (case 2). When the contrast material has been mostly absorbed from the peritoneal cavity, a reasonably satisfactory excretory urogram can be obtained. This may show an abnormal kidney position, possibly in association with a diaphragmatic defect or intrinsic renal pathology.

REFERENCES

1. Meyers, M. A.: Peritoneography, Am. J. Roentgenol. **117:** 353, 1973.
2. Oh, K. S., Dorst, J. P., White, J. J., Haller, J. A., Jr., Heller, R. M., James, A. E., Jr., Johnson, B. A., and Strife, J. L.: Positive contrast peritoneography and herniography, Radiology **108:** 647, 1973.
3. White, J. J., Haller, J. A., Jr., and Dorst, J. P.: Congenital inguinal hernia and inguinal herniography, Surg. Clin. North Am. **50:** 823, 1970.
4. White, J. J., Shaker, I. J., Oh, K. S., Murphy, J., Engel, R., and Haller, J. A., Jr.: Herniography: A diagnostic refinement in the management of cryptorchidism, Am. Surg. **39:** 624, 1973.

Effect of ethanol, acetylsalicylic acid, acetaminophen, and ferrous sulfate on gastric mucosal permeability in man

Michael J. Gordon, M.D., John J. Skillman, M.D., Bruce G. Edwards, B.S., *and* **William Silen, M.D.,** *Boston, Mass.*

Permeability of the human gastric mucosa was assessed in 25 studies performed in 19 fasting healthy male subjects after instillation of ethanol (20 percent, v/v), acetylsalicylic acid (20 mEq. per liter), acetaminophen (24 mEq. per liter), or ferrous sulfate (300 mg. per 225 ml. solution). An acid-free (NaCl-LiCl) solution was used to assess the effects of the first three substances on gastric mucosal permeability and the effect of ferrous sulfate was tested with an acid (HCl-LiCl) solution. Ethanol produced the expected increase in gastric mucosal permeability. The experiments with ethanol support the concept that the use of the acid-free solution is a safe and valid method for assessment of gastric mucosal permeability. The experiments with acetylsalicylic acid suggest that an acid environment is necessary for the continuance and detection of aspirin-induced barrier disruption in man. Support for the use of antacid therapy in aspirin-induced gastric bleeding is provided by these data. Intragastric instillation of acetaminophen mixed with the acid-free solution was not followed by any changes in gastric mucosal permeability. This suggests that acetaminophen may be a satisfactory substitute for aspirin in clinical situations where one would be concerned about aspirin-induced gastric mucosal bleeding. Ferrous sulfate, a drug which occasionally produces clinically significant gastric irritation, caused a decrease in gastric mucosal permeability, although acid secretion by the stomach was significantly increased after instillation of this drug.

From the Department of Surgery, Harvard Medical School, and the Beth Israel Hospital, Boston, Mass.

CURRENT TECHNIQUES to assess changes in human gastric mucosal permeability employ strongly acid solutions, the use of which may cause bleeding from the stomach.[22] This uncommon, but potentially serious complication stimulated us to investigate the applicability of an acid-free sodium chloride–lithium chloride technique to assess changes in gastric mucosal permeability.[12, 13]

This work was supported by United States Public Health Service Grant No. AM 15681 and by a grant from the John A. Hartford Foundation.

Accepted for publication April 15, 1974.

Reprint requests: John J. Skillman, M.D., Associate in Surgery, Beth Israel Hospital, 330 Brookline Ave., Boston, Mass. 02215.

The first purpose of the study was to establish in man that the acid-free technique was reliable in reflecting alterations in gastric mucosal permeability similar to those detected by previous techniques employing solutions containing acid in high concentration.[23] This was achieved by the addition to the acid-free solution of either ethanol or acetylsalicylic acid, agents which are known to increase gastric mucosal permeability in acidic solutions. The second purpose was to test the effect of acetaminophen, a drug which is often used as a substitute for aspirin, on gastric mucosal permeability in the acid-free solution. The third purpose was to assess the effects of ferrous sulfate, an agent which frequently produces clinically significant gastric irritation[14] on gastric mucosal permeability. This latter part of the study was performed by adding ferrous sulfate to the acid solution, since this medication usually produces its irritative effects in the stomach of patients who are producing acid.

METHODS

Twenty-five studies were performed in 19 fasting healthy male subjects (age range, 18 to 33 years). None of the subjects had a history of gastrointestinal disease. Each was interviewed and fully informed of the protocol details prior to acceptance for study. A 14 gauge nasogastric tube was positioned in the stomach to allow free instillation and recovery of control and test solutions. Although fluoroscopic control of the nasogastric tube position was not employed, the tube was advanced and withdrawn frequently during the aspiration period to ensure maximal recovery of these solutions. Experience by two groups has indicated that fluoroscopic control of the nasogastric tube position is unnecessary to obtain adequate recovery during tests of gastric secretion.[15, 18] In addition, previous experiments in which this technique of tube placement has been used in combination with the acid-lithium test solution indicated excellent recovery of test solutions which contained acetylsalicylic acid or ethanol.[23] Studies were performed with the subjects in the supine position and saliva was expectorated continuously. Gastric contents were aspirated and the stomach was washed by instillation and withdrawal of 225 ml. of an acid-free isosmotic sodium chloride–lithium chloride (NaCl-LiCl) test solution, containing 150 mEq. per liter of NaCl, 5 mEq. per liter of LiCl, and 100 mg. per 100 ml. of polyethylene glycol (PEG—Carbowax 4000) or 200 ml. of an isosmotic hydrochloric acid–lithium chloride (HCl-LiCl) solution containing 140 mEq. per liter of HCl, 15 mEq. per liter of NaCl, 5 mEq. per liter of LiCl, and 100 mg. per 100 ml. of PEG. The pH of the acid-free solution was 6.8 and the pH of the acid solution was 1.0. All solutions were at ambient temperature when instilled. The first aliquot of either the acid-free (225 ml.) or acid (200 ml.) wash solution was then instilled, mixed gently by hand aspiration for one minute, and left in the stomach for 30 minutes. After its removal, three 10 minute washes were performed in a similar manner. The composition of the wash solution and baseline test solution was identical for each individual study. The purpose of these instillations was to cleanse the stomach thoroughly and allow maximal adsorption of PEG to the gastric mucosa.[16] Then 225 ml. of wash solution was instilled and immediately withdrawn (quantitative wash). Following these washes, flux measurements were started. Baseline values were obtained by the performance of four identical serial 15 minute flux measurements, each separated by a quantitative wash. Each flux period was initiated by the instillation of 225 ml. of the acid-free (NaCl-LiCl) test solution or 200 ml. of the acid (HCl-LiCl) solution. The solution was mixed gently for one minute. After mixing, an "initial" 40 to 50 ml. sample was withdrawn, and a flux period commenced. Exactly 15 minutes later, the residual gastric contents were aspirated as the "final" sample for that flux period. A rapid quantitative wash was then repeated, and the second of four similar baseline flux periods was commenced.

Five studies were performed to assess the effects of the acid-free (NaCl-LiCl) test solution with the addition of 20 percent (v/v) ethanol (ETOH) on gastric mucosal permeability. The mean pH of this solution was 5.4. Following baseline flux determinations with the standard NaCl-LiCl test solution, three additional flux periods were performed in each of the five subjects with the NaCl-LiCl-ETOH solution. Blood alcohol levels were drawn at the completion of each study.

The residual effect of acetylsalicylic acid (ASA) on gastric mucosal permeability in an acid-free milieu was assessed in five studies. ASA (pKa 3.5) will not affect significantly gastric mucosal permeability when it is instilled in a neutral solution.[3, 7] It was necessary, therefore, to instill the ASA in an acid solution. Following baseline fluxes with the

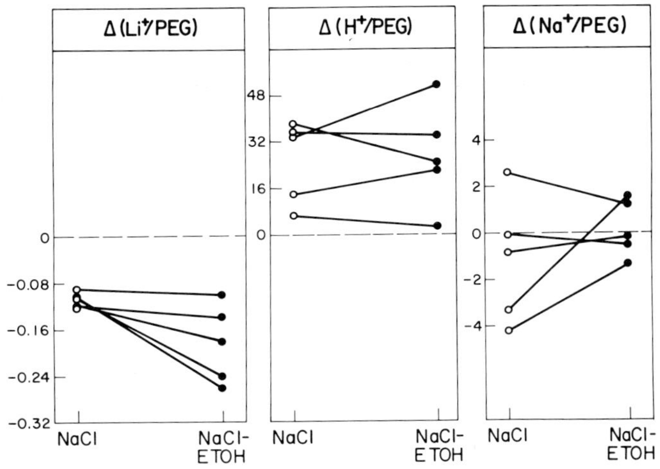

Fig. 1. Individual ion flux data in five subjects after NaCl-LiCl baseline was followed by NaCl-LiCl-ETOH instillations. Significantly increased gastric mucosal permeability [$\Delta(Li^+/PEG)$] ($p < 0.05$), which occurred with NaCl-LiCl-ETOH instillations, was accompanied by an increased flux of sodium ion from mucosa to lumen [$\Delta(Na^+/PEG)$] ($0.1 > p > 0.05$). There was no significant change in the [$\Delta(H^+/PEG)$] ratio.

acid-free solution, each subject had three consecutive 20 minute instillations of 225 ml. of a solution containing 150 mEq. per liter of HCl, 5 mEq. per liter of LiCl, 100 mg. per 100 ml. of PEG, and 20 mEq. per liter of ASA, the equivalent of two 5 grain ASA tablets in each 225 ml. of solution instilled. After a 5 minute wash with the NaCl-LiCl solution, four flux periods were repeated with the acid-free technique. These flux periods were performed in the same manner as the baseline flux periods.

Five studies were performed to assess the effect of acetaminophen on gastric mucosal permeability. Following baseline flux periods, four additional 15 minute flux periods were performed in each subject by the instillation of 225 ml. of the NaCl-LiCl solution to which 24 mEq. per liter of acetaminophen had been added, the equivalent of two 5 grain acetaminophen tablets in each 225 ml. of test solution. The pH of the NaCl-LiCl- acetaminophen solution was 4.0. The pKa of acetaminophen is 9.5.

Ten additional studies were performed to assess the effect of ferrous sulfate ($FeSO_4$) on gastric mucosal permeability in eight additional subjects. Two of the subjects were studied twice. Following the four baseline flux periods with the acid solution, four additional 15 minute flux periods were performed by instilling 225 ml. of the HCl-LiCl solution to which had been added 300 mg. of $FeSO_4$ per 225 ml. of acid solution.

All samples were analyzed for the concentration of hydrogen (H^+), lithium (Li^+), sodium (Na^+), potassium (K^+), chloride (Cl^-), pepsin, and PEG. The concentration of H^+ was determined by electrometric titration to pH 7.0 with 0.1N sodium hydroxide. The concentration of Li^+ was determined by atomic absorption spectrophotometry (model 205B Perkin-Elmer spectrophotometer). The concentrations of Na^+ and K^+ were determined by flame photometry with the use of a lithium standard. The concentration of chloride ion was assessed by the Buchler-Cotlove chloridometer. The concentration of pepsin was determined by a modification of the method of Anson.[1] The concentration of PEG was assessed by the turbidimetric method of Malawer and Powell.[19]

Changes in gastric mucosal permeability were inferred from changes in the ratio of the concentration of ion to the concentration of PEG [Δ(ion/PEG)] from the initial to the final sample.[2, 23] The Δ(ion/PEG) ratios for the serial replicate 15 minute flux periods were averaged for each patient. An increase in the change of this ratio represents a posi-

Table I. *Changes in intraluminal ion/PEG ratios after NaCl-LiCl baseline instillations were followed by NaCl-LiCl-ETOH solution**

Solution	No. of subjects	Δ(ion/PEG)					
		Δ(Li^+/PEG)	Δ(H^+/PEG)	Δ(Na^+/PEG)	Δ(K^+/PEG)	Δ(Cl^-/PEG)	Δ(pepsin/PEG)
Baseline (NaCl)	5	−0.11 ± 0.01	25.9 ± 6.3	−1.2 ± 0.4	4.9 ± 1.2	31.3 ± 7.4	239.0 ± 47.7
Test (ETOH)	5	−0.19 ± 0.03	26.6 ± 7.9	0.2 ± 0.3	3.9 ± 0.9	31.6 ± 9.4	226.0 ± 57.9
p value		< 0.05	N. S.†	0.1 > p > 0.05	N. S.	N. S.	N. S.

*All values are mean ± S.E.M. of five studies.
†N.S. = not significant.

Table II. *Changes in intraluminal ion/PEG ratios after NaCl-LiCl baseline solution and HCl-LiCl-ASA washes were followed by instillation of NaCl-LiCl baseline solution**

Solution	No. of subjects	Δ(ion/PEG)					
		Δ(Li^+/PEG)	Δ(H^+/PEG)	Δ(Na^+/PEG)	Δ(K^+/PEG)	Δ(Cl^-/PEG)	Δ(pepsin/PEG)
Baseline (NaCl)	5	−0.15 ± 0.02	20.6 ± 5.7	0.9 ± 1.2	3.3 ± 0.7	25.7 ± 5.9	170.0 ± 36.0
Test (p̄ ASA)†	5	−0.13 ± 0.01	14.2 ± 4.1	−1.0 ± 0.5	1.8 ± 0.9	15.6 ± 5.6	211.7 ± 43.7
p value		N. S.‡	N. S.	N. S.	N. S.	N. S.	N. S.

*All values are mean ± S.E.M. of five studies.
†(p̄ ASA) = after aspirin.
‡N.S. = not significant.

Table III. *Changes in intraluminal ion/PEG ratios after NaCl-LiCl baseline solution was followed by NaCl-LiCl-ACET (acetaminophen) instillations**

Solution	No. of subjects	Δ(ion/PEG)					
		Δ(Li^+/PEG)	Δ(H^+/PEG)	Δ(Na^+/PEG)	Δ(K^+/PEG)	Δ(Cl^-/PEG)	Δ(pepsin/PEG)
Baseline	5	−0.15 ± 0.02	12.6 ± 4.3	−0.8 ± 1.0	1.7 ± 0.5	15.6 ± 4.0	132.7 ± 29.2
Test (acetaminophen-NaCl)	5	−0.17 ± 0.02	18.2 ± 6.8	−0.4 ± 1.5	2.5 ± 0.9	19.7 ± 7.2	130.4 ± 46.7
p value		N. S.†	N. S.	N. S.	N. S.	N. S.	N. S.

*All values are mean ± S.E.M. of five studies.
†N.S. = not significant.

Table IV. *Changes in intraluminal ion/PEG ratios after HCl-LiCl baseline solution was followed by HCl-$FeSO_4$ instillations**

Solution	No. of subjects	Δ(ion/PEG)					
		Δ(Li^+/PEG)	Δ(H^+/PEG)	Δ(Na^+/PEG)	Δ(K^+/PEG)	Δ(Cl^-/PEG)	Δ(pepsin/PEG)
Baseline (HCl)	10	−0.16 ± 0.04	0.54 ± 1.5	4.9 ± 1.0	1.8 ± 0.34	8.39 ± 2.5	145.1 ± 15.2
Test ($FeSO_4$)	10	−0.09 ± 0.06	3.62 ± 1.2	4.0 ± 0.5	2.1 ± 0.5	10.9 ± 1.7	160.3 ± 14.0
p value		< 0.005	< 0.005	N. S.†	N. S.	N. S.	N. S.

*All values are mean ± S.E.M. of 10 studies.
†N.S. = not significant.

tive ion flux (net gain of ion into the lumen) and a decrease in the Δ(ion/PEG) ratio represents a negative ion flux (net loss of ion from the lumen). A more negative value for the mean $\Delta(Li^+/PEG)$ ratio after adding ethanol, ASA, acetaminophen, or $FeSO_4$ reflects an increased loss of lithium ion from the lumen, and, therefore, increased gastric mucosal permeability.[23] A change in intraluminal fluid volume produces an equal change in the concentration of ions and PEG, and, therefore, does not affect the ratio. Similarly, pyloric loss of intraluminal content does not alter the ratio of ion to PEG.

Paired t tests were performed by a computer program.

RESULTS

The addition of ethanol to the acid-free solution resulted in a decrease in the $\Delta(Li^+/PEG)$ ratio from -0.11 ± 0.01 to -0.19 ± 0.03 ($p < 0.05$), a change which indicates increased gastric mucosal permeability (Table I, Fig. 1). The $\Delta(Na^+/PEG)$ ratio increased from -1.2 ± 0.04 to $\pm 0.2 \pm 0.3$ ($0.1 > p > 0.05$) after ethanol. No significant changes in the fluxes of hydrogen, potassium, chloride, or pepsin were observed. The mean blood alcohol level of the five subjects at the conclusion of the ethanol instillations was 181 ± 4 mg. per 100 ml.

Instillation of HCl-LiCl solution to which ASA had been added was followed by an insignificant change in the $\Delta(Li^+/PEG)$ ratio, when compared to baseline values (Table II). This suggests that there was no residual ASA-induced alteration of gastric mucosal permeability detectable by the subsequent instillation of the acid-free NaCl-LiCl solution. In addition, there were no significant changes in the $\Delta(H^+/PEG)$, $\Delta(Na^+/PEG)$, $\Delta(K^+/PEG)$, or Δ(pepsin/PEG) ratios in this particular group of experiments.

Instillation of acetaminophen had no significant effect on gastric mucosal permeability (Table III). Although there were small increases in $\Delta(H^+/PEG)$, $\Delta(Na^+/PEG)$, $\Delta(K^+/PEG)$, and $\Delta(Cl^-/PEG)$ ratios, these changes were not statistically significant.

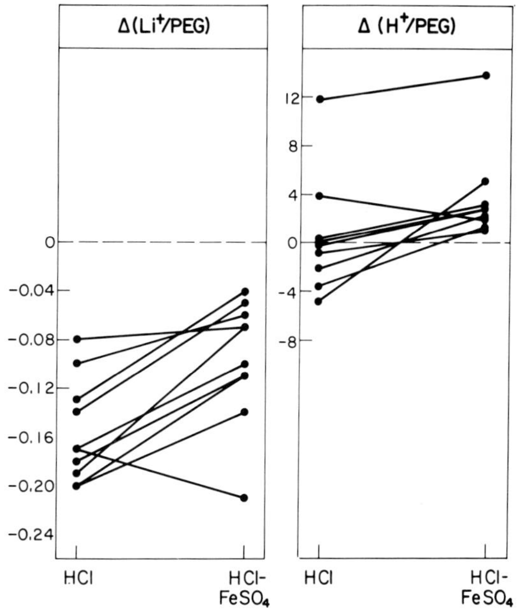

Fig. 2. Individual ion flux data in 10 subjects after HCl-LiCl baseline was followed by HCl-$FeSO_4$ instillations. Gastric mucosal permeability [$\Delta(Li^+/PEG)$] decreased significantly ($p < 0.005$) with the instillation of HCl-$FeSO_4$ solution. This was accompanied by a significant increase in hydrogen ion secretion [$\Delta(H^+/PEG)$] ($p < 0.005$).

The mean $\Delta(Li^+/PEG)$ was -0.16 ± 0.04 in the baseline period before iron sulfate and increased to -0.09 ± 0.06 after iron sulfate ($p < 0.005$) (Table IV, Fig. 2). The mean baseline $\Delta(H^+/PEG)$ was 0.54 ± 1.5 and increased to 3.62 ± 1.2 after iron sulfate ($p < 0.005$) (Table IV, Fig. 2). No significant changes were observed in the $\Delta(Na^+/PEG)$, $\Delta(K^+/PEG)$, $\Delta(Cl^-/PEG)$, and Δ(pepsin/PEG) ratios when mean baseline values were compared to the mean values after iron sulfate instillation (Table IV).

Samples from all studies either were visibly clear with variable amounts of mucus or were lightly bile stained. Significantly more mucus was observed in the solutions which were recovered after a 15 minute flux period in those studies performed with the acid-free technique. Previous experiments performed with acid-lithium test solutions in man have demonstrated that traces of bile in the aspirated samples occured in approximately one third of the initial and final 15 minute samples.[23] Bile-stained samples were not excluded from our statistical analyses, since this previous work[23] indicated that inclusion of such samples produced no statistical differences in either the ion flux or transmural gastric mucosal potential difference data. If the concentration of bile in such samples was high enough to alter gastric mucosal permeability, one would have expected abrupt changes to occur in the transmural potential difference.[11] This effect was not observed in these previous experiments.[23]

DISCUSSION

Ethanol-acid solutions produce increased gastric mucosal permeability (GMP) when these mixtures are instilled into the stomach of human subjects[23] and dogs.[6] When ETOH is instilled into the canine gastric pouch in a neutral solution, changes consistent with increased GMP are also observed.[7] The present data indicate that instillation of ETOH in a neutral solution into the stomach of man is also associated with an increased lumen-to-mucosa flux of lithium ion. Ethanol is a known stimulus to the secretion of acid by the stomach.[6] Although an increase of acid secretion (an increase of the $\Delta(H^+/PEG)$ ratio after ethanol could not be proved in these experiments, it is possible that the acid secretory effect of ethanol may have been masked by a concomitant increase in hydrogen ion back diffusion, an effect which would decrease the $\Delta(H^+/PEG)$ ratio. This suggestion is supported by the increase in the flux of sodium from mucosa to lumen and the significant increase in the disappearance of lithium from the lumen. The significantly more negative $\Delta(Li^+/PEG)$ ratio after ethanol suggests that this agent did produce an increase of gastric mucosal permeability. Disruption of the gastric mucosal barrier by other agents has been reported to be associated with an increased intraluminal concentration of pepsin.[17] This effect was not observed in the present study. Alcohol is known to decrease substantially the apparent activity of pepsinogen and pepsin.[20] Therefore, it is possible that the actual secretion of pepsin may have been greater than our data suggest.

The pKa of acetylsalicylic acid is 3.5. It has been shown that ASA must be instilled in a strongly acid solution to affect GMP.[4, 7] In weakly acid or neutral solutions, virtually all the acetylsalicylic acid is ionized. In this dissociated form the ions are water soluble, and it has been suggested that passage of these dissociated ions through the gastric mucosa is restricted to water-filled channels.[5] The undissociated form of ASA which occurs at a pH less than 3.5 is soluble in lipid and is rapidly absorbed directly through the mucosa of the stomach. Instillation of an HCl-LiCl-ASA mixture in man is associated with a marked increase in GMP, a change which is indicated by a significant decrease in the $\Delta(Li^+/PEG)$ ratio.[23] In the present experiments, when instillation of the HCl-ASA solution was followed by its removal with a neutral NaCl-LiCl solution, no residual alterations in GMP were observed in subsequent test periods in which the acid-free solution was employed. Increased flux of sodium from mucosa to lumen, a reflection of increased GMP,[9] has been observed in man after the instillation of HCl-ASA solutions.[20] In this study, washout of the HCl-ASA solution was associated with a more negative $\Delta(Na^+/PEG)$ ratio, a finding which further supports the suggestion that alterations in GMP associated with the instillation of HCl-ASA solutions appear to be abolished by removal of HCl-ASA solutions and substitution by a neutral NaCl-LiCl solution. It is possible that repeated washings of the stomach with the acid-free solution totally eliminated the effect of the HCl-ASA solution.

The present study suggests that an acid milieu is necessary for the continuance or detection of ASA-induced disruption of the gastric mucosal barrier in man. This observation has been made also in isolated segments of rabbit gastric mucosa in vitro which were exposed to neutral solutions containing ASA.[10] Instillation of HCl-ASA solutions into canine pouches has resulted in residual changes in permeability only in an acid milieu.[3, 7] Davenport[7] reported that bleeding from HCl-ASA-ETOH instillations continued and usually became worse if acid was left in contact with the mucosa of the pouch. If the pouch was perfused with a neutral solution, bleeding usually stopped. The observations made by Davenport in animals are extended by our data obtained in man and support the use of aggressive antacid therapy (titration of stomach contents to a neutral pH) in ASA-induced gastritis.

Acetaminophen (pKa 9.5) is unionized in a solution of neutral pH. This drug is readily absorbed when it is instilled with the acid-free NaCl-LiCl test solution. There was no significant change in the $\Delta(Li^+/PEG)$ ratio after instillation of this agent. The absence of changes in any of the Δ(ion/PEG) ratios suggests strongly that acetaminophen produces no alteration in gastric mucosal permeability. It is possible that acetaminophen may be a safer drug to use than aspirin in clinical situations where one would be concerned about the possibility of gastric mucosal bleeding.

The significantly less negative $\Delta(Li^+/PEG)$ ratio after iron sulfate instillations implies that there was a decrease in the permeability of the gastric mucosa. The increased $\Delta(H^+/PEG)$ ratio suggests that an increased secretion of H^+ was stimulated by iron sulfate, a conclusion which is strengthened by the observation that the permeability of the stomach to lithium was decreased. When the gastric mucosa is secreting H^+, one would expect to see a decreased influx of Na^+ into the lumen.[3] In the presence of $FeSO_4$ there was a small, but statistically insignificant decrease in the $\Delta(Na^+/PEG)$ ratio, an observation which supports further the contention that the instillation of $FeSO_4$ decreases the permeability of the human gastric mucosa. These data suggest that $FeSO_4$ produces gastric irritation by a mechanism other than a change in mucosal permeability.

Activation of pepsinogen to pepsin is almost instantaneous at pH 2.[8] The Δ(pepsin/PEG) ratio of the gastric juice samples seen in the experiments with iron sulfate in an acidic solution should be a reflection of pepsinogen secretion. The absence of a significant increase in the Δ(pepsin/PEG) ratio in the presence of an increase of the $\Delta(H^+/PEG)$ ratio suggests the possibility that pepsinogen release may have been inhibited by $FeSO_4$.

REFERENCES

1. Anson, M. L.: The estimation of trypsin, papain, and cathepepsin with hemoglobin, J. Gen. Physiol. **22:** 79, 1932.
2. Chung, R. S. K., Field, M., and Silen, W.: Permeability of gastric mucosa to hydrogen and lithium, Gastroenterology **64:** 593, 1973.
3. Davenport, H. W.: Damage to the gastric mucosa: Effects of salicylates and stimulation, Gastroenterology **49:** 189, 1965.
4. Davenport, H. W.: Fluid produced by the gastric mucosa during damage by acetic and salicylic acids, Gastroenterology **50:** 487, 1966.
5. Davenport, H. W.: Salicylate damage to the gastric mucosal barrier, N. Engl. J. Med. **276:** 1307, 1967.
6. Davenport, H. W.: Ethanol damage to canine oxyntic glandular mucosa, Proc. Soc. Exp. Biol. Med. **126:** 657, 1967.
7. Davenport, H. W.: Gastric mucosal hemorrhage in dogs: Effects of acid, aspirin and alcohol, Gastroenterology **56:** 439, 1969.
8. Davenport, H. W.: Physiology of the digestive tract, ed. 3, Chicago, 1971, Year Book Medical Publishers, Inc., pp. 97-98.
9. Davenport, H. W., Warner, H. A., and Code, C. F.: Functional significance of gastric mucosal barrier to sodium, Gastroenterology **47:** 142, 1964.
10. Fromm, D., Schwartz, J. H., and Quijano, R.: Effects of salicylates and bile salt on ion transport across isolated mammalian gastric mucosa, Gastroenterology **64:** 729, 1973.
11. Geall, M. G., Phillips, S. F., and Summerskill, W. H. J.: Profile of gastric potential difference in man: Effects of aspirin, alcohol, bile and endogenous acid, Gastroenterology **58:** 437, 1970.
12. Gordon, M. J., Skillman, J. J., and Silen, W.: An acid-free technique to study human gastric mucosal permeability: Effect of ethanol and acetylsalicylic acid, Surg. Forum **23:** 384, 1972.
13. Gordon, M. J., Skillman, J. J., and Silen, W.: Assessment of human gastric mucosal permeability by an acid-free technique, Gastroenterology **62:** 846, 1972.
14. Hallberg, L., Harwerth, H. G., and Vannotti, A.: Iron deficiency—pathogenesis, clinical aspects, therapy, New York, 1970, Academic Press, Inc.
15. Hassan, M. A., and Hobsley, M.: Positioning of subject and of nasogastric tube during a gastric secretion study, Br. Med. J. **1:** 458, 1970.

16. Ivey, K. J., and Shedl, H.: Gastric nonabsorbable indicators for studies in man, Gastroenterology **59:** 234, 1970.
17. Johnson, L. R.: Pepsin secretion during damage of the gastric mucosa by ethanol and acetylsalicylic acid, Gastroenterology **62:** 412, 1972.
18. Lawrie, J. H., Smith, G. M. R., and Forrest, A. P. M.: The histamine infusion test, Lancet **2:** 270, 1964.
19. Malawer, S. J., and Powell, D. W.: An improved turbidimetric analysis of polyethylene glycol utilizing an emulsifier, Gastroenterology **53:** 520, 1967.
20. Neumann, H., and Shinitzky, M.: Reversible inactivation of the potential pepsin activity of pepsinogen by alcohols, Biochemistry **10:** 4335, 1971.
21. Overholt, B. F., and Pollard, H. M.: Acetylsalicylic acid and ion fluxes across the gastric mucosa of man, Gastroenterology **54:** 538, 1968.
22. Skillman, J. J., Gould, S. A., Chung, R. S. K., and Silen, W.: The gastric mucosal barrier: Clinical and experimental studies in critically ill and normal man, and in the rabbit, Ann. Surg. **172:** 564, 1970.
23. Smith, B. M., Skillman, J. J., Edwards, B. G., and Silen, W.: Permeability of the human gastric mucosa: Alteration by acetylsalicylic acid and ethanol, N. Engl. J. Med. **285:** 716, 1971.

Axillo-axillary bypass with cephalic vein for correction of subclavian steal syndrome

Herbert Dardik, M.D., *and* **Irving Dardik, M.D.,** *Englewood, N. J., and Bronx, N. Y.*

Case reports are presented which describe experience with the use of the contralateral axillary artery as the donor vessel for correction of symptomatic subclavian steal.

From the Departments of Surgery of the Englewood Hospital, Englewood, N. J., and Montefiore Hospital and Medical Center, Albert Einstein College of Medicine, Bronx, N. Y.

SYMPTOMATIC subclavian steal syndromes can be corrected by a variety of operative approaches. Advocates of a particular procedure have pointed out the deficiencies of the alternatives but, in fact, no single approach is completely devoid of complications. Attention has recently been focused on the possibility of increasing the perfusion pressure in the distal subclavian-vertebral complex by avoiding both thoracotomy and use of the carotid artery. Such a procedure would avoid the hazards of a major intrathoracic operation and negate any possibility of carotid artery steal or thrombosis. The following case reports describe our experience using the contralateral axillary artery as the donor vessel for correcting symptomatic subclavian steal.

CASE REPORTS

Case 1. A 44-year-old white man was hospitalized for evaluation of severe claudication of the lower extremities and the left upper extremity and frequent episodes of dizziness. Three years previously the patient had been told that pulses could be felt only in the right upper extremity and that no blood pressure could be obtained from the left upper extremity. During the interval the patient became impotent and, with progression of his symptoms, sought medical attention.

Arteriography. Retrograde right brachial arteriography demonstrated (1) occlusion of the first portion of the left subclavian artery with retrograde flow in the left vertebral artery supplying the circulation to the left upper extremity (Figs. 1*A* and 1*B*), (2) stenosis at the origin of the right vertebral artery, and (3) severe bilateral iliac artery stenosis with marked atheromatous involvement of the distal abdominal aorta.

Surgery. Attention was initially directed toward correction of the patient's symptomatic subclavian steal. Operation was performed under general anesthesia by exploring both axillary arteries by the infraclavicular approach. The pectoralis major was divided in line with its fibers. The clavipectoral fascia was incised and the entire first portion of the axillary artery mobilized. Division of the pectoralis minor facilitated the dissection of the axillary artery. The right cephalic vein was 5 mm. in diameter. By dissecting a sufficient length, the vein was employed as the arterial substitute with appropriate orientation of the valves and placement in a presternal subcutaneous tunnel. The anastomosis was performed with 5-0 Prolene suture material. Excellent flow was obtained through the graft and intraoperative angiography confirmed flow proximally into the subclavian artery and up the vertebral as well as distally into the upper extremity (Figs. 2*A* and 2*B*). Pulses at the wrist level were immediately palpable. The postoperative course was unevent-

Accepted for publication May 20, 1974.

Reprint requests: Herbert Dardik, M.D., 1555 Center Ave., Fort Lee, N. J. 07024.

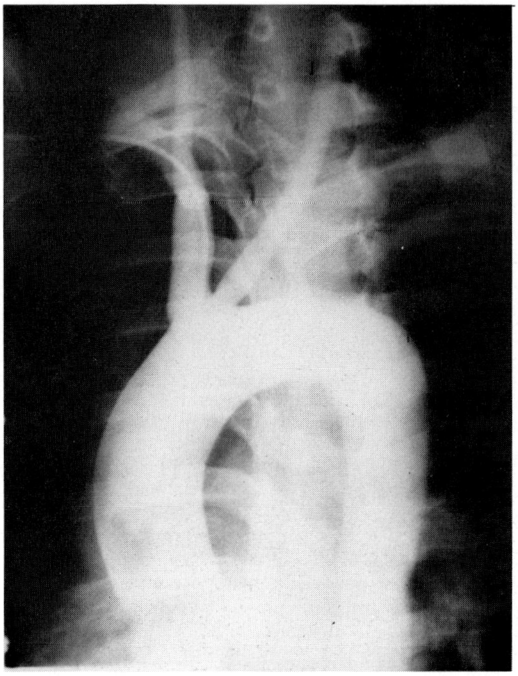

Fig. 1A. Early arterial phase demonstrating intact right innominate arterial system and occlusion of left subclavian artery at its origin (case 1).

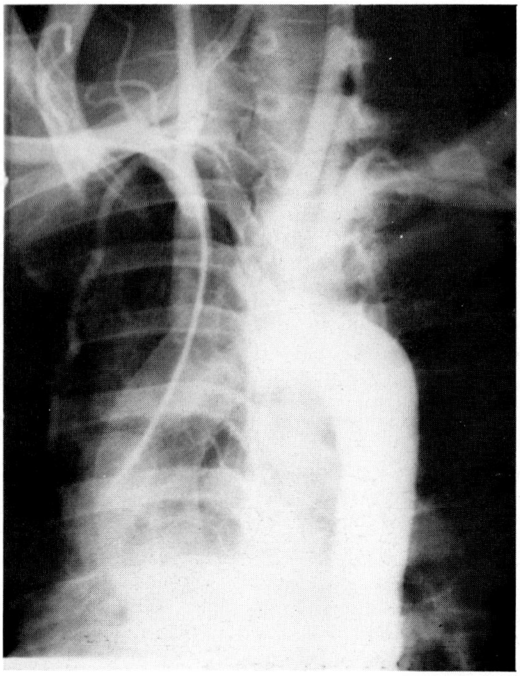

Fig. 1B. Later film showing retrograde filling of left vertebral and distal left subclavian arteries.

ful. Ten days later the patient underwent a successful aortic bifurcation bypass graft. The patient has remained asymptomatic with respect to his previous cerebral and upper and lower extremity symptoms on follow-up during the past year.

Case 2. A 77-year-old white man was hospitalized following an episode of loss of vision, aphasia, and "heaviness" of the right leg that lasted approximately 25 minutes. There were no residual neurologic deficits but on examination the blood pressure in the left upper extremity was 90 mm. Hg systolic compared to 120/70 mm. Hg for the right upper extremity. Arterial pulses in the left upper extremity were barely palpable.

Arteriography. Retrograde right brachial arteriography showed (1) segmental occlusion of the left subclavian artery with retrograde flow in the left vertebral artery into the left subclavian artery (Fig. 3), (2) mild stenosis at the origin of the right vertebral artery, and (3) 30 and 40 percent stenosis of the right and left internal carotid arteries, respectively. It was felt that the subclavian steal was the significant hemodynamic lesion, perhaps compounded by the moderate degree of carotid stenosis.

Surgery. Under general anesthesia, an axillo-axillary bypass was performed by the infraclavicular approach with a presternal tunnel. The right cephalic vein was employed as the bypass graft. The anastomosis was constructed with 6-0 Prolene. Intraoperative angiography confirmed flow through the graft into the distal left subclavian artery and retrograde into the proximal left subclavian artery and up the vertebral artery (Fig. 4). The postoperative course was uneventful. The pulses and blood pressure in the left upper extremity returned to normal levels. The patient has remained asymptomatic on follow-up over the past eight months.

DISCUSSION

The direct approach for the surgical treatment of the subclavian steal syndrome involves thoracotomy and consequently carries an increased risk, particularly when so many of these patients have diffuse vascular problems. One of the simplest extrathoracic procedures is ligation of the vertebral artery.[3, 18] Obviously, complete restoration of cerebral blood flow does not occur with this operation and therefore may not be indicated where the cerebral circulation is already marginal. On the right side, vertebral artery ligation might in fact precipitate or aggra-

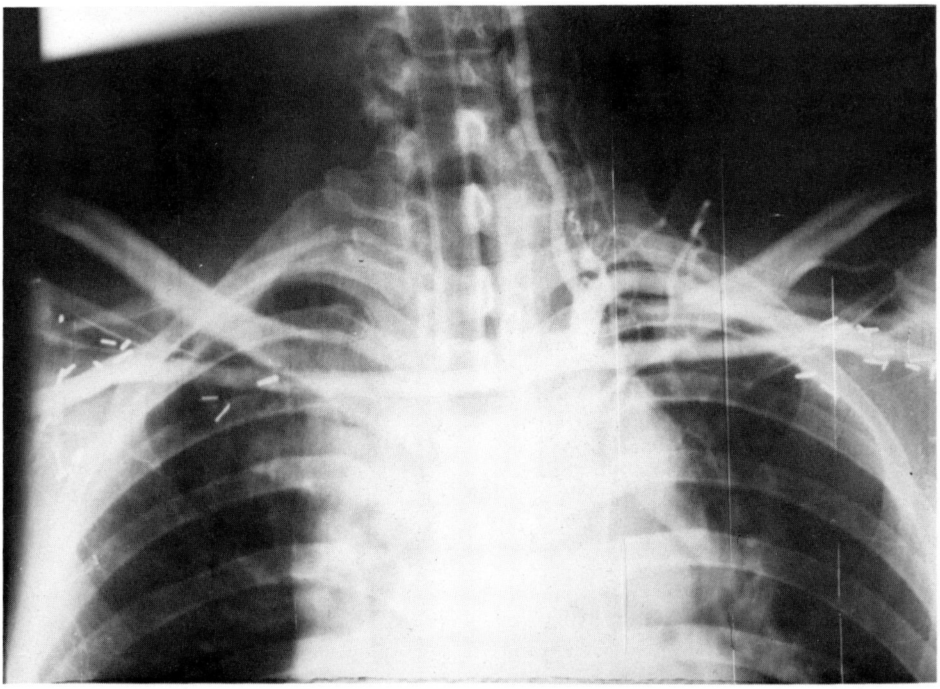

Fig. 2A. Intraoperative angiogram depicting position of venous axillo-axillary bypass graft with opacification of left vertebral and subclavian arteries (case 1).

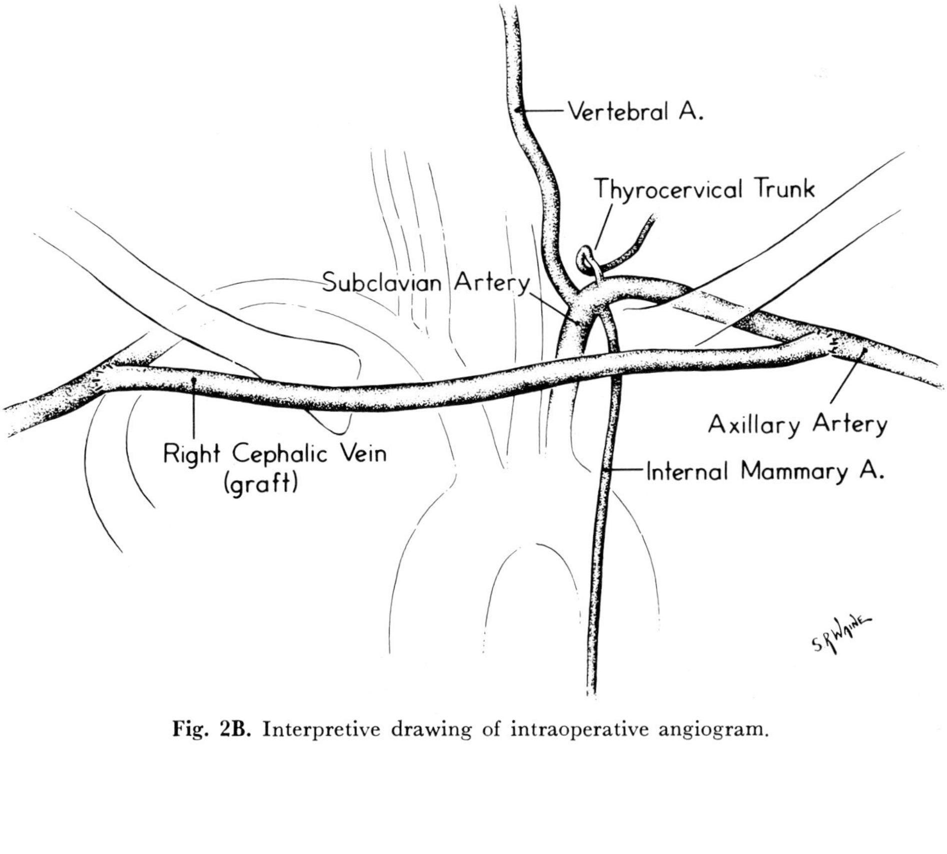

Fig. 2B. Interpretive drawing of intraoperative angiogram.

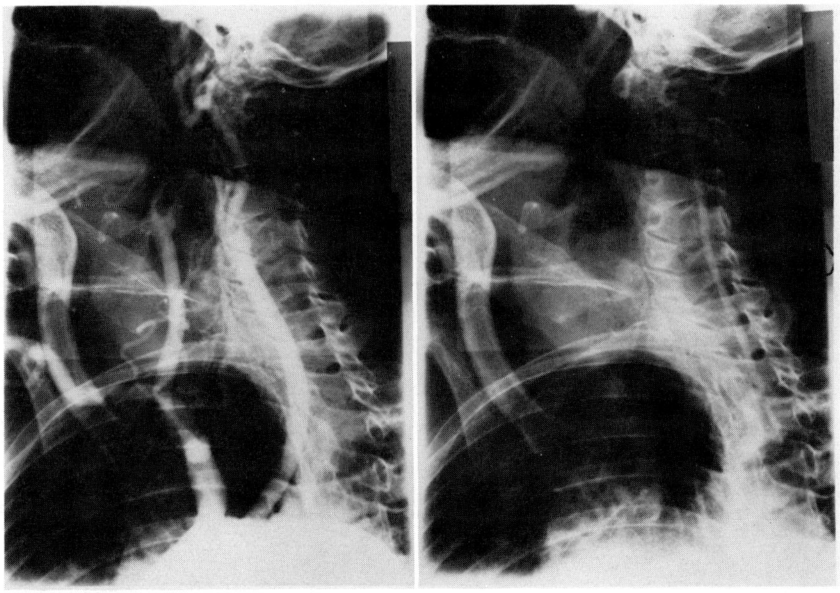

Fig. 3. Sequential films demonstrating initial opacification of the innominate and left carotid arterial systems with occlusion of the left subclavian artery and subsequent retrograde flow in the left vertebral artery (case 2).

Table I. *Axillo-axillary bypass*

Author	*Pathology*	*Bypass material*
Myers et al.[15]	Subclavian block	Dacron
Myers et al.[16]	Tracheal–innominate artery fistula	Dacron
Mozersky et al.[14]	Left subclavian artery occlusion (case 1)	Dacron
	Innominate artery occlusion (case 2)	Dacron
	Innominate artery occlusion, S.P. ligation of right vertebral artery (case 3)	Dacron
Jacobson et al.[10]	Left subclavian artery occlusion	Autogenous saphenous vein
LeVeen et al.[11]	Left subclavian artery occlusion	Autogenous saphenous vein
Dardik and Dardik (present report)	Left subclavian artery occlusion (case 1)	Autogenous cephalic vein
	Left subclavian artery occlusion (case 2)	Autogenous cephalic vein

vate reverse flow in the right carotid artery.

The indirect cervical approach of carotid-subclavian bypass was initially also suggested to obviate the need for thoracotomy.[13] Considerable effort has since been expended in an attempt to delineate instances where further steal via the carotid circulation might occur. The evidence is debatable but most investigators now feel that blood from the carotid would be siphoned off into the axillary-brachial system in the presence of a significant stenosis of the proximal or distal carotid artery or if there is diminished resistance in the upper extremity vasculature.[1, 2, 4, 12] Carotid-subclavian bypass or anastomosis has become the primary extrathoracic procedure with modifications including clavicular resection, transposition, and extension to the axillary artery.[5, 6, 17, 19] Nevertheless, partial or complete occlusion of the carotid artery, albeit of short duration, is of concern particularly where a cerebral circulatory deficit is already known to exist. Additionally, the right carotid artery cannot serve as a donor vessel where the steal syndrome is based on occlusion of the innominate artery.

An alternative to the problems posed by

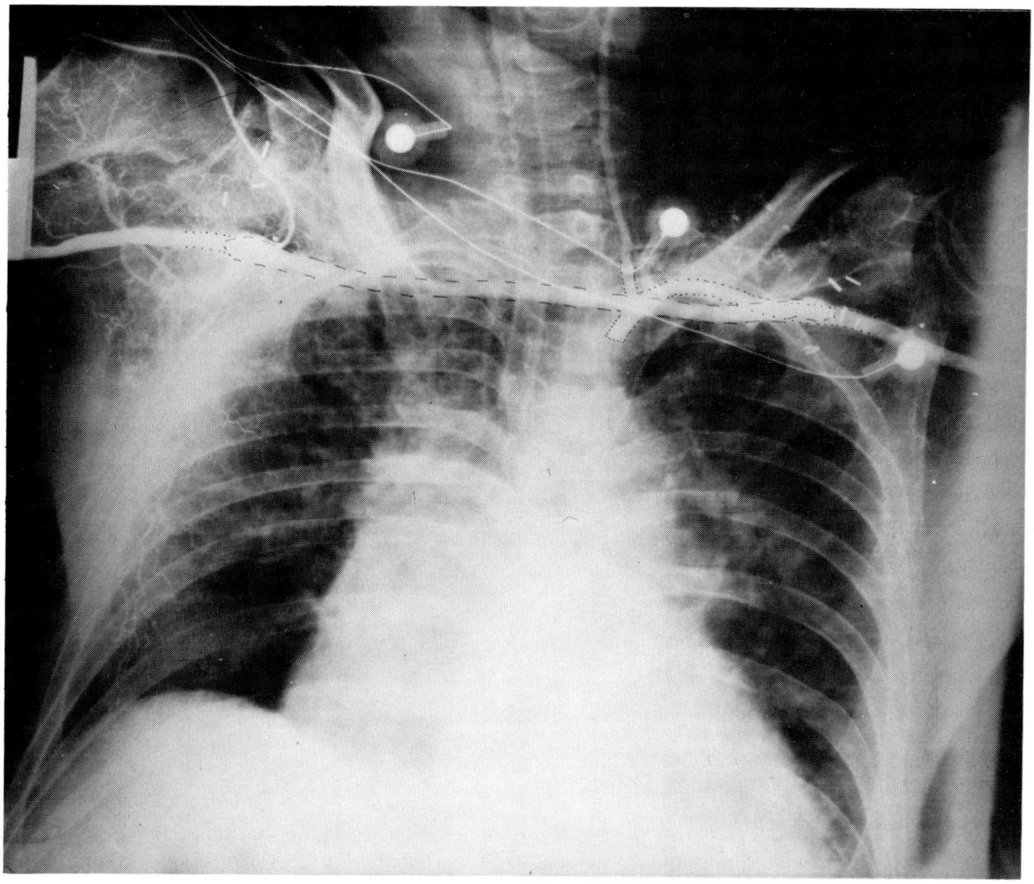

Fig. 4. Intraoperative angiogram confirming flow into the left vertebral and subclavian arteries via the axillo-axillary bypass (case 2).

the direct approach via thoracotomy or by using the carotid artery is the subclavian cervical crossover.[7-9] This procedure has been documented to be hemodynamically effective. A meticulous cervical dissection is required, including isolation of the phrenic nerves bilaterally. Perhaps an easier alternative to this procedure is the axillo-axillary bypass, first employed by Myers and associates[15, 16] and subsequently by Mozersky,[14] Jacobson,[10] and Le Veen[11] and their colleagues (Table I). This operation can be performed under local as well as general anesthesia and entails a relatively easier dissection of the vessels. Though any segment of the axillary artery can be employed for anastomosis, an infraclavicular approach to the first part of the axillary artery as we have described enables one to employ a shorter segment of graft. To date, the total experience with autogenous veins and prosthetic grafts in this location has been minimal, but we feel that based on the experience gained in other areas of peripheral vascular surgery autogenous tissue will ultimately prove to be superior.

The subcutaneous presternal tunnel may be objectionable on a theoretical basis and perhaps the graft can be tunneled into the retrosternal position analogous to the retropubic femoral crossover graft. However, the accumulated experience with a variety of extra-anatomic bypasses in the subcutaneous position supports the continued use of the simpler subcutaneous tunnel. Excision of a wedge of pectoralis major muscle adjacent to where the graft rises up to the sternum was performed in our cases with the intent to prevent any possibility of extrinsic compression.

Still another alternative to cerebral revascularization is the femoral-axillary bypass.[20] The experience gained thus far with the axillo-femoral bypass for lower extremity revascularization suggests that long-term patency would be inferior to what might be obtained with the axillo-axillary bypass. This may be related to the shorter length of graft for the axillo-axillary route as well as a lesser likelihood of kinking due to flexion or traction forces.

The authors gratefully acknowledge the assistance of Dr. Sam Shapiro in the management of these cases.

REFERENCES

1. Barner, H. B., Kaiser, G. C., and Willman, V. L.: Hemodynamics of carotid-subclavian bypass, Arch. Surg. **103:** 248, 1971.
2. Barner, H. B., Rittenhouse, E. A., and Willman, V. L.: Carotid subclavian bypass for "subclavian steal syndrome," J. Thorac. Cardiovasc. Surg. **55:** 773, 1968.
3. Cameron, D. J., and Wright, I. S.: Subclavian steal with olfactory hallucinations, Ann. Intern. Med. **61:** 128, 1964.
4. Cook, C. H., Stemmer, E. A., and Connolly, J. E.: Effect of peripheral resistance on carotid blood flow after carotid-subclavian bypass, Arch. Surg. **105:** 9, 1972.
5. Crawford, E. S., De Bakey, M. E., Morris, G. C., and Howell, J.: Surgical treatment of the occlusion of the innominate, common carotid and subclavian arteries: A one-year experience, SURGERY **65:** 17, 1969.
6. Edwards, W. H., and Wright, R. S.: Surgical therapy in subclavian occlusive disease, Am. J. Surg. **123:** 689, 1972.
7. Ehrenfeld, W. K., Levin, S. M., and Wylie, E. J.: Venous crossover bypass grafts for arterial insufficiency, Ann. Surg. **167:** 287, 1968.
8. Finkelstein, N. M., Byer, A., and Rush, B. F.: Subclavian-subclavian bypass for the subclavian steal syndrome, SURGERY **71:** 142, 1972.
9. Forestner, J. E., Ghosh, S. K., Bergen, J. J., and Conn, J., Jr.: Subclavian-subclavian bypass for correction of the subclavian steal syndrome, SURGERY **71:** 136, 1972.
10. Jacobson, J. J., Mozersky, D. J., Mitty, H. A., and Brothers, M. J.: Axillary-axillary bypass for the "subclavian steal" syndrome, Arch. Surg. **106:** 24, 1973.
11. LeVeen, H. H., Piccone, V. A., Jr., Diaz, C., Christoudias, G., Slade, W., and Norstrand, I.: A simplified correction of subclavian steal syndrome, SURGERY **75:** 299, 1974.
12. Lord, R. S. A., and Ehrenfeld, W. K.: Carotid-subclavian bypass: A hemodynamic study, SURGERY **66:** 521, 1969.
13. Lyons, C., and Galbraith, G.: Surgical treatment of atherosclerotic occlusion of the internal carotid artery, Ann. Surg. **146:** 487, 1957.
14. Mozersky, D. J., Sumner, D. S., Barnes, R. W., and Strandness, P. E., Jr.: Subclavian revascularization by means of subcutaneous axillary-axillary graft, Arch. Surg. **106:** 20, 1973.
15. Myers, W. O., Lawton, B. R., and Sautter, R. D.: Axillo-axillary bypass graft, J. A. M. A. **217:** 826, 1971.
16. Myers, W. O., Lawton, B. R., and Sautter, R. D.: An operation for tracheal-innominate artery fistula, Arch. Surg. **105:** 269, 1972.
17. Parrot, J. C.: The subclavian steal syndrome, Arch. Surg. **88:** 661, 1964.
18. Rob, C.: Subclavian occlusive disease and reversal of flow in ipsilateral vertebral artery, *in* Treatment in cerebral vascular diseases: Fourth Conference, New York, 1965, Grune & Stratton, Inc., p. 122.
19. Shumacker, H. B.: Carotid axillary bypass grafts for occlusion of the proximal portion of the subclavian artery, Surg. Gynecol. Obstet. **136:** 447, 1973.
20. Sproul, G.: Femoral-axillary bypass for cerebral vascular insufficiency, Arch. Surg. **103:** 746, 1971.

Gastrin concentrations in upper gastrointestinal mucosa in dogs*

Larry C. Watson, M.D., David D. Reeder, M.D., Horst D. Becker, M.D., Lavenia LaGrone, *and* **James C. Thompson, M.D.,** *Galveston, Texas*

The major source of gastrin in dogs is the antral mucosa; four percent of total mucosal gastrin was extracted from fundic and small bowel mucosa. The major portion of gastrin in the fundic and antral mucosa is in the small heptadecapeptide molecular form. The fundus and small bowel require consideration as sources of gastrin in physiologic studies of the hormone; extra-antral sites in the dog do not contain as great a concentration of gastrin as has been reported in man.

From the Department of Surgery, The University of Texas Medical Branch, Galveston, Texas

THE MAJOR humoral stimulus of gastric secretion is the hormone gastrin. It was initially identified from mucosal extracts of the gastric antrum[4] and was first isolated and purified by Gregory and Tracy[6] from extracts of hog antral mucosa. For many years, gastrin was considered to be a hormone which arose only from the gastric antrum.[13]

Recent observations suggest that mucosal sites in the gastrointestinal tract other than the antrum possess significant potential as sources of gastrin. Substantial concentrations of circulating gastrin have been measured in dogs in which total gastrectomy was performed[10]; antrectomy has been found to alter neither basal serum gastrin nor food-stimulated gastrin values[2, 12]; the concentration of gastrin in the duodenal mucosa of man has been reported to be equal to the concentration in antral mucosa[11]; and acute elevations of gastrin concentrations in the duodenal vein have been measured in response to acetylcholine applied topically to the duodenal mucosa.[1]

The present studies were designed to measure the mucosal concentration of gastrin and to calculate the total gastrin content present in mucosa at different levels of the canine gastrointestinal tract.

MATERIAL AND METHODS

Nine healthy mongrel dogs, weighing 20 to 25 kilograms, were used in these studies. Each dog received Histalog (betazole HCl), 1 mg. per kilogram, intravenously 45 minutes before being killed by a captive-bolt pistol. The abdomen was quickly opened, and the stomach and entire small bowel were removed rapidly and opened longitudinally. The total mucosa of the upper gastrointestinal tract was removed in segments (Fig. 1). The junction of the antrum and the acid-secreting fundus was defined circumferentially with pH-sensitive paper. The antral and fundic mucosae were dissected separately from the muscular wall of the stomach and the mucosae of the various segments of small bowel

Supported by grants from the National Institutes of Health (No. AM 15241) and by a grant from The John A. Hartford Foundation, Inc.

Accepted for publication April 18, 1974.

*A preliminary report of this work has been published.[14]

Reprint requests: James C. Thompson, M.D., Department of Surgery, The University of Texas Medical Branch, Galveston, Texas 77550.

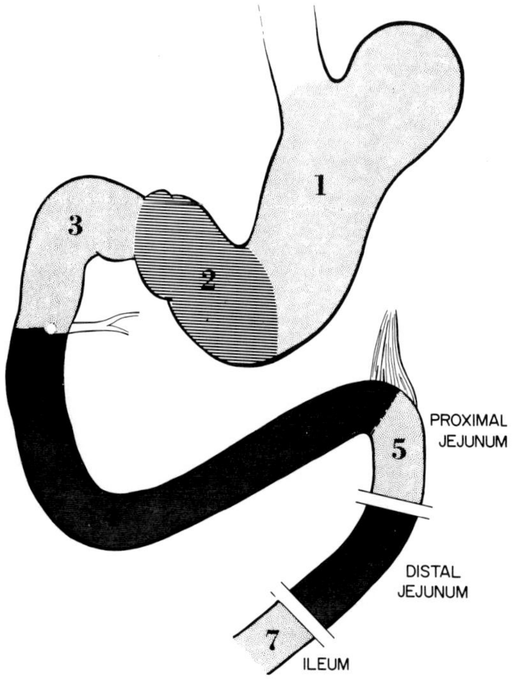

Fig. 1. Division of the gastrointestinal tract for measurement of mucosal content of gastrin.

Table I. *Average mucosal gastrin content (nine dogs)*

Mucosa	*Average weight (Gm.)*	*Average total gastrin content (ng.)*
Fundus	76	4,028
Antrum	14	296,800
Proximal duodenum	8	1,072
Distal duodenum	23	1,308
Proximal jejunum	53	1,892
Distal jejunum	76	2,207
Ileum	81	1,138

were carefully and totally removed by scraping. The demarcation between proximal and distal duodenum was the entrance of the main pancreatic duct; the division between distal duodenum and jejunum was the ligament of Treitz. The proximal two fifths of the small bowel distal to the ligament of Treitz was considered arbitrarily to be jejunum; the distal three fifths, ileum. The jejunum was divided into two segments of equal length.

Mucosa from each segment was immediately weighed, diluted with nine parts distilled water, and placed in a boiling water bath for 30 minutes. After centrifugation at 20,000 r.p.m. for 20 minutes, the supernatant was stored at –20° C. for subsequent gastrin measurement. The concentrations of gastrin present in the mucosa of the fundus, antrum, proximal and distal duodenum, proximal and distal jejunum, and ileum were measured by radioimmunoassay.[7] The total gastrin content of each segment of mucosa was calculated by multiplying the weight by the gastrin concentration of each segment.

Extracts of each mucosa were submitted to starch-gel electrophoresis in order to separate gastrin into the "big" (33 amino acid) and "little" (17 amino acid) forms.[3] Thirty microliters of the supernatant were spotted at the cathode end of a sheet of starch gel. Electrophoresis was performed for 16 hours, and the starch gel was then divided into 1 cm. squares. The squares were pulverized in phosphate buffer solution and centrifuged at 6,000 r.p.m. for 15 minutes. The eluate was assayed for gastrin.[7]

RESULTS

The highest concentration of gastrin was found in antral mucosa (Fig. 2). The mean concentration of gastrin in the antral mucosa of nine dogs was 21,200 ng. per gram tissue. This was almost 500 times the concentration of gastrin in the fundic mucosa (53 ng. per gram). As tissue more distal to the stomach was extracted, the concentration of gastrin became progressively smaller.

Total gastrin contents of the mucosa of various segments are shown in Table I. The average total content of gastrin extracted from antral mucosa was about 0.3 mg. Gastrin content for all other mucosa ranged from 1 to 4 μg.

The distribution of gastrin from the antral extract and fundic extract on the starch gel is shown in Fig. 3. Approximately 70 percent of the total gastrin in the antrum and approximately 90 percent of the total gastrin in the fundus is the small (17 amino acid) form. The largest portion of gastrin in both segments migrates ahead of the free

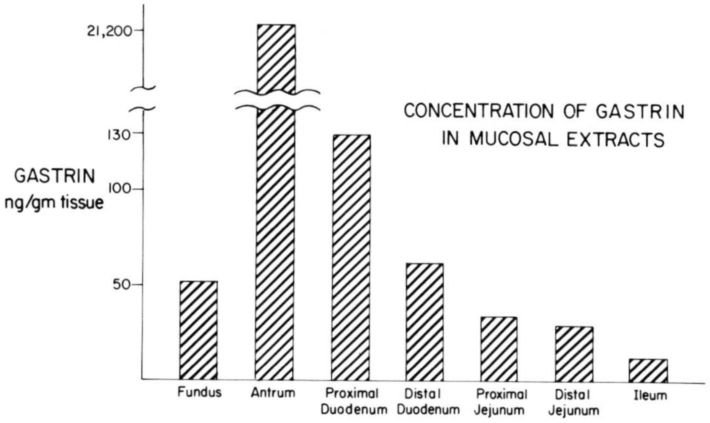

Fig. 2. Concentrations of gastrin, measured by radioimmunoassay, found in mucosa of the upper gastrointestinal tract of dogs.

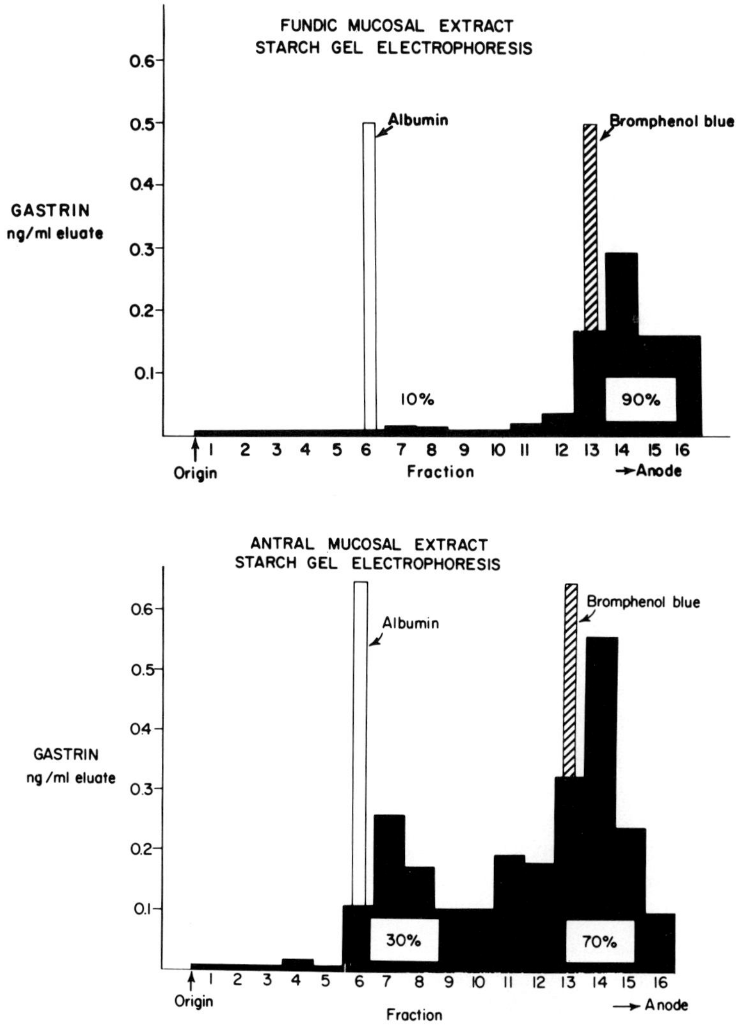

Fig. 3. Distribution of immunoreactive gastrin on starch-gel electrophoresis in extract of dog antral and fundic mucosa.

bromphenol blue; this portion has been identified previously as heptadecapeptide-like, or "little," gastrin.[3] The amounts of gastrin in segments of small bowel mucosa were insufficient to allow accurate partitioning into big and little fractions.

DISCUSSION

The highest concentration of gastrin was found, as expected, in the antral mucosa. Gastrin has been assumed to arise nearly exclusively from the antrum and the majority of studies of gastric physiology have been based on that assumption. We have previously reported a high degree of correlation between non–acid-secreting gastric mucosa and the area of mucosa containing the highest concentrations of gastrin.[8] The concentration of gastrin in the antral mucosa of the dog as measured by radioimmunoassay in this study is in agreement with values reported previously.[8, 9]

The concentration of gastrin in duodenal mucosa approximated that of fundic mucosa in the dog. The amount of gastrin in the duodenal mucosa of the dog is apparently much less than in man, in whom the concentration of gastrin in the duodenal mucosa has been reported to be equal to that of antral mucosa.[11] Emås and associates[5] estimated that in man the duodenal content is approximately 35 percent that found in the antrum by bioassay. In dogs, the total gastrin content in the entire small bowel mucosa plus the gastric fundic mucosa is only four percent of the total amount of gastrin measured in the gastric antral mucosa by radioimmunoassay.

While the content of gastrin in extra-antral mucosa in the dog is not nearly as large as in man, there is a need to evaluate carefully all future experimental designs in studies of gastric physiology, recognizing that extra-antral sources of gastrin exist and are of physiologic importance.[1]

The distribution of gastrin present in the fundic and antral mucosa as measured by starch-gel electrophoresis is similar to that reported by Berson and Yalow.[3] We found approximately the same ratio of "little" to "big" gastrin in both fundic and antral mucosae. The concentration of gastrin in intestinal mucosa was too small to fractionate accurately.

REFERENCES

1. Becker, H. D., Reeder, D. D., Evans, J. C. W., and Thompson, J. C.: Gastrin release from duodenum and jejunum in dogs, Surg. Forum **23:** 314, 1972.
2. Becker, H. D., Reeder, D. D., and Thompson, J. C.: Effect of truncal vagotomy with pyloroplasty or with antrectomy on food-stimulated gastrin values in patients with duodenal ulcer, SURGERY **74:** 580, 1973.
3. Berson, S. A., and Yalow, R. S.: Nature of immunoreactive gastrin extracted from tissue of gastrointestinal tract, Gastroenterology **60:** 215, 1971.
4. Edkins, J. S.: The chemical mechanism of gastric secretion, J. Physiol. **34:** 133, 1906.
5. Emås, S., Borg, I., and Fyrö, B.: Antral and duodenal gastrin activity in nonulcer and ulcer patients, Scand. J. Gastroenterol. **6:** 39, 1971.
6. Gregory, R. A., and Tracy, H. J.: The constitution and properties of two gastrins extracted from hog antral mucosa, Gut **5:** 103, 1964.
7. Jackson, B. M., Reeder, D. D., and Thompson, J. C.: Dynamic characteristics of gastrin release, Am. J. Surg. **123:** 137, 1972.
8. Jackson, B. M., Reeder, D. D., Searcy, J. R., Watson, L. C., Hirose, F. M., and Thompson, J. C.: Correlation of the surface pH, histology and gastrin concentration of gastric mucosa, Ann. Surg. **176:** 727, 1972.
9. McGuigan, J. E.: Gastric mucosal intracellular localization of gastrin by immunofluorescence, Gastroenterology **55:** 315, 1968.
10. Miller, J. H., Jackson, B. M., and Thompson, J. C.: Effect of total gastrectomy and partial evisceration on circulating gastrin concentration, Surg. Forum **21:** 295, 1970.
11. Nilsson, G., Yalow, R. S., and Berson, S. A.: Distribution of gastrin in the gastrointestinal tract of human, dog, cat and hog, *in:* Andersson, S., editor: Nobel Symposium 16: Frontiers in gastrointestinal hormone research, Stockholm, 1973, Almqvist and Wiksell, p. 95.
12. Stern, D. H., and Walsh, J. H.: Gastrin release in postoperative ulcer patients: Evidence for release of duodenal gastrin, Gastroenterology **64:** 363, 1973.
13. Thompson, J. C.: Gastrin and gastric secretion, Ann. Rev. Med. **20:** 291, 1969.
14. Watson, L. C., Reeder, D. D., Becker, H. D., LaGrone, L., and Thompson, J. C.: Gastrin concentrations in upper gastrointestinal mucosa, Physiologist **15:** 298, 1972.

Effect of ischemia on hepatic parenchymal and reticuloendothelial function in the baboon

Klaus Holper, M.D., Isik Olcay, M.D., Akio Kitahama, M.D., Robert H. Miller, M.D., Lawrence Brettschneider, M.D., Theodore Drapanas, M.D., Rafael A. Trejo, M.D., PhD., *and* **Nicholas R. Di Luzio, Ph.D.,** *New Orleans, La.*

The influence of prolonged (90 minutes) hepatic ischemia on the reticuloendothelial system (RES) and hepatocellular function was evaluated to relate functional alterations to subsequent mortality patterns. RES activity and hepatic blood flow were measured at varying intervals by the use of appropriate doses of the ^{131}I-labeled RE test lipid emulsion. The hepatic-intestinal ischemic insult in 11 baboons resulted in a 72 hour mortality rate of 55 percent. Alterations in bilirubin, Bromsulphalein (BSP), plasma glutamic oxalacetic transaminase (GOT), ornithine carbamyl transferase, lactic dehydrogenase (LDH), and alkaline phosphatase did not distinguish survivors from nonsurvivors. In contrast, the degree of depression of phagocytic activity significantly distinguished nonsurvivors from survivors. Whereas the intravascular clearance rate of the RE test lipid emulsion was only slightly prolonged 24 hours following insult in survivors, profound depression in phagocytic function occurred in nonsurvivors. Hepatic blood flow, which was significantly depressed immediately following ischemia, was essentially normal at 24 hours, denoting that impaired vascular clearance of the lipid emulsion was not due to reduced liver blood flow. These results demonstrate that impaired phagocytosis and possibly other functional alterations of Kupffer cells play a significant role in pathophysiology of acute hepatic failure since derangement in RE function was most indicative of the final outcome of hepatic ischemia.

From the Departments of Surgery and Physiology, Tulane University School of Medicine, New Orleans, La.

THE TEMPORARY interruption of hepatic blood flow is sometimes desirable in the surgical management of acute hepatic trauma and obligatory during hepatic transplantation.[6, 20, 22, 25, 32, 35] In both instances the ischemic interval may induce injury to the two major cell populations of the liver, i.e., the parenchymal and the Kupffer cells. Although functional changes of hepatocytes following partial or complete occlusion of hepatic blood flow have been studied extensively,[1, 2, 15, 18, 26] there is little information available relating functional alterations of Kupffer cells.

Among the multiple responsibilities of the liver in homeostasis are the phagocytic activity and detoxifying capacity of the Kupffer cells.[12, 13, 36] By virtue of these qualities the liver has been postulated to play an important role in the maintenance of cardiovascular integrity by removing gut-derived vasoactive substances, bacteria, and their endo-

Reprint requests: N. R. Di Luzio, Ph. D., Department of Physiology, Tulane University School of Medicine, New Orleans, La. 70112.

Accepted for publication April 18, 1974.

Supported, in part, by the American Heart Association, the Louisiana Heart Association, and National Institutes of Health grant AM 13935.

toxins.[11, 17, 21] The frequent development of gram-negative bacteremia and sepsis following a variety of hepatic insults including hepatic transplantation[5,19] could be due, in part, to a depression of the RES with resulting impairment in host-defense mechanisms.

The purpose of this study was to investigate the effects of ischemia induced by prolonged hepatic occlusion without portal-systemic decompression in the subhuman primate on survival and hemodynamic and hepatic cellular function. In an effort to establish what functional tests would be of predictive value, specific alterations of parenchymal and Kupffer cell function were correlated with the subsequent mortality pattern. This correlation was possible since the ischemic insult selected produced an approximate 50 percent mortality rate. The comparative and simultaneous evaluation of reticuloendothelial and parenchymal cell functions of the liver following ischemia contributes to the assessment of the relative role and importance of specific liver cell populations in the reversibility or irreversibility of acute hepatic failure induced by an ischemic insult.

MATERIALS AND METHODS

Nineteen healthy *Papio papio* baboons of either sex, weighing between 10 and 14 kilograms, were fasted overnight but allowed free access to water. They were immobilized with Sernalyn (piperidine hydrochloride, 1 mg. per kilogram) intramuscularly and proper anesthesia was maintained with minimal amounts of intravenous pentobarbital. Catheters were placed in the femoral vein and artery for infusion and blood sampling as well as continuous monitoring of blood pressures by use of a pressure transducer. Following a 30 minute normalization interval, baseline measurements of arterial blood pressures and heparinized blood samples were obtained. Under sterile conditions the abdomen was opened with a midline incision and the liver exposed. All structures leading to and coming from the liver were carefully dissected and all tissue and ligaments adjacent to the liver and the right gastric artery ligated and divided. In an effort to achieve complete hepatic devascularization, all collateral circulation to the liver was interrupted since Farkouh and associates[16] have reported that the presence of a collateral circulation to the liver could significantly modify the ischemic insult. Loops of umbilical tape were passed around the portal triad including the common hepatic artery, portal vein, and common bile duct, and around the supra- and infra-hepatic inferior vena cava. Total normothermic hepatic ischemia was produced by pulling the tapes tightly through rubber tubings, occluding all hepatic blood flow for a period of 90 minutes. Since occlusion of the portal vein is well tolerated in nonhuman primates,[24] a portal-systemic shunt was not performed. The sham operation was identical to the operative procedure with the exception that the occlusion of the vessels was not conducted.

Phagocytic activity of the RES was determined in experimental and in sham-operated animals by measuring the intravascular clearance of a gelatinized ^{131}I-labeled RE test lipid emulsion.[10] This method is based on the ability of cells of the RES to phagocytize circulating foreign particulates.[3, 4] It has been extensively used in animals[8, 29] and man[9, 30] and was performed as described in detail elsewhere.[28] Briefly, the test material consisted of a ^{131}I-triolein labeled gelatinized RE test lipid emulsion administered in a dose of 0.5 Gm. per kilogram of body weight. The RE test lipid emulsion was freshly prepared and autoclaved prior to use. Following rapid intravenous injection, the intravascular disappearance rate was ascertained by measuring the radioactivity of serial blood samples taken over a period of 30 minutes. The values were plotted in percent of injected dose semilogarithmically against time in minutes and the intravascular half-time ($T_{1/2}$) was determined. The circulating blood volume was calculated by extrapolating the curve back to zero time. Plasma volumes were determined using a corrected hematocrit.[23]

Hepatic blood flow was estimated also by means of an intravascular colloid tech-

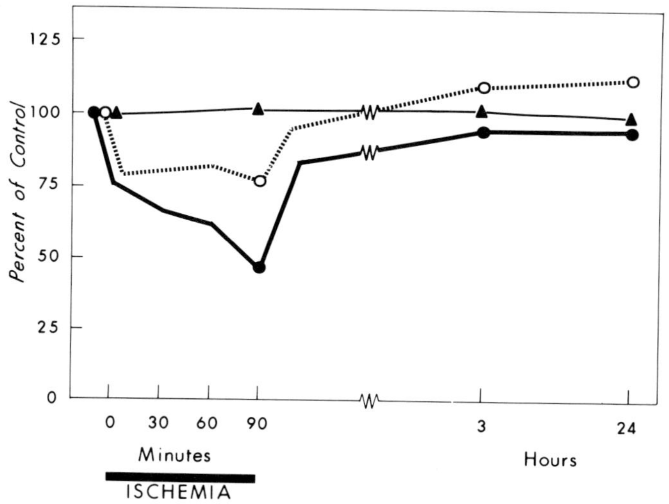

Fig. 1. Mean arterial blood pressure, expressed as a percent of control, of the sham-operated (n = 8, ▲——▲) and hepatic ischemic group. The latter group is subdivided into survivor (n = 5, ○ - - - - ○) and nonsurvivor (n = 6, ●——●) populations.

nique.[28] The amount of gelatinized ^{131}I-labeled lipid emulsion used was 0.04 Gm. per kilogram of body weight, a dose which is below the "critical colloid dose" and thus dependent on liver blood flow for its intravenous clearance. Baseline determinations of hepatic blood flow and reticuloendothelial function were performed one day prior to the experimental procedure.

At specific intervals, arterial pH and blood gases were analyzed by means of a blood-gas analyzer. Plasma total bilirubin was determined by the Diazo reaction. Plasma alkaline phosphatase, plasma GOT, and plasma LDH were measured with the use of commerically available test kit combinations (Sigma). Ornithine carbamyl transferase (OCT) activity of plasma was determined with a microdiffusion NH_3 technique by Reichard and Reichard.[27] Plasma activities of alkaline phosphatase are expressed in Bodansky units, GOT in Sigma-Fraenkel units (SFU) per milliliter, LDH in Berger-Broida units (BBU) per milliliter, and OCT in Reichard units (RU), expressed as micromoles of ammonia formed per 0.5 ml. of plasma in 24 hours (Sigma Tech. Bulletin No. 108). All determinations were made prior to occlusion and at 3, 24, and 48 hours following restoration of hepatic blood flow. In all instances the volume of withdrawn blood was replaced by infusion of sterile saline.

Eleven baboons were randomly selected for the ischemic insult; RE function studies were undertaken in seven while hepatic blood flow was measured in the remaining four baboons. Eight sham-operated animals were utilized, four for each respective determination. Upon completion of the experiments the data of surviving and nonsurviving baboons were analyzed separately to permit a comparison between survivors, nonsurvivors, and the sham-operated controls. Statistical significance between various groups was ascertained according to Student's t test.

RESULTS

Ninety minutes of normothermic hepatic ischemia without venous decompression resulted in a survival of 45 percent. The animals which survived the insult awoke rapidly from anesthesia and recovered to normal physical appearance within a few days, although a slight loss in body weight occurred. In animals which succumbed to the insult, death occurred at a time ranging from 28 to 70 hours, with a mean time of 43 hours. Postoperative recovery in these baboons appeared somewhat delayed. The reduction in

Table I. *Alterations in plasma BSP retention following 90 minutes of total hepatic occlusion*

Time* (hr.)	Sham-operated group (4 baboons) (mg./100 ml.)	Hepatic occluded group: Survivors (4 baboons) (mg./100 ml.)	Hepatic occluded group: Non-survivors (3 baboons) (mg./100 ml.)
0	0.06 ± 0.02	0.05 ± 0.01	0.10 ± 0.06
3	0.08 ± 0.05	2.36 ± 0.93	3.68 ± 0.70
24	0.37 ± 0.15	3.27 ± 0.42	3.05 ± 1.77
48	0.13 ± 0.04	2.57 ± 0.57	—

*The time intervals are following the restoration of hepatic blood flow.

Table II. *Plasma GOT elevations following hepatic ischemia*

Time (hr.)	Sham-operated group (4 baboons) (SFU/ml.)	Hepatic occluded group: Survivors (4 baboons) (SFU/ml.)	Hepatic occluded group: Nonsurvivors (3 baboons) (SFU/ml.)
0	107 ± 70	291 ± 156	166 ± 75
3	155 ± 101	1,811 ± 700	3,374 ± 1,537
24	181 ± 42	1,235 ± 533	2,640 ± 957
48	285 ± 150	970 ± 213	—

Table III. *Plasma LDH in sham-operated and hepatic ischemic baboons*

Time (hr.)	Sham-operated group (4 baboons) (BBU/ml.)	Hepatic occluded group: Survivors (4 baboons) (BBU/ml.)	Hepatic occluded group: Nonsurvivors (3 baboons) (BBU/ml.)
0	958 ± 461	1,425 ± 551	883 ± 286
3	868 ± 381	6,352 ± 2,106	7,496 ± 2,318
24	870 ± 275	6,641 ± 2,565	9,278 ± 2,548
48	1,477 ± 52	4,537 ± 751	—

body core temperature was more pronounced. All sham-operated animals survived.

Mean arterial blood pressure (MABP). with the onset of hepatic occlusion the MABP decreased 21 percent within 5 minutes (Fig. 1). In animals which subsequently survived, blood pressure was maintained throughout the remainder of the occlusive interval. In contrast, a steady decline in MABP occurred in the animals which did not survive the insult. The 54 percent decrease of MABP in the nonsurviving group during the period of ischemia was significantly different ($p < 0.02$) from that of surviving animals. Following restoration of hepatic blood flow, the MABP recovered to 95 and 108 percent of control values at 30 minutes and 3 hours, respectively, in the survivors. Recovery of MABP was also observed in the group which ultimately succumbed, although MABP values were slightly below normal (Fig. 1).

Acid-base status. The blood-gas changes in surviving as well as nonsurviving animals were minimal and similar to those of the sham-operated group. Three hours after occlusion, the arterial pH fell slightly from a control of 7.35 to 7.32 in the surviving group. A more pronounced acidosis developed in nonsurvivors with a pH of 7.28 at the same time interval. This group continued to be slightly acidotic at 24 hours with a mean value of 7.32 while the arterial pH of survivors was normal.

Hepatocellular alterations. The biochemical changes in relation to hepatocellular function are presented in Tables I to VI. Plasma BSP retention was significantly elevated in the group undergoing the ischemic insult. The degree of BSP retention did not, however, significantly distinguish the survivors from the nonsurvivors (Table I), as comparable plasma concentrations were observed. Likewise, the elevations in plasma GOT, LDH, and bilirubin (Tables II to IV) were not significantly different in the baboons which survived or succumbed from the ischemic insult. In essential agreement with these observations, the plasma elevation of the highly liver-specific enzyme, OCT, was essentially identical in survivors as well as in nonsurvivors (Table V). Plasma alkaline phosphatase was not altered in either of the groups undergoing hepatic ischemia. Thus, the degree of impairment of parenchymal cell function, as reflected by various indices, did not correlate with survival or nonsurvival. Alterations in the activity of plasma enzymes and BSP retention in the sham-operated animals were minimal.

Table IV. *Plasma total bilirubin concentration following hepatic ischemia*

Time (hr.)	Sham-operated group (4 baboons) (mg./100 ml.)	Hepatic occluded group: Survivors (4 baboons) (mg./100 ml.)	Hepatic occluded group: Non-survivors (3 baboons) (mg./100 ml.)
0	0.04 ± 0.03	0.37 ± 0.02	0.34 ± 0.03
3	0.44 ± 0.07	0.87 ± 0.21	1.25 ± 0.29
24	0.64 ± 0.10	1.21 ± 0.18	1.39 ± 0.53
48	0.40 ± 0.06	0.96 ± 0.09	—

Table V. *Comparable elevation in plasma ornithine carbamyl transferase activity following hepatic ischemia in surviving and nonsurviving baboons*

Time (hr.)	Sham-operated group (4 baboons) (RU)	Hepatic occluded group: Survivors (4 baboons) (RU)	Hepatic occluded group: Non-survivors (3 baboons) (RU)
0	0.07 ± 0.03	0.06 ± 0.02	0.13 ± 0.14
3	0.24 ± 0.10	1.67 ± 0.07	1.75 ± 0.42
24	0.87 ± 0.22	4.50 ± 1.10	4.43 ± 0.82
48	0.36 ± 0.15	2.20 ± 0.74	—

Table VI. *Plasma alkaline phosphatase concentrations in control and experimental baboons*

Time (hr.)	Sham-operated group (4 baboons) (Bodansky U.)	Hepatic occluded group: Survivors (4 baboons) (Bodansky U.)	Hepatic occluded group: Non-survivors (3 baboons) (Bodansky U.)
0	28.5 ± 4.9	11.7 ± 1.2	13.1 ± 1.5
3	17.5 ± 4.2	11.7 ± 1.0	17.4 ± 3.7
24	23.2 ± 3.9	11.4 ± 1.3	17.5 ± 2.4
48	18.5 ± 5.7	13.6 ± 3.0	—

Table VII. *Enhanced phagocytic dysfunction in baboons which succumb to hepatic ischemic injury**

Time (hr.)	Sham-operated group (4 baboons) (M. ± S.E.)	Hepatic occluded group: Survivors (4 baboons) (M. ± S.E.)	Hepatic occluded group: Death (3 baboons) (M. ± S.E.)
0	27.4 ± 5.1	18.8 ± 4.9	19.4 ± 4.4
3	25.0 ± 6.0	25.2 ± 4.9	38.0 ± 7.6
24	29.4 ± 12.3	41.3 ± 8.0	141.0 ± 49.0
48	31.3 ± 11.6	33.8 ± 5.8	—

*The intravascular half-time of the gelatinized ^{131}I-triolein labeled RE test lipid emulsion was measured prior to and at varying intervals following 90 minutes of total hepatic ischemia. Comparable studies were made in sham-operated baboons.

Relative to zero time values, the only significantly different plasma enzyme alteration in the sham-operated group was the OCT concentration 24 hours postoperatively.

Reticuloendothelial function. The intravascular half-time of the gelatinized ^{131}I-labeled test lipid emulsion in 17 normal baboons averaged 21.7 ± 2.8 minutes. The repeated daily injection of the test lipid emulsion over a period of 4 consecutive days, i.e., one day prior to, and 3, 24, and 48 hours following operative procedures, was well tolerated by all animals. Repeated administration of the RE test lipid emulsion did not significantly modify RE function as the intravascular half-time in the sham-operated group remained essentially unaltered (Table VII).

In the group which survived the ischemic insult, the intravascular half time was slightly increased at 3 hours and significantly increased at 24 hours (Table VII). In the group which did not survive the insult a slight impairment was observed at 3 hours and the half-time was significantly prolonged to a mean of 141 minutes at the 24 hour interval. This latter value differs significantly from the 41 minute half time observed in the surviving group.

Hepatic blood flow (HBF). The mean HBF in seven normal baboons was 21.2 ml. per minute per kilogram of body weight. Hepatic blood flow was essentially unaltered 3 hours following sham operation and decreased slightly below control values at 24 hours (Fig. 2). In contrast, in baboons subjected to hepatic ischemia, HBF decreased approximately 50 to 60 percent at the 3 hour postocclusion period. The decrease in HBF was essentially restored to normal values at 24 hours in both experimental groups.

Blood volume. The mean circulating

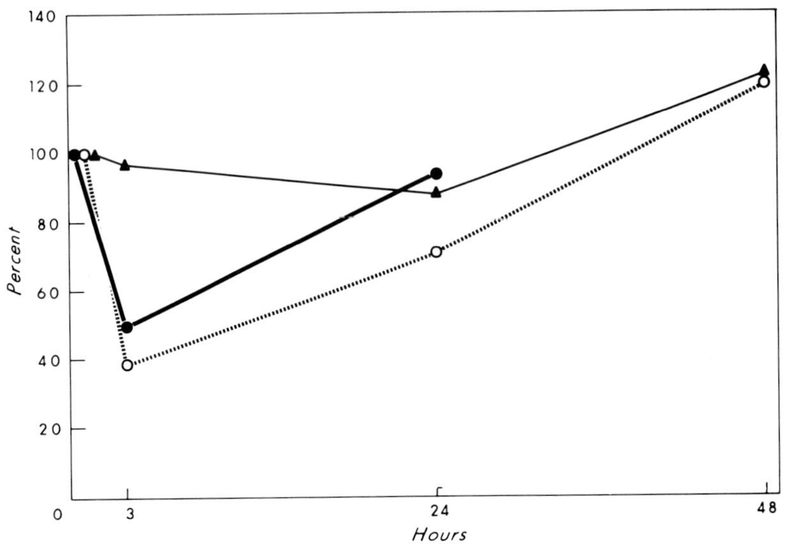

Fig. 2. Liver blood flow, presented as percent of control values, in sham-operated (n = 2, ▲——▲) and ischemic baboons. The latter is presented as a surviving (n = 2, O - - - - O) and nonsurviving (n = 2, O——O) population.

blood volume of 17 normal baboons was 98.1 ± 2.8 ml. per kilogram of body weight. Three hours following the ischemic insult a significant decrease in circulating blood volume occurred (Fig. 3). A further reduction in circulating blood volume in surviving and nonsurviving animals was observed at 24 hours with decreases of 33 and 48 percent, respectively. The hypovolemia was significantly greater in the nonsurviving group. Sham-operated animals maintained normovolemia throughout the experimental period.

DISCUSSION

Our results demonstrate that 90 minutes of normothermic hepatic ischemia, coupled with the simultaneous occlusion of the splanchnic outflow and infrahepatic caval return, was associated with a 45 percent survival in the subhuman primate. This finding is in essential accord with observations of other investigators that hepatic ischemia of considerable duration is compatible with survival. Drapanas and associates[14] reported that a period of hepatic ischemia of 75 minutes or less was nonlethal to dogs. A 33 percent survival was observed with 90 minutes of ischemia. Farkouh and associates[15, 16] studied the influence of a 30 to 110 minute hepatic ischemic insult and observed that all dogs survived a 40 minute ischemic insult, 60 percent survived a 50 to 70 minute occlusion, and 100 percent died with an ischemic insult of 80 minutes or longer. Both Selkurt[31] and Backlund and associates[2] also observed that a 2 hour deprivation of liver blood flow produced a 100 percent mortality rate in dogs. Rangel and associates[26] showed the same fatal outcome in portacaval-shunted rhesus monkeys after 120 minutes of hepatic ischemia.

In an effort to ascertain the mechanism of death following acute portal vein occlusion in dogs, Tanturi and associates[34] stated that a marked reduction in circulating blood volume occurred following the occlusion of the portal vein. During the period of occlusion, electrocardiographic patterns of subendocardial ischemic lesions were observed in all animals.[34] Although we did not record electrocardiographic changes, the reduction in circulating blood volume which was noted by Tanturi and associates[34] in the dog was also seen in the baboon.

Farkouh and associates[15] measured various biological substances to ascertain their

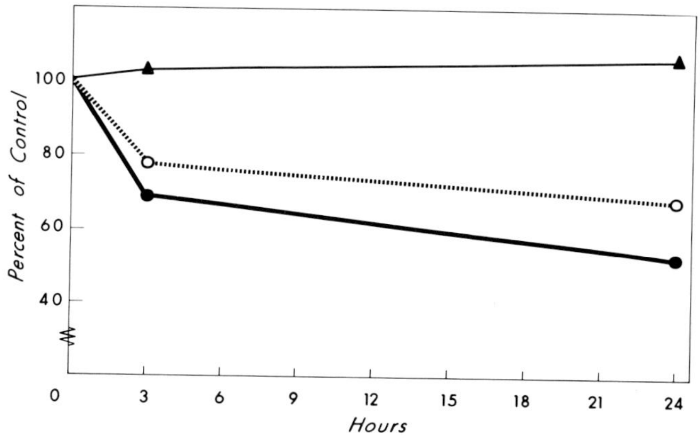

Fig. 3. Circulating blood volume, expressed as percent of control of the sham-operated (n = 4, ▲——▲) and normothermic hepatic ischemic groups. The ischemic group is subdivided into a surviving (n = 5, O - - - - O) and nonsurviving (n = 6, ●——●) population.

possible prognostic value following ischemic injury to the liver in dogs. Marked metabolic changes in the liver occurred due to temporary occlusion of the hepatic circulation. Liver lactate and phosphate were significantly elevated shortly following the ischemic insult while adenine nucleotides were significantly decreased. The hepatic concentrations of ATP, ADP, and AMP were all significantly decreased. Hepatic cytoplasmic enzymes such as GOT, GPT, and LDH were markedly elevated in plasma after ischemic injury to the liver and increased in proportion to the period of ischemia. Farkouh and associates[15] reported that the degree of elevation in liver lactate concentration was the only finding which related to the final fate of the animal, as no dog survived when the liver lactate concentration was 17 mM. per gram, while levels below 15 mM. per gram were associated with excellent prognosis.

Our findings are in essential agreement with those of Farkouh and associates[15] that classical liver function tests, which essentially reflect the integrity of parenchymal cells, did not correlate with the subsequent mortality pattern. Furthermore, our observations that plasma OCT concentrations were nearly identical in survivors and nonsurvivors indicate that the hepatocellular response to the ischemic hepatic injury was similar in the surviving and nonsurviving groups. These findings denote that the damage of the parenchymal cells, although of considerable magnitude in both groups, is apparently still compatible with survival.

Similar observations of alterations in hepatic function following liver ischemia were made by Rangel and associates[26] in *Macaca mulatta* monkeys and by Flock and Gilquist[18] in dogs. Ultrastructural studies made by Flock and Gilquist revealed that significant ultrastructural changes occur in hepatic parenchymal cells following a 20 minute period of ischemia. The major cellular events were the disruption of parenchymal cells and the appearance of cellular organelles in the space of Disse. These morphological changes were associated with an elevation in serum OCT levels.

Rangel and associates[26] observed elevations of acid phosphatase and beta glucuronidase in monkeys following 2 hours of hepatic ischemia. In their studies SGOT and SGPT as well as elevation in alkaline phosphatase increased upon revascularization of the liver. Similar to the observations of Flock and Gilquist,[18] electron miscrocopic studies revealed alterations in mitochondria, endoplasmic reticulum, and lysosomes. Pretreatment of the animals with phenoxybenzamine significantly reduced the ultrastructural alterations which characterized the ischemic group. Since a reduction in plasma enzyme levels and prolongation in survival time were seen in the treated group, the authors suggested that the beneficial effect of phenoxybenzamine may be due to its membrane stabilizing properties.

Dinbar and Fonkalsrud[11] reported that neomycin-treated macaca monkeys, which underwent one hour of hepatic ischemia one week after a side-to-side portacaval shunt was performed, did not show a significant elevation in SGPT and acid phosphatase values. In contrast, these animals had progressive increases in both enzymes after the shunt procedure alone. The authors stated that hepatic cellular injury, which occurred after first operation, i.e., the portacaval shunt, and was not observed following the ischemic insult, was due to the regenerative ability of the liver and its adaptation to the new hemodynamic state.

In portasystemic shunted dogs, Swenson and associates[33] showed moderate to marked alkaline phosphatase alterations after 1.5 to 4 hours of liver ischemia. The authors stated that routine liver function tests, other than alkaline phosphatase, were not significantly changed. Alkaline phosphatase levels were increased in all experimental animals. It would appear, based upon the studies of Dinbar and Fonkalsrud[11] and Swenson and associates,[33] that shunting of the portal blood reduces or eliminates the functional alterations observed following total hepatic ischemia. The mechanism of the possible protective effect of portal shunting remains to be ascertained but could well be related to the avoidance of congestive episodes in the mesenteric-splenic system.

In contrast to the lack of correlation of the classical hepatic parenchymal function tests to the final outcome of the animal following ischemic insult, the degree of impairment of reticuloendothelial function appeared to correlate with survival or nonsurvival. Hepatic blood flow, which can influence phagocytic clearance,[13] was significantly depressed only in the initial postocclusive phase. The approximate twofold prolongation of the intravascular clearance half-time in survivors as well as nonsurvivors at that time interval may be possibly explained by the observed reduction of hepatic blood flow. At 24 hours, however, where major depression in RE function was observed, hepatic blood flow was essentially normalized. Thus, impaired intravascular clearance of the lipid emulsion seen in the nonsurviving group could not be due to reduced hepatic blood flow. Since the status of RE function following ischemia in our experimental model was the only parameter in a variety of biological determinations which correlated with subsequent mortality patterns, RE function may play a significant role in the pathophysiology of hepatic failure. In view of the role of the RES in the phagocytosis and detoxification of endotoxin as well as in the inactivation of other vasoactive preparations,[7] the loss of RES function following ischemia could be of major significance.

The fact that both survivors and nonsurvivors exhibited a similar degree of hepatic parenchymal cell injury allows one to conclude that the existence of hepatic parenchymal cell lesions induced in the baboon by an ischemic interval of 90 minutes is compatible with survival if it is associated with adequate RE function. Recovery did not occur when RE function was significantly and conjointly inhibited. While the mechanism by which ischemic insult to the liver induces R5 dysfunction is yet to be ascertained, the further evaluation of RE function tests as a prognostic expression of hepatic injury appears warranted.

REFERENCES

1. Almersjö, O., Benkmark, S., Domellöf, L., and Hafström, L.: Immediate effects of short-term hepatic and splanchnic ischemia in pigs, Am. J. Surg. **122:** 91, 1971.
2. Backlund, W. M., Stevens, T. J., Hamit, H. F., and Jorden, G. L.: Hepatic ischemia in dogs, J. A. M. A. **194:** 214, 1965.
3. Benacerraf, B., Biozzi, G., Halpern, B. N., and Stiffel, C.: Physiology of phagocytosis by the RES, *in* Halpern, B. N., editor: Physiology of the reticuloendothelial system. Oxford, 1957, Blackwell Scientific Publications, pp. 52-79.
4. Biozzi, G., and Stiffel, C.: The physiopa-

thology of the reticuloendothelial cells of the liver and spleen, in Popper, H., and Schaffner, F., editors: Progress in liver disease, New York, 1965, Grune & Stratton, Inc., pp. 166-191.
5. Brettschneider, L., Tong, J. L., Bosse, D. S., Daloze, P. M., Smith, G. V., Huguet, C., Blanchard, H., Groth, C. G., and Starzl, T. E.: Specific bacteriologic problems after orthotopic liver transplantation in dogs and pigs, Arch. Surg. **97:** 313, 1968.
6. Calne, R. Y., Yoffa, D. E., White, H. J. O., and Maginn, R. R.: A technique of orthotopic liver transplantation in the pig, Br. J. Surg. 55: 203, 1968.
7. Cuevas, P., and Fine, J.: Production of fatal endotoxic shock by vasoactive substances, Gastroenterology **64:** 285, 1973.
8. Di Luzio, N. R., and Riggi, S. J.: The development of a lipid emulsion for the measurement of reticuloendothelial function, J. Reticuloendothel. Soc. **1:** 136, 1964.
9. Di Luzio, N. R., Salky, N. K., Riggi, S. J., and Ladman, A. J.: Experimental and clinical evaluation of reticuloendothelial function by means of a specific lipid emulsion, *in* The reticuloendothelial system, morphology, immunology, and regulation, Japan, 1965, Nissha Printing Co., pp. 389-404.
10. Di Luzio, N. R., Pisano, J. C., and Saba, T. M.: Evaluation of mechanism of glucan-induced stimulation of the reticuloendothelial system, J. Reticuloendothel. Soc. **7:** 731, 1970.
11. Dinbar, A., and Fonkalsrud, E. W.: Enzymatic and histologic effects of side-to-side portacaval anastomosis on the primate liver, Surg. Gynecol. Obstet. **133:** 35, 1971.
12. Dobson, E., and Jones, H.: The behavior of intravenously injected particulate matter. Its rate of disappearance from the blood stream as a measure of liver blood flow, Acta Med. Scand. Suppl. 273, 1952.
13. Dobson, E. L.: Factors controlling phagocytosis, *in* Halpern, B. N., editor: Physiopathology of the reticuloendothelial system, Oxford, 1957, Blackwell Scientific Publications.
14. Drapanas, T., Becker, D. R., Alfano, G. S., Potter, W. H., and Steward, J. D.: Some effects of interrupting hepatic blood flow, Ann. Surg. **142:** 831, 1955.
15. Farkouh, E. F., Daniel, A. M., Beaudoin, J. G., and MacLean, L. D.: Predictive value of liver biochemistry in acute hepatic ischemia, Surg. Gynecol. Obstet. **132:** 832, 1971.
16. Farkouh, E. F., Daniel, A. M., and MacLean, L. D.: The effect of collateral circulation on survival in liver ischemia, J. Surg. Res. **11:** 130, 1971.
17. Filkins, J. P.: Hepatic vascular response to endotoxin, Proc. Soc. Exp. Biol. Med. **131:** 1235, 1969.
18. Flock, A., and Gilquist, J.: Changes of the ultrastructure of liver cells after shortlasting liver ischemia in dogs, Acta Clin. Scand. **136:** 405, 1970.
19. Gans, H., Mori, K., Lindsey, E., Kaster, B., Richter, D., Quinlan, R., Dineen, P. A., and Tan, B. H.: Septicemia as a manifestation of acute liver failure, Surg. Gynecol. Obstet. **132:** 783, 1971.
20. Garnier, H., Clot, J. P., and Chomette, G.: Orthotopic transplantation of the porcine liver, Surg. Gynecol. Obstet. **130:** 105, 1970.
21. Greene, R., Wiznitzer, T., Rutenberg, S., Frank, E., and Fine, J.: Hepatic clearance of endotoxin absorbed from the intestine, Proc. Soc. Exp. Biol. Med. **108:** 261, 1961.
22. Madding, G. F., and Kennedy, P. A.: Trauma to the liver, Philadelphia; 1965, W. B. Saunders Company.
23. McGovern, J. J., Jones, A. R., and Steinberg, A. G.: The hematocrit of capillary blood, N. Engl. J. Med. **253:** 308, 1955.
24. Milnes, R. F., and Child, C. G.: Acute occlusion by ligature of the portal vein in the Macacus rhesus monkey, Proc. Soc. Exp. Biol. Med. **70:** 332, 1949.
25. Pappas, G., Plamer, W. M., Martineau, G. L., Penn, I., Halgrimson, C. G., Groth, C. G., and Starzl, T. E.: Hemodynamic alterations caused during orthotopic liver transplantation in humans, SURGERY **70:** 872, 1971.
26. Rangel, D. M., Bruckner, W. L., Byfield, J. E., Adomian, G. E., Dinbar, A., and Fonkalsrud, E. W.: Enzymatic and ultrastructural evaluation of hepatic preservation in primates, Arch. Surg. **100:** 284, 1970.
27. Reichard, H., and Reichard, P.: Determination of ornithine carbamyl transferase in serum, J. Lab. Clin. Med. **52:** 709, 1958.
28. Saba, T. M., and Di Luzio, N. R.: Surgical stress and reticuloendothelial function, SURGERY **65:** 802, 1969.
29. Saba, T. M., and Di Luzio, N. R.: Reticuloendothelial blockade and recovery as a function of opsonic activity, Am. J. Physiol. **216:** 197, 1969.
30. Salky, N. K., Di Luzio, N. R., Levin, A. G., and Goldsmith, H. S.: Phagocytic activity of the reticuloendothelial system in neoplastic disease, J. Lab. Clin. Med. **70:** 393, 1967.
31. Selkurt, E. E.: Intestinal ischemic shock and the protective role of the liver, Am. J. Physiol. **197:** 281, 1959.
32. Starzl, T. E. (with the assistance of Putman, C. W.): Experience in hepatic transplantation, Philadelphia, 1969, W. B. Saunders Company.

33. Swenson, O., Grana, L., Inouye, T., and Donnella, W. L.: Immediate and long-term effects of acute hepatic ischemia, Arch. Surg. **95:** 451, 1967.
34. Tanturi, C., Mejia, R. H., Canepa, J. F., and Gomez, O. T.: Electrocardiographic and humoral changes in transient occlusion of the portal vein in the dog, Surg. Gynecol. Obstet. **110:** 537, 1960.
35. Waltuck, T. L., Crow, R. W., Humphrey, L. J., and Kauffman, H. M.: Avulsion injuries of the vena cava following blunt abdominal trauma, Ann. Surg. **171:** 67, 1970.
36. Zweifach, W., and Benacerraf, B.: Effect of hemorrhagic shock on the phagocytic function of Kupffer cells, Circ. Res. **6:** 83, 1958.

British surgery today: Perspective of a James IV surgical traveler

Keith A. Kelly, M.D., *Rochester, Minn.*

A 6 week visit to Scotland and England, sponsored by the James IV Association of Surgeons, presented an opportunity for a brief but close view of British surgery today. Both patients and surgeons seem pleased with this government-sponsored health system and the high standards of medical care it affords the population. Potential problem areas are government direction of research funds and projects, fixed salaries for surgeons, and little economic encouragement for specialization.

From the Mayo Clinic and the Mayo Foundation, Rochester, Minn.

In 1957, the James IV Association of Surgeons was founded by three noted surgeons—one from the United States, one from England, and one from Scotland. Their purpose was to "foster the exchange of knowledge among the distinguished surgeons of those countries of the world wherein the English language is freely spoken." In 1973, when the society had expanded to include 87 active members from 16 different countries, four Surgical Travelers were awarded honoraria to cross an ocean and to share knowledge with their surgical colleagues in other English-speaking countries. A Canadian travelled to England, Ireland, and Scotland, an Australian as well as an Englishman visited the United States and Canada, and an American (myself) journeyed to Scotland and England.

I began my itinerary in Prestwick, Scotland, where my plane landed on May 27 at 7:00 A.M. The sunshine was streaming through the morning mist, and the clean smell of the sea drifted across the links. It was a great day! For 6 weeks I travelled from Scotland down through the Midlands to London, taking several side trips along the way. I left Heathrow for "the States" on another bright day, July 9.

Accepted for publication April 18, 1974.

Reprint requests: Keith A. Kelly, M.D., Mayo Clinic, 200 First Street SW, Rochester, Minn. 55901.

During my trip, I met scores of surgeons, physicians, basic scientists, house officers, students, and other medical personnel, visited many hospitals and laboratories, and attended several surgical and scientific meetings. The people I visited were affiliated primarily with academic centers emphasizing gastroenterology, my major interest, but I obtained a perspective of British surgery in general.

I found a number of current forces influencing surgery in Britain, which sorted themselves out into the patterns described below.

SOCIALIZATION

The government-sponsored health scheme (National Health Service, NHS) is in full swing throughout Britain. In general, it is working well and there was little talk of withdrawing from the system or abandoning it in favor of a free-enterprise or privately financed plan.

The patients are pleased with the NHS.

The standard of care is high and the patients have ready access to the system, especially for acute or emergent illnesses. Although the waiting lists for elective surgery still tend to be long in rural areas, they are attractively short in metropolitan areas. I was told that elective operations could be scheduled within a few days at several London hospitals.

The British patient, who obtains his care "free" from the NHS, may feel somewhat more a captive of the system than his American counterpart. For instance, he may be more likely to submit to investigational study if the staff asks him to do so. However, I encountered no instances in which the position of the patient was compromised.

Despite the success of the National Health Service, a definite demand for private health care still exists. Some patients feel the need to have their operation (1) at the time they want it, (2) by a surgeon of their choice, and (3) in the surroundings they choose. They believe that care will be more personalized, more attentive, and more carefully delivered in the private sector than in the public domain. A private insurance scheme is available to deal with this need.

The surgeons, for the most part, are also content with the professional aspects of the NHS. They have the senior directive position in surgery. The hospitals are pleasant places in which to work, and the equipment is good. They have adequate junior staff to assist them. They can maintain a high standard of practice and often develop expertise in a certain area, attracting patients from their region to their unit. Receiving their salary from the NHS allows them to be objective in their recommendations for operation. Yet, they show a great interest in their patients and a devotion to them.

The medical students believe that the government-sponsored system of health care is the best system available. Indeed, they have difficulty understanding why all sick people should not have access to high-quality medical care regardless of their ability to pay.

Government sponsorship covers not only health care but also the vast majority of research. Investigators submit proposals to the Medical Research Council, where they are given a just peer review. The system has worked well and fairly, and in the past adequate funds have been available for good projects. But investigators sometimes complain about the short term of the awards and the need for excessively frequent progress reports. Moreover, the government recently decided that a greater proportion of medical research (25 percent) should be oriented toward patient care, and it has directed that awards be made in these areas. This "contract" research resembles that becoming more common in the United States—with its attending hazards. Government direction of the nature and type of research can destroy individual initiative, imagination, and creativity. Moves in this direction may provide temporary gains but may ultimately destroy the originality so essential to research.

The research in Britain is largely sponsored by the government, but some hospitals also have endowments that have enabled them to fund work within their own departments. These endowments are now in danger of being confiscated by the government, again possibly leading to increased central direction of research.

INFLATIONARY ECONOMY

Almost every surgeon with whom I spoke referred to the economy at some time during our visit, reflecting great concern in this area. Surgeons in Britain are paid a fixed salary by the government for their services. Most consultants either work full time for the government or 9/11 of their time, collecting 9/11 of a full-time salary. Those who choose the latter can use the remaining 2/11 of their work week for private practice. Academic people essentially do full-time surgery. Nonacademic surgeons are more likely to engage in private practice, although opportunities for this are limited outside the large metropolitan areas.

As prices rise, surgeons on a fixed salary are at an increasing disadvantage. Their purchasing power decreases, bringing down their standard of living. The cost of living is especially high in London. Young surgeons think twice about accepting a post in London, since their purchasing power there is less than in other parts of Britain.

In order to supplement their income, some surgeons unwillingly focus increasing attention on the 2/11 of their time used in private practice. Their energies are thus directed away from their NHS work, or away from research or educational objectives they might otherwise have pursued.

The salutary effect of private practice on the over-all income of surgeons throughout Britain is small. The NHS salaries set the standard. The gap between the salaries of physicians and persons in other occupations is narrowing, leaving fewer economic incentives to enter medicine.

Yet increased investment in the health care system by the government is apparent. Perhaps the greatest period of building hospitals and clinics is taking place since the Victorian era. New medical schools, outpatient clinics, beautiful modern hospitals, and new research facilities are going up. Construction was under way in every center I visited.

On the other hand, the main arrangement for in-hospital care is still the open ward, with about 20 patients in one room. The patients can be screened off from one another when privacy is required. The nurses have a central work area in the room that gives them ready access to the patients. Although lack of privacy is sometimes a disadvantage, this common room does allow easy monitoring of the sick by the staff. Certainly there is less opportunity for such oversights as an intravenous infusion running out unobserved. These units are not too dissimilar from open intensive-care areas in hospitals in the United States.

EXPLOSION OF KNOWLEDGE

The explosion of knowledge has forced surgeons to specialize. In order to become expert in one area, they have had to compartmentalize and specifically direct their interests. Because one surgeon cannot know it all, teams of people, each with special talents, have been amassed in departments of surgery. Almost all departments have several, and sometimes numerous, full-time nonsurgical faculty. Nor is the team approach limited to members of a single department, hospital, or university. Researchers from Leeds, Liverpool, Manchester, and Sheffield with varied backgrounds but with a mutual interest in gastroenterology are working together on common problems.

This team approach to problem solving offers greater depth and versatility. But the system has disadvantages, too, especially for the nonsurgical members of a department of surgery. The traditional avenues of promotion and advancement in their own specialties are not easily available to the nonsurgeons. In some cases the jobs in surgical departments seem to be "dead ends."

Rapid growth of knowledge has increased the need for meetings and for communication of advances. The local and national meetings at which I was a guest were avidly attended. They were of a high standard and the presentations were excellent. I liked the way the chairmen of sessions often made a comment or an interpretation at the end of a presentation to allow the audience time to prepare a question and to give the speaker a chance to recover. It also meant that the presentations were not marred by the embarrassing period of silence that sometimes follows when the chairman says simply, "Any questions?"

The placement of academic departments of surgery in general hospitals also seemed to me an excellent system for allowing advances in research to readily diffuse into the nonacademic group, while at the same time forcing the academic surgeons to be as good as their colleagues in the care of patients.

The rapid advances in the various sciences have not wrought substantial curriculum changes in the medical schools nor altered the material used on tests by the Royal Colleges and Faculties. The Colleges and Faculties still emphasize anatomy, physiology, and pathology, with less stress on subjects such as immunology, statistics, and genetics. Surgeons are satisfied with the fellowship system, which they believe offers a challenge to the neophyte and assures a certain academic excellence in those who pass.

INTERNATIONALISM

British surgery has been "international" for years in that it possesses a long history of influx of faculty and students from the Commonwealth countries. The fellowships of the various Royal Colleges have set a standard of surgery throughout the world, and much evidence supports the fact that English is the international language.

I was especially curious about whether these international exchanges would be increased in this day when travel to and communication with other countries are easier. Also I wondered whether the British entry into the European economic community would affect medical practice.

No major additional international influences were apparent. A commission to explore international recognition of surgical training among English-speaking surgeons has met, but no alteration in recognition has yet occurred. The four Royal corporations of Glasgow, Edinburgh, England, and Ireland are still autonomous, and I was told of no plans for amalgamation. British surgeons have not moved toward practice in Common Market countries, nor did I encounter surgeons from the continent who have recently come to practice in Britain.

On the other hand, international societal cooperation seems to be increasing. The Surgical Research Society (SRS) meets with its European and American counterparts, and I met surgeons from the continent at the SRS meeting. Language is still a major barrier, however.

British medical students strongly consider a period of study in a foreign country. Several schools have regular programs of exchange. Students gain sponsorship from their families, their schools, and the government. Inexpensive international flights have also helped make these trips possible.

POPULATION SHIFTS

The population in Britain is rather stable geographically and patients tend to remain in one region, often in one town, throughout their lives. The pattern of medical care within a region is also stable. The patients generally go to the same doctors and hospitals for years. Allegiance to hospitals is strong and the desire to seek medical care in a distant center is weak. The patients are confident in and loyal to their doctors and are inclined to take their advice without question.

The emphasis on regional medical care means that patients often are not sent long distances to see experts in a particular discipline, even though the patient would bear little additional expense and the official restrictions on such movements would be few.

This stability offers great advantage for the study of populations of patients. The patient can easily be contacted, and he returns for outpatient visits and examinations reliably. Indeed, patients are happy to return because of their loyalty to their doctors and hospitals. Moreover, because of the socialized system, fewer economic restraints are placed on investigational studies. Controlled clinical trials are extremely well done in Britain, emphasizing the need for improvement of efforts in this area in other countries.

The few shifts in population that have occurred have been to and within metropolitan areas. Suburbanization is on the upswing. The center of a large city like London has become a place for work, while suburbia has become the place to live, shop, and spend one's leisure time. The move to the suburbs has meant that patients now prefer to have their medical treatment in the suburbs. This has resulted in a drift of patients away from the centrally located London teaching hospitals and toward the suburban hospitals. The number of patients in the London teaching hospitals has declined to the point where the waiting lists are short or nonexistent in some. In fact, the staff are actively recruiting patients.

The move of patients to the suburbs is facilitated by the emergence of excellent suburban hospitals staffed by well-trained surgeons and physicians. The quality of care in suburban hospitals is apparently beginning to rival that available in central London. However, it is difficult to believe that the care in suburban hospitals will replace completely that available at the well-established, central medical centers.

Some London teaching hospitals have developed a satellite or sponsorship arrangement with a suburban hospital that includes exchange of registrars. At least one hospital, Charing Cross, has left its central location and moved into new facilities located in Fulham.

The surgeons, too, tend to remain in the region of the country where they grew up. The uniform regional background of some surgical staffs must mean that the selection of staff is greatly influenced by the local people—no doubt in an effort to achieve harmonious relationships. I encountered few foreign graduates in consultant positions, although there were some.

The greater ease of transportation and communication between the various parts of the country has meant that surgeons do not feel they are "in mothballs" if they do not work in the center of a metropolitan area. In fact, many prefer the slower pace and more pleasant life of the small towns. Younger surgeons are inclined toward small towns for economic reasons.

Once a surgeon is established as a consultant in a hospital, there is little likelihood of his moving to another hospital. This is conducive to good follow-up of his patients over the years. On the other hand, one wonders whether movement of consultants should not be encouraged in some instances. Professional needs and goals change with personal growth, and moves are not unreasonable. Shifts in the academic medical community are more frequent. Perhaps they would be healthy in the nonacademic medical community as well.

THE YOUTH MOVEMENT

Medicine is still an attractive career for young people in Britain. There is keen competition for places in the medical schools. Students are anxious to enter medicine for humanitarian reasons, but they are also attracted because of the economic stability of the profession.

The students are less outspoken and quieter than those in the United States. They agitate less and criticize their surroundings and teachers less. There also seem to be more female students.

The standards at the various medical schools are similar, and the schools are generally considered equal. This uniformity may have resulted partly from government sponsorship and partly from the close communication among schools. Professors from one school move to other schools to conduct examinations, a system that fosters exchange of ideas in teaching and promotes a uniform standard.

The increase in knowledge has altered the curriculum in medical schools to some extent, but most professors and students believe that the time allotted to surgery (about one year) is satisfactory. Certainly surgery is still a major subject in the clinical years. Surgeons teach not only surgery but also general medicine.

Emphasis is still placed on bedside teaching and lectures. The students do not spend a great deal of time in the operating rooms. Teaching aids ("hardware" and "software") are not commonly used, although some faculty members take advantage of newer teaching techniques. For example, a computer in Leeds shows students what criteria they should apply in making a diagnosis, among other things.

The medical students are anxious to shorten their period of training. Some schools are considering a change from a 6 to 5 year program.

After medical school, about 50 percent of the graduates enter general practice. The decision against specialization is influenced by the long training required in fields such as surgery, as well as by the uncertainties of finishing and of obtaining a position as a consultant. Financially, too, there is an incentive toward general practice. The salaries of a surgeon and a general practitioner are comparable, but one can become a general practitioner without additional training. The working conditions of general practitioners are also improving. They are banding together in clinics where calls during off hours and responsibilities are shared, making practice more pleasant. These clinics also allow part-time work, an attractive feature to female physicians with family responsibilities. I met very few women who were training in surgery and none who were consultants.

Still, a large number of the good students and many surgeons believe that the best students are attracted to surgery. I encountered no surgical department unable to recruit house staff.

Young surgeons of today can expect to obtain a consultant post after about 10 years of postgraduate training, at about age 35. Once one has reached the senior registrar post, a consultantship is virtually assured.

My experiences between May 27 and July 9, 1973, convinced me that the personal contacts and exchanges between the James IV Surgical Traveler and the hosts provide a depth of communication that no other method would make possible.

I sincerely thank the James IV Association of Surgeons for giving me the opportunity to travel in Britain as their Surgical Traveler, the Mayo Foundation for allowing me to accept the award, and the British people for offering their warm and wonderful hospitality during my 6 week stay there.

Body responses and recovery after 2½ hour hypothermic circulatory arrest

Yoshio Kondo, M.D., M. Don Turner, Ph.D., Jose Bebin, M.D., *and* **James D. Hardy, M.D.,** *Jackson, Miss.*

With a modified method of hypothermia, body responses and recovery pattern were studied in 13 puppies after 2½ hours of circulatory arrest at 11° C. Body temperature was lowered by surface and limited left-heart bypass cooling. Pluronic F-68, methylprednisolone, and low-molecular-weight dextran were administered. Before circulatory arrest, an intracellular-type solution was infused into the arteries of the brain, heart, and lungs. All animals were successfully resuscitated and resumed proper cardiac function. Three were put to death acutely for in vitro microrespirometry. Four of the remaining 10 puppies died of respiratory insufficiency within 48 hours, one died of pneumonia at 5 days, and the other five resumed normal daily activity until killed at 14 to 150 days. Metabolic derangements, such as lactic acidosis, serum electrolyte changes, and impaired insulin response with hyperglycemia, were severe but transient. Recovery of many animals was complicated by hind-leg weakness and loss of vision; most of these symptoms disappeared within 3 weeks, but various degrees of pathologic lesions remained in the central nervous system. These results indicate that 2½ hours of circulatory arrest is still beyond the "safe time limits." However, the "intracellular-type" solution used protects the function of vital organs so well that resuscitation is uniformly possible and long-term survival rates are acceptably high.

From the Departments of Surgery and Pathology, The University of Mississippi Medical Center, Jackson, Miss.

A NEW method of deep hypothermia with surface cooling and limited cardiopulmonary bypass has been developed recently as a useful adjunct to open-heart surgery for correction of congenital defects in infants.[1, 9] However, duration of circulatory arrest has been restricted to 90 minutes or less. In an attempt to prolong the permissible duration of circulatory arrest, we have modified the method by applying recent innovations in ischemic organ preservation techniques. Details on developmental studies of the modification have been described in a separate paper.[12] This report is mainly concerned with body response and reversibility of the resultant changes after 2½ hours of total circulatory arrest under our modified method of hypothermia.

METHODS

Two groups of preliminary experiments were performed with 16 puppies. These studies were followed by a final group of 13 experiments, which have provided the principal material for this study. As shown in Fig. 1,

Work supported by United States Public Health Service Grants HL 06163 and HL 11730.

Accepted for publication May 13, 1974.

Reprint requests: Yoshio Kondo, M.D., Department of Surgery, The University of Mississippi Medical Center, 2500 N. State St., Jackson, Miss. 39216.

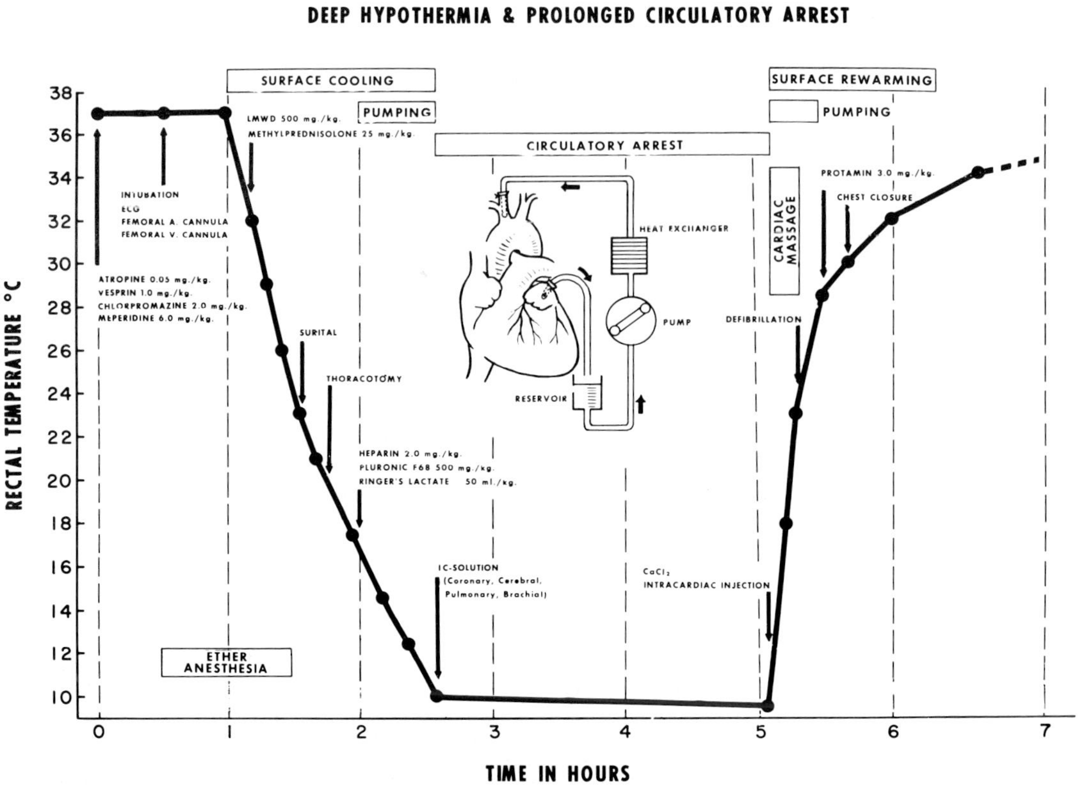

Fig. 1. Typical time course and body temperature change of the experimental procedure. A schematic insertion shows the left-heart bypass circuit.

puppies weighing 3 to 8 kilograms were premedicated with triflupromazine (Vesprine), atropine, meperidine, and chlorpromazine. Following intravenous administration of methylprednisolone and low-molecular-weight dextran, surface cooling by ice-water immersion was carried out under ether anesthesia. When the rectal temperature was lowered to 20° C., heparin and Pluronic F-68 were given intravenously, and both pleural cavities were opened through the fourth intercostal space. Left-heart bypass cooling was begun at 16 to 18° C. by cyclic perfusion through a left atrial cannula, a reservoir, a Sarns' pump, a stainless steel tube coil heat exchanger immersed in ice water and a cannula inserted into the aortic arch from the right carotid artery. The extracorporeal circuit was primed with 300 ml. of Ringer's lactate solution. The pump flow was adjusted to the range of 40 to 60 ml. per kilogram per minute, depending upon the return flow to the reservoir. Cooling was stopped at a rectal temperature of 11° C. The coronary and brachiocephalic arteries were flushed with 30 ml. of 4° C. solution with an electrolyte concentration similar to that of intracellular fluid (IC-solution). This solution contains 107 mEq. per liter of potassium, 9 mEq. per liter of sodium, 28 mEq. per liter of magnesium, 14 mEq. per liter of chloride, 54 mEq. per liter of phosphate, 9 mEq. per liter of bicarbonate, 28 mEq. per liter of sulfate, and 25 Gm. per liter of glucose.[5] The flushing procedure was accomplished by clamping the descending aorta and injecting the solution from the carotid artery cannula. The heart beat was stopped immediately by this procedure. Then, 40 to 50 ml. of IC-solution were infused in the pulmonary artery of the inflated lung by puncture of the right ventricle and by recovery of the perfusate from the atrial cannula. The animal was left at room temperature with no supportive measures. After 2½ hours of total circulatory arrest, rewarming was started by left-heart bypass and immersion in a warm bath. Overdistention of the heart was avoided by manual cardiac massage until ventricular fibrillation converted to a regular beat by electric shock. The left-heart bypass was ended at 32° C. rectal temperature and the pleural cavities were closed in three layers with a chest tube on each side for drainage. Sodium bicarbonate was used to regulate blood pH, and protamine to neutralize heparin.

Recovery course and survival record were followed in 10 of 13 puppies. In the remaining three puppies, open biopsies of the liver and kidney tissue were obtained before and one hour after the procedure for in vitro microrespirometry; the technique was described previously.[18]

Blood samples were obtained before, one hour after, and 24 hours after hypothermia, and later in the convalescent period. Laboratory studies included arterial blood-gas analysis with a Corning Blood Gas Analyser, plasma insulin by radioimmunoassay, blood glucose by the hexokinase method, blood lactate and pyruvate by lactate dehydrogenase. Serum electrolytes, blood urea nitrogen (BUN), uric acid, bilirubin, cholesterol, total protein, albumin/globulin ratio, alkaline phosphatase, lactic dehydrogenase (LDH), and serum glutamic oxalacetic transaminase (SGOT) were determined with a Multichannel Technicon AutoAnalyzer.

All animals were autopsied after they either died or were killed up to five months after operation for routine pathological study. Before the brain was removed a carotid artery was cannulated and perfused with isotonic saline followed by 10 percent formalin. Then the brain and segments of the spinal cord were further fixed in 10 percent formalin and stained with hematoxylin-eosin and luxol fast blue-cresyl violet for microscopy.

In a series of preliminary studies (in which the method described above was used except that the left-heart bypass was not performed and the lung was not perfused with IC-solution), one puppy recovered completely from the operation; this animal was put to death after six months. In another series of preliminary studies in which the lung was not perfused with IC-solution, all animals had severe respiratory distress and died within 48 hours. Some of the laboratory data on these dogs have been included in this report for comparison.

RESULTS

Four of 10 puppies in the final group died within 48 hours (nonsurvivors), and six survived for more than 48 hours (survivors). Of these survivors, one died of pneumonia 5 days postoperatively and the other five were killed at 14, 88, 135, 136, and 150 days, respectively.

Hemodynamic response. Resuscitation of the heart was achieved in all cases at between 20 and 24° C. rectal temperature without remarkable difficulty. The heart resumed regular sinus rhythm with normal rate and blood pressure. Transient atrioventricular dissociation was observed in two puppies. So far, no remarkable damage has been noted in the cardiovascular system.

Respiratory function. Spontaneous respiratory movement reappeared uniformly between 24 and 28° C. in the rewarming process. The respiration was assisted for at least 3 hours by a Bird Mark 8 respirator supplying 40 percent O_2 and air mixture. During this interval, arterial blood-gas studies revealed apparently intact gas exchange in 6 dogs; Po_2 over 150 mm. Hg (mean ± standard error of mean, 258.3 ± 5.1), Pco_2 under 45 mm. Hg (40.2 ± 2.4), and pH between 7.30 and 7.40 (7.34 ± 0.07). These dogs were able to sustain self-respiration after being disconnected from the respirator, although two of them showed moderate dyspnea for about 48 hours. One puppy died of severe bilateral pneumonia 5 days postoperatively and another showed thoracic empyema when killed at 14 days. The remaining survivors revealed no remarkable change in the autopsied lungs. The other four dogs manifested low Po_2 and high Pco_2 even with respiratory assistance. These dogs suffered from persistent dyspnea after being disconnected from the respirator, and died within 48 hours. Microscopic findings of the lungs from these dogs were consistent, exhibiting pulmonary con-

Table I. *Hepatorenal function in 2½ hour hypothermic circulatory arrest*

	Control	After hypothermia 1 hr.	After hypothermia 24 hr.	After hypothermia 3 wk.
	(n = 7)	(n = 10)	(n = 8)	(n = 5)
BUN (mg. per 100 ml.)	11.7 ± 2.3	14.2 ± 1.2	12.9 ± 3.0	17.2 ± 2.2
Uric acid (mg. per 100 ml.)	0.6 ± 0.1	1.9 ± 0.2*	0.8 ± 0.1	0.5 ± 0.0
Cholesterol (mg. per 100 ml.)	143 ± 12	119 ± 8	156 ± 12	157 ± 9
Total protein (mg. per 100 ml.)	5.3 ± 0.1	4.1 ± 0.2*	4.8 ± 0.4	5.5 ± 0.3
Bilirubin (mg. per 100 ml.)	0.13 ± 0.03	0.12 ± 0.02	0.17 ± 0.04	0.12 ± 0.02
Alkaline phosphatase (U./L.)	193 ± 33	316 ± 37**	292 ± 41	176 ± 21
LDH (U./L.)	203 ± 36	377 ± 48**	522 ± 156	254 ± 81
SGOT (U./L.)	58 ± 10	333 ± 44*	699 ± 296	61 ± 28

All results are the means ± S.E.M.

*p < 0.01 compared to "control" value. **p < 0.05 compared to "control" value. "p" refers to a probability of falsely rejecting the null hypothesis by Student's t test.

Table II. *Metabolic responses in 2½ hour hypothermic circulatory arrest*

	Control	After hypothermia 1 hr.	After hypothermia 24 hr.	After hypothermia 3 wk.
	(n = 15)	(n = 20)	(n = 10)	(n = 5)
Lactate (mg. per 100 ml.)	32.0 ± 5.6	114.3 ± 5.6*	33.1 ± 14.8	19.5 ± 1.7
Pyruvate (mg. per 100 ml.)	1.4 ± 0.2	3.5 ± 0.2*	1.6 ± 0.5	1.0 ± 0.1
	(n = 8)	(n = 9)	(n = 5)	(n = 5)
Insulin (μU/ml.)	32.4 ± 8.2	21.8 ± 5.8	19.6 ± 8.1	11.0 ± 4.7
Glucose (mg. per 100 ml.)	148.9 ± 11.3	324.6 ± 30.9*	127.0 ± 8.8	94.1 ± 2.6
	(n = 8)	(n = 10)	(n = 8)	(n = 5)
Potassium (mEq./L.)	5.3 ± 0.5	3.5 ± 0.2*	3.7 ± 0.1*	5.6 ± 0.3
Sodium (mEq./L.)	148.1 ± 0.3	153.0 ± 1.0*	149.8 ± 3.5	151.4 ± 1.2
Magnesium (mEq./L.)	2.3 ± 0.1	2.3 ± 0.1	2.1 ± 0.2	2.9 ± 0.6
Calcium (mEq./L.)	10.4 ± 0.3	9.3 ± 0.2**	9.1 ± 0.4**	10.1 ± 0.3
Chloride (mEq./L.)	112.2 ± 2.1	115.5 ± 0.9	111.4 ± 1.9	116.2 ± 1.6
Bicarbonate (mEq./L.)	23.6 ± 1.1	15.1 ± 1.3*	28.2 ± 1.1**	23.8 ± 2.0
Inorganic phosphorus (mEq./L.)	6.5 ± 0.9	8.6 ± 0.6**	5.8 ± 0.6	6.6 ± 0.1

All results are the mean ± S.E.M.

*p < 0.01 compared to "control" value. **p < 0.05 compared to "control" value. "p" refers to a probability of falsely rejecting the null hypothesis by Student's t test.

gestion, edema, and moderate to severe intra-alveolar hemorrhage; similar changes were seen uniformly in the animals of the preliminary series which died of respiratory failure.

Hepatorenal function. All puppies showed increased diuresis after the procedure. As summarized in Table I, laboratory studies of the blood indicated no significant change in BUN, cholesterol, and bilirubin levels. There were modest increases in uric acid, alkaline phosphatase, LDH, and SGOT, and there was a decrease in total serum protein at one hour after hypothermia. These values returned to normal in the later studies.

Pathologic studies of the liver in the nonsurvivors showed focal areas of early central necrosis in one and rather extensive cytoplasmic vacuolization in another. The kidneys of the nonsurvivors and the livers and kidneys of the survivors were not remarkable.

In vitro microrespirometry of the biopsied kidney and liver tissue (cell suspensions) revealed no detectable post-hypothermia changes from control in oxygen consumption in the presence of pyruvate or succinate.

Metabolic response. As shown in Table II, blood lactate and pyruvate increased significantly immediately after hypothermia, but returned to normal within 24 hours. A dog showing satisfactory recovery exhibited normal lactate and pyruvate levels in 6 hours

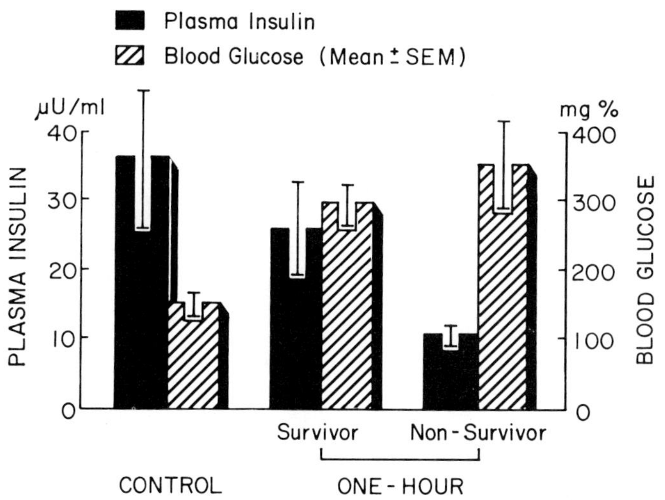

Fig. 2. The plasma insulin and blood glucose variations in the survivors and nonsurvivors.

after hypothermia, whereas these values remained higher for 24 hours in two nonsurvivors. Blood glucose showed a marked increase after the procedure. In contrast, blood insulin declined somewhat from the control level; the decrease was not statistically significant. The increase in glucose and decrease in insulin were more pronounced in the nonsurvivors than in the survivors (Fig. 2). These values returned to normal within 24 hours. There were significant decreases at one hour post-hypothermia in serum potassium, calcium, and bicarbonate, and significant increases in sodium and inorganic phosphorus. Magnesium and chloride did not change significantly. All abnormal values returned to normal gradually within 3 weeks. The long-term survivors gained weight normally.

Central nervous system. All puppies resumed intact pupillary reflexes shortly after resuscitation. Three puppies showed mild to moderate convulsions and fasciculations in the upper half of the body, but these symptoms usually disappeared within 12 hours. Four had loss of vision, in three instances due to an opacity within the eyes; however, their vision returned within 3 weeks. Another had loss of vision until killed after 3 months. All survivors evidenced various degrees of hind-leg weakness, from which they gradually recovered over a period of 3 to 15 days. Thereafter, these dogs resumed normal activity.

Histologic findings on the central nervous system of two long-term survivors (killed at 135 and 88 days) showed diffuse cerebral cortical damage with loss of neurons, increase in astrocytes (gliosis), and focal necrosis. The cerebellar cortex was also damaged with laminar necrosis, loss of Purkinje cells, gliosis, and atrophy of foliae. These dogs had no convulsions or muscular fasciculations postoperatively; loss of vision occurred in both animals. Sight was recovered in 2 weeks in one dog but not in the other. Milder lesions of a similar nature were seen in two dogs which were killed at 14 and 136 days, and minimal changes in another long-term survivor (killed at 150 days). One animal which died of pneumonia at 5 days showed marked neuronal damage in the caudate nucleus with increase of microglia and proliferation of newly formed capillaries. Another dog which died of respiratory failure on the second day showed edema and acute neuronal degeneration in both the cerebrum and the cerebellum. A long-term survivor from a preliminary series (killed at 196 days) had no lesion. Another dog of a preliminary series, which died of brain damage and respiratory failure on the second day, showed diffuse cerebral and cerebellar edema and degeneration of Purkinje cells.

DISCUSSION

The theoretical and practical advantages of the new hypothermia technique using surface cooling and limited cardiopulmonary bypass have been stressed by many investigators.[1, 9] (1) This method retains all the advantages of classic hypothermia, namely, dry operating field, completely relaxed heart, and less injury to the blood elements. (2) Initial surface cooling decreases oxygen demand of the peripheral tissue efficiently before the functional depression of vital organs occurs due to low temperature. (3) Limited cardiopulmonary bypass for the last phase of cooling shortens the critical period of cooling; during that time depressed cardiac function impairs peripheral perfusion and delays the cooling process. (4) Bypass rewarming obviates the necessity for cardiac massage. (5) Rapid rewarming of the circulating blood resumes the function of vital organs before oxygen demand of the peripheral tissue increases markedly. (6) Total body circulation can be assisted mechanically until the resuscitated heart regains complete performance.

In this study, we have further modified the method in several aspects.

Application of left-heart bypass. This modification simplifies the extracorporeal circuit by eliminating the oxygenator and reducing the priming volume, thus emphasizing the advantages of hypothermia. Distention of the right heart chambers was easily avoided by periodic gentle compression of the right ventricle.

Anesthesia. We use ether anesthesia with a lytic cocktail premedication, based upon our previous experiences in heart transplantation.[10] Ether anesthesia has been recommended by several investigators[14, 16] because of its vasodilating and minor cardiorespiratory depressing effects.

Initial flushing of the heart, lung, and brain with intracellular-type solution during circulatory arrest. We consider this procedure as the most important modification of our hypothermia technique. The advantages of such a perfusate for ischemic kidney protection have been reported by Collins[5] and Sacks[17] and their associates. Recently we have confirmed the efficacy of this solution for protection of the heart[10] and the lung[11] from ischemic damage. Loss of potassium and magnesium and gain of sodium and chloride are the well-recognized changes during cold ischemia of the mammalian cells.[21] The blood-brain barrier might be affected by hypothermic circulatory arrest in a similar way.[20] IC-solution would decrease cellular energy requirements utilized to maintain the active-transport mechanism of the membrane by reduction of sodium and elevation of potassium concentrations in the extracellular fluid. Other investigators stressed the importance of high magnesium concentration.[5, 7] Therefore, it seems logical to protect the vital organs—the brain, the heart, and the lung—during hypothermic circulatory arrest by temporal flushing with IC-solution. Total body perfusion with IC-solution, although theoretically desirable, requires too much perfusate, and results in uncontrollable hyperkalemia during the rewarming process.

Other protective measures. Low-molecular-weight dextran was used to prevent intravascular sludging or coagulation,[15] and methylprednisolone to protect against ischemic injury to the lung and other tissue. Pluronic F-68 was used to lessen the formation of fat emboli and hemolysis by stabilizing the lipoproteins in the plasma and red cell membranes.[6] The lungs were kept inflated during circulatory arrest based on the knowledge acquired in lung preservation studies.[11, 19] Although theoretically advantageous, it was difficult to separate the effect of each protective measure from that of others.

With these modifications, we designed this series of experiments to seek body responses and recovery after total circulatory arrest for 2½ hours, approximately twice the so-called "safe time limits" of conventional hypothermia. The results indicate that IC-solution protects the heart completely from ischemic injury. On the other hand, hypothermia lung,[13] characterized by alveolar collapse, alveolar hemorrhage, and interstitial edema, remained as the serious problem and caused the early death of four animals even after flushing with IC-solution. The liver and the kidney tolerated the procedure well. Metabolic derangements were severe but transient. They included severe lactic acidosis, indicating significant O_2 debt during circulatory arrest, significant decrease in serum potassium, calcium, and bicarbonate, and increase in sodium and inorganic phosphorus. Plasma insulin decreased even in the presence of hyperglycemia. This finding agrees with the reports of other investigators.[2-4] Damage of the central nervous system was relatively mild so far as physical signs and symptoms were concerned; our impression was that IC-solution protected the brain from ischemic insult. Many long-term survivors have behaved like normal puppies after they recovered from the initial complications. However, pathologic studies of the brain revealed various grades of permanent destruction caused by ischemia and possible thrombi or air embolism.[8]

In summary, 2½ hours of circulatory arrest is certainly beyond the "safe time limits" even with our modified method of hypothermia. However, IC-solution protects the function of vital organs so well that resuscitation is uniformly possible and recovery with long-term survival is acceptably high.

REFERENCES

1. Barratt-Boyes, B. G., Simpson, M., and Neutze, J. M.: Intracardiac surgery in neonates and infants using deep hypothermia with surface cooling and limited cardiopulmonary bypass, Circulation (Suppl. I) **43-44:** 25, 1971.
2. Baum, D., Dillard, D. H., and Porte, D., Jr.: Inhibition of insulin release in infants undergoing deep hypothermic cardiac surgery, N. Engl. J. Med. **279:** 1309, 1968.
3. Blackard, W. G., Nelson, N. C., and Labat, J. A.: Insulin secretion in hypothermic dogs, Am. J. Physiol. **212:** 1185, 1967.
4. Brown, T. C. K., Dunlop, M. E., Stevens, B. J., Clarke, C. P., and Shanahan, E. A.: Biochemical changes during surface cooling for deep hypothermia in open-heart surgery, J. Thorac. Cardiovasc. Surg. **65:** 402, 1973.
5. Collins, G. M., Hartley, L. C. J., and Clunie, G. J. A.: Kidney preservation for transplantation: Experimental analysis of optimal perfusate composition, Br. J. Surg. **59:** 187, 1972.
6. Danielson, G. K., Dubilier, L. D., and Bryant, L. R.: Use of Pluronic F-68 to diminish fat emboli and hemolysis during cardiopulmonary bypass, J. Thorac. Cardiovasc. Surg. **59:** 178, 1970.
7. Downes, G., Hoffman, R., Huang, J., and Belzer, F. O.: Mechanism of action of washout solutions for kidney preservation, Transplantation **16:** 46, 1973.
8. Edmunds, L. H., Jr., Folkman, J., Snodgrass, A. B., and Brown, R. R. B.: Prevention of brain damage during profound hypothermia and circulatory arrest, Ann. Surg. **157:** 637, 1963.
9. Hikasa, Y., Shirotani, H., Satomura, K., Muraoka, R., Abe, K., Tsushimi, K., Yokota, Y., Miki, S., Kawai, J., Mori, A., Okamoto, Y., Koie, H., Ban, T., Kanzaki, Y., Yokota, M., Mori, C., Kamiya, T., Tamura, T., Nishii, A., and Asawa, Y.: Open heart surgery in infants with the aid of hypothermic anesthesia, Arch. Jap. Chir. **36:** 495, 1967.
10. Kondo, Y., Grogan, J. B., Cockrell, J. V., Kuramochi, T., Smith, G. V., and Hardy, J. D.: Comparison of the efficacy of immunosuppressive regimens on orthotopic heart allografts, J. Thorac. Cardiovasc. Surg. **67:** 612, 1974.
11. Kondo, Y., Turner, M. D., Cockrell, J. V., and Hardy, J. D.: Ischemic tolerance of the lung: Immediate and total functional dependence studied by bilateral allotransplantation, To be published.
12. Kondo, Y., Turner, M. D., Kuwahara, O., and Hardy, J. D.: Prolonged suspended animation in puppies, Cryobiology (in press).
13. Lesage, M. A., Tsuchioka, H., Young, W. G., Jr., and Sealy, W. C.: Tolerance of dogs to deep hypothermia, Arch. Surg. **89:** 677, 1964.
14. Mohri, H., Dillard, D. H., and Merendino, K. A.: Hypothermia: Halothane anesthesia and the safe period of total circulatory arrest, SURGERY **72:** 345, 1972.
15. Mohri, H., Hessel, E. A., Nelson, R. J., Matano, I., Anderson, H. N., Dillard, D. H., and Merendino, K. A.: Use of Rheomacrodex and hyperventilation in prolonged circulatory arrest under deep hypothermia induced by surface cooling: Method for open heart surgery in infants, Am. J. Surg. **112:** 241, 1966.
16. Okamura, H., Nakamura, T., Sagara, T., Matsuoka, S., Sezaki, T., Yamashita, J., Kobayashi, H., Hosoi, Y., Kobayashi, N., Okamoto, T., and Okita, M.: Total correction of tetralogy of Fallot under simple profound hypothermia, Heart **1:** 806, 1969.
17. Sacks, S. A., Petritsch, P. H., and Kaufman,

J. J.: Canine kidney preservation using a new perfusate, Lancet **1:** 1024, 1973.
18. Turner, M. D., Neely, W. A., and Pitts, H. R.: Polarographic respirometer for the isolated perfused rat kidney, J. Appl. Physiol. **24:** 102, 1968.
19. Veith, F. J., Sinha, S. B. P., Graves, J. S., Boley, S. J., and Dougherty, J. C.: Ischemic tolerance of the lung: The effect of ventilation and inflation, J. Thorac. Cardiovasc. Surg. **61:** 804, 1971.
20. Wells, L. A.: The effects of low body temperatures on deposition of tracers in the mammalian brain, Cryobiology **9:** 367, 1972.
21. Willis, J. S.: The possible roles of cellular K for survival of cells at low temperature, Cryobiology **9:** 351, 1972.

Ischemic tolerance of the canine autotransplanted lung

Yoshio Kondo, M.D., M. Don Turner, Ph.D., John V. Cockrell, M.D., *and*
James D. Hardy, M.D., *Jackson, Miss.*

The ischemic tolerance of the lung has been studied by subsequent bilateral allotransplantation which provides a means of placing total functional dependence on the grafts from the time of operation. A total of 62 donor dogs were divided into a control group, four cold-ischemia groups, and six warm-ischemia groups. Survival record, respiratory patterns, blood-gas analyses, and pathologic studies in each group clearly reflected the grades of ischemic injury. Initial flushing of the excised lungs with Ringer's lactate permitted 2 hours, but not 5 hours, of cold ischemia (4° C.) prior to bilateral allotransplantation, which required at least one additional hour of ischemia. Initial flushing with cryoprecipitated homologous plasma did not significantly improve the results, whereas Sacks' solution protected the lung from 5 hours of cold ischemia prior to bilateral allotransplantation. One hour of warm ischemia (body temperature) in a heparinized cadaver was permissible prior to bilateral allotransplantation, but the results were not consistent after 2 hours of warm ischemia, and 3 hours or more of warm ischemia were not tolerated. Replacement of the blood in the pulmonary vasculature with Sacks' solution prolonged the permissible warm ischemia time in a cadaver to 3 hours, but not to 4 hours or more.

From the Department of Surgery, The University of Mississippi Medical Center.

In spite of exhaustive attempts by many investigators[1, 2, 4-6, 8-11, 14-16, 18-22] to protect the lung from ischemic injury, preservation of this organ still remains one of the most difficult problems to study. There are two main reasons for the slow progress in this field. First, the unique, delicate architecture of the lung does not always allow one to apply the same techniques profitable in the study of other organs. For example, no encouraging results have been reported[6, 8, 15] with continuous perfusion of the isolated lung; this method has been widely used as the standard procedure in kidney and liver storage. Second, the lack of a good experimental preparation, which provides a means of placing total functional dependence on the transplant, obscures the objective judgment of the stored lung function. Ischemic injury of the lung, if it is not severe, often results in early and reversible impairment of pulmonary function; this neither precludes the survival of animals having unilateral transplants nor demonstrates severe depression of the late function.[1, 2, 20, 22] However, such lungs would not be acceptable in clinical situations, since patients undergoing transplantation operations usually have advanced bilateral pulmonary insufficiency.

Work supported by United States Public Health Service Grant No. HL 11730.

Accepted for publication May 13, 1974.

Reprint requests: Yoshio Kondo, M.D., Department of Surgery, University of Mississippi Medical Center, 2500 N. State St., Jackson, Miss. 39216.

Technical accomplishment of one-stage bilateral lung allotransplantation in our laboratory[13] facilitates the study of the lung preservation problem since the one-stage procedure requires immediate and total respiratory function of the transplants. After an initial flush with different solutions, the lungs were subjected to various regimens of warm or cold ischemia (1 to 5 hours) without further perfusion before they were tested by bilateral transplantation.

METHODS

Sixty-two donor-recipient pairs of mongrel dogs, weighing 15 to 30 kilograms, were divided into a group of controls, four groups with cold ischemia, and six groups with warm ischemia.

Group I (control study, six transplants). In this group procurement of the lungs from a living donor, initial flushing with Ringer's lactate (4° C.), temporary refrigeration, and bilateral allotransplantation were carried out consecutively; thus no ischemia time was deliberately added to the unavoidable period of ischemia during anastomoses. This time amounted to approximately one hour of ischemia for transplantation as described below.

Group II (six transplants). The grafts were initially flushed with Ringer's lactate, stored for 2 hours in a refrigerator (cold ischemia), and then bilaterally allotransplanted, with an additional hour of ischemia during transplantation.

Group III (six transplants). In this group there was an initial flush with Ringer's lactate and then there were 5 hours of cold ischemia plus 1 hour of ischemia for transplantation.

Group IV (four transplants). This group had initial flush with homologous plasma (4° C.) and 5 hours of cold ischemia plus 1 hour of ischemia for transplantation. Homologous plasma was prepared from pooled dog plasma by cryoprecipitation according to the method of Belzer and associates.[3]

Group V (six transplants). This group had initial flush with Sacks' solution (4° C.) and 5 hours of cold ischemia plus 1 hour of ischemia for transplantation. Sacks' solution is an intracellular-type solution prepared as Sacks and associates[17] did in renal preservation studies. It has 126 mEq. per liter of potassium ion, 14 mEq. per liter of sodium ion, 120 mEq. per liter of phosphate ion, 16 mEq. per liter of chloride ion, 20 mEq. per liter of bicarbonate ion, 16 mEq. per liter of magnesium ion, 37.5 Gm. per liter of mannitol, and an osmolarity of 430 mOsm. per liter.

Group VI (six transplants). In this group the lung grafts were left for 1 hour in a heparinized cadaver (warm ischemia) and then procured and bilaterally allotransplanted as in the control study.

Group VII (six transplants). This group had 2 hours of warm ischemia plus 1 hour of ischemia for transplantation.

Group VIII (six transplants). This group had 3 hours of warm ischemia plus 1 hour of ischemia for transplantation.

Group IX (four transplants). This group had 4 hours of warm ischemia plus 1 hour of ischemia for transplantation.

Group X. (six transplants). In this group the lungs were flushed in situ with Sacks' solution and then underwent 3 hours of warm ischemia plus 1 hour of ischemia for transplantation.

Group XI (six transplants). This group had 4 to 5 hours of warm ischemia after Sacks' solution plus 1 hour of ischemia for transplantation.

Procurement and ischemia of the grafts. In Groups I to V, the donor dog was premedicated with 1 mg. of atropine and anesthetized with 20 mg. per kilogram of intravenous Pentothal sodium. Respiration was controlled by a Bird respirator delivering a 40 percent oxygen-air mixture. The animal was heparinized (3 mg. per kilogram) systemically. The right lung was excised through a lateral thoracotomy in the fifth intercostal space by dissecting the bronchus, the pulmonary artery, and the left atrial cuff containing the orifices of the right pulmonary veins. The excised lung, which was kept inflated by clamping the distal stump of bronchus, was immediately flushed through the pulmonary artery with 500 ml. of perfusate (6 to 10° C.) with a pressure head

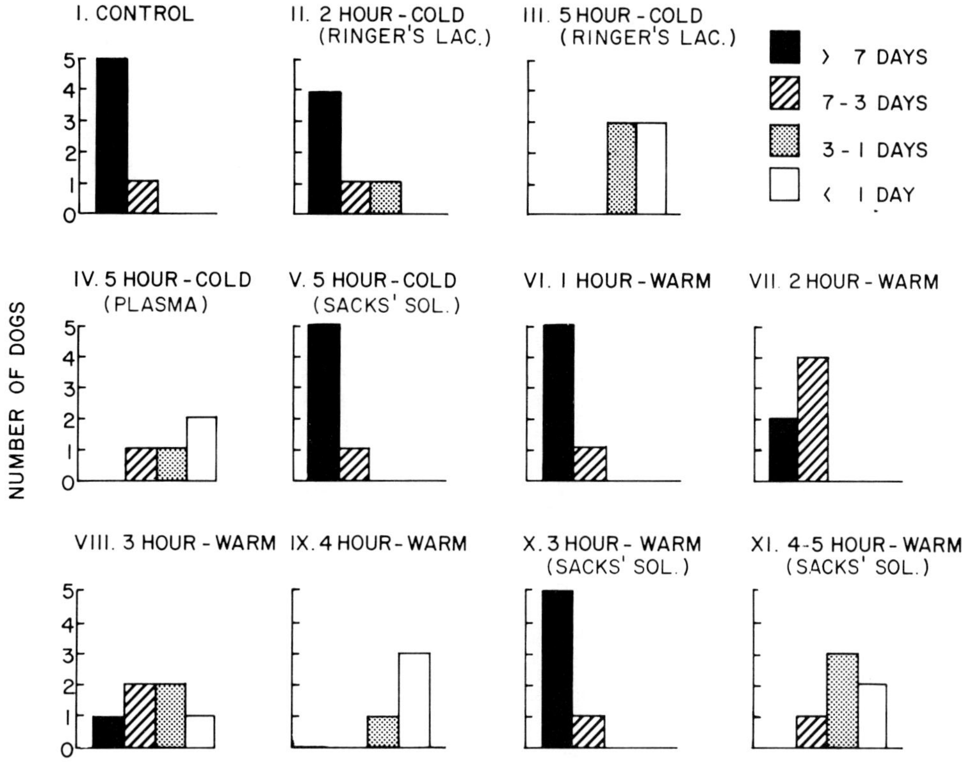

Fig. 1. Survival record in experimental groups showing distribution in four different categories.

of 40 cm. H_2O. In the meantime, the left lung together with the heart was divided from the pulmonary ligament, the mediastinum, the aorta, then venae cavae, and the trachea, and excised *en bloc* through the same thoracotomy. After quick removal of the pericardium and the major parts of the heart, the inflated lung was similarly flushed with perfusate. Then excess tissue was trimmed off, leaving adequate amounts of the bronchus, the pulmnoary artery, and the left atrial cuff for anastomosis. These inflated lungs were put in a metal container holding a small amount of perfusate and kept in a refrigerator (4° C.) until transplantation.

In the warm-ischemia series (Groups VI to XI) the donor dog, prepared as described above, was kept in the prone position and 30 ml. per kilogram of blood was shed acutely from a cannula inserted into the femoral artery. In Groups VI to IX the tracheal tube was then externally occluded during inspiration. Death due to suffocation occurred within 5 to 10 minutes as confirmed by monitoring the electrocardiogram (ECG). In Groups X and XI a catheter was inserted through the right jugular vein into the right ventricle, and 500 ml. of Sacks' solution (10° C.) were infused through it into the inflated lungs with a pressure head of 60 cm. H_2O. The ECG recording indicated unequivocal cardiac standstill within a minute. Temperature of the midesophagus declined to between 30 and 32° C. by the end of this perfusion and then increased slightly during the ischemic period. At the conclusion of the warm ischemia period the lungs were excised, flushed, and kept in a refrigerator as outlined above.

Bilateral allotransplantation of the lungs. Although the procedures of graft procurement and ischemia time differed among the groups, the technique of transplantation was the same for all groups. The recipient dog was anesthetized with atropine and intermittent doses of thiamylal sodium. Bilateral allotransplantation of the lung was carried out through the separate thoracotomies, the right side first, according to the method detailed elsewhere.[13] During anastomosis of the atrial cuff and the pulmonary artery, the graft was held in convenient position in the chest cavity, and no special effort was made to maintain a constant temperature. After circultaion had been restored to the graft, the bronchial anastomosis was performed with a continuous mattress suture. The ischemia time for the right lung was approximately 30 minutes in the refrigerator and 30 minutes in the thoracic cavity, and for the left lung was 90 to 120 minutes in the refrigerator plus 30 minutes in the chest. Since the lung transplants in this study were unavoidably burdened with at least an hour of ischemia for the right lung and with a somewhat longer period of ischemia for the left, we have estimated it as "1 hour of ischemia for transplantation."

Postoperative management and laboratory studies. The animal was kept in a cage that supplied an oxygen-enriched atmosphere overnight, and given 500 ml. of Ringer's lactate with 5 percent glucose solution intravenously. Penicillin-streptomycin and/or chloromycetin were administered daily for 2 weeks. All animals were treated with a combination of imunosuppressive drugs; 2.5 to 3.0 mg. per kilogram of azathioprine was given daily for the first week, 2 mg. per kilogram daily for the next 2 weeks, and 1 mg. per kilogram daily or less as the maintenance dosage. Methylprednisolone was administered at a level of 6 to 7 mg. per kilogram on the day of operation, and in the same dosage as azathioprine thereafter. Antilymphocyte serum was given intramuscularly (0.5 mg. per kilogram daily) starting 2 days before transplantation and continuing for 3 weeks with gradually decreasing regularity.

Postoperatively, the recipient dogs were observed closely for respiratory pattern and arterial blood samples obtained in a conscious state were analyzed for pH, Po_2, and Pco_2. Chest x-ray films, white cell counts with hemograms, and measurements of pulmonary artery pressure were performed as indicated. Systematic postmortem examination and routine histologic studies were performed on all dogs as soon as possible after death.

RESULTS

Since early death of the animal seemed to be the best indicator of ischemic injury in our experimental model, all animals were tentatively classified into four categories: (A) survival less than 24 hours, (B) between 1 and 3 days, (C) between 3 and 7 days, and (D) more than 7 days. Fig. 1 shows the number of dogs in the various groups which fell into each category. The survival records for Groups II, V, VI, and X were comparable to that of the control group, whereas Groups III, IV, IX, and XI had poor survival records.

All animals in Category A demonstrated various grades of dyspnea and cyanosis after the respirator had been disconnected. Some showed incipient lung edema, as indicated by a frothy, hemorrhagic bronchial exudate, slow stereotyped respiration, and decreased ventilation while still on the operating table. The mean pulmonary artery pressure in such animals rose to 30 to 40 mm. Hg. Autopsy of the lung revealed severe congestion, diffuse intraalveolar hemorrhage, patchy atelectasis, and various grades of edema. These changes were mostly attributable to ischemic injury of the lung, since such changes were not observed in the control animals (Group I) and very rarely in our large series of immediate bilateral lung allotransplants.[12]

Animals in Category B showed fewer symptoms immediately after transplantation; however, their general condition did not improve appreciably before respiratory insufficiency caused death in a relatively short time. Histologic study of these lungs showed acute pneumonia in many specimens, and edema, hemorrhage, and congestion in others. Again, ischemic insult seemed to be an important promoting factor in these changes, since they were observed mainly in the groups which had suffered a severe grade of ischemia.

The postoperative progress, survival records, and postmortem examination findings for most animals in Categories C and D resembled those of the control group. They

Table I. *Summary of data in experimental groups*

Group	No. of dogs	No. dying in < 3 days	No. showing early dyspnea	Median survival time (days)	Longest survival time (days)	Pathologic changes: Rejection	Pneumonia	Ischemic injury*	Others†
I	6	0	0	10	59	3	2	0	1
II	6	1	1	8	28	1	3	1	1
III	6	6	6	1	2	0	1	5	0
IV	4	3	3	1.5	5	0	1	3	0
V	6	0	0	9	37	4	2	0	0
VI	6	0	1	8	34	2	4	0	0
VII	6	0	3	5.5	35	0	5	0	1
VIII	6	3	3	3	51	1	2	3	0
IX	4	4	4	1	2	0	0	3	1
X	6	0	1	11	49	2	3	0	1
XI	6	5	5	2	4	0	3	3	0

*Intra-alveolar hemorrhage, congestion, and edema without significant indication of rejection or pneumonia.
†Atrial thromboembolism, atelectasis, severe anemia, and multiple granulomatous disease.

resumed daily activity as a successful bilateral lung transplant dog should, and the arterial blood gases and pulmonary artery pressure remained within normal limits. Many long-term survivors (up to 59 days) were obtained; most of these died from rejection and/or pneumonia. It was impossible to separate by any means the ill effects of ischemic injury from those of rejection or infection.

In Table I are listed the number of experiments, the number of dogs dying within 3 days (Categories A and B), the number of dogs exhibiting dyspnea shortly after transplantation, the median and the longest survival times, and the frequency of major pathologic findings in the transplants for each group. There is a significant correlation between the number of dogs dying within 3 days and the number of dogs showing dyspnea shortly after transplantation ($r = 0.87$, $p < 0.01$). Also, good correlation was obtained between the number of dogs dying within 3 days and the pathologic findings suggesting ischemic injury ($r = 0.87$, $p < 0.01$). Dogs dying within 3 days had an average arterial blood oxygen tension of 65.9 ± 3.7 mm. Hg (S.E.), whereas dogs surviving longer averaged 75.0 ± 2.1 mm. Hg ($N = 24$); this difference was not statistically significant. Arterial blood carbon dioxide tension did not show any significant changes in these dogs.

These data indicate that initial flushing of the lungs obtained from a living donor dog with Ringer's lactate permits 2 hours, but not 5 hours, of cold ischemia (4° C.) prior to bilateral allotransplantation, which requires at least one additional hour of ischemia. Initial flushing with cryoprecipitated homologous plasma did not significantly improve the results, whereas initial flushing with Sacks' solution protected the lung from 5 hours of cold ischemia prior to bilateral allotransplantation. Further extension of cold-ischemia time has not been studied. One hour of warm ischemia (body temperature) in a heparinized cadaver is permissible prior to bilateral allotransplantation, but the results are not consistent after 2 hours of warm ischemia. Three or more hours of warm ischemia cannot be tolerated. Replacement of the blood in the pulmonary vasculature with Sacks' solution prolongs the permissible warm ischemia time for the lung in a cadaver to 3 hours, but not to 4 hours or more.

DISCUSSION

Several unique features of this study deserve to be emphasized. Aside from species differences, all the knowledge obtained from this study should be applicable to clinical cadaver donors. For example, the results indicate that the lung can tolerate warm ischemia unexpectedly well compared to cold ischemia, especially when Sacks' solution is perfused in situ. This encouraging finding provides some leeway in the critical timing between death of the donor and procurement of the graft. The theoretical advantages of an intracellular-type solution for temporary perfusion of the ischemic organ has been discussed by several investigators.[7, 17] A perfusate approximating intracellular electrolyte composition apparently mitigates the changes in ion distribution on both sides of the cell membrane; it helps prevent both potassium and magnesium loss from—and sodium, chloride, and water uptake by—the cell. Mannitol probably exerts its effect by countering the Donnan and osmotic influence of the negatively charged nondiffusible intracellular protein molecules, thereby not only preventing movement of water into the cells but even slightly dehydrating the cells. The beneficial effects of keeping the lung inflated during the period of storage have also been stressed by several investigators.[4, 18, 20, 22]

In this series, the effects of various grades of ischemia on the lung were evaluated by bilateral allotransplantation. The results of such evaluation will provide the most important basic knowledge for predicting the behavior of human lung transplants since in patients the grafts must maintain the total pulmonary function immediately after insertion. Undoubtedly, this model re-establishes the most physiologic post-transplant condition for the graft, and unequivocal judgment of subsequent function can be made simply by following the respiratory pattern, survival record, and a few noninvasive studies such as blood-gas analyses.

Many investigators working on unilateral lung transplantation or its sham operation models have attempted to isolate the effects of ischemia on the lung in a number of ways. Although bronchospirometry[1, 2, 9, 14, 16, 21] was used to demonstrate the ultimate function of such lung transplants, the technique itself was inaccurate and cumbersome, and adequacy of early function was not known. Results of delayed contralateral pneumonectomy[1, 11, 18] or pulmonary artery ligation[9] in such animals were usually disappointing. Normothermic ischemia of unilateral in situ lung has been successfully evaluated by immediate contralateral pulmonary artery ligation by Veith and associates.[22] Their report is one of few attempts to study immediate performance by placing the total respiratory function on the lung subjected to ischemia. However, the method must be modified to determine the effects of cold ischemia. Also, their method creates very abnormal hemodynamics since the entire flow of the pulmonary circulation suddenly shifts to a single lung from the moment of contralateral artery ligation. Nevertheless, the results of their study correspond well with our results for warm ischemia in many respects.

Our study indicates that the lung can be stored at least 5 hours in a refrigerator or can be left in the cadaver for 3 hours, with subsequent bilateral allotransplantation. Although this is considered a most severe test, the duration of permissible ischemia is not comparable with today's kidney preservation, which now extends to several days. Further development in this area is very desirable.

REFERENCES

1. Ardekarni, R. G., Faber, L. P., and Beattie, E. J.: Pulmonary function after various periods of ischemia in the canine lung, J. Thorac. Cardiovasc. Surg. **59:** 607, 1970.
2. Arnar, O., Andersen, R. C., Hitchcock, C. R., and Haglin, J. J.: Reimplantation of the baboon lung after extended ischemia, Transplantation **5:** 929, 1967.
3. Belzer, F. O., Ashby, B. S., Huang, J. S., and Dunphy, J. E.: Etiology of rising perfusion pressure in isolated organ perfusion, Ann. Surg. **168:** 382, 1968.
4. Blumenstock, D. A., Hechtman, H. B., and Collins, J. A.: Preservation of the canine lung, J. Thorac. Cardiovasc. Surg. **44:** 771, 1962.
5. Brownlee, R. T., and Couves, C. M.: Factors concerned in the maintenance of viability in pulmonary transplants, Ann. Thorac. Surg. **5:** 112, 1968.
6. Castagna, J. T., Shors, E., and Benfield, J. R.: The role of perfusion in lung preservation, J. Thorac. Cardiovasc. Surg. **63:** 521, 1972.
7. Collins, G. M., Bravo-Shugarman, M., and Terasaki, P. I.: Kidney preservation for transplantation: Initial perfusion and 30 hours' ice storage, Lancet **2:** 1219, 1969.
8. Fonkalsrud, E. W., Stevens, G. H., Rangel, D. M., Joseph, W. L., Yakeishi, Y., and Tocornal, J. A.: Physiologic evaluation of allogeneic canine lung transplants from living

donors, J. Thorac. Cardiovasc. Surg. **57:** 607, 1969.

9. Garzon, A. A., Cheng, C., Pangan, J., and Karlson, K. E.: Hypothermic hyperbaric lung preservation for twenty-four hours with replantation, J. Thorac. Cardiovasc. Surg. **55:** 546, 1968.
10. Hardy, J. D., Eraslan, S., Dalton, M. L., Jr., Alican, F., and Turner, M. D.: Re-implantation and homotransplantation of the lung: Laboratory studies and clinical potential, Ann. Surg. **157:** 707, 1963.
11. Hino, K., Grogan, J. B., and Hardy, J. D.: Viability of stored lungs, Transplantation **6:** 25, 1968.
12. Kondo, Y., Cockrell, J. V., Kuwahara, O., and Hardy, J. D.: Histopathology of one-stage bilateral lung allografts, Ann. Surg. In press.
13. Kondo, Y., Isin, E., Cockrell, J. V., and Hardy, J. D.: One-stage bilateral allotransplantation of canine lungs: Further studies: Early rejection and prolonged survival with immunosuppression, J. Thorac. Cardiovasc. Surg. **64:** 897, 1972.
14. Largiader, F., Manax, W. G., Lyons, G. W., and Lillehei, R. C.: In vitro preservation of canine heart and lung, Arch. Surg. **91:** 801, 1965.
15. Otto, T. J., Trenkner, M., Stopczyk, A., Gawdzinski, M., and Chelstowska, B.: Perfusion and ventilation of isolated canine lungs, Thorax **23:** 645, 1968.
16. Rangel, D. M., Stevens, G. H., Yakeishi, Y., Sanchez, M., and Fonkalsrud, E. W.: Physiologic evaluation of canine lung allografts from cadaver donors, SURGERY **66:** 863, 1969.
17. Sacks, S. A., Petritsch, P. H., and Kaufman, J. J.: Canine kidney preservation using a new perfusate, Lancet **1:** 1024, 1973.
18. Stevens, G. H., Sanchez, M. M., Chapell, G., Bennett, L. R., Gyepes, M. T., and Fonkalsrud, E. W.: Prolonged lung-allograft preservation using inbred beagles, J. Surg. Res. **12:** 246, 1972.
19. Theodorides, Th., Webb, W. R., Nakae, S., and Sugg, W. L.: Prolonged survival of the anoxic lung with metabolic inhibitors in normothermic and hypothermic conditions, Ann. Thorac. Surg. **5:** 411, 1968.
20. Thomas, P. A., and Buchman, R. J.: Successful 20 hour preservation of ischemic canine lung by hypothermia combined with minimal ventilation, J. Thorac. Cardiovasc. Surg. **62:** 176, 1971.
21. Veith, F. J., Panossian, A., Bogartz, L., and Koerner, S.: Immediate and early functional adequacy of transplanted lungs, Surg. Gynecol. Obstet. **129:** 493, 1969.
22. Veith, F. J., Sinha, S. B. P., Graves, J. S., Boley, S. J., and Dougherty, J. C.: Ischemic tolerance of the lung: The effect of ventilation and inflation, J. Thorac. Cardiovasc. Surg. **61:** 804, 1971.

A model for cardiogenic shock by coronary artery microembolization in calves

Richard M. Satava, Jr., M.D., *and* **Dwight C. McGoon, M.D.,** *Rochester, Minn.*

A model for severe cardiogenic shock was produced by selective microembolization of the left coronary artery in calves. Criteria were established for shock so severe that death routinely followed within one half hour. A review of the literature and a critique of previous models are presented. Although requiring close monitoring and several precautions, this model permits assessment of various cardiac-assist devices with respect to their ability to support life.

From the Department of Surgery, Mayo Clinic and Mayo Foundation, Rochester, Minn.

In order to study the complexities of alterations in cardiac performance in cardiogenic shock from myocardial ischemia and to evaluate the efficacy of cardiac-assist devices in supplementing this impaired performance, a consistently reproducible model of cardiogenic shock, which closely resembles the clinical situation, is necessary. In 1952, Agress and associates[1, 3, 4] proposed a model in dogs using embolization of plastic microspheres to the coronary arteries. Subsequently, Monroe[27] and LaFarge[19] and their coworkers adapted this technique to calves; however, their experiments were designed to investigate the efficacy of a cardiac-assist device rather than to establish a model of lethal cardiogenic shock. The purpose of our study is to delineate the methods and criteria for establishment of a dependable model of lethal cardiogenic shock secondary to myocardial ischemia, by selective microembolization of the left coronary artery in the calf.

Accepted for publication May 23, 1974.

Reprint address: Dr. Richard M. Satava, c/o Section of Publications, Mayo Clinic, 200 First Street SW, Rochester, Minn. 55901.

MATERIALS AND METHODS

Divinyl benzene microspheres with a mean diameter of 10 μ (6 to 14 μ) were purchased commercially.* They were supplied in a 30 percent solution, which was diluted with normal saline to a 3 percent solution (30 mg. of microspheres per milliliter).

The plastic microspheres were contained within a closed system of syringes and stopcocks to avoid air embolism to the coronary artery. This was accomplished by having three syringes in a parallel circuit attached to right-angled stopcocks. The syringes contain microspheres, normal saline for flushing the microspheres from the catheter after each injection, and radiopaque dye for identifying the coronary arteries between injections of microspheres.

All of the hemodynamic parameters were recorded on light-sensitive paper by a visual recorder (Honeywell 12 channel Visicorder 1508). All pressure measurements were transmitted to the recorder by fluid-filled strain-gauge transducers (Statham P23D).

*Particle Information Service, 600 S. Springer Rd., Los Altos, Calif. 94022.

Cardiac output was determined by using the indocyanine green dye-dilution technique. The dye was injected into the pulmonary artery, with sampling from the carotid artery through a densitometer (Waters XT250).

Male Holstein-Friesian calves that were 5 to 6 weeks old and 120 to 160 pounds (approximately 60 kilograms) were selected. The calves were fasted overnight and were given 0.4 mg. of atropine intramuscularly at the time of the procedure. Anesthesia was induced with an open-drop ether technique, followed by endotracheal intubation and maintenance in a lightly anesthetized state by a combination of oxygen and halothane (Fluothane)* in concentrations that varied from 0.5 to 4.0 percent.[20, 21] Ventilation was controlled throughout the procedure by an automatic respirator. The calf was positioned on the table in the left lateral thoracotomy position with legs "spread eagle" to allow easy access to the femoral vessels. Both carotid arteries and the right femoral artery were exposed; the caliber of the carotid artery was too small to permit the easy manipulation of more than one cardiac catheter. A 14 gauge polyethylene catheter was inserted into the left jugular vein for intravenous fluid and drug administration, and the calf was systemically heparinized with 0.5 mg. per kilogram. An open-ended No. 8 cardiac catheter was inserted into the femoral artery and advanced to lie within the left ventricular cavity. A 12 gauge polyethylene catheter was inserted into the left carotid artery to monitor blood pressure during thoracotomy.

Two categories of calves were studied: an intact closed-chest group and an open thoracotomy group. In the intact calf, the procedure was identical to that for the thoracotomy group, except that cardiac catheterization techniques were utilized under fluoroscopy to position the recording catheter in the pulmonary artery via the right jugular vein. All hemodynamic parameters (except left atrial pressure, which was not recorded in the closed-chest group) and the microembolization protocol were identical for both groups.

For the open-chest model, a generous left thoracotomy was made in the sixth intercostal space. The pericardium was incised, and the pulmonary artery was cannulated by a transmural puncture technique, by use of a No. 12 needle through which a length of No. 120 polyethylene catheter was advanced. The left atrium was cannulated in an identical manner through the tip of the left auricular appendage.

Before proceeding to microembolization, each preparation was allowed to stabilize for 10 minutes. Baseline hemodynamic parameters were then recorded. These included the following pressures: left atrial, left ventricular, pulmonary arterial, and carotid arterial. In addition, cardiac output was determined by the dye-dilution technique, 10 mg. of dye being injected into the pulmonary artery and samples taken from the left carotid artery.

Cardiogenic shock secondary to microsphere injection was accomplished in the following manner. A standard No. 7 coronary catheter (Sones) with three holes (two side holes and an end hole) was advanced via the right carotid artery to lie within the left coronary ostium. A small injection of contrast material (Renovist-N-76) readily identified the bifurcating left coronary artery system, and variations in coronary anatomy were noted. The catheter was attached to the stopcock device and flushed with 5 ml. of saline. The microspheres were injected as 1 ml. boluses 3 to 5 minutes apart, followed immediately by 3 to 5 ml. of a saline flush. The microsphere solution was shaken before each injection because the microspheres have a tendency to settle. Before each injection, the position of the catheter was noted by fluoroscopy, and, if necessary, its position in the left coronary artery was confirmed by the use of an injection of contrast medium. Both the systolic arterial pressure and the left ventricular end-diastolic

*Generously supplied by the Ayerst Laboratories, New York, N. Y.

Table I. *Effect* of microembolization of the left coronary artery in calves*

Group	No. of calves	Cardiac output (ml./Kg./min.)		Peak systemic systolic blood pressure (mm. Hg)		Left ventricular end-diastolic pressure (mm. Hg)	
		Before	After	Before	After	Before	After
Closed chest†	10	246 (±73)	103 (±30)	138 (±11)	77 (±13)	4 (±4)	20 (±7)
Closed chest‡	5	161 (±58)	37 (±18)	171 (±13)	48 (±6)	8 (±2)	27 (±6)
Open thoracotomy	23	172 (±54)	65 (±34)	127 (±17)	55 (±8)	6 (±5)	26 (±6)

*Mean ± S.D.

†End point in relation to peak systemic systolic blood pressure: $\leq$ 80 mm. Hg.

‡End point in relation to peak systemic systolic blood pressure: $\leq$ 60 mm. Hg.

pressure were closely monitored; these two parameters determined the point at which microsphere embolization was terminated. Initially in our experiment, we adhered to the criterion of a peak systemic systolic blood pressure of less than 80 mm. Hg as representing profound cardiogenic shock. However, further experimentation in our calves demonstrated that a few of these animals could recover spontaneously from a blood pressure of 80 mm. Hg. Therefore, we have utilized a systolic blood pressure of 60 mm. Hg as more accurately representing "irreversible shock." The importance of the left ventricular end-diastolic pressure was that, once this pressure rose above 25 mm. Hg, further injection of microspheres caused a precipitous decrease in systolic blood pressure, associated with an exponential increase in left ventricular end-diastolic pressure, and ventricular fibrillation invariably occurred. Therefore, when the peak systemic systolic blood pressure was less than 80 mm. Hg or as the left ventricular end-diastolic pressure approached 20 mm. Hg, longer times or smaller amounts of microspheres were allowed between the injections of microspheres, until the systolic pressure of 60 mm. Hg or less was reached. Once this level was attained, hemodynamic parameters were measured.

RESULTS

Cardiogenic shock secondary to microembolization of the coronary artery was produced in 54 calves. Sixteen of the calves developed ventricular fibrillation before postembolization hemodynamics could be measured. Of the remaining 38 calves, 15 were in the closed-chest group and 23 in the thoracotomy group.

In 10 calves of the close-chest group, the criteria of Agress and associates[2-4] were applied, that is, the end point was a decrease in systolic blood pressure to approximately 80 mm. Hg—a point that those investigators found reduced the cardiac output to approximately one third. In our study, the mean peak systolic blood pressure decreased from 138 to 77 mm. Hg and the mean cardiac output decreased from 246 to 103 ml. per minute per kilogram (Table I). Of these 10 calves, five died within one half hour, two within 4 hours, one at 48 hours, and one at 72 hours. One calf survived 6 weeks, at which time it was killed. Thus, the mortality rate was 70 percent in 4 hours and 90 percent within 3 days.

To produce a more lethal preparation, profound cardiogenic shock was produced in five calves of the closed-chest group by using a peak systolic pressure of 60 mm. Hg or less as the end point. This resulted in a concomitant cardiac output reduction to less than one third of baseline cardiac output, and a mean survival time of 18 minutes. From the time at which blood pressure decreased to 60 mm. Hg or less, the systemic arterial blood pressure gradually decreased until ventricular fibrillation ensued. The mean peak systolic blood pressure decreased from 171 to 48 mm. Hg and the mean cardiac output decreased from 161 to 37 ml. per kilogram per minute. The mean left ventricular end-diastolic pressure increased from 8 to 27 mm. Hg after microembolization (Table I).

In the group of calves that had undergone thoracotomy, an intraventricular balloon was inserted prior to production of cardiogenic shock for temporary short-term cardiac assist. In this group, the mean systolic blood pressure decreased from 127 to 55 mm. Hg and the mean cardiac output decreased from 172 to 65 mg. per kilogram per minute. The mean left atrial pressure increased from 6 to 26 mm. Hg after embolization (Table I). Within 5 minutes of production of cardiogenic shock, cardiac assist with the intraventricular balloon was instituted, with an immediate improvement in all parameters. However, when cardiac assist was momentarily discontinued at regular intervals for the recording of systemic blood pressure, left atrial pressure, and cardiac output, these parameters returned simultaneously to the same level of cardiogenic shock as immediately after microembolization. Seventeen of the 23 calves died during the 5 minute intervals when cardiac assist was discontinued in order that hemodynamic parameters could be measured. In six calves, cardiac assist was terminated at 3 hours; all calves died in less than one half hour. Thus, none of the 23 calves survived longer than one half hour without cardiac assist.

The average volume of microspheres required to decrease the systolic blood pressure to 60 mm. Hg or less was 7.0 ml. in the closed-chest group and 8.7 ml. in the thoracotomy group. All but two of the calves required from 6 to 11 ml. of microspheres; one required 5 ml. of microspheres, and one required 14 ml.

Pathologic study of the hearts of the first group of calves (in which less severe shock was produced), which survived 48 hours, 72 hours, and 6 weeks, revealed punctate infarcts (0.5 to 2.0 mm.) circumferentially distributed equally from the subendocardial to the epicardial layers. Histologic sections in every heart confirmed the presence of microspheres in all layers of the heart. The microspheres were embedded between the myocardial fibers (Fig. 1, *A*) or within the terminal capillaries (Fig. 1, *B*); rarely, there was capillary blockage with a plug of microspheres (Fig. 1, *C*). In four calves, microspheres were demonstrated in the right ven-

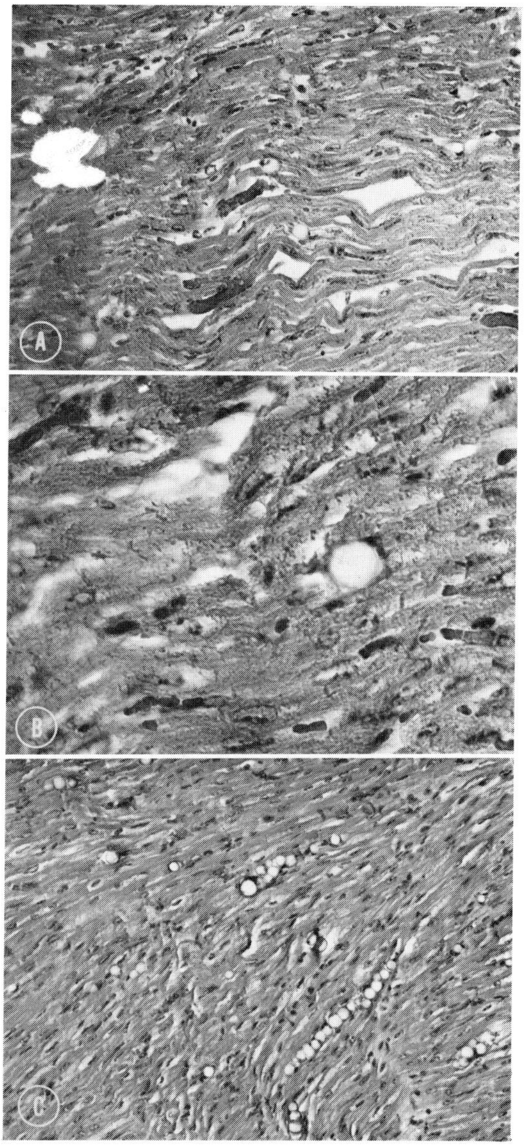

Fig. 1. *A,* Microspheres located between myocardial fibers. (Hematoxylin and eosin; ×270.) *B,* Microsphere located in terminal capillary; note capillary endothelial cell stretched around circumference of the microsphere. (Hematoxylin and eosin; ×670.) *C,* Plugs of microspheres in capillaries. (Hematoxylin and eosin; ×43.)

tricular wall; in three of these, a single coronary artery was present; all four calves had fibrillated before hemodynamics could be measured.

DISCUSSION

Nearly 100 years ago, Cohnheim and von Schulthess-Rechberg[8] reported the results of the effect of ligating the coronary artery in dogs. In the same year, Sée and associates[33] studied the effect of injecting lycopodium spores into the coronary circulation of dogs and noted identical results: death by ventricular fibrillation. Since these pioneering experiments, investigators have devised innumerable techniques to study the influence of coronary occlusion and its sequelae. In 1896, Porter[30] produced occlusion of the left coronary ostia with a glass rod and accurately concluded that the changes in the heart beat produced by rapid closure of the coronary artery was a consequence of sudden interruption of the nutrition of the heart. In 1926, Hamburger and associates[13] reviewed the existing literature on methods of producing coronary occlusion and detailed their technique of direct injection of the left anterior descending or the circumflex coronary artery with lycopodium spores, ". . . with the view that the injection of minute solid particles into the coronary circulation with subsequent lodgment of these small particles (emboli) in the capillaries and arterioles, would more nearly approximate the clinical findings of coronary embolus than the ligation of larger branches."

The next major advance in investigating cardiogenic shock was presented by Agress and associates[3] in 1951. In the closed-chest animal, a balloon catheter was used to occlude the aorta while plastic microspheres were injected into the root of the aorta, with resultant dispersion throughout the coronary circulation. From these studies, Agress proposed the following criteria for cardiogenic shock: mean arterial blood pressure reduced by approximately one third for a minimum of 30 minutes, electrocardiographic evidence of severe myocardial ischemia, and absence of arrhythmias. Numerous investigators have based their studies of the various aspects of cardiogenic shock on this model,[5-7, 9, 14, 24, 25, 28, 34, 36, 37] but mortality rates in these studies have ranged from 40 to 100 percent. Noting this variability, Lluch and associates[22] devised a preparation in the unanesthetized dog using selective injection of the circumflex branch of the left coronary artery of dogs with 0.2 ml. of mercury. Even though systemic blood pressure returned to normal soon after the initial episode of shock, this model results in a mortality rate of 100 percent in 5 to 48 hours. Other investigators[10, 23, 26] have not demonstrated this consistent mortality rate.

In 1972, LaFarge and associates[19] proposed the selective embolization of plastic microspheres into the left coronary artery of calves. Their criteria were elevation of left ventricular end-diastolic pressure from 30 to 45 mm. Hg and a concomitant decrease in systemic blood pressure to between 55 and 75 mm. Hg. Investigations with this model centered around evaluating a cardiac-assist device in chronic congestive failure rather than around validating the preparation of cardiogenic shock.

Results of techniques based on intraluminal stimulation of coronary thrombosis with wires,[12, 16] steel cylinders,[29] or electrocoagulation[32] have varied. External compression of the coronary artery with ameroid constrictors,[35] inflatable cuffs,[18] and classic ligation techniques[11, 15, 17, 31] also has been used.

Despite this array of techniques, the need remained for a model of cardiogenic shock so severe as to be lethal in the absence of some circulatory support system, and in an animal comparable in size to the adult human. The LaFarge model[19] of cardiogenic shock most closely approaches this need; however, by establishing a more severe end point for cardiogenic shock (a peak systolic block pressure of 60 mm. Hg or less), we have demonstrated that a uniformly lethal preparation can be achieved with a maximal survival time of one half hour. In the group of calves with reduction of systolic blood pressure to 80 mm. Hg, the model was less consistent and the survival time was longer (70 percent death at 4 hours, 90 percent death at 72 hours). As stressed by LaFarge, close monitoring of left ventricular end-diastolic pressure is important because, when this value increases to greater than 25 mm. Hg, further embolization causes very rapid and dramatic deterioration of cardiac performance. As the systolic blood pressure is reduced to 60 mm. Hg, there is a concomitant decrease in cardiac output to approximately one third of the baseline cardiac output.

The apparent importance of avoiding embolization to the right coronary artery is to be noted. Four of the calves had microembolization to the right coronary system; three of these had a single coronary ostium, and in one, the coronary artery was incorrectly identified. All of these calves died from ventricular fibrillation.

Our experience has led us to adopt the following guidelines and precautions for producing a reliable, reproducible model of lethal cardiogenic shock: reduction of peak systemic systolic blood pressure to approximately 60 mm. Hg or less; as the peak systemic systolic blood pressure decreases below 80 mm. Hg or as the left ventricular end-diastolic pressure increases toward 20 mm. Hg, the interval of time between microsphere injections should be prolonged from 5 to 15 minutes and smaller doses of microspheres should be used; microspheres should not be injected into the right coronary artery.

REFERENCES

1. Agress, C. M., and Estrin, H. M.: Mechanism and management of coronary shock, Biochem. Clin. **1:** 181, 1963.
2. Agress, C. M., Glassner, H. F., Binder, M. J., and Fields, J.: Hemodynamic measurements in experimental coronary shock, J. Appl. Physiol. **10:** 469, 1957.
3. Agress, C. M., Rosenburg, M. J., Binder, M. J., Schneiderman, A., and Clark, W. G.: Blood volume changes in protracted shock resulting from experimental myocardial infarction, Am. J. Physiol. **166:** 603, 1951.
4. Agress, C. M., Rosenburg, M. J., Jacobs, H. I., Binder, M. J., Schneiderman, A., and Clark, W. G.: Protracted shock in the closed-chest dog following coronary embolization with graded microspheres, Am. J. Physiol. **170:** 536, 1952.
5. Bing, R. J., Castellanos, A., Gradel, E., Lupton, C., and Siegel, A.: Experimental myocardial infarction: circulatory, biochemical and pathologic changes, Am. J. Med. Sci. **232:** 533, 1956.
6. Bloch, J. H., Pierce, C. H., Manax, W. G., and Lillehei, R. C.: Treatment of experimental cardiogenic shock, SURGERY **58:** 197, 1965.
7. Bloch, J. H., Pierce, C. H., Manax, W. G., Lyons, G. W., and Lillehei, R. C.: Experimental cardiogenic shock: effect of low molecular weight dextran, Arch. Surg. **91:** 77, 1965.
8. Cohnheim, J., and von Schulthess-Rechberg, A.: Ueber die Folgen der Kranzarterienverschliessung für das Herz, Virchows Arch. (Pathol. Anat.) **85:** 503, 1881.
9. Cronin, R. F. P., and Zsotér, T.: Hemodynamic effects of rapid digitalization in experimental cardiogenic shock, Am. Heart J. **69:** 233, 1965.
10. Edelman, N. H., Gorfinkel, H. J., Lluch, S., Gottschalk, A., Hirsch, L. J., and Fishman, A. P.: Experimental cardiogenic shock: Pulmonary performance after acute myocardial infarction, Am. J. Physiol. **219:** 1723, 1970.
11. Feola, M., Haiderer, O., and Kennedy, J. H.: Experimental graded "pump failure" of the left ventricle, J. Surg. Res. **11:** 325, 1971.
12. Gage, A. A., Olson, K. C., and Chardack, W. M.: Experimental coronary thrombosis in the dog: description of a method, Ann. Surg. **143:** 535, 1956.
13. Hamburger, W. W., Priest, W. S., and Bettman, R. B.: Experimental coronary embolism, Am. J. Med. Sci. n.s. **171:** 168, 1926.
14. Jacobey, J. A., Taylor, W. J., Smith, G. T., Gorlin, R., and Harken, D. E.: A new therapeutic approach to acute coronary occlusion. I. Production of standardized coronary occlusion with microspheres, Am. J. Cardiol. **9:** 60, 1962.
15. Kennedy, J. H., Bailas, N., Rasch, C., Hajdu, S., Beyer, A. J., and Sarap, N.: Left heart bypass in left ventricular failure due to experimental coronary artery ligation, J. Thorac. Cardiovasc. Surg. **51:** 797, 1966.
16. Kordenat, R. K., Kezdi, P., and Stanley, E. L.: A new catheter technique for producing experimental coronary thrombosis and selective coronary visualization, Am. Heart J. **83:** 360, 1972.
17. Kralios, A. C., Zwart, H. H. J., Wu, Y., Moulopoulos, S. S., and Kolff, W. J.: Coronary flow supplementation in experimental

myocardial infarction with shock, Chest **61:** 365, 1972.
18. Kumar, R., Hood, W. B., Jr., Joison, J., Norman, J. C., and Abelmann, W. H.: Experimental myocardial infarction. II. Acute depression and subsequent recovery of left ventricular function: Serial measurements in intact conscious dogs, J. Clin. Invest. **49:** 55, 1970.
19. LaFarge, C. G., Carr, J. E., Coleman, S., and Bernhard, W. F.: The maintenance of circulatory competence during chronic microsphere-induced myocardial failure, J. Thorac. Cardiovasc. Surg. **64:** 652, 1972.
20. Larson, R. E., and McGoon, D. C.: Experimental cardiac surgery in calves. II. Management for aortic valve surgery, J. Surg. Res. **3:** 104, 1963.
21. Larson, R. E., Moffitt, E. A., and McGoon, D. C.: Experimental cardiac surgery in calves. I. Anesthesia, J. Surg. Res. **3:** 101, 1963.
22. Lluch, S., Moguilevsky, H. C., Pietra, G., Shaffer, A. B., Hirsch, L. J., and Fishman, A. P.: A reproducible model of cardiogenic shock in the dog, Circulation **39:** 205, 1969.
23. Lumicao, B. G., Russell, R. O., Jr., and Rackley, C. E.: Left ventricular performance in dogs with selective coronary embolization with mercury, Am. J. Med. Sci. **261:** 27, 1971.
24. MacFarlane, J. K., Scott, H. J., and Cronin, R. F. P.: Effects of left heart bypass in experimental cardiogenic shock, J. Thorac. Cardiovasc. Surg. **57:** 214, 1969.
25. Marcus, E., Katz, L. N., Pick, R., and Stamler, J.: The production of myocardial infarction, chronic coronary insufficiency and chronic coronary heart disease in the dog, Acta Cardiol. **13:** 190, 1958.
26. Misra, S. N., Stanley, E. L., and Kezdi, P.: Hemodynamic determinants of cardiogenic shock, J. Surg. Oncol. **2:** 245, 1970.
27. Monroe, R. G., LaFarge, C. G., Gamble, W. J., Kumar, A. E., and Manasek, F. J.: Left ventricular performance and coronary flow after coronary embolization with plastic microspheres, J. Clin. Invest. **50:** 1656, 1971.
28. Munro, G., Balchum, O. J., Owens, J. C., and Swan, H.: Experimental chronic myocardial insufficiency produced by coronary artery embolization, Surg. Forum **6:** 204, 1956.
29. Nakhjavan, F. K., Shedrovilsky, H., and Goldberg, H.: Experimental myocardial infarction in dogs: Description of a closed chest technique, Circulation **38:** 777, 1968.
30. Porter, W. T.: Further researches on the closure of the coronary arteries, J. Exp. Med. **1:** 46, 1896.
31. Rushmer, R. F., Watson, N., Harding, D., and Baker, D.: Effects of acute coronary occlusion on performance of right and left ventricles in intact unanesthetized dogs, Am. Heart J. **66:** 522, 1963.
32. Salazar, A. E.: Experimental myocardial infarction: induction of coronary thrombosis in the intact closed-chest dog, Circ. Res. **9:** 1351, 1961.
33. Sée, G., Bochefontaine, and Roussy: Arrêt rapide des contractions rythmiques des ventricules cardiaques sous l'influence de l'occlusion des artères coronaires, C. R. Acad. Sci. (Paris) **92:** 86, 1881.
34. Stone, H. L., Bishop, V. S., and Guyton, A. C.: Cardiac function after embolization of coronaries with microspheres, Am. J. Physiol. **204:** 16, 1963.
35. Vineberg, A., Mahanti, B., and Litvak, J.: Experimental gradual coronary artery constriction by ameroid constrictors, SURGERY **47:** 765, 1960.
36. West, J. W., Kobayashi, T., and Anderson, F. S.: Effects of selective coronary embolization on coronary flow and coronary sinus venous blood oxygen saturation in dogs: With special reference to coronary reflexes, Circ. Res. **10:** 722, 1962.
37. Wong, M., Escobar, E. E., Martinez, G., and Rapaport, E.: Effect of coronary artery embolization on ventricular volumes, Circ. Res. **16:** 518, 1965.

Results of renal transplantation in 100 children

Claude V. DeShazo, M.D., Richard L. Simmons, M.D., Dorothy M. Bernstein, M.D., Maureen M. DeShazo, Justine Willmert, R.N., Carl M. Kjellstrand, M.D., *and* John S. Najarian, M.D., *Minneapolis, Minn.*
Minneapolis, Minn.

Over a 10 year span ending in 1973, 125 kidney transplants were carried out in 100 children. Omitting only four infants under one year of age, all of whom died, the 10 year patient survival rate with related donor transplants was 77 percent and with cadaver donor allografts 63 percent. The 10 year success rate of the first transplant was 74 percent for related kidneys and 44 percent for cadaver kidneys. When the results of multiple allografts were added to the initial transplant statistics, the ultimate success rate since 1968 has been 93 percent for related and 87 percent for cadaver organs. After successful transplantation, most children showed important gains in physical growth as well as in cognitive and perceptual mental ability.

From the Department of Surgery, University of Minnesota Health Sciences Center, Minneapolis, Minn.

CHILDREN are not readily accepted for treatment by most renal transplant programs, despite some encouraging results.[4, 5, 7] Concern over psychological management and the technical difficulties attendant to hemodialysis and the transplant operation are partly responsible for this attitude, as is the lack of certainty about the prospects for near-normal growth and long-term success. In 1973, a 10 year period ended in which 125 renal transplants were performed in 100 children from 6 weeks to 16 years of age. Six months after transplant the records of each of these 100 children were reviewed for cumulative data on the patient population, transplant success, and subsequent growth and psychological adjustment.

Accepted for publication May 23, 1974.

Reprint requests: Claude V. DeShazo, M.D., Department of Surgery, University of Washington School of Medicine, Seattle, Wash. 98195.

METHODS AND MATERIALS

The basic protocols for patient evaluation, management of hemodialysis, techniques of kidney placement, and postoperative management were established in 1968.[7] Recent advances in hemodialysis techniques allow infants as small as 4 kilograms to be supported for months, if necessary, until kidney transplants can be performed.[1, 2, 6] The data on 26 patients transplanted prior to 1968 and the four infants under one year of age were analyzed separately. We did not reject any child referred to us for evaluation of end-stage renal failure on the basis of disease diagnosis.

Transplantations in children over 20 kilograms in weight are routinely carried out by an adult-type approach. The kidney is placed in the right false pelvis with anastomosis of the renal artery to the recipient's hypogastric artery and the renal vein end-to-side into the

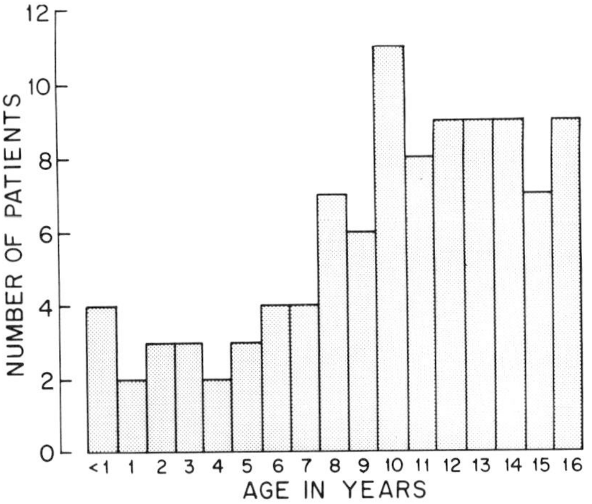

Fig. 1. Age at time of transplant in 100 pediatric patients.

recipient's iliac vein. The donor ureter is implanted with a submucosal tunnel technique. In children weighing less than 20 kilograms transplantation is carried out through a midline incision, usually in conjunction with bilateral nephrectomy, splenectomy, and appendectomy. In these instances disproportionate vessel size is managed by anastomosis of the renal vessels to the recipient's aorta and vena cava.[7]

The immunosuppressive regimen is begun 48 hours prior to transplant with prednisone, 1 mg. per kilogram per day, and decreased to 0.2 to 0.3 mg. per kilogram per day in about one month. For cadaver donor kidney transplants the diminishing dose of prednisone begins at 2 mg. per kilogram per day. Azathioprine is given, 5 mg. per kilogram per day, until the third postoperative day, when it is decreased stepwise to a maintenance dose of 3 to 2 mg. per kilogram per day. In addition three daily doses of methylprednisolone are given, 20 mg. per kilogram per day, starting on the day of transplant. Antilymphoblast globulin (ALG) is given in a dose of 20 mg. per kilogram per day (30 mg. for cadaver donor recipients). It is administered through a central vein or by A-V shunt over a 6 hour period. Fourteen infusions of ALG are given, beginning 2 days prior to operation when possible. To minimize possible thrombocytopenia no ALG is given on the day of transplantation.

Local irradiation of the graft is used only as a component of antirejection therapy. When a rejection episode is diagnosed the patient is given 150 rads per day every other day for three doses. The prednisone dosage is also increased to 2 mg. per kilogram per day, then decreased by 0.5 mg. per kilogram every three days to 0.5 mg. per kilogram per day. Methylprednisolone, 20 mg. per kilogram per day intravenously for 3 days, is also given. ALG therapy is not repeated during a rejection episode.

RESULTS

Age at time of transplant. In this study the pediatric age group was defined as infants and children up to and including the age of 16. Fig. 1 shows the age of all patients at the time of their first transplant. More than half (62 patients) were 10 years of age or older at that time. In the majority of instances a diagnosis of renal disease and failure to grow had been already made by age 4 or 5, and these children had been managed conservatively. For some children hemodialysis became mandatory, but often it was used as an adjunct to improve status and to stop proteinuria and the other effects of renal failure in preparation for transplant. As our experience grew, it became possible to perform transplants sooner after the diagnosis of end-stage renal disease had been made. We performed 32 transplants in the younger age group (2 to 10 years of age) during the last 2 years. Two children were 1 year old when transplantation was done; one died 2 months later of rejection and the other had hyperacute rejection of a first transplant and died of sepsis after receiving a second kidney.

Transplantation in infants. Four infants less than 1 year of age (12 months, 5 months, 4 months, 6 weeks) have had transplants. Their small size necessitated waiting for cadaver organs from other children. Although one of these children survived long enough to receive a second kidney, three died after rejecting their transplants and one died of respiratory arrest. The operations in these infants, who were as small as 4 kilo-

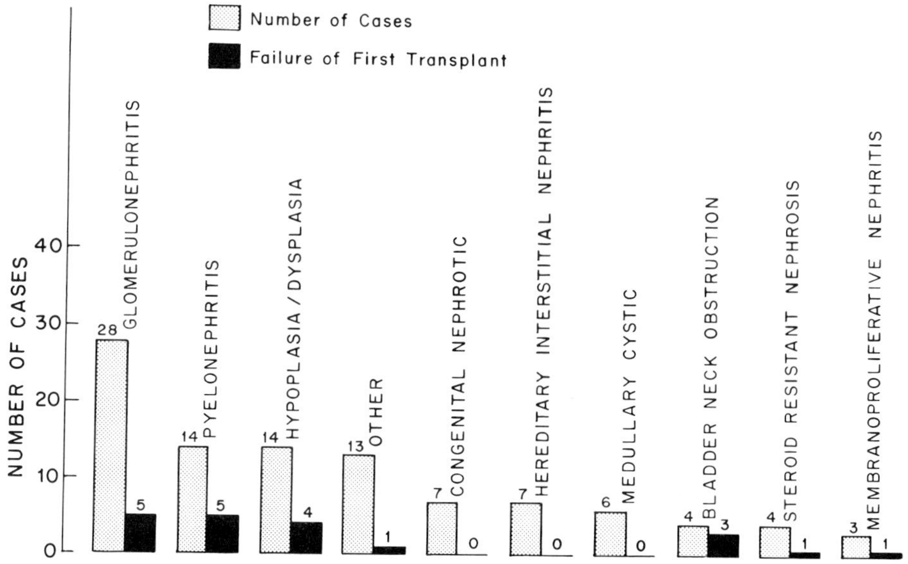

Fig. 2. Incidence of diseases leading to end-stage renal failure and transplant among 100 pediatric patients. Also shown is the number of first transplants in each group that ultimately failed.

grams in weight, were technical successes from the viewpoints of dialysis and surgical procedure. The lack of survivors, however, has led us to re-evaluate transplantation in this age group and exclude these four infants from most computations in this paper.

Renal diseases leading to transplantation. Fig. 2 shows the incidence of various diseases which led to transplantation in these 100 patients. The leading causes of renal failure were chronic glomerulonephritis (28 percent), pyelonephritis (14 percent), and hypoplasia/dysplasia (14 percent). The diversity of the next largest group of end-stage renal failure (13 cases) caused it to be grouped into an "Other" category. It included: cystinosis, anaphylactoid purpura, Wilms' tumor, lupus erythematosus, polycystic disease, and meningomyelocele with neurogenic bladder. Only one kidney was lost in this group, and that patient received a second transplant. Five first transplants failed in the 28 children with chronic glomerulonephritis.

The most complex dysfunction, and the one with the highest failure rate, was obstructive uropathy. This was a common diagnosis leading to transplant prior to 1968, and these patients have been dealt with individually.[7] A number of these cases now have been placed in the pyelonephritis category.

Since the 1971 report,[7] four additional ileal loop bladders have been done: two of these patients are dead, a third lost the first kidney but is well following a second transplant, and the fourth is well two years after transplant.

Source of donor organs. Living related donors were preferred when they were available for pediatric transplantation. It was often possible to use living related kidneys because of the parents' willingness to donate; 59 of the 100 first transplants were parental donors and 10 of the second transplants were from the parents (55 percent of 125 operations). Siblings are the most nearly ideal group of organ donors, comprising about 30 percent of donors in the total Minnesota experience. Among the pediatric transplant patients, however, siblings were of adult age and able to donate in only six instances (5 percent). Three aunts and one grandmother were the other related kidney donors. Before 1968 cadaver organs had to be used more often (12 of 32 transplants—37 percent) than after that date (19 of 93 cases—20 percent). Pediatric cadaver allografts must still be used when the small abdominal size of

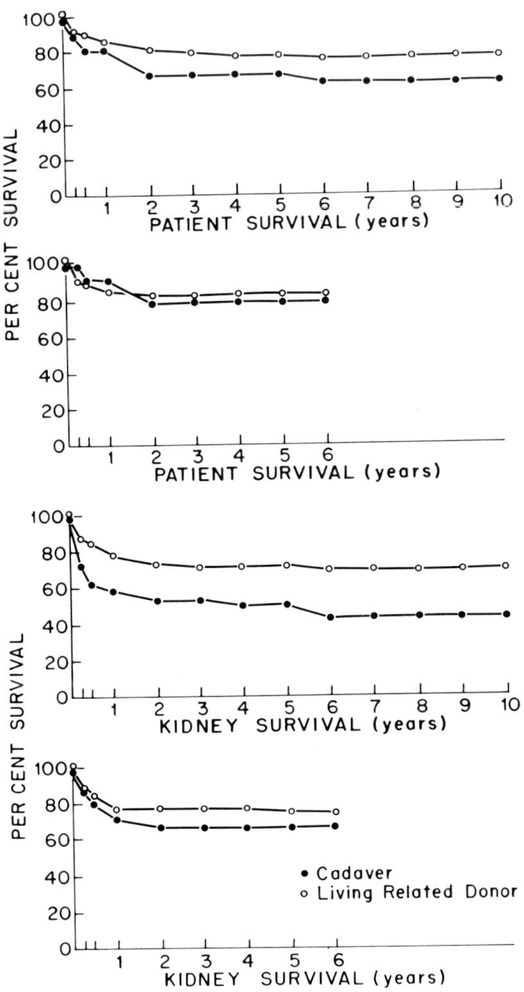

Fig. 3. Upper two panels show survival, or percent of patients living (minus four infants) following related and cadaver renal allografts in the over-all series since 1963 (96 cases) and since the present transplant team was formed in 1968 (70 cases). The lower two panels show kidney survival, or success of the initial allograft, for the entire series and since 1968.

a child causes too much disparity to accommodate a parent's kidney.

Transplant success and patient survival. Fig. 3 shows the results of renal transplantation in 100 consecutive children, omitting only the four infants described earlier. Our 10 year study allows an uncommon opportunity for long-term follow-up of transplant patients. This represents almost all pediatric patients with end-stage renal disease referred for transplantation. For clarity the results were divided into patient survival of the entire group and kidney survival of the first transplant. Further subdivision was made between the total 10 year experience of 120 transplants in 96 patients and that of the 6 years since the present transplant team was formed in 1968 (87 transplants, 70 pediatric patients). From the entire series of 100 patients, including the four infants, 24 patients (24 percent) are now dead. Thirteen of the 31 who received first transplants from cadaver donors (42 percent) are dead while only 11 of 69 who received living related donor first transplants (16 percent) are dead.

The over-all patient survival rate of recipients of living related donor kidneys was 86 percent at one year, 82 percent at 2 years, 80 percent at 3 years; thereafter it stabilized at 77 percent out to 10 years. Since 1968 the figures are 88 percent survival for one year and 86 percent survival from 2 to 6 years. When a cadaver kidney was used in the first transplant, the over-all figures are 82 percent at one year, 67 percent at 2 to 5 years, and 63 percent out to 10 years.

The success with the first transplant for the entire series is shown in the third panel of Fig. 3. For living related donor transplants, the success rate was 79 percent at one year, 76 percent at 2 years, 75 percent at 3 years, and 74 percent out to 10 years. Since 1968 the figures are 78 percent for the first through fourth years and 76 percent for years 5 and 6. Cadaver transplant success rate for the whole series was 59 percent at one year, 52 percent at 2 and 3 years, and 44 percent at 10 years. Since 1968 the cadaver results were 73 percent at one year and 66 percent from 2 to 6 years.

Growth following transplantation. There were only 37 patients (17 girls and 20 boys) on whom we had sufficient data for in-depth evaluation. Table I lists the reasons for not including the other 63 patients. Fig. 4 shows the growth in months since transplant when these 37 patients were divided into four groups. Each sex was divided into children ages 2 to 10 at time of transplant and those ages 11 years or older. Boys of 2 to 10 years

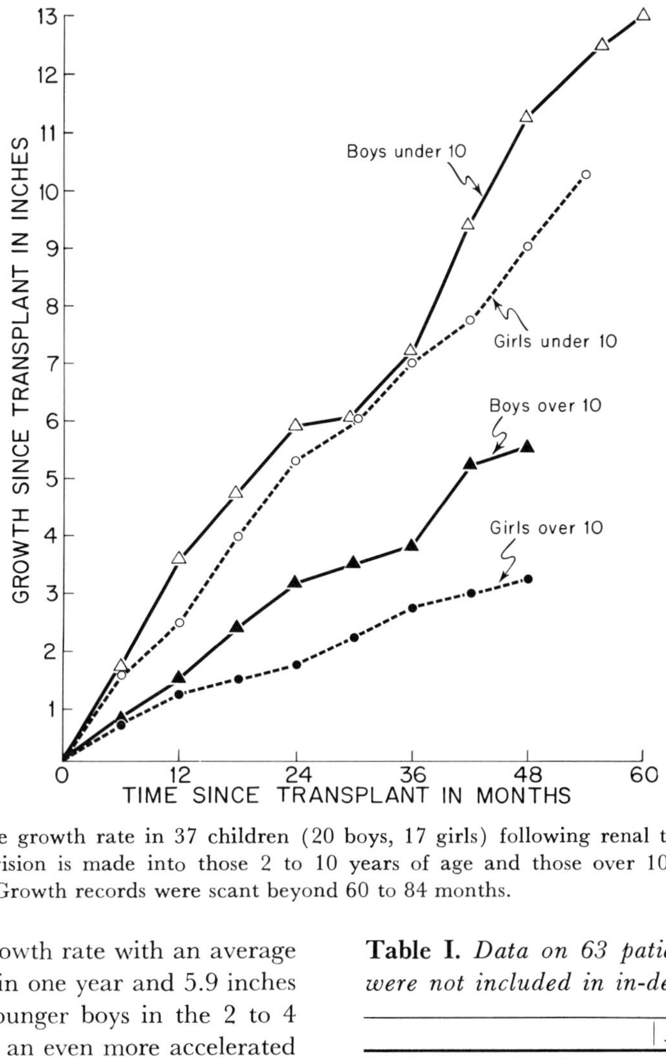

Fig. 4. Average growth rate in 37 children (20 boys, 17 girls) following renal transplantation. Further subdivision is made into those 2 to 10 years of age and those over 10 years at time of transplant. Growth records were scant beyond 60 to 84 months.

showed a steady growth rate with an average total of 3.6 inches in one year and 5.9 inches by 2 years. The younger boys in the 2 to 4 year range grew at an even more accelerated rate, averaging over 5 inches in the first year, but follow-up is relatively short (unreported data). The growth in girls 2 to 10 years varied more and averaged slightly less than the boys of comparable age, with 2.5 inches average at one year and 5.3 inches in 2 years.

Boys who received transplants after age 10 showed a considerably reduced growth rate: 1.5 inches at one year and 3.2 inches at 2 years. The girls over 10 years grew even more slowly: 1.25 inches at one year and 1.75 inches at 2 years. There was a surprisingly good correlation within these subgroups, but each had exceptions. Some children continued growing until their late teen years. One boy who had his transplant at age 12 grew 13 inches at a steady rate over a 7 year period. All but one of the patients who received more than one transplant grew significantly, almost as well as others of the same age group. This is interesting since retransplant almost always means a difficult clinical course. One patient had no growth

Table I. *Data on 63 patients of 100 who were not included in in-depth evaluation*

	Male	*Female*	*Total*
Dead at time of study	11	13	24
Followed less than one year	7	3	10
Growth one inch or less	2	1	3
Fully grown at transplant	3	2	5
Incomplete data			
Transplant to initial recording	7	3	10
Last two years	1	3	4
No height data	2	5	7
Total			63

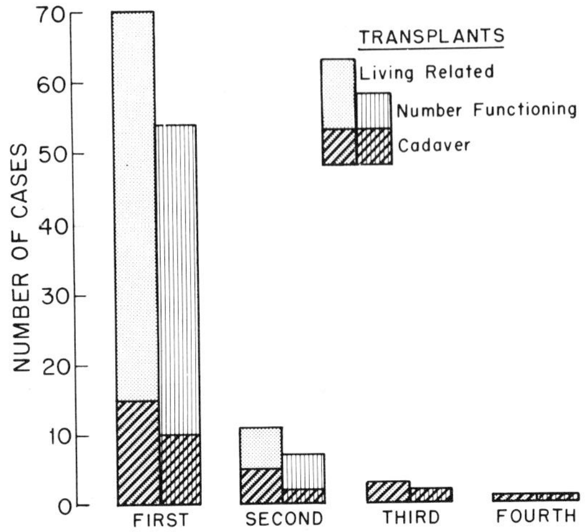

Fig. 5. Success of initial and subsequent allografts in 70 children receiving transplant since 1968. The 70 patients are divided into living related (55) and cadaver origin (15) of graft with the number still functioning in the adjacent bar. Eleven patients went on to second transplant with success in five of the six receiving related grafts and two of the five receiving cadaver allografts. Three children received third grafts. In the one failure here the patient went on to receive a fourth graft that is still functioning after 2 years.

for 24 months, until he received his third transplant.

Growth was evaluated in the first 58 patients in this series in a previous report.[7] At that time the over-all one-year growth rate for all patients averaged only 1.32 inches for girls and 1.59 inches for boys. Of the patients added in the present report on whom any data were available (not those with complete follow-up described above) the one-year growth was 2.0 inches for girls and 1.8 inches for boys. Average growth following living related donor transplant for both sexes and all ages was 2.25 inches at one year. Growth in this more heterogeneous group after cadaver transplant was 1.56 inches.

Multiple transplants. Fig. 5 shows the fate of first and subsequent transplants, both living and cadaver donors, since 1968. Prior to that time seven multiple transplants had been done. The first bar shows that of the 70 first transplants, 55 were living related and 44 successful (80 percent). Of 15 cadaver first transplants, 10 were successful (67 percent). Of the first transplant failures, 11 children received a second kidney, six from a relative (five parents, one brother) with 83 percent success. Two of five patients (40 percent) who received cadaver kidneys still have functioning grafts. Three patients received third transplants, two of which are functioning. The only patient who required a fourth graft has a functioning kidney (creatinine, 1.4 mg. per 100 ml.) after two years.

Emotional outcome. Success is measured in pediatric transplantation by the degree of physical and mental rehabilitation that takes place in addition to physical growth. Children who receive transplants at this center are examined psychiatrically prior to transplantation and 6 days, 6 months, and one year after transplantation.

Characteristically these children lacked any energy for play prior to transplantation. They had regressed into earlier behavior and thinking levels and choice of play activities. Interactional skills were poorly developed. Contact with peers was minimal or only with younger children. Although their behavior was usually passive and conforming, transplant patients often presented difficulties in adhering to dietary restrictions.

When the child first returned home after transplantation he still bore the image of a sick child. Parents and siblings handled him with uncertainty. The family assumed responsibility for administering the patient's medications, a role previously filled by a complex medical center. These children also were overly cared for upon returning to school. Younger children were open with their peers about their operations while adolescents hid their operative scars and did not volunteer information about the transplant. Steroid facies and short body stature were distressful to the older children and may have led to their identity crisis. By the end of the first posttransplant year, however, better adjustment had taken place both outside and in the home. Among the patients with successful transplants, only one has failed to return to school or some other appropriate role. Only six showed notable emotional reaction in readjusting.

The most prominent change seen in a successful transplant recipient was the child's energy level. The children became highly active, playing continuously, and this play became more age congruent. Peer interaction, which had been regressed or absent, also became age specific. Adolescents also noted an increase in well-being and showed less lag in emotional development. Mental growth, both cognitive and perceptual, took place at an accelerated rate during the first posttransplant year. This is notable since many young children with chronic renal disease also show a lag in mental development as well as stunted physical growth. Indications are that mental growth after transplant will be more rapid for the young child than for the adolescent.

DISCUSSION

The present study gives results of 125 consecutive renal transplants performed in 100 children since 1963 at the University of Minnesota Hospitals. Additional data are given to complement an earlier description of the management of 58 of these patients.[7] The minimum follow-up is 6 months and assessment after a 10 year span gives encouragement in dealing with a difficult patient population.

Virtually all children evaluated for end-stage renal disease were accepted for transplantation regardless of diagnosis. The only qualification made to the statistical analysis of these 100 patients was the omission of four infants under the age of 1 year who all died. The technical obstacles in these infants have been mastered[1, 2, 6, 7] but long-term success has not been achieved. Transplantation in this age group and even up to 2 years must continue to be approached cautiously. Above the age of 2 years the results continue to improve. This is especially true when living related organs are available for transplantation.

The 10 year patient survival rate with related donor allograft was 77 percent and the 10 year success with the first transplant alone was 74 percent. In children receiving a cadaver kidney in the first transplant the 10 year survival rate was 63 percent and 10 year graft success 44 percent. Since 1968 over-all cadaver graft success has improved significantly to 66 percent. After the second year patient and allograft loss were both relatively rare. This emphasizes that factors which really affect transplant success, such as over-all surgical management, technical expertise, and the host-graft adaptation, manifest themselves in the early months. They largely predict ultimate outcome. This observation is in agreement with conclusions from a series of pediatric transplants reported from Denver.[5] In that report no patients were lost after 19 months with follow-up as long as 7½ years.

If the first transplant fails, the situation is far from hopeless. Fifteen patients in our series received second grafts. If a kidney from a related donor is available, chances for success with the *second* transplant can be as high as 83 percent. This is in close agreement with Fine's 11 functioning allografts in 13 second transplants in children.[3] Another important computation can be made on the basis of repeated transplantation when the initial graft is lost. In the 55 patients who received related first transplants since 1968, repeated transplantation accounts for 15 of the children having functioning allografts at the present time. When this success is added to that of the initial transplant procedure, it gives an over-all success rate of 93 percent. A similar commitment to retransplantation in the 15 patients whose first allograft was of cadaver origin resulted in 13 having functioning kidneys (87 percent success).

Postoperative technical failures have been rare in recent years and the use of ALG has diminished the incidence of allograft loss due to rejection. When rejection does occur we feel the best policy is vigorous immunosuppressive therapy according to our protocol. A total of three courses can be given. Young children do not seem to be as susceptible as adults to opportunistic infections even if the courses of antirejection therapy are given in rapid succession. If these measures fail and transplant damage appears irreparable, our success with multiple transplants and a consideration for the patient's long-term well-being have led us to accept this initial setback and to advocate retransplantation as soon as possible.

Dealing with children in chronic renal failure can be a disappointment to all involved. Renal transplantation offers a real opportunity to reverse the psychological regression, decreased activity, stunted growth, and dietary controls imposed by the uremic state. For very small children (under 20 kilograms) dialysis and supportive management may be helpful in allowing growth to 7 to 10 kilograms prior to transplantation. For children over the age of 2, however, we feel that transplantation is advantageous as soon as a diagnosis of irreversible renal disease is made. True "catch-up" growth probably does not occur. The younger the child at the age of transplantation, however, the greater the amount of growth and greater the chance a child has to re-enter the normal growth curve. Height advances of 4 inches in the first year are common, as is total growth of one foot or more. The full height attained by the large number of small children transplanted in the past 3 years will be needed before a final evaluation can be made, but this interim assessment is most promising.

REFERENCES

1. Buselmeier, T. J., Santiago, E. A., Simmons, R. L., Najarian, J. S., and Kjellstrand, C. M.: Arteriovenous shunts for pediatric hemodialysis, Surgery **70:** 638, 1971.
2. Buselmeier, T. J., and Kjellstrand, C. M.: A-V shunts and fistulas for hemodialysis in neonates, infants, and small children, Proc. Eur. Dial. Trans. Soc. June 1973.
3. Fine, R. N., Korsch, B. M., Riddell, H., Stiles, Q. R., Edelbrock, H. H., Brennan, L. P., Heuser, E., and Grushkin, C. M.: Second renal transplants in children, Surgery **73:** 1, 1973.
4. Fine, R. N., Korsch, B. M., Brennan, L. P., Edelbrock, H. H., Stiles, Q. R., Riddell, H. I., Weitzman, J. J., Mickelson, J. C., Tucker, B. L., and Grushkin, C. M.: Renal transplantation in young children, Am. J. Surg. **125:** 559, 1973.
5. Lilly, J. R., Giles, G., Hurwitz, R., Schroter, G., Tagaki, H., Gray, S., Penn, I., Halgrimson, C. G., and Starzl, T. E.: Renal homotransplantation in pediatric patients, Pediatrics **47:** 548, 1971.
6. Mauer, S. M., Shideman, J. R., Buselmeier, T. J., and Kjellstrand, C. M.: Long-term hemodialysis in the neonatal period, Am. J. Dis. Child. **125:** 269, 1973.
7. Najarian, J. S., Simmons, R. L., Tallent, M. B., Kjellstrand, C. M., Buselmeier, T. J., Vernier, R. L., and Michael, A. F.: Renal transplantation in infants and children, Ann. Surg. **174:** 583, 1971.

In vitro demonstration of altered antigenicity of metastases from a primary methylcholanthrene-induced sarcoma

Robert P. Faraci, M.D., *Bethesda, Md.*

Antigenic differences between a primary methylcholanthrene-induced fibrosarcoma (MCA-P) and two of its pulmonary metastases (MCA-M-1 and MCA-M-2) were observed. C57B1 mice immunized against any one of the three tumors rejected single-cell challenge of the tumor to which they were immunized, whereas low-grade tumor incidence followed challenge with single-cell suspensions of either of the other tumors to which mice were not immune. Lymphocyte-mediated cytotoxicity tests amplified the differences seen in vivo. Lymphocytes from animals immune to the MCA-P sarcoma were cytotoxic to all three tumor cell lines whereas, at the other extreme, lymphocytes from animals immune to the MCA-M-2 metastasis were cytotoxic only to MCA-M-2 target cells. The results suggest that, although the metastases share some antigens with the primary tumor, they also contain "neoantigens" which make them immunologically distinct from the primary, and possibly allow the metastases to escape the immune surveillance of the host.

From the Surgery Branch, National Cancer Institute, Bethesda, Md.

SINCE THE demonstration of tumor-specific antigens (TSA's) by Prehn and Main[10] and the discovery of the phenomenon of concomitant immunity,[3, 6] investigators have been concerned over the apparent paradoxical development of metastases in animals in which immunity to the primary cancer could be demonstrated. Many plausible explanations for the above findings have been proposed.

One explanation is that circulating tumor cells are often coated with microthrombi which may prevent their being destroyed by host defenses and, therefore, allow them to become metastatic implants in distant organs.[2, 5, 11] Another area in which attention has focused is that of immunologic enhancement.[1, 9] Evidence has accumulated which suggests that serum blocking factors (antibody or antigen-antibody complexes) develop in tumor-bearing animals and man and take up antigenic sites on circulating tumor cells, thus preventing recognition of TSA's by cytotoxic antibody and immune lymphocytes. Another factor which may be responsible for metastatic spread of a tumor is the generalized immunosuppressed state characteristically seen in the tumor-bearing host.[4]

One explanation for the development of metastases in an animal which has immunity to the primary tumor has received little attention. This possibility is that the cells which ultimately form metastases have undergone antigenic modulation and, therefore, escape the host's immune surveillance because they are no longer immunologically identical to the primary tumor from which they arose.

The present experiments were designed to

Accepted for publication May 29, 1974.

Reprint requests: Dr. Faraci, 10N111, National Cancer Institute, Bethesda, Md. 20014.

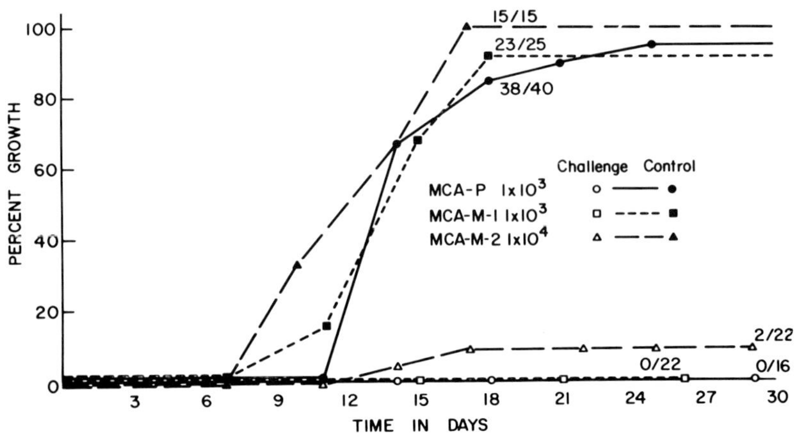

Fig. 1. Tumor incidence following challenge of MCA-P immune mice with single-cell suspensions of MCA-P, MCA-M-1, and MCA-M-2 sarcomas.

determine if antigenic differences existed between a primary MCA-induced fibrosarcoma in C57B1 mice and two of its pulmonary metastases. To accomplish this goal, in vivo tumor challenge studies and in vitro lymphocyte-mediated cytotoxicity tests were conducted.

MATERIALS AND METHODS

Mice used in all experiments were adult C57B1/6N mice obtained from the Laboratory Aids Division, National Institutes of Health. The tumor used was a primary methylcholanthrene-induced fibrosarcoma (MCA-P) and two of its pulmonary metastases (MCA-M-1 and MCA-M-2 occurring simultaneously in the same mouse). The primary tumor and the metastases were maintained by serial trocar passage of tumor bits in C57 mice. All tumors were found to be highly immunogenic, as shown by absence of tumor growth following amputation of established tumors and challenge with tumor suspensions.

Single-cell suspensions were prepared by mincing solid tumors and agitating in 0.25 percent trypsin for 20 minutes three times. Supernatants from the second and third trypsinizations were centrifuged at 1,500 r.p.m. for 10 minutes at 4° C., washed twice with Hank's solution, and counted in a hemocytometer. By this method, cell suspensions of 85 to 90 percent viability, judged by 0.05 percent trypan blue exclusion, were obtained.

Lymphocyte-mediated cytotoxicity tests were performed according to the method of Takasugi and Klein.[13] Tumor cells were plated out in Microtest tissue culture plates (Falcon Plastics, Oxnard, Calif.) (approximately 100 cells per well); 24 hours later, lymphocytes were added at a ratio of 100:1 to target cells. Following this, the plates were incubated at 37° for 48 hours in a 5 percent CO_2 atmosphere. After incubation, the lymphocytes were washed from the wells, and the plates were stained with crystal violet and counted. Thirty-six replicate wells were included for each group of immune lymphocytes. Cytotoxic indices for each well were calculated by the following method:

$$\text{Cytotoxic index} = \frac{\text{no. of viable control cells} - \text{no. of viable test cells}}{\text{no. of viable control cells}}$$

A cytotoxic index of greater than 0.20 was statistically significant ($P < 0.05$).

EXPERIMENTAL DESIGN

Adult C57 mice were divided into three groups, and each group was immunized, using the method described above, with either the primary methylcholanthrene-induced fibrosarcoma (MCA-P) or one of the metastases (M-1 or M-2). The three groups of immune animals which resulted were then

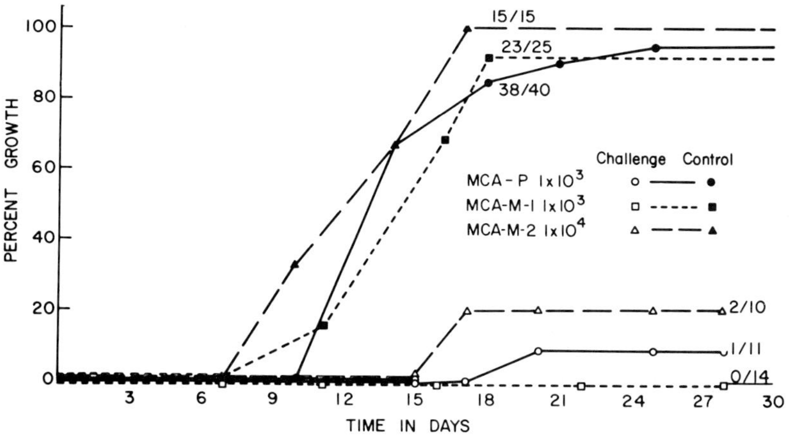

Fig. 2. Tumor incidence following challenge of MCA-M-1 immune mice with single-cell suspensions of MCA-P, MCA-M-1, and MCA-M-2 sarcomas.

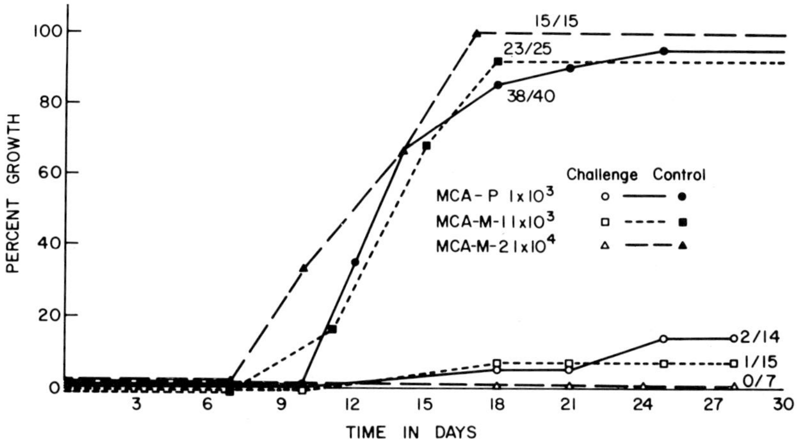

Fig. 3. Tumor incidence following challenge of MCA-M-2 immune mice with single-cell suspensions of MCA-P, MCA-M-1, and MCA-M-2 sarcomas.

subdivided. Animals immune to the primary tumor were divided into three groups, one to be challenged with primary tumor, one to be challenged with M-1 metastasis, and one to be challenged with M-2 metastasis. Animals immunized to M-1 and M-2 tumors were similarly cross-challenged. Control animals received similar challenges with each of the three tumors. The animals were observed twice weekly for tumor growth.

Just prior to tumor challenge, splenic lymphocytes were harvested from representative mice immune to each of the three tumors and from control mice for use in the cytotoxicity assay. Target cells from each of the tumor lines were tested against lymphocytes from animals immune to each of the three tumors.

RESULTS

Figs. 1, 2, and 3 show the results of the in vivo challenge. From these data it can be seen that mice immune to each of the three tumor lines were completely resistant to challenge of the respective tumors against which they were immunized. However, when a group of animals immune to one of the tumors was challenged with either of the other two sarcomas, tumor growth could be detected (except in MCA-P immune mice which were completely resistant to MCA-M-1 challenge). Immunity to the MCA-P

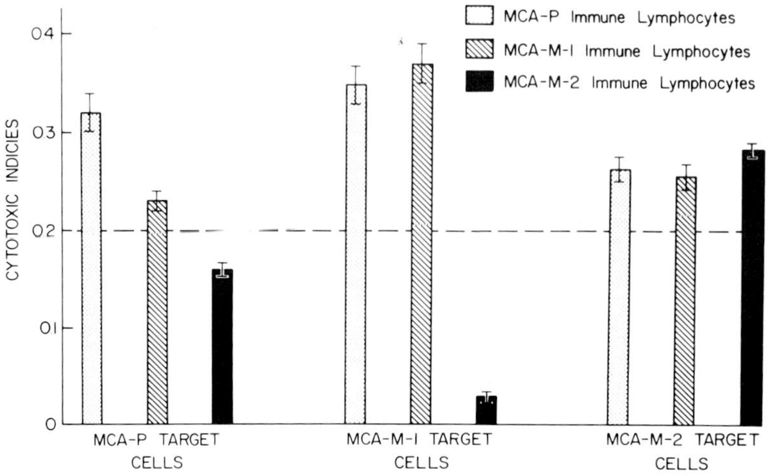

Fig. 4. Cytotoxic effect of immune lymphocytes against all three tumor target cell lines.

sarcoma produced the best protection against cross-challenge with either of the other two tumors, whereas the MCA-M-2 tumor was the least well recognized by animals immune to either the MCA-P or MCA-M-1 tumors.

Results of the lymphocyte-mediated cytotoxicity test correlate well with the in vivo challenge data. The greatest cytotoxicity seen against each tumor target cell line was manifested by lymphocytes from mice immune to that respective tumor (Fig. 4). However, lymphocytes from animals immune to the MCA-P sarcoma were cytotoxic to all three cell lines. Similarly, MCA-M-1 immune lymphocytes were cytotoxic to all three target cell lines although they were significantly less cytotoxic to MCA-P target cells than were MCA-P immune lymphocytes ($P < 0.05$). Finally, lymphocytes immune to the MCA-M-2 tumor were cytotoxic only to the MCA-M-2 target cell line.

DISCUSSION

The results indicate that significant differences in antigenicity exist between a primary sarcoma and its metastases. Previous reports have suggested that altered antigenicity of cells from the primary tumor is responsible for the very development of metastases.[7, 8] That is, metastatic cells antigenically different from those of the primary tumor could escape the surveillance of antibody and lymphocytes immune to primary tumor cells and implant in distant organs. In support of this theory, Sugarbaker and Cohen[12] have shown, in vivo, that significant antigenic differences exist between a primary sarcoma in C57 mice and its metastases. In addition, they showed that antigenic differences existed between the metastases themselves.

The present study corroborates the above findings and the in vitro cytotoxicity results add insight into the mechanism of metastasis formation. From the data, it is clear that lymphocytes from animals immune to the MCA-P sarcoma immunologically recognize all three tumor target cell lines, while lymphocytes immune to the MCA-M-2 sarcoma are able to immunologically recognize only MCA-M-2 target cells. MCA-M-1 immune lymphocytes recognize all three tumor target cell lines but less well than MCA-P immune lymphocytes. Therefore, a pattern of immunologic cross-recognition exists with the greatest cross-reactivity demonstrated by MCA-P immune lymphocytes and the poorest seen with MCA-M-2 immune lymphocytes.

These findings suggest that the metastatic tumors share antigens with the primary tumor from which they arose, and that these antigens allow the metastatic cells to be recognized by lymphocytes immune to the primary. However, the metastatic cells have also developed "neoantigens" which have made them immunologically distinguishable from the primary tumor. Furthermore, these neoantigens must play a significant role in the host's immune response to the metastases, since they confer complete immunity against the metastases, while they may produce no immunity against the primary tumor or another metastasis (as in the case of the MCA-M-2 metastasis). Further experiments are currently under way using humorally mediated cytotoxicity tests in order to further delineate the antigenic differences between the MCA-P sarcoma and its metastases.

REFERENCES

1. Bansal, S. C., and Sjogren, H. O.: Effects of BCG on various facets of the immune response against polyoma tumors in rats, Int. J. Cancer **11:** 162, 1973.
2. Brown, J. M.: A study of the mechanism by which anticoagulation with warfarin inhibits blood-borne metastases, Cancer Res. **33:** 1217, 1973.
3. Cohen, A. M., Millar, R. C., and Ketcham, A. S.: Host immunity to a growing transplanted methylcholanthrene-induced guinea pig sarcoma, Cancer Res. **32:** 2421, 1972.
4. Eilber, F. R., and Morton, D. L.: Impaired immunologic reactivity and recurrence following cancer surgery, Cancer **25:** 362, 1970.
5. Fisher, B., and Fisher, E. R.: Experimental studies of factors which influence hepatic metastases. VIII. Effect of anticoagulants, SURGERY **50:** 240, 1961.
6. Fisher, B., Saffer, E. A., and Fisher, E. R.: Comparison of concomitant and sinecomitant tumor immunity, Proc. Soc. Exp. Biol. Med. **135:** 68, 1970.
7. Fisher, B.: The present status of tumor immunology, Adv. Surg. **5:** 189, 1971.
8. Kim, U.: Metastasizing mammary carcinomas in rats: Induction and study of their immunogenicity, Science **167:** 72, 1970.
9. Moller, G.: Effect on tumor growth in syngeneic recipients of antibodies against tumor-specific antigens in methylcholanthrene-induced mouse sarcomas, Nature (London) **204:** 846, 1964.
10. Prehn, R. T., and Main, J. M.: Immunity to methylcholanthrene-induced sarcomas, J. Natl. Canc. Inst. **18:** 769, 1957.
11. Ryan, J. J., Ketcham, A. S., and Wexler, H.: Warfarin therapy as an adjunct to the surgical treatment of malignant tumors in mice, Cancer Res. **29:** 2191, 1969.
12. Sugarbaker, E. V., and Cohen, A. M.: Altered antigenicity in spontaneous pulmonary metastases from an antigenic murine sarcoma, SURGERY **72:** 155, 1972.
13. Takasugi, M., and Klein, E.: A microassay for cell-mediated immunity, Transplantation **9:** 219, 1970.

Role of endotoxin and bacteria in long-term survival of preserved small-bowel allografts

Luis H. Toledo-Pereyra, M.D., Leopoldo Raij, M.D., Richard L. Simmons, M.D., *and* **John S. Najarian, M.D.,** *Minneapolis, Minn.*

Endotoxins are potent immunological adjuvants that can accelerate the death of unprepared canine small bowels perfused for 12 hours and then allotransplanted. Hemorrhagic necrosis was a consistent finding in the endotoxin-positive dogs. This represented either an accelerated type of rejection or intravascular coagulation-like phenomenon. The preparation of the small bowel with antibiotics led to prolongation of survival.

From the Departments of Surgery and Pediatrics, University of Minnesota, Minneapolis, Minn.

TRANSPLANTATION of the small bowel entails the transplantation of an organ laden with bacteria and endotoxin into an immunosuppressed host. If the organ is damaged in the process of donor death or during organ preservation, the bacteria and/or endotoxin will be released into the recipient. Not only are these substances toxic in themselves, but they are also known to be immunological adjuvants[9, 10] which might, under some circumstances, augment the rejection response.

We have previously noted that orthotopic whole small intestinal allografts which had been preserved by hypothermic perfusion were sometimes destroyed by hemorrhagic necrosis soon after allotransplantation.[22] The presence of bacteria and endotoxin in the perfusate was suggested as a potential cause of this problem. The present study was designed to evaluate the role of intraluminal bacteria and endotoxins in the long-term survival of small intestinal allografts which had been preserved by hypothermic perfusion.

This work was supported by Grant No. AM13083 from the United States Public Health Service.

Accepted for publication May 29, 1974.

Reprint requests: Dr. Toledo-Pereyra, Box No. 223, University of Minnesota Hospitals, Minneapolis, Minn. 55455.

METHODS

Experimental model. Adult mongrel dogs weighing between 15 and 24 kilograms were anesthetized with sodium methohexital for induction and halothane for maintenance. The entire small bowel was resected and flushed through the superior mesenteric artery with cold (4° C.) Ringer's lactate solution containing procaine (1 Gm. per liter) and heparin (10,000 U. per liter) until the venous effluent was clear. Immediately thereafter the intestine was preserved by pulsatile perfusion in the modified Mox-100 system as previously described.[14, 22] This perfusion system was primed with 750 ml. of human plasmanate (Cutter Laboratories) containing $MgSO_4$ (1 Gm. per liter), regular insulin (80 U. per liter), PSP indicator (2 ml. per liter), methylprednisolone (500 mg. per liter), chlorpromazine (50 mg. per liter), ampicillin (1 Gm. per liter) and kanamycin (1 Gm. per liter). The proximal and distal ends of the small bowel were cannulated and the fluid excretion was collected and measured every four hours. Fresh perfusate was added if serious reduction in the level of perfusate was observed in the perfusion system.

During preservation (7° C.; pH 7.4; Po_2, 200 mm. Hg; pulse rate, 60 per minute; systolic pressure 60 mm. Hg) perfusate flow rate and organ weights were determined. Samples of perfusate were removed periodically (every 2 hours) in order to determine Po_2, Pco_2, pH, Na^+ concentration, K+ concentration, CO_2 concentration, osmolarity, and the levels of lysosomal enzymes (lactic dehydrogenase [LDH], serum glutamic oxalacetic transaminase [SGOT], and β-glucuronidase).

Operative technique and recipient treatment. Following 12 hours of preservation, the entire small intestine was transplanted orthotopically into an unrelated dog according to standard technique.[21] Biopsy specimens were taken from the preserved bowel after revascularization. Posttransplant intravenous fluids were given for 7 days depending on hydration, fluid loss, and general recovery. Azathioprine (2.5 mg. per kilogram per day) was given intravenously until death. Oral fluids were begun by the fifth postoperative day and solid food was started 2 days thereafter. All animals were examined daily until they died. Hematocrit, electrolytes, total proteins, and albumin were determined twice weekly in all dogs. *d*-Xylose absorption tests were performed at weekly intervals postoperatively in all groups according to standard techniques.[1, 19] Postmortem examinations were performed in all animals.

Groups of animals. Two groups of dogs with small bowel transplanted after 12 hour perfusion were compared. The differences between these groups were standard small bowel preparation before operation, treatment of the donor's bowel with antibiotics during perfusion, steroid therapy after transplant revascularization, and antibiotic treatment following grafting.

Group I (12 dogs). No dietary or antibiotic preparation of the donor dog was made before operation, no antibiotics were added during perfusion, and no antibiotics of steroids were given to the recipient after transplantation.

Group II (12 dogs). In this group, the donor and recipient dogs were prepared for four days prior to operation with oral fluids, Fleet enemas daily, and oral kanamycin (500 mg.) and neomycin (1 Gm.) three times a day. The small bowel was shortened by six inches in the proximal and distal ends prior to transplantation. Immediately after the clamps were released at the mesenteric anastomosis, methylprednisolone (1 Gm.) was given intravenously to the recipient. In addition, a catheter was placed in the abdominal cavity for drainage and irrigation with kanamycin (500 mg.) in 250 ml. of normal saline every 12 hours. Three days postoperatively the catheter was removed. Kanamycin (500 Gm. intramuscularly twice a day) and chloramphenicol (500 mg. intravenously every 8 hours) were given for one week after transplantation.

Bacteriological studies; bacterial cultures. Recipient dog blood cultures (5 ml. of blood in 50 ml. of culture media) were performed on enriched trypticase soy broth (TSB) and in thioglycolate broth. Samples were obtained before anesthesia, after anesthesia, before opening the mesenteric vascular clamps, from the mesenteric vein immediately after transplantation, five minutes after opening the clamps from a peripheral vein, and then every 4 hours for 3 days. The samples were incubated at 37° C. and observed for a period of one week. Cultures from the peritoneal cavity, inside the bowel, and the distal-free border of the proximal and distal ends (2 ml. of the sample in 10 ml. of culture media) were performed on TSB and were plated on the blood agar, eosin–methylene blue, and 1 percent sodium azide blood agar plates. TSB cultures were also taken from the perfusate: control, 5 minutes following the placement of the organ, and every 2 hours until the end of perfusion.

Endotoxin studies. Samples for determination of endotoxin were obtained from the perfusate, recipient dog blood, and the peri-

Table I. *Bacteriological and endotoxin findings during perfusion and after transplantation in nontreated and sterilized-bowel dogs*

	Bacteria		Endotoxin	
Sample	*Group I, no bowel prep.*	*Group II, bowel prep.*	*Group I, no bowel prep.*	*Group II, bowel prep.*
Perfusate:				
Control	0/12	0/12	0/12	0/12
5 min.	2/12	0/12	4/12	2/12
2 hr.	2/12	0/12	5/12	4/12
6 hr.	3/12	3/12	8/12	6/12
12 hr.	3/12	3/12	8/12	6/12
	p = 0		p = 0.40	
Recipient blood:				
Control	0/12	0/12	1/12	0/12
5 min. after transplant	4/12	0/12	6/12	2/12
4 hours after transplant	5/12	0/12	6/12	2/12
	p = 0.003		p = 0.06	
Peritoneal fluid:				
After transplant	10/12	2/12	9/12	5/12
	p < 0.001		p = 0.01	
Intestinal lumen:				
After transplant	8/12	6/12	11/12	8/12
	p = 0.4		p = 0.1	

Table II. *Bacteriological spectra* in two groups of dogs*

	Groups†	
Specific bacteria	*I‡*	*II‡*
Pseudomonas sp.	2	1
P. fluroescens	1	0
P. maltophilia	3	1
P. putida	2	1
E. coli	2	0
Anaerobic gram-negative rod	1	1
Clostridium	1	0
Staphylococcus, coagulase negative	1	1
Mean ± S.E.	1.6 ± 0.5	0.6 ± 0.2

*Bacterias were cultured from one or more of the following places: perfusion system, mesenteric or peripheral vein after transplantation, peritoneal fluid, or distal ends of the small bowel.

†In small dogs there was more than one type of bacteria present at the same time.

‡p < 0.01 when dogs of Groups I vs. II are compared.

toneal cavity at the same time that the specimens were taken for cultures.

Endotoxin was measured by the method described by Levin and associates.[11, 13] Their method is based on the observation that endotoxin induces the gelation of the lysate obtained from the amebocytes of the horseshoe crab, *Limulus polyphemus*. The possibility that the Limulus test could be positive in the presence of substances other than endotoxin has not been absolutely excluded, but the experience available so far seems to indicate that this test is specific for endotoxin. Fever *per se*,[12] gram-positive bacteria, derivative products of gram-positive bacteria,[18] or vasoactive amines[20] have not been found to give a positive reaction.

A plasma standard was made by suspending endotoxin lipopolysaccharide (*E. coli* endotoxin, Bacto lipopolysaccharide, *E. coli* 055:B5) (Difco Laboratories), in a pool of normal plasma from normal donors, in a concentration of 1 mg. per milliliter. The standard, the normal plasma without endotoxin, and the dog's plasma were each extracted with chloroform for 4 hours. After centrifugation at 1,100 × G for 10 minutes, 0.2 ml. of the middle layer was withdrawn. From this sample, 0.1 ml. was directly mixed with the Limulus lysate and 0.1 ml. was serially diluted tenfold with sterile saline; 0.1 ml. of the diluted plasma was then mixed with 0.1 ml. of the Limulus lysate. All the samples were incubated in a water bath at 37° C. for a minimum of 4 hours and a

Table III. *Survival after preservation and allotransplantation of unprepared small bowel (Group I)*

Survival (days)	Cause of death	Endotoxemia in recipient 5 min. after transplant
0.5	Hemorrhagic necrosis	+
0.8	Hemorrhagic necrosis	+
1.5	Hemorrhagic necrosis	+
2.0	Early vascular thrombosis	+
2.0	Hemorrhagic necrosis	–
3.0	Early vascular thrombosis	+
4.0	Generalized sepsis	+
6.0	Generalized sepsis	–
8.0	Peritonitis	–
11.0	Intussusception	–
12.0	Late vascular thrombosis	–
15.0	Bowel perforation	–
5.5 ± 1.4*		Total 6/12

*Mean ± S.E.

Table IV. *Dog survival after preservation and allotransplantation of prepared small bowel (Group II)*

Survival* (days)	Cause of death	Endotoxemia in recipient 5 min. after transplant†
2	Hemorrhagic necrosis	+
4	Early vascular thrombosis	+
6	Generalized sepsis	–
16	Late vascular thrombosis	–
18	Intussusception	–
20	Late vascular thrombosis	–
28	Bowel perforation	–
35	Intussusception	–
42	Bowel atrophy	–
44	Rejection	–
45	Cachexia	–
50	Rejection	–
25.8 ± 4.9		Total 2/12

*$p < 0.001$ when survival of dogs in Groups I vs. II compared.

†$p = 0.06$ when endotoxemia of dogs in Groups I vs. II compared.

maximum of 24 hours. An obvious increase in viscosity or gelation, as read by two independent observers, was interpreted as a positive test. The test proved to be reproducible with a sensitivity for the lipopolysaccharide used as standard of 10^{-1} ng. of endotoxin per milliliter of plasma or a dilution of 10^{-6} of the original plasma standard. The results are expressed as nanograms of endotoxin per milliliter of plasma, which are calculated from the maximal dilution of the dog's plasma that is able to effect gelation. The dilutions were then multiplied by the minimal concentration of endotoxin that could be detected by these methods (10^{-1} ng. per milliliter) in order to give the final concentration. The same methods were used for calculating the concentration of endotoxin in the perfusate. Concentration of endotoxin in plasma and perfusate between 1.0 and 1×10^{-1} ng. per milliliter were considered as positive.

Technical failure. Eight dogs which died due to perfusion or technical errors were excluded from this study. The errors included hemorrhage from the vascular anastomosis (three), anesthetic overdosage (two), small bowel leakage at the anastomosis (two), and air emboli in the perfusion system (one). The analysis includes all dogs (12 per group) in whom transplantation was technically successful.

RESULTS

Table I summarizes the results of endotoxin determinations and cultures of perfusates and recipient blood of animals receiving bowel transplants after 12 hours of preservation.

Group I. Unprepared bowel.

Perfusate studies. Prior to perfusion the perfusate was sterile and contained no bacteria or endotoxin. Soon after the perfusion began, bacteria and endotoxin appeared on the perfusate. There were 3/12 perfusate samples contaminated with bacteria and 8/12 samples contained endotoxin by the end of the 12 hour perfusion.

Recipient blood studies. Prior to transplantation there was no bacteria detected in the blood samples and only one recipient dog had detectable endotoxemia. Within 5

Table V. *Results of postoperative follow-up of treated dogs until death occurred (mean values*

Postop. time	Weight loss (% from initial)	Hb (Gm./100 ml.)	Total proteins (Gm./100 ml.)	Albumin (Gm./100 ml.)
1 day	6.5 ± 2.3	10.5 ± 1.7	4.7 ± 1.2	3.0 ± 0.9
1 wk.	13.3 ± 3.7	10.8 ± 1.2	3.9 ± 0.9	2.9 ± 0.3
2 wk.	15.6 ± 6.1	10.0 ± 1.1	4.0 ± 1.0	2.8 ± 0.9
3 wk.	17.2 ± 7.4	11.2 ± 1.0	4.2 ± 0.9	2.7 ± 1.0
4 wk.	24.6 ± 11.2	10.8 ± 0.9	4.6 ± 0.8	3.1 ± 1.1
5 wk.	30.5 ± 9.7	10.9 ± 0.7	5.1 ± 0.8	3.2 ± 0.9
6 wk.	39.3 ± 10.2	11.0 ± 1.1	4.4 ± 1.0	2.8 ± 1.0

*Serum concentration at indicated time interval after oral *d*-xylose administration.

minutes after transplantation 4/12 recipients experienced bacteremia and 6/12 endotoxemia. The same results were obtained 4 hours later. Table II documents the type of bacteria found in blood or perfusate in the various dogs. The most common organism was one of the species of Pseudomonas. Several types were found in the same animal on samples taken from different places.

Survival after transplantation. Dogs which had transplants with unprepared small intestine perfused for 12 hours survived only an average of 5.5 days. Causes of death in this group are shown in Table III. Endotoxemia had been found in six dogs immediately after transplantation with unprepared bowel; five of these dogs died with either hemorrhagic necrosis of the bowel in the first three days or earlier vascular thrombosis. One dog died of generalized sepsis on the fourth day. Of the seven dogs in this group that died prior to the fourth day after transplantation, six had endotoxemia immediately after transplantation. The dogs without endotoxemia immediately after transplantation survived for significantly longer periods of time.

Group II. Prepared bowel.

Perfusate studies. There were no positive perfusate samples prior to small bowel perfusion. Two hours later 3/12 samples were contaminated with bacteria and 6/12 samples contained endotoxin (Table I). Species of Pseudomonas were the most frequent gram-negative microorganisms found (Table II).

Recipient blood studies. Recipient dogs of prepared bowel had no bacteremia and only 2/12 developed endotoxemia. The peritoneal fluid was positive in 2/12 for bacteria and 5/12 for endotoxin. The intestinal lumen had 6/12 positive bacteria cultures and endotoxin was obtained in 8/12 samples (Table I).

Survival after transplantation. Dogs that had transplants with prepared small intestine survived for an average of 26 days. The causes of death and survival times are noted in Table IV. Only two dogs in this group had demonstrated endotoxemia immediately after transplantation and both of these dogs died of hemorrhagic necrosis or early vascular thrombosis in the first 4 days following transplantation. Of the 10 dogs in this group without endotoxemia, all but one survived for at least 16 days and 4/10 survived for more than 40 days.

Comparison of Groups I and II. There was a slightly earlier appearance of bacteria and endotoxin in the perfusate samples of the unprepared bowel (Group I). The recipient dogs of prepared bowel (Group II) transplants had no bacteremia and only rare endotoxemia whereas, of the dogs that received unprepared bowel, almost half experienced endotoxemia and bacteremia. Similarly contaminated peritoneal fluid was found in the recipients of unprepared bowel far more often than the prepared bowel. Prolonged survival was observed in the dogs with prepared bowels (Table IV). Dogs that received unprepared bowel had an average of less than one week of survival (Table III).

Functional characteristics of long-term survivors. Table V demonstrates that pro-

± S.E.)

d-Xylose*					
30 min.	60 min.	120 min.	180 min.	240 min.	300 min.
—	—	—	—	—	—
1.2 ± 0.3	2.0 ± 1.1	2.4 ± 1.0	2.2 ± 1.1	1.7 ± 0.5	0.6 ± 0.7
2.1 ± 1.2	2.3 ± 0.9	2.9 ± 1.4	2.1 ± 1.3	1.5 ± 0.8	0.9 ± 0.4
1.8 ± 0.7	2.1 ± 0.6	3.7 ± 1.1	2.8 ± 0.9	1.1 ± 0.3	0.4 ± 0.1
1.6 ± 0.4	2.9 ± 0.9	4.2 ± 0.9	2.7 ± 1.2	1.4 ± 0.6	0.3 ± 0.1
1.9 ± 0.6	3.1 ± 1.0	5.9 ± 1.3	2.9 ± 0.8	1.7 ± 0.4	0
1.5 ± 0.6	2.8 ± 0.9	3.7 – 0.9	2.7 ± 0.6	2.0 ± 0.8	0

gressive weight loss, persistent moderate anemia, hypoproteinemia, and hypoalbuminemia were present in all long-term surviving dogs. *d*-Xylose absorption from the transplanted intestine was maximal five weeks after grafting, but in all cases the *d*-xylose absorption was inferior to that seen preoperatively.

DISCUSSION

The endotoxins of gram-negative bacteria are complex lipopolysaccharides cleared from the circulatory system by cells of the reticuloendothelial system (RES) of the liver, spleen, and other reticuloendothelial organs. It is also known that these lipopolysaccharides (LPS) can interact with complement in vitro in the absence of added antibody, resulting in loss of hemolytic activity.[6] Furthermore, LPS from gram-negative bacteria have certain immunological characteristics that distinguish them from other antigens. These unique features of LPS concern its immunogenicity as well as its tolerogenicity.[2, 5, 6] In addition, it has recently been found that LPS acts as mitogen capable of stimulating DNA systhesis in subpopulations of lymphocytes from various species.[15, 16]

The endotoxins have a general and particular immunological adjuvant effect.[11, 13] They can stimulate the RES and antibody production but the degree of stimulation will depend on the amount of endotoxin used.

When the endotoxin is not inactivated or removed from the body, other physiopathological effects could be seen: pyrogenesis, tolerance, Schwartzman-like phenomenon, and lethal endotoxin shock.[8] Furthermore, animals made resistant to the pyrogenic effects of gram-negative endotoxin by repeated daily intravenous administration showed evidence of stimulated general immunological function.[4] These animals showed increased resistance to pyrogenic organisms and increased RES phagocytic activity. These animals are also more resistant to viral infections.[4]

Generally, the clinical effect of gram-negative bacteremia with endotoxin release is to impair the immune system. First, by producing a granulocytopenia followed by lymphocytopenia, and later on, the phagocytic activity of the RES is reduced. Another property is the ability to produce local and generalized Schwartzman phenomenon.[7] These reactions could readily be visualized during the early phases following graft implantation. Changes in the vascular endothelium of the grafted organ rendered it hypersusceptible to the effects of endotoxins. This would make an acceptable model to the deposit of leukocytes, platelets, thrombin, and fibrinoid, remaniscence of the reaction seen in the bilateral cortical necrosis of the generalized Schwartzman reaction. It was common to observe that practically no long-term survivors were obtained in the nonprepared small-bowel dogs. Most of the dogs that were endotoxemia positive died with hemorrhagic necrosis. A similar phenomenon was noted in the endotoxin-positive dogs of the treated group.

Whether the hemorrhagic necrosis of the small bowel in the endotoxemic dogs was related to intravascular coagulation or a form of rejection is difficult to differentiate at the present time. The endotoxins are excellent antigens that stimulate the formation of agglutinating and precipitating antibody to high titer. If the antibody, however, fails to neutralize the toxicity to more than a minor extent, the endotoxin thus resembles an active azoantigen whose activity is not neutralized by antibody, though they combine.[3] This mechanism could be involved in the production of hemorrhagic bowel. However, gram-negative bacteria are also potent stimulators of the mechanisms participating in intravascular coagulation. Further studies of small bowel contaminated during perfusion with endotoxin will allow a better clarification of this phenomenon. A known dose of endotoxin could be added to the perfusate (LD_{25}) and then the transplant could be followed up. In addition, unprepared bowel could be perfused for 24 hours, the perfusate tested for bacteria and endotoxin, and later on given intravenously to a dog to observe the immunological and general response of the dog. Ultimately, another problem remains whether the small bowel could be properly prepared in the perfusion machine, since the preparation of cadaver donors will be difficult in clinical practice.

REFERENCES

1. Benson, J. A., Jr., Culver, P. A., Ragland, S., Drummey, C. D., and Bougas, E.: The d-xylose absorption test in malabsorption syndromes, N. Engl. J. Med. **256:** 335, 1957.
2. Britton, S., and Möller, G.: Regulation of antibody synthesis against *Escherichia coli* endotoxin. I. Suppressive effect of endogenously produced and passively tranferred antibodies, J. Immunol. **100:** 1326, 1968.
3. Burrows, W., editor: Textbook of microbiology, ed. 9, Philadelphia, 1968, W. B. Saunders Company, p. 269.
4. Condie, R. M., Staab, E. V., and Good, R. A.: Studies on the biologic relationship of endotoxin and other toxic proteins. I. Comparison of the properties of snake venom and endotoxin, J. Exp. Med. **115:** 563, 1962.
5. Galanos, C., Rietschel, E. T., Lüderitz, O., and Westphal, O.: Interaction of lipopolysaccharides and lipid A with complement, Eur. J. Biochem. **31:** 230, 1972.
6. Gewurz, H., Snyderman, R., Mergenhasen, S. E., and Shin, H. S.: Effects of endotoxic lipopolysaccharides on the complement system, *in* Kadis, S., Weinbaum, G., and Ajl, S. J., editors: Microbial toxins, New York, 1971, Academic Press, Inc., vol. 4, pp. 127-149.
7. Horn, R. G.: Evidence for participation of granulocytes in the pathogenesis of the generalized Schwartzman reaction: A review, *in* Kass, E. H., and Wolff, S. M., editors: Bacterial lipopolysaccharides, Chicago, 1973, Chicago Press, pp. 126-135.
8. Jawetz, E., Melnick, J. L., and Adelberg, E. A., editors: Review of medical microbiology, ed. 9, Los Altos, Calif., 1970, Lange Medical Publishers, pp. 193-194.
9. Johnson, A. G.: The adjuvant action of bacterial endotoxins on the primary antibody response, *in* Landy, M., and Braun, W., editors: Bacterial endotoxins, New Brunswick, N. J., 1964, Rutgers University Press, p. 252.
10. Johnson, A. G., Gaines, S., and Landy, M.: Studies on the O-antigen of *Salmonella typhosa*. V. Enhancement of antibody response to protein antigens by the purified lipopolysaccharide, J. Exp. Med. **103:** 225, 1956.
11. Levin, J., and Bang, F. B.: Clottable protein in Limulus: Its localization and kinetics of its coagulation by endotoxin, Thromb. Diath. Haemorrh. **19:** 186, 1970.
12. Levin, J., Poore, T. E., Zauber, N. P., and Oser, R. S.: Detection of endotoxin in the blood of patients with sepsis due to gram-negative bacteria, N. Engl. J. Med. **283:** 1313, 1970.
13. Levin, J., Tomasulo, P. A., and Oser, R. S.: Detection of endotoxin in human blood and demonstration of an inhibitor, J. Lab. Clin. Med. **75:** 903, 1970.
14. Moberg, A. W., Mozes, M. F., Santiago, E. A., Campos, R., Mason, R., and Najarian, J. S.: A new transportable organ perfusion system. Experimental and clinical experience, Lancet **2:** 1403, 1971.
15. Peavy, D. L., Adler, W. H., and Smith, R. J.: The mitogenic effects of endotoxin and staphylococcal enterotoxin B on mouse spleen cells and human peripheral lymphocytes, J. Immunol. **105:** 1453, 1970.
16. Möller, G., editor: Immunological tolerance. Effect of antigen on different cell populations, Transplant. Rev. **8:** 3, 1972.
17. Möller, G., Sjöberg, O., and Andersson, J.: Immunogenicity, tolerogenicity and mitogenicity of lipopolysaccharides, *in* Kass, E. H., and Wolff, S. M., editors: Bacterial lipopolysaccharides, Chicago, 1973, Chicago Press, pp. 44-48.
18. Reinhold, R. B., and Fine, J.: A technique

for quantitative meaurement of endotoxin in human plasma, Proc. Soc. Exp. Biol. Med. **137:** 334, 1971.
19. Roe, J. H., and Rice, E. W.: Photometric method for determination of free pentoses in animal tissues, J. Biol. Chem. **173:** 307, 1948.
20. Rojas-Corona, R. R., Skarnes, R., Tamakuma, S., and Fine, J.: The Limulus coagulation test for endotoxin. A comparison with other assay methods, Proc. Soc. Exp. Biol. Med. **132:** 599, 1969.
21. Ruiz, J. O., Uchida, H., Schultz, L. S., and Lillehei, R. C.: Problems in absorption and immunosuppression after entire allotransplantation, Am. J. Surg. **123:** 297, 1972.
22. Toledo-Pereyra, L. H., and Najarian, J. S.: Small bowel preservation: Comparison of perfusion and nonperfusion systems, Arch. Surg. **107:** 875, 1973.

Coronary blood flow and myocardial reactive hyperemia in the ischemic dog heart

William E. Elzinga, Ph.D., David B. Skinner, M.D., F.A.C.S., Mary F. Dutka, B.S., R.N., *and* **Vincent L. Gott, M.D., F.A.C.S.,** *Baltimore, Md., and Chicago, Ill.*

Restoring blood flow may or may not reverse ischemic myocardial injury, depending on the duration and severity of ischemia. To investigate methods for predicting reversibility of myocardial damage, coronary blood flow and reactive hyperemic responses (RHR) were assessed after the left circumflex coronary artery was reopened following 20, 60, or 120 minutes of occlusion in 45 anesthetized dogs. After a 20 minute occlusion, cell injury was reversible. Blood flow and RHR were high initially and stabilized near preocclusion levels. After 60 or 120 minute occlusions, which caused irreversible infarction, initial coronary flows were also high. However, 2 hours after revascularization flow averaged only 65 percent of preocclusion levels and fell to 55 percent after 4 hours. In 80 percent of these dogs flow patterns became nonpulsatile and reached zero flow in several. RHR measured within minutes of vessel reopening following 60 or 120 minute occlusions was greatly reduced and returned to an average of only 36 percent of control values one hour after reopening compared to 80 percent in the 20 minute occlusion group. RHR predicted the eventual recovery of the myocardium within minutes after restoration of flow, whereas this could not be detected by coronary flow measurements alone.

From the Department of Surgery, The Johns Hopkins University, School of Medicine, Baltimore, Md., and the Department of Surgery, The University of Chicago, Pritzker School of Medicine, Chicago, Ill.

NEW SURGICAL procedures such as aorta–coronary artery bypass grafts and the use of circulatory support devices as intra-aortic balloon augmentation offer therapeutic approaches to reversing cell damage in the severely ischemic or infarcting myocardium.[2, 5, 8] Although histological and histochemical alterations may be present in the ischemic myocardium, restoration of adequate blood flow to the tissue before too much time elapses will result in rapid and nearly complete recovery of the myocardial cells. On the other hand, if a portion of myocardium is permitted to be ischemic for long periods, it will suffer irreversible injury and die whether or not the blood supply is restored. Valid indices of irreversible injury are needed before it can be determined whether corrective vascular surgery or heart support should be employed in an effort to reverse myocardial ischemia. Experiments were performed to study the sequential changes in coronary artery blood flow and myocardial reactive hyperemia after an acutely occluded coronary vessel was reopened in dogs in which the vessel was

Accepted for publication May 29, 1974.

This work was supported by National Institutes of Health Grants HL-11831 and HE-09997, Department of Health Education, and Welfare.

Reprint requests: David B. Skinner, M.D., Department of Surgery, University of Chicago, 950 E. 59th St., Chicago, Ill. 60637.

reopened either prior to irreversible ischemic injury or after irreversible damage had occurred.[1]

MATERIALS AND METHODS

This investigation was performed on 45 heart-worm–negative mongrel dogs of varying age and sex, ranging in weight from 20 to 30 kilograms. Anesthesia was induced with sodium pentobarbital (30 mg. per kilogram) and maintained with intermittent intravenous injections (6 mg. per kilogram). After endotracheal intubation, positive pressure ventilation was maintained by a Harvard respirator using room air. Fluid was given at the rate of 50 c.c. per hour of 5 percent dextrose solution into the femoral vein. Blood pressure in the descending aorta was measured (in millimeters of mercury) by a polyethylene catheter (PE 140, length 50 cm.) inserted through the left femoral artery. The catheter was connected to a Statham P23Db pressure transducer. The electrocardiogram was monitored from the limb leads.

A left fifth intercostal space thoracotomy was done and the pericardium opened. A 2.5 cm. segment of the left circumflex coronary artery (LCCA) was isolated. A Biotronex electromagnetic flow probe was positioned around the LCCA near its origin. The probe was connected to a Biotronex model BL-612 electromagnetic flowmeter. Mean flow was obtained by a resistor-capacitor circuit damping of the pulsatile signal. Zero flow was determined at intervals by brief distal vessel occlusion. The flow probes were calibrated directly on the coronary artery at the termination of most experiments. In six dogs a Teflon probe (length 8 in., diameter 1.5 mm.) was inserted apex to base into the left ventricular wall. The length of the probe in the myocardium was approximately 2 cm. The probe was connected to a model MS-8 mass spectrometer for continuous measurements of intramyocardial Po_2 and Pco_2.[4]

Three groups of animals were studied. In seven dogs the LCCA was occluded for 20 minutes, in 22 dogs for 60 minutes, and in 16 dogs for 120 minutes. In each group, ECG (Lead II), arterial pressure, coronary flow,

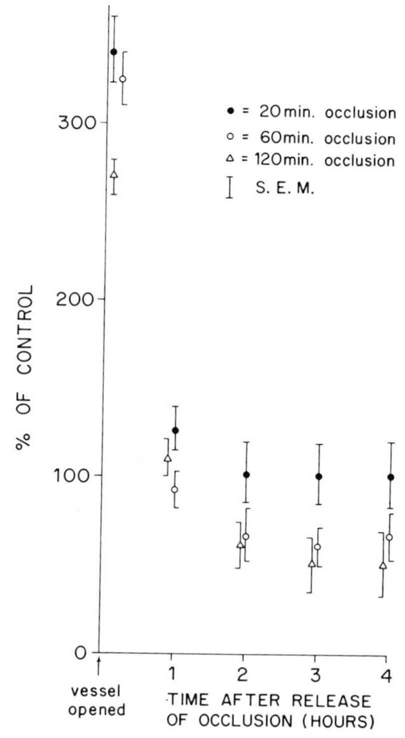

Fig. 1. LCCA flow at various times after vessel reopening, expressed as a percentage of the mean preocclusion LCCA flow. No divergence in flow among the three groups is seen until the second hour. The difference between the 20 minute group and the other two groups is significant ($p < 0.05$ or less) for the second, third, and fourth hours.

and two 10 second reactive hyperemic measurements were recorded just prior to occlusion. A 10 second reactive hyperemic response (RHR) was performed by occluding the LCCA with a bulldog clamp distal to the flow probe for exactly 10 seconds and then releasing it.[1] The maximum (peak) mean flow and the area under the mean flow tracing were both employed to describe the RHR. All measurements were recorded on a multichannel Mark 200 brush recorder. Measurements were again recorded just prior to vessel reopening, just after vessel reopening, and on an hourly basis 4 hours after flow was reinstated. If fibrillation occurred either during the occlusion or upon restoration of flow, hearts were immediately defibrillated.

In the 20 minute occlusion group the myocardium supplied by the occluded LCCA was severely ischemic but still reversible at the

Table I. *Mean left circumflex coronary artery flow (cubic centimeters per minute)*

	20 min. occlusion			60 min. occlusion			120 min. occlusion		
	Mean	*No.*	*S. D.*	*Mean*	*No.*	*S. D.*	*Mean*	*No.*	*S. D.*
Baseline	71.4	5	31.1	57.1	20	17.1	64.7	14	38.4
At opening	243.3*	3	54.6	152.6*‡	18	86.3	196.6*	14	76.2
1 hour	90.2	5	32.4	62.0	17	27.6	61.6	14	37.7
2 hours	76.8	5	32.1	36.0*†	17	19.3	46.6‡	14	26.5
3 hours	76.2	5	28.3	31.4*†	16	18.9	44.2†	13	19.7
4 hours	77.4	5	30.4	30.6*†	13	21.0	46.9‡	12	22.6

*Significant change from baseline ($p < 0.001$).
†Significant decrease from 20 minute occlusion value at same time ($p < 0.01$).
‡Significant decrease from 20 minute occlusion value at same time ($p < 0.05$).

Table II. *Peak reactive hyperemic response expressed as percentage compared to coronary flow prior to the 10 second occlusion*

	20 min. occlusion			60 min. occlusion			120 min. occlusion		
	Mean	*No.*	*S. D.*	*Mean*	*No.*	*S. D.*	*Mean*	*No.*	*S. D.*
Baseline	210.0	5	66.1	171.7	20	57.0	220.6	14	75.7
1 hour	200.8	5	73.7	99.8*	17	48.6	128.9*	14	54.9
2 hours	179.0	5	63.4	73.9*	17	44.1	108.1*	14	52.4
3 hours	180.2	5	58.9	71.6*	16	41.6	101.9*	13	51.5
4 hours	179.4	5	49.6	62.4*	13	47.8	98.9*	12	56.4

*Significant decrease from baseline ($p < 0.001$) and from 20 minute occlusion value at same time ($p < 0.05$ or less).

time blood flow was restored. In the 60 and 120 minute occlusion groups the myocardium deprived of blood was considered to be frankly infarcted and restoration of flow was not expected to restore muscle viability.[1]

RESULTS

Revascularization prior to irreversible ischemic damage. When the LCCA was occluded for 20 minutes, the hearts of three of the seven dogs fibrillated during the occlusion. Two could not be revived. The ECG changes were characterized by prominent ST segment elevations which were more pronounced in hearts which had fibrillated. When the LCCA was reopened and flow restored to the ischemic myocardium, four of the five dogs' hearts fibrillated immediately but were easily defibrillated and maintained normal rhythm throughout the rest of the study.

The mean blood flow through the reopened LCCA was very high immediately upon reopening. It went directly from zero to a peak mean flow of 243 c.c. per minute or 342 percent of control values (Fig. 1, Table I). From the pulsatile flow tracings at this time it was evident that flow was equally elevated during both diastole and systole (Fig. 2). One hour after opening the LCCA the mean flow returned to 127 percent of the preocclusion control, and after 2 hours it was back to control levels, where it remained. There were no changes in mean arterial blood pressure throughout the experiments.

The normal RHR of the myocardial vascular bed following a 10 second arterial occlusion was somewhat reduced in the animals which had the LCCA blocked for 20 minutes. Shortly after reopening the occluded vessel, a RHR was noted in the 20 minute occlusion group (Fig. 2). After the flow had been restored for one hour, the peak RHR was 80 percent of preocclusion control, and after 2 hours 75 percent of the control (Figs. 3 and 4, and Table II). No improvement in RHR was seen for the next 2 hours.

Fig. 5 shows the changes in intramyocardial P_{O_2} and P_{CO_2} in the posterior ventricular wall in response to a 20 minute occlusion of the LCCA. The P_{O_2} was 8 mm. Hg and P_{CO_2} was 188 mm. Hg and still increasing

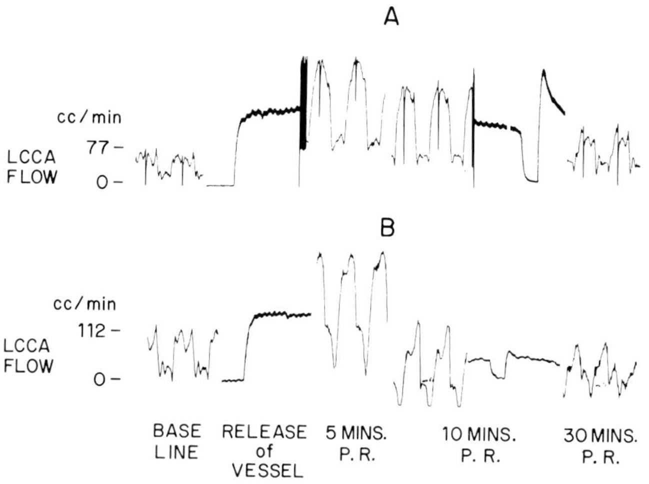

Fig. 2. Composites of pulsatile and mean LCCA flows at various times following release of LCCA occlusion of 20 minutes (dog A) or 120 minutes (dog B). Mean flows are elevated in both initially as are diastolic and systolic components. A reactive hyperemic test at 10 minutes post release (P. R.) shows a high response in *A* but almost no response in *B*.

after 20 minutes of occlusion. Thirty minutes sions had returned to normal values. following restoration of flow, both gas ten-

Revascularization after irreversible ischemic damage. When the LCCA was occluded for 60 or 120 minutes, the hearts of 11 of the 38 dogs fibrillated during the occlusion period. Four could not be promptly defibrillated and were not used in the study. When the LCCA was reopened, five out of 20 in the 60 minute group immediately fibrillated, and five out of 14 in the 120 minute group fibrillated. All these hearts were successfully defibrillated. In the 60 minute group, normal rhythm was maintained throughout the remainder of the experiment. In the 120 minute group, 11 dogs developed ventricular arrhythmias in the third and fourth hours after the vessel was reopened.

As in the 20 minute occlusion group, mean blood flow through the reopened LCCA was initially very high in both the one and 2 hour occlusion groups (Fig. 1, Table I). In the one hour occlusion group, mean flow was 273 percent of control values. In the 2 hour group it was 325 percent of control shortly after vessel reopening. Both systolic and diastolic flow components were elevated (Fig. 2).

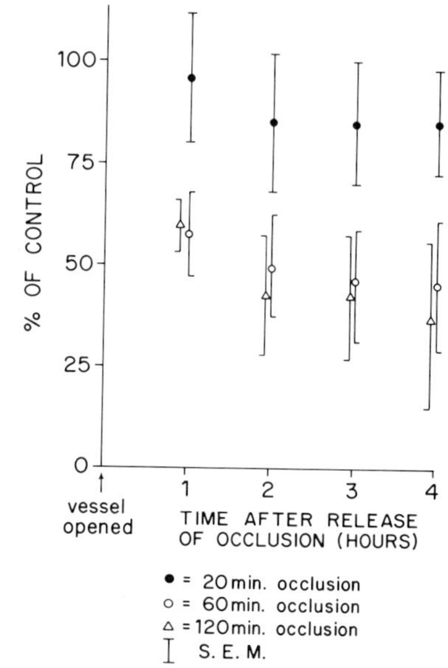

Fig. 3. Peak reactive hyperemic responses at hourly intervals after vessel reopening, expressed as a percentage of the mean preocclusion peak RHR. The differences between the 20 minute group and the other two groups are significant ($p < 0.05$ or less).

Within the first hour after opening the LCCA, the mean flow had returned to preocclusion values in both groups. Two hours after reopening, the mean flow in all animals in both groups was below the preocclusion value averaging 65 percent of control. Four

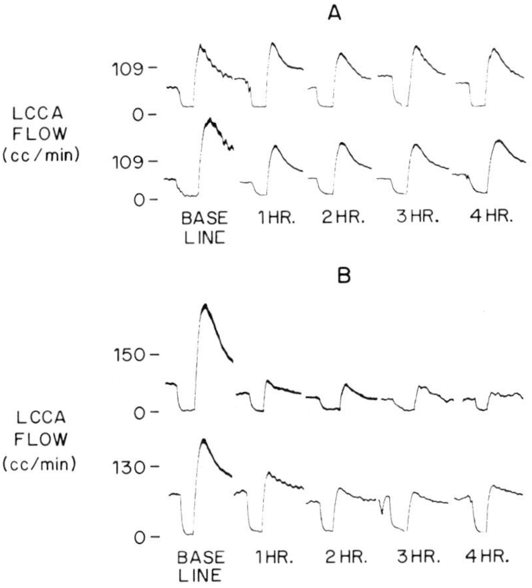

Fig. 4. Mean LCCA flow tracings showing RHR at intervals after vessel reopening. Tracings for two dogs in the 20 minute occlusion group are shown in *A* and for two dogs in the 60 minute occlusion group in *B*.

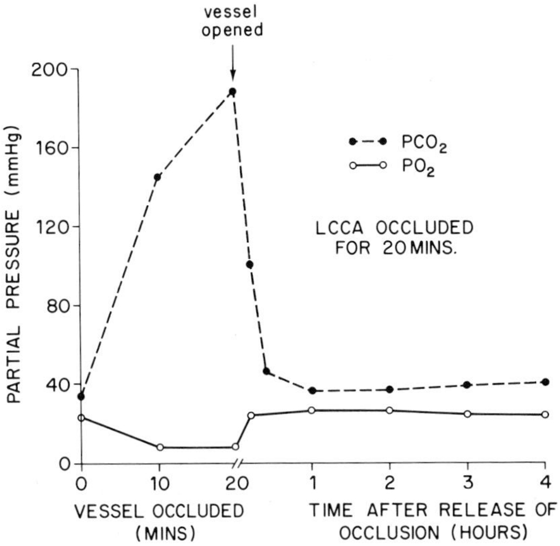

Fig. 5. Intramyocardial gas tensions in a dog undergoing a 20 minute LCCA occlusion.

hours after LCCA reopening, mean flow for all animals averaged only 55 percent of control levels. In several dogs the LCCA flow 4 hours after opening the vessel was near zero (Fig. 6). In 80 percent of the dogs in both groups, the normal pulsatile flow pattern progressed to a nonpulsatile pattern by the fourth hour. There was a great reduction of LCCA flow during cardiac diastole. In some animals flow was retrograde during cardiac systole.

In the one-hour occlusion group, baseline mean arterial blood pressure averaged 111 mm. Hg (S. D. 16). After reopening the vessel mean blood pressure declined to an average of 99 mm. Hg (S. D. 21) ($p < 0.05$), and a further decline to 94 mm. Hg (S. D. 15) ($p < 0.01$) was observed 4 hours later. In the 2 hour occlusion group, baseline mean arterial blood pressure was 115 mm. Hg (S. D. 15) which declined to 109 mm. Hg (S. D. 14) after vessel reopening. After 4 hours arterial pressure averaged 91 mm. Hg (S. D. 17) which was significantly lower than baseline or reopening values ($p < 0.01$).

In the one and 2 hour occlusion groups, RHR to a 10 second arterial test occlusion could not be elicited shortly after vessel reopening. One hour after opening of the vessel, the peak mean RHR was reduced to 36 percent of control values. After 4 hours the peak mean RHR averaged only 29 percent of preocclusion control values (Figs. 3 and 4, Table II). The total volume as well as peak RHR were severely depressed in the one and 2 hour occlusion groups (Fig. 7). Four hours after vessel reopening, it averaged only 15 percent of control values.

Changes in intramyocardial Po_2 and Pco_2 for both the one and 2 hour occlusion groups are shown in Figs. 8 and 9. Myocardial Po_2 dropped to 7 mm. Hg during occlusion in both groups. After LCCA opening, Po_2 returned to baseline in the animal studied after 2 hours of occlusion. However, in the one-hour group, myocardial Po_2 was abnormally elevated 4 hours after restoration of flow. Myocardial Pco_2 peaked about 30 to 40 minutes after vessel occlusion and slowly declined for the next 30 or 90 minutes until the vessel was reopened. In both groups, the Pco_2 returned to control levels within one hour after LCCA opening.

DISCUSSION

Previous studies in our laboratory have shown that LCCA occlusions of 15 minutes'

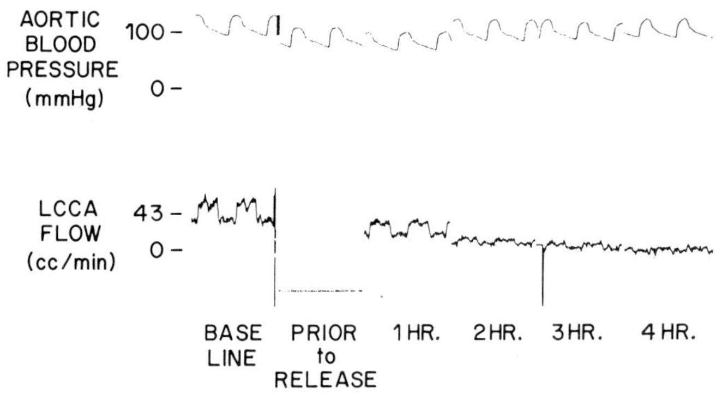

Fig. 6. Composite of blood pressure and pulsatile LCCA flow tracings at intervals before, during, and after an LCCA occlusion of 120 minutes duration. Note that LCCA flow is nearly zero and apulsatile in the third and fourth hours.

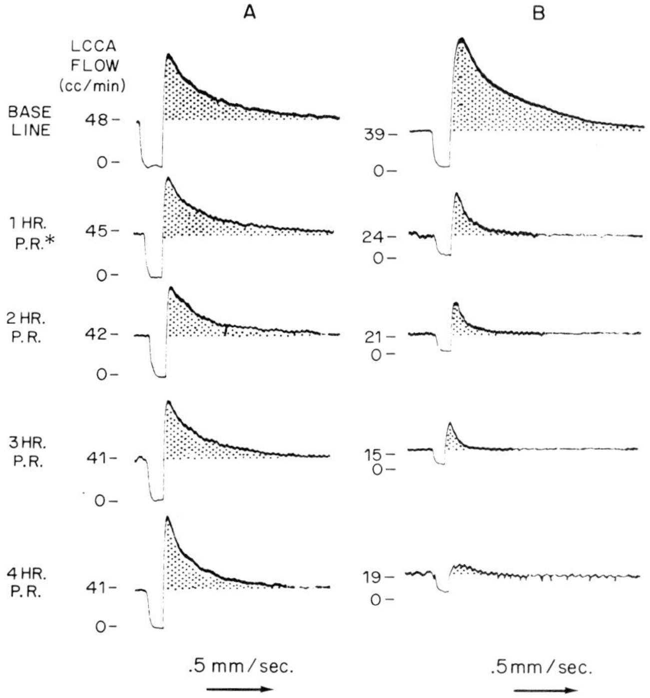

Fig. 7. Mean LCCA flow tracings showing RHR at intervals following LCCA occlusions of 20 minutes (dog A) or 60 minutes (dog B). Shaded areas represent total volume of flow increase during RHR.

duration caused no microscopic abnormality of the myocardium when the hearts were examined 7 days later. Thirty-minute occlusions caused patchy necrosis and 60 minute occlusions caused an extensive infarction.[1] In a subsequent study (unpublished data), 10 of 11 dogs had developed a definite infarction involving the posterolateral myocardial wall, the posterior papillary muscle, and a portion of the ventricular septum when their hearts were examined at autopsy 2 weeks after a 60 minute LCCA occlusion.

In this study when flow was interrupted to the myocardium for 20, 60, or 120 minutes and then restored, it was high compared to preocclusion levels. The high phasic flow pattern during cardiac diastole indicated that the vessels were dilated.[10] High flow was

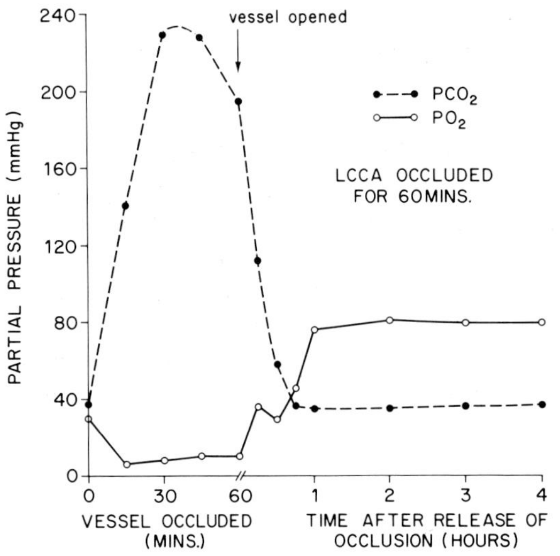

Fig. 8. Intramyocardial gas tensions in a dog undergoing a 60 minute LCCA occlusion.

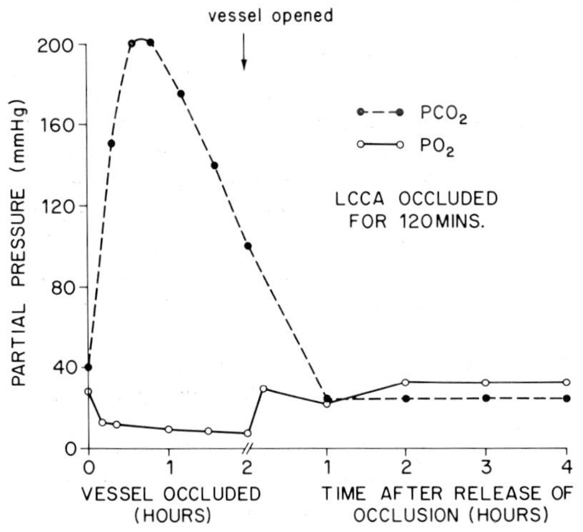

Fig. 9. Intramyocardial gas tensions in a dog undergoing a 120 minute LCCA occlusion.

also observed during cardiac systole which suggested that the vigor of contraction and intramyocardial pressure was decreased immediately after restoration of flow.

The subsequent rapid return to baseline mean flow in the 20 minute occlusion group indicated that the vascular resistance to flow returned to preocclusion levels rapidly. The drop in both peak diastolic and systolic flow gave further evidence of the return to normal vascular tone and an increase in contraction.

The rapid return within minutes of the RHR in the 20 minute occlusion group strongly suggested that the ischemic injury in this group was reversible. The RHR of the vascular bed to a brief 10 second anoxic test period indicated that the vessels were no longer maximally dilated and that metabolic byproducts were being produced by functioning viable myocardial cells. There appeared to be some deterioration in the RHR during the first 2 hours after restoration of blood flow in the 20 minute occlusion group, but in the third and fourth hours the RHR improved.

In the 60 and 120 minute occlusion groups, coronary flow fell to 65 percent of control values within 2 hours after revascularization. No improvement was seen in flow for the next 2 hours. The LCCA flow in 80 percent of the animals in these groups became nearly apulsatile by the fourth hour. Although there was some decrease in mean arterial blood pressure in these groups, these findings strongly suggested that intramyocardial resistance rapidly increased after restoration of blood flow to the ischemic area. This agreed with the findings of Yokoyama[10] who showed that peripheral coronary artery pressure increased after revascularization of severely damaged myocardium. Jennings and associates[3] and Sobel[9] have shown that restoration of flow to the severely ischemic myocardium promoted rapid and severe disorganization of the cells and produced tissue edema.

The inability of the myocardial vascular bed in the 60 and 120 minute occlusion groups to respond significantly to a 10 second test occlusion shortly after LCCA opening indicated that one or both of the following had occurred. The myocardial extravascular resistance was too high preventing normal dilatation of the vessels, or metabolic products were not being produced and the cells were dead. The slight decline in blood pressure noted at this time was not sufficient to account for the marked decline in RHR. In the 60 and 120 minute occlusion groups, it was not possible to ascertain whether the ischemic cells were irreversibly injured at the end of the anoxic period, or whether the restoration of blood flow in some way caused the damage.

Early measurement of coronary blood flow after reopening the occluded vessel failed to predict the subsequent course. However, the RHR test predicted the eventual outcome very early after the vessel was opened. If the RHR was low, coronary blood flow gradually diminished over the following hours. If the RHR was high shortly after vessel opening, satisfactory coronary perfusion continued.

It has been previously reported and also noticed in this study that the incidence of ventricular fibrillation was high upon reinstating blood flow after 20 minutes of flow interruption. In both the 60 and 120 minute occlusion groups, fibrillation was less frequent. During the initial 20 to 30 minute interval of flow interruption, intramyocardial Pco_2 increased rapidly. However, after 30 minutes of anoxia, the tissue Pco_2 plateaued and began a slow decline. The rapid drop of intramyocardial Po_2 when blood flow was suddenly interrupted for 5 or 10 minutes indicated that aerobic metabolism quickly ceased. Po_2 values of 3 to 7 mm. Hg have been suggested to be a critical level for transfer of oxygen across the cell membrane.[7] The rapid changes in myocardial metabolism early after coronary occlusion probably predisposed to ventricular fibrillation.

CONCLUSIONS

Myocardial blood flow and RHR to a 10 second test occlusion follow definite distinctive patterns when the LCCA is reopened after 20, 60, or 120 minutes of vessel occlusion. In the ischemic myocardium, in which the cell injury is still reversible after 20 minutes of occlusion, blood flow and RHR quickly return to near normal preocclusion values. In the irreversibly damaged myocardium after 60 or 120 minutes of anoxia, flow and myocardial RHR were generally severely depressed even after 4 hours of flow restoration. Early measurements of blood flow to an ischemic myocardium up to one hour after revascularization give little or no information concerning viability and eventual recovery. Flow measurements 2 to 3 hours after revascularization do give such information concerning viability of the myocardium. Delays of this length are not practical clinically in assessing the effectiveness of revascularization. The myocardial reactive hyperemic test to a 10 second occlusion gives information concerning the viability of the vascular bed within minutes after restoration of blood flow to an anoxic area. The myocardial RHR test would appear to have clinical value in predicting the outcome from revascularization of an acute myocardial infarction.

REFERENCES

1. Brantigan, J. W., Gott, V. L., and Martz, M. N.: A Teflon membrane for measurement of blood and intramyocardial gas tensions by mass spectrometer, J. Appl. Physiol. **32:** 276, 1972.
2. Favaloro, R. G., Effler, D. B., Groves, L. K., Sheldon, W. C., Shirley, E. K., and Sones, F. M., Jr.: Severe segmental obstruction of the left main coronary artery and its divisions, J. Thorac. Cardiovasc. Surg. **60:** 469, 1970.
3. Jennings, R. B., Sommers, H. M., Smyth, G. A., Flack, H. A., and Linn, H.: Myocardial necrosis induced by temporary occlusion of a coronary artery in the dog, Arch. Pathol. **70:** 82, 1960.
4. Johnson, W. D., and Lepley, D.: An aggressive surgical approach to coronary disease, J. Thorac. Cardiovasc. Surg. **59:** 128, 1970.
5. Matthews, H. R., Skinner, D. B., and Pitt, B.: Reactive hyperemia following coronary occlusion as a measurement of myocardial viability, Curr. Top. Surg. Res. **3:** 39, 1971.
6. Rakusan, K.: Oxygen in the heart muscle, Springfield, Ill., 1971, Charles C Thomas, Publisher.
7. Reneman, R. S., and Spencer, M. P.: The use of diastolic reactive hyperemia to evaluate the coronary vascular system, Ann. Thorac. Surg. **13:** 477, 1972.
8. Sanders, C. A., Buckley, M. J., Leinbach, R. C., and Mundth, E. D.: Mechanical circulatory assistance, Circulation **14:** 1292, 1972.
9. Sobel, B. E.: Biochemical and morphologic changes in infarcting myocardium, Hosp. Pract. **7:** 59, 1972.
10. Yokoyama, M.: National increase in the distal coronary pressure following acute ligation, Bull. Heart Inst. (Japan) 35, 1969.

A chickenpox epidemic in a pediatric burn unit

W. H. Weintraub, M.D., J. R. Lilly, *and* **J. G. Randolph,** *Washington, D. C.*

A case of chickenpox (varicella) developed in a child 36 hours after admission to our burn unit. Of 20 children exposed to the disease, six who had not previously had chickenpox developed it. The varicella lesions in these children had a greater predilection for areas of partial-thickness injuries than for healthy skin, and were not seen in areas of full-thickness burn. In addition to the increased numbers of vesicles in partial-thickness burns, the individual vesicles were more virulent, extending deep into the dermis. They were punched out, hemorrhagic, prone to secondary infection, and frequently left permanent scars. Areas of full-thickness burn that had undergone successful skin grafting 2 weeks or longer before the child developed chickenpox also showed these same virulent varicella lesions. Particularily disturbing was the extensive eruption of vesicles in nonburned skin that had been used for donor sites. Also, skin grafts applied just prior to the outbreak of the vesicles did not take, presumably because of vesicular lesions developing under the graft. Despite these serious cutaneous manifestations, no child developed systemic complications of varicella, and zoster-immune globulin was not used.

From the Burn Unit, Children's Hospital National Medical Center, Washington, D. C.

DURING THE SPRING of 1973, an epidemic of chickenpox occured in the burn unit of the Children's Hospital National Medical Center. Before subsiding, 20 children in the burn unit were exposed to the virus and seven burned children suffered through the entire clinical course of chickenpox. The purpose of this communication is to discuss the clinical manifestations of varicella infection in burn injury, the problems relating to its management in the burned child, and the logistic complications of an outbreak of chickenpox in a children's burn unit.

Accepted for publication May 31, 1974.

Reprint requests: William H. Weintraub, M.D., Department of Pediatric Surgery, C. S. Mott Hospital, University of Michigan Medical Center, Ann Arbor, Mich. 48104.

CASE MATERIAL

Patient 1. The index case (Table I) was a 1-year-old black girl with a 18 percent second-degree scald burn of the face, chest, and shoulders. Thirty-six hours after injury, she developed the classical varicella rash with lesions concentrated in the area of her burn. She was treated with Sulfamylon and her burns healed primarily without skin grafts. Several pox scars remained in the area of the burn, but no scars appeared in the nonburned skin.

Patient 2. A 7-year-old black boy developed chickenpox 2 months after his burn injury and one month after his first contact with Patient 1. He had been grafted one month prior to developing chickenpox and in the areas of healed second-degree burn surrounding the skin graft, as well as in the graft of the right anterior lower leg, he developed unusual, punched-out, hemorrhagic lesions that were different from his other vesicles which were the classical clear type. Many lesions left permanent scars.

Patient 3. A 4-year-old black girl had second-

Vol. 76, No. 3, pp. 490-494

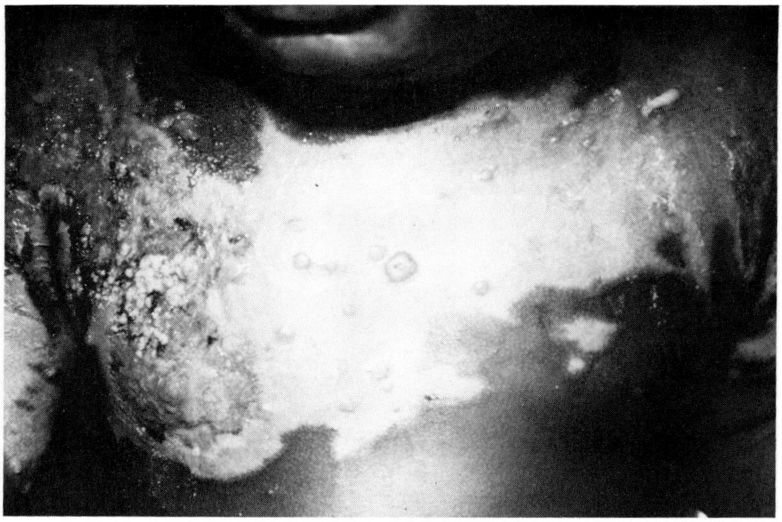

Fig. 1. Patient 7: No vesicles appear in third-degree areas. Several pox scars remained in the sternal area.

Table I. *Varicella in a burn unit—seven cases*

Patient No.	*Age (yr.)*	*Burn*	*Incubation of varicella (days)*	*Sequelae*
1	1	18% first and second degree of face and chest	Index case	Permanent scars in site of second-degree burn
2	7	5% second and third degree of anterior leg	34	Pox scars in second-degree burn; 30-day-old graft affected
3	4	10% second and third degree of legs	13	Pox scar in skin graft and adjacent second-degree burn
4	2	2% third degree of sole of foot	12	Skin graft failed; epithelialization without second graft
5	5	22% second and third degree of chest and arms	22	Partial loss of skin graft; regraft successful; permanent scars in donor site
6	1	15% second and third degree of trunk and feet	23	Pox scars in second-degree area; partial loss of graft
7	1	12% second and third degree of chest and shoulders	31	Pox scars in second-degree area; grafted after varicella; 100% take

and third-degree scald burns of both lower extremities. She had been successfully grafted 16 days prior to developing chickenpox. In the skin graft, the donor sites, and second-degree burn area, unusual, punched-out, hemorrhagic, 4 to 6 mm. vesicles developed. These lesions subsequently healed with minor scarring.

Patient 4. A 2-year-old white girl was burned on the plantar aspect of the foot. Postage stamp grafts were placed 3 days prior to development of chickenpox. The donor site and sole of her foot were completely covered with lesions and the grafts did not take. Subsequent healing occured by epithelialization.

Patient 5. A 5-year-old black girl had been grafted on the chest 5 days prior to developing chickenpox. Approximately 20 percent of the split-thickness graft did not take. Varicella lesions which were hemorrhagic and punched out appeared on the donor site and these healed with some residual scarring. She was regrafted successfully 2 weeks later.

Patient 6. A 1-year-old black boy developed chickenpox 3 days after postage stamp grafts were placed on a grease burn of the dorsum of the foot. The varicella lesions appeared prominently in areas of second-degree burns. In addition, several of the postage stamp grafts did not survive, but healing occured by epithelialization from surrounding skin.

Patient 7. A 1-year-old black boy had second-

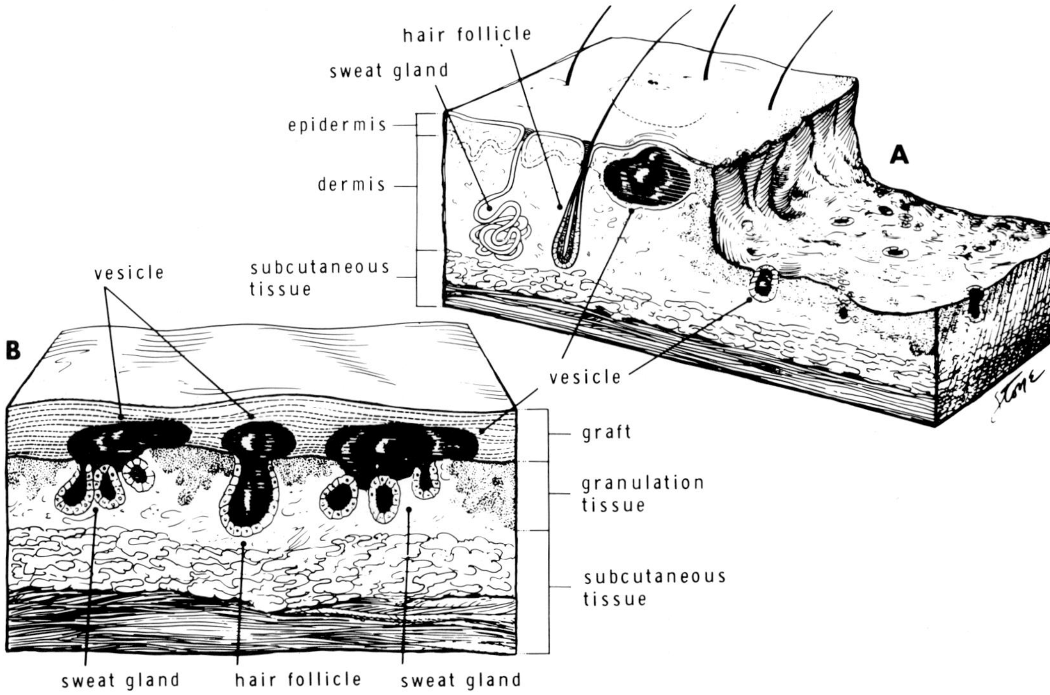

Fig. 2. Upper right: Represents a third degree burn with several surviving skin appendages. Lower left: A skin graft applied over areas where vesicles have released fluid and lifted the graft.

and third-degree grease burns of the shoulder and chest. He was the last patient to develop chickenpox and the eruption was allowed to subside before grafting. The graft took well and the child had only an occasional pox scar in the area of his original second-degree burn.

DISCUSSION

Varicella is usually a mild acute vesicular disease of childhood.[3] The varicella-zoster organism is highly contagious but invades only the prickle-cell layer of the epidermis. The disease spreads by direct contact from one individual to another but third-party transmission has been reported in hospitalized patients. The incubation period is 11 to 14 days and the patient can transmit the disease 24 hours before the rash appears and continues to shed the virus for 6 days afterward. The vesicles are much more common on the trunk than on the extremities. The lesions are usually clear, raised vesicles with minimal surrounding reaction. After a short, febrile illness associated with moderate discomfort from pruritus, the disease resolves with serious sequelae occurring only rarely.

Of the 20 patients exposed to the index case of chickenpox, only six had never had the disease and all six developed varicella. This is not surprising since the infection rate in exposed, susceptible individuals is extremely high.[3] The cases developed sequentially over a 30 day period following the epidemiologic pattern of chickenpox that has been described in hospitalized patients.[3] No subsequent cases developed in the burn unit over the following 6 months.

Although it was not possible to distinguish symptoms referable to chickenpox from those associated with burn discomfort, the acute clinical course of chickenpox did not appear to affect the children adversely. None of our patients developed severe complications of varicella, i.e., pneumonia, glomerulonephritis, or encephalitis,[2] and zoster-immune globulin was not administered. An increased incidence of systemic complications of chickenpox has been reported in immunosuppressed patients,[1, 4, 5, 8-11] but this has not yet been noted in patients with major burns. The lesions of varicella have a predilection for injured skin.[6] In our experience, areas of second-degree burn were particularly susceptible, demonstrating an increase in the absolute number of vesicles. Unfortunately, these vesicles were hemorrhagic, punched out, and unusually deep in contrast to the more commonly seen clear, raised vesicles found in nonburned areas. These unusual vesicles often became secondarily infected from the nearby burn surface which resulted in further deepening of the lesion to full-thickness injury and consequently in permanent scarring.

Since no epidermis remains in a third-degree burn, these areas were not expected to develop obvious vesicles and none were seen (Fig. 1). Despite this fact, it became apparent that in children who were skin grafted up to 2 weeks before the appearance of the varicella eruption, the grafts took poorly. A plausible explanation for this phenomenon might be that minute areas of partial-thickness burn present in a full-thickness injury might develop varicella lesions and the resultant inflammation prevent adherence of the grafts and their subsequent loss (Fig. 2).

Varicella shows the same predilection for skin autografts as it does for partial-thickness burn injury. Identical lesions that were hemorrhagic and punched out appeared in greater than expected numbers in grafts 3 to 4 weeks old. Finally, skin-graft donor sites also developed increased numbers of these severe chickenpox lesions. These donor areas in our patients were uniformly covered with the abnormal vesicles (Fig. 3) which left residual scars if they became infected.

CONCLUSIONS

Chickenpox is not a benign disease in the burned child. A child with partial-thickness burn injury develops unusual vesicles which frequently leave scars. Areas of full-thickness burn do not take skin grafts well during an attack of chickenpox. Skin-graft donor sites which normally heal without scar formation become covered with chickenpox lesions which frequently scar. Chickenpox can be expected to affect every susceptible child

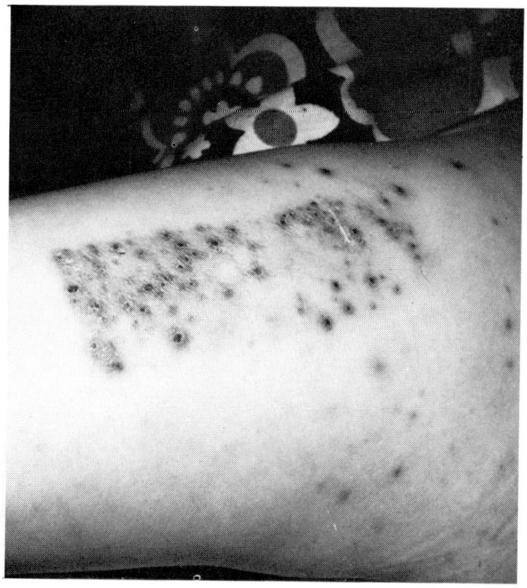

Fig. 3. Donor site (Patient 4) selectively covered with vesicles.

who is exposed to it during an epidemic.

Because of the epidemiologic consequences and severe cutaneous sequelae in a number of the burned children, we propose the following guidelines in the event of a varicella outbreak in a pediatric burn unit. (1) Children susceptible to chickenpox should not be admitted to a burn unit where a case of varicella is present. (2) All susceptible children in the unit who have unwittingly been exposed to chickenpox should continue with their routine daily burn care. (3) If feasible, skin grafting procedures should be postponed until the vesicular eruption of chickenpox has subsided. (4) In milder burns, zoster-immune globulin to prevent or modify the disease is probably unnecessary.

REFERENCES

1. Aceto, T., Beckhorn, G. D., Mattimore, J. M., and Kenny, F. M.: Cortisol secretion in children with varicella or rubeola, Am. J. Dis. Child. **117:** 294, 1969.
2. Blair, A. W., Jamieson, W. M., and Smith, G. H.: Complications and death in chickenpox, Br. Med. J. **2:** 981, 1965.
3. Brunnell, P. A., Krugman, S.: *In* Barnett, H. L., and Einhorn, A. H., editors: Pediatrics, New York, 1972, Appleton-Century-Crofts.
4. Brunnell, P. A., and Gershon, A. A.: Passive

immunization against varicella-zoster infections and other modes of therapy, J. Infect. Dis. **127:** 415-23, 1973.
5. Brunnell, P. A., Ross, A., Miller, L. H., and Kuo, B.: Prevention of varicella by zoster immune globulin, N. Engl. J. Med. **280:** 1191, 1969.
6. Castrow, F. F., and Wolf, J. E.: Photolocalized varicella, Arch. Dermatol. **107:** 628, 1973.
7. Foley, F. D., Greenawald, K. A., Nash, G., and Pruitt, B. A.: Herpesvirus infection in burned patients, N. Engl. J. Med. **282:** 652, 1970.
8. Janeway, C. A.: Passive immunization against chickenpox, N. Engl. J. Med. **280:** 1237, 1969.
9. Judelsohn, R. G.: Prevention and control of varicella-zoster infections, J. Infect. Dis. **125:** 82, 1972.
10. Movassaghi, N.: The prevention and treatment of varicella-zoster infection in patients at high risk, Clin. Pediatr. **12:** 299, 1973.
11. Torstenson, O. L., Meyer, W. J., and Quie, P. G.: Burn wound infection with viruses, N. Engl. J. Med. **282:** 1272, 1970.

Intestinal absorption of intake antigenic protein

Andrew L. Warshaw, M.D., *and* W. Allan Walker, M.D., *Boston, Mass.*

Antigenic quantities of proteins from ingested food, bacterial breakdown products, and secreted enzymes can be absorbed intact from the adult small intestine. In our previous studies, measurable quantities of absorbed protein could be detected in both intestinal lymph and systemic blood. This study was designed to determine if the appearance of protein in the mesenteric lymph reflects direct and independent transport into the intestinal lymphatics or only a recirculation of protein from the portal blood. Tritiated bovine serum albumin (^{3}H-BSA) was injected into the duodenal lumens of six rats prepared with cannulas in the intestinal lymphatics and portal veins; sequential samples of portal blood and intestinal lymph were collected and assayed for ^{3}H-BSA. The results clearly show that intact albumin is transported independently into both intestinal lymphatics (0.76 percent) and portal blood (1.11 percent) in the rat. This observation may help to explain the pathogenesis of numerous intestinal and systemic immune states and may be used in further studies that investigate the role of local intestinal antibodies in controlling soluble antigen absorption from the small intestine.

From the Departments of Surgery and Pediatrics, Harvard Medical School, and the General Surgical Services and Pediatric Gastrointestinal Unit, Massachusetts General Hospital, Boston, Mass.

ALTHOUGH it has been widely accepted that the mature gut does not absorb undigested proteins, there is increasing evidence that small amounts of intact protein can and regularly do reach the circulation from the intestinal lumen.[2, 6, 7, 23, 24] A detailed discussion of the implications of this phenomenon in a wide variety of local and systemic allergic and autoimmune diseases has recently appeared.[21] Of particular interest is a proposed role for absorption of antigenic protein in the pathogenesis of inflammatory bowel disease,[16] a theory which would be strengthened by the demonstration of antigens within the submucosa of the bowel and in the regional lymphatics.

Molecules traversing the intestinal mucosa can pass either into the portal bloodstream or into the intestinal lymphatics.[9] Most small molecules, including amino acids, are transported into the portal blood.[1] Uptake into the intestinal lymphatics occurs primarily during absorption of long-chain fatty acids.[4] Using bovine serum albumin labelled with tritium (^{3}H-BSA), a protein known to cause human atopic intestinal disease[8, 11] and a proved immunogen when administered orally to the rat,[19] we have previously reported that approximately 2 percent of the albumin placed in the intestinal lumen of the rat appeared intact in aliquots of peripheral blood and intestinal lymph.[24] Because lymph is a

Accepted for publication May 29, 1974.

Reprint requests: Andrew L. Warshaw, M.D., General Surgical Services, Massachusetts General Hospital, Boston, Mass. 02114.

Table I. *Absorption of ^{3}H-BSA into intestinal lymph and portal blood*

Animal No.	Dose given (mg.)	Protein absorbed: Lymph µg	Lymph %	Blood µg	Blood %	Total µg	Total %
1	23.5	564	2.40	682	2.90	1,246	5.30
2	23.7	225	0.95	201	0.85	426	1.80
3	21.0	32	0.15	332	1.58	364	1.73
4	23.5	35	0.15	94	0.40	129	0.55
5	21.0	74	0.35	132	0.63	206	0.98
6	26.5	148	0.56	77	0.29	225	0.85
Mean			0.76		1.11		1.87

derivative of plasma, however, these studies did not prove that BSA was transported directly into lymph, rather than appearing there secondarily after recirculation of the portal blood.

In this study, using cannulation of both the mesenteric lymphatic and the portal vein of rats to allow for the separate but simultaneous measurement of ^{3}H-BSA uptake into the intestinal lymph and portal blood, we show that macromolecular antigens can be transported across the intestine directly into both the lymphatic and portal circulations.

MATERIALS AND METHODS

These experiments were performed upon six albino male Charles River rats (Charles River Breeding Laboratories, Wilmington, Mass.), weighing 400 to 500 grams, and maintained on a standard laboratory diet (Ralston-Purina, St. Louis, Mo.). The mesenteric lymphatic, the portal vein, and the duodenum were cannulated with PE-50 polyethylene tubing as previously described.[22] The venous cannula was kept free of clot by constant saline perfusion with a Harvard pump. After the preparative operation, animals were placed in a restraint cage, allowed to awaken, and given free access to 5 percent dextrose in normal saline. Experiments were performed on the following day upon unanesthetized animals whose intestinal lymph flow exceeded 1 ml. per hour.

^{3}H-BSA was prepared by exchange-labelling of crystalline BSA (Nutritional Biochemicals, Cleveland, Ohio), with tritium gas under increased pressure (New England Nuclear Corp., Boston, Mass.) according to the Wilzbach[26] method. The ^{3}H-BSA was further purified by gel diffusion on a G-25 Sephadex column and by dialysis in saline to remove extraneous radioactivity and denatured protein. Unlabelled crystalline BSA was added to produce protein concentrations equal to 5 mg. per milliliter of normal saline.

Each animal received 50 mg. per kilogram of BSA, instilled into the duodenum after collection of control lymph and portal blood samples. Intestinal lymph was collected in heparinized vessels in 30 minute aliquots. Then 1 ml. samples of portal blood were taken at 30 minute intervals and replaced with 2 ml. of saline. Experiments were terminated at 3 hours, at which time a sample of mixed peripheral blood was obtained by direct cardiac puncture.

All samples were dialyzed against large volumes of saline to remove labelled protein fragments and free isotope; aliquots (1.0 ml.) in 10 ml. of Bray's solution[3] were assayed for radioactivity in a Beckman liquid scintillation counter. Protein concentrations were determined by the method of Lowry and associates.[13] Using techniques of gel filtration (G-50 Sephadex, Pharmacia Inc., Piscataway, New Jersey), and radioimmunodiffusion against monospecific rabbit anti-BSA as previously described,[23, 24] we have shown that the assayed radioactive material appearing in the lymph and blood in these experiments is intact BSA.[24]

The amount of BSA absorbed via the intestinal lymphatics was calculated directly from the specific activity of the administered protein and the volume and postdialysis specific activity of the lymph. Because all intestinal lymph was diverted from the animal,[12] the amount of BSA absorbed into the portal blood could be estimated from the specific activity of the peripheral plasma at 3 hours, the hematocrit, and the blood volume (considered to be 7 percent of body weight).[24]

RESULTS

Transmission of ^{3}H-BSA into intestinal lymph and portal blood occurs regularly within the first 30 minutes after instillation of the labelled protein into the duodenum. As shown in Table I, there is some variation from animal to animal in the total amount of protein absorbed in the 3 hour experimental period, with the average being 0.76 percent of the administered dose appearing in the lymph and 1.11 percent in the bloodstream. However, in all experiments BSA was present in both lymph and serum samples in amounts easily detected by our techniques.

As exemplified in Fig. 1, the specific activity of intestinal lymph was quite unrelated to the specific activity of portal plasma over the course of these experiments. The levels of radioactivity in lymph rose considerably higher than in portal plasma and returned almost to baseline levels, whereas portal plasma levels rose in a sigmoid curve to a plateau. This observation clearly demonstrates that the ^{3}H-BSA appearing in the lymph does not get there via re-circulation of the portal plasma, but must be transmitted directly from intestinal lumen into intestinal lymph.

Similarly the data show that uptake into the portal blood is a genuine route of absorption of BSA. In all experiments, the specific activity of portal plasma at the 3 hour end-point was 25 to 100 percent greater than the specific activity of peripheral plasma (Table II). This increment in radioactivity as blood perfuses the intestine represents protein continuing to pass into the portal blood from the intestine, even 3 hours after instillation.

The amount of absorption of protein into the lymph appears to be independent of the amount absorbed into the portal blood, further suggesting separate routes of absorption. Of the total ^{3}H-BSA absorbed by each animal, the relative fractions transmitted into lymph versus blood were quite unpredictable, ranging between 9 and 65 percent into lymph.

DISCUSSION

This report confirms and extends our previous studies[6, 23, 24] showing uptake of protein by mature mammalian intestine and its

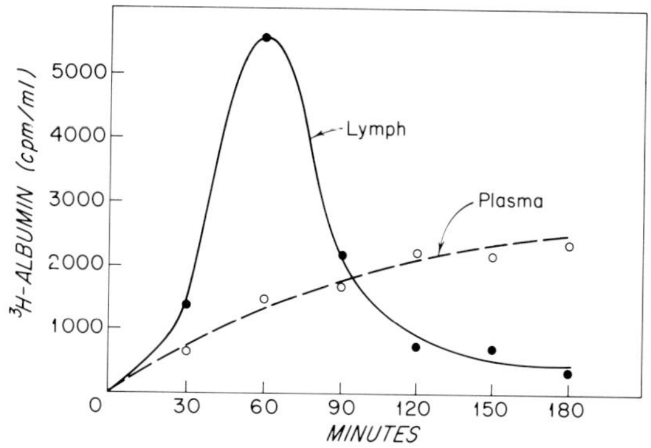

Fig. 1. Specific activities of dialyzed intestinal lymph and portal plasma at intervals after infusion of ^{3}H-BSA into the duodenal lumen.

Table II. *Specific activity of dialyzed portal plasma and systemic plasma 3 hours after infusion of ^{3}H-BSA into the duodenal lumen*

Animal No.	*Specific activity (c.p.m./ml.)*	
	Portal plasma	*Systemic plasma*
1	2,320	1,220
2	6,320	4,560
3	4,630	3,320
4	3,030	2,400
5	1,180	760
6	890	720

transmission into the intestinal lymph and portal blood. We have shown that approximately 2 percent of the protein available in the lumen remains physically and immunologically intact during absorption.[24] An appreciably greater amount of the protein is, of course, broken down within the lumen or within the cell by lysosomal enzymes,[25] but the radioactivity of labelled polypeptides, amino acids, and free ^{3}H resulting from digestion of ^{3}H-BSA does not appear amid the macromolecule fraction we assay.[24]

In the experimental model used there is total diversion of intestinal lymph, uncontaminated by other lymph, and simultaneous cannulation of the portal vein, allowing sampling of portal blood without interference to flow. This arrangement has enabled us to show that absorption into the lymphatic and portal circulations are each *bona fide* pathways for the uptake of intact protein macromolecules from the gut. While transmission of absorbed protein into lymphatics has been suggested because of detection in intestinal lymph of BSA,[24] horseradish peroxidase,[6, 23] elastase,[10] α-chymotrypsin,[27] and Salmonella flagellar antigen,[5] the present observations establish conclusively that most of the absorbed protein appearing in the intestinal lymph gets there directly from the intestinal lumen and not via the portal system.

The amount of protein absorbed intact under these experimental conditions is estimated to be almost 2 percent of the dose presented. Although nutritionally insignificant, more than enough protein gets across the intestinal mucosal barrier to become hormonally effective,[17] toxigenic,[15, 17] and antigenic.[14] In particular, the fact that antigenic protein reaches the lymphatics from the intestinal lumen provides a mechanism for the direct sensitization of the regional lymphoid tissue of the gut and this supports the hypothesis that inflammatory bowel diseases, especially Crohn's disease and ulcerative colitis, may be the result of an immunologic reaction to absorbed sensitizing antigens.[16] Since absorption of antigen may vary from one area to another,[18] depending in part on local factors affecting the integrity of the mucosal barrier, the concept of antigen access to limited areas of lymphoid tissue could explain the tendency of Crohn's disease to involve segments of intestine. In addition, since more lymphoid tissue is available in the ilium and colon, uptake of antigen from the gut may result in more prominent reactions by these areas of intestine.

If protein can be absorbed intact under the conditions of these experiments (i.e., bypassing the stomach), we must ask whether intact protein absorption is in fact a normal and usual phenomenon. If it is, sensitization to the absorbed protein may also be normal and usual, and not lead routinely to disease. Evidence from this laboratory[19, 20] suggests that ingested proteins induce formation of antibodies which inhibit further absorption of those proteins, thus buttressing the mucosal barrier to transmucosal passage of intact protein. Factors which disturb that barrier are under investigation.

REFERENCES

1. Alpers, D. H., and Isselbacher, K. J.: Protein synthesis by rat intestinal mucosa. The role of ribonuclease, J. Biol. Chem. **242:** 5617, 1967.
2. Bernstein, I. D., and Ovary, Z.: Absorption of antigens from the gastrointestinal tract, Int. Arch. Allergy Appl. Immunol. **33:** 521, 1968.
3. Bray, G.: A simple efficient liquid scintillator for counting aqueous solutions in a liquid scintillation counter, Anal. Biochem. **1:** 279, 1960.
4. Cardell, R. R., Badenhausen, S., and Porter, K. R.: Intestinal triglyceride absorption in the rat, J. Cell Biol. **34:** 123, 1967.
5. Cooper, G. N., Halliday, W. J., and Thonard, J. C.: Immunological reactivity associated with antigens in the intestinal tracts of rats, J. Pathol. Bacteriol. **93:** 223, 1967.
6. Cornell, R., Walker, W. A., and Isselbacher, K. J.: Small intestinal absorption of horseradish peroxidase: A cytochemical study, Lab. Invest. **25:** 42, 1971.
7. Danforth, E., Jr., and Moore, R. O.: Intestinal absorption of insulin in the rat, Endocrinology **65:** 118, 1959.
8. Gerrard, J. W., MacKenzie, J. W. A., Goluboff, N., et al.: Cow's milk allergy: Prevalence and manifestations in an unselected series of newborns, Acta Pediatr. Scand. (Suppl.) **234:** 1, 1973.
9. Graney, D.: The uptake of ferritin by ileal absorptive cells in suckling rats. An electron microscopic study, J. Anat. **123:** 227, 1968.
10. Katayama, K., and Fujita, T.: Studies on biotransformation of elastase: II. Intestinal absorption of ^{131}I-labeled elastase in vivo, Biochem. Biophys. Acta **288:** 181, 1972.
11. Korenblat, R. E., Rothberg, R. M., Murden, P., et al.: Immune response of human adults after oral and parenteral exposure to bovine serum albumin, J. Allergy **41:** 226, 1968.
12. Lambert, R.: Surgery of the digestive system in the rat, Springfield, Ill., 1965, Charles C Thomas, Publisher.
13. Lowry, O. H., Rosebrough, N. J., Farr, A. L., et al.: Protein measurement with Folin phenol reagent, J. Biol. Chem. **193:** 265, 1951.
14. Rothberg, R. M.: Immunoglobulin and specific antibody synthesis during the first weeks of life of premature infants, J. Pediatr. **75:** 391, 1969.
15. Serebro, H. A., McGonagle, T., Iber, F. L., et al.: An effect of cholera toxin on small intestine without direct mucosal contact, Johns Hopkins Med. J. **125:** 229, 1968.
16. Shorter, R. G., Huizenga, K. A., and Spen-

cer, R. J.: A working hypothesis for the etiology and pathogenesis of non-specific inflammatory bowel disease, Dig. Dis. **17:** 1024, 1972.

17. Vaughn-Williams, E. M., and Dohadwalla, A. N.: Experimental cholera: Observations relevant to toxin-absorption hypothesis, J. Infect. Dis. **120:** 652, 1969.
18. Walker, W. A., Cornell, R., Davenport, L. M., and Isselbacher, K. J.: Macromolecular absorption: Mechanism of horseradish peroxidase uptake and transport in adult and neonatal rat intestine, J. Cell Biol. **54:** 195, 1972.
19. Walker, W. A., Isselbacher, K. J., and Bloch, K. J.: Intestinal uptake of macromolecules: Effect of oral immunization, Science **177:** 608, 1972.
20. Walker, W. A., Isselbacher, K. J., and Bloch, K. J.: Intestinal uptake of macromolecules. II. Effect of parenteral immunization, J. Immunol. **111:** 221, 1973.
21. Walker, W. A., and Isselbacher, K. J.: Uptake and transport of macromolecules by the intestine: possible role in clinical disorders, Gastroenterology **67:** 1974.
22. Warshaw, A. L.: A simplified method of cannulating the intestinal lymphatic of the rat, Gut **13:** 66, 1972.
23. Warshaw, A. L., Walker, W. A., Cornell, R., et al.: Small intestinal permeability to macromolecules: Transmission of horseradish peroxidase into mesenteric lymph and portal blood, Lab. Invest. **25:** 675, 1971.
24. Warshaw, A. L., Walker, W. A., and Isselbacher, K. J.: Protein uptake by the intestine: evidence for absorption of intact macromolecules, Gastroenterology **66:** 987, 1974.
25. Weissman, G.: Lysosomes, N. Engl. J. Med. **273:** 1084 and 1143, 1965.
26. Wilzbach, K. E.: Tritium-labeling by exposure of organic compounds to tritium gas, J. Am. Chem. Soc. **79:** 1013, 1957.
27. Yamaguchi, K., Moriwaki, C., and Moriya, H.: Abstr. 91st Ann. Meet. Pharm. Soc. Japan, 230, 1971 (cited in ref. 10).

Dissolution of gallstones with bile salts, lecithin, and heparin

Laurence Y. Cheung, M.D., Edwin Englert, Jr., M.D., Frank G. Moody, M.D., *and* **Eugene E. Wales,** *Salt Lake City, Utah*

The solubility of human cholesterol gallstones in the individual bile salts in physiological concentration with and without the addition of lecithin and heparin was studied in in vitro experiments. Unconjugated deoxycholate (100 mM.) with lecithin solution (100 mM.) was the most effective solution for dissolving human cholesterol gallstones. The addition of heparin at a concentration of 1,000 U. per 10 ml. did not increase the solubilizing capacity of deoxycholate. Optimal dissolution of gallstones required renewal of the solutions. These results indicate that unconjugated deoxycholate with lecithin has potential use as an effective solution for chemical dissolution of retained bile duct stones via T-tube infusion. However, its safety and toxicity by T-tube continuous infusion are unknown and warrant further study.

From the Departments of Surgery and Medicine, University of Utah Medical Center, and Veterans Administration Hospital, Salt Lake City, Utah.

HUMAN CHOLESTEROL gallstones can be dissolved in vitro in micellar bile salt solutions[5, 9, 11, 13] and in vivo in the gallbladder of the dog, pig, and sheep[13] and in man by feeding bile salts.[2-4, 6, 15] Recently Way and associates[17] have reported that retained bile duct stones were eliminated in 12 of 22 patients by continuous infusion of cholic acid via T tube. However, 10 to 14 days of therapy were required in most of the cases. Its effectiveness may be improved if a more potent solution could be used. Solubilizing capacities of several individual bile salts have been reported,[5, 9, 12, 14] but the results were not uniform. The purpose of this investigation was to systematically evaluate the solubility of human cholesterol gallstones in the various bile salt solutions in physiological concentration with and without the addition of lecithin and heparin.

MATERIAL AND METHODS

Gallstones were collected at operation with a sterile technique and placed in the patient's own bile. Stones were grossly typical of mixed cholesterol gallstones and were analyzed qualitatively to assure cholesterol content.[10] Gallstones of similar size and weight obtained from the same patient were placed in 10 ml. of 150 mM. sodium phosphate buffer solution (pH 8) containing one of the bile salts* (100 mM.) with and

Accepted for publication June 18, 1974.

This work was supported in part by research Grants 5356 and AM14584 from the NIAMDD, National Institutes of Health, Bethesda, Md.

Presented at the Annual Meeting of the Western Section of American Federation for Clinical Research, Carmel, Calif., Feb. 7, 1974.

Reprint requests: Laurence Y. Cheung, M.D., Department of Surgery and Medicine, University of Utah Medical Center and Veterans Administration Hospital, Salt Lake City, Utah 84112.

*Pure bile salts were supplied by Kolir and Karas Laboratory, Plainview, N. Y., and Steraloids, Inc., Pawling, N. Y.

Table I. *Human cholesterol gallstone dissolution in various bile salt solutions (mean ± S.D.)*

Solutions#	No.	Original wt. (mg.)	Wt. at 7 days (mg.)	Difference in wt. (mg.)	Wt. loss (%)
Saline	9	155.1 ± 85.4	149.3 ± 57.0	5.7 ± 5.4	3.8 ± 3.4
Buffer§	9	170.4 ± 44.4	161.5 ± 44.3	9.0 ± 7.3	5.4 ± 4.6
Deoxycholate*	17	158.2 ± 43.5	124.7 ± 41.9	33.4 ± 8.5	21.9 ± 6.8†
Taurodeoxycholate	5	152.7 ± 37.7	133.5 ± 35.1	19.2 ± 6.1	12.8 ± 4.0
Glycodeoxycholate	5	162.7 ± 48.9	141.8 ± 44.9	20.8 ± 6.3	13.1 ± 3.4
Chenodeoxycholate*	5	158.4 ± 40.7	130.8 ± 9.4	27.8 ± 6.4	18.0 ± 3.9
Cholate*	5	171.3 ± 29.5	153.0 ± 26.8	18.3 ± 4.8	10.7 ± 2.2
Deoxycholate‖ plus lecithin	6	160.7 ± 26.2	117.3 ± 22.3	43.3 ± 4.2	27.2 ± 2.4‡
Deoxycholate plus heparin¶	5	163.8 ± 15.7	130.3 ± 17.6	33.4 ± 2.8	20.6 ± 3.3

*$P < 0.005$ if compared to saline and buffer solution.

†$P < 0.005$ if compared to cholate, and $P < 0.025$ to taurodeoxycholate and glycodeoxycholate (Student's t test).

‡$P < 0.05$ if compared to deoxycholate solution alone.

§0.15M sodium phosphate buffer (pH 8).

‖Deoxycholate 100 mM. and lecithin 100 mM.

¶Deoxycholate 100 mM. and heparin 1,000 U. per 10 ml.

#All solutions were not changed.

without lecithin* and heparin and incubated at 37° C. Stones were removed every other day, dried at 70° C. for 90 minutes, and weighed. At the end of each experiment, cholesterol content in each solution was measured.[1]

RESULTS

Table I shows the differences in the capacity of the individual bile salt to dissolve cholesterol gallstones. Deoxycholate was the most effective bile salt ($p < 0.001$ by Student's t test when compared to saline or buffer solution) and was more effective than cholate ($p < 0.005$) and chenodeoxycholate. The addition of lecithin in six experiments produced a significant increase in the rate of gallstone dissolution. Unconjugated deoxycholate was more effective than its conjugates, but there was no significant difference between taurine and glycine conjugates. Spontaneous fragmentation of stones occurred in several experiments at 7 days in deoxycholate solution. The addition of heparin at concentrations of 1,000 units per 10 ml., suggested by Gardner and associates[8] in the clinical patients, did not increase solubilizing capacity.

*Lecithin (Dipalmitoyl) was supplied by Kolir and Karas Laboratory, Plainview, N. Y.

Fig. 1 illustrates the mean accelerated stone weight loss which occurred when deoxycholate was changed every other day compared to that in the same solution which was not changed at all ($p < 0.005$).

DISCUSSION

In this study, unconjugated deoxycholate was found to be the most effective bile salt to dissolve human cholesterol gallstones. This result agrees with those reported by Earnest and Admirand[5] and Way.[16] In contrast to their results and those of Neiderhiser and Roth[14] and Hegardt and Dam,[9] there was no significant difference between taurine and glycine conjugates. This discrepancy may be methodological, since the first group did not state that uniform stones from the same patient were studied and the second and third groups used crystalline cholesterol.

As previously reported with crystalline cholesterol,[13, 14] we have also shown with human cholesterol gallstones that the addition of lecithin at 100 mM. concentration enhanced the rate of dissolution.

As expected, size affected the rate of dissolution. Small stones lost relatively less absolute weight but showed a greater percent of weight change than large stones. This has been reported in human feeding experi-

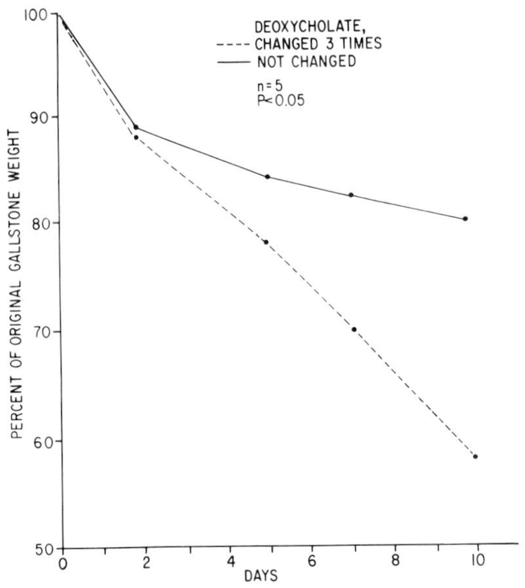

Fig. 1. The rate of gallstone weight loss in a solution of unchanged deoxycholate 100 mM. as compared to that in three changes of the same solution in 10 days.

ments as well.[2] At the end of each experiment, the relative amount of cholesterol solubilized in each solution correlated well with stone weight loss.

Fig. 1 shows that the mean stone weight loss in five experiments was accelerated significantly when deoxycholate solution was changed every other day. This result disagrees with those of Lutton and Large[13] who found uniform weight loss of stones for a period of 9 days whether or not the bile salt solution was changed. However, their experiment utilizing animal bile was not comparable to ours with a pure bile salt. From our experiment, it was concluded that saturation of pure bile salt solutions with cholesterol diminished further gallstone dissolution and that optimum dissolution required renewal of the bile salt solution.

Lahana and associates[12] have reported that cholic acid with heparin was the most effective solution to dissolve human cholesterol gallstones. However, gentle stirring and continuous bile flow were used in the preparation of their experiments. This discrepancy in results could be due to the methodological difference. Evans and Cussler[7] have demonstrated that gallstone dissolution varied widely with the rate of bile flow. At low flow it is controlled by the properties of the solution, at high flow, by the characteristics of the cholesterol surface. In patients with retained bile duct stones, bile flow varies according to the degree of obstruction by the retained stones and is not exactly known. Our previous experience in T-tube infusion of various solutions has been that only slow flow of infusion can be tolerated by most patients with retained bile duct stones. Therefore, we suggest that unconjugated deoxycholate with lecithin has the potential for use as an effective infusate for retained bile duct stones. However, its toxicity by T-tube infusion at this concentration is unknown and is currently being studied in our laboratory.

REFERENCES

1. Abell, L. L., Levy, V. V., Brodie, B. B., and Kendall, F. E.: A simplified method for the estimation of total cholesterol in serum and demonstration of its specificity, J. Biol. Chem. **195:** 357, 1952.
2. Bell, G. D., Whitney, B., and Dowling, R. H.: Gallstone dissolution in man using chenodeoxycholic acid, Lancet **2:** 1213, 1972.
3. Cole, W. H., and Harridge, W. H.: Disappearance of "stone" shadow in postoperative cholangiograms, J. A. M. A. **164:** 238, 1957.
4. Danzinger, R. G., Hofmann, A. F., Schoenfield, L. J., and Thistle, J. L.: Dissolution of cholesterol gallstones by chenodeoxycholic acid, N. Engl. J. Med. **286:** 1, 1972.
5. Earnest, D. L., and Admirand, W. H.: The effects of individual bile salts in cholesterol solubilization and gallstones dissolution, Gastroenterology **60:** 722, 1971.
6. Englert, E.: Gallstones: Production and shrinkage by diet, Actas Del X Congresson Panamericano de Gastroenterologia, Lima, Peru, 1967.
7. Evans, D. F., and Cussler, E. L.: Physiochemical considerations in gallstone pathogenesis, Hosp. Pract. **135:** 133, 1974.
8. Gardner, B., Ostrowitz, A., and Masur, R.: Reappraisal of possible role of heparin in dissolution of gallstones, SURGERY **69:** 854, 1971.
9. Hegardt, F. G., and Dam, H.: The solubility of cholesterol in aqueous solution of bile salts and lecithin, Z. Ernahrungswiss. **10:** 223, 1971.
10. Holt, P. E., and Tarnoky, A. L.: The analy-

sis of calculi using microchemical methods, J. Clin. Path. **6:** 114, 1953.
11. Johnson, C., and Nakayama, F.: Solubility of cholesterol gallstones in metabolic material, Arch. Surg. **75:** 436, 1957.
12. Lahana, A., Bonorris, G. G., and Schoenfield, L. J.: Dissolution of gallstone in vitro by bile acids, heparin, and quanternary amines (abst.), Gastroenterology **65:** 555, 1973.
13. Lutton, R. G., and Large, A. M.: Gallstones: Solubility studies, SURGERY **42:** 488, 1957.
14. Neiderhiser, D. H., and Roth, H. P.: Cholesterol solubilization by solutions of bile salts and bile salts plus lecithin, Proc. Soc. Exp. Biol. Med. **128:** 221, 1968.
15. Rewbridge, A. G.: The disappearance of gallstone shadows following the prolonged administration of bile salts, SURGERY **1:** 395, 1937.
16. Way, L. W.: In vitro dissolution of cholesterol gallstones, Surg. Forum **14:** 412, 1973.
17. Way, L. W., Admirand, W. H., and Dunphy, J. E.: Management of choledocholithiasis, Ann. Surg. **176:** 347, 1972.

Brief clinical reports

A technique for in situ repair of bipolar transvenous pacemaker electrode

Michael L. Gelfand, M.D., *and* **Robert M. Blumenberg, M.D.,** *Schenectady, N. Y.*

A simple method of pacemaker lead repair is described which uses readily available materials. There is no change or loss in pacemaker activity.

From the Departments of Surgery, Ellis Hospital, Schenectady, N. Y., and the Albany Medical College, Albany, N. Y.

IMPROVED materials and techniques in the preparation of transvenous endocardial pacemaker electrodes have obviated electrode replacement when the wires become fractured. This was recently demonstrated in the case of a patient who experienced acute flexion of the pacemaker lead with erosion through the skin. Two fractures developed in the silicone rubber coating with exposure of both electrodes at two points, even though the bipolar wires were intact. This report describes a method by which satisfactory repair of the silicone rubber defect was accomplished.

J. V., aged 85 years, initially underwent permanent pacemaker implantation on Nov. 11, 1970, at which time a Medtronic-Chardack 5816 lead and 5842 pacemaker were employed for complete heart block. The lead was introduced into the right ventricle via the right external jugular vein. On July 19, 1972, the pacemaker was replaced because it had ceased to function. The threshhold at that time was in excess of the maximum measurable 5 milliamperes. The right external jugular vein was not reusable, and the right cephalic was fibrosed secondary to previous cannulation attempts. As the left cephalic vein was extremely small and unsuitable, the left external jugular vein was the only available route for transvenous cannulation, other than the internal jugular veins. A Medtronic-Chardack 5818 bipolar lead and 5942 pacemaker were inserted. A pacemaker pouch seroma was drained on Aug. 11, 1972, which cultured coagulase-negative *Staphylococcus aureus*. Complete healing ensued in this extremely thin patient but, on Jan. 24, 1973, the pacemaker electrode was noted to have eroded through the skin in the left prepectoral region. Debridement of the area and secondary closure were performed; however, shortly after removal of the sutures, the exposed lead was again noted to have eroded through the chest wall. On Feb. 13, 1972, the patient underwent repair of the electrode in the manner described below and the lead was repositioned via the creation of a pectoral muscle flap transfer. The patient was discharged on Feb. 25, 1973, all wounds having healed cleanly with maintenance of excellent pacemaker electrode function. At the date of this writing, there have been no further wound or pacemaker electrode problems.

Accepted for publication May 23, 1974.

Reprint requests: Michael L. Gelfand, M.D., 1412 Union St., Schenectady, N. Y. 12308.

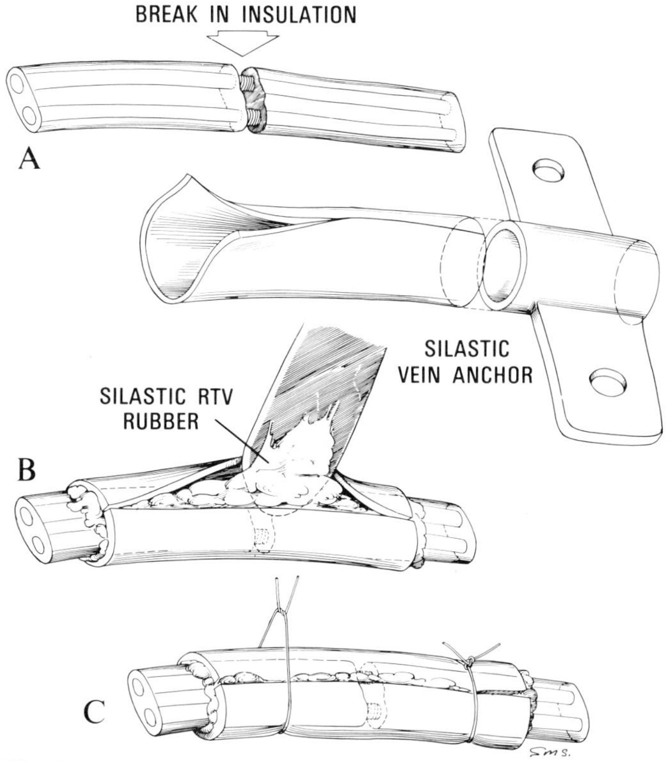

Fig. 1. Diagrammatic representation of the technique. See text.

TECHNIQUE OF REPAIR

A U-shaped portion of the bipolar electrode was noted to protrude through the site of erosion on the anterior chest wall. At the most acute point of flexion of the electrode there were two fractures in the silicon-rubber. Both wires were completely exposed in two areas approximately 1 cm. apart (Fig. 1, *A*). Although satisfactory pacing continued with the wire exposed, replacement of the exposed wires into a milieu rich in electrolyte fluid might induce either pacing of the chest wall muscles or short-circuiting of the lead with the loss of endocardial pacing. As the patient's only remaining available superficial vein—the left external jugular—might on removal of the electrode prove to be unusable, an attempt at electrode repair was begun. This was done in the following fashion: The protruding electrode was cleansed with acetone and patted dry. Silastic Brand Medical Adhesive Silicone Type A (Dow-Corning Corp.) was generously placed between and around the electrode wires and the adjacent damaged silicone rubber (Fig. 1, *B*). The Medtronic Silicone Rubber Lead Anchoring Sleeve was trimmed to an appropriate length, placed over the lead such that it extended proximal and distal to the points of fracture, and tied in place with interrupted sutures of 3-0 Tedvek (Fig. 1, *C*). During the course of opening the pacemaker pouch and the creation of the pectoral muscle flap transfers, the adhesive and the rubber became dry and intimately adherent. The lead was then placed in an area away from the site of previous erosion and a flap of pectoral muscle was sewn over it. No alteration or loss in pacemaker activity was noted at any time during the procedure. The pacemaker and lead have continued to function well to the date of this writing.

This simple method of pacemaker lead repair preserves an electrode with a damaged sheath in which the wires are exposed but intact. The readily available materials spared the changing of an otherwise well-functioning bipolar electrode.

Subclavian artery aneurysm; sequela of thoracic outlet syndrome

Stephen J. Mathes, M.D., *and* **Atef A. Salam, M.D.,** *Atlanta, Ga.*

A case of subclavian aneurysm secondary to thoracic outlet syndrome causing gangrene of the upper extremity is reported. The pathophysiology and the surgical treatment of this serious complication are discussed. The supraclavicular approach is recommended whenever a need for vascular reconstruction is anticipated.

From the Department of Surgery, Emory University School of Medicine, Atlanta, Ga.

SUBCLAVIAN aneurysm associated with thoracic outlet syndrome was recognized as early as 1831 by Mayo.[7, 20] Serious ischemia of the upper extremity may occur as a result of distal embolization or local thrombosis of the aneurysm itself. Recently we had the opportunity to document, clinically and angiographically, the natural course of this disease for a period of three years in a patient who initially refused surgical treatment.

CASE REPORT

A 53-year-old woman presented for treatment of severe, constant, rest pain in the entire right upper extremity. She had first noted the pain 3 years prior to this admission, following blunt trauma to her right wrist. Evaluation in the hospital at that time revealed complete bilateral cervical ribs[13] and absent right radial and ulnar pulses. An arteriogram then showed occlusion of the distal brachial artery with reconstitution in the distal one third of the forearm. The diagnosis of thoracic outlet syndrome was made and surgical treatment advised, but she declined. The patient was lost to follow-up until she presented for this admission with sloughing of the fingernails, extreme sensitivity to temperature changes, pregangrenous changes in hand and arm, and constant

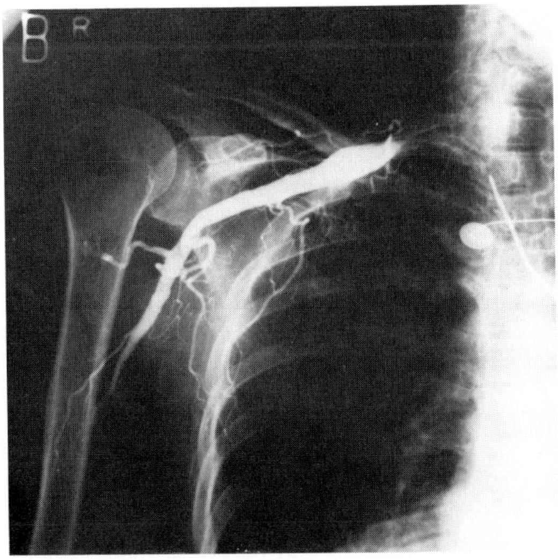

Fig. 1. Arteriogram revealing subclavian artery aneurysm with cervical rib.

rest pain which was no longer relieved by holding the arm in the dependent position. A pulsatile mass was felt in the right supraclavicular space, and brachial pulsations were present in the axillae, but they disappeared when Adson's[2] maneuver was performed. The right upper extremity was cyanotic, with gangrenous ulcers on two digits and extensive atrophy of the intrinsic hand muscles. Angiographic study of the upper extremity revealed an aneurysm of the subclavian artery, thrombosis of the entire brachial artery, and multiple filling defects in the profunda brachial artery

Accepted for publication May 23, 1974.

Reprint requests: Stephen J. Mathes, M.D., Department of Surgery, Emory University School of Medicine, 69 Butler St., S.E., Atlanta, Ga. 30303.

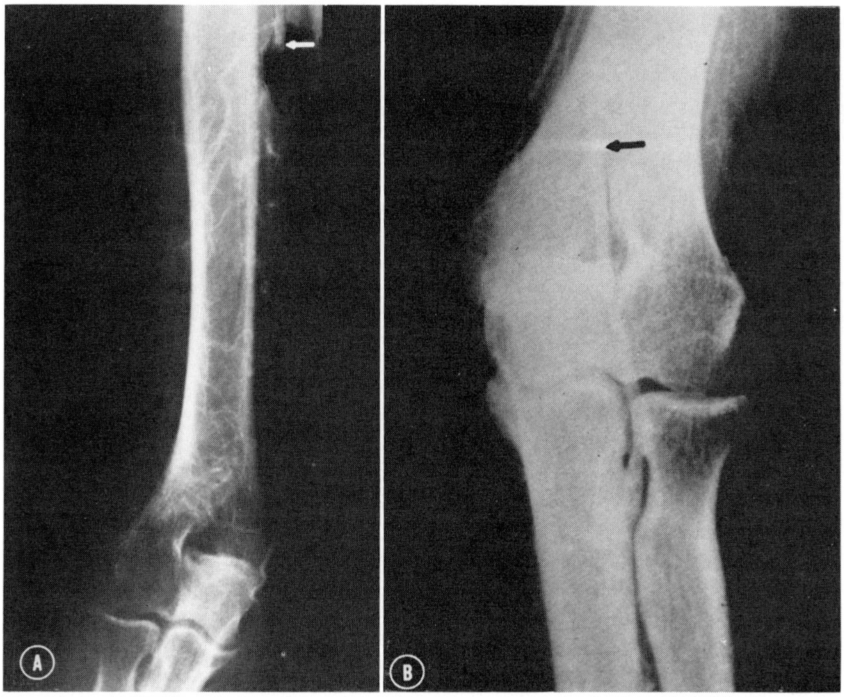

Fig. 2. *A,* Brachial artery occlusion level on first hospitalization at level of proximal brachial artery. *B,* Brachial artery occlusion level 3 years later at level of profunda brachial artery.

(Fig. 1). The cervical rib was excised with a supraclavicular approach[9, 29] and the subclavian aneurysm resected. The artery was repaired by end-to-end anastomosis. An attempt to use a saphenous vein bypass graft from the brachial to the radial artery failed because of the poor runoff. Ischemia persisted postoperatively, and 2 months later the hand was amputated.

COMMENTS

Major vascular complications due to thoracic outlet syndrome have received considerable interest in the English literature. In 1956, Schein and Haemocici[28] reviewed 29 cases; and in 1972, Judy and Heymann[16] collected 53 cases from the literature and added seven cases of their own. These authors' reviews indicate that major and minor amputations are not infrequently required in advanced thoracic outlet compression syndromes.

In 1916 Halsted[14] collected 27 cases of cervical rib with associated subclavian artery aneurysm. The majority of these had severe circulatory disturbances. In 1962 Wickham and Martin[33] brought the number of such cases to 57. Since that time, 16 more cases have been reported.[3, 4, 8, 15-17, 19, 21, 28, 30]

Murphy,[22] and later Schein and Haemocici,[28] described those events which regularly attend the vascular scalene tunnel due to either cervical rib or anomalous first rib wherein there is intermittent positional compression of the subclavian artery. The mechanism by which this mechanical compression leads to aneurysm formation is not exactly known. In 1917 Halsted[14] noted that blood in a vessel beyond a constriction streams in whirlpool effect. Later he produced poststenotic aortic dilatation experimentally in dogs' aortas, concluding that these aneurysms resulted from turbulent flow. Bruns and associates[5] confirmed this thesis, showing that structural fatigue resulting from turbulent flow beyond the arterial constriction may cause aneurysm formation. A combination of the turbulent flow and repeated mechanical trauma to the subclavian artery can lead to aneurysmal formation and/or intramural thrombosis. Another mechanism for the development of subclavian artery aneurysm was

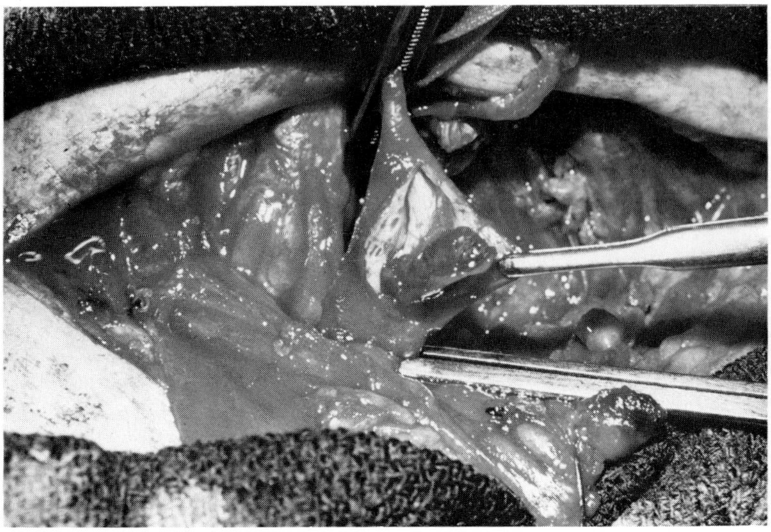

Fig. 3. Subclavian aneurysm arteriotomy revealing thrombus (not seen in arteriogram in Fig. 2).

described by Todd[32] in 1911 and Telford[31] in 1931. They proposed that irritation of sympathetic fibers in the thoracic outlet caused contraction and thrombosis of vasa vasorum. This thesis is not widely accepted; in our case no such abnormality was detected on microscopic study of the aneurysmal wall.

Emboli from subclavian artery aneurysm associated with cervical rib causing vascular symptoms were first recognized[8] by Symonds. His case demonstrated proximal spread of thrombosis, reaching the bifurcation of the innominate artery and causing hemiplegia. The natural tendency of distal embolization to recur and to cause progressive vascular ischemia is well demonstrated by the case history of our patient (Fig. 2). Similar experience has been reported by other investigators.[8, 23, 28]

The findings in our case support the observation of Rob and Standeven[23] that once the occlusive process involves the bifurcation of the brachial artery, the danger of limb loss becomes very imminent. Unlike more proximal brachial artery occlusion, this area is seldom able to develop satisfactory collateral support. As a result, further progression of the clotting process distally may occur.

At the onset of thoracic outlet syndrome, postural compression of the subclavian artery can be detected clinically by certain provocative maneuvers. These maneuvers employ actions by the patient to decrease the interscalene space and increase existing compression of the subclavian artery. They include having the patient hold his breath with his neck extended and his chin turned to the symptomatic side.[1] The radial pulse may also decrease or disappear if the involved extremity is abducted and externally rotated, or if the patient is placed in the exaggerated military position.[10, 34] It should be emphasized that obliteration of the radial pulse by these provocative maneuvers can be elicited frequently in asymptomatic patients.[34] Arteriography is the only reliable means for differentiating between extrinsic arterial compression and such arterial lesions as aneurysms or arterial thrombosis. Since the latter lesions require arterial reconstruction, the surgeon should be aware of their presence preoperatively so he will choose an approach that is adequate for this purpose. In addition, he will be able to plan the reconstructive procedure according to the arteriographic appearance of the arteries distally. It should be emphasized that a sizable thrombus may be present in the aneurysm in the absence of any filling defects in the arteriogram (Figs. 1 and 3).

The presence of ischemic symptoms, which are unrelated to posture, in a patient with demonstrable subclavian aneurysm secondary to thoracic outlet syndrome should be considered as an indication for urgent surgical treatment. These symptoms are manifestations of recurrent thromboembolism and, because of their progressive nature, undue delay of the operation may lead to loss of the extremity, as is clearly demonstrated in our case.

Four main approaches have been described for the surgical correction of the thoracic outlet syndrome. These are the supraclavicular,[9, 29] infraclavicular,[12] posterior (periscapular),[6, 11, 18, 24] and transaxillary[25, 27] approaches. There is general agreement that the operative treatment must include division of the scalenus anticus and medius, as well as resection of the offending rib. The axillary approach which was originally described by Roos[26] offers an excellent exposure for the excision of the first rib. It requires minimal dissection and offers the best cosmetic result. The use of this approach for the excision of a cervical rib may, however, be less satisfactory. Roos[25] has stated in his original article that the axillary approach could be used for the surgical correction of subclavian artery aneurysm associated with thoracic outlet syndrome. Conversely, we recommend the supraclavicular route whenever the need for vascular reconstruction is anticipated. The latter approach provides direct access to the subclavian artery and, should more proximal exposure of the artery be required, the incision can readily be extended to reflect a costosternal flap.

REFERENCES

1. Adson, A. W.: Cervical ribs: Symptoms, differential diagnosis for section of the insertion of the scalenus anticus muscle, J. Int. Coll. Surg. **16:** 546, 1951.
2. Adson, A. W.: Surgical treatment of symptoms produced by cervical ribs and scalenus anticus muscle, Surg. Gynecol. Obstet. **85:** 687, 1947.
3. Billington, W.: Excision of subclavian aneurysm associated with cervical rib, Br. J. Surg. **19:** 334, 1931.
4. Bretelsen, S., Mathiesen, F. R., and Ohlenschlager, H. H.: Vascular complications of cervical rib, Scand. J. Thorac. Cardiovasc. Surg. **2:** 133, 1968.
5. Bruns, D. L., Connolly, J. E., Holman, E., and Stofer, R. C.: Experimental observations on post-stenotic dilatation, J. Thorac. Cardiovasc. Surg. **38:** 662, 1959.
6. Clagett, O. T.: Presidential address: Research and prosearch, J. Thorac. Cardiovasc. Surg. **44:** 153, 1962.
7. Coote, H.: Exostosis of the left transverse process of the seventh cervical vertebrae surrounded by blood vessels and nerves; successful removal, Lancet **1:** 360, 1861.
8. Cunning, A. J.: Mural thrombosis of the subclavian artery and subsequent embolism in cervical rib, Q. J. Med. **33:** 133, 1964.
9. Falconer, M. A., and Li, F. W.: Resection of first rib in costoclavicular compression of the brachial plexus, Lancet **1:** 59, 1962.
10. Falconer, M. A., and Weddel, G.: Costoclavicular compression of the subclavian artery and vein: Relation to the scalenus anticus syndrome, Lancet **2:** 539, 1943.
11. Ferguson, T. B., Burford, T. H., and Roper, C. L.: Neurovascular compression at the superior thoracic aperature: Surgical management, Ann. Surg. **167:** 573, 1968.
12. Gol, A., Patrick, D. W., and McNeal, D. P.: Relief of costoclavicular syndrome by infraclavicular removal of first rib, J. Neurosurg. **28:** 81, 1968.
13. Gruber, W.: Ueber die Halsrippen des Menschen mit vergluchend anatomischen Bermerkunken, Mem. Acad. Imp. Sci. (St. Petersburg) **12:** 1869.
14. Halsted, W. S.: An experimental study of circumscribed dilation of an artery immediately distal to a partially occluding band and its bearing on the dilation of the subclavian artery observed in certain cases of cervical rib, J. Exp. Med. **24:** 271, 1916.
15. Harris, J. D., and Jepson, R. P.: Vascular complications of cervical ribs, Aust. N. Z. J. Surg. **34:** 269, 1964.
16. Judy, K., and Haymann, R. L.: Vascular complications of thoracic outlet syndrome, Am. J. Surg. **123:** 521, 1972.
17. Lindskog, G. E., and Howes, E. L.: Cervical rib with aneurysm of subclavian artery, Arch. Surg. **34:** 310, 1937.
18. Longo, M. F., Clagett, O. T., and Fairbarn, T. F.: Surgical treatment of thoracic outlet syndrome, Ann. Surg. **171:** 538, 1970.
19. Lord, J., Jr.: Thoracic outlet syndrome, current management, Ann. Surg. **173:** 700, 1971.
20. Mayo, H.: Exostosis of the first rib with strong pulsations of the subclavian artery, London Med. Phys. J. (N.S.) **11:** 40, 1831.
21. Moore, C. A.: A case of subclavian aneurysm with cervical rib, Lancet **1:** 1045, 1922.

22. Murphy, J. B.: Case of cervical rib with symptoms resembling subclavian aneurysm, Ann. Surg. **41:** 399, 1905.
23. Rob, C. G., and Standeven, A.: Arterial occlusion complicating thoracic outlet compression syndrome, Br. Med. J. **2:** 709, 1958.
24. Roeder, D. K., Mills, J. J., McHale, B. M., et al.: First rib resection in the treatment of thoracic outlet syndrome, Am. Surg. **178:** 49, 1973.
25. Roos, D. B.: Experience with first rib resection for thoracic outlet syndrome, Ann. Surg. **173:** 429, 1971.
26. Roos, D. B.: Transaxillary approach for first rib resection to relieve thoracic outlet syndrome, Ann. Surg. **163:** 354, 1966.
27. Roos, D. B., and Owens, J. C.: Thoracic outlet syndrome, Arch. Surg. **93:** 71, 1966.
28. Schein, C. J., Haemocici, J., and Young, H.: Arterial thrombosis associated with cervical ribs: Surgical considerations, SURGERY **40:** 420, 1956.
29. Schein, C. J.: Technique for cervical rib resection, Am. J. Surg. **121:** 623, 1971.
30. Shucksmith, H. S.: Cerebral and peripheral emboli caused by cervical ribs, Br. Med. J. **2:** 835, 1963.
31. Telford, E. D.: Two cases of cervical rib with vascular symptoms, Lancet **2:** 1116, 1913.
32. Todd, T. W.: The relations of the thoracic operculum considered in reference to the anatomy of cervical ribs of surgical importance, J. Anat. Physiol. (London) 1911.
33. Wickham, J. E. A., and Martin, P.: Aneurysm of the subclavian artery in association with cervical abnormality, Br. J. Surg. **50:** 205, 1963.
34. Wright, I. S.: The neurovascular syndrome produced by hyperabduction of the arms, Am. Heart J. **29:** 1, 1945.

Cystic adventitial degeneration of the common femoral artery

Daniel K. Lowe, M.D., Frederick G. Winegarner, M.D., *and* **John E. Jesseph, M.D.,**
Indianapolis, Ind.

This is a rare case of cystic adventitial degeneration occurring in the common femoral artery. All but five reported cases of this disease were located in the popliteal artery. The cause is unknown. Simple cyst evacuation is effective in most cases but the diagnosis must be made early. The long-term prognosis is good.

From the Department of Surgery, Indiana University School of Medicine, Indianapolis, Ind.

An adventitial cyst involving the external iliac artery was first recognized and reported in 1946 by Atkins and Key.[1] Since then 50 other cases have been reported in the literature, 42 involving the popliteal artery and the others the radial and ulnar arteries. Most of the case reports and descriptions of the lesion have come from the British and Australian literature. This article reports a case of adventitial degeneration involving the common femoral artery. This lesion is a rare cause of claudication in the young and can be corrected simply if detected early. More and more cases of this lesion are being reported now that arteriography is more common, and this disease entity should be included in the differential diagnosis of claudication. An incidence has been suggested of one per 1,000 studies.

CASE REPORT

A 27-year-old Caucasian man presented with right leg claudication on walking 100 yards. There was no past history of hypertension, heart disease, generalized arterial disease, diabetes mellitus, or renal disease. In August of the same year, four months previously, he had required emergency oversewing of a duodenal ulcer with vagotomy and pyloroplasty for massive upper gastrointestinal hemorrhage.

Distal pulses were normal at that time and during his hospital stay he did not have any arterial or venous punctures in his legs or groins. He made an uneventful recovery but soon after hospitalization noticed the onset of claudication. Physical examination on this admission showed a blood pressure of 120/80 mm. Hg and a pulse of 80 per minute. The only positive physical findings were related to the right lower extremity. A bruit was heard over the right common femoral artery but the pulse was strong. The right popliteal, dorsalis pedis, and posterior tibial pulses were diminished. Findings in the left leg were normal. Exercise caused marked diminution of distal pulses in the right leg but none in the left. Dependent rubor appeared in the right foot after elevation of both legs for 5 minutes.

Laboratory studies showed normal fasting and 2 hour postprandial blood sugar, serum cholesterol, triglycerides, and serum lipoprotein electrophoresis. An electrocardiogram was normal. An aortogram showed concentric narrowing of the right common femoral artery with 50 percent occlusion. There was no evidence of any other lesions.

Impression at this time was that he had a significant occlusion of the right common femoral artery, but after the arteriogram the pulses were

Accepted for publication May 27, 1974.

Reprint requests: Frederick G. Winegarner, M.D., Department of Surgery, Indiana University School of Medicine, 1100 W. Michigan St., Indianapolis, Ind. 46202.

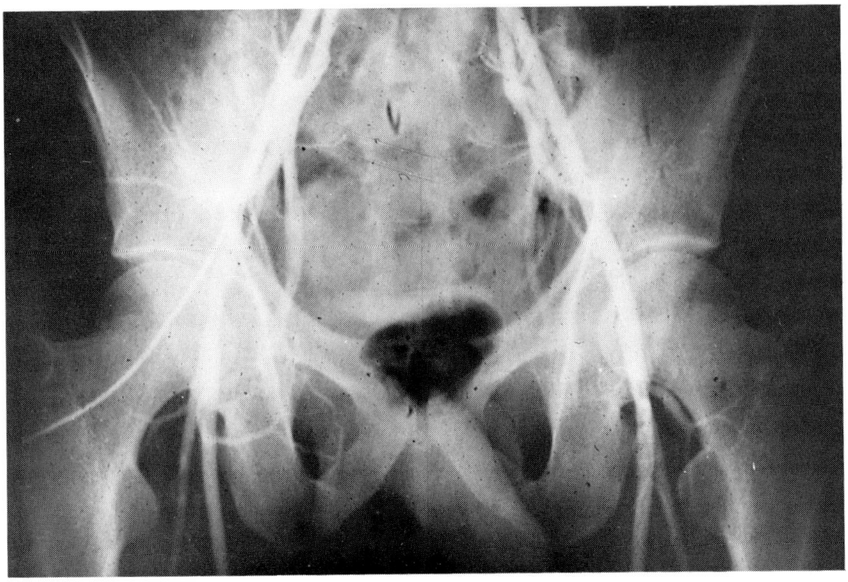

Fig. 1. Angiogram showing 3 cm. stenotic area in distal right common femoral artery.

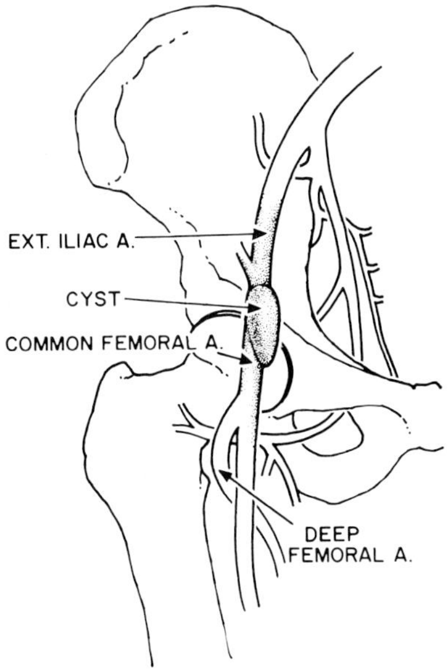

Fig. 2. Diagram showing location of common femoral arterial cyst, 1 by 3 by 1 cm.

improved. For this reason the patient was sent home, but he continued to have symptoms and subsequently was readmitted.

The right common femoral artery was explored through a vertical incision. Just proximal to the deep profunda femoral artery a cystic structure was seen enveloping the anterior and medial aspect of the common femoral artery, 3 cm. long and 1.5 cm. wide (Fig. 1). The arterial lesion appeared to be at the level of narrowing seen on the radiograph and was located directly anterior to the hip joint (Fig. 2). The cyst was dissected free from the media of the artery and was excised without entering the artery. Postoperatively the patient had good femoral, popliteal, dorsalis pedis, and posterior tibial pulses. Following uneventful wound healing exercise stress no longer caused diminished pulses. Presently he is able to walk unlimited distances without complaints.

DISCUSSION

This young man presented with the acute onset of ischemic symptoms due to an unusual cause of claudication—cystic adventitial degeneration. This case has many typical features of this rare disease: acute onset of symptoms of ischemia in a man between the ages of 30 and 50, a bruit heard over the involved artery, decreased pulses found with exercise, a positive "scimitar sign" seen on angiograph, and a cyst filled with clear gelatinous material partially occluding the artery. The region involved in this case is atypical. Of the 50 cases reported in the literature since 1946, 43 involved the popliteal artery and seven others involved the following arteries: two, the radial artery; one, the ulnar artery, three, the external iliac artery, and one, the common femoral.

Surgical exploration typically reveals a unilocular cyst arising from the media and adventitia. The cyst usually contains a clear, gelatinous fluid much like that of the ganglia associated with tendon sheaths and joints. Chemical analysis of the fluid suggests that the material might be derived from degenerated collagen because of the significant amount of hydroxyproline as analyzed by Harris and Jepson.[10] Others have not been able to confirm these findings and suggest that, because of the glucosamine and amino acid concentrations found, the fluid is a mucoprotein.

Theories of the pathogenesis of the cyst formation have been trauma, a generalized connective tissue disorder, and a developmental inclusion of mucin-secreting cells within the arterial wall. The cysts are located most commonly in the popliteal artery, which suggests trauma as an etiology. The rare occurrence of this entity, however, rules out minor trauma as the cause and major trauma is rarely coincident by history. The disorder is not secondary to any generalized disorder in connective tissue because of the usual localization to the popliteal artery and the paucity of other signs or symptoms. Developmental inclusion of mucinous cells in the wall of the artery is an attractive theory because of the closeness of the cyst to joint spaces. Trauma may initiate production of the mucin by these included cells. As the cyst enlarges, mucin production continues, with even minor trauma accelerating cyst enlargement. This may account for the rapid production of symptoms.

The natural history of the lesion has been described by Hierton and others.[11] The cyst begins in the adventitia and enlarges, causing pressure injury to the media and intima. With significant stenosis the onset of claudication occurs which precedes eventual thrombosis and occlusion. The time span of these events is not known but radiographically few collaterals are seen with the stenotic or occluded vessel and the onset of symptoms is characteristically acute, suggesting a rapid course.

Diagnosis of the condition is primarily by angiographic means with a curvilinear stenosis seen in the involved artery—the scimitar sign. The artery frequently is involved over a length of several centimeters, with skip areas of involvement seen at times from multiple cysts. Surgical correction has been recently well discussed by Haid and colleagues,[8] with numerous follow-up findings from cases previously reported. The conclusion reached was that conservative measures, such as cyst evacuation or simple excision without resection of the artery, are effective in the majority of cases. With extensive medial or intimal damage and occlusion of the vessel, excision and reconstruction becomes necessary. Long-term prognosis is excellent. Haid reported that no amputations were necessary even with graft failure and no other cystic degeneration occurred in any other arteries in the cases reported.

REFERENCES

1. Atkins, H., and Key, J.: A case of myxomatous tumour arising in the adventitia of the left external iliac artery, Br. J. Surg. **34:** 426, 1946.
2. Bäckström, C., Linell, F., and Östberg, G.: Cystic, myxomatous adventitial degeneration of the radial artery with development of ganglion in the connective tissue, Acta Chir. Scand. **129:** 447, 1965.
3. Barnett, A., Dugdale, L., and Ferguson, I.: Disappearing pulse syndrome due to myxomatous degeneration of the popliteal artery, Med. J. Aust. **2:** 355, 1966.
4. Bliss, B., Rhodes, J., and Harding Rains, A.: Cystic myxomatous degeneration of popliteal artery, Br. Med. J. Oct. **5:** 847, 1963.
5. Campbell, R., McCluskey, B., and Andrews, M.: A case of polycystic adventitial disease of the left external iliac and femoral artery, Br. J. Surg. **57:** 865, 1970.
6. Chandler, J., and Burks, W.: Popliteal artery occlusion by subadventitial pseudocyst: Case report and summary of world literature, SURGERY **69:** 474, 1971.
7. Flanc, C.: Cystic degeneration of the popliteal artery, Aust. N. Z. J. Surg. **36:** 243, 1967.
8. Haid, S., Conn, J., and Bergan, J.: Cystic adventitial disease of the popliteal artery, SURGERY **101:** 765, 1970.
9. Hamming, J., and Vink, M.: Obstruction of the popliteal artery at an early age, J. Cardiovasc. Surg. **6:** 516, 1965.
10. Harris, J., and Jepson, R.: Cystic degeneration of the popliteal artery, Aust. N. Z. J. Surg. **34:** 265, 1965.
11. Hierton, T., Lindberg, K., and Rob, C.: Cystic

degeneration of the popliteal artery, Br. J. Surg. **44:** 348, 1957.
12. Holmes, J.: Cystic adventitial degeneration of the popliteal artery, J. A. M. A. **173:** 654, 1960.
13. Ishikawa, K., Mishima, Y., and Kobayashi, S.: Cystic adventitial disease of the popliteal artery, Angiology **12:** 357, 1961.
14. Lambley, D.: Intermittent claudication due to cystic degeneration of the popliteal artery, Br. Med. J. **2:** 849, 1963.
15. Leaf, G.: Addendum: Ammino-acid analysis of protein present in a popliteal artery cyst, Br. Med. J. **3:** 415, 1967.
16. Lewis, G., Douglas, D., Reid, W., and Kennedy Watt, J.: Br. Med. J. **3:** 411, 1967.
17. Little, J., and Goodman, A.: Cystic adventitial disease of the popliteal artery, Br. J. Surg. **57:** 708, 1970.
18. Milliken, J.: Cystic degeneration of the popliteal artery in a female, Br. Med. J. **2:** 769, 1971.
19. Powis, S., Morissey, D., and Jones, E.: Cystic degeneration of the popliteal artery, SURGERY **67:** 891, 1970.
20. Robb, D.: Obstruction of popliteal artery by synovial cyst, Br. J. Surg. **48:** 221, 1960.
21. Weston, T., Thompson, H., and Ardagh, J.: Cystic myxomatous degeneration of the popliteal artery, Aust. Radiol. **13:** 383, 1969.

Pathogenesis of peptic ulcer: A selective review

John J. Skillman, M.D., *Boston, Mass.*

All benign acute and chronic peptic ulcers of the stomach and duodenum are acid-peptic dissolutions of the gastric and duodenal mucosa. The underlying pathophysiological mechanisms involved appear to be distinctly different, however, in the various forms of this disease. This selective review examines the mechanisms involved in these related disorders.

From the Department of Surgery, Harvard Medical School, and the Beth Israel Hospital, Boston, Mass.

THE PATHOGENESIS of benign peptic ulcer of the stomach and duodenum remains a controversial subject. In this brief review, I will examine selectively some of the earlier work together with recent new information which provide insight into the etiology of chronic benign gastric and duodenal ulcer and acute stress ulcer. I should emphasize at the outset that this review is a highly selective critique of a large amount of material and will, therefore, exclude contributions by many excellent workers.

A. GASTRIC ULCER

Considerable difference of opinion still exists concerning the origin of gastric ulcer. Dragstedt and associates[25] originally proposed the hypothesis in 1954 that gastric ulcers develop because of stasis in the stomach which results in hypersecretion of antral gastrin. The conclusion that this hypothesis explains the development of chronic gastric ulcer can now be challenged.

1. Dragstedt's theory. The ingenious series of experiments performed by Dragstedt and his coworkers[24] were stimulated by careful clinical evaluation of patients who were treated for duodenal ulcer. Dragstedt observed that five of 131 patients who were observed after supradiaphragmatic vagotomy developed new gastric ulcers in the postoperative period, but gastric ulcer did *not* develop in more than 800 patients with duodenal ulcer who were treated by vagotomy and gastroenterostomy to prevent stasis. This observation was followed by an investigation of gastric secretion in dogs prepared with Heidenhain pouches (devoid of vagus nerve innervation). When these animals were subjected to vagus nerve section performed within the chest or immediately below the diaphragm, a marked and long-continued increase in the output of gastric juice from the Heidenhain pouch was observed.[29] Gastroenterostomy prevented the increase in

This work was supported by United States Public Health Service Grant No. AM15681 and by a grant from the John A. Hartford Foundation.

This article is based on a discussion presented at the Postgraduate Course in Gastrointestinal Physiology, American College of Surgeons Meeting, Chicago, Ill., October, 1973.

Accepted for publication May 15, 1974.

Reprint requests: John J. Skillman, M.D., Department of Surgery, Beth Israel Hospital, Harvard Medical School, Boston, Mass. 02215.

gastric secretion seen in similarly prepared animals. Dragstedt and associates[26] then observed that when the antrum of a dog was transplanted as a diverticulum into the side of the transverse colon, a profound increase in gastric secretion of the separated isolated stomach developed and ulceration of the stomach regularly occurred. In other experiments in which the antrum was transplanted into the colon and the gastric remnant was drained into the duodenum or jejunum, the ulcers developed not in the stomach, but in the vicinity of the gastroenterostomy stoma, invariably on the intestinal side.

These observations formed the basis for Dragstedt's concept that gastric ulcers are caused by exessive release of gastrin during the digestive phase of acid secretion, a concept which has dominated the thinking of surgeons interested in this field for at least 15 years. However, the consistent finding of low acid secretion (both of volume and concentration[3, 49]) in patients with gastric ulcer has never been adequately explained. Only in patients with pyloric stenosis due to concomitant duodenal ulcer has it been possible to demonstrate that patients with gastric ulcer have antral stasis.[11] Even if hypergastrinemia were unequivocally established in patients with gastric ulcer, a point over which there is controversy,[10, 73] such a correlation would not necessarily establish a causal relationship between increased serum gastrin levels and the presence of ulceration. Patients with pernicious anemia and total achlorhydria have severe hypergastrinemia[53] but no ulcers. Hypergastrinemia in such patients may simply be the result of an absence of antral inhibition by acid. Studies by Trudeau and McGuigan[73] suggest an inverse relation between fasting serum gastrin concentrations and the secretion of hydrochloric acid.

2. Relationships between the gastric mucosal barrier, back-diffusion of acid, bile reflux, and gastritis and pyloric sphincter dysfunction in patients with gastric ulcer. The low acid concentration found in the stomachs of patients with gastric ulcer has been explained by hyposecretion of gastric acid, but Davenport[21] suggested in 1965 that the hyposecretion might be more apparent than real, and that excessive loss of secreted acid might be occurring by "back-diffusion" of secreted hydrogen ion into a gastric mucosa which had developed an abnormal permeability to acid. Although the existence of a barrier in the stomach resistant to the diffusion of hydrogen ion from lumen to mucosa was proposed over 35 years ago by Teorell,[71] experiments by Davenport beginning in 1964 stimulated new investigation of this important concept in laboratory animals and in man. Teorell[69, 70] proposed that there was a continuous exchange diffusion of hydrogen for sodium in the stomach, a process he called "back-diffusion," which accounted for the reduction of acidity. Although Teorell recognized that there might be a "certain degree of influence from a diluting and slightly neutralizing mucus secretion," particularly in normal subjects with small acidic gastric volumes, he rejected the importance of Hollander's[43-45] two-component theory of gastric secretion as being an unnecessary assumption of the mechanism of regulation of acidity and variation of chloride.

Teorell's work was largely forgotten until the recent classic work of Davenport, which stimulated new investigation of the gastric mucosal barrier. Davenport re-explored the important question asked by many previous physiologists, such as Claude Bernard and Pavlov, namely, why doesn't the normal stomach digest itself? In order to answer this question he studied the nature of the gastric mucosal barrier, a barrier which normally maintains a concentration gradient of hydrogen ion with respect to plasma of 1,000,000:1. Davenport[17-20] investigated the effect of a variety of agents which were instilled into the stomach and were associated with an increased lumen-to-mucosa movement of hydrogen ions. He postulated that the effect of these agents on the gastric mucosa was related to their ability to attack the lipoprotein layer of cell walls. He showed in canine fundic pouches that aspirin,[20] alcohol,[19] bile,[17] and pancreatic juice[18] all result in an increased permeability of the stomach to acid. Support to Davenport's[21] concept that the low acid secretion seen in patients with gastric ulcer might be at least in part related to an abnormal permeability of the gastric mucosa to hydrogen ion was provided by the studies of Chapman, Werther, and Janowitz[13] and Overholt and Pollard.[58] These two groups showed that the stomachs of patients with pernicious anemia, gastritis, and gastric ulcer do show an increased permeability to an instilled acid load in comparison to those of patients without these diseases. An abnormal gastric mucosal barrier appears to be one important factor in the pathogenesis of gastric ulcer. It seems most likely, however, that this is a secondary phenomenon which results from the effect of injurious agents such as bile and pancreatic juice which often bathe the stomach in excess amounts in patients with this disease.

The almost universal occurrence of chronic gastritis in the stomachs of patients with gastric ulcer has received a great deal of attention in recent years.[11, 28] Du Plessis[28] studied the occurrence of chronic atrophic gastritis in 18 patients with duodenal ulcer and 75 patients with gastric ulcer and found that there was severe chronic gastritis in 61 of 75 stomachs resected for gastric ulcer. This process was more severe in the pyloric gland area than in the fundic gland area. Gastric ulcers occurred in the area affected by chronic gastritis and were located in the zone of atrophic mucous membrane abutting on normal acid and pepsin-secreting fundic mucosa. The studies of Oi and co-workers[57] indicate that essentially all chronic benign gastric ulcers are found in an area of mucosa incapable of secreting acid.

A large body of evidence is now available which strongly suggests that the reflux of bile and pancreatic juice into the stomach is causally related to the development of chronic gastritis and the subsequent development of gastric ulcer. This evidence may be summarized as follows.

1. Gastric ulcer is invariably associated with chronic atrophic gastritis.[28]

2. Drainage of duodenal content into the stomach of dogs, either by reflux or directly, can produce a chronic superficial gastritis which is most pronounced in the antrum.[52]

3. Du Plessis[28] investigated the fasting resting gastric juice for the presence of bile acid conjugates in patients with a variety of gastrointestinal diseases and found that there was a high concentration of these conjugates in patients with gastric ulcer and after gastrectomy, but a low concentration was observed in patients without dyspepsia and in patients with dyspepsia unrelated to ulcer disease.

4. Dragstedt and associates[27] examined in dogs the question of bile regurgitation as a cause for the development of gastric ulcer by various modifications of the McCann experimental procedure, in which duodenal content is drained into the fundic portion of the stomach and intestinal continuity is reestablished by gastrojejunostomy. Dragstedt reported that ulcers did not occur in the stomach or at the gastroduodenostomy when duodenal juices were diverted into the stomach of these animals by an anastomosis between the lower duodenum and antral border of the stomach. Intestinal continuity was restored in these animals by an anastomosis between the distal end of divided duodenum and the pyloric end of the stomach. In other modifications of the McCann procedure, in which bile and pancreatic juice were diverted into the lower esophagus by either an end-to-side esophagoduodenostomy or an end-to-side esophagojejunostomy, Dragstedt reported that ulcers occurred in some animals in the duodenum near the gastroduodenostomy or in the jejunum near the gastrojejunostomy, but ulcers were never found in the esophagus or stomach. Microscopic examination of the stomachs in many of the animals were reported to show gastritis of varying extent. Dragstedt concluded that these experiments provided no support for the theory that gastric ulcers are caused by regurgitation of bile and pancreatic juice into the stomach.

These conclusions may be criticized, however, because no measurements of the pH of the gastric content in these experiments were reported. Although it is known that increased gastric mucosal permeability may occur after exposure to bile salts at a pH of 8.0,[7] back-diffusion of acid is quantitatively less at this high pH than at a low pH (pH 2.0). The absence of dectectable gross ulceration of the stomach in Dragstedt's experiments may, therefore, be related to the small quantity of hydrogen ion which was available for back-diffusion because of neutralization of gastric acid by bicarbonate from bile and pancreatic juice. If, on the other hand, the gastric contents were extremely acid, the bile acids may have precipitated and, therefore, been rendered inactive by virtue of their insolubility in the gastric content. Also, since gastritis was observed in many of the animals, it may be that there was not enough time for bile and pancreatic juice to produce grossly detectable gastric ulceration.

5. Ivey and co-workers[47] have shown that when a mixture of hydrochloric acid (160 mEq. per liter) and taurine-conjugated bile salts (84 percent taurocholic acid, 14 percent taurodeoxycholic acid, and 2 percent taurochenodeoxycholic acid) is instilled into the normal human stomach in concentrations equal to those found in the stomach of patients with gastric ulcers (5.5 mM.),[61] a significant increase in the back-diffusion of hydrogen ion occurs.

6. When food or acid is ejected by the stomach into the duodenum of normal man, the pyloric sphincter closes to prevent reflux of duodenal juices into the stomach. Fisher and Cohen[31] reported recently that pyloric sphincter dysfunction is responsible for increased duodenogastric reflux in patients with gastric ulcer. These investigators studied 10 patients with gastric ulcer before and after healing and 10 normal patients matched for age and sex. Basal pyloric pressure did not differ significantly between those patients with a normal stomach and patients who had a gastric ulcer. However, duodenal acidification with 0.1N hydrochloric acid was associated with an increased pyloric pressure and diminished duodenogastric reflux in normal subjects, but not in patients with gastric ulcer. Stimulation of endogenous hormone release by the intraduodenal instillation of olive oil and amino acids or exogenous administration of secretin and cholecystokinin also failed to produce a rise in plyloric pressure in patients with gastric ulcer. After healing of the ulcer, the pyloric sphincter still showed no response to hormonal stimulation. Wormsley[76] has reported similar results in patients with gastric ulcer and this investigator also showed that patients with duodenal ulcer have a pyloric mechanism which is near normal. One may conclude from these studies that an important reason for reflux of duodenal juices in patients with gastric ulcer has been clarified.

All these lines of evidence strongly support the concept of a causal relationship between an abnormal pyloric sphincter mechanism resulting in increased bile reflux, chronic gastritis, an increased permeability of the gastric mucosa to hydrogen ion, and the subsequent development of gastric ulcer.

B. DUODENAL ULCER

Although individual patients with duodenal ulcer may have normal acid secretion, most patients with this disease, and especially those whose duodenal ulcer is a severe clinical problem, have increased gastric acid secretion[78] and an increased parietal cell mass.[12] Although increased vagal activity was considered by Dragstedt to be the cause of increased gastric acid secretion in patients with duodenal ulcer, the fact that vagotomy abolishes the hypersecretion does not necessarily support such a cause-and-effect relationship.[39] It is known, for example, that vagotomy decreases the gastric secretory response to all stimuli of gastric acid secretion. Since the maximal capacity of the stomach to secrete acid is not diminished by vagotomy (although the maximal acid-forming capacity must be restored by drugs which restore cholinergic tone),[9, 39] it appears that increased vagal activity is not the cause of increased gastric secretory capacity. Grossman[39] has also pointed out that the percentage reduction in acid secretion seen after vagotomy in patients with duodenal ulcer is only slightly less in those patients with high acid secretion in comparison to patients with low preoperative acid secretion.

New information concerning the hormonal relationships in patients with duodenal ulcer and the mechanism of acid disposal by the duodenum appear to be importantly related to the development of duodenal ulcer.

1. Hypergastrinemia. Jaffe, McGuigan, and Newton[48] and Becker, Reeder, and Thompson[4] have confirmed the earlier classical observations of Uvnäs[74] and Thein and Schofield[72] that vagal stimulation does indeed release gastrin. Jaffe and co-workers[48] showed in dogs that vagal stimulation induced by insulin hypoglycemia initiates the release of gastrin at blood glucose concentrations of 43 ± 11 mg. per 100 ml. Although Trudeau and McGuigan[73] found an inverse correlation between fasting serum gastrin concentrations and the secretion of hydrochloric acid by the stomach and also noted normal serum gastrin levels in patients with duodenal ulcer disease, Brynes and co-workers[10] and Reeder and associates[60] showed that patients with duodenal ulcer have increased levels of serum gastrin, both in the fasting and fed states, in comparison to normal patients or patients with gastric ulcer. The discrepancies in these reports may represent differences in the immunoassay system, since Trudeau and McGuigan[73] used an antiserum raised against human gastrin 1,[38] while Brynes and co-workers[10] used an antiserum prepared against pentagastrin. In addition, Brynes and co-workers showed that patients with duodenal ulcer had a larger incremental secretion of gastrin after protein digestion than normal patients or patients with gastric ulcer. These recent observations suggest that caution is justified in the acceptance of the validity of Dragstedt's hypothesis of vagal overactivity as a primary causal mechanism in the etiology of chronic benign duodenal ulcer.

2. Disposal of acid by the duodenum. Secretin and cholecystokinin are released by the duodenal mucosa when hydrochloric acid enters the duodenum. These hormones stimulate the flow of bicarbonate-rich pancreatic juice, bile, and Brunner's gland secretion, all of which dilute and neutralize the acid. Recent investigations of the disposal of acid by the human duodenum indicate that there is a marked capacity of the duodenal mucosa to dispose of acid by the combined mechanisms of neutralization, dilution, and insorption directly through the duodenal mucosa.[75] Winship and co-workers[75] found that the disposal of acid by the proximal 1 cm. of human duodenum is a saturable process which is probably related to a limitation of the secretion of bile and pancreatic juice. In the more distal 15 cm. portion of duodenum studied by these workers it appeared that hydrogen ion absorption directly through the duodenal mucosa might be an important mechanism of acid removal, although the possibility that bicarbonate was entering the lumen by the mechanisms of diffusion or secretion could not be excluded. Another exploration of these important duodenal protective mechanisms was performed in dogs by Dorricott, Fiddian-Green, and Silen.[23] These investigators studied distal duodenal Thiry pouches chronically excluded from the intestinal stream. A constant circulation technique using isosmolor solutions containing 60 to 120 mM. hydrochloric acid was employed in these experiments. This preparation excluded the pancreatic and proximal duodenal bicarbonate contribution to duodenal acid disposal. These workers found that the duodenum can dispose of a large amount of acid by a mechanism which is independent of the alkaline secretions of the biliary tract, pancreas, and Brunner's glands. The acid disposal seen in these experiments appeared to be dependent on the concentration of hydrogen ion in the perfusate, data which are consistent with the experimental findings of King and Schloerb.[51] In the experiments of Dorricott and co-workers about two thirds of the disappearance of acid was related to neutralization by bicarbonate and the remainder of the acid was lost by back-diffusion by a one-to-one transmural exchange of hydrogen for sodium. In these experiments chronic distal duodenal pouches disposed of less acid than similarly prepared acute pouches, an effect which may be related to repeated episodes of acid exposure. This observation may possibly be relevant to the pathogenesis of chronic duodenal ulcer in man, where a defective response to the removal of acid in the duodenum has been suggested.[77]

Hypergastrinemia, increased acid secretion, and defective acid disposal appear to be involved in the pathogenesis of duodenal ulcer disease, but one can only speculate on the precise role that each of these factors contribute to the digestion of the duodenal mucosa.

C. ACUTE STRESS ULCERS

Acute gastrointestinal ulceration may occur with a variety of systemic conditions such as trauma,[32, 33, 40] operation,[5, 34] central nervous system disease,[16] burns,[15, 63] hypertension, sepsis, respiratory failure, uremia, and jaundice.[30, 64] Although acute ulcerations which develop in all of these conditions are commonly grouped together as stress ulcers, many features of these ulcers suggest a varied pathogenesis.[66, 67]

1. Gastric mucosal permeability. Davenport[17-20] has shown that damage to canine gastric mucosa induced by a variety of chemical agents results in increased lumen-to-mucosa back-diffusion of hydrogen ions. Many critically ill patients and patients with diseases of the stomach have similarly been found to have greatly increased gastric mucosal permeability to hydrogen ion.[13, 58, 65] Excess intake of aspirin or alcohol, agents which also produce an increased back-diffusion of acid in man,[68] is definitely associated with clinically significant drug-induced erosive gastritis.[1, 37, 59] This latter condition should be sharply distinguished from true stress ulceration, however, since the clinical course of drug-induced gastritis is usually less severe than that seen in sick postoperative patients who develop acute ulceration. Steroids potentiate the increased permeability of the gastric mucosa to hydrogen ions which is caused by bile salts, aspirin, and acetic acid, while alone they do not cause disruption of the gastric mucosal barrier.[2, 14]

2. Effects of ischemia. An episode of shock almost invariably precedes the development of acute gastric ulceration in man. A decrease in mucosal blood flow seems to be the underlying mechanism for the development of experimentally induced acute gastric ulceration in rats (pyloric occlusion plus intraperitoneal epinephrine,[62] rabbits (hemorrhagic shock),[42, 65] and pigs (hemorrhagic shock).[35] All studies of hemorrhagic shock[22, 54] have shown that ulceration occurs only when acid is present in the stomach. Although back-diffusion of acid was not detected by the experimental technique employed by Moody and Aldrete,[54] it is significant that ulcers developed in these experiments *only* when acid was present. Studies of hemorrhagic shock in the dog show a high incidence of multiple gastric ulcerations.[41] In these latter experiments the gastric lesions were invariably preceded by reflux of duodenal content into the stomach. Inhibition of the trypsin in the chyme prevented the associated intestinal lesions and also prevented the development of acute gastric ulceration. Alternatively, pyloric occlusion, which excluded duodenal chyme from the stomach, also significantly reduced the incidence and severity of the gastric ulcerations. These experiments strongly suggest that in hemorrhagic shock, the gastric mucosal barrier may be disrupted by reflux of duodenal content into the stomach. This factor may be operative in many sick patients with ileus. In addition, experiments performed in canine vagally denervated fundic pouches have shown that gastric mucosal blood flow (studied by the aminopyrine clearance technique) is decreased by acid solutions containing 10 or 40 mM. solutions of sodium taurocholate or 20 mM. solutions of aspirin.[56] This suggests that these agents may be damaging to the gastric mucosa not only by causing back diffusion of hydrogen ion but also by producing mucosal ischemia.

Large quantities of pepsin are released by many agents which produce disruption of the gastric mucosal barrier.[50] In the presence of ischemia and acid, release of pepsin may be an additional potent ulcerative factor in these patients. Even a small amount of acid appears to be capable of producing these lesions in the presence of ischemia. Although anoxia by itself does not produce a large increase in back-diffusion in experimental in vitro preparations of gastric mucosa,[6] the combined effects of ischemia and other damaging agents regularly produce ulceration.[22]

A recent study[36] of gastric mucosal permeability in a group of 13 patients with general surgical problems and nine patients with neurological disease confirmed an earlier report[65] that gastric mucosal permeability was increased when multiple complications (hypotension, sepsis, respiratory and renal failure, and jaundice) were present. The neurosurgical patients had normal gastric mucosal permeability but greatly increased gastric acid secretion and pepsin secretion in comparison to the sickest group of general surgical patients. Patients from this study who bled (gastric aspirate greater than 2+ guaiac for three consecutive hours in the 12 hour period prior to study) had a significantly increased gastric mucosal permeability and higher incidence of clinical complications in comparison to the patients who did not bleed. A relationship between increased gastric mucosal permeability and bleeding was strongly supported by this latter study. A study of serum gastrin levels in patients injured in Vietnam indicates that patients with central nervous system injury have significantly higher levels of serum gastrin than those without injury of the nervous system,[8] although there was no relationship between the levels of serum gastrin and the subsequent development of stress ulcer in these patients. It is possible that the higher levels of serum gastrin seen in these patients with central nervous system injury are related to increased vagal activity. Support for this suggestion is provided by several studies of patients with head injury which show elevated gastric acid secretion[36, 55] and elevated concentrations of acid and pepsin in the gastric juice.[46]

Circumstantial evidence seems reasonably strong that ischemia, the presence of even small amounts of acid, and disruption of the gastric mucosal barrier which leads to increased back-diffusion of hydrogen ion are all key factors in the genesis of acute gastrointestinal ulceration. Bile reflux into the stomach may aid the development of this form of peptic ulcer in the same way that it produces a problem in patients with chronic benign gastric ulcer, namely, by increasing the back-diffusion of hydrogen ion and possibly also by producing mucosal ischemia.

REFERENCES

1. Alvarez, A. S., and Summerskill, W. H. J.: Gastrointestinal hemorrhage and salicylates, Lancet **2:** 920, 1958.
2. Aubrey, D. A., and Burns, G. P.: Topically administered prednisolone and the antral phase of gastric secretion, Arch. Surg. (Chicago) **105:** 467, 1972.
3. Baron, J. H.: An assessment of the augmented histamine test in the diagnosis of peptic ulcer, Gut **4:** 243, 1963.
4. Becker, H. D., Reeder, D. D., and Thompson, J. C.: Direct measurement of vagal release of gastrin, SURGERY **75:** 101, 1974.
5. Beil, A. R., Jr., Mannix, H., Jr., and Beal, J. M.: Massive upper gastrointestinal hemorrhage after operation, Am. J. Surg. **108:** 324, 1964.
6. Birkett, D., and Silen, W.: Effect of severe anoxia and sodium taurocholate on H^+ loss from luminal surface of in vitro gastric mucosa, Surg. Forum **24:** 421, 1973.
7. Black, R. B., Hole, D., and Rhodes, J.: Bile damage to the gastric mucosal barrier: the influence of pH and bile acid concentration, Gastroenterology **61:** 178, 1971.
8. Bowen, J. C., Fleming, W. H., and Thompson, J. C.: Elevated serum gastrin levels in Vietnam casualties with CNS injury, Surg. Forum **24:** 351, 1973.
9. Broome, A.: Mechanism of vagotomy-induced suppression of the maximal acid response to histamine in antrectomized duodenal ulcer patients, Scand. J. Gastroenterol. **2:** 275, 1967.
10. Brynes, D. J., Young, J. D., Chisholm, D. J., and Lazarus, L.: Serum gastrin in patients with peptic ulceration, Br. Med. J. **2:** 626, 1970.
11. Capper, W. M.: Factors in the pathogenesis of gastric ulcer, Ann. R. Coll. Surg. (Eng.) **40:** 21, 1967.
12. Card, W. I., and Marks, I. N.: The relationship between acid output of the stomach following "maximal" histamine stimulation and the parietal cell mass, Clin. Sci. **19:** 147, 1960.
13. Chapman, M. A., Werther, J. L., and Janowitz, H. D.: Responses of the normal and pathological human gastric mucosa to an in-

stilled acid load, Gastroenterology **50:** 344, 1968.

14. Chung, R. S. K., Field, M., and Silen, W.: Gastric mucosal permeability to H^+: Effects of prednisolone and acetylsalicylic acid on the co-efficient of H^+ diffusion, Gastroenterology **58:** 1038, 1970.
15. Curling, T. B.: On acute ulceration of the duodenum in cases of burn, Med. Chir. Trans. **25:** 260, 1842.
16. Cushing, H.: Peptic ulcers and the interbrain, Surg. Gynecol. Obstet. **55:** 1, 1932.
17. Davenport, H. W.: Destruction of the gastric mucosal barrier by detergents and urea, Gastroenterology **54:** 175, 1968.
18. Davenport, H. W.: Effects of lysolecithin, digitonin and phospholipase A upon the dog's gastric mucosal barrier, Gastroenterology **59:** 505, 1970.
19. Davenport, H. W.: Ethanol damage to canine oxyntic glandular mucosa, Proc. Soc. Exp. Biol. Med. **126:** 657, 1967.
20. Davenport, H. W.: Gastric mucosal injury by fatty and acetylsalicylic acids, Gastroenterology **46:** 245, 1964.
21. Davenport, H. W.: Is the apparent hyposecretion of acid by patients with gastric ulcer a consequence of a broken barrier to diffusion of hydrogen ions into the gastric mucosa? Gut **6:** 513, 1965.
22. Den Besten, L., and Hamza, K. N.: Effect of bile salts on ionic permeability of canine gastric mucosa during experimental shock, Gastroenterology **62:** 417, 1972.
23. Dorricott, N. J., Fiddian-Green, R. G., and Silen, W.: Mechanisms of acid disposal in canine duodenum, Am. J. Physiol. In press.
24. Dragstedt, L. R., Camp, E. H., and Fritz, J. M.: Recurrence of gastric ulcer after complete vagotomy, Ann. Surg. **30:** 843, 1949.
25. Dragstedt, L. R., Oberhelman, H. A., Jr., Evans, S. O., and Rigler, S. P.: Antrum hyperfunction and gastric ulcer, Ann. Surg. **140:** 396, 1954.
26. Dragstedt, L. R., Oberhelman, H. A., Jr., and Smith, C. A.: Experimental hyperfunction of the gastric antrum with ulcer formation, Ann. Surg. **134:** 332, 1951.
27. Dragstedt, L. R., Woodward, E. R., Seito, T., Isaza, J., Rodriguez, J. R., and Samiian, R.: The question bile regurgitation as a cause of gastric ulcer, Ann. Surg. **174:** 548, 1971.
28. Du Plessis, D. J.: Pathogenesis of gastric ulceration, Lancet **1:** 974, 1965.
29. Evans, S. O., Jr., Zubiran, J. M., McCarthy, J. D., Ragins, H., Woodward, E. R., and Dragstedt, L. R.: Stimulating effect of vagotomy on gastric secretion in Heidenhain pouch dogs, Am. J. Physiol. **174:** 219, 1953.
30. Fischer, R. P., and Stremple, J. F.: Stress ulcers in post-traumatic renal insufficiency in patients from Vietnam, Surg. Gynecol. Obstet. **134:** 790, 1972.
31. Fisher, R. S., and Cohen, S.: Pyloric-sphincter dysfunction in patients with gastric ulcer, N. Engl. J. Med. **288:** 273, 1973.
32. Fletcher, D. G., and Harkins, H. N.: Acute peptic ulcer as a complication of major surgery, stress or trauma, SURGERY **36:** 212, 1954.
33. Fogelman, J. J., and Garvey, J. M.: Acute gastrointestinal ulceration incidence to surgery and disease: Analysis and review of 88 cases, Am. J. Surg. **112:** 651, 1966.
34. Goodman, A. A., and Frey, C. F.: Massive upper gastrointestinal hemorrhage following surgical operations, Ann. Surg. **167:** 180, 1968.
35. Goodman, A. A., and Osborne, M. P.: An experimental model and clinical definition of stress ulceration, Surg. Gynecol. Obstet. **124:** 563, 1972.
36. Gordon, M. J., Skillman, J. J., Zervas, N. T., and Silen, W.: Divergent nature of gastric mucosal permeability and gastric acid secretion in sick patients with general surgical and neurological disease, Ann. Surg. **178:** 285, 1973.
37. Goulston, K., and Cooke, A. R.: Alcohol, aspirin and gastrointestinal bleeding, Br. Med. J. **4:** 664, 1968.
38. Gregory, R. A., Hardy, P. M., Jones, D. S., Kenner, G. W., and Shepperd, R. C.: The antral hormone gastrin: Structure of gastrin, Nature (London) **204:** 931, 1964.
39. Grossman, M. I.: Some minor heresies about vagotomy, Gastroenterology. In press.
40. Grosz, C. R., and Wu, K. T.: Stress ulcers: A survey of the experience of a large general hospital, SURGERY **61:** 853, 1967.
41. Guilbert, J., Bounous, G., and Gurd, F. N.: Role of intestinal chyme in the pathogenesis of gastric ulceration following experimental hemorrhagic shock, J. Trauma **9:** 723, 1969.
42. Harjola, P. A., and Sivula, A.: Gastric ulcerations following experimentally induced hypoxia and hemorrhagic shock: In vivo study in pathogenesis in rabbits, Ann. Surg. **163:** 21, 1966.
43. Hollander, F.: Bicarbonate in mucinous secretions from canine gastric pouches, *in* XXII International Congress of Physiological Science, Sept. 10-17, 1962, Abstracts of Free Communication, Amsterdam, 1973, Excerpta Medica Foundation, abst. No. 392.
44. Hollander, F.: Gastric secretion of electrolytes, Fed. Proc. **11:** 706, 1952.
45. Hollander, F.: Studies in gastric secretion.

IV. Variations of the chlorine content of gastric juice and their significance, J. Biol. Chem. **97:** 585, 1932.
46. Idjadi, F., Robbins, R., Stahl, W. M., and Essiet, G.: Prospective study of gastric secretion in stressed patients with intracranial injury, J. Trauma **11:** 681, 1971.
47. Ivey, K. J., Den Besten, L., and Clifton, J. A.: Effects of bile salts on ionic movement across the human gastric mucosa, Gastroenterology **59:** 683, 1970.
48. Jaffe, B. M., McGuigan, J. E., and Newton, W. T.: Immunochemical measurement of vagal release of gastrin, SURGERY **68:** 196, 1970.
49. James, A. H., and Pickering, G. W.: The role of the gastric acidity in the pathogenesis of peptic ulcer, Clin. Sci. **8:** 181, 1949.
50. Johnson, L. R.: Pepsin secretion during damage by ethanol and salicylic acid, Gastroenterology **62:** 412, 1972.
51. King, C. R., and Schloerb, P. R.: Gastric juice neutralization in the duodenum, Surg. Gynecol. Obstet. **135:** 22, 1972.
52. Lawson, H. H.: Effect of duodenal contents on the gastric mucosa under experimental conditions, Lancet **1:** 469, 1964.
53. McGuigan, J. E., and Trudeau, W. L.: Serum gastrin concentrations in pernicious anemia, N. Engl. J. Med. **282:** 358, 1970.
54. Moody, F. G., and Aldrete, J. S.: Hydrogen permeability of canine gastric secretory epithelium during formation of superficial erosions, SURGERY **70:** 154, 1971.
55. Norton, L., Greer, J., and Eisemen, B.: Gastric secretory response to head injury, Arch. Surg. **101:** 200, 1970.
56. O'Brien, P., and Silen, W.: Effect of bile salts and aspirin on the gastric mucosal blood flow, Gastroenterology **64:** 246, 1973.
57. Oi, M., Oshida, K., and Sugimara, S.: The location of gastric ulcer, Gastroenterology **36:** 45, 1959.
58. Overholt, B. F., and Pollard, H. M.: Acid diffusion into the human gastric mucosa, Gastroenterology **54:** 182, 1968.
59. Palmer, E. D.: Gastritis: A re-evaluation, Medicine (Baltimore) **33:** 199, 1954.
60. Reeder, D. D., Jackson, J., Ban, J. L., Davidson, W. D., and Thompson, J. C.: Effect of food on serum gastrin concentrations in duodenal ulcer and control patients, Surg. Forum **21:** 290, 1970.
61. Rhodes, J., Barnado, D. E., Phillips, S. F., Rovelstad, R. A., and Hoffman, A. F.: Increased reflux of bile into the stomach in patients with gastric ulcer, Gastroenterology **57:** 241, 1969.
62. Sethbhakdi, S., Pfeiffer, C. J., and Roth, J. L. A.: Gastric mucosal ulceration following vasoactive agents: A new experimental model, Am. J. Dig. Dis. **15:** 1055, 1970.
63. Sevitt, S.: Duodenal and gastric ulceration after burning, Br. J. Surg. **54:** 32, 1967.
64. Skillman, J. J., Bushnell, L. S., Goldman, H., and Silen, W.: Respiratory failure, hypotension, sepsis and jaundice: A clinical syndrome associated with lethal hemorrhage from acute ulceration of the stomach, Am. J. Surg. **117:** 523, 1969.
65. Skillman, J. J., Gould, S. A., Chung, R. S. K., and Silen, W.: The gastric mucosal barrier: Clinical and experimental studies in critically ill and normal man, and in the rabbit, Ann. Surg. **172:** 564, 1970.
66. Skillman, J. J., and Silen, W.: Acute gastrointestinal "stress" ulceration: Barrier disruption of varied pathogenesis, Gastroenterology **59:** 478, 1970.
67. Skillman, J. J., and Silen, W.: Stress ulcers, Lancet **2:** 87, 1972.
68. Smith, B. M., Skillman, J. J., Edwards, B. G., and Silen, W.: Permeability of the human gastric mucosa: Alteration by acetylsalicylic acid and ethanol, N. Engl. J. Med. **285:** 716, 1971.
69. Teorell, T.: On the permeability of the stomach mucosa for acids and some other substances, J. Gen. Physiol. **23:** 263, 1939.
70. Teorell, T.: On the primary acidity of the gastric juice, J. Physiol. (Lond.) **97:** 308, 1940.
71. Teorell, T.: Untersuchungen über die magensaftsekretion, Scand. Arch. Physiol. **66:** 225, 1933.
72. Thein, M. P., and Schofield, B.: Release of gastrin from the pyloric antrum following vagal stimulation by sham feeding in dogs, J. Physiol. (Lond.) **148:** 291, 1959.
73. Trudeau, W. L., and McGuigan, J. E.: Relations between srum gastrin levels and rates of gastric hydrochloric acid secretion, N. Engl. J. Med. **284:** 408, 1971.
74. Uvnäs, B.: The part played by the pyloric region in the cephalic phase of gastric secretion, Acta Physiol. Scand. (Suppl. 13) **4:** 1, 1942.
75. Winship, D. H., Caflisch, C. R., and Schulte, W. J.: Acid loss in the human duodenum, J. Appl. Physiol. **32:** 585, 1972.
76. Wormsley, K. G.: Aspects of duodeno-gastric reflux in man, Gut **13:** 243, 1972.
77. Wormsley, K. G.: Reactions to acid in the intestine in health and disease, Gut **12:** 67, 1971.
78. Wormsley, K. G., and Grossman, M. I.: Maximal histalog test in control subjects and patients with peptic ulcer, Gut **6:** 427, 1965.

Letters to the editors

Lower abdominal tenderness following traumatic rupture of the spleen

To the Editors:

Many patients, especially the young, who have sustained a rupture of the spleen are not in overt hemorrhagic shock when first seen. A period of observation follows during which one may look for a shift in the pattern of abdominal tenderness while other examinations are taking place.

If the tenderness, originally in the left upper quadrant, extends to the lower abdomen, this is strong evidence that a fluid material irritating to the peritoneum is flowing downward. Cases reported attest to the value of this sign.

Case 1. A 14-year-old boy was struck in the left side while playing football 6 hours prior to admission to the hospital. He complained of mild upper abdominal pain. The pulse and blood pressure were within normal limits. Slight tenderness was found in the left upper abdominal quadrant. The hemoglobin was 12.7 Gm. and the hematocrit 37.5 percent. X-rays of the thorax and an intravenous pyelogram were negative. Four hours later there was marked tenderness in the left lower abdominal quadrant accompanied by rectal tenderness. Surgery revealed a rent on the diaphragmatic surface of the spleen with blood in the left colic gutter and pelvis as well as in the left upper quadrant.

Case 2. A 12-year-old boy also was injured in a football game. After supper he had begun his evening studying when his father, a physician, discovered the boy had left upper quadrant pain and admitted him to the hospital. The boy's pulse and blood pressure were normal on admission. He was tender in the left upper abdominal quadrant. The hemoglobin was 13.4 Gm. and the hematocrit 37 percent. X-rays of the chest and abdomen were negative. Four hours later, the maximum tenderness was in the left groin, accompanied by rectal tenderness. At surgery, a laceration of the diaphragmatic surface of the spleen was found with clots in the subphrenic space and a large amount of blood in left colic gutter and pelvis.

Case 3. A 36-year-old man was stabbed in the left lower chest with a small knife. He was admitted to the hospital for observation with slight tenderness in the left upper quadrant. Twenty-four hours later he developed a right upper and mid-abdominal tenderness without any drop in the hematocrit. He was explored and found to have a tear in his splenic capsule. A large amount of blood had migrated over the left lobe of the liver beneath the ligamentum teres and into the subhepatic space.

Case 4. A 34-year-old man who was being treated for infectious mononucleosis was awakened one morning by sneezing followed by pain and tenderness in his right scrotum. Blood came from a spontaneous rupture of the spleen.

It is well known that over half of the deaths following splenic rupture are due to hemorrhage.[7] For this reason, there is need for early recognition and treatment. As has been demonstrated in the above cases, repeated examinations were rewarded by the appearance of physical findings in the lower quadrants, indicating that there had been free bleeding into the peritoneal cavity with migration to the pelvic peritoneum.

The nature of the symptoms and signs depends upon the amount of bleeding and the course that the blood takes within the peritoneal cavity. Most of the blood may be retained in the left upper quadrant by the adjacent viscera and peritoneal reflexions. When this occurs, pain and local tenderness and a positive Kehr's sign may be present. Kehr's sign of left shoulder pain has long been taught to be the hallmark of splenic rupture.[1, 3, 4, 6, 9, 11] However, in literature, the frequency of this sign is reported to vary from uncommon to occurring in half of the patients. We have found that looking for additional symptoms in the reverse direction from that to which Kehr called attention is also rewarding.

Usually, the blood is not confined to the left upper quadrant, but flows downward toward the pelvis. The distance it travels and where it may lodge depend upon the configuration of the viscera; symptoms and signs will be present where the greatest quantity of blood pools. Lazaro and associates[2] have given a fascinating description of this phenomenon in a report of three cases of splenic rupture masquerading as appendicitis in which blood was found upon entering the abdominal cavity through a McBurney incision. Mansfield[5] found rectal tenderness in 14 out of 16 patients with splenic rupture.

In conclusion, one should maintain careful surveillance of patients suspected of having splenic rupture, paying particular attention to the valuable sign of downward migration of pain and tenderness into the pelvic area.

John L. Butsch, M.D.
Winfield L. Butsch, M.D.
Department of Surgery
Medical School
State University of New York at Buffalo
Buffalo, N. Y. 14214

REFERENCES

1. Boley, S. J., McKinnon, W. M. P., and Schwartz, S. S.: Traumatic rupture of the spleen in children, Surg. Gynecol. Obstet. **109:** 78, 1959.
2. Lazaro, E. J., Flaviano, O. F., and Parmer, L. P.: Splenic rupture masquerading as acute appendicitis, Am. Surg. **36:** 706, 1970.
3. Lieberman, R. S., and Welch, C. S.: A study of 248 instances of traumatic rupture of the spleen, Surg. Gynecol. Obstet. **127:** 961, 1968.
4. Magee, R. B., and D'Suzansky, J. J.: Acute blunt traumatic rupture of the spleen, Arch. Surg. **99:** 121, 1969.
5. Mansfield, R. D.: Traumatic rupture of the normal spleen, Am. J. Surg. **89:** 759, 1955.
6. Pender, B. W. T.: Traumatic rupture of the normal spleen in children, Lancet **2:** 544, 1953.
7. Shirkey, A. L., Wukasch, D. C., Beall, A. C., Jr., et al.: Surgical management of splenic injuries, Am. J. Surg. **108:** 630, 1964.
8. Slate, R. W., Getzen, L. C., and Laning, R. C.: One hundred cases of traumatic rupture of the spleen, Arch. Surg. **99:** 498, 1969.
9. Terry, J. H., Self, M. N., and Howard, J. M.: Injuries of the spleen: A report of 102 patients and a review of the literature, SURGERY **40:** 615, 1956.
10. Touloukian, R. J.: Abdominal trauma in childhood, Surg. Gynecol. Obstet. **127:** 561, 1968.
11. Upadhyaya, P., and Simpson, J. S.: Splenic trauma in children, Surg. Gynecol. Obstet. **126:** 781, 1968.

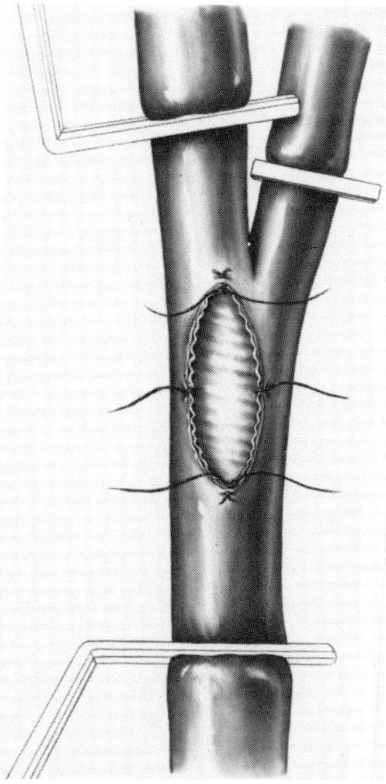

Fig. 1. The edges of the patch fall naturally into the everted position.

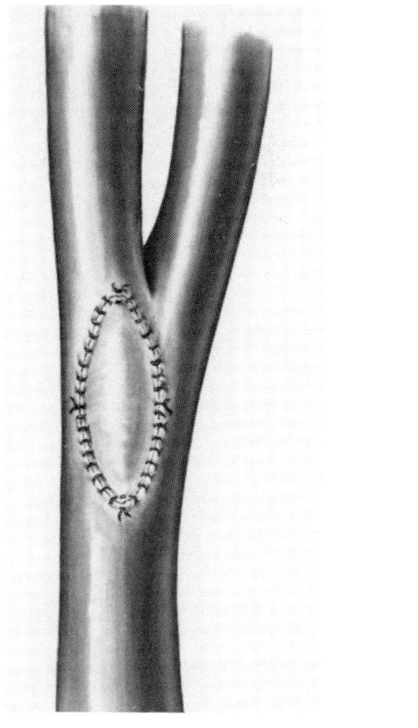

Fig. 2. The patch springs into the convex position when the arterial clamps are released.

An inverted Dacron patch graft

To the Editors:

The Dacron patch graft is used frequently to avoid compromise of the arterial lumen following endarterectomy. A common technique is to cut an elliptical patch from a tubular Dacron graft of appropriate diameter. The patch is then sutured into place with the concave side down so that the curve of the patch matches the curve of the vessel wall. However, this presents some problems as the edges of the patch tend to curl under and it may be difficult to achieve a proper everted suture line. This is especially important since the edges of the cut patch are irregular and are a potential site for thrombus formation.

The author has been using a technique which simplifies placement of the Dacron patch. The patch is cut in the usual fashion but it is sutured into place with the concave side up. The edges of the patch will then fall naturally into the everted position (Fig. 1). Not only is it easier to perform the anastomosis but the patch can also be trimmed more accurately during the procedure. The inverted position of the patch does not compromise the lumen, as the patch springs into the convex position when the arterial clamps are released (Fig. 2).

Frank W. Lo Gerfo, M.D.
Department of Surgery
University of Maryland Hospital
Baltimore, Md. 21201

Volume 76 Number 4

SURGERY

OCTOBER, 1974

Original communications

Evaluation of pulmonary function in the ischemic, nonventilated canine lung

Eric W. Fonkalsrud, M.D., Isao Higashijima, M.D., Abdel K. Sarwat, M.D., Eitoku Arima, M.D., *and* **Manuel Sanchez,** *Los Angeles, Calif.*

Twenty-three dogs underwent left pulmonary hilar occlusion with the lung in the deflated state to determine the period of lung ischemia that can be tolerated before consistent pulmonary edema and congestion develop after lung revascularization. Hilar occlusion for 6 hours or longer under these conditions results in a twofold increase in pulmonary vascular resistance for more than 1 week that decreases to nearly normal levels after 3 weeks in dogs that survive. Pulmonary ventilation scans show a fourfold decrease in uptake during the first week after 6 hours of hilar occlusion that returns to values which are one-half the preoperative values at three weeks. Hilar occlusion for shorter periods does not produce a significant increase in pulmonary vascular resistance. Occlusion for 8 hours or longer resulted in death of the dog within 6 hours after the occlusion clamps had been released, despite respiratory and vascular support. Lungs occluded for 4 hours or less developed mild-to-moderate pulmonary edema within 10 minutes after vascularity was restored to the lung. Longer periods of hilar occlusion produced severe pulmonary edema that caused death in many dogs. Differential pulmonary ventilation with a Carlens tube indicates that pulmonary edema does not occur in the contralateral lung. The present studies suggest that the immediate increased pulmonary vascular resistance observed after lung allografting may be largely the result of vascular compression produced by pulmonary edema and vascular congestion.

From the Department of Surgery, UCLA School of Medicine, Los Angeles, Calif.

Supported by United States Public Health Service Grant No. HL 14333-02.

Accepted for publication April 4, 1974.

Reprint requests: Eric W. Fonkalsrud, M.D., Department of Surgery, School of Medicine, The Center for the Health Sciences, University of California, Los Angeles, Calif. 90024.

Vol. 76, No. 4, pp. 527-532

CAREFUL documentation of the deleterious effects of lung ischemia and nonventilation is a necessary prerequisite to evaluation of techniques of pulmonary preservation. In contrast to the salutary effects of organ per-

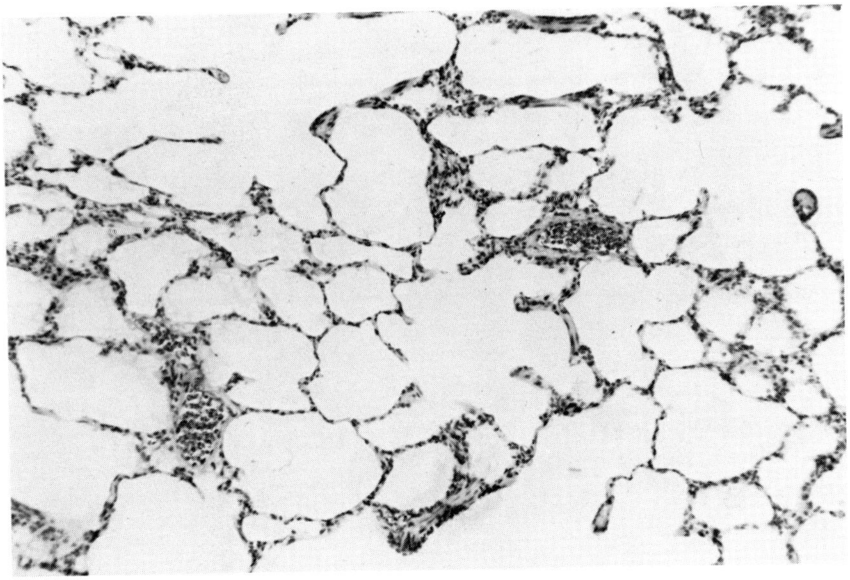

Fig. 1. Lung from dog in Group 2 (hilar occlusion for 3 hours) taken 2 hours after vascularization. Note thin alveolar septae.

Table I. *Pulmonary artery pressure changes after pulmonary ischemia (mm. Hg)*

Group	*No. of dogs*	*Period of hilar occlusion (hr.)*	*Control*		*Postocclusion*		*Postocclusion: 1 wk.*		*Postocclusion: 3 wk.*	
			Main PA	*Left PA*	*Main PA*	*Left PA*	*Main PA*	*Left PA*	*Main PA*	*Left PA*
1	3	2	13/6	31/15	14/9	30/20	16/8	33/18	13/5	30/9
2	2	3	12/5	32/15	17/7	35/17	19/10	40/18	18/8	35/15
3	4	4	14/5	26/9	15/6	29/15	18/8	33/17	17/8	28/10
4	6	5	13/4	24/11	14/5	26/13	13/5	28/15	12/5	23/10
5	4	6	14/6	25/9	16/8	45/38	29/15	50/40	18/10	36/20
6	2	8	12/5	20/10	14/7	42/35				
7	2	10	14/7	27/15	15/8	54/41				

fusion for renal preservation,[2] similar perfusion of the isolated canine lung has been shown to be harmful rather than helpful.[3, 5] Pulmonary edema and microvascular congestion commonly occur after transplantation of a canine lung that has been perfused for 2 to 4 hours; in contrast, histologic evidence of these conditions has been found to be much less severe when a lung graft has been ventilated but not perfused for a similar period. Previous studies from this laboratory suggest that ventilation of a cadaveric canine lung in vivo prior to harvesting may be a satisfactory and practical method of short-term lung graft preservation.[6] The present investigation was undertaken to determine the maximum period that a lung can tolerate ischemia with nonventilation in vivo without consistent pulmonary edema and alveolar congestion occurring after the lung is revascularized.

MATERIALS AND METHODS

Twenty-three conditioned dogs, weighing 12 to 16 kilograms, were anesthesized with intravenous sodium pentobarbital and intubated with endotracheal tubes. Ventilation at 14 to 18 breaths per minute was provided with metaphane and oxygen by means of a Bird respirator, and body temperatures were

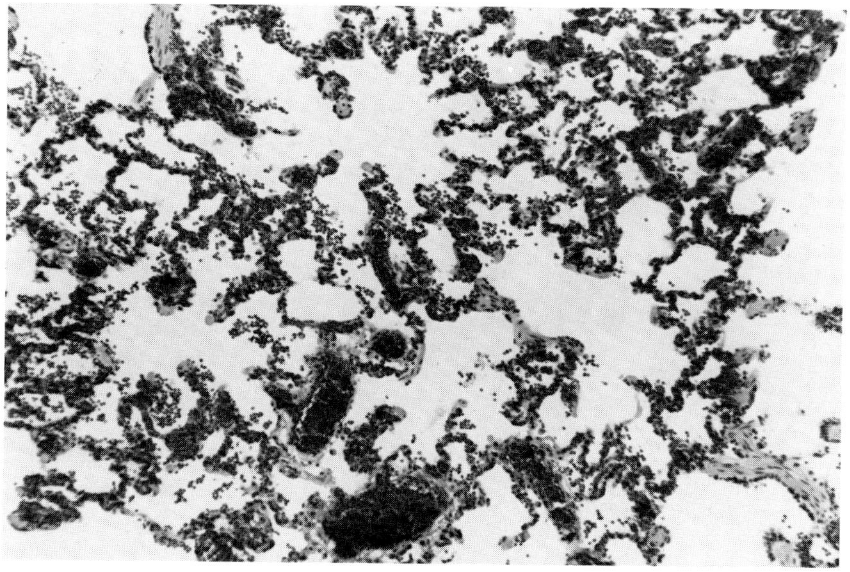

Fig. 2. Lung from dog in Group 4 (hilar occlusion for 5 hours) taken 3 hours after revascularization. Note alveolar thickening and cellular extravasation. Alveolar edema fluid was removed during fixation.

maintained at 37° C. In each dog, a left thoracotomy was performed through the fourth intercostal space, the left main pulmonary artery (PA) was mobilized, and the pulmonary veins from the left lung were isolated. Noncrushing occlusion clamps were then placed on the left PA and the pulmonary veins. The left mainstem bronchus was clamped with the lung in the deflated state.

The dogs were divided into seven experimental groups: Group 1 (three dogs), hilar occlusion for 2 hours; Group 2 (two dogs), hilar occlusion for 3 hours; Group 3 (four dogs), hilar occlusion for 4 hours; Group 4 (six dogs), hilar occlusion for 5 hours; Group 5 (four dogs), hilar occlusion for 6 hours; Group 6 (two dogs), hilar occlusion for 8 hours; and Group 7 (two dogs), hilar occlusion for 10 hours.

Pressures from the main PA and left PA were measured (with right PA occluded) before the experimental period of left hilar occlusion, again immediately after the period of occlusion, and then 1 and 3 weeks later through a right thoracotomy and direct PA puncture. Biopsies of the left lung were taken immediately after the period of left hilar occlusion and 3 weeks later. Single breath, equilibrium, washout ventilation scans with xenon-133, and perfusion scans with ^{99m}technetium sulfate–labeled albumin macroaggregates were performed 3 days, 1 week, and 3 weeks after the period of left hilar occlusion.

RESULTS

The main PA pressure remained very close to normal immediately after the period of left hilar occlusion in the first four groups; however, it increased in Groups 5, 6, and 7 to approximately the same degree as that observed when the right PA was occluded prior to the experimental period of left hilar occlusion (Table I). Similarly, the left PA pressure (with the right PA clamped) did not increase significantly after experimental occlusion of the left hilum for up to 5 hours; however, it did increase appreciably in Groups 5, 6, and 7. These changes in PA pressure suggest an increase in pulmonary vascular resistance and reduction in blood flow through the left lung after a period of hilar occlusion of 6 hours or more. The main PA pressure and left PA pressure in dogs from Groups 1 to 4, when remeasured 1 week after experimental left hilar occlusion, had increased very slightly over the immediate

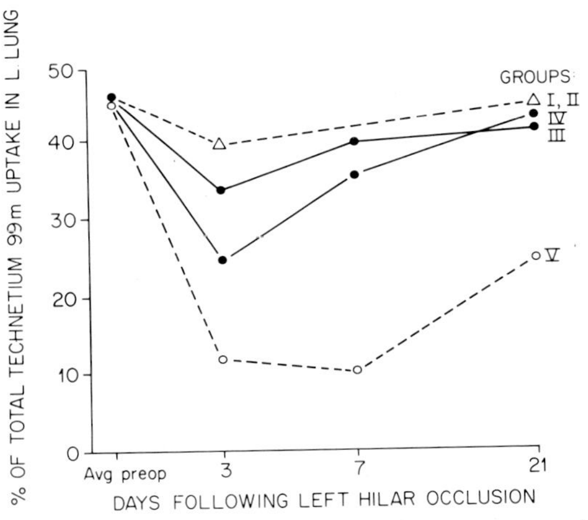

Fig. 3. Average ventilatory uptake as measured on xenon-133 ventilation scans in dogs from Groups 1 through 5.

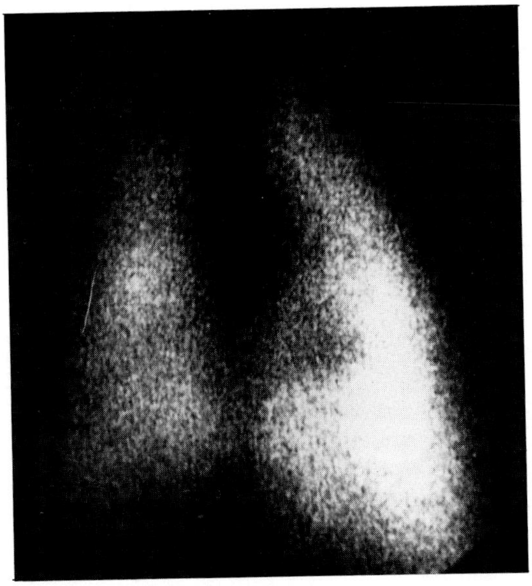

Fig. 4. Perfusion scan from dog in Group 4, 1 week after revascularization.

posthilar occlusion values, but at 3 weeks had returned to approximately that of preocclusion levels.

All dogs in Groups 1 and 2 survived during the study (Fig. 1). One of four dogs from Group 3 experienced empyema of the left chest and was killed 7 days after hilar occlusion. Mild pulmonary edema, which persisted for 2 to 6 hours, was experienced by all four dogs from this group during the first 10 minutes after release of the occlusion clamps. One of the six dogs from Group 4 died within 72 hours with pulmonary edema that involved both lungs and intra-alveolar hemorrhage, primarily of the left lung (Fig. 2). The remaining five dogs all experienced pulmonary edema within 5 to 10 minutes after release of the hilar occlusion clamps that gradually subsided during the subsequent 48 hours. In three of these dogs, pneumonia developed in the left lung within 2 weeks after hilar occlusion. All four dogs from Group 5 experienced severe pulmonary edema and pneumonia in the left lung; however, ventilation was accomplished with a Carlens double-lumen endotracheal tube for 24 hours after the period of occlusion, and three dogs survived for at least 2 weeks. All dogs from Groups 6 and 7 manifested a similar clinical syndrome: massive pulmonary edema that became apparent within 5 to 10 minutes of release of the hilar occlusion clamps; production of massive quantities of bloody edema fluid; and death within 6 hours, despite prolonged mechanical ventilatory support with standard endotracheal tubes.

The histologic sections of lung biopsies obtained within 1 hour after revascularization demonstrated alveolar wall thickening, with progressively more filling of alveolar spaces by edema fluid in dogs undergoing longer periods of hilar occlusion. Interstitial and intra-alveolar hemorrhage was prominent in lungs anoxic for 6 or more hours. Some sections revealed complete loss of any recognizable histologic pattern and severe necrosis.

Both ventilatory and perfusion pulmonary scans in dogs from Groups 1 and 2 showed a decrease in isotope uptake in the left lung from a preocclusion value of 46 percent uptake to an average of 39 percent uptake 3 days postoperatively (Fig. 3). Three weeks after the period of occlusion, the average left lung uptake was 44 percent. The changes that occurred in perfusion and ventilatory scans were almost identical in these dogs. Three days after occlusion, the ventilation isotope uptake in the left lung decreased to 33 percent of total in dogs from Group 3 and to 24 percent of total in those from Group 4. One week after occlusion, the average left pulmonary ventilatory isotope uptake was 39 percent in dogs from Group 3 and 35 percent in those from Group 4. Three weeks after occlusion, the average ventilatory uptake in the left lung was 42 percent for dogs in Group 3 and 43 percent for dogs in Group 4. The average ventilation isotope uptake in the left lung was 45 percent for dogs in Group 5 before occlusion, 12 percent after three days, ten percent after one week, and 24 percent in the three dogs that survived for this period. Scans were not performed on dogs from Groups 6 and 7 because their conditions were critical after hilar occlusion. Perfusion scans were consistently better than the corresponding ventilation scans in dogs from Groups 3, 4, and 5 (Fig. 4).

Dogs from Groups 1 and 2 that underwent right pneumonectomy 3 weeks after hilar occlusion survived for 1 week or more. Dogs from Groups 3 and 4 died within 48 hours after contralateral pneumonectomy.

Dogs in both Groups 6 and 7 experienced severe hypotension and generalized bleeding in the wound within 15 minutes after release of the hilar occlusion clamps. This was accompanied by progressive pulmonary congestion and hypotension that resulted in death within 2 to 6 hours. Fibrin split products were elevated in the circulation in the two dogs from Group 6 in which they were measured, suggesting the presence of disseminated intravascular coagulopathy.

DISCUSSION

Differentiation of the chronic manifestations of anoxic pulmonary injury from rejection in the transplanted canine lung has been difficult since both processes involve alveoli, blood vessels, interstitial tissues, and bronchi. The pathologic changes resulting from anoxia occur immediately after injury, in contrast to the latent period of a few days seen with rejection; nonetheless, there is considerable overlap. The histologic and angiographic appearance of pulmonary rejection has been well summarized by Veith and associates.[7] The early appearance of intra-alveolar edema in unmodified recipients is similar to that observed in lungs made anoxic from 2 to 4 hours in the present study. As the time after revascularization increases, both round and polymorphonuclear cells are observed in the interstitial tissues, and pneumonia frequently ensues. Perivascular thickening is commonly observed in lungs that have been made anoxic for four to six hours, and pulmonary angiograms show rapid tapering of the major branches of the main pulmonary arteries within one week after the period of hilar occlusion, similar to the changes observed in the rejecting lung allograft.[7]

Pulmonary anoxia in dogs for 2 to 3 hours produces mild edema of the alveolar wall that does not significantly interfere with perfusion or ventilation as measured by scans. Dog survival is common, and the histologic appearance of the lung is almost normal one week later. When pulmonary anoxia is extended to 4 hours, intra-alveolar edema is more severe and persistent. Lung scans show a reduction in both perfusion and ventilation for more than a week. Infection occurs in a few lungs after several days, but almost all dogs may survive with suitable supportive care. Five hours of pulmonary anoxia produced severe interstitial and alveolar edema with mild congestion and hemorrhage and was fatal in 17 percent of dogs within the first few days. When pulmonary anoxia was extended to 6 hours, edema and congestion were more severe and caused death within a few hours in one of the four dogs. Severe infection, scarring, contraction, and diminished function almost invariably developed in the left lungs from dogs that survived this period of ischemia.

Anoxia for 8 or more hours produces severe cellular injury that results in hypotension immediately after revascularization, presumably because of release into the circulation of cellular breakdown products similar to that observed when hepatic effluent blood is released into the circulation after periods of hepatic ischemia. Anoxia of this duration produces coagulation disorders and is uniformly fatal within a few hours in the animal preparation utilized in this study.

As observed by Ardekarni and associates,[1] pulmonary edema occurs in both lungs of most dogs when hilar occlusion of one lung is extended to four hours or more. In four dogs from Group 5 in the present study, ventilation of the left lung separate from the right with a modified Carlens double-lumen endotracheal tube during and after left hilar occlusion clearly demonstrated that the normal right lung does not produce edema and, further, that any intrabronchial fluid that develops in the normally perfused (right) lung is produced by aspiration from the contralateral nonperfused (left) lung. The edema subsided in the previously occluded left lung after 2 to 3 hours, permitting extubation at that time.

In previous pulmonary autotransplantation studies,[6] it has been observed that the pulmonary vascular resistance increases acutely after periods of hilar occlusion of more than 4 hours. In the present studies, the PA pressure did not increase until after 6 hours of hilar occlusion. However, pulmonary artery pressure, even with the contralateral PA occluded, is only a crude measurement of the severity of pulmonary injury after anoxia. The left atrial pressure increased only as a late phenomenon when the hilum had been occluded for 6 or more hours and progressive hypotension occurred. These studies suggest that the immediate increased pulmonary vascular resistance in the transplanted lung that has been anoxic for extended periods is largely the result of vascular injury and compression of the intrapulmonary vascular bed by edema and congestion, although it is likely that the vascular obstruction in a grafted lung may be further compounded by rejection.

The pulmonary edema and congestion that appear after 4 to 6 hours of hilar occlusion are comparable in severity to that observed after lung autotransplantation when the anoxic period is less than 2 hours, although the onset of pulmonary edema may be delayed somewhat in autotransplants when the graft is kept inflated. The reason that the transplanted lung is more vulnerable to anoxia than is the in situ lung is not clearly apparent. There is remarkable return of pulmonary function in ischemic lungs three weeks later if suitable respiratory support is provided during the early postischemic period.

A knowledge of the pathologic changes that occur after varying periods of pulmonary anoxia should be of benefit in future evaluation of preservation techniques.

REFERENCES

1. Ardekarni, R. G., Faber, L. P., and Beattie, E. J., Jr.: Pulmonary function after various periods of ischemia in the canine lung, J. Thorac. Cardiovasc. Surg. **59:** 607, 1970.
2. Belzer, F. O., Ashby, B. S., and Dunphy, J. E.: Twenty-four hour and 72-hour preservation of canine kidneys, Lancet **2:** 536, 1967.
3. Castagna, J. T., Shors, E., and Benfield, J. R.: The role of perfusion in lung preservation, J. Thorac. Cardiovasc. Surg. **63:** 521, 1972.
4. Daicoff, G. R., Allen, P. D., and Streck, C. J.: Pulmonary vascular resistance following lung reimplantation and transplantation, Ann. Thorac. Surg. **9:** 569, 1970.
5. Stevens, G. H., Rangel, D., Yakeishi, Y., Sanchez, M., and Fonkalsrud, E. W.: Evaluation in dogs of various techniques of perfusion to preserve the lung, *in* Norman, J. E.: editor: Organ perfusion and preservation, New York, 1968, Appleton-Century Crofts, Inc.
6. Stevens, G. H., Rangel, D. M., Yakeishi, Y., Sanchez, M. M., and Fonkalsrud, E. W.: The relationship of ventilation to preservation of the ischemic canine lung graft, J. Surg. Res. **7:** 246, 1972.
7. Veith, F. J., Sinha, S. B. P., Blümcke, S., Dougherty, J. C., Becker, N. H., Siegelman, S. S., and Hagstrom, J. W. C.: Nature and evolution of lung allograft rejection with and without immunosuppression, J. Thorac. Cardiovasc. Surg. **63:** 509, 1972.

Impaired gluconeogenesis in dogs with *E. coli* bacteremia

A. C. Groves, M.D., F.R.C.S.(C), L. I. Woolf, Ph.D., P. J. O'Regan, M.B., C. Beach, B.Sc.(Oxon.), C. Hasinoff, B.Sc., *and* W. H. Sutherland, M.D., F.R.C.S.(C), *Vancouver, B. C., Canada*

Exhaustion of hepatic glycogen, hypoglycemia, increased arterial plasma alanine and glycine, and decreased serum insulin were found in fasting dogs receiving 2.4×10^9 viable E. coli bacteria per kilogram intravenously. The findings suggest impaired gluconeogenesis from amino acids. The simultaneous rise of arterial lactate and fall of plasma glucose in these dogs also suggests impaired gluconeogenesis from lactate. Since both lactate and alanine must be converted to pyruvate as the first step in gluconeogenesis, increasing arterial lactate, pyruvate, and alanine concentrations combined with decreasing plasma glucose implies a block in gluconeogenesis between pyruvate and glucose. Except for the rise of serum urea concentration, the metabolic changes observed in this experiment closely resemble those seen following hepatectomy and provide evidence that deranged liver metabolism is a cause of death in the dog with E. coli bacteremia and hyperlactacidemia.

From the Department of Surgery, Shaughnessy Hospital and University of British Columbia, Kinsmen Laboratory of Neurological Research, and the Department of Psychiatry, University of British Columbia, Vancouver, B. C., Canada

In previous studies, Griffiths and associates[11] demonstrated that hypoglycemia, hypertriglyceridemia, and hypoinsulinemia occur in dogs with *E. coli* bacteremia of 12 hours' duration. A rise of serum triglyceride was found to correlate with a rise of plasma norepinephrine, and this observation suggested that hypertriglyceridemia was a result of excessive lipid mobilization induced by increased endogenous norepinephrine release. The hypoglycemia and hypoinsulinemia suggested that the bacteremic dogs had impaired gluconeogenesis.

Supported by grants from British Columbia Medical Services Foundation and Medical Research Council of Canada.

Accepted for publication April 4, 1974.

Reprint requests: Alan C. Groves, M.D., Department of Surgery, Shaughnessy Hospital, Vancouver 9, B. C., Canada V6H 3N1.

The key gluconeogenic amino acid, alanine, is deaminated to pyruvate, which subsequently is converted to glucose.[9] Impaired hepatic utilization of alanine is thought to cause the hyperalaninemia which has been observed in lactic acidosis.[16]

Decreased oxidation of lactate via pyruvate in the tricarboxylic acid cycle is generally considered responsible for the lactic acidosis of shock.[23] However, gluconeogenesis from lactate in the Cori cycle is an additional pathway for removal of lactate from the blood.[5] After an overnight fast, approximately one fifth of endogenous glucose production is derived from lactate, but after starvation for three days, gluconeogenesis from lactate may account for one third of glucose production.[13] Medalle and associates[18] observed three patients with serious sepsis who had lactic

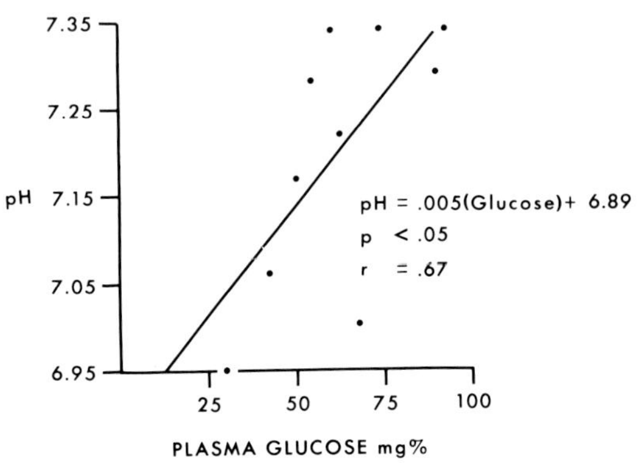

Fig. 1. These data obtained at 6 hours show that the dogs with the lowest blood sugars were the most acidotic.

acidosis and hypoglycemia; they suggested that hypoglycemia resulted from impaired hepatic uptake of lactate. During perfusion of livers removed from rats given *E. coli* endotoxin, Williamson and co-workers[26] observed impaired gluconeogenesis from lactate.

In an attempt to determine if there was evidence of impaired gluconeogenesis in serious gram-negative sepsis, changes of arterial amino acids, lactate, pyruvate, and gases, and venous serum creatinine, urea nitrogen, and insulin were studied in relationship to changes of plasma glucose following the intravenous injection of viable *E. coli* bacteria into dogs.

MATERIAL AND METHODS

Ten adult mongrel dogs, weighing 15 to 20 kilograms, were fasted for 72 hours prior to the experiment because, in postabsorptive dogs, catecholamine-induced hepatic glycogenolysis would obscure or attenuate a fall in blood sugar resulting from impaired gluconeogenesis. They were anesthetized with 20 to 25 mg. per kilogram of intravenous pentobarbital, intubated, and given an intravenous injection of 2.4×10^9 living *E. coli* bacteria per kilogram. Arterial and venous blood was obtained before and two, four, and six hours after the injection of the bacteria. Also, blood was obtained at the same intervals from ten similarly starved and anesthetized control dogs which did not receive bacteria.

With the use of the ferricyanide method for glucose, the diacetyl monoxime method for urea, and the alkaline picrate method for creatinine, plasma glucose and serum urea nitrogen and creatinine were measured on an AutoAnalyzer.* Arterial blood lactate and pyruvate were measured by enzymatic techniques and arterial blood gases were measured on Radiometer blood gas analyser. The double antibody direct precipitation method was used to measure serum insulin.†

Individual amino acids from arterial blood were determined quantitatively by using sodium citrate buffers on a Beckman 120C amino acid analyzer. Glutamine cannot be measured on an ordinary amino acid analyzer with conventional buffers because asparagine migrates with glutamine and glutamine is considered unstable. Therefore, 0.7 ml. of plasma was incubated for 30 minutes at pH 5.0 and 37° C. with 0.125 U. of glutaminase obtained from *E. coli* bacteria,‡ in order to convert glutamine to glutamic acid, which then was measured on the amino acid analyzer. Each batch of glutaminase was tested for freedom of any effect on glutamic acid. On another portion of plasma, the free glutamic acid content was determined with the use of the enzyme glutamic dehydrogenase.[1]§ The concentration of glutamine was calculated by subtracting the amount of free glutamic acid from the amount of glutamic acid measured after glutaminase treatment. Further incubation with asparaginase converted asparagine to aspartic acid and confirmed the complete conversion of glutamine.

After six hours, all the dogs were killed with an overdose of pentobarbital and approximately 5 Gm. of liver were removed and frozen immediately in liquid nitrogen. Following extraction by alkaline hydrolysis,[12] the liver glycogen was washed in 70 and 95 percent ethanol and finally acetone. The amount of dry glycogen in each specimen was weighed.

RESULTS

Glucose. Mean fasting plasma glucose before the intravenous injection of *E. coli* bac-

*Technicon Instruments Corp., Tarrytown, N. Y.
†Amersham Searle, Des Plaines, Ill.
‡Grade V, Sigma Chemical Co., St. Louis, Mo.
§Boehringer Mannheim Corp., Montreal, Quebec.

Table I. *Metabolic changes in dogs with E. coli bacteremia*

	0 hr.	*2 hr.*	*p**	*4 hr.*	*p**	*6 hr.*	*p**
Glucose (mg. per-cent)							
Experi-mental	102.2 ± 8.0	93.8 ± 36.2	N.S.	58.9 ± 20.0†	< 0.001	62.4 ± 20.0†	< 0.001
Control	100.8 ± 9.0	104.9 ± 8.2	N.S.	105.0 ± 10.7	N.S.	108.9 ± 7.7	< 0.05
Urea nitro-gen (mg./100 ml.)							
Experi-mental	14.2 ± 3.3	20.1 ± 3.2†	< 0.001	24.8 ± 3.5†	< 0.001	29.3 ± 4.4†	< 0.001
Control	13.0 ± 2.3	12.6 ± 2.0	N.S.	12.3 ± 2.2	N.S.	11.9 ± 2.3	N.S.
Creatinine (mg./100 ml.)							
Experi-mental	0.9 ± 0.1	1.4 ± 0.3†	< 0.001	1.7 ± 0.3†	< 0.001	2.0 ± 0.4†	< 0.001
Control	0.9 ± 0.2	0.8 ± 0.2	< 0.01	0.8 ± 0.2	< 0.01	0.8 ± 0.1	< 0.01
Lactate (mg./100 ml.)							
Experi-mental	9.3 ± 3.4	36.2 ± 14.8†	< 0.001	46.1 ± 13.6†	< 0.001	48.5 ± 16.3†	< 0.001
Control	8.2 ± 2.8	7.4 ± 3.6	N.S.	6.4 ± 2.8	< 0.01	6.4 ± 3.1	< 0.01
Pyruvate (mg./100 ml.)							
Experi-mental	0.33 ± 0.10	1.80 ± 0.61†	< 0.01	1.78 ± 0.71†	< 0.01	1.73 ± 0.81†	< 0.01
Control	0.40 ± 0.10	0.39 ± 0.21	N.S.	0.32 ± 0.66	N.S.	0.29 ± 0.11	N.S.
Insulin (μU./ml.)							
Experi-mental	18.1 ± 4.6	13.9 ± 7.2	< 0.05	10.5 ± 5.3†	< 0.01	10.6 ± 3.7‡	< 0.001
Control	19.6 ± 6.9	16.9 ± 2.8	N.S.	17.0 ± 4.4	N.S.	14.3 ± 4.0	< 0.05
pH							
Experi-mental	7.36 ± 0.06	7.27 ± 0.11	< 0.01	7.25 ± 0.10	< 0.01	7.20 ± 0.15‡	< 0.01
Control	7.38 ± 0.05	7.33 ± 0.07	< 0.01	7.32 ± 0.09	< 0.05	7.32 ± 0.08	< 0.01
P_{CO_2} (mm. Hg)							
Experi-mental	39.5 ± 6.5	29.2 ± 12.8‡	< 0.01	28.3 ± 11.5†	< 0.01	28.5 ± 11.6†	< 0.01
Control	37.5 ± 6.0	42.7 ± 9.5	N.S.	44.9 ± 11.8	< 0.05	41.9 ± 9.0	N.S.
P_{O_2} (mm. Hg)							
Experi-mental	84.1 ± 10.0	94.7 ± 12.3‡	< 0.01	94.9 ± 7.1†	< 0.01	92.4 ± 9.2†	< 0.01
Control	85.5 ± 7.7	78.7 ± 14.0	N.S.	76.6 ± 12.4	< 0.05	80.4 ± 14.4	N.S.
HCO_3 (mEq./L.)							
Experi-mental	22.2 ± 2.2	15.9 ± 2.2†	< 0.001	14.7 ± 1.9†	< 0.001	14.0 ± 2.6†	< 0.001
Control	22.8 ± 2.1	22.0 ± 1.5	N.S.	21.7 ± 1.9	N.S.	21.8 ± 2.0	N.S.

*Probability that the difference from zero time occurred by chance (paired t test).

†p < 0.01—Probability that the differences between the experimental and control groups are caused by chance (Student's t test).

‡p < 0.05—Probability that the differences between the experimental and control groups are caused by chance (Student's t test).

Table II. *Changes of plasma amino acids in experimental and control dogs at 6 hours:—Mean arterial plasma concentration (μM/L.)*

Amino acid	Experimental 0	Experimental 6 hr.	Experimental p*	Control 0	Control 6 hr.	Control p*
Taurine	67.7 ± 35.3	342.9 ± 180.9	< 0.001	48.8 ± 27.6	110.4 ± 111.9	N.S.
Aspartic acid	22.6 ± 9.5	30.6 ± 9.7	< 0.05	21.1 ± 9.7	24.1 ± 6.7	N.S.
Threonine	175.1 ± 61.9	190.9 ± 83.1	N.S.	221.8 ± 136.3	186.8 ± 95.3	N.S.
Serine	122.0 ± 30.1	100.1 ± 31.0	N.S.	126.7 ± 31.4	112.9 ± 13.5	N.S.
Asparagine	53.1 ± 27.3	53.9 ± 27.1	N.S.	33.3 ± 16.9	28.8 ± 14.2	N.S.
Citrulline	25.7 ± 11.2	27.6 ± 18.4	N.S.	39.2 ± 8.2	30.0 ± 7.7	< 0.01
Glycine	138.7 ± 53.5	254.6 ± 77.5	< 0.01	160.6 ± 50.7	131.5 ± 26.1	< 0.05
Alanine	277.4 ± 70.4	1129.2 ± 590.3	< 0.01	326.2 ± 64.1	177.8 ± 42.9	< 0.001
α-Aminobutyrate	62.0 ± 21.3	38.4 ± 21.6	< 0.05	76.0 ± 23.4	62.8 ± 29.2	< 0.05
Valine	234.9 ± 46.6	305.6 ± 100.4	N.S.	215.5 ± 45.8	265.0 ± 25.4	< 0.05
Methionine	44.0 ± 11.0	51.4 ± 14.8	N.S.	49.3 ± 25.6	51.8 ± 16.2	N.S.
Isoleucine	86.2 ± 21.2	119.2 ± 28.1	< 0.05	79.8 ± 17.5	119.2 ± 16.4	< 0.001
Leucine	161.2 ± 36.1	228.5 ± 60.3	< 0.05	142.1 ± 29.8	202.8 ± 31.2	< 0.001
Tyrosine	33.2 ± 10.4	58.2 ± 15.8	< 0.001	33.0 ± 9.9	36.4 ± 4.2	N.S.
Phenylalanine	62.9 ± 13.5	102.6 ± 29.5	< 0.01	52.2 ± 14.2	74.8 ± 6.6	< 0.001
Ornithine	18.7 ± 10.8	220.3 ± 66.7	< 0.001	46.9 ± 25.9	35.4 ± 25.6	N.S.
Lysine	153.5 ± 43.4	257.8 ± 115.9	N.S.	159.4 ± 64.8	111.6 ± 30.9	N.S.
Histidine	36.2 ± 18.3	91.5 ± 62.1	< 0.05	36.4 ± 17.3	41.9 ± 22.9	N.S.
3-Methyl histidine	12.3 ± 8.7	15.0 ± 10.5	N.S.	11.2 ± 8.7	9.8 ± 7.6	N.S.
Carnosine	27.3 ± 11.8	98.6 ± 49.1	< 0.01	28.6 ± 18.5	21.8 ± 14.9	N.S.
Arginine	70.0 ± 14.0	3.0 ± 9.0	< 0.001	93.1 ± 41.3	58.4 ± 19.1	< 0.05
Glutamine	698.4 ± 176.3	723.6 ± 244.9	N.S.	577.5 ± 261.9	451.5 ± 213.9	< 0.01
Glutamic acid	46.2 ± 13.9	97.5 ± 53.3	< 0.01	58.5 ± 29.8	62.8 ± 33.4	N.S.

*p (paired t test).

teria was 102.2 ± 8.0 mg. per 100 ml. (Table I). Two hours after bacteremia was established, three of the 10 dogs developed transient hyperglycemia (126, 129, and 164 mg. per 100 ml.) and the other seven dogs were hypoglycemic; consequently there was no significant change of *mean* plasma glucose at this time (93.8 ± 36.2 mg. per 100 ml.). At four hours, mean plasma glucose in the experimental group had decreased to 58.9 ± 20.0 mg. per 100 ml. ($p < 0.001$) and at six hours remained decreased at 62.4 ± 20.0 mg. per 100 ml. ($p < 0.001$). Six hours after the injection of bacteria, the lowest plasma glucose concentrations were seen in the most acidotic dogs (Fig. 1). Two dogs developed profound hypoglycemia (28 and 42 mg. per 100 ml.) at 6 hours. In contrast, at 6 hours mean plasma glucose had increased in the control dogs from 100.8 ± 9.0 to 108.9 ± 7.7 mg. per 100 ml. ($p < 0.05$).

Serum urea nitrogen and creatinine. Serum urea nitrogen and creatinine increased in a linear manner. Mean serum urea nitrogen before bacteremia (14.2 ± 3.3 mg. per 100 ml.) rose to 29.3 ± 4.4 mg. per 100 ml. ($p < 0.001$, Table I) at 6 hours. Similarly, mean serum creatinine before bacteremia (0.9 ± 0.1 mg. per 100 ml.) increased to 2.0 ± 0.4 mg. per 100 ml. ($p < 0.001$) at 6 hours. Mean serum urea nitrogen and creatinine did not rise in the control animals.

Lactate and pyruvate. Mean arterial lactate and pyruvate rose quickly and remained elevated at 6 hours but did not increase in control dogs (Table I). There was no correlation between arterial Pco_2 and lactate at any time.

Serum insulin. In the experimental dogs, mean serum insulin declined from 18.1 ± 4.6 μU to 13.9 ± 7.2 μU per milliliter at 2 hours ($p < 0.05$, Table I) and remained significantly decreased at 4 hours (10.5 ± 5.3 μU per milliliter ($p < 0.01$) and at 6 hours (10.6 ± 3.7 μU per milliliter, $p < 0.001$) after the intravenous injection of *E. coli* bacteria. Although mean serum insulin had fallen by 6 hours in the control dogs ($p < 0.05$), mean serum insulin at 4 and 6 hours was significantly lower in the bacteremic dogs

Table III. *Comparison of plasma amino acids in experimental and control dogs at 6 hours:—Mean arterial plasma concentration (μM/L.)*

Amino acid	*Experimental*	*Control*	*p**
Taurine	342.9 ± 180.9	110.4 ± 111.9	< 0.01
Aspartic acid	30.6 ± 9.7	24.1 ± 6.7	N.S.
Threonine	190.9 ± 83.1	186.8 ± 95.3	N.S.
Serine	100.1 ± 31.0	112.9 ± 13.5	N.S.
Asparagine	53.9 ± 27.1	28.8 ± 14.2	< 0.05
Citrulline	27.6 ± 18.4	30.0 ± 7.7	N.S.
Glycine	254.6 ± 77.5	131.5 ± 26.1	< 0.001
Alanine	1129.2 ± 590.3	177.8 ± 42.9	< 0.001
α-Aminobutyrate	38.4 ± 21.6	62.8 ± 29.2	< 0.05
Valine	305.6 ± 100.4	265.0 ± 25.4	N.S.
Methionine	51.4 ± 14.8	51.8 ± 16.2	N.S.
Isoleucine	119.2 ± 28.1	119.2 ± 16.4	N.S.
Leucine	228.5 ± 60.3	202.8 ± 31.2	N.S.
Tyrosine	58.2 ± 15.8	36.4 ± 4.2	< 0.01
Phenylalanine	102.6 ± 29.5	74.8 ± 6.6	< 0.05
Ornithine	220.3 ± 66.7	35.4 ± 25.6	< 0.01
Lysine	257.8 ± 115.9	111.6 ± 30.9	< 0.01
Histidine	91.5 ± 62.1	41.9 ± 22.9	N.S.
3-Methyl histidine	15.0 ± 10.5	9.8 ± 7.6	N.S.
Carnosine	98.6 ± 49.1	21.8 ± 14.9	< 0.01
Arginine	3.0 ± 9.0	58.4 ± 19.1	< 0.01
Glutamine	723.6 ± 244.9	451.5 ± 213.9	< 0.05
Glutamic acid	97.5 ± 53.3	62.8 ± 33.4	N.S.

*p (Student's t test).

than in the control animals ($p < 0.01$, $p < 0.05$).

Blood gases. In the bacteremic dogs, the arterial pH fell continually from 7.36 ± 0.06 to 7.20 ± 0.15 ($p < 0.01$, Table I) by 6 hours. Arterial pH also declined slightly in the control dogs, but at 6 hours the experimental dogs were more acidotic ($p < 0.01$). Although five dogs developed severe metabolic acidosis at 6 hours, the arterial pH in the other five bacteremic dogs at this time was 7.28 or greater (Figs. 1 and 3).

Liver glycogen. Very small amounts of glycogen were found in the livers of three bacteremic dogs (0.05, 0.10, and 0.22 Gm. per 100 Gm. of liver), and none was found in the livers of the others. Mean liver glycogen in the fasted control dogs (0.63 ± 0.45 Gm. per 100 Gm. of liver) was greater than in the experimental group ($p < 0.01$). Surprisingly, three control dogs had a liver glycogen content greater than 1 Gm. per 100 Gm. of liver despite starvation for 3 days prior to the experiment.

Amino acids. A marked increase of alanine which occurred in all bacteremic dogs was the most striking change observed. Mean arterial plasma alanine increased from 277.4 ± 70.4 to 1,129 ± 590.3 μM per liter ($p < 0.01$, Table II) at 6 hours. At this time, increased arterial alanine correlated inversely with decreased plasma glucose (Fig. 2) and decreased arterial pH (Fig. 3). Conversely, arterial plasma alanine decreased in all control dogs from a mean of 326.2 ± 64.1 to 177.8 ± 42.9 μM per liter ($p < 0.001$) at 6 hours. Similarly, another gluconeogenic amino acid, glycine, rose from 138.7 ± 53.5 to 254 ± 77.5 μM per liter ($p < 0.01$, Table II) in the experimental dogs but fell in the controls from 160.6 ± 50.7 to 131.5 ± 26.1 μM per liter ($p < 0.05$).

At 6 hours, mean plasma tyrosine, phenylalanine, taurine, lysine, glutamic acid, and carnosine in the experimental dogs were higher than in the control animals (Table III). Isoleucine and leucine had risen by 6 hours in both the bacteremic and control dogs (Table II), but between the two groups, there was no significant difference in the concentrations of these amino acids (Table III). After 6 hours, mean plasma glutamine was unchanged in the bacteremic dogs but had decreased in the control dogs ($p < 0.01$,

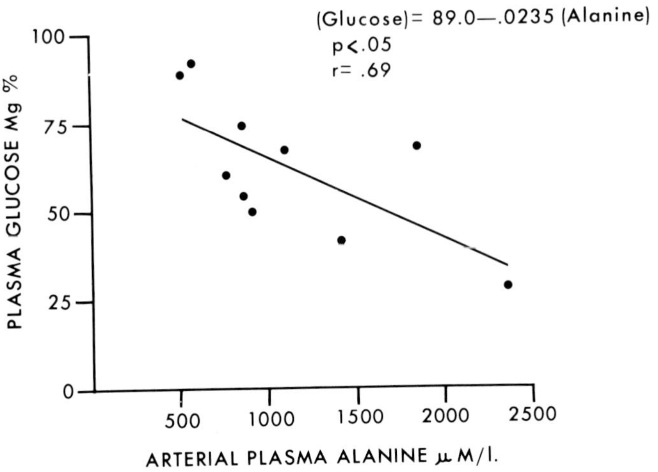

Fig. 2. At 6 hours, decreased plasma glucose correlated inversely with increased arterial alanine.

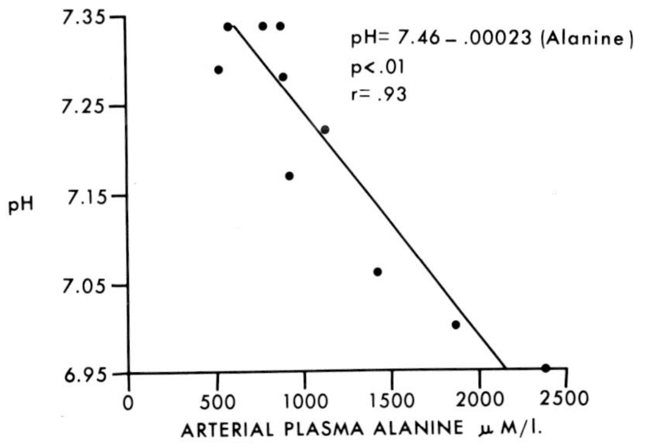

Fig. 3. Six hours after the injection of bacteria, the dogs with the most profound acidosis had the highest arterial alanine concentrations.

Table II). At this time, plasma glutamine was significantly greater in the experimental group ($p < 0.05$, Table III). Although decreased at 6 hours in both groups, α-aminobutyrate was significantly lower in the experimental dogs ($p < 0.05$, Table III).

DISCUSSION

The onset of sepsis causes changes in the plasma concentrations of many hormones which influence gluconeogenesis. In previous studies, dogs receiving an intravenous dose of *E. coli* bacteria comparable to that used in this experiment were found to have increased plasma norepinephrine and epinephrine.[11] Both these hormones inhibit insulin release,[19, 20] and therefore, increased circulating concentrations of these hormones may be partly responsible for the decreased serum insulin seen in the bacteremic dogs in this experiment. Plasma glucagon is greatly elevated in serious bacterial infection.[21] Hypoglycemia, observed in the bacteremic dogs, also causes increased plasma glucagon and growth hormone.[22] Plasma cortisol is elevated in gram-negative bacteremia,[11] but recent studies indicate that cortisol has a permissive rather than direct role in gluconeogenesis.[8]

Glucose synthesis is increased when serum insulin is low, but Unger[24] has suggested that a decline of the insulin:glucagon molar ratio rather than just the insulin concentration in the blood causes increased gluconeogenesis. Thus, the hormonal changes previously found in bacteremic dogs and patients with serious infection would tend to increase the rate of gluconeogenesis. When there is increased gluconeogenesis from amino acids, as in inadequately treated diabetes, there is a fall of the arterial plasma concentrations of the important glucogenic amino acids alanine and glycine.[25] In the control dogs, serum insulin and arterial plasma alanine and glycine declined, whereas plasma glucose rose, suggesting increased gluconeogenesis. However, the experimental dogs, despite having significantly lower serum insulin than the control dogs, had increased arterial plasma alanine and

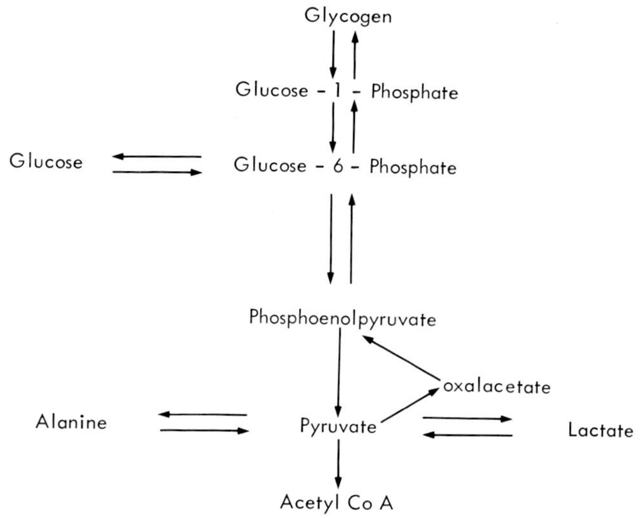

Fig. 4. Metabolic pathways of gluconeogenesis and glycolysis.

glycine associated with hypoglycemia. These metabolic changes could have occurred only if gluconeogenesis from amino acids were impaired. Also, at 6 hours, the highest arterial alanine and lowest plasma glucose concentrations were found in the most acidotic dogs; the latter finding is consistent with the earlier report of Berk and associates.[2]

Exton and Park[7] showed that epinephrine and glucagon cause a marked increase of hepatic glucose production from lactate. In both sepsis and hypoglycemia, the plasma concentrations of epinephrine and glucagon are elevated; therefore, the association of increasing arterial blood lactate and falling plasma glucose concentrations implies impaired gluconeogenesis from lactate.

Since both lactate and alanine must be converted to pyruvate as the first step in gluconeogenesis (Fig. 4), the accumulation of lactate, pyruvate, and alanine in the blood, together with falling plasma glucose concentrations and exhaustion of hepatic glycogen reserves in the dogs with *E. coli* bacteremia, strongly suggests that there was a block in gluconeogenesis between pyruvate and glucose.

The energy required for gluconeogenesis is derived from aerobic metabolism.[4] Inadequate tissue oxygenation secondary to decreased blood flow, which occurs in the dog with *E. coli* endotoxin shock,[6] would impair both oxidation of lactate to CO_2 and gluconeogenesis from lactate. The relative importance of impaired oxidation and gluconeogenesis as causes of elevated arterial lactate cannot be determined from this experiment. Hyperventilation increases arterial blood lactate,[27] but the lack of correlation in this experiment between arterial P_{CO_2} and lactate confirms earlier observations indicating that the hyperlactacidemia of sepsis is not related to the rate of breathing.[6]

In patients with refractory shock, many of whom were septic, LaBrosse and associates[14] found increased plasma amino acids, particularly alanine, and Marliss and co-workers[16] found similar changes in a group of patients with lactic acidosis. Their observations are in agreement with the data in this experiment.

Increased utilization of glucose is a potential cause of hypoglycemia. However, decreased serum insulin found in this investigation combined with increased plasma concentrations of growth hormone,[22] glucagon,[21] and cortisol,[11] which occur during hypoglycemia and sepsis, would tend to decrease glycolysis. Hence, increased glycolysis is unlikely to be the cause of the hypoglycemia.

In dogs receiving varying doses of *E. coli* endotoxin intravenously, Berk and associates[2] found that some dogs developed early transient hyperglycemia followed by hypoglycemia, whereas in others blood glucose declined immediately and remained low. Studying tranquilized dogs receiving 10^9 viable *E. coli* bacteria per kilogram intravenously, a dose similar to that used in this investigation, Griffiths and associates[11] observed transient hyperglycemia at two hours in some dogs, but plasma glucose subsequently declined in all animals; most dogs survived twelve hours despite persisting hypoglycemia.

In this study, the livers of some control dogs still contained moderate amounts of glycogen after a three-day fast, although mean liver glycogen was decreased considerably from levels seen postabsorptively. In the bacteremic dogs, only trace amounts of glycogen were found in the livers of three and none was found in the livers of the other seven. Since glucagon is a potent glycogenolytic as well as gluconeogenic hormone, the findings are consistent with the concept that increased circulating concentrations of glucagon occurring in sepsis cause glycogenolysis of residual liver glycogen and the early transient rise of blood glucose seen in some dogs. Epinephrine causes glycogenolysis of liver glycogen but possibly only indirectly since epinephrine increases plasma glucagon.[10]

During starvation combined with uncomplicated renal failure, blood urea nitrogen and serum creatinine increase only 10 and 1 mg. percent per day, respectively,[3] and therefore, the rapid elevation of these metabolites in the experimental dogs is a result of increased synthesis rather than renal insufficiency. Epinephrine and glucagon also stimulate ureagenesis,[15] and the increased rate of urea synthesis observed in this investigation is in accord with previously described elevations of these hormones in sepsis. The simultaneous fall of blood glucose and progressive rise of serum urea nitrogen observed in all bacteremic dogs suggest that the dose of bacteria used in this experiment caused liver dysfunction sufficient to impair gluconeogenesis but insufficient to prevent increased ureagenesis.

Hypoglycemia and increased circulating concentrations of lactate, pyruvate, alanine, glycine, tyrosine, phenylalanine, and taurine as well as decreased α-aminobutyrate, which were seen in the bacteremic dogs, are seen in the dog immediately following hepatectomy.[17] Thus, except for the rise of serum urea the findings in the present study suggest that there is severe impairment of liver metabolism in dogs with hyperlactacidemia following the intravenous injection of *E. coli* bacteria.

REFERENCES

1. Bergmeyer, H.-U.: Methods of enzymatic analysis, Weinheim, Germany, 1965, Verlag Chemie, p. 384.
2. Berk, J. L., Hagen, J. F., Beyer, W. H., and Gerber, M. J.: Hypoglycemia of shock, Ann. Surg. **171:** 400, 1970.
3. Black, D. A. K.: Renal disease, Oxford and Edinburgh, 1967, Blackwell Scientific Publications, p. 321.
4. Cahill, G. F.: Starvation in man, N. Engl. J. Med. **282:** 668, 1970.
5. Cori, C. F.: Mammalian carbohydrate metabolism, Physiol. Rev. **11:** 143, 1931.
6. Duff, J. H., Groves, A. C., McLean, A. P. H., Lapointe, R., and MacLean, L. D.: Defective oxygen consumption in septic shock, Surg. Gynecol. Obstet. **128:** 1051, 1969.
7. Exton, J. H., and Park, C. R.: The stimulation of gluconeogenesis from lactate by epinephrine, glucagon, and cyclic 3′,5′ adenylate in the perfused rat liver, Pharmacol. Rev. **18:** 181, 1966.
8. Exton, J. H., Friedmann, N., Wong, E. H., Brineaux, J. P., Corbin, J. D., and Park, C. R.: Interaction of glucocorticoids with glucagon and epinephrine in the control of gluconeogenesis and glycogenolysis in the liver and of lipolysis in adipose tissue, J. Biol. Chem. **247:** 3579, 1972.
9. Felig, P., and Wahren, J.: Amino acid metabolism in exercising man, J. Clin. Invest. **50:** 2703, 1971.
10. Gerich, J. E., Karam, J. H., and Forsham, P. H.: Stimulation of glucagon secretion by epinephrine in man, J. Clin. Endocrinol. Metab. **37:** 479, 1973.
11. Griffiths, J. C., Groves, A. C., and Leung, F. Y. T.: Hypertriglyceridemia and hypoglycemia in gram negative sepsis in the dog, Surg. Gynecol. Obstet. **136:** 897, 1973.
12. Hildes, J. A., Sherlock, S., and Walshe, V.: Liver and muscle glycogen in normal subjects, in diabetes mellitus, and in acute hepatitis. Part 1. Under basal conditions, Clin. Sci. **7:** 287, 1949.
13. Kreisberg, R. A., Siegal, A. M., and Owen, W. C.: Glucose-lactate interrelationships: Effect of ethanol, J. Clin. Invest. **50:** 175, 1971.
14. LaBrosse, E. H., Beech, J. A., McLaughlin, J. S., Mansberger, A. R., Keene, W. D., and Cowley, R. A.: Plasma amino acids in normal humans and patients with shock, Surg. Gynecol. Obstet. **125:** 516, 1967.

15. Mallette, L. E., Exton, J. H., and Park, C. R.: Control of gluconeogenesis from amino acids in the perfused rat liver, J. Biol. Chem. **244:** 5713, 1969.
16. Marliss, E. B., Aoki, T. T., Toews, C. J., Felig, P., Connon, J. J., Kyner, J., Huckabee, W. E., and Cahill, G. F.: Amino acid metabolism in lactic acidosis, Am. J. Med. **52:** 474, 1972.
17. McMenamy, R. H., Vang, J., and Drapanas, T.: Amino acid and α-keto acid concentrations in plasma and blood of the liverless dog, Am. J. Physiol. **209:** 1046, 1965.
18. Medalle, R., Webb, R., and Waterhouse, C.: Lactic acidosis and associated hypoglycemia, Arch. Intern. Med. **128:** 273, 1971.
19. Porte, D.: A receptor mechanism for inhibition of insulin release by epinephrine in man, J. Clin. Invest. **46:** 86, 1967.
20. Porte, D., and Williams, R. H.: Inhibition of insulin release by norepinephrine in man, Science **152:** 1248, 1966.
21. Rocha, D. M., Santeusanio, F., Faloona, G. R., and Unger, R. H.: Abnormal pancreatic alpha-cell function in bacterial infections, N. Engl. J. Med. **288:** 700, 1973.
22. Roth, J. Glick, S. M., Yalow, R. S., and Berson, S. A.: Hypoglycemia: A potent stimulus to secretion of growth hormone, Science **140:** 987, 1963.
23. Schumer, W.: Localization of the energy pathway block in shock, SURGERY **64:** 55, 1968.
24. Unger, R. H.: Glucagon and the insulin:glucagon ratio in diabetes and other catabolic illness, Diabetes **20:** 834, 1971.
25. Wahren, J., Felig, P., Cerasi, E., and Luft, R.: Splanchnic and peripheral glucose and amino acid metabolism in diabetes mellitus, J. Clin. Invest. **51:** 1870, 1972.
26. Williamson, J. R., Refino, C., and LaNoue, K.: Effects of *E. coli* lipopolysaccharide B treatment of rats on gluconeogenesis, *in* Porter, R., and Knight, J., editors: Energy metabolism in trauma, London, 1970, J. & A. Churchill, Ltd., p. 145.
27. Zborowska-Sluis, D. T., and Dossetor, J. B.: Hyperlactatemia of hyperventilation, J. Appl. Physiol. **22:** 746, 1967.

Accumulation of lymphotoxin-secreting lymphoid cells in rat heart allografts

Gale A. Granger, Ph.D., *Irvine, Calif.,* and **Thomas C. Moore, M.D.,** *Los Angeles, Calif.*

Lymphocyte-rich preparations were prepared from minced autologous and allografted hearts of heterotopic heart allografted rats at intervals of 3 to 19 days after grafting. The number of lymphocytes which were extractable from autologous hearts remained constant at about 3 to 5 × 10^6 cells per heart. These cells, upon morphologic observation, appeared to be primarily small lymphocytes, which, when placed in culture, did not undergo any spontaneous LT secretion. However, the lymphocytes which could be extracted from allografted hearts began to increase in number at about 3 days after grafting, reaching a maximum at about 10 days and slowly declining thereafter. The morphologic appearance of these cells was primarily of medium to large lymphocytes. In addition, the cells extracted from the allograft were spontaneously involved in LT secretion, which reached a peak at about 10 days and then slowly declined thereafter. The data indicate that lymphoid cells removed from the rejecting allograft were activated, indicating their medium to large size, and involved in spontaneous LT secretion.

From the Department of Molecular Biology and Biochemistry, School of Biological Sciences, University of California, Irvine, and the Department of Surgery (Harbor General Hospital Campus), School of Medicine, University of California, Los Angeles.

LYMPHOKINES are a family of effector molecules which are produced by activated lymphocytes which may function as mediators of cellular immunity.[1, 4, 9] Lymphocytes are stimulated to produce lymphokines in vitro by several methods: (1) specific—addition of the sensitizing antigen to immune lymphoid cells in tissue culture, or (2) by coculture of histoincompatible lymphocytes, and (3) nonspecific—when nonimmune lymphocytes are cultured with mitogenic agents known to induce blast cell formation and DNA synthesis.[4] The latter (mitogenic agents) include substances such as phytohemagglutinin (PHA) and concanavalin A (Con-A).

Lymphotoxin (LT) is a lymphokine which has been shown to cause a concentration-dependent, nonspecific destruction of nonlymphoid cells in culture.[2, 12] LT has been identified in the cell-free culture media following activation of lymphocytes by all of the above treatments,[3] and inhibitors of protein synthesis reversibly inhibit its release by activated human lymphocytes.[11] The precise chemical composition of LT has not been established. It is known that human and mouse LT are proteins which differ from each other and from certain of the other lymphokines which have molecular weights in the 70,000 to 30,000 range.[1]

Accepted for publication June 6, 1974.

This work was supported by grants from the National Institutes of Health (AM-10373 and AI-09460), the Los Angeles County Heart Association, and the John A. Hartford Foundation.

Reprint requests: Thomas C. Moore, M.D., University of California, Harbor General Hospital, 1000 W. Carson St., Torrance, Calif. 90509.

Prior studies of LT have been concerned largely with in vitro activated lymphoid cells. The present brief report is concerned with in vivo stimulation of lymphoid cells in rats which received heterotopic heart allografts. The numbers of lymphocytes accumulating in the grafts, their microscopic appearance, and their capacity to secrete LT in vitro was assessed in the autologous ("native") and allografted hearts at various intervals after grafting.

MATERIALS AND METHODS

Inbred male Brown Norway (BN) rats* weighing approximately 300 grams were used as heart donors and inbred male Lewis rats* weighing approximately 300 grams were used as heterotopic heart allograft recipients. The ascending aorta of the donor heart was anastomosed end-to-side into the abdominal aorta of the ether-anesthetized recipient animal. The pulmonary artery of the donor heart was anastomosed end-to-side into the inferior vena cava of the recipient animal.

The heterotopic heart allograft was selected for these studies because it was possible to have the native and allografted organs in two separate body cavities to avoid possible difficulties resulting from adjacent study organs being involved in varying degrees of inflammatory reaction. BN and Lewis rats were employed because of their use in prior studies by one of us (T. C. M.) relating to the role of vasoactive substances in afferent and efferent arch of cellular immunity.

Recipient rats were killed at intervals from 3 to 19 days after grafting. The "native" and allografted hearts were removed for study. The hearts were rinsed in Eagle's minimal essential medium (MEM)† + 10 percent newborn calf serum (NBCS), then minced into fine fragments and centrifuged at 50 × g to remove tissue debris. The cells in the supernatant were pelleted by further centrifugation at 250 × g and rewashed in complete MEM culture medium. The suspension was

*BN and Lewis rats were obtained from Microbiological Associates, Walkersville, Md.

†Eagle's MEM and the NBCS were obtained from Grand Island Biological Company, Grand Island, N. Y.

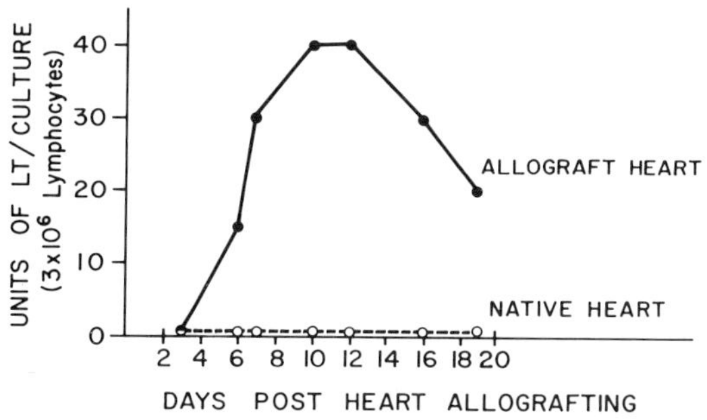

Fig. 1. Secretion of LT by lymphoid cells (3×10^6 per 1 ml. of culture) extracted from autologous and allografted hearts of heterotopic (abdominal) heart allografted rats at various intervals after grafting.

glass absorbed at 37° C. for 1 hour in 16 oz. prescription bottles at a cell density of 10 to 70×10^6 cells per bottle to remove polymorphonuclear cells and monocytes. Total viable and differential cell counts were performed. This method produced relatively pure (95 to 99 percent) concentrations of lymphocytes admixed with red blood cells and a few graft cells. The cell suspensions were cultured in MEM plus 10 per cent NBCS at a density of 3×10^6 lymphoid cells per milliliter for 72 hours. The culture medium was collected and cleared of cells and debris by centrifugation at 30 × g for 15 minutes. The supernatant fluid was diluted with fresh medium and tested in our standard (G. A. G.) tube culture titration technique, which has been previously described, to determine the levels of LT present.[10] Briefly, varying dilutions of test and control supernatant are tested for cytotoxic activity on 100,000 mouse L cells in 1.0 ml. MEM. At the end of 48 hours' incubation, the viable cells are removed from the monolayer by trypsinization and enumerated in a Coulter counter. The percent of destruction for each dilution titer of test or control supernatant is obtained by the formula

$$\% \text{ destruction} = \frac{\text{control-test}}{\text{control}} \times 100.$$

The dilution titer of test supernatant killing 50 percent of the target cells is designated as one unit of LT activity. Each assay was run in duplicate (i.e., two complete assays of 3

Table I. *In vitro secretion of LT by lymphoid cells extracted from allografted and autologous hearts from recipient Lewis rats at various intervals after grafting*

Supernatant Dilution	*Percent of traget L-cell destruction at various intervals after transplantation**							
	3 days		*6 days*		*10 days*		*19 days*	
	Allograft heart	*Native heart*	*Allograft heart*	*Native heart*	*Allograft heart*	*Native heart*	*Allograft heart*	*Native heart*
1:5	0	0	100	5	100	0	100	3
1:10	0	0	80	0	100	4	80	13
1:20	3	2	30	3	100	10	40	5
1:40	1	5	5	0	60	0	5	9
Units of LT activity†	0	0	<15	0	>40	0	<20	0

*Lymphoid cell suspensions were cultured at a density of 3×10^6 cells per milliliter for 72 hours. Dilutions of the cell-free culture supernatants were placed on L-cell monolayer tube cultures containing 100,000 cells per tube. After 48 hours, the number of intact cells remaining in the culture and the degree of target cell destruction was determined as described in "Materials and methods."

†Amount of LT activity is the dilution producing 50 percent destruction of target L Cells.

$\times 10^6$ ml. cultures of test lymphocytes). Four dilutions were assayed for cytotoxic activity for each culture medium.

RESULTS

Animals were put to death at 3, 6, 7, 10, 12, 16, and 19 days after heart allografting. Twenty-six hearts, native and allograft, from 13 animals were studied. Three animals were studied at 3 days and two at 6, 10, and 16 days.

There were variable numbers of lymphocytes extractable from the grafts at different times after grafting. A constant number of lymphocytes (3 to 5×10^6 cells) was extracted from the native or syngeneic heart of heart-allografted animals at all postgrafting intervals studied. These cells were predominantly of the small lymphocyte type. Assay of the supernatant derived from cultures of these cells for LT activity revealed zero units of LT at all postgrafting intervals.

From 3 to 5×10^6 lymphocytes, predominantly of the small lymphocyte type, were also obtained from each of the three allografted hearts studied at 3 days after grafting. The levels of LT in cultures of lymphoid cells obtained from native and allograft hearts at various intervals after grafting is presented in Table I. There was no detectable LT activity present in six of the culture supernatants obtained from these cells. However, at 6 days after grafting, the number of extractable lymphocytes in the allograft heart had increased to 30×10^6 cells per heart. The cells in this population appeared to be largely of the medium to large lymphocyte type. Fifteen units of LT activity per milliliter of supernatant were found in lymphocyte cultures obtained from allograft hearts 6 days after grafting (Fig. 1).

LT activity increased to 30 units per milliliter per 3×10^6 lymphocytes cultured from an allografted heart at 7 days after grafting. LT levels reached a maximum of 40 LT units per milliliter per 3×10^6 lymphocytes at 10 and 12 days after grafting. At 10 days after grafting, 50 to 70×10^6 lymphocytes were extracted from each allografted heart. At these intervals lymphocytes extracted from the allografted hearts were largely of the medium to large lymphocyte type. LT activity in units per 3×10^6 lymphocytes cultured from allografted hearts and the total number of lymphoid cells extractable decreased after 12 days after grafting.

DISCUSSION

The rat heart allograft model provides an opportunity to study in vivo stimulation of lymphocytes with respect to their relative levels of accumulation in the graft, their morphologic types (small, medium, or large), and amount of lymphokine secretion as measured by LT production. These studies were carried out in similar organs—one native and one allograft heart, in different body cavities (thoracic and abdominal) in the same animal and presumably exposed to the same cellular elements in circulating blood at intervals after grafting.

Essentially no change was found in the numbers of cells which accumulated, their morphology, or their LT-secretory activity of lymphocytes from native syngeneic hearts of allografted animals at all intervals after grafting. There was no difference between test and control allografted hearts at 3 days after grafting. However, at 6 days after grafting, the numbers of lymphocytes extractable from the graft increased as did their ability to secrete LT. The numbers of cells and their LT-secretory activity increased at intervals after grafting to a maximum at 10 days after grafting, with a gradual decline in LT after 12 days after grafting.

The 10 day maximums in relative numbers of harvestable lymphocytes from allografted hearts and in LT-secretory activity of these cells correlate to the 10 days postgrafting peak increase in Lewis rat allograft (skin and kidney) activity of histidine decarboxylase (HDC), the histamine-forming enzyme.[6, 7] It has been theorized that the activity of vasoactive substances such as histamine, the kinins, and prostaglandin E^1 may be involved in the vascular component of the recruiting, release, and attraction of immunocompetent lymphocytes to and from lymphoid organs and to the allograft target of the cellular immune response.[5]

In another study still in progress, we have observed that direct-vision (laporatomy) injection into Lewis rat spleens both of the mitogenic agent Con-A in control culture medium and of the lymphokines in the cell-free culture medium supernatant of 5 day Con-A activated lymphocytes has been associated with significantly higher splenic HDC activity at death after 4 days than that produced by control direct injections of physiologic saline solution. In vitro exposure of PHA and Con-A stimulated lymphocyte culture medium supernatants to lymphoid and nonlymphoid rat tissues produced variable results with respect to HDC activity, some stimulating and some inhibiting, but was associated with significant release of histamine into the incubating supernatant.[8]

REFERENCES

1. Granger, G. A.: Lymphokines, mediators of cellular immunity, Ser. Haemato. **4:** 8, 1972.
2. Hessinger, D. A., Daynes, R. A., and Granger, G. A.: The binding of human lymphotoxin to target cell membranes and its relation to cell-mediated cytodestruction, Proc. Nat. Acad. Sci. USA **11:** 3082, 1973.
3. Kolb, W. P., Williams, T. W., and Granger, G. A.: Lymphocyte activation and lymphotoxin production, *in* Bloom, B. R., and Glade, P. R., editors: In vitro methods in cell-mediated immunity New York, 1971, Academic Press, Inc., p. 333.
4. Lawrence, L. H., and Landy, M., editors: Mediators of cellular immunity, New York, 1969, Academic Press, Inc.
5. Moore, T. C.: A theory of the role of histamine metabolism in transplant rejection, Surg. Gynecol. Obstet. **132:** 489, 1971.
6. Moore, T. C., and Schayer, R. W.: Histidine decarboxylase activity of autografted and allografted rat skin, Transplantation **7:** 99, 1969.
7. Moore, T. C., Sinclair, M. C., and Lemmi, C. A. E.: Elevation in host splenic and allograft parenchymal and capsular histidine decarboxylase activity and weights following renal allografting in rats, SURGERY **75:** 203, 1974.
8. Moore, T. C., Granger, G. A., and Lemmi, C. A. E. In vivo elevation in rat splenic histidine decarboxylase activity by intra-splenic injection of con A and con A activited lymphokines, Int. Res. Comm. Sys. Med. Sci. Submitted for publication.
9. Ruddle, N. H.: Approaches to the quantative analysis of delayer hypersensitivity, Curr. Top. Microbiol. Immunol. **57:** 75, 1972.
10. Spofford, B., Daynes, R. A., and Granger, G. A.: Cell mediated immunity in vitro: New, highly sensitive assays for human lymphotoxin, J. Immunol. **112:** 2111, 1974.
11. Williams, T. W., and Granger, G. A.: Lymphocyte in vitro cytoxicity. Correlation of derepression with release of lymphotoxin from human lymphocytes, J. Immunol. **103:** 170, 1969.
12. Williams, T. W., and Granger, G. A.: Mechanisms of human lymphotoxin induced cell destruction, Cell. Immunol. **6:** 171, 1973.

Experience with autotransfusion in the surgical management of trauma

George J. Reul, Jr., M.D., R. Thomas Solis, M.D., S. Donald Greenberg, M.D., Kenneth L. Mattox, M.D., *and* **Hartwell H. Whisennand, M.D.,** *Houston, Texas*

Intraoperative autotransfusion or the salvage and immediate infusion of shed blood during surgery is a potential solution to the problems of blood procurement and the toxicity of blood transfusion. In order to evaluate the safety of this procedure, 25 selected trauma patients were studied. Most injuries were the result of penetrating trauma. Two techniques of autotransfusion were utilized: (1) the Bentley Autotransfusion System (ATS) consisting of a roller pump and infusion chamber, similar to the cardiotomy reservoir used during cardiopulmonary bypass; and (2) a device of our design consisting of an external vacuum exerted on a standard blood donor bag. We salvaged 105 units of blood in 25 patients. Coagulation studies were within normal limits except for fibrinogen, which was markedly decreased both in the reservior and in the immediate postoperative period. Most studies returned to normal within 2 days following autotransfusion. There were four deaths in the series. Some patients would not have survived without ATS, due to acute blood shortage. By limiting the selection of patients for autotransfusion and utilizing proper suction techniques with local anticoagulation, most of the complications previously reported with autotransfusion have been avoided. Autotransfusion is recommended as an adjunct to the treatment of the trauma patient and is especially useful in the patient receiving not massive transfusions but a moderate amount of blood.

From the Cora and Webb Mading Department of Surgery, Department of Medicine, and the Department of Pathology, Baylor College of Medicine and the Ben Taub General Hospital, Houston, Texas

BECAUSE of the increasing severity and frequency of trauma necessitating emergency surgery and the addition of complex elective surgical procedures, a seemingly insatiable demand for homologous blood has evolved. As large amounts of homologous blood are transfused, the inherent complications resulting from its administration have affected increasing numbers of patients. In the important recuperative period, serum hepatitis has delayed many satisfactory recoveries and eliminated some excellent surgical results. In addition, a significant group of patients have acute transfusion reactions or cannot obtain cross-matched blood readily because of complex antibodies. Because of unpredictable needs, a large supply of blood must be constantly available in an active trauma center.

Autotransfusion, or the salvage of acute blood loss and immediate reinfusion, is a potential solution to homologous blood toxicity and blood availability problems. Autotransfusion was proposed over 150 years ago.[8] Watson and Watson[30] reviewed the experience with autotransfusion in the era prior to homologous blood transfusion. Since that time, autotransfusion has been applied to

Accepted for publication June 6, 1974.

Reprint requests: Dr. George J. Reul, Jr., Texas Heart Institute, P.O. Box 20345, Houston, Texas 77025.

numerous surgical procedures.[1, 12-14, 16, 17, 27-29, 31] Recently, vast experience has been gained in the technique of cardiopulmonary bypass and the retrieval of large volumes of blood by cardiotomy suction during open-heart procedures. The importance of microfiltration of blood and a better understanding of shock and organ failure have evolved. These principles have been adapted to autotransfusion for further refinement of the existing techniques, thereby rendering a broader application. This report concerns our experience with the application of intraoperative autotransfusion to a selected group of trauma patients and the introduction of a new device for retrieval of blood from the chest cavity of patients with hemothorax.

CLINICAL MATERIAL

From January, 1973, through June, 1973, 25 patients, all victims of trauma, had acute reinfusion of their own shed blood by autotransfusion. There were 20 male and 5 female patients, ranging from 13 to 44 years of age. Injuries resulted from gunshot wounds in 15 patients, stab wounds in 7, and motor vehicular accidents in three. The chest was the most frequently injured area, accounting for 18 of the primary injuries. Twelve of these patients underwent exploratory thoracotomy and repair of their wounds. Four of the 12 patients had accompanying intra-abdominal repair through separate abdominal incisions for treatment of combined thoracoabdominal trauma. Six of the 18 patients with chest trauma did not have surgery but underwent chest tube thoracostomy with retrieval of blood solely through the chest tube. One patient underwent exploration of a groin wound with subsequent femoral artery repair. The remaining six patients had primary abdominal injuries and underwent intra-abdominal operations (Tables I and II).

MATERIALS AND METHOD

One of two types of autotransfusion was used, depending upon the type of injury and the subsequent treatment. In the emergency center, a device of our design was utilized for salvage of blood from hemothorax patients (Fig. 1). It consisted of a pump which was regulated to exert vacuum in a transparent sealed container into which a standard blood collection bag* had been inserted (Viavac unit†). Because of the larger lumen of the chest tube, a urological irrigating tubing† was attached to the standard blood collection bag which contained the standard anticoagulant citrate-phosphate-dextrose (CPD). At the time of insertion of the chest tube, it was clamped to minimize blood loss. The chest tube was then connected to the autotransfusion device by a standard rubber connecting tube and the clamp released, allowing blood to drain by gravity or vacuum applied

Table I. *Primary source of hemorrhage in patients receiving autotransfusion*

Source	*No.*
Thoracic:	
Lung	4
Chest wall	2
Thoracic spine	2
Liver (through diaphragm)	2
Heart	1
Pulmonary artery	1
Total	12
Abdominal:	
Spleen	3
Lumbar spine	1
Iliac vein	1
Portal vein	1
Total	6
Extremities: Femoral artery	1
Chest (hemothorax reinfusion only)	6
Total	25

Table II. *Secondary sources of hemorrhage in 19 patients receiving ATS*

Source	*No.*
Lung	4
Liver	3
Diaphragm	2
Inferior vena cava	2
Pancreas	2
Small bowel	2
Colon	1
Stomach	1
Subclavian vein	1
Kidney	2

*Fenwal Laboratories, Morton Grove, Ill.

†Travenol Laboratories, Morton Grove, Ill.

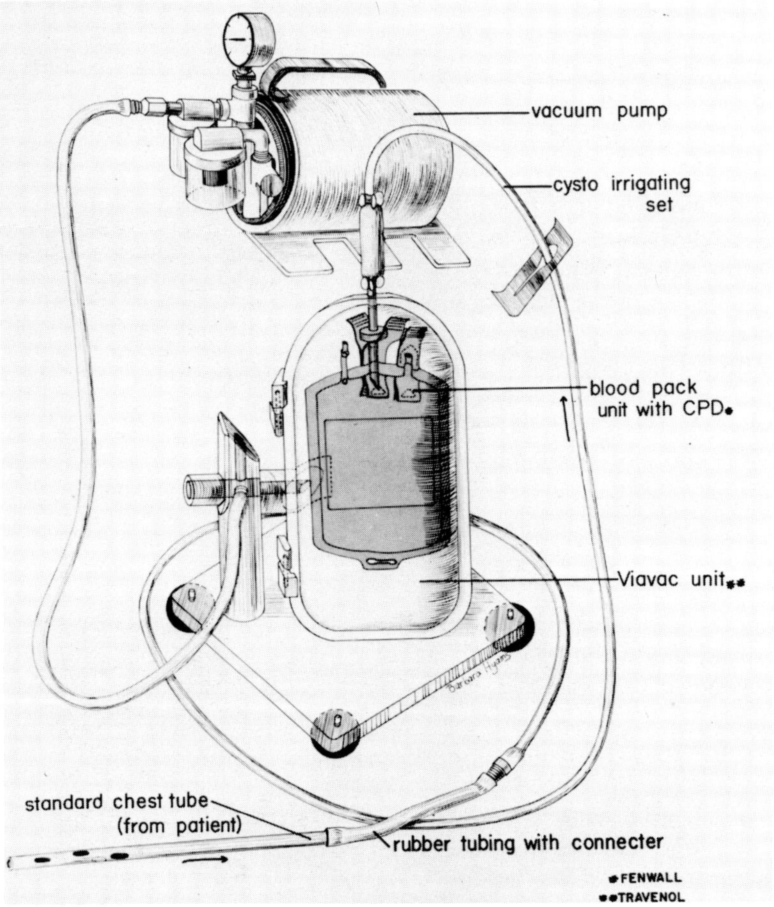

Fig. 1. Diagrammatic representation of the Viavac Autotransfusion Unit which is utilized for draining hemothorax into a standard blood collection bag. The bag is inverted and its contents reinfused into the patient through a fine-screen filter. External vacuum regulated by the vacuum pump is applied to the blood bag. The air must be expelled from the bag prior to transfusion.

to the blood bag by regulating the vacuum pump to the pressure desired. Generally suction of from 5 to 10 mm. Hg was required. This was well within the safe range for prevention of hemolysis but higher levels could be utilized. The blood was mixed with the CPD solution in the bag and the collecting tubing clamped. A standard blood tubing was inserted along with a Pall Ultipor* fine-screen filter to prevent the infusion of particulate matter. The bag was then placed on a stand and the blood reinfused through a large venous cannula. If air entered the bag at the time of suctioning, the air was bled out either through a separate vent created by inserting a needle into the tubing or through blood tubing prior to administration to the patient. If this is not done, there is a potential complication of air embolus when the blood is returned to the patient by utilizing an external pressure pump for infusion.

The second device was the Bentley Autotransfusion System (ATS),* which has been previously described[16, 17] (Fig. 2). The ATS is available commercially and consists of a cardiotomy reservoir and a roller pump similar to the suction unit employed during cardiopulmonary bypass. The blood was suctioned from the patient into the cardiotomy

*Pall Corporation, Glen Cove, L. I., N. Y.

*Bentley Autotransfusion System, ATS 100, Bentley Laboratories, Inc., Santa Ana, Calif.

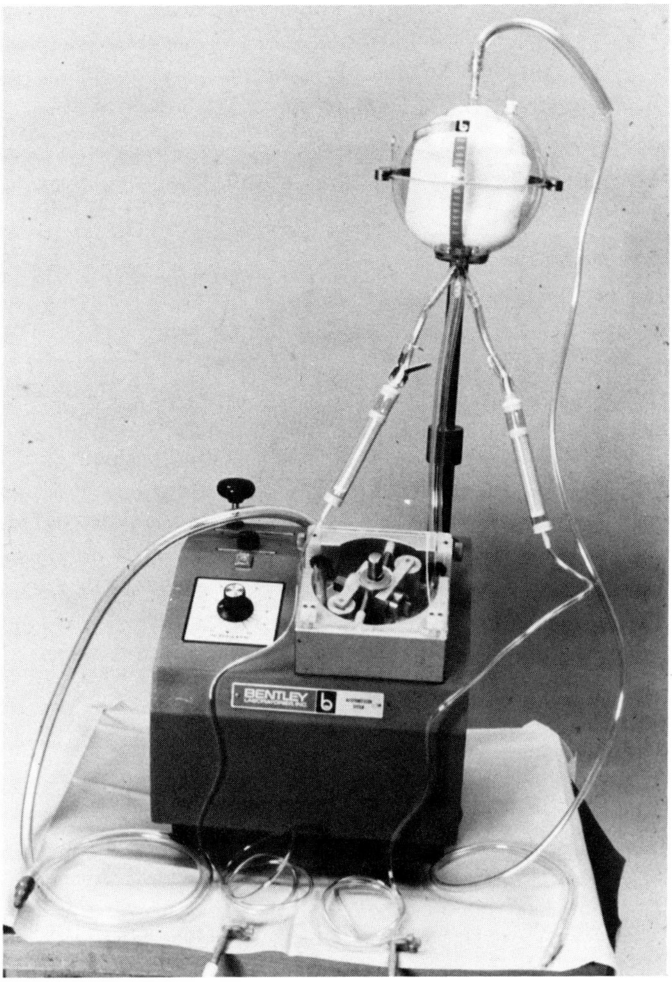

Fig. 2. Photograph of the Bentley Autotransfusion System (ATS) employed. The blood is suctioned by way of the suction tube into the cardiotomy reservoir and returned to the patient through the two intravenous lines. The rolled pump controls the speed of suctioning and blood return.

reservoir and returned to the patient by two separate lines. A 125 micron pore nylon filter was in the cardiotomy reservoir. The maximum infusion rate under pressure through a 15 gauge needle was approximately 900 ml. per minute. In the latter part of the series, a 40 micron fine screen filter* was placed in the suction (effluent) line.

Our technique in utilizing the ATS was established by first suctioning the blood into collection bags and analyzing the components. After adequate assurance of its safety, we proceeded with direct infusion into the patient. Clotted blood was not retrieved. The blood was suctioned with the suction tip always below the blood level to prevent an air-fluid interface, which causes hemolysis. Because of the risk of hemolysis, all shed blood was not salvaged. Most of the blood was suctioned with a roller pump speed not in excess of 160 r.p.m. The roller pump was turned off immediately when suctioning or blood infusion was not in progress. The blood was administered under pressure exerted in the cardiotomy reservoir through one or two intravenous lines. A percutaneous subclavian catheter and a peripheral vein

*Barrier Filter, Johnson & Johnson, New Brunswick, N. J.

cannula were used. Three-way stopcocks were placed at the level of the intravenous cannula so that other medications or homologous blood could be administered when the ATS was not infusing in both lines. Large clamps were used to stop the flow of blood in the ATS. Care was taken to avoid air embolus by maintaining a constant level of 200 c.c. in the cardiotomy reservoir until the last portion of blood was infused, at which time the blood was slowly returned to the patient and the tubing clamped as the cardiotomy reservoir was evacuated of blood. Almost all the actual autotransfusion times were less than 15 to 30 minutes since, in most cases, bleeding was controlled in that time period. In only two patients did the time exceed one hour.

Total-body heparinization or partial heparinization as described by others[6] was not employed because most of our trauma patients had multiple injuries. Furthermore, the use of local heparinization of the tubing and blood reservoir could be harmful because of the formation of platelet aggregates associated with partial heparinization.[7] The use of acid-citrate-dextrose (ACD) in the priming solution has been suggested by Klebanoff.[18] CPD is similar to ACD but less volume is required and it is less acidic. Therefore, CPD solution was used as the anticoagulant in both ATS and Viavac procurement of blood.

Stored blood contains 67 c.c. of CPD in each unit (500 c.c.). The basic anticoagulation solution we utilized in ATS consisted of 200 c.c. of CPD solution mixed with 800 c.c. of normal saline, totaling 1,000 c.c. Thus, in every 100 c.c. increment of prime solution, there were 20 c.c. of CPD. This was mixed and suctioned into the lines filling the cardiotomy reservoir and tricot filter priming the cardiotomy reservoir and bleeding the infusion lines of air. Once all the air was removed from the system, the remainder of the CPD solution was removed so that a level of 200 c.c. of the priming solution was maintained in the cardiotomy reservoir. The shed blood was then suctioned into the device until a total of at least 1,000 c.c. (800 c.c. of blood and 200 c.c. of prime with 40 c.c. of CPD) were obtained. The solution was then mixed and readministered to the patient. After each additional 1,000 c.c. had been suctioned into the cardiotomy reservoir, an additional 200 c.c. of the CPD solution was suctioned into the tubing to prevent washout of the CPD solution. We did not see clot on the tricot filter and the blood did not clot in the tubing.

SELECTION OF PATIENTS

The first category of patients especially ideal for autotransfusion were the noncontaminated cases with acute continuing blood loss treated by operation immediately after injury. Most patients with simple perforating wounds of the chest or blunt trauma to the chest requiring thoracotomy were ideal candidates, since only large wounds of the trachea, bronchus, or esophagus can cause internal contamination, and the blood loss is usually significant since we use the estimated acute loss of 1,500 c.c. from a chest wound as an indication for thoracotomy. Autotransfusion in the operating room was also applicable to the patients with moderate injury and acute blood loss from simple penetrating wounds of the abdomen which did not involve the hollow viscera. Wounds of the liver and pancreas were not contraindications. A second category of patients resulted from immediate need. These were patients without massive blood loss (that is, over one blood volume) in whom no homologous blood was available because of the urgency of the situation, blood shortage, or a difficult crossmatch. In these patients, autotransfusion was the only available method of maintaining a blood volume compatible with survival. It was utilized despite the type of injury. Proper precautions were taken by packing of grossly contaminated areas. A third category of candidates for ATS were the patients with massive injury resulting in blood loss of over one blood volume in whom ATS was used as a supplement to the massive blood replacement.

The external vacuum device was applied to patients who presented with hemothorax which occurred approximately 1 to 2 hours prior to admission and which was not as-

Table III. *Blood salvaged by ATS*

	Average (ml.)	*Range (ml.)*	*Total (ml.)*	*No. of patients*
Bentley Autotransfusion System	1,637	600-3,700	31,100	19
Travenol Viavac unit	1,340	350-4,000	21,500	11
Total			52,600	25*

*Five patients received both ATS and Viavac autotransfusion.

sociated with contaminated wounds. Intactness of the diaphragm was likewise assumed, although in one patient this was not true. Return of blood into the unit was limited in some cases and if a large amount of air was mixed with the blood or small amounts of blood were obtained, the blood was discarded.

General contraindications to the use of autotransfusion were: (1) the presence of malignant lesions, (2) gross contamination including colon injury with fecal spillage, small bowel injury with significant drainage, and stomach wounds, (3) wounds over 4 hours old, and (4) known hepatic or renal insufficiency. The presence of any of these contraindications was occasionally overruled by the lack of available blood. Thus, the autotransfusion unit was always on standby for every potentially serious trauma case.

RESULTS

The ATS alone was utilized in 14 patients (Table III). The ATS plus the Viavac unit was used in five other patients. The Viavac unit alone was used in six patients who did not undergo surgery and had drainage of penetrating wounds of the chest through the chest tube. The Viavac unit was utilized in 11 patients and an average of 1,340 ml. was salvaged. The ATS was utilized in a total of 19 patients and an average of 1,637 ml. was salvaged. Thus, in 25 patients, approximately 105 units of blood were salvaged by application of the two autotransfusion devices.

Because of the nature of their injuries, 16 of the 19 patients who underwent operations received homologous blood. Of the six patients who underwent Viavac drainage alone, one patient received 2 units of blood in addition to 1,400 ml. of autotransfused blood.

There were four deaths in the series. Two patients with massive injuries died in the operating room because of failure to control hemorrhage. One patient had a high-velocity gunshot wound to the abdomen with transection of the spinal cord and lumbar spine along with perforation of the inferior vena cava, aorta, and small bowel. He received 2,900 c.c. total autotransfusion and died because of failure to control hemorrhage from the lumbar spine. The other patient received 3,000 c.c. of autotransfused blood following blunt trauma which resulted in a complete disruption of the diaphragm and avulsion of the liver into the right chest.

Of the two patients who died in the postoperative period, one was a 15-year-old girl who had multiple injuries from a motor vehicular accident. She underwent exploratory laparotomy, splenectomy, and repair of liver wounds, receiving only 1,500 c.c. of autotransfused blood and over 20 units of homologous blood. In the postoperative period, she developed disseminated intravascular coagulation (DIC), severe pulmonary insufficiency, and renal failure. The other patient died following two 0.357 magnum gunshot wounds to the chest which resulted in perforation of the hilum of the right lung. She received 4,000 c.c. of blood by the Viavac unit in the emergency room and 2,200 c.c. of blood in the operating room from the autotransfusion unit. She also received 10 units of homologous blood. On the first postoperative day she developed severe pulmonary edema and DIC and died. At autopsy, transmission electron and light microscopy of the lung showed the characteristic picture of posttraumatic pulmonary insufficiency. Unfortunately, fat stains were not done, although the electron microscopy coincided with the classical picture of fat embolization. A microfilter was not in the suction line; it could have possibly prevented the dissemi-

Table IV. *Blood studies in 19 patients with ATS*

	Normal (mean/range)	Infusion line (mean/range)	First postop. day (mean/range)
Hematocrit (%)	43 (42-47)	26 (18-42)	—
White blood cell count (×1,000 mm.^{3})	75 (5-10)	10.9 (2.2-18.5)	13.7 (7.6-22.5)
Plasma free hemoglobin (mg./100 ml.)	0 —	49 (4-106)	63 (11-218)
Total bilirubin (mg./100 ml.)	(0.1-0.9)	0.8 (0.2-1.9)	0.8 (0.2-2.7)
Prothrombin time (sec.)	10.8 (10-13)	13.1 (10.9-15.2)	12.2 (10.4-14.7)
Partial thromboplastin time (sec.)	28.6 (25-40)	31.1 (25.3-40.2)	32.8 (27.7-42)
Fibrinogen (Gm./100 ml.)	300 (200-400)	170 (112-224)	203 (135-392)
Total protein (Gm./100 ml.)	7 (6-8)	4.2 (3.3-5.1)	4.8 (4.1-5.6)
Albumin (Gm./100 ml.)	3.9 (3.2-4.5)	2.5 (1.9-3.1)	3.1 (2.7-3.7)
Calcium	9.8 (9-11)	7.1 (6.2-10)	7.9 (6.6-8.7)
Cholesterol	225 (150-300)	91 (53-130)	156 (70-493)

nation of microaggregates, although none were seen in the precapillary arterioles.

Thus, of the 25 patients receiving autotransfusion, two patients died in the operating room because of mortal wounds and a third patient died of multiple blunt trauma where there was only minimal use of ATS. The last death may have represented a complication of autotransfusion, although many other factors were operative, including massive homologous blood infusion, loss of one lung, and hypothermia. These two patients were the only possible cases of DIC in the series of autotransfusion. There were no other serious complications such as renal failure, pulmonary insufficiency, hemorrhage, or infection in the surviving patients.

LABORATORY FINDINGS

In each patient, blood studies were measured in the following time periods: (1) from the infusion lines during the autotransfusion, (2) immediately postoperatively, and (3) once a day for the next four days following surgery. The studies were: blood hemoglobin, hematocrit, white blood cell count, platelet count, prothrombin time, partial thromboplastin time, fibrinogen level, plasma free hemoglobin, bilirubin, total protein, albumin, globulin, cholesterol, alkaline phosphatase, serum glutamic oxalacetic transaminase, serum glutamic pyruvic transaminase, amylase, creatinine, blood urea nitrogen, serum carbon dioxide content, sodium, potassium, calcium, and phosphorous. Blood cultures were taken if the patient was febrile postoperatively.

The studies obtained from the infusion line generally reflected the effects of hemodilution (Table IV). There was a hemodilution factor of from 5 to 20 percent, with the prime solution depending on the amount of autotransfusion, since a level of at least 200 c.c. of prime was used. Hemolysis was also apparent, although the levels were not as high as expected. Serum calcium levels in the cardiotomy reservoir probably reflected the hemodilution factor and low albumin levels. Denaturation of the protein may have accounted for some of the low protein and albumin levels. Blood coagulation studies were abnormal but not in excess of the values obtained in the first 24 hours following ATS. Most individual values were not in the coagulopathy range. Unfortunately, platelet counts were not obtained in a significant number of patients since most of the autotransfusion was done when platelet counts were not available. However, others have shown thrombocytopenia to be dependent on the volume of autotransfusion.[5, 6]

Some of the blood chemistry results measured immediately postoperatively and in the first through the fourth postoperative days were difficult to interpret since homologous blood was administered to most of the patients. The plasma free hemoglobin levels were significantly elevated but not to harmful levels. In the immediate postoperative period, the average plasma free hemoglobin was 63 mg. per 100 ml., the range being from 22 to 218 mg. per 100 ml. The fibrinogen levels were decreased in almost all the patients in the immediate postoperative period. Mild bilirubin elevations correlated with the amounts of blood autotransfused and the homologous blood administered. Bilirubin levels were somewhat higher on the third and fourth postoperative day (highest value, 4.2 mg. per 100 ml.). Serum protein and albumin gradually returned to normal in all patients. The postoperative mean total protein (4.8 mg. per 100 ml.) appears low when compared to the albumin (3.1 percent). The reason for this discrepancy was not apparent. Blood coagulation studies returned to normal in the survivors after the first 24 hours.

In patients who did not receive autotransfused blood from the ATS, i.e., the patients with hemothorax only who underwent autotransfusion from the Viavac unit, there were no significant alterations in blood chemistry studies obtained postoperatively. Usually no more than 1,500 c.c. of blood was given to these patients because of the nature of their injuries, and therefore any dose-related effects did not occur.

COMMENTS

The effects of autotransfusion have been studied rather extensively.[4, 5, 17, 27-29] Thrombocytopenia, hypofibrinogenemia, and hemolysis are the principal complications. These complications appear to be dose-related and are similar to those which occur with the administration of homologous blood.[19, 21, 24] Platelets lose their viability within a few days of storage in ACD and the clotting factors are altered.[2] Thus, even though the platelet count of the reinfused blood may be low, it is probably higher than most units of stored blood. Hypofibrinogenemia is a natural sequela after blood clots and may also result when the blood is in contact with the peritoneal serosa or pleural cavity. The presence of plasma free hemoglobin is inevitable for many reasons. Trauma to the blood cells at the time of suctioning results in the generation of plasma free hemoglobin because of the increased air-blood interface, high vacuum pressure of suction, blood contact with tubing, or clot formation. A safe plasma free hemoglobin level is difficult to determine. It has become obvious that dehydration and acidosis may render harmless levels of plasma free hemoglobin dangerous to the kidney tubule, resulting in acute tubular necrosis.[3, 10, 11, 32] Thus, if dehydration and acidosis are avoided by proper blood volume replacement and administration of sodium bicarbonate when needed, the potential harmful effects of plasma free hemoglobin may be avoided. Moderately high levels of plasma free hemoglobin are relatively well tolerated following cardiopulmonary bypass. In our series, there was no evidence of acute tubular necrosis from the autotransfusion.

The possibility of air embolism by both the Bentley Autotransfusion System and the Viavac unit is a potentially lethal but avoidable problem. The warning photoelectric alarm in the ATS should not be relied upon since a clot on the tricot may obscure the cell and silence the alarm. Strict observation of the fluid level is therefore mandatory. Air infusion may also result from the Viavac unit if air is in the blood collection bag at the time of reinfusion under pressure, but this may easily be avoided by bleeding air from the blood bag prior to forcing the blood into the patient.

Unavoidable formation of platelet microaggregates occurs during collection and infusion or during the clotting process prior to retrieval. The effects of these aggregates on the microvasculature following homologous blood administration have been well described.[9, 15, 20, 22, 25, 26] Employment of a filter with smaller pore size than the cardiotomy tricot filter of 125 microns appears to be essential to avoid at least platelet aggregate infusion along with infusion of particulate matter, cell membranes, foreign material from the wound, and possibly fat emboli.[23] The type of aggregates which form appears to be dependent somewhat on the type of anticoagulation used in the ATS unit.[7] The chelating effect of locally employed ACD or CPD appears to cause less aggregate formation than partial heparinization locally or systemically or total body heparinization with large doses of heparin.[7]

With local anticoagulation with CPD, the problems of heparinization can be avoided. Harmful effects of CPD solution are well tolerated even in large amounts, as evidenced during rapid infusion of homologous blood. The dosage of CPD utilized in our series results in a volume of approximately 40 c.c. of CPD for every 800 c.c. of blood obtained. This is approximately one half the amount of CPD used when whole blood is collected and stored (67 c.c. of CPD per each 500 c.c. unit of blood).

Further techniques to avoid clotting in the ATS are the confinement of autotransfusion to short periods, administering the blood retrieved immediately after adequate dilution with the priming solution, and avoiding the introduction of old clotted blood into the system. Even though the microfilter will filter most of the clot from the blood, its potentials for toxicity, in addition to the microaggregates, are high plasma free hemoglobin, low fibrinogen and platelet levels, and the possible presence of fibrinolysins. These potentially harmful effects of microaggregates and clot infusion may be diminished by adhering to the techniques described.

In vivo red cell survival of the autotransfused blood was not measured but changes in red cell survival have not occurred after infusion from hemothorax[29] or in experimental administration of autotransfused blood in large amounts.[5] Serial hematocrits on our patients remained stable after the initial period of hemostasis.

After following all these precautionary measures, the major question is: is autotransfused blood better than, the same as, or more harmful than similar amounts of homologous blood? Unfortunately, because of the selectivity employed in this study, the number of patients available for autotransfusion did not allow a randomized controlled study. With the wide variety of trauma injuries and surgical repairs possible, a large number would have to be studied. Like homologous blood, the toxicity of the autotransfused blood is dose related. There appeared to be no harmful effects of infusion of 1,500 c.c. or less of autotransfused blood with the technique used. When the seriously injured patient requires massive amounts of autotransfused blood and homologous blood, many factors determine the outcome and it is difficult to single out autotransfusion as the cause of a complication such as disseminated intravascular coagulation, pulmonary and renal insufficiency, hypothermia, or other system failure. Thus, it would seem that the technique of autotransfusion is most applicable not to the patient requiring massive blood transfusion but to the patient who may require 3 or 4 units of blood during the operative treatment of trauma. In these patients, the complications are minimal and homologous blood may be completely avoided. On the other hand, ATS may not increase survival in massive blood transfusion but it will certainly decrease the drain on the blood bank in these sometimes hopeless mortal injuries. The need for a controlled series of randomly selected patients comparing autotransfusion to homologous blood transfusion is obvious.

REFERENCES

1. Backer-Grondahl, N.: Autotransfusion of blood, Acta Chir. Scand. **3:** 105, 1953.
2. Baldini, M., Costea, N., and Pameshek, W.: The viability of stored human platelets, Blood **16:** 1669, 1960.
3. Barrett, J. O. W., and York, W.: An investigation into mechanism of production of blackwater fever, Ann. Trop. Med. **3:** 1, 1909.
4. Bennett, S. H., Hoye, R. C., and Riggle, G. C.: Intraoperative autotransfusion: Preliminary report of a new blood suction device for

anticoagulation of autologous blood, Am. J. Surg. **123:** 257, 1972.
5. Bennett, S. H., Geelhoed, G. W., Gralnick, H. R., and Hoyde, R. C.: Effects of autotransfusion on blood elements, Am. J. Surg. **125:** 273, 1973.
6. Brener, B. J., Raines, J., and Darling, R. C.: The use of intraoperative autotransfusion in abdominal aortic resections, Arch. Surg. **107:** 78, 1973.
7. Brener, B. J.: *In* First Annual Bentley Autotransfusion Seminar, Bentley Laboratories, Inc., 1973.
8. Blumdell, J.: Experiments on the transfusion of blood, Med. Chir. Trans. **9:** 56, 1918.
9. Connell, R. S., and Swank, R. L.: Pulmonary fine structure after hemorrhagic shock and transfusion of ageing blood, *in* Microcirculatory approaches to current therapeutic problems, 6th European Conference on Microcirculation, Aalborg, 1970, Basel, 1971, S. Karger AG, pp. 49-58.
10. DeGowin, E. L., Osterhagen, H. F., and Andersch, M.: Renal insufficiency from blood transfusion relation to urinary acidity, Arch. Intern. Med. **59:** 432, 1937.
11. DeGowin, E. L., Warner, E. D., and Randall, W. L.: Renal insufficiency from blood transfusion. II. Anatomical changes in man compared with those dogs with experimental hemoglobinuria, Arch. Intern. Med. **61:** 609, 1938.
12. Dorang, L. A., Klebanoff, G., and Kemmerer, W. T.: Autotransfusion in long-segment spinal fusion, Am. J. Surg. **123:** 686, 1972.
13. Dyer, R. H., Jr., Alexander, J. T., and Brighton, C. T.: Atraumatic aspiration of whole blood for intraoperative autotransfusion, Am. J. Surg. **123:** 510, 1972.
14. Griswold, R. A., and Ortner, A. B.: The use of autotransfusion in surgery of the serous cavities, Surg. Gynecol. Obstet. **77:** 167, 1943.
15. Jenevein, E. P., and Weiss, D. L.: Platelet microemboli associated with massive blood transfusion, Am. J. Pathol. **45:** 313, 1964.
16. Klebanoff, G.: Early clinical experience with a disposable unit for the intraoperative salvage and reinfusion of blood loss (intraoperative autotransfusion), Am. J. Surg. **120:** 718, 1970.
17. Klebanoff, G., Phillips, J., and Evans, W.: Use of a disposable autotransfusion unit under varying conditions of contamination, Am. J. Surg. **120:** 351, 1970.
18. Klebanoff, G.: *In* First Annual Bentley Autotransfusion Seminar, Bentley Laboratories, Inc., 1973.
19. Kovaric, J. J., and Hamit, H. F.: The use of fresh blood to correct coagulation defects associated with trauma and shock, Milit. Med. **133:** 534, 1968.
20. Reul, G. J., Greenberg, S. D., Lefrak, E. A., McCollum, W. B., Beall, A. C., Jr., and Jordan, G. L., Jr.: Prevention of post-traumatic pulmonary insufficiency: Fine screen filtration of blood, Arch. Surg. **106:** 386, 1973.
21. Simmons, R. L., Collins, J. A., Heisterkamp, C. A., Mills, D. E., Ancrea, R., and Phillips, L. L.: Coagulation disorders in combat casualties. I. Acute changes after wounding. II. Effects of massive transfusion. III. Postresuscitative changes, Ann. Surg. **169:** 455, 1969.
22. Solis, R. T., and Gibbs, M. B.: Filtration of the microaggregates in stored blood, Transfusion **12:** 245, 1972.
23. Solis, R. T., et al.: Filtration of microaggregates formed in vivo, *in* First Annual Bentley Autotransfusion Seminar, Bentley Laboratories, Inc., B7-45, 1973.
24. Sunada, T., Sugihara, H., Sato K., Sakato, M., and Sato, T.: Hemorrhagic tendency after massive transfusion of preserved blood, SURGERY **50:** 437, 1961.
25. Swank, R. L.: Alteration of blood on storage: Measurement of adhesiveness of "aging" platelets and leukocytes and their removal by filtration, N. Engl. J. Med. **265:** 728, 1961.
26. Swank, R. L., and Porter, G. A.: Disappearance of microemboli transfused into patients during cardiopulmonary bypass, Transfusion **3:** 192, 1963.
27. Symbas, P. N., Levin, J. M., Ferrier, F. L., Muse, A. D., and Sybers, R. G.: Autotransfusion and its effects upon the blood components and the recipient, *in* Zuidema, G. C., and Skinner, D. B., editors: Current topics in surgical research, New York and London, 1969, Academic Press, Inc., vol. 1, p. 387.
28. Symbas, P. N., Levin, J. M., Ferrier, F. L., and Sybers, R. G.: A study on autotransfusion from hemothorax, South. Med. J. **62:** 671, 1969.
29. Symbas, P. N.: Autotransfusion from hemothorax: Experimental and clinical studies, J. Trauma **12:** 689, 1972.
30. Watson, C. M., and Watson, J. R.: Autotransfusion: Review of American literature with report of two additional cases, Am. J. Surg. **33:** 232, 1936.
31. Wilson, J. D., Utz, D. C., and Taswell, H. F.: Autotransfusion during transurethral resection of the prostate: Technique and preliminary clinical evaluation, Mayo Clin. Proc. **44:** 374, 1969.
32. York, W., and Nauss, R. W.: The mechanism of the production of suppression of urine in blackwater fever, Ann. Trop. Med. **5:** 287, 1911.

Thymectomy in the young pig: Effects on the level of circulating thymic hormone

M. Lacombe, M.D., F. Perner, M.D., M. Dardenne, M.D., *and* **J. F. Bach, M.D.,** *Paris, France*

Thymectomy in the young pig induces a rapid decrease in the level of a serum factor active on mouse rosette-forming cells. Conversely, this activity, which is also found in thymic extracts, is not altered by sham thymectomy.

From Hôpital Necker, Paris, France.

SURGICAL THYMECTOMY has been performed on a number of animal species, including the dog,[6] mouse,[7] rat,[5] and chicken[12] and in human subjects.[8] Few data are available on thymectomy in pigs.[6, 9] This is, however, an interesting matter since the pig has now proved to be an important species for many immunological studies, including transplantation. A swine leukocyte-antigen system has even recently been developed (S.L.A.).[10, 11]

The particular problems raised by thymectomy in the pig are linked to the size of the animal and the general problems of thoracic surgery in this species and also to the particular morphology of the thymus in the pig.

The porcine thymus consists of two parts, one in the neck and the other in the thorax (Fig. 1). The cervical part is made of two lobes. Each lobe is located laterally along the cervical vessels between the laryngotracheal axis and thyroid posteriorly, the subhyoid muscles anteriorly, the vascular axis deep, and the sternomastoid muscle superficially. Each lobe occupies most of the neck's length beginning at the base of the mouth, in contact with the twelfth cranial nerve pair, down to the cervicothoracic junction. At this level the two lobes meet on the median line to continue to the thoracic part. Vascularization is made by multiple vessels coming from and going to the carotid-jugular axis. The thoracic part is located in the anterosuperior part of the mediastinum in front of the pericardium and is more developed on the left side where it reaches the phrenic nerve.

Facing such a complicated anatomy, the problem arises of leaving behind some functional tissue after thymectomy, which may be detrimental for a number of studies. To check the quality of the thymectomy we have not only carefully examined the pigs at the time of death but have also measured the level of the circulating thymic hormone recently described in several other animal species including the mouse and in human subjects.[1, 2, 3] In all cases, the hormone disappeared after thymectomy whereas sham thymectomy did not induce any change in its level.

MATERIAL AND METHODS

Animals. Pigs were large white pigs with an average weight of 25 kilograms and an average age of 6 weeks (4 to 10 weeks).

Accepted for publication June 6, 1974.

Reprint requests: J. F. Bach, M.D., Clinique Nephrologique, Hôpital Necker, 161 rue de Sèvres—75730, Paris France.

Arteriovenous shunt. A silicone rubber arteriovenous shunt was placed between the common carotid artery and the jugular vein 2 to 5 days before thymectomy. This shunt allowed repeated blood samples, facilitated the pressure surveillance during the operation, and permitted easy postoperative care.

Thymectomy. The operation was preceded by the injection 90 minutes before anesthesia of atropine sulfate (0.25 mg. intramuscularly) and acepromazine maleate (10 mg. intramuscularly). Anesthesia was obtained by inhalation of a mixture of halothane, nitrogen protoxide, and oxygen. An endotracheal tube was inserted and ventilation was performed with a volumetric respiratory (R.P.R.). Anesthesia was maintained by varying the percentage of halothane in the mixture.

Follow-up of the pig during the operation was performed by evaluating blood pressure through the arterial cannula of the shunt connected to an electric manometer (Telco). Saline was infused through the venous cannula of the shunt. Nothing else was administered in order to avoid any interference with the biological tests to be performed later.

A long cervicosternal incision from the base of the mouth to the xiphoid process was performed with median total sternotomy. Thymectomy began by ablation of the two cervical lobes of the thymus, the dissection of which was relatively easy. Hemostasis of the thymic vessels was obtained by coagulation. The most difficult part of the operation was the ablation of the higher part of each lobe, which was in direct contact with the base of the mouth and the twelth cranial nerves.

The ablation of the thoracic part was performed afterwards. The thoracic thymus was dissected from the pericardium, the pleura, and the phrenic nerves. Thymectomy ended with the dissection of the gland at the level of the cervicothoracic junction. In all cases particular care was taken to remove the entire gland intact, without leaving separated fragments.

When the pleura were open the lung was reinflated before the end of the operation by increasing the gas output of the respirator. No drain was necessary. The sternum was closed at three points with nonresorbable thread. Skin was closed hermetically.

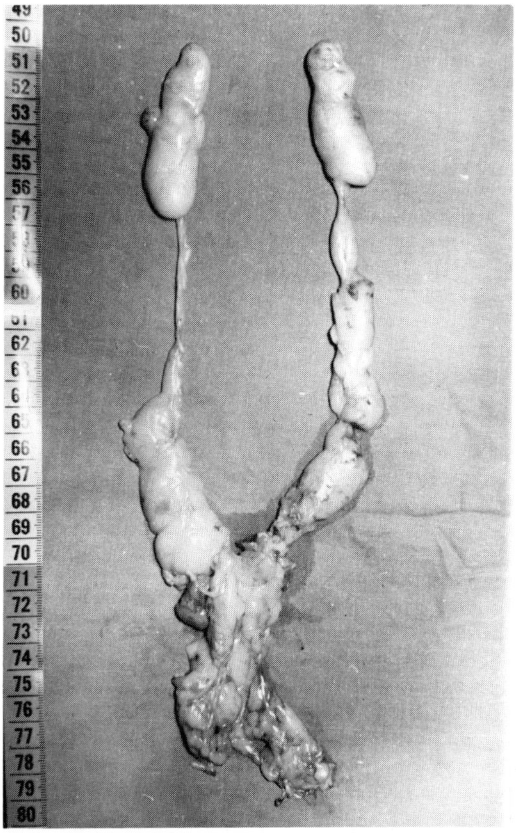

Fig. 1. Pig thymus after surgical thymectomy.

Postoperative care. Artificial ventilation was continued until the animal was completely awake. As soon as the animal breathed spontaneously, the endotracheal tube was removed. No infusion or antibiotics were given after the operation.

Sham thymectomy. Sham thymectomies were performed as controls for the thymectomy. The operation was the same as that described above with the only difference being that the thymus was dissected completely but was not removed. The vessels were carefully identified and inspected, but not ligated.

Serum thymic hormone determination. Serum was collected and stored at –20° C. before testing. It was ultrafiltered through Amicon membranes CF 50 and then incubated for 90 minutes at 37° C. with spleen

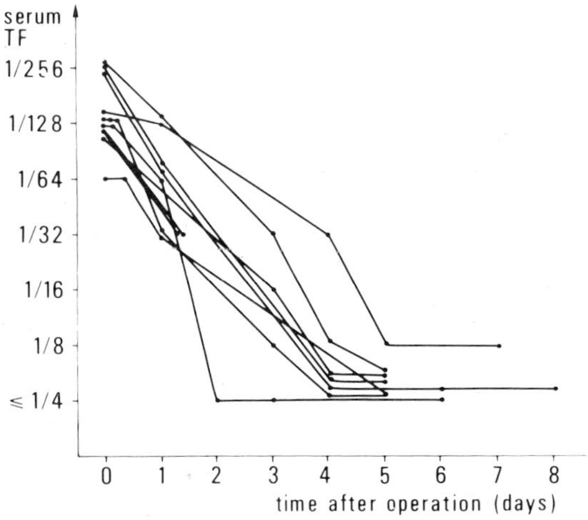

Fig. 2. Effects of thymectomy on serum thymic factor (TF) level in 9 pigs.

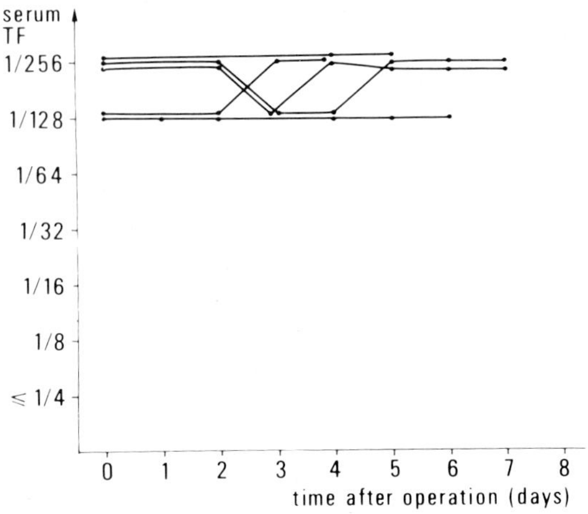

Fig. 3. Effects of sham thymectomy on serum TF level in 5 pigs.

cells from C57/B16 mice thymectomized 10 to 15 days earlier. Thymic hormone evaluation was performed as described previously.[1-3]

Serum thymic factor (TF) was detected by incubating the filtered serum in a hemolysis tube with 3×10^6 spleen cells from adult C57/B16 mice thymectomized 10 to 20 days earlier. The incubation lasted for 90 minutes at 37° C. in the presence of azathioprine (Az) at a concentration of 10 μg per milliliter. Such a concentration is intermediate between the AZ minimal concentration inhibiting 50 percent spleen RFC from normal mice (1 μg per milliliter) and from adult thymectomized mice (25 to 10 μg per milliliter). At the end of the incubation period, 12×10^6 sheep red blood cells (SRBC) were added to the cells which were then centrifuged and resuspended by rotation on a roller (10 cm. in diameter) at low speed (10 r.p.m.). RFC were counted in a hemocytometer. In the absence of TF, the number of RFC was $1210/10^6 \pm 120$ (S. D.). In the presence of LTF, the RFC level was lowered to 200 to $400/10^6$ cells. In the absence of AZ, normal serum induced no inhibition of RFC except at the highest concentrations (1/1 to 1/2).

RESULTS

Pig survival. Twenty pigs were operated on. There were 15 thymectomies and 5 sham thymectomies. Among the 15 thymectomized pigs were three early postoperative deaths in the 12 hours following the operation: one by cardiac arrest at the end of the procedure, one by respiratory failure (improper intubation), and one by accidental opening of the shunt which induced a rapid air embolus. The 12 surviving pigs were bled systematically at different times after the operation and were killed between 9 and 14 days after the operation in order to collect the blood.

Among the 5 sham thymectomized pigs all were in good health before death, which was induced between 10 and 20 days.

Thymectomy control. Macroscopic examination of the operated area prior to death showed that no thymus remnants could be found in the thorax or the neck of the thymectomized pigs.

Serum level of circulating thymic hormone in normal pigs. The level of serum thymic hormone was studied systematically in 20 pigs before any operation. The level was regularly between 1/64 and 1/128 (the maximum dilution of serum, giving to the spleen cells from adult thymectomized mice sensitivity to azathioprine). This level was comparable to that found in human or mouse serum. It confirmed the absence of species specificity of the rosette assay for thymic hormone.

Effect of thymectomy. In all cases thymectomy induced a very rapid disappearance of the serum thymic factor. The half-life was less than 24 hours, and 4 to 6 hours in the few pigs in which it could be studied accurately. There was no recovery of the serum factor level up to 14 days after thymectomy. Fig. 2 shows the curves of disappearance of the thymic hormone from pig serum in all the animals studied.

Sham thymectomy. The level of circulating thymic hormone was never altered by sham thymectomy, as shown in Fig. 3.

DISCUSSION

This paper presents a technique for thymectomy in young pigs which has proved to be reliable and which produced a high survival rate in the animals. The mortality rate was low and became nil after the fifth pig of the series—once a few technical problems had been solved. The quality of the thymectomy could be confirmed in this particular study by the dosage of the circulating thymic hormone. A total disappearance of the hormone after thymectomy indicated that there was no ectopic functional thymus in the pig, since, if it had been the case, one should have still seen a significant activity after removal of the main gland. The pig may thus prove to be an interesting tool in the future for the study of the effect of thymectomy, as has been already stressed by Binns.[4]

The discovery of the presence of the thymic hormone in the pig extends the findings already made in other animal species. It confirms, as mentioned above, the absence of species specificity of the rosette assay for thymic hormone, which might suggest that the pig is an interesting species in which to test the activity of thymic extracts prepared in other species. Moreover, it provides direct proof of the existence of the thymic hormone in the pig, and eventually it establishes the basis for a fractionation of pig thymic hormone, either from thymus gland or from serum as we have been doing recently (unpublished results).

REFERENCES

1. Bach, J. F., and Dardenne, M.: Thymus dependency of rosette-forming cells. Evidence for a circulating thymic hormone, Immunology **4:** 345, 1973.
2. Bach, J. F., and Dardenne, M.: Studies on thymus products. II. Demonstration and characterization of a circulating thymic hormone, Immunology **25:** 353, 1973.
3. Bach, J. F., Dardenne, M., Papiernik, M., Barois, A., Levasseur, P., and Le Brigand, H.: Evidence for a serum factor secreted by the human thymus, Lancet **22:** 1056, 1972.
4. Binns, R. M.: Cellular immunology in the pig, Proc. R. Soc. Med. **66:** 1155, 1973.
5. Folch, H., and Waksman, B. H.: In vitro responses of rat lymphocytes following adult thymectomy. I. Rapid decrease and recovery of responses to mitogens and hemiallogeneic cells, J. Immunol. **109:** 1046, 1972.
6. Kisken, W. A.: Skin allograft survival in the thymectomized azathioprine-treated adult mongrel dogs, Arch. Surg. **92:** 386, 1966.
7. Miller, J. F. A. P.: Studies on leukaemic mice. The role of the thymus in leukaemia genesis by cell-free leukaemic filtrates, Br. J. Cancer **14:** 93, 1960.
8. Papatestas, A. E., Alpert, L. I., Osserman, K. E., Osserman, R. S., and Kark, A. E.: Studies in myasthenia gravis: effects of thymectomy. Results on 185 patients with non thymomatous myasthenia gravis, 1941-1969, Am. J. Med. **50:** 465, 1971.
9. Pestana, C., Hallenbeck, G. A., and Shorter, R. G.: Thymectomy in newborn pigs, J. Surg. Res. **5:** 306, 1965.
10. Vaiman, M., Renard, C., Lafage, P., Ameteau, J., and Nizza, P.: Evidence for a histocompatibility system in swine (SL-A), Transplantation **10:** 155, 1970.
11. White, D. J. G., Bradley, B., Calne, R. Y., and Binns, R. M.: The relationship of the histocompatibility locus in the pig to allograft survival, Transplant. Proc. **5:** 317, 1973.
12. Wick, G., Kite, J. H., and Witerbsky, E.: Spontaneous thyroiditis in the obese strain of chickens. IV. The effect of thymectomy and thymo-bursectomy on the development of the disease, J. Immunol. **104:** 54, 1970.

Cardiopulmonary effects of volume loading of primates in endotoxin shock

Lazar J. Greenfield, M.D., Richard H. Jackson, Ronald C. Elkins, M.D., Jacqueline J. Coalson, Ph.D., *and* **Lerner B. Hinshaw, Ph.D.,** *Oklahoma City, Okla.*

Myocardial performance was evaluated in rhesus monkeys after endotoxin shock, and the responses to fluid loading with colloid were measured in both anesthetized control and experimental groups. Minute work and cardiac output (CO) were decreased in five monkeys after 6 hours endotoxin to levels significantly below control values. Infusing colloid to a mean left ventricular end-diastolic pressure (LVEDP) of 12 to 15 mm. Hg increased both CO and minute work significantly but they remained one half that of the control group of four primates after fluid loading. Improved cardiac performance persisted after infusion through a 30 minute recovery stage when LVEDP returned to normal. Simultaneous pulmonary arterial wedge (PAW) pressures showed some correlation with LVEDP reading up to 6 mm. Hg, but above that level the PAW underestimated the LVEDP by 3 to 6 mm. Hg. Microscopic study showed that fluid loading produced comparable pulmonary edema in both groups, but endotoxin produced ultrastructural capillary lesions. A normal PAW pressure after fluid administration can occur after transient overloading of the left ventricle. Since interstitial pulmonary edema is not readily reversible, persistent respiratory insufficiency may result and the cause be unsuspected unless ventricular filling pressures are monitored during fluid administration.

From the Departments of Surgery, Pathology, Physiology, and Biophysics, University of Oklahoma Health Sciences Center, and the Veterans Administration Hospital, Oklahoma City, Okla.

VARIABLE observations have been reported on the relationship between pulmonary arterial wedge (PAW) pressures and left atrial (LA) pressures measured consecutively in patients with valvular or congenital heart disease, or simultaneously in experimental animals.[3, 6, 24] Since LA pressure is the same as left ventricular pressure during diastole in the absence of mitral valve disease, it is usually assumed that left ventricular end-diastolic pressure (LVEDP) has the same relationship to PAW pressure as to the LA pressure during ventricular diastole. Consequently the ready accessibility of pulmonary arterial pressure measurement with the development of flow-directed balloon catheters can provide an indirect bedside approach to assessment of left ventricular function. However, variability of these measurements, particularly in shock, has concerned the clinician attempting to improve cardiac output by volume loading without producing pulmonary edema.

Cardiac output (CO) usually shows a steady decline in human septic shock[18] but

Accepted for publication June 12, 1974.

This work was supported in part by United States Public Health Service Grant HL 15037, the Office of Naval Research Contract N 00014-68-A-0496, and the Markle Foundation (Dr. Greenfield).

Reprint requests: Lazar J. Greenfield, M.D., Department of Surgery, Medical College of Virginia, P. O. Box 786, Richmond, Va. 23298.

there is disagreement regarding the pathogenesis of cardiac failure in man[7] or the nonhuman primate.[8] The development of early myocardial failure in clinical sepsis could account for the lowered CO but a significant decrease in venous return to the heart is the more likely explanation and has been confirmed in the dog[23] and rhesus monkey.[2] Studies using the primate model[14, 19] indicate that its hemodynamic characteristics make it particularly suitable as a shock model.

The present study was designed to evaluate primate myocardial performance in endotoxin shock and the cardiopulmonary response to fluid loading with colloid. Also tested was the validity of using PAW pressure to assess left ventricular filling pressure as opposed to direct catheterization of the left ventricle to measure LVEDP.

METHODS

Eleven healthy adult rhesus monkeys *(Macaca mulatta)* of both sexes were selected for study. They were anesthetized by intravenous administration of 20 to 25 mg. of pentobarbital per kilogram of body weight. A No. 5 Lehman catheter was threaded into the left ventricle and a No. 5 balloon-tipped catheter was positioned in the left pulmonary artery from the femoral artery and vein. A No. 19 Teflon needle was introduced into the opposite femoral artery and a No. 6 Goodale-Lubin catheter was advanced into the right atrium. All catheters were positioned under direct fluoroscopic control. A cuffed endotracheal tube was inserted and the cuff inflated to permit the collection of expired gases and allow for periodic positive pressure ventilation to prevent atelectasis. The endotracheal tube was connected to a Sierra valve with an 8 ml. dead space, and expired gases were collected in a water-sealed spirometer. Expired gases and arterial and mixed venous blood were analyzed for pH, P_{CO_2} and P_{O_2} on an analyzer (Instrumentation Laboratories Model 113) calibrated with known gas mixtures prior to each determination. Oxygen content of arterial and mixed venous blood was measured directly (Lexington Instruments, Lex-O_2-Con). Oxygen consumption ($\dot{V}_{O_2}$) was calculated using these data and cardiac output (CO) was calculated by the Fick method. Left ventricular end-diastolic pressure (LVEDP) and pulmonary arterial wedge pressure (PAW) were recorded with a single Statham P23Db transducer. Systemic arterial pressure (SAP) was recorded with a separate transducer on a multichannel oscillographic recorder. Minute work was calculated from the formula

$$\frac{(\text{MSAP} - \text{LVEDP})\ \text{CO}\ (1.36)}{100}$$

which is a modification of Ross' formula for stroke work[20] where MSAP and LVEDP are in millimeters of mercury, CO is in liters per minute, and minute work is expressed in kilogram-meters. All pressure measurements were recorded simultaneously.

After baseline hemodynamic, respiratory, and blood gas data had been obtained, five monkeys were injected with 6 mg. of purified *E. coli* endotoxin (Difco, Detroit) per kilogram of body weight and four monkeys were given a saline blank of equal volume over a 15 minute period. Six hours after the injections of endotoxin or saline, a second set of baseline measurements was obtained and the colloid infusion started (Plasmanate, Cutter Laboratories). The colloid was administered in increments of 5 ml. per kilogram of body weight until an LVEDP of 12 to 15 mm. Hg was reached, with measurements taken after each increment. The time of infusion of each increment was approximately 10 minutes. After an LVEDP of 12 to 15 mm. Hg was reached, the animal was allowed to recover for a period of 30 minutes and measurements were repeated.

Five to 10 minutes before being killed with an overdose of pentobarbital, the animals were injected with 1 ml. per kilogram of Pelikan ink. A thoracotomy was performed and samples were taken from one lung and the left ventricle for examination by light and electron microscopy. For light microscopic studies specimens were placed in Carnoy's fixative and sections were stained by hematoxylin and eosin, phosphotungstic acid, hematoxylin, and Van Gieson elastica. Specimens

Table I. *Alterations in heart rate (HR) in control and endotoxin-shock primates following coll*

	Saline control						
	No. 3	*No. 4*	*No. 5*	*No. 9*	$\overline{M}$	*S.D.*	*S.E.*
Control	170	155	107	185	154.2	33.8	17
+6 hr.	210	170	200	220	200	21.6	10.8
5 c.c. Pl*/kg.	200	165	220	210	199	24	12
10 c.c. Pl/kg.	200	165	210	205	195	20.4	10.2
15 c.c. Pl/kg.	190	160	210	205	191	22.5	11.2
20 c.c. Pl/kg.			200	205	202.5	3.5	2.5
25 c.c. Pl/kg.			200		200		
30 c.c. Pl/kg.			200		200		
35 c.c. Pl/kg.			195		195		
40 c.c. Pl/kg.							
Recovery		165		230	197.5	46	32.5

*Plasmanate, Cutter Laboratories, Inc., Berkeley, Calif.

Table II. *Alterations in mean systemic arterial pressure (MSAP) in control and endotoxin-sho*

	Saline control						
	No. 3	*No. 4*	*No. 5*	*No. 9*	$\overline{M}$	*S.D.*	*S.E.*
Control	135	130	145	135	136.2	6.3	3.1
+6 hr.	115	140	130	135	130	10.8	5.4
5 c.c. Pl*/kg.	155	145	140	150	147.5	6.4	3.2
10 c.c. Pl/kg.	135	140	150	145	142.5	6.4	3.2
15 c.c. Pl/kg.	145	150	145	145	146.2	2.5	1.2
20 c.c. Pl/kg.			150	145	147.5	3.5	2.5
25 c.c. Pl/kg.			140		140		
30 c.c. Pl/kg.			140		140		
35 c.c. Pl/kg.			130		130		
40 c.c. Pl/kg.							
Recovery		160		115	137.5	31.8	22.5

*Plasmanate, Cutter Laboratories, Inc., Berkeley, Calif.

obtained for ultrastructural study were placed in Zeterqvist's fixative, dehydrated in ascending grades of ethanol, and embedded in Epon 812 and Araldite. Thin sections were stained with Reynold's lead citrate and uranyl acetate and examined with an RCA EMU 3-S or Hitachi HS-7 electron microscope.

Whole inflated lung samples were blotted dry and wet/dry weight ratios obtained after oven drying for a minimum of 48 hours. Two Gm. samples of lung tissue also were minced in saline for determination of pulmonary surfactant on the surfactometer as described previously.[9]

RESULTS

Classical signs of endotoxin shock were observed in the injected group of monkeys 6 hours after endotoxin administration.[2, 4, 25] Mean heart rate (HR) had increased from control values of 180 per minute to 234 per minute after 6 hours ($p < 0.05$). Mean hematocrit had increased from 41.4 percent to 45.8 percent ($p < 0.05$) after 6 hours and mean HCO_3^- fell from 25.8 to 17.0 mEq. per liter ($p < 0.05$). In addition, the mean cardiac output (CO) had dropped from 0.120 to 0.082 L. per minute per kilogram ($p < 0.05$) and mean systemic arterial pressure (MSAP) had dropped from 157 to 112 mm. Hg, although the latter change was not significant. Minimal changes occurred in these parameters in the control monkeys and none was significant statistically.

The effects produced by infusion of colloid were compared immediately after infusion and after the recovery period in controls and in the endotoxin groups. The mean HR in the endotoxin monkeys decreased from 234 per minute at 6 hours to 205 per minute *usion and recovery for 30 minutes*

			Endotoxin				
No. 3	*No. 7*	*No. 8*	*No. 10*	*No. 11*	$\overline{M}$	*S.D.*	*S.E.*
175	185	170	190	180	180	7.906	3.536
230	245	235	240	220	234	9.618	4.301
220	225	230	230	215	224	6.519	2.915
210	225	220	220	215	218	5.701	2.549
205	210	215	220	220	214	6.519	2.915
200	210	210	215	215	210	6.124	2.739
200	210	205	210	215	208	5.701	2.549
	205	205	210	200	205	4.082	2.041
	200	195			197.5	3.536	2.500
		190			190		
	195	190	210	200	198.7	8.539	

mates following colloid infusion and recovery for 30 minutes

			Endotoxin				
No. 6	*No. 7*	*No. 8*	*No. 10*	*No. 11*	$\overline{M}$	*S.D.*	*S.E.*
165	150	120	205	145	157	31.3	14.0
135	70	90	145	120	112	31.3	14.0
115	80	100	150	120	113	25.9	11.6
135	85	90	150	120	116	28.1	12.6
130	80	70	160	115	111	36.8	16.5
120	75	75	150	110	106	31.9	14.3
110	75	65	150	105	101	33.4	14.9
	70	65	145	95	93.7	36.6	18.3
	70	60			65	7.1	5.0
		55			55		
	80	70	145	90	96.2	33.5	16.8

after fluid loading ($p < 0.05$) and fell further to 199 per minute after the 30 minute recovery period ($p < 0.05$). This rate was still significantly faster than the initial control rate. No decrease in mean heart rate occurred after fluid loading in the control monkeys, and after recovery the rate had not changed (Table I).

Mean hematocrit in the endotoxin group of monkeys dropped from 45.8 percent at 6 hours to 30.0 percent after fluid loading ($p < 0.05$) and remained at 31 percent after the recovery period ($p < 0.05$). This was still significantly below the control value of 41.4 percent. The mean hematocrit for the control monkeys fell from 42 to 34.5 percent ($p < 0.05$) after fluid loading and continued to fall to 33.5 percent after the 30 minute recovery period. This also was significantly below the control value (Fig. 1).

The mean HCO_3^- for the endotoxin group fell significantly after 6 hours from the control value of 25.8 mEq. per liter and then increased slightly from 17 to 19.2 mEq. per liter after fluid loading but the change was not significant and no significant change occurred after the 30 minute recovery period. The mean HCO_3^- for the control monkeys showed no significant change from the initial or 6 hour period values. The mean arterial pH was elevated slightly in control animals after 6 hours but did not change significantly in the endotoxin group. Values in the endotoxin group, however, were significantly lower than in the control group after loading and the recovery period (Fig. 2). Control animals increased their alveolar-arterial (A-a) O_2 gradient from control values of 17.7 ± 7.0 to 39.9 ± 7.6 mm. Hg after 6 hours of anesthesia and further to 55.8 ± 2.2 mm.

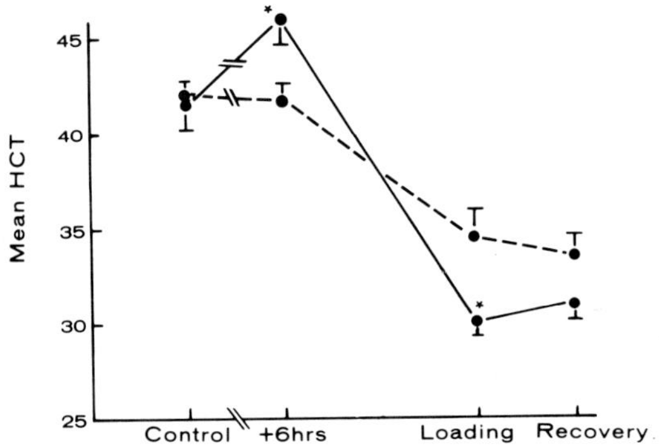

Fig. 1. Changes in mean hematocrit (Hct) in endotoxin-shocked (solid line) and control (dashed line) primates after 6 hours and following colloid infusion. The recovery measurement was made 30 minutes after cessation of infusion. Statistically significant differences (*, $p < 0.05$) were observed in the endotoxin group at 6 hours and after loading when compared to control.

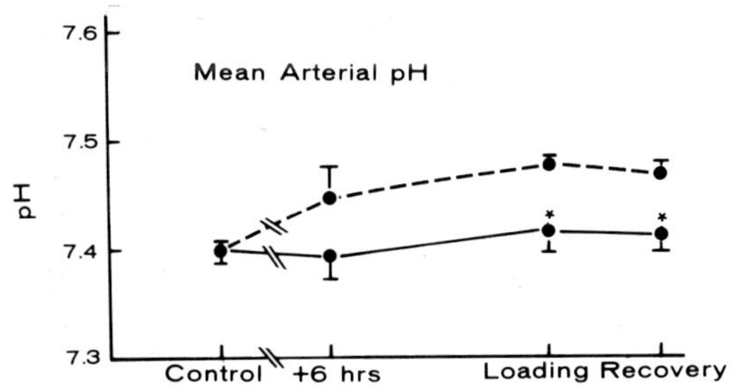

Fig. 2. Changes in mean arterial pH in endotoxin-shocked (solid line) and control (dashed line) primates after 6 hours and following fluid loading by colloid. Statistically significant (*, $p < 0.05$) differences between groups were observed after loading and following a 30 minute recovery period.

Hg after loading with depression of the Pa_{O_2} to 49 mm. Hg. This hypoxia was felt to be secondary to atelectasis but was also associated with hyperventilation and decreased Pa_{CO_2}. No significant change in A-a gradient was noted in the endotoxin group. Arterial Po_2 was slightly higher in the endotoxin group after 6 hours and associated with a greatly increased respiratory rate and reduced Pa_{CO_2} (Fig. 3) although the differences were not statistically significant.

The endotoxin group showed further depression of average MSAP from 112 mm. Hg at 6 hours to 94 mm. Hg after loading with 30 c.c. of colloid per kilogram of body weight and then remained at 96 mm. Hg after the 30 minute recovery period (Table II and Fig. 4). This pressure was significantly lower than the average control value of 157 mm. Hg. Control monkeys experienced a significant rise in average MSAP from 130 to 147.5 mm. Hg after loading with 20 c.c. of colloid per kilogram of body weight, but after recovery MSAP averaged 138 mm. Hg, which was comparable to the control pressure (136 mm. Hg). The PAW was found to be a relatively inaccurate method for determining LVEDP, tending to overestimate slightly up to 6 mm. Hg and progressively to underestimate the true LVEDP at higher values, so that above an LVEDP of 10 mm. Hg the error was 4 to 6 mm. Hg (Fig. 5).

Mean CO per kilogram for the endotoxin group showed a significant fall at 6 hours compared to control animals but increased from 0.082 L. per minute per kilogram at 6 hours to 0.158 L. per minute per kilogram after fluid loading, and showed a slight further rise to 0.189 L. per minute per kilogram after the 30 minute recovery period (Fig. 6). This level of CO was greater than the initial mean value in the endotoxin group (0.120 L. per minute per kilogram) and not significantly different from the control group. Fluid loading increased the CO of the control monkeys from 0.148 to 0.233 L. per minute per kilogram, which returned after recovery to 0.182 L. per minute per kilogram.

Fluid loading with 20 c.c. of colloid per kilogram of body weight raised the LVEDP to 12 to 15 mm. Hg in all but one of the control monkeys while the same volume of infusion in the endotoxin monkeys failed uniformly to increase the LVEDP above 10 mm. Hg (Table III). Three of the five endotoxin-treated monkeys finally reached an LVEDP of 15 mm. Hg after infusion of a total of 30 c.c. of colloid per kilogram of body weight, while one required 35 c.c. per kilogram and the other one 40 c.c. per kilogram before reaching an LVEDP of 15 mm. Hg. After fluid loading the endotoxin group

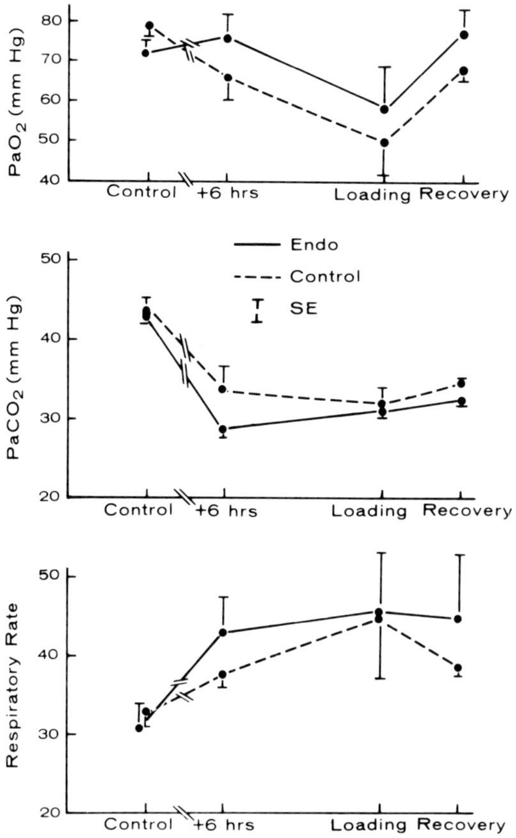

Fig. 3. Alterations in respiratory rate and arterial blood gases (Pa_{O_2} and Pa_{CO_2}) in endotoxin-shocked (solid line) and control (dashed line) primates after 6 hours and following colloid fluid loading and recovery. The endotoxin group showed higher respiratory rates and Pa_{O_2} with lower Pa_{CO_2} although the differences were not statistically significant.

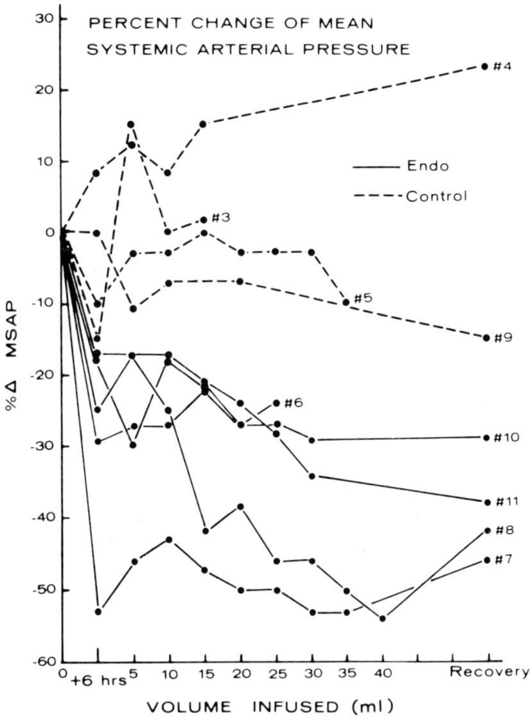

Fig. 4. Alterations in mean systemic arterial pressures expressed as percent control measured after 6 hours in endotoxin-shocked (solid line) and control (dashed line) primates. The response to fluid infusion with colloid to an LVEDP of 15 mm. Hg is shown for each animal (Nos. 3 to 11) during infusion and after a recovery period of 30 minutes.

to an LVEDP of 15 mm. Hg, recovery for 30 minutes resulted in a mean LVEDP of 4.2 mm. Hg, which was not significantly different from the control value of 2.6 mm. Hg. Similarly the control monkeys recovered after infusion to a mean LVEDP of 3 mm. Hg, which did not differ from the control value of 2.1 mm. Hg. The correlation between PAW and LVED pressures was significant with a coefficient of $R = 0.89$ ($p < 0.005$). No significant difference was noted between the groups but the correlation was significantly different from unity (Fig. 5).

Calculated minute work per kilogram of the heart fell significantly from 0.247 Kg.-M. per kilogram at control to 0.117 Kg.-M. per kilogram after 6 hours in the endotoxin group, while it rose insignificantly from 0.221 to 0.262 Kg.-M. per kilogram in the control monkeys. Fluid loading raised the minute work of the endotoxin monkeys to 0.190 Kg.-M. per kilogram and it rose further to 0.198 Kg.-M. per kilogram after the recovery period. Fluid loading raised the minute work of the control monkeys from 0.262 to 0.406 Kg.-M. per kilogram after which it decreased to 0.336 Kg.-M. per kilogram (Fig. 6). Calculated pulmonary arterial input resistance increased in both groups in response to fluid loading by an average of 67 percent in the endotoxin animals and 84 percent in the controls. The measured wet/dry weight ratios of excised lung were abnormally elevated in both groups to 6.17 ± 2.3 in controls and 6.35 ± 0.70 in the endotoxin group but the difference between the groups was not statisti-

Table III. *Alterations in left ventricular end-diastolic pressure (LVEDP) in control and*

	Saline control					
	No. 3	*No. 4*	*No. 5*	*No. 9*	$\overline{M}$	*S.E.*
Control	2.5	2	1	1	2.1	0.43
+6 hr.	1	1.5	1	1	1.1	0.12
5 c.c. Pl*/kg.	1	2	1	1	1.2	0.25
10 c.c. Pl/kg.	7	4	1		4	1.73
15 c.c. Pl/kg.	17	8	2	5	8	3.2
20 c.c. Pl/kg.		12	1	15	8	7
25 c.c. Pl/kg.			4		4	
30 c.c. Pl/kg.			14		14	
35 c.c. Pl/kg.			15		15	
40 c.c. Pl/kg.						
Recovery		4		2	3	1

*Plasmanate, Cutter Laboratories, Inc., Berkeley, Calif.

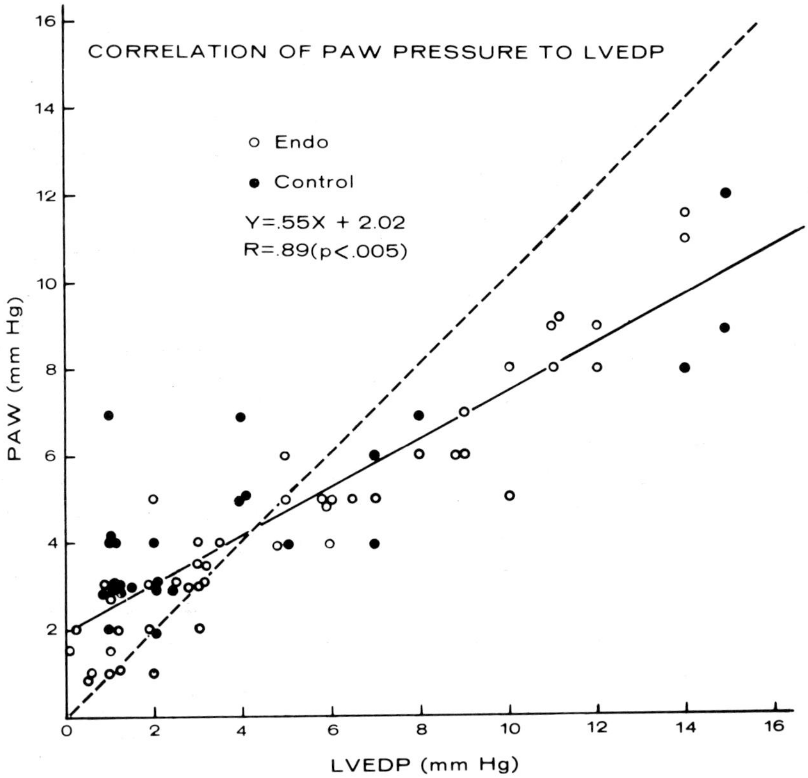

Fig. 5. Correlation of PAW and LVEDP pressures shows a tendency for PAW to exceed slightly the measured LVEDP up to pressure of 6 mm. Hg beyond which the PAW tends to underestimate the LVEDP.

cally significant. The minimum surface tensions of lung extracts were also abnormally high in both groups, averaging 23.6 dynes per centimeter in the controls and 22.8 dynes per centimeter in the endotoxin group. Hysteresis loop areas were similarly depressed to 1.10 sq. in. in the endotoxin group.

Light microscopically, the Pelikan ink was noted to fill extensively the vascular beds in both the normal and experimental animals. In heart sections both the control and the endotoxin-treated groups showed comparable degrees of perinuclear edema. In lung sections, endotoxin-treated animals showed *toxin-shock primates following colloid infusion and recovery for 30 minutes*

Endotoxin						
No. 6	No. 7	No. 8	No. 10	No. 11	$\overline{M}$	S.E.
3	1	3	6	0	2.6	1.03
3	1	0.5	1	1	1.3	0.44
5	0.5	2	0	1	1.7	0.89
5	2	2	1	3	2.6	0.68
8	3	2.5	6	3	4.5	1.1
10	6	3.5	9	6	6.9	1.2
12	9	6.5	11	10	9.7	0.94
	11	9	14	12	11.5	1.04
	14	11			12.5	1.50
		12			12	
	3	7	5	2	4.2	1.11

more alveolar space rounding, alveolar wall collapse, and pulmonary edema (Fig. 7). Ultrastructural changes in the lung in the endotoxin-treated specimens showed more extensive endothelial swelling when compared to loaded controls (Fig. 8), occasional endothelial cell lifting from the underlying basement membrane, and an abundance of white blood cells and platelets within the lumina of the capillaries (Fig. 9). Varying degrees of perivascular space edema were seen in both the control and experimental groups and this feature was not helpful in distinguishing the two groups. The ink tracer was noted infrequently in the alveolar space transudate but the method of transfer across the endothelial barrier could not be defined. The intercellular junctions between the endothelial cells only occasionally showed increased granularity, and no Pelikan ink could be seen within the pinocytotic vesicles of the endothelial cytoplasm.

In ultrastructural sections of the heart, the control group showed mild perinuclear edema, lack of mitochondrial swelling, normal interfiber spaces, and normal capillary endothelium (Fig. 10). The presence of ink was noted in the capillary lumina and only rarely outside the vascular lumina. At no time could the ink be found in the pinocytotic vesicles or within the intercellular spaces.

When compared to the control group, the endotoxin-treated hearts showed more extensive edematous changes. Most prominently seen was an endothelial lesion consisting of marked edema with resultant swelling of the capillary endothelium projecting into the vascular lumen (Fig. 11). The edema was seen as individual cell swelling but quite frequently the entire endothelial lining would show marked edematous change. Occasional bleblike structures were seen in the edematous endothelial myocardial cells (Fig. 12). Free blebs were seen frequently in the capillary lumina. Multiple low-power micrographs revealed more extensive fluid accumulations within the interfiber spaces with marked separation of the perivascular bundles of collagen. In addition, there was marked intrafiber edema with separation of the myofibrils. Many animals showed focal mitochondrial swelling but no marked disruption of mitochondrial membranes was noted and the mitochondrial changes would ordinarily be considered reversible.

DISCUSSION

Both groups of monkeys demonstrated significant interstitial pulmonary edema following fluid loading to a transient LVEDP of 12 to 15 mm. Hg which did not resolve after the recovery period with return of LVEDP to normal levels. In the group administered endotoxin plus fluid loading the pulmonary edema was more pronounced histologically, presumably due to the endothelial damage seen ultrastructurally. The perivascular space edema in both groups as well as the white blood cells and platelets in the capillaries of the endotoxin group as found by other in-

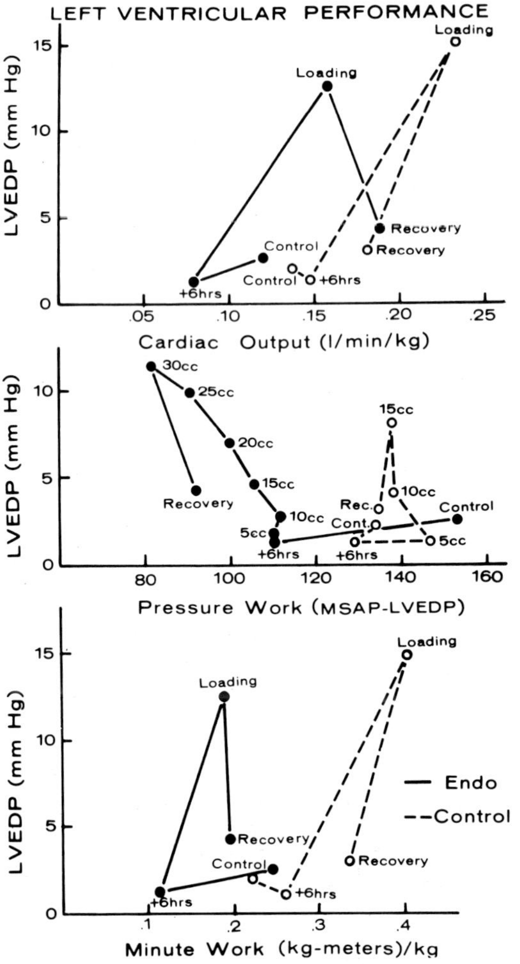

Fig. 6. Alterations in cardiac output (CO) and LVEDP shown for endotoxin-shocked (solid line) and control (dashed line) primates after 6 hours and following colloid infusion and a 30 minute recovery period. As shown at the top, the response to left ventricular loading is less in the endotoxin groups than in controls but continues to improve during the recovery period. The pressure work performed, shown in the center graph, shows a greater discrepancy between the groups with less recovery after loading, and comparable depression of minute work and response to loading is observed below.

vestigators[5, 13, 15, 19] may account for increased resistance to flow in the pulmonary capillaries in both groups, and may explain the pressure gradient between the values of the PAW and LVEDP observed at higher LVEDP during the fluid loading. The observed increase in pulmonary arterial input resistance in both groups supports this hypothesis and explains

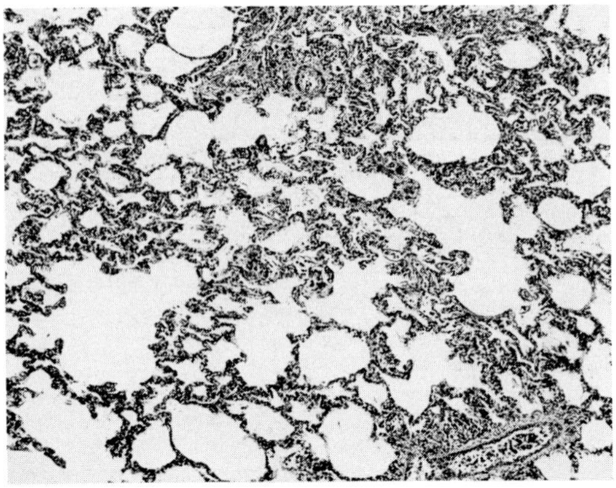

Fig. 7. Endotoxin lung specimen. Low-power micrograph depicting moderate alveolar wall collapse with focal pulmonary edema. The walls appear to be hypercellular. (Hematoxylin and eosin; ×63.)

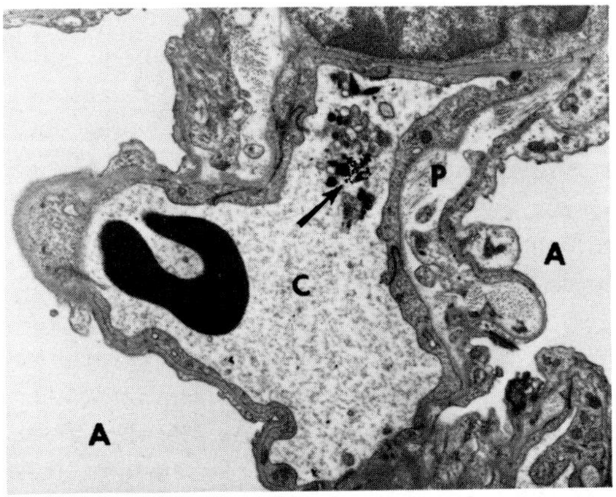

Fig. 8. Control lung specimen. Low-power electron micrograph in which the capillary *(C)* contains cellular remnants intermingled with the Pelikan ink (arrow). There is minimal edema noted within the perivascular space *(P)*. The alveolar spaces *(A)* are free from transudate. (Lead citrate and uranyl acetate; ×7300.)

the uniformity of the relationship between PAW and LVEDP in both groups.

In a recent publication, Kusajima and associates[16] reported early small pulmonary vein constriction representing active occlusion and later capillary obstruction representing passive occlusion of vessels in dogs after hemorrhagic shock. These findings were associated with a 5 mm. Hg pressure gradient between the PAW and small pulmonary vein. Hinshaw and associates[15] observed massive

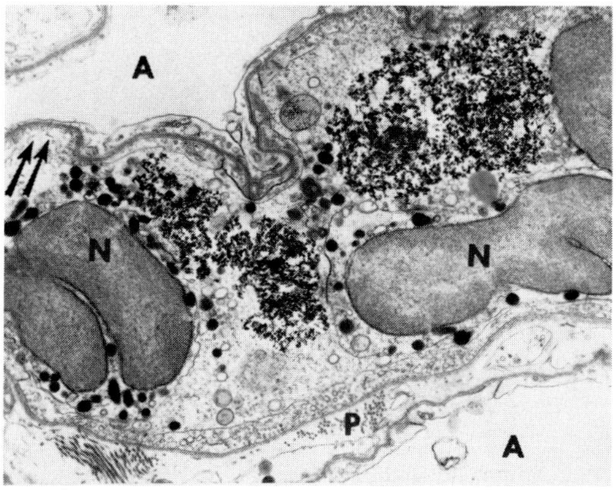

Fig. 9. Endotoxin lung specimen. The capillary is filled with polys *(N)*, one of which has lost its cytoplasmic membrane integrity. The plasma transudate contains free specific granules and cellular debris associated with the Pelikan ink. The endothelium shows focal cytoplasmic disruption (double arrows). There is minimal perivascular space *(P)* edema. The alveolar spaces *(A)* are free from transudate. (Lead citrate and uranyl acetate; ×7300.)

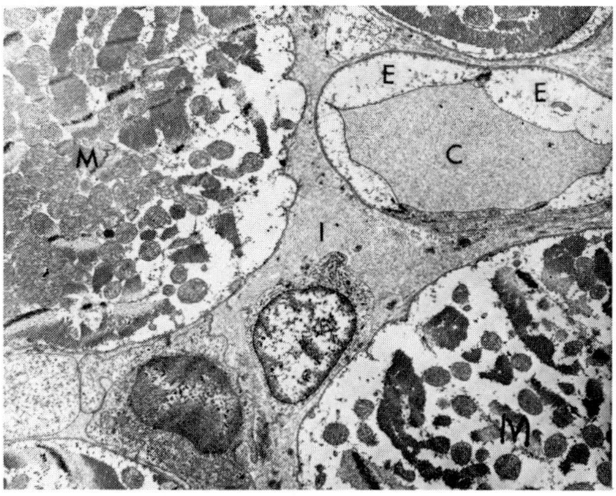

Fig. 11. Endotoxin heart specimen. The muscle fibers *(M)* noted in cross section show the presence of intrafiber edema with separation of the myofibrils and mitochondria. Within the interfiber spaces *(I)*, there is an edematous transudate. The capillary *(C)* within this connective tissue compartment shows severe edema *(E)* in two of the three endothelial cytoplasmic portions. Several Pelikan ink particles are noted within the capillary lumen. (Lead citrate and uranyl acetate; ×6900.)

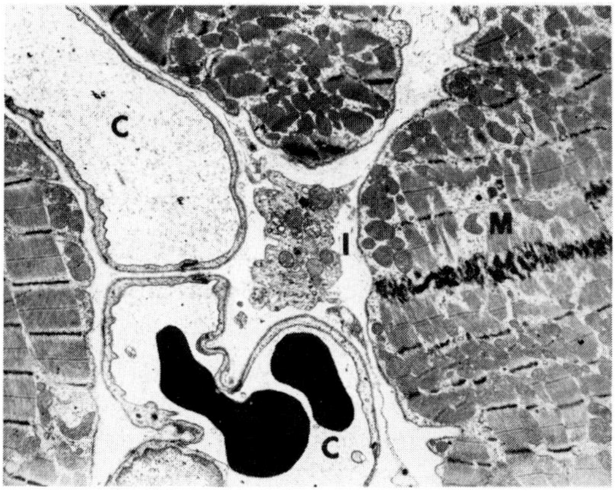

Fig. 10. Control heart specimen. Low-power electron micrograph shows the presence of several myocardial fibers *(M)* and capillaries *(C)*. Note that the endothelium of the capillary is thin with distinct intercellular junctions. There are multiple Pelikan ink particles present. The interfiber space *(I)* is normal in contents and width. (Lead citrate and uranyl acetate; ×4540.)

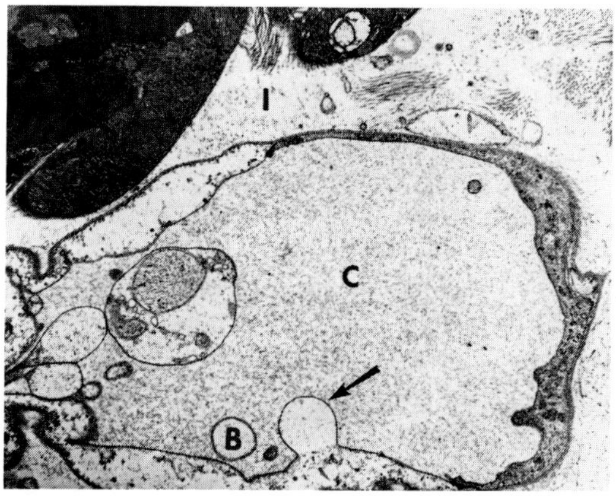

Fig. 12. Endotoxin heart specimen. The endothelial cytoplasm of the myocardial capillary *(C)* shows edema with focal bleblike formations (arrow). Several blebs *(B)* are free in the plasma. The interfiber space *(I)* contains increased amounts of fluid. (Lead citrate and uranyl acetate; ×8000.)

sequestration of polymorphonuclear leukocytes in pulmonary capillaries which produced passive obstruction to blood flow and active pulmonary venous constriction in adult anesthetized Rhesus monkeys with intravenously administered lethal doses of *E. coli* endotoxin. Both of these studies suggest that the effects of shock on the pulmonary vascular bed have both a passive and active occlusive action which can dampen the transmission of LVEDP to the PAW catheter tip and may explain the observed pressure gradient. Clinical studies in patients with mitral stenosis or bronchogenic carcinoma[6]

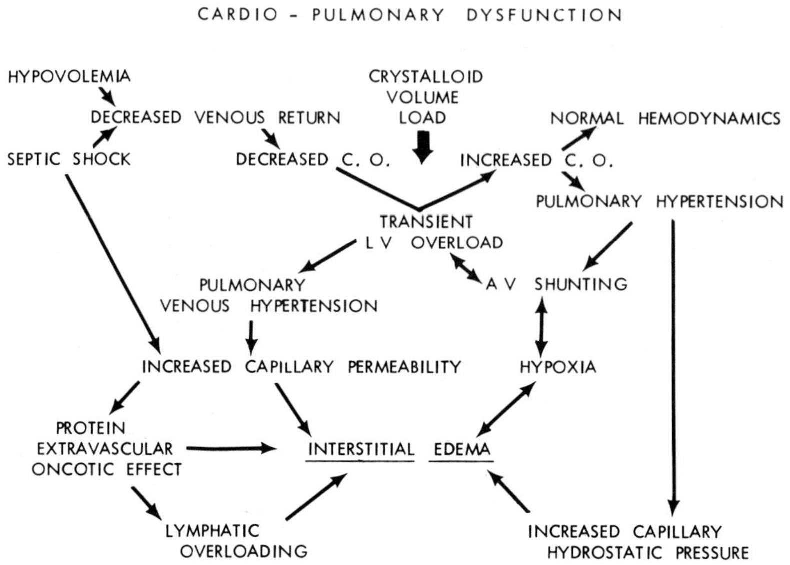

Fig. 13. Schematic representation of the possible effect of volume loading with fluid to a point of transient ventricular overloading. The resulting development of interstitial pulmonary edema would tend to be self perpetuating while the hemodynamics returned to normal.

showed a direct correlation between PAW and LVEDP and similar reliability has been demonstrated between PA end-diastolic pressure (PAEDP) and LVEDP in patients in shock.[21] When there is left ventricular dysfunction, however, the LVEDP is observed to be consistently higher than PAEDP and the disparity is further exaggerated by increasing systemic pressure with methoxamine.[1] The data from this study indicate a linear relationship of the PAW to the LVEDP, but it differs from unity and shows that the PAW pressure tends to be 3 to 6 mm. Hg lower than the LVEDP at higher ventricular filling pressures in this preparation These observations suggest that the validity of PAW and PAEDP in resuscitation may be questioned and may not insure the avoidance of fluid overloading and transient left ventricular dysfunction.

The interstitial pulmonary edema induced in both control and endotoxin groups resulted in comparable increases in wet/dry weight ratios and reductions in pulmonary surfactant. Since colloid was used rather than a crystalloid, it is not necessary to consider the added deleterious effects of hemodilution and alteration of the Starling capillary relationship, although the measured osmolality of the colloid used was slightly less than isooncotic (202 mOsm. per liter). The fact that the LVEDP returned to normal levels 30 minutes after fluid infusion has interesting implications. Obviously a single measurement of a normal LVEDP cannot reflect a previously elevated LVEDP, during which time pulmonary venous hypertension and edema could have occurred. Thus the transient ventricular overloading can initiate pulmonary edema which is not readily reversible, as has been demonstrated in isolated lungs made edematous by hydrostatic pressure.[11] The interstitial pulmonary edema produced in this manner remains even when pulmonary venous pressure is restored to normal or negative values. It seems reasonable then to suggest that many cases of the "wet-lung syndrome" associated with shock and resuscitation may in fact have been initiated by fluids administered rapidly for resuscitation, producing transient ventricular overload not excluded by a subsequently measured normal PAW pressure (Fig. 13).

The significantly lower CO for the endotoxin monkeys after 6 hours as compared to control monkeys could reflect either decreased venous return, as demonstrated by other investigators,[2, 23] or myocardial depression, or both. Even though the endotoxin monkeys received an average of almost twice as much colloid as the control monkeys, their CO increased to only half the CO of the control monkeys. This suggests that myocardial performance was impaired directly as a result of the 6 hour endotoxin insult in addition to the decreased venous return corrected by volume repletion (Fig. 6).

The significant drop in calculated minute work of the heart after 6 hours exposure to endotoxin and the average minute work response to volume loading performed by the endotoxin-treated hearts was less than half the minute work performed by the control hearts after fluid loading with colloid (Figs. 6 and 7). This decrease in myocardial performance has been shown for septic shock in man[22] but was not reported previously in monkeys.[2]

Another factor which may have contributed to the myocardial dysfunction is metabolic acidosis, although there was adequate compensation with constant pH throughout the study. Hypoxia also can be eliminated since the Pa_{O_2} of the endotoxin monkeys was greater than the Pa_{O_2} of the control monkeys for the duration of the experiment. The mean hematocrit for the endotoxin monkeys was significantly higher after 6 hours than in the control monkeys, which may have influenced capillary perfusion but was likely to be less significant than the generalized circulatory impairment which resulted from pooling. Although a myocardial depressant factor[17] or some other circulating factor or abnormal metabolite released during shock could also influence myocardial function in the endotoxin group, this has been shown to be of no significance in the early or intermediate stages of shock.[10]

From observations made after the recovery stage, it appears that fluid loading with colloid improves cardiac output in endotoxic shock to levels above control in the subhuman primate while the minute work improves to a level just slightly lower than normal. This benefit however can be costly in terms of pulmonary function if the rate of infusion produces transient overloading of the left ventricle.

REFERENCES

1. Bouchard, R. J., Gault, J. H., and Ross, J., Jr.: Evaluation of pulmonary arterial end-diastolic pressure as an estimate of left-ventricular and diastolic pressure in patients with normal and abnormal left-ventricular performance, Circulation **44:** 1072, 1971.
2. Brockman, S. K., Thomas, C. S., Jr., and Vasko, J. S.: The effect of *Escherichia coli* endotoxin on the circulation, Surg. Gynecol. Obstet. **125:** 763, 1969.
3. Burton, A. C.: Peripheral circulation, Annu. Rev. Physiol. **15:** 213, 1953.
4. Cavanagh, D., Rao, P. S., Sutton, D. M. C., dev Bhagat, B., and Bachmann, F.: Pathophysiology of endotoxin shock in the primate. Am. J. Obstet. Gynecol. **108:** 705, 1970.
5. Coalson, J. J., Hinshaw, L. B., and Guenter, C. A.: The pulmonary ultrastructure in septic shock, Exp. Mol. Pathol. **12:** 84, 1970.
6. Connolly, D. C., Kirklin, J. W., and Wood, E. H.: The relationship between pulmonary artery wedge pressure and left atrial pressure in man, Circ. Res. **2:** 434, 1954.
7. Gilbert, R. P.: Mechanisms of the hemodynamic effects of endotoxin, Physiol. Rev. **40:** 245, 1960.
8. Gilbert, R. P.: Endotoxin shock in the primate, Proc. Soc. Exp. Biol. Med. **111:** 328, 1962.
9. Greenfield, L. J., Duncan, R. C., and Parker, D. E.: Response surface analysis of pulmonary surfactant hysteresis loops, J. Surg. Res. **9:** 671, 1969.
10. Greenfield, L. J., McCurdy, J. R., Hinshaw, L. B., and Elkins, R. C.: Preservation of myocardial function during cross-circulation in terminal endotoxin shock, SURGERY **72:** 111, 1972.
11. Greenfield, L. J., Reif, M. E., Coalson, J. J., McCurdy, J. R., and Elkins, R. C.: Comparative effects of interstitial pulmonary edema produced by venous hypertension or hemodilution in perfused lungs, SURGERY **71:** 857, 1972.
12. Guenter, C. A., Fiorica, V., and Hinshaw, L. B.: Cardiorespiratory and metabolic responses to live *E. coli* and endotoxin in the monkey, J. Appl. Physiol. **26:** 780, 1969.
13. Harrison, L. H., Beller, J. J., Hinshaw, L. B., Coalson, J. J., and Greenfield, L. J.: Effects of endotoxin on pulmonary capillary permeability, ultrastructure and surfactant, Surg. Gynecol. Obstet. **129:** 723, 1969.

14. Hinshaw, L. B., Solomon, L. A., Reins, D. A., and Fiorica, V.: Sympathoadrenal system and renal response to endotoxin in the primate, Nephron **4:** 394, 1967.
15. Hinshaw, L. B., Shanbour, L., Greenfield, L. J., and Coalson, J. J.: Mechanism of decreased venous return, Arch. Surg. **100:** 600, 1970.
16. Kusajima, K., Webb, W. R., Wax, S. D., Parker, F. B., Jr., and Ozdemir, I. A.: Hemodynamic effects of methylprednisolone on pulmonary microcirculation in hypovolemia, Physiologist **16:** 369, 1973.
17. Lefer, A. M., and Glenn, T. M.: Role of the pancreas in the pathogenesis of circulatory shock, *in* Hinshaw, L. B., editor: The fundamental mechanisms of shock, New York, 1972, Plenum Press, pp. 326-330.
18. MacLean, L. D., Mulligan, W. G., McLean, A. P. H., and Duff, J. H.: Patterns of septic shock in man: A detailed study of 56 patients, Ann. Surg. **166:** 543, 1967.
19. McKay, D. G., Margaretten, W., and Csavossy, I.: An electron microscope study of endotoxin shock in rhesus monkeys, Surg. Gynecol. Obstet. **125:** 825, 1967.
20. Ross, J., Jr., Sonnenblick, E. H., Kaiser, J. A., Frommer, P. L., and Braunwald, E.: Electroaugmentation of ventricular performance and oxygen consumption by repetitive application of paired electrical stimuli, Circ. Res. **16:** 332, 1965.
21. Scheinman, M., Evanes, C. T., Weiss, A., and Rapaport, E.: Relationship between pulmonary artery end-diastolic pressure and left ventricular filling pressure in patients in shock, Circulation **47:** 317, 1973.
22. Siegel, J. H., Greenspan, M., and Del Guercio, L. R. M.: Abnormal vascular tone, defective oxygen transport, and myocardial failure in human septic shock, Ann. Surg. **165:** 504, 1967.
23. Weil, M. H., MacLean, L. D., Visscher, M. B., and Spink, W. W.: Studies on the circulatory changes in the dog produced by endotoxin from gram-negative microorganisms, J. Clin. Invest. **35:** 1191, 1956.
24. Wiggers, C. J.: Pulmonary wedged catheter pressures (Editorial), Circ. Res. **1:** 371, 1953.
25. Wyler, F., Forsyth, R. P., Nies, A. S., Neutze, J. M., and Melmon, K. L.: Endotoxin-induced regional circulatory changes in the unanesthetized monkey, Circ. Res. **24:** 777, 1969.

Anti–HL-A antibodies: Failure to correlate with renal allograft rejection

Clive O. Callender, M.D., Richard L. Simmons, M.D., Edmund J. Yunis, M.D., Luis H. Toledo-Pereyra, M.D., Maureen T. M. DeShazo, B.S., *and* **John S. Najarian, M.D.,** *Minneapolis, Minn.*

Previous work has shown that the presence of anti–HL-A lymphocytotoxic antibodies (not donor specific) are correlated with renal allograft rejection. From May, 1971, through December, 1972, 185 renal allotransplants were done. None of these patients has been lost to follow-up and all have been observed for a minimum period of 10 months. Thirty-two transplants were carried out in the presence of anti–HL-A antibodies but in the absence of a positive antidonor crossmatch. These patients were compared with a similar number of patients without cytotoxic antibodies, who were matched as to sex, age of the recipient, time of the transplant, and relationship to donor as well as with the total transplant population. There was no statistically significant difference between renal allograft survival in any of these groups. Thus, in a group of transplant recipients at one center, there appears to be no correlation between the presence of lymphocytotoxic antibodies and renal allograft rejection in the absence of a positive crossmatch.

From the Department of Surgery and Laboratory Medicine, University of Minnesota, Minneapolis, Minn.

THE PRESENCE of preformed cytotoxic antibodies against donor leukocytes will almost always result in the rapid rejection of human renal allografts.[20] A number of investigators have recently demonstrated that the presence of serum antibodies directed against histocompatibility antigens were correlated with early loss of renal allotransplants, even if there were no demonstrable antibodies directed against donor tissue itself.[2, 3, 10-13, 15, 17-19, 25, 27]

A potential defect in the latter studies is that the clinical data have been pooled from a number of transplant centers, each of which has different criteria of patient selection and different modes of patient care. In some cases even the typing, antibody screening, and crossmatching were performed by slightly different techniques at different laboratories. It is our purpose to evaluate the role of cytotoxic antibodies on renal transplants performed at a single large center where clinical follow-up is complete and where knowledge of the presence or absence of cytotoxic antibodies againt nondonors was not known by the clinician at any time. It will be shown that, in the presence of a negative crossmatch, patients with lymphocytotoxic antibodies did as well following kidney allografting as did patients without lymphocytotoxic antibodies.

Accepted for publication June 13, 1974.

This work was supported by Grant No. 5 PO2AM 13083-04 from the United States Public Health Service.

Reprint requests: Dr. Simmons, P. O. Box 185, Mayo Memorial Building, University of Minnesota, Minneapolis, Minn. 55455.

MATERIALS AND METHODS

The serum of prospective kidney transplant recipients was examined for the presence of cytotoxins by the simple microtoxicity test of Amos and associates[1] plus the modification instituted at the National Institutes of Health, which requires a cell washing before addition of complement. Reactivity against lymphocytes of more than 15 percent of the donor cells was taken to indicate the presence of cytotoxins.

The prospective kidney transplant recipients were screened for lymphocytotoxins monthly while awaiting transplantation. Each recipient was screened one to 19 times. Patients were considered to have cytotoxic antibiotics if at any time during the pretransplant screening they had greater than a 15 percent response to the cell panel. The screening panel consisted of cells from 18 persons selected from 120 donors to include all the HL-A and W specificities known, as follows:

First-locus antigens: HL-A1 on the leukocytes of five panel members, HL-A2 in eight, HL-A3 in six, HL-A9 in four, HL-A10 in four, HL-A11 in three, W28 in one, and W19 in four.

Second-locus antigens: HL-A7 in three, HL-A8 in four, HL-A12 in four, HL-A13 in one, W5 in four, W10 in three, W14 in one, W15 in two, W16 in one, W17 in two, W18 in one, W22 in two, and W27 in one.

The match between donor and recipient was measured in several ways by comparing (1) the haploidentities in the related group, (2) the number of common HL-A antigens, (3) the number of common first- and second-locus antigens, and (4) the net histocompatibility ratio (NHR). The NHR was computed by the method of Rappaport and Dausset.[21] The ratio of the antigenic similarities (common antigens) and dissimilarities (uncommon antigens) at each of the known HL-A (first and second) loci were determined. When all four antigens were detectable the following formula was used:

$$\text{NHR} = 1/4\left(\frac{\text{total antigenic identities}}{\text{total antigenic incompatibilities}}\right).$$

When less than four antigens were detected the following formula was used:

$$\text{NHR} = 1/4\left(\frac{\text{avg. total antigenic identities}}{\text{total antigenic incompatibilities}}\right)$$

taking each probable different antigen into consideration as either an identity or incompatibility. The similar, dissimilar, and presumptively different antigens were compared in each group and the NHR derived. NHR's ranged from zero to one. In no case, however, was this technique used for donor-recipient selection prior to transplant. The only immunologic contraindication to transplantation was a positive crossmatch between recipient sera and donor cells.

From May, 1971, through December, 1972, 185 consecutive renal allotransplants in 172 patients were performed. Thirty-two recipients had developed antibodies to the HL-A antigens on the panel prior to transplant. No transplants were carried out to recipients with cytotoxic antibodies against donor leukocytes. All patients have been followed for at least 10 months. No patients was lost to follow-up. Our procedures for the selection of donors and recipients, the techniques of transplantation, and the standard immunosuppressive regimes have been previously described.[23] All patients received antilymphocyte globulin, azathioprine, and prednisone as initial immunosuppressive therapy and have been maintained on azathioprine and prednisone for the life of the graft. The clinical laboratory records of every patient were reviewed in detail in addition to the laboratory records from the tissue-typing laboratory. The tissue-typing laboratory was not aware of the results of transplantation in these patients until this study was performed, nor were the transplant physicians influenced or aware of the presence of cytotoxic antibodies against the leukocytes of panel members. This lack of knowledge allowed us to avoid the "self-fulfilling prophecy" of removing a "badly matched kidney" in a patient with cytotoxic antibodies during a rejection episode because of the "known" poor prognosis in such patients.

In order to define the prognostic implica-

Table I. *Renal transplant survival with and without HL-A antibodies*

Donor*	No. of transplant	Matched control patients: With HL-A antibodies No.	%	Without HL-A antibodies No.	%	All patients without anti–HL-A antibodies
LRD	1	11/12	92	9/12	75	81/99 = 81% kidney survival 93/99 = 93% patient survival
CAD	1	9/11	82	8/11	73	39/54 = 72% kidney survival 44/54 = 83% patient survival
LRD	2	1/2	50	—	—	8/10 = 80% kidney survival
CAD	2	4/7	55	—	—	6/9 = 67% kidney survival
Total kidney survival		25/32	78	17/23	74	120/153 (77%)
Total patient survival		27/32	84	19/23	80	137/153 (90%)

*LRD = related donor; CAD = cadaver donor.

tions of anti HL-A cytotoxic antibodies not directed to donor cells, the choice of control patients is crucial. If one compares only the prognosis of patients with antibodies with that of the total group of transplant recipients, no account will be taken of changes in recipient and donor selection, in personnel, or in immunosuppressive regimen, all of which take place inevitably with time. Therefore, the controls for the 32 patients who had antibodies against HL-A antigens were carefully chosen by matching each patient who had antibodies with another patient who had not developed antibodies. The matching criteria were (1) sex and age of the recipient (±15 years), (2) time of the transplant (±2 months), and (3) relationship to donor (related or cadaver). In order to fulfill the important matching criteria of age and time of transplant, three recipients were matched to a recipient of the opposite sex. Certain recipients with antibodies who received kidneys from relatives could not be matched with the recipients without antibodies who received kidneys from a donor with the exact same relationship to the recipient. In these cases matched controls were selected who received kidneys from a donor with a different relationship to the recipient. Recipients of related kidneys were always compared with recipients of related kidneys.

RESULTS

The functional survival rate of kidneys transplanted into patients with and without preformed cytotoxic antibodies is shown in Table I. Three groups are compared in this table. Those with anti–HL-A antibodies are matched with those patients of similar age, sex, time of transplant, and relationship to donor without HL-A antibodies. In addition, all patients transplanted during the period of time from May, 1971, through December, 1972, without anti–HL-A antibodies—regardless of age, sex, or time of transplant—are also listed to demonstrate that the matched control patients without HL-A antibodies are typical of all the patients without HL-A antibodies.

The effect of preformed cytotoxic antibodies on related transplant survival. Table II lists the pertinent characteristics of the 12 patients (Group 1) who had preformed lymphocytotoxic antibodies prior to receiving a transplant from a relative. No recipient had detectable antibodies to lymphocytes of the donor at the time of transplant. Matched control patients who had not developed preformed cytotoxic antibodies are compared in Table II, Group 2. Eleven of the 12 patients with cytotoxic antibodies are well with normal renal function from 10 to 28 months after transplantation. Nine of the 12 matched control patients without cytotoxic antibodies are well with functioning kidneys for a similar period of time. Certain differences between the patients with preformed cytotoxic antibodies and those without cytotoxic antibodies may be important. The ages, sex, original diagnosis, number of pretransplant trans-

Table II. *Effect of preformed cytotoxic antibodies on first transplants*

Group no.	No. of patients	Relation to donor	Antibodies to panel	Mean age (± S.E.)	Mean no. of similar antigens (± S.E.)	Mean no. of dissimilar antigens (± S.E.)	Mean no. of probable different antigens (± S.E.)	Mean no. of NHR (± S.E.
1	12	Relative	Yes	32 ± 5	2.3 ± 0.3	0.8 ± 0.2	1.0 ± 0.1	0.6 ± 0.
2	12	Relative	No	29 ± 4	2.0 ± 0.3	1.5 ± 0.2	0.4 ± 0.1	0.4 ± 0.
3	11	Cadaver	Yes	41 ± 2	0.8 ± 0.3	1.9 ± 0.5	1.1 ± 0.4	0.3 ± 0.
4	11	Cadaver	No	36 ± 2	0.9 ± 0.2	2.5 ± 0.3	0.5 ± 0.3	0.5 ± 0.

Table III. *Effect of preformed cytotoxic antibodies on second transplants*

Group no.	No. of patients	Relation to donor	Antibodies to panel	Age (± S.E.)	Similar antigens (± S.E.)	Dissimilar antigens (± S.E.)	Probable different antigens (± S.E.)	NHR (± S.E.
5	7	Cadaver	Yes	33 ± 5	0.9 ± 0.4	2.0 ± 0.5	1.0 ± 0.4	0.3 ± 0.
6	9	Cadaver	No	32 ± 5	0.6 ± 0.2	2.6 ± 0.2	0.6 ± 0.3	0.1 ± 0.
7	2	Relative	Yes	25 ± 13	1.5 ± 0.5	1.5 ± 0.5	1.0 ± 1.0	0.4 ± 0.
8	10	Relative	No	23 ± 3	2.1 ± 0.3	1.4 ± 0.3	0.6 ± 0.1	0.5 ± 0.

*Only one patient living.

fusions and dialyses were comparable (Table II, Groups 1 and 2). All of the female patients with cytotoxic antibodies had been pregnant whereas six of the eight women without cytotoxic antibodies had not.

The net histocompatibility ratio (NHR) revealed a high degree of mismatch in both groups of patients, but patients with cytotoxic antibodies were significantly better matched than those without cytotoxic antibodies ($p \leq 0.05$). The recipients with anti–HL-A antibodies were particularly well matched at the second HL-A (or, alternatively, the four) locus. The major difference between the groups in this regard was the inclusion of five patients with cytotoxic antibodies who received kidneys from phenotypically identical siblings. However, eight of eight recipients with cytotoxic antibodies who received kidneys from phenotypically nonidentical relatives are well with good function, and nine of 11 phenotypically nonidentical recipients without cytotoxic antibodies are well. Thus the excellent results in the patients with cytotoxic antibodies cannot be attributed to excellent matches alone.

Opelz and associates[15] have noted that patients with a large percentage of cytotoxic antibodies against panel leukocytes have a worse prognosis than those with lesser numbers of antibodies against members of the panel. Of five patients with antibodies against more than 50 percent of a panel in Table II, Group 1, four are well with good function from 10 to 24 months, and only one patient has died. Of patients with less than 50 percent antibodies, all are well. Of patients without antibodies, nine of 12 are well.

The effect of preformed anti–HL-A cytotoxic antibodies on cadaver transplant survival. Table II lists 11 patients (Group 3) who had preformed antibodies directed against HL-A antigens prior to receiving a first transplant from a cadaver. Matched control patients who had not developed preformed cytotoxic antibodies are listed in Table II, Group 4. Nine of the 11 patients with cytotoxic antibodies are well with normal renal function; eight of the 11 patients without cytotoxic antibodies are well. No patient with preformed cytotoxic antibodies rejected a kidney, but two died. Despite similar survival data, patients without cytotoxic anti-

Mean no. of HLA second-locus identities (± S.E.)	*No. of cytotoxic antibodies to panel (± S.E.)*	*Mean no. of rejection episodes/ patient*	*Mean no. of pretransplant dialyses (± S.E.)*	*Mean no. of pretransplant transfusions (± S.E.)*	*Mean current serum creatinine level (mg.% ± S.E.)*
1.5 ± 0.2	7.5 ± 1.2	0.5	118 ± 64	24 ± 5	1.0 ± 0.1
1.0 ± 0.2	0	0.3	73 ± 44	31 ± 6	1.0 ± 0.1
0.2 ± 0.1	10.8 ± 1.4	0.1	278 ± 83	39 ± 13	1.1 ± 0.1
0.5 ± 0.2	0	0.8	102 ± 53	28 ± 5	1.2 ± 0.1

H-LA second-locus identities (± S.E.)	*No. of cytotoxic antibodies to panel (± S.E.)*	*Mean no. of rejection episodes/ patient*	*Mean no. of pretransplant dialyses (± S.E.)*	*Mean no. of pretransplant transfusions (± S.E.)*	*Mean current serum creatinine level (mg.% ± S.E.)*
0.3 ± 0.2	10.4 ± 2.3	0.5	233 ± 80	85 ± 19	1.6 ± 0.5
0.8 ± 0.2	0	1.0	90 ± 21	65 ± 18	1.2 ± 0.2
1.0 ± 0.1	3.0 ± 1.0	0.1	120 ± 60	38 ± 3	1.0*
1.0 ± 0.1	0	1.0	107 ± 39	51 ± 9	1.1 ± 0.1

bodies had significantly more reversible rejection episodes than did patients with cytotoxic antibodies. One patient without cytotoxic antibodies underwent transplant rejection and two died. There were no significant differences in age, sex, original diagnosis, number of pretransplant transfusions, or tissue typing results. Only three patients had less than 50 percent cytotoxic antibodies against the panel. All patients were poorly matched with respect to the HL-A antigens of the donor, including second-locus antigens. The patients with cytotoxic antibodies had a greater number of pretransplant dialyses. Of the eight women with cytotoxic antibodies, all but one had been pregnant, but only two of six women without cytotoxic antibodies had been pregnant.

The effect of preformed cytotoxic antibodies on second or subsequent transplants. Table I and Table III, Group 5, characterize nine patients who had previously lost one or more transplants. Each had developed cytotoxic antibodies prior to the subsequent transplantation. Of the seven cadaver kidney recipients only four are well with adequate renal function. In this group, two kidneys were rejected (one soon after transplantation) and one patient lost a kidney due to local infection.

This group can be compared with nine patients who received second or third kidneys from cadaver donors (Table III, Group 6). These patients cannot be matched for age and sex, but do repreesnt all of the second, third, or fourth transplants performed during the same period of time to patients without cytotoxic antibodies. Six out of nine of these control patients are well (Table I). There are no differences between these groups with respect to age, number of rejection episodes, or number of transfusions (Table III). There were more females in the sensitized group and the sensitized patients had received more dialyses. All patients were poorly matched at both the first and second HL-A loci, but those with antibodies were slightly better matched.

There were two additional patients who lost their first transplants, developed cytotoxic antibodies, and later received a second related transplant (Table III, Group 7). One of these patients is well 11 months later, but one underwent hyperacute rejection. This was the only obvious hyperacute rejection during the period studied. It occurred in a woman who had rejected two previous transplants. The second transplant was not removed. Her third kidney was donated by her son against whose cells antibodies had been demonstrated prior to her second transplant. With the second rejected transplant in situ, the antibodies against her son had disappeared, but her son's kidney was rejected immediately.

Ten patients with second transplants from related donors representing all such transplants performed during this period are characterized in Table III, Group 8. Eight of 10 of these patients are well with normal renal function despite a high degree of mismatch in HL-A typing at both loci.

DISCUSSION

Opelz, Mickey, and Terasaki[15] have shown that failure after renal transplantation is best predicted by the presence of anti HL-A antibodies in the serum of the recipient, even if these antibodies do not react with the cells of the donor. They interpret these findings to suggest that some patients are nonresponsive to HL-A despite multiple transfusions of blood during hemodialysis. The difficulties with these studies as well as with other cooperative studies which have been performed[4, 13, 14, 16, 26, 28] are that despite that precision of antibody detection there is no precision in the accuracy of recording clinical data nor is there consistency of clinical management. We have, therefore, compared 32 kidney transplants in 30 recipients with preformed anti–HL-A antibodies with a group of patients carefully matched with respect to age, sex, time of transplant, and donor relationship, who did not have preformed anti–HL-A antibodies. The physicians and surgeons in charge of the patient were not aware of the presence of lymphocytotoxic antibodies in any of the recipients except when antibodies directed against the donor cells (positive crossmatch) were noted. No patients were transplanted across a positive crossmatch in this series. Similarly, the typing laboratory personnel were not made aware of the clinical results until this analysis was completed.

We found no evidence to support the idea that "responder" or "nonresponder" patients react differently to their grafts. Patients who developed antibodies against allogeneic histocompatibility antigens within the population had an equally good prognosis when compared to those who did not. No clear-cut correlation could be made between kidney function of allotransplants and the number of transfusions (all patients were transfused multiple times) or number of dialyses (all patients were dialyzed numerous times). Similarly, there seemed to be no correlation between kidney function of allotransplants and the degree of histocompatibility matching at either HL-A locus within the small numbers of patients within this subpopulation. Neither could we see in these groups of matched control patients any difference between results of living, related-donor transplantation and cadaver transplantation.

There are a number of limitations to this study. The patients have been followed for only 10 to 28 months following transplantation. The matched control groups tend to compensate for the defect of short-term follow-up since the matched control patients have been similarly followed for only a relatively short period of time. Short-term follow-up appears to be inherent in any study of this type at present since the laboratory techniques involved in tissue typing are still evolving and the typing sera are constantly changing so that recent transplants have more complete HL-A typings than those performed previously.

Although we have developed even more sensitive methods to detect lymphocytotoxins, two standard techniques have been used for this study: that of Amos and associates[1] and the NIH technique which requires a cell washing before addition of complement. With these techniques hyperacute rejection was avoided in every case but one, in which a previously rejected kidney in situ may have absorbed detectable anti–HL-A antibodies which had been found against the donor son.

The implications of these data may be very

important. If Opelz and associates[15] are correct that patients who are "responders" have a worse prognosis than "nonresponders," a different strategy should be employed with respect to choosing recipients for available kidneys. Recipients would then be chosen for the nonresponders first since the prognosis in these patients is so much better. Conversely, if our data are correct, one should transplant "responders" first, if kidneys are available to which the potential recipient does not have preformed antibodies.

The reasons for the differences in these results and those of the cooperative groups are not clear. Our patients are fewer in number than any cooperative group but clinical management is more uniform. All our patients receive a standard immunosuppressive regimen which includes splenectomy (which may decrease serologic antibody formation) and two weeks of posttransplant high-dose antilymphocyte globulin.[24] ALG has recently been shown capable of diminishing the humoral antibody response to certain antigens.[5-9, 22] One would not expect, however, that ALG would have a great effect on preformed but undetected antibodies against graft donors, although it may have an effect on patients who are immunocompetent, i.e., those who are "responders." We tend to favor this latter explanation. Of the 32 kidneys transplanted to patients with anti–HL-A cytotoxic antibodies, only three were rejected, although four other patients died with intact kidneys. It appears that the immuosuppressive regimen which involves high dose ALG suppresses rejection sufficiently so that even "responders" can be immunosuppressed. An alternative explanation may be that the use of two uniform sensitive crossmatch techniques in a single laboratory could possibly eliminate "responders" who have low titers of antidonor serum, undetectable by the use of a single crossmatch technique.

REFERENCES

1. Amos, D. B., Bashir, A., Boyle, W., MacQueen, M., and Tullikainen, A.: A simple microtoxicity test, Transplantation **7:** 220, 1969.
2. Beleil, O. M., Mickey, M. R., and Terasaki, P. I.: Comparison of male and female kidney transplant survival rates, Transplantation **13:** 493, 1972.
3. Braun, W. E., Straffon, R. A., Nakamoto, S., Popowniak, K. L., Gifford, R. W., Kuruvila, C, and Zachany, A. A.: Mismatched M.-A haplotypes with antigens HL-A1, 3, and II associated with excellent renal allograft function, Transplantation **15:** 86, 1973.
4. Dausset, J., and Hors, J.: Analysis of 221 renal transplants: Influence of cross-reactions between donor and recipient HL-A antigens, Transplant. Proc. **III:** 1004, 1971.
5. James, K.: Anti lymphocyte antibody—a preview, Clin. Exp. Immunol. **2:** 615, 1967.
6. James, K., and Anderson, N. F.: Parallel studies on the effect of anti lymphocyte antibody on cell mediated and humoral antibody responses in the rat, Clin. Exp. Immunol. **3:** 227, 1968.
7. James, K., and Jubb, V. S.: Effect of anti rat lymphocyte antibody on humoral antibody formation, Nature (Lond.) **215:** 367, 1967.
8. Kerbel, R. S., Eidinger, D.: Variable effects of anti lymphocyte serum on humoral antibody formation. Role of thymus dependency on antigen, J. Immunol. **106:** 917, 1971.
9. Monaco, A. P., Wood, M. L., Gray, J. G., and Russell, P. S.: Studies on heterologous antilymphocyte serum in mice. II. Effect on the immune response, J. Immunol. **96:** 229, 1966.
10. Morris, P. J., and Ting, A.: Leukocyte antigens on renal transplantation: Matching for the HL-A system and the early course of cadaveric renal grafts, Med. J. Aust. **1:** 517, 1970.
11. Morris, P. J., Williams, G. M., Hume, D. M., Mickey, M. R., and Terasaki, P. I.: Serotyping for homotransplantation. XII. Occurrence of cytotoxic antibodies following kidney transplantation in man, Transplantation **6:** 392, 1968.
12. Oh, J. H., McLean, L. D., Mackinnon, K. J., Gaile, M. H., and Dossetor, J. B.: Significance of a negative cross match in recipients with a wide spectrum of lymphocytotoxic antibodies, Transplantation **11:** 92, 1971.
13. Oliver, R. T. D., Sachs, J. A., and Festenstein, H.: A collaborative scheme for tissue typing and matching in renal transplantation. VI. Clinical relevance of HL-A matching in 349 cadaver renal transplants, Transplant. Proc. **5:** 245, 1973.
14. Oliver, R. T. D., Sachs, J. A., Festenstein, H., Pegrum, J. D., and Morrehead, J. F.: Influence of HL-A matching antigenic strength and immune responsiveness on outcome of 349 cadaver renal grafts, Lancet **2:** 1381, 1972.

15. Opelz, G., Mickey, M. R., and Terasaki, P. I.: Identification of unresponsive kidney-transplant recipients, Lancet **1:** 868, 1972.
16. Opelz, G., Sengar, D. P. S., Mickey, M. R., and Terasaki, P. I.: Effect of blood transfusion on subsequent kidney transplants, Transplant. Proc. **5:** 253, 1973.
17. Opelz, G., and Terasaki, P. I.: Effect of splenectomy on human renal transplants, Transplantation **15:** 605, 1973.
18. Patel, R., Merrill, J. P., and Briggs, W. A.: Comparison in recipients with and without preformed antileukocyte antibodies, New Engl. J. Med. **285:** 274, 1971.
19. Patel, R., Mickey, M. R., and Terasaki, P. I.: Serotyping for homotransplantation. XVI. Analysis of kidney transplants from unrelated donors, New Engl. J. Med. **279:** 501, 1968.
20. Patel, R., and Terasaki, P. I.: Significance of the positive crossmatch test in kidney transplantation, New Engl. J. Med. **280:** 735, 1969.
21. Rappaport, F. T., and Dausset, J.: Ranks of donor-recipient histocompatibility for human transplantation, Science **167:** 1260, 1969.
22. Rethy, L., and Padanyi, M.: Suppression of the primary immune response by anti-lymphocyte serum, Separatum Experientia **25:** 747, 1969.
23. Simmons, R. L., Kjellstrand, C. M., and Najarian, J. S.: Kidney transplantation: Technique, complications, and results, *in* Najarian, J. S., and Simmons, R. L., editors: Transplantation, Philadelphia, 1972, Lea & Febiger, Publishers.
24. Simmons, R. L., Condie, R., and Najarian, J. S.: Anti lymphoblast globulin for renal allograft prolongation, Transplant. Proc. **4:** 487, 1972.
25. Terasaki, P. I., Kreisler, M., and Mickey, R. M.: Presensitization and kidney transplant failures, Postgrad. Med. J. **47:** 89, 1971.
26. van Hooff, J. P., van der Steen, G. J., Schipper, H. M. A., and van Rood, J. J.: Efficacy of HL-A matching in eurotransplant, Lancet **2:** 1385, 1972.
27. van Rood, J. J.: Tissue typing and organ transplantation. Lancet **1:** 1142, 1969.
28. van Rood, J. J., Koch, C. T., van Hooff, J. P., van Leeuwen, A., van den Tweel, J. G., Frederiks, E., Schippers, H. M. A., Hendriks, G., and van der Steen, G. J.: Graft survival in unrelated donor-recipient pairs matched for MLC and HL-A. Transplant. Proc. **5:** 409, 1973.

Follow-up study of the endorectal pull-through operation for the treatment of Hirschsprung's disease, with special reference to intestinal anastomosis

Kisaku Satomura, M.D., Zheng Hang-Long, M.D., Satoshi Ohnishi, M.D., Kaoru Kumada, M.D., Yoshihiko Kisaka, M.D., Hidehiro Yamazaki, M.D., Katsuhiko Komaki, M.D., Nobuhiko Tanigawa, M.D., *Kyoto, Japan,* **Keibun Hara, M.D.,** *Shiga, Japan,* **Sumio Tominaga, M.D.,** *Kobe, Japan, and* **Kenichi Kinoshita, M.D.,** *Ehime, Japan.*

Endorectal pull-through operation without resection of mucosal cuff has been found to be a simple and safe operation in 20 cases. Endoscopic study revealed that the telescoping anastomosis used in the operation formed a smooth, anastomotic stoma. Histologic study of the anastomosis in dogs revealed that the unity between oral and anal segments consisted of proliferation of connective tissue. Also marked proliferation of the submucosal tissue at the end of the invaginated segment was observed.

From the Second Surgical Division, School of Medicine, Kyoto University, Kyoto, and the Nagahama Red Cross Hospital, Shiga, and Kobe Seiko Hospital, Kobe, and Uwajima City Hospital, Ehime, Japan

IN A PREVIOUS article,[9] we reported a simplified endorectal pull-through method for the treatment of Hirschsprung's disease. Principles of the method are as follows. (1) Resection of the aganglionic segment is done in almost the same way as in the method of Rehbein and associates,[8] except that the oblique distal transection line is higher anteriorly at the level of the peritoneal floor to preserve the prerectal nerve plexus (Fig. 1, *A*). (2) Limited resection of the aganglionic segment is compensated for by a longitudinal division of the posterior midline of the anorectal canal and placement of the ganglionic colon into this presacral space (Fig. 1, *B*). (3) Leakage from the anastomosis is prevented by exteriorization of the pulled-through colon. The need for resection of the mucosal cuff is eliminated, unlike Soave's[10] method, while spontaneous retraction of the exteriorized colon is expected (Fig. 1, *D*).

In reference to our method some questions have been raised. (1) Does suture insufficiency never occur at the site of the anastomosis? The anterior semicircular mucosal surface of the anorectal canal faces the serosal surface of the pulled-through colon (Fig. 1, *D*), and between these two layers adhesion is not expected to occur. (2) Does the exteriorized colon retract spontaneously in every case? Some authors feared that the anterior wall of the pulled-through colon would remain in the anorectal canal forming a "curtain-like pendulum."

In order to answer these questions and to clarify the details of the method, we are

Accepted for publication June 17, 1974.

Reprint requests: Kisaku Satomura, M.D., Second Surgical Division, Kyoto University School of Medicine, 54-Kawara-Cho, Shogoin, Sakyo-Ku, Kyoto, Japan.

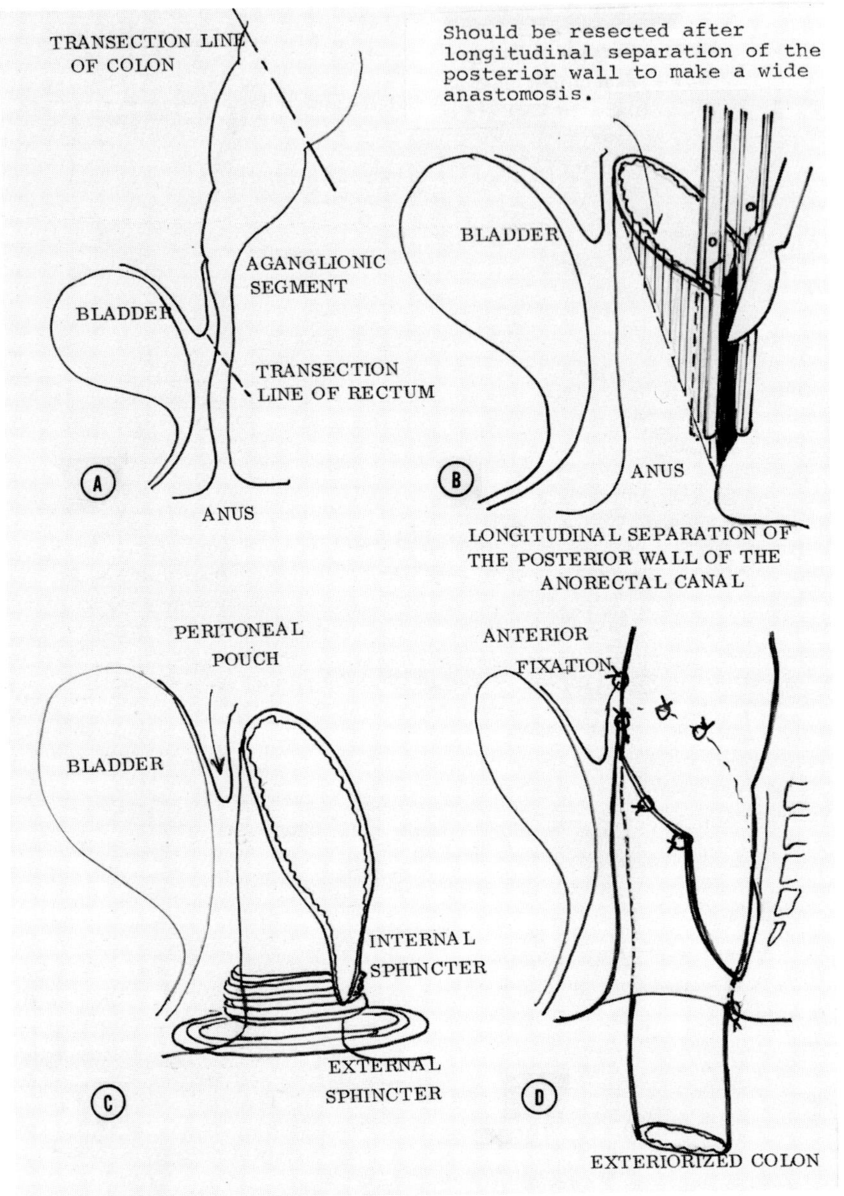

Fig. 1. Procedure for endorectal pull-through operation.

reporting the development of our clinical and experimental studies on the anastomosis.

MATERIALS AND METHOD

Twenty patients who had been treated by our method were observed for follow-up study. Their ages ranged from 3 months to 16 years. The aganglionic segment in all cases extended to the sigmoid colon and the lower part of the descending colon, namely 10 to 18 cm. above the anocutaneous line.

Roentgenographic and endoscopic examinations were carried out 2 weeks to 2 years after the operation.

Prior to radiologic examination, physiological saline solution enema was administered, but purgation was not employed. Endoscopic study was done without any

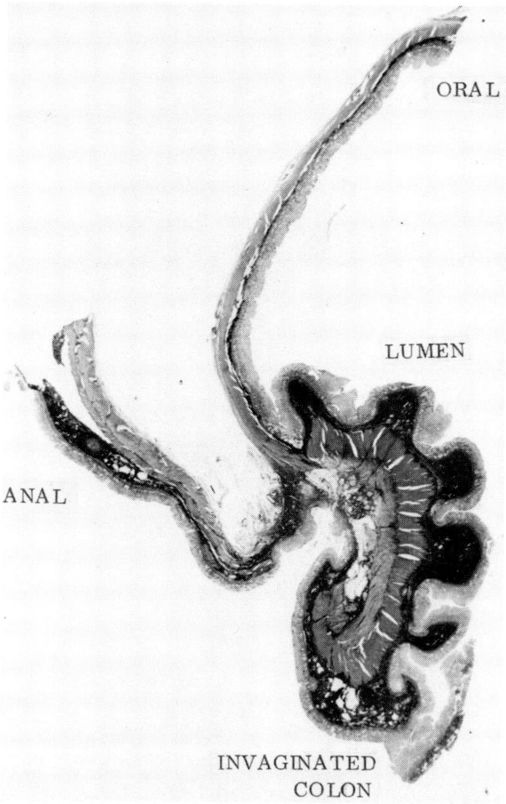

Fig. 2. Ten weeks after telescoping anastomosis of the descending colon in a dog, the retracted anterior wall of the colon has curled back on itself to heal mucosa-to-mucosa to the upper end of the anal segment, much as an ileostomy or colostomy matures on the abdominal wall turning itself over and healing to the skin. Note the proliferation of the submucosal connective tissue of the distal end of the pulled-through colon. This flap is usually large enough to require or to justify subsequent resection. (Van Gieson stain; ×10.)

anesthesia using Olympus Colonofiberscope Model CS-Type LB, at intervals of 2, 4, and 8 weeks and 2 years after operation.

RESULTS

Seventeen out of 20 patients had uneventful convalescence and their postoperative courses were uncomplicated (Tables I, II, and III). Retraction of the exteriorized colon into the anorectal canal usually occurred within 2 weeks.

Nine patients had no special postoperative treatment; all were less than one year of age. Eight others received finger or metal bougie dilation for a period of one to 8 weeks. The oldest child, a 16-year-old girl, needed forcible bouginage for 20 weeks postoperatively.

Complications occurred in three patients, of whom two required colostomy. Resection of the exteriorized colon was done in two patients in whom edematous swelling of the gut, which was covered with purulent fibrinous membrane, was considered to be responsible for fever.

Table I. *Age at radical operation*

	3 to 6 mo.	*7 to 12 mo.*	*1 to 3 yr.*	*> 3 yr.*
No. of patients	6	6	5	3

Table II. *Postoperative course and complications*

	Uneventful		*Long-term bouginage required*	*Colostomy after the radical operation to relieve colitis*
	Required no bouginage	*1 to 8 wk. bouginage*		
No. of patients	9	8	1	2*

*Patient 1 died of strangulation ileus one year after the operation.

Table III. *Fecal continence after operation*

	Excellent	*Fair*	*Poor*
No. of patients	16	2	2*

*Patient 1 died of strangulation ileus one year after the operation.

CASE REPORTS

Case 1. A 16-month-old boy had severe colitis after the pull-through operation. The anterior wall of the pulled-through colon remained in the rectal canal, and septotomy, which is routinely required in Duhamel's[1] procedure, was done 8 weeks after the radical operation.

This procedure temporarily improved the symptoms of colitis; however, recurrence of the same burden and retardation in general development necessitated transverse colostomy. After improvement of the colitis, the colostomy was closed. One

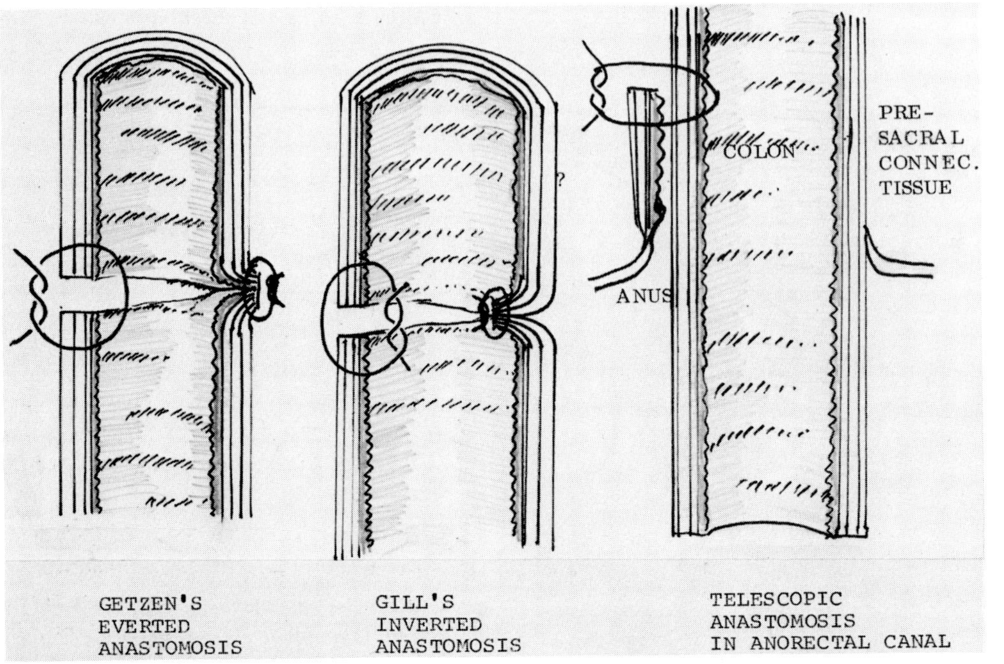

Fig. 3. Getzen's everted, Gill's inverted intestinal anastomosis, and our telescoping anastomosis.

year later the patient died of ileus. Autopsy revealed strangulation of the ileum, but smooth passage of the anastomotic area.

Case 2. A 14-month-old boy underwent laparotomy 10 days after the pull-through operation because of moderate abdominal distention, fever (38 to 38.5° C.), and vomiting, which had started on the fourth postoperative day. At the reoperation paralytic ileus due to peritonitis was suspected and fleck-wise suggillation and purulent membrane on the serosal surface of the descending colon above the anastomosis were found. Stenosis at the level of anterior fixation (anastomosis) was considered to be responsible for these complications. Transverse colostomy successfully relieved the symptoms.

Case 3. In a 2-year-old girl, necrosis of the pulled-through colon in its full length distal to the anastomosis was found on the second postoperative day. Forceful dilatation of the anal sphincter prevented anastomotic leakage; however, bouginage was required for as long as 12 weeks.

Patients 2 and 3 are presently doing very well.

Endoscopic findings. The condition of the pulled-through colon depended mostly on the blood supply through the mesocolic vessels. In other words, the length of the mesocolon and sufficiency of blood flow decided the biological reaction of the transected distal end of the pulled-through colon.

Two weeks. After retraction of the pulled-through colon, either spontaneously or by resection of the exteriorized part, the anterior wall remained as a "curtain-like pendulum." The posterior wall was almost fixed to the presacral space. The transected distal end was found to be granulomatous, and this swelling increased in the following 2 weeks.

Four weeks. The granulomatous proliferation of the transected end of the colon reached its maximum and forceful bouginage caused bleeding from the crushed mucosa.

Eight weeks. A sufficient stoma was insured by this time, but the transitional zone between the mucosa of the pulled-through colon and anorectal canal was still granulomatous and easily bled after bouginage.

Two years. Complete fixation of the pulled-through posterior wall was found and the mucosa of the gut merged into the anorectal mucosa. This was so smooth that the transition to the ganglionic segment was almost unidentified except for the slight swelling from the proliferation of submucosal layer.

EXPERIMENTAL STUDY

Five mongrel dogs weighing 6 to 13 kilograms were used for experimental study to elucidate the fate of the pulled-through colon and the nature of the distal transected end of the gut which formed valvular mechanism.

The animals were anesthetized with intravenous injections of Nembutal (25 mg. per kilogram). The same anastomotic technique was applied as in the clinical method. One layer of interrupted silk sutures was used to make a telescoping anastomosis at the large intestine and 3 to 6 cm. of the proximal transected end was invaginated into distal intestine. Ten weeks later the anastomotic area was resected and fixed in 20 percent neutral formalin, and a 10 μ paraffin section was made. Hematoxylin-eosin stain, Van Gieson's stain, and Mallory Azan stain were used for histological study.

Histological findings. The unity of the oral and anal colon was achieved chiefly by the proliferation of connective tissue. The continuity of any layer of the two colons was hardly seen at the tenth postoperative week (Fig. 2).

Both the circular and longitudinal muscular layer thickened considerably. The most distinguishing finding was the marked proliferation of the submucosal tissue, which was the main component of the granulomatous proliferation seen at the distal end of the invaginated colon. Though the mucosal layer of the anal colon showed considerable upward extension, the mucosal continuity of the oral and anal colon have not yet taken place.

The valvular mechanism[9] of the telescoping anastomosis consisted of marked proliferation of the submucosal connective tissue coupled with the thickened muscular layers. The excessive length of the invaginated segment naturally resulted in severe intestinal obstruction.

DISCUSSION

The anastomotic technique of colorectostomy plays an important role in the operative treatment of Hirschsprung's disease. Leakage from an insufficient anastomosis may cause abscess and stricture, which sometimes terminate in death. Furthermore, anastomosis at the level of the minor pelvic floor is difficult to perform. Since the first report of exteriorization of the intestine by Hochenegg,[7] many surgeons, including Duhamel,[1] have tried the method as a solution for the difficulty of anastomosis.

For reconstruction of the alimentary tract following intestinal resection, two layer suture, through-and-through suture covered by seromuscular suture, is standardly used in the anastomosis.

Halsted[6] demonstrated that the anastomotic strength of the intestine is mostly dependent on the anastomotic continuity of the submucosal layer, and seromuscular suture is only a minor supplement. From this standpoint, many surgeons hold the opinion that one-layer suture is sufficient for the anastomosis.

Getzen and associates[3, 4] recognized that one-layer through-and-through suture is more effective for the prevention of stricture when everted rather than inverted, and demonstrated that everted anastomoses were always stronger than were inverted ones until the twenty-first postoperative day (Fig. 3).

Gill and associates,[5] on the other hand, proved more incidence of microfistula and microabscess with everted anastomoses than with inverted ones, and mostly employed the method of through-and-through suture with inverted anastomosis.

Although our previously reported endorectal pull-through method is not literally a single layer suture, the main concept of the anastomosis is the same.

The pathogenesis of Hirschsprung's disease naturally requires avoidance of stricture of the anastomosis. Everted anastomosis has some advantage in reference to the prevention of the stricture of the anastomosis. Our method has the advantages of both everted and inverted anastomosis due to its structure.

The following precautions should be taken to make the endorectal pull-through operation successful: (1) Exteriorized colon should be well vascularized. To insure firm adhesion of the ganglionic colon to the presacral space, even the exteriorized part of the colon should have mesocolon. (2) Septotomy (V-form crushing of the anterior wall of the pulled-through colon) is recommended 10 to 14 days after the pull-through operation, when the fixation of the posterior wall to the presacral space is established. This procedure minimizes granulomatous proliferation at the distal end of the colon. (3) Energetic bouginage is essential to insure wide anastomosis and fixation of incarcerated ganglionic colon to the presacral space.

REFERENCES

1. Duhamel, B.: A new operation for the treatment of Hirschsprung's disease, Arch. Dis. Child. **35:** 38, 1960.
2. Ehrenpreis, T.: Hirschsprung's disease, Chicago, 1970, Year Book Medical Publishers, Inc.
3. Getzen, L. C.: Clinical use of everted intestinal anastomosis, Surg. Gynecol. Obstet. **123:** 1027, 1966.
4. Getzen, L. C., Roe, R. G., and Holloway, C. K.: Comparative study of intestinal anastomotic healing in inverted and everted closures, Surg. Gynecol. Obstet. **123:** 1219, 1966.
5. Gill, W., Fraser, Sir J., Carter, D. C., and Hill, R.: Everted intestinal anastomosis, Surg. Gynecol. Obstet. **128:** 1297, 1969.
6. Halsted, W. S.: Circular suture of the intestine—an experimental study, Am. J. Med. Sci. **94:** 436, 1887.
7. Hochenegg, J.: Beiträge zur chirurgie des rectum und der beckenorganc, Wien. Klin. Wochenschr. **2:** 515, 1889, cited from reference 2.
8. Rehbein, F., Morger, R., Kundert, J. G., and Meier-Ruge, W.: Surgical problems in congenital megacolon, J. Pediatr. Surg. **1:** 526, 1966.
9. Satomura, K., Nagamine, S., Kisaka, Y., Ueki, S., Masuda, M., Hara, K., and Kimura, C.: A simplified endorectal pull-through operation for the treatment of Hirschsprung's disease, SURGERY **71:** 345, 1972.
10. Soave, F.: Hirschsprung's disease; clinical evaluation and details of a personal technique, Z. Kinderchir. (Suppl.) 66, 1966.

Combined use of ^{131}I hippurate blood clearance and bladder/kidney ratio data in the early detection, classification, and management of accelerated rejection of human renal transplants

Thomas C. Moore, M.D., *and* **Michael Hayes, M.D.,** *Torrance, Calif.*

The combined use of ^{131}I hippurate blood isotope clearance (BIC) data and of bladder/kidney (B/K) ratios of isotope intensity information calculated from isotope counts obtained by a scintillation camera detector with area-of-interest capability proved to be of considerable value in the early detection, type classification, and early treatment of accelerated rejection in 11 cases of accelerated rejection of human renal allografts from a group of 79 transplant recipients studied on a frequent, generally daily, basis following transplantation. The combined use of BIC and B/K ratio data provided evidence of accelerated rejection malfunction of the allograft from one to 5 days earlier than other monitoring data—urine output, serum creatinine (Cr), and blood urea nitrogen (BUN)—in all cases studied.

From the Divisions of Pediatric Surgery and Renal Transplantation and of Nuclear Medicine, UCLA–Harbor General Hospital, Torrance, Calif., and the Departments of Surgery and Radiology, University of California, Los Angeles.

PROCEDURES utilizing radionuclides have been found to be useful in the study of experimental and clinical renal transplant function and in the early detection of rejection. The renogram, the hippurate blood clearance index, and sequential renal scintigraphy have been used by many investigators.

Renographic abnormalities observed during rejection are flattening of the second segment, prolongation of the peak time, and flattening of the third segment. In 1966 Sharpe and associates[15] proposed the use of the half-time of the third segment of the renogram as an index of renal allograft rejection malfunction. In 1968 Magnusson and associates[9] observed that a flattening of the third segment of the renogram was the first renogram alteration to occur during rejection. In 1969 Staab and associates[16] proposed the use of a ratio based on the renographic height at 20 minutes divided by the height at peak time for the detection of rejection.

In 1965 Kountz and associates[6] observed the blood clearance rate of ^{131}I hippurate to be a sensitive means of detecting renal allograft rejection. Their findings have been corroborated by Awad and associates,[1] Egelston and associates,[2] and Weiss and associates.[17]

Renal imaging also has been employed as an aid in the study of renal transplant patients. In 1965 Figueroa and associates[3] reported on the usefulness of sequential renal

Accepted for publication June 27, 1974.

This study was supported by the John A. Hartford Foundation, National Institutes of Health Grant No. AM-10373, the Los Angeles County Heart Association, and Contract AT (04-1) GEN-12 between the United States Atomic Energy Commission and the University of California at Los Angeles.

Reprint requests: Thomas C. Moore, M.D., Department of Surgery, UCLA–Harbor General Hospital, 1000 W. Carson St., Torrance, Calif. 90509.

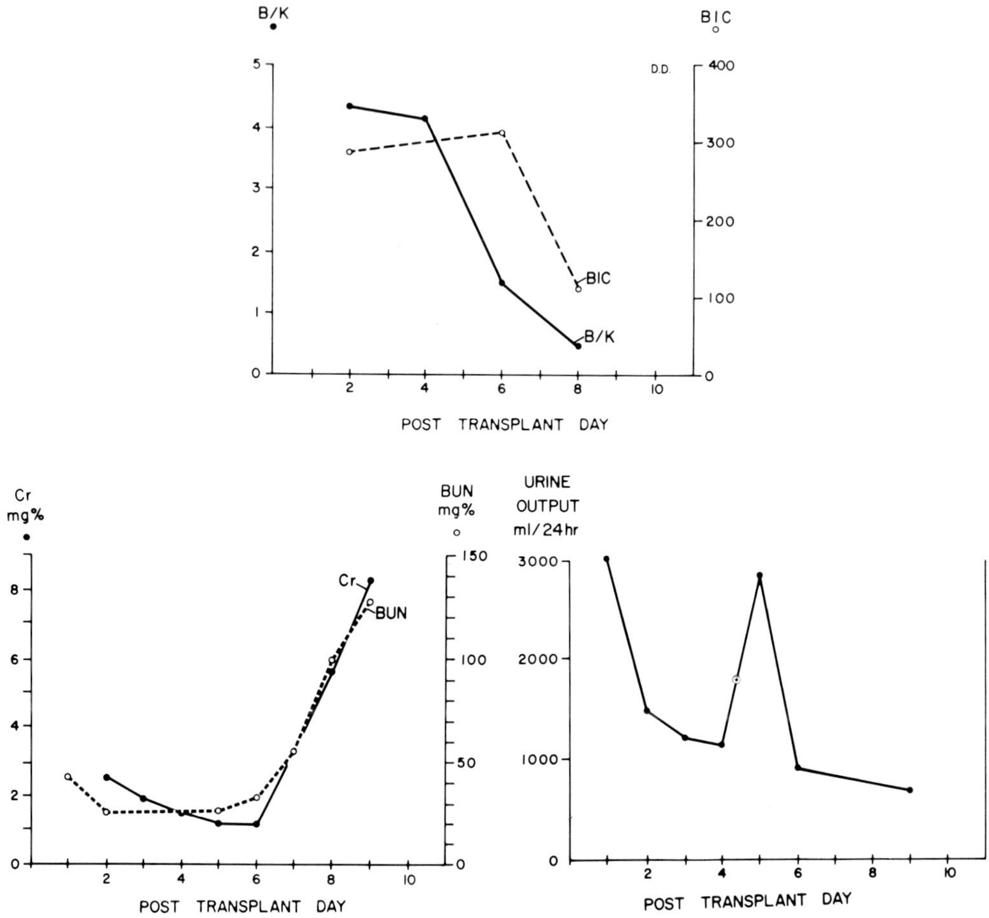

Fig. 1. Graph showing temporal correlation in post-transplant isotope study (B/K ratio and blood isotope clearance [BIC]) and nonisotope study (BUN, serum creatinine [Cr], and 24 hour urinary output) data in Case 1. B/K ratios were falling mildly on the fourth day and sharply on the sixth day, while BIC increased. Despite every-other-day isotope studies, B/K ratio changes provided evidence of transplant malfunction at least one day prior to BUN and Cr changes and aided in the interpretation of urinary output alterations.

scintigraphy and in 1968 Lubin and associates[8] described their experience with the use of the rectilinear scanner.

We have found blood clearance of ^{131}I hippurate to be misleading at times with respect to early rejection changes. A transient rise in blood clearance of ^{131}I hippurate has been found as an initial change on daily study when renal transplants are performed on nonimmunosuppressed and bilaterally nephrectomized dogs.[11] This transient increase in blood isotope clearance was found to be associated temporally with an increase in the urinary excretion of histamine. The true significance of this change as a bad rather than a good sign with respect to allograft function and the early onset of rejection could be determined by the use of a scintillation camera detector with area-of-interest capability and the calculation of bladder/kidney (B/K) concentrations of isotope. Increased clearance of isotope into the kidney rather than into the urinary bladder (a decreased B/K ratio) was found to be an early indication of acute rejection in these nonsensitized and nonimmunosuppressed dogs despite the transient increase in blood clearance of ^{131}I hippurate.[5] The transient increase in blood isotope clearance was followed by a sharp fall in clearance. These allografted canine kid-

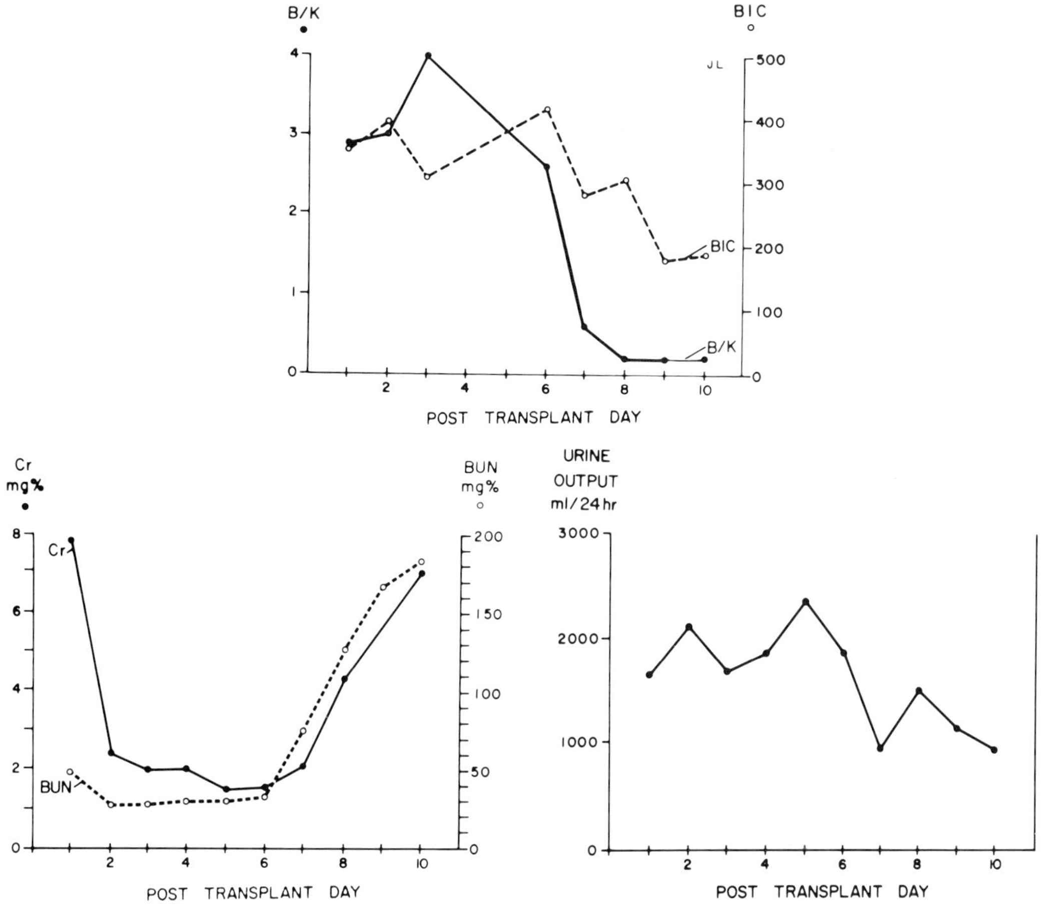

Fig. 2. Graph presenting isotope study and nonisotope study data post-transplant in Case 2, a second transplant. On the sixth post-transplant day, the B/K ratio fell sharply as the BIC was rising. The B/K ratio change occurred one day before BUN change, 2 days before an elevation in Cr, and during a period when urinary output changes were unclear in significance.

neys increased threefold in weight during rejection and it is probable that the increased isotope which was cleared from the blood early in rejection was cleared into the accumulating allograft edema fluid of rejection.

We have found the combined use of blood isotope clearance of ^{131}I hippurate and B/K ratios obtained on a daily basis after transplant to be quite useful in the early detection of renal allograft rejection in nonimmunosuppressed dogs and in immunosuppressed human patients.[4, 5] We consider this to be the most important information available for the early post-transplant clinical monitoring of renal transplant patients. These data are obtained daily (including weekends and holidays) and are recorded immediately on the clinical transplant flow sheets for immediate evaluation by the house staff and faculty.

Frequent, generally daily, studies of ^{131}I hippurate blood isotope clearance (BIC) and B/K ratios have been carried out in 79 patients following renal transplantation during the past 5 years. This report is concerned with B/K ratio and BIC alterations in 11 recipients who experienced accelerated rejection malfunction of their transplants in the early post-transplant period.

METHOD OF STUDY

Transplant recipients were given 300 μCi of ^{131}I hippurate just prior to the initiation

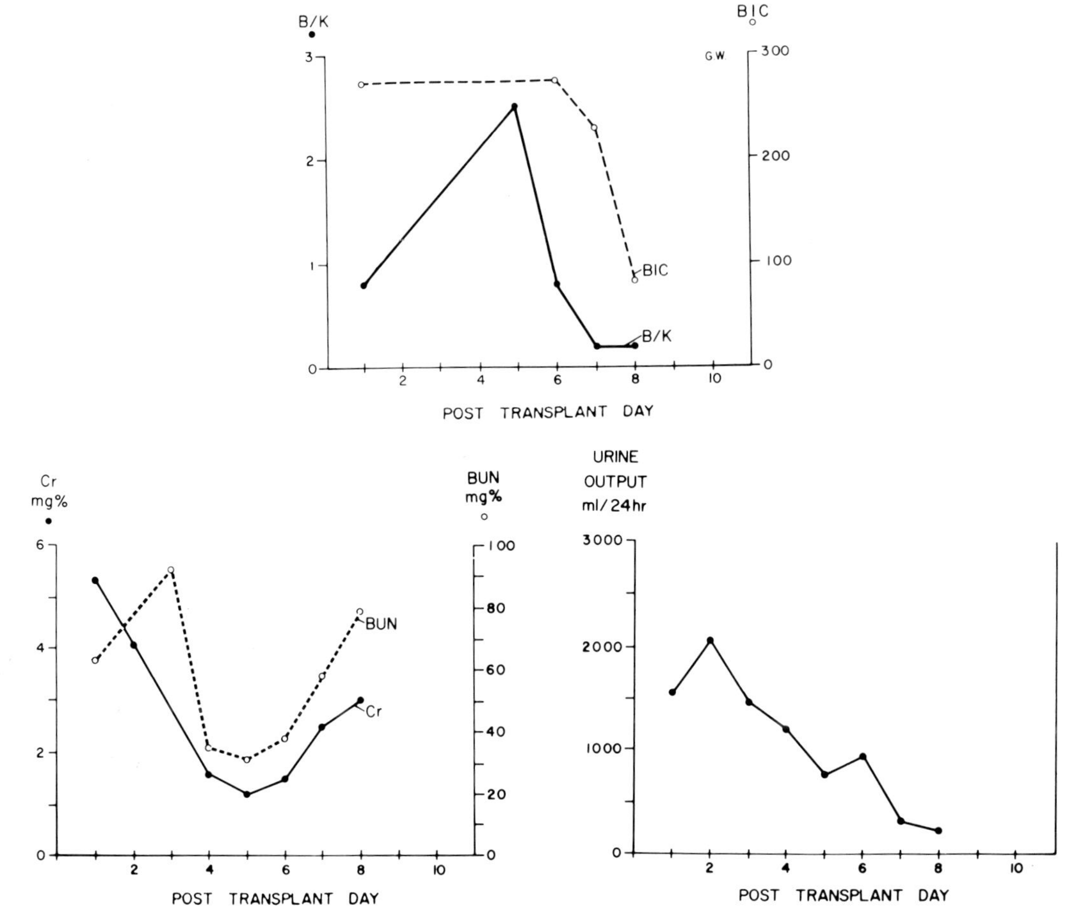

Fig. 3. Graph demonstrating post-transplant isotope study and nonisotope study data changes in Case 3 during the initial 8 days after transplant. The B/K ratio fell sharply before BIC. This occurred one day before BUN, Cr, and urinary output changes of transplant malfunction. These changes were observed despite a 4 day hiatus in BIC and a 3 day hiatus in B/K studies early after transplant.

of study. Patients were studied in supine position with a large crystal scintillation camera detector (Picker Dynacamera II) which visualized both the transplanted kidney and the urinary bladder and had area-of-interest capability. Serial one-minute studies were carried out up to 20 minutes following isotope injection. Once scintigraphs were obtained, the kidney and bladder were localized with "areas of interest" selected during replay of scintigraphic data recorded on magnetic tape. Bladder/kidney (B/K) ratios at 20 minutes after injection were calculated from these data. BIC indices were calculated from the slope of the external cardiac probe isotope clearance curve by the method of Awad and associates[1] and are expressed as the log of the isotope count at 10 minutes divided by the count at 20 minutes times 10^3.[1, 11]

RESULTS OF STUDY

In five cases, the initial pattern of change which suggested the onset of accelerated rejection transplant malfunction from the combined use of daily isotope study BIC and B/K ratio data was that of a decrease in B/K ratio as the BIC was rising (or stable, as in one case with a 4 day hiatus in BIC information during the critical observation period). In three cases, the initial pattern of daily change was that of a decrease in BIC as the B/K ratio was rising. In three cases, the BIC and B/K ratio fell together.

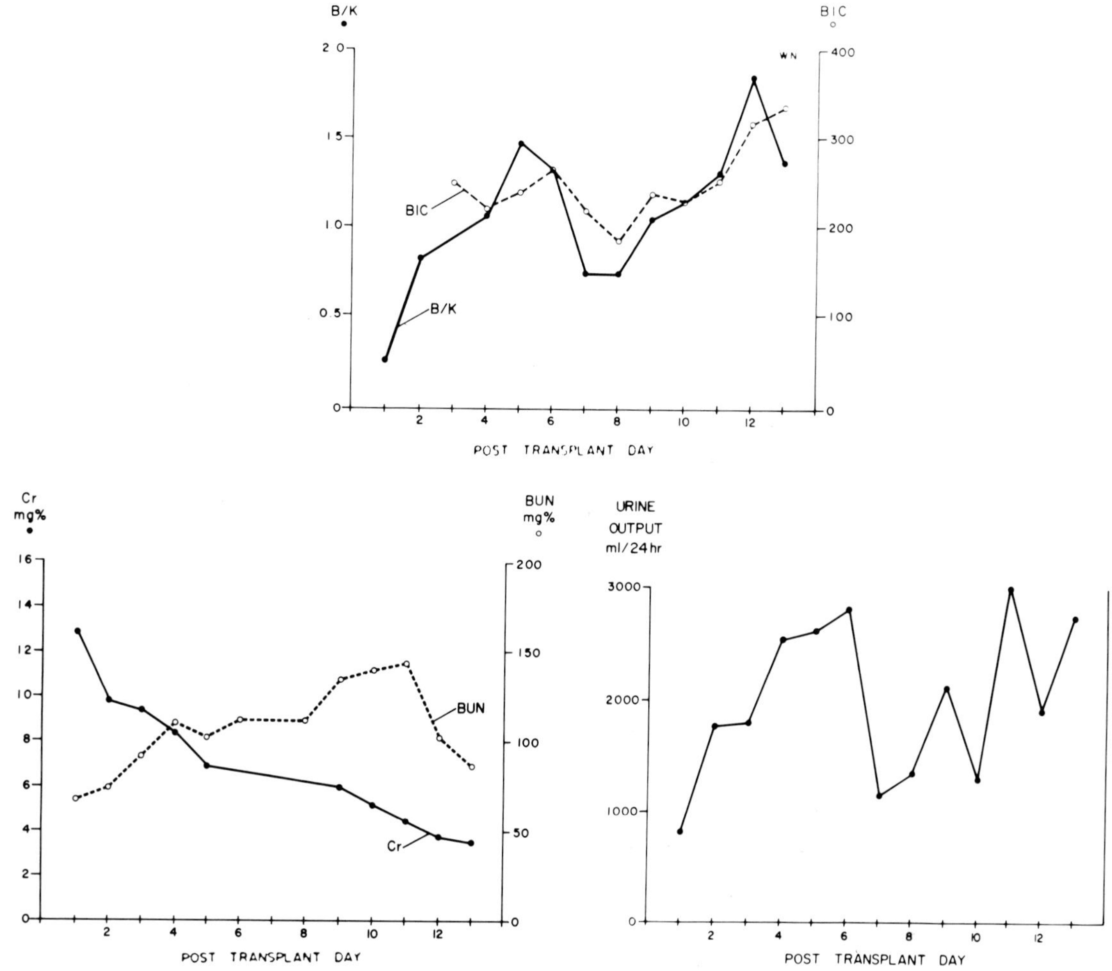

Fig. 4. Graph showing post-transplant monitoring data during the initial 13 days after transplant in Case 4. On day 6, the B/K ratio fell as the BIC was increasing. A sharp fall in B/K ratio and a decrease in BIC on day 7 led to high dose methylprednisolone therapy which reversed the isotope study evidence of transplant malfunction. The only nonisotope study index of function to change was the urinary output and this improved with treatment.

The cases are presented according to the nature of the observed pattern of BIC and B/K ratio changes on frequent (generally daily) isotope studies.

BIC INCREASE AS B/K RATIO FALLS

Case 1. D. D., a 19-year-old male patient, received a cadaveric-donor (CD) first renal transplant. The transplant functioned immediately with a good output of urine and prompt fall in blood urea nitrogen (BUN) and serum creatinine (Cr) levels (Fig. 1). He had an excellent B/K ratio on the second day following transplantation. A slight fall in the B/K ratio occurred on the fourth day and there was a marked fall on the sixth day. The BIC on the sixth day, after a lapse of three days, was elevated above the second-day level. Although urine output fell on the sixth day, BUN and Cr levels at this time were essentially unchanged. Transplant function failed rapidly thereafter and the transplant was removed.

Case 2. J. L., a 31-year-old man who had promptly rejected an RLD first transplant, received a CD second transplant. The transplant functioned immediately with a good output of urine and a prompt fall in BUN and Cr levels. He had an excellent B/K ratio on the third day following transplantation (Fig. 2). Three days later, after a 2 day weekend hiatus without isotope studies, the B/K ratio had fallen sharply and the BIC was elevated over the prior levels. At this time, the BUN, Cr, and urinary output were un-

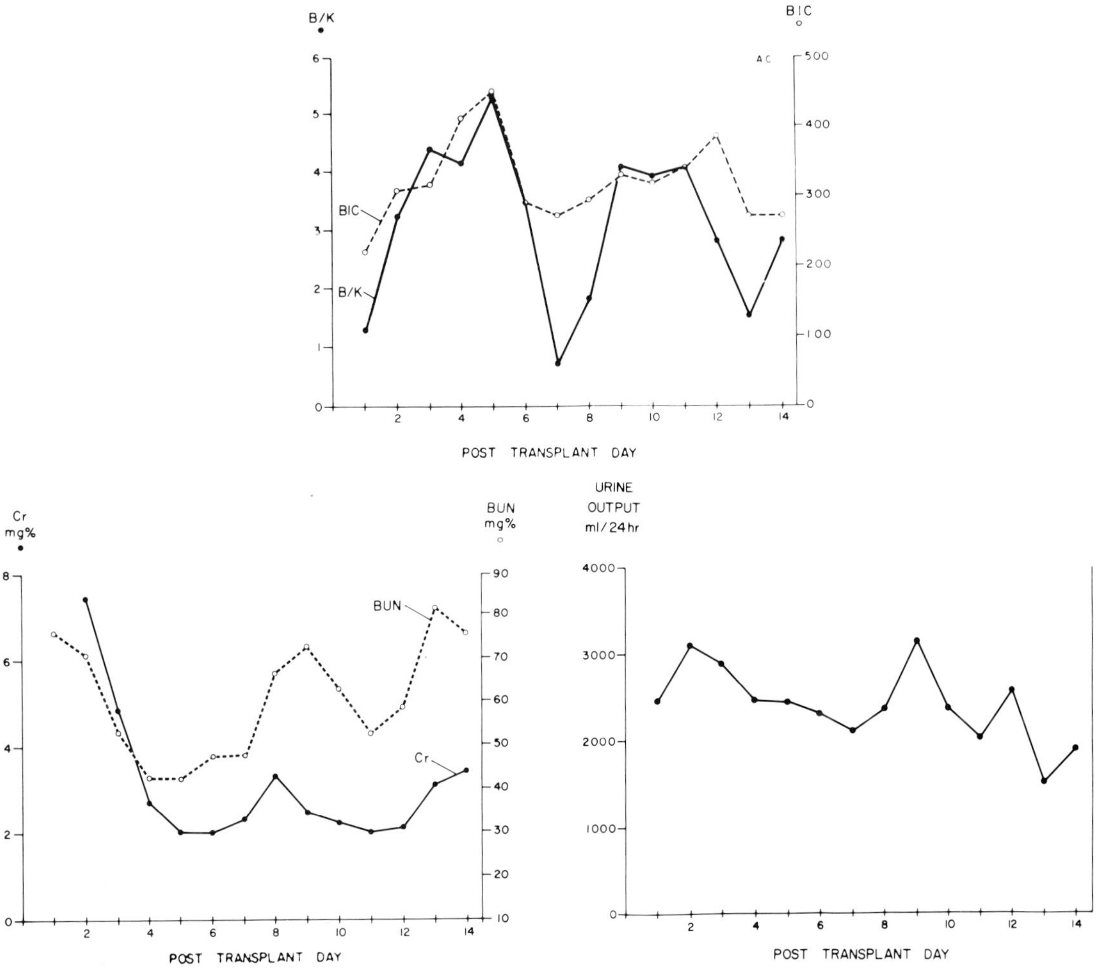

Fig. 5. Graph demonstrating post-transplant isotope study and nonisotope study monitoring data in Case 5. On the fourth day, the B/K ratio fell as the BIC was rising. BIC fell sharply on day 6. Improvement with high dose methylprednisolone therapy on day 8 is shown.

changed. On the next day further marked deterioration in the B/K ratio and BIC indices was associated with a stable Cr and a mild increase in BUN with a fall in urinary output. Transplant failure was rapid. The transplant became quite tender and transplant nephrectomy was scheduled. The tenderness disappeared within a short time following the initiation of antihistamine and antiserotonin therapy (cyproheptadine and Chlor-trimeton). Transplant function improved slowly and hemodialysis, carried out four times, was discontinued on the twenty-third post-transplant day. The transplant later was removed because of chronic rejection (at 5 months).

Case 3. G. W., a 34-year-old woman who had malignant hypertension which had complicated the third trimester of a recent pregnancy, received a CD first transplant. The transplant functioned immediately with a good output of urine. On the fifth day, after a 3 day weekend and holiday hiatus in isotope studies, the B/K ratio was 2.5 (Fig. 3). It fell precipitiously on the next day with no change in the BIC from the initial level. There was a mild increase in BUN and Cr and a stable urinary output. Methylprednisolone (1 Gm. per day) was started at this time and continued for 5 days. The patient suffered a massive cerebrovascular accident on the tenth day following transplantation. Her BUN rose to 123 and her Cr to 3.6 on the eleventh day. She received peritoneal dialysis on the thirteenth day. Her neurological condition deteriorated rapidly as her transplant function improved. When she died on the sixteenth day following transplantation, her BUN was 48 and her Cr was 1.8.

Case 4. W. N., a 40-year-old man, received a CD first-transplant kidney. Early urine output was adequate. The B/K ratio and BIC were at com-

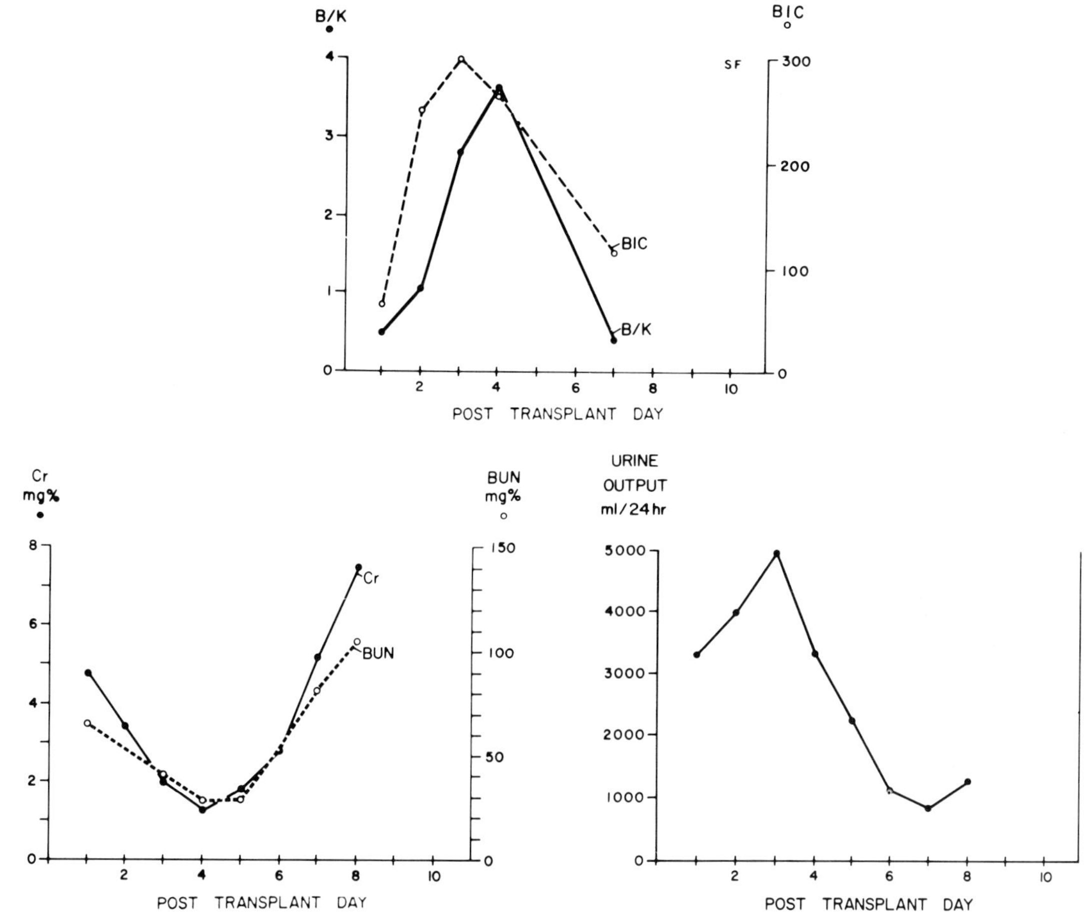

Fig. 6. Graph demonstrating alterations in isotope study and nonisotope data after transplant in Case 6. On day 4, the BIC fell as the B/K ratio was rising. This was 2 days prior to BUN and Cr changes, and 2 days prior to a fall in urinary output below the 2,000 ml. per day level.

paratively low levels. The B/K ratio fell on the sixth day while the BIC was rising. On the seventh day, the B/K ratio fell sharply with a fall in BIC, and the urine output fell to one half that of the previous day (Fig. 4). Methylprednisolone (2 Gm. per day for 3 days and one Gm. per day for 2 days) was given with some improvement in function. By the eighteenth day, the BUN was 37 and the Cr. was 2.2. Two additional rejection episodes led to the removal of the transplant.

Case 5. A. C., a 29-year-old patient, received a first-transplant CD kidney. The transplant functioned immediately with a good output of urine and a prompt fall in BUN and Cr levels (Fig. 5). A transient fall in the B/K ratio occurred on the fourth day while the BIC was rising. A sharp fall in B/K ratio and BIC occured on the sixth day and a greater fall on the seventh day. Urine output and BUN and Cr levels were not altered significantly at this time. BUN and Cr levels were increased on the eighth day. At this time methylprednisolone (2 Gm. per day for 3 days) was started with lowering of BUN and Cr and improvement in B/K ratios and BIC. A second episode of transplant malfunction followed discontinuation of methylprednisolone therapy but was reversed by a retinstitution of this therapy. Repeated rejection episodes led to the removal of the transplant 5 months after transplant.

BIC DECREASE AS B/K RATIO RISES

Case 6. S. F., a 45-year-old woman, received a CD first transplant. She had had eight pregnancies, all terminated by spontaneous abortions or miscarriages. The transplant functioned immediately with good output of urine and a prompt fall in BUN and Cr levels (Fig. 6). On the fourth day following transplantation, a fall in the BIC occurred at a time that the B/K ratio was still

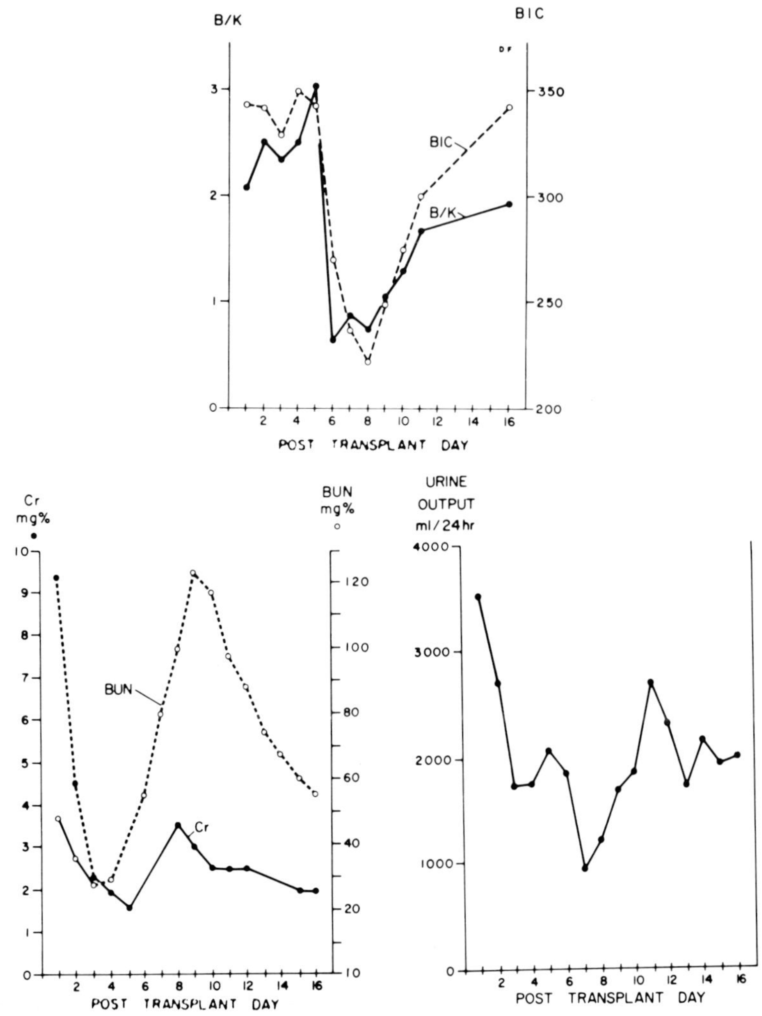

Fig. 7. Graph showing isotope study and nonisotope study monitoring data in Case 7. On day 5 a mild fall in BIC occurred as the B/K ratio was rising. On day 6 a sharp fall in both B/K ratio and BIC occurred, while urinary output remained good and as a fall in Cr and an increase in BUN were taking place. Improvement in function with heparin therapy is indicated.

rising. Other signs of function were good at this time. A mild increase in Cr occurred on the next day, while the BUN remained unchanged, and urinary output was good. BUN was elevated and urinary output depressed on the sixth day. Isotope studies on the seventh day, after a 2 day weekend lapse, showed marked deterioration in transplant function. The transplant was removed on the twenty-fourth day after transplant. A second CD transplant, avoiding HL-A antigens of both the first transplant and the husband, has functioned well for 3 years with a recent BUN of 22 and Cr of 1.2 mg. percent.

Case 7. D. F., a 31-year-old man received a CD first transplant. The transplant functioned immediately with a good output of urine and a prompt lowering of BUN and Cr levels (Fig. 7). The BIC started to fall on the fifth day following transplantation as the B/K ratio was rising. A precipitious fall in the B/K ratio on the sixth day and a sharp decrease in BIC led to the initiation of heparin therapy (20,000 units per day for 8 days) despite a good urine output and unclear or absent BUN and Cr determinations at this time. During the period of heparin therapy, the patient's blood histamine levels were one tenth of normal. Urinary output fell to one half the prior day's level on the seventh day. The BUN rose to 123 and the Cr to 3.5 before the accelerated rejection malfunction process was reversed. The transplant was functioning well 1½ years after transplantation with a BUN of 22 and a Cr of 1.3. Daily isotope studies indicated both deterioration of transplant function and subsequent recovery.

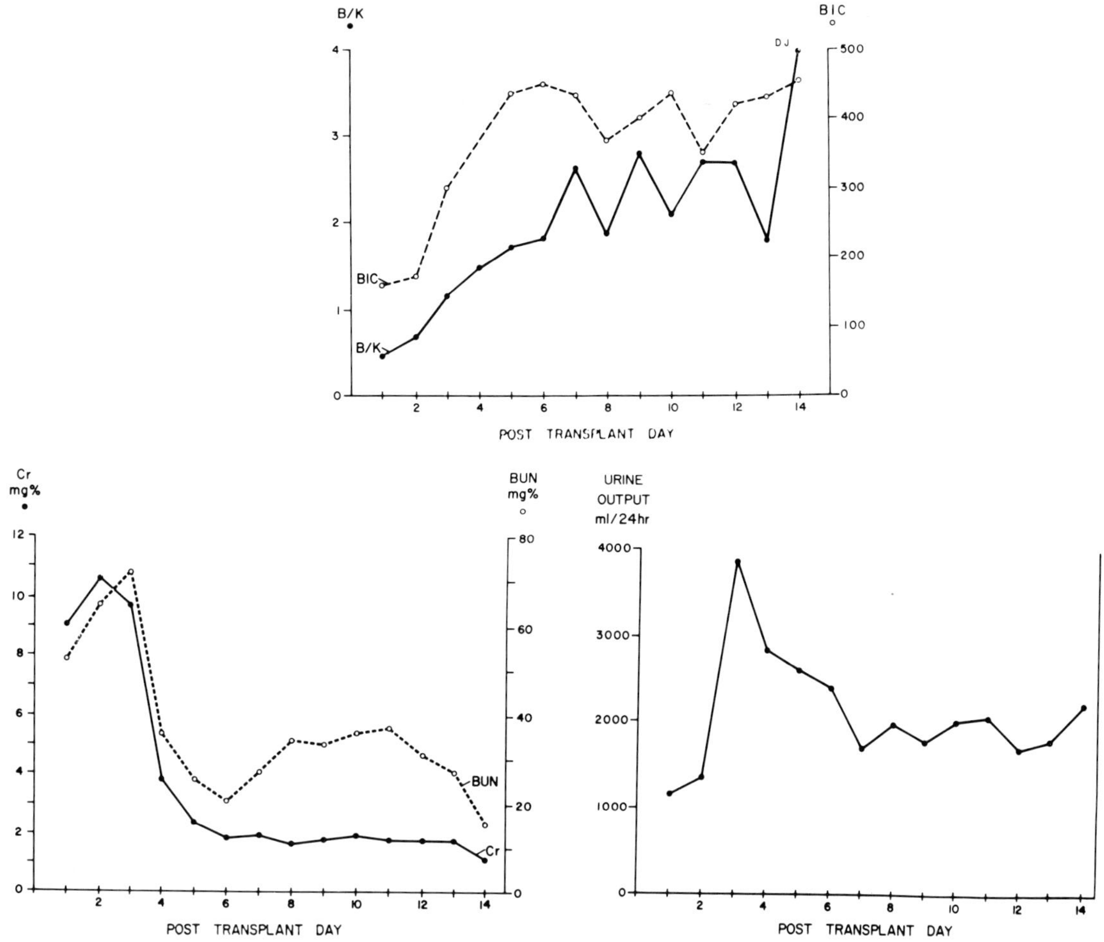

Fig. 8. Graph showing post-transplant monitoring data in Case 8. The BIC decreased as the B/K ratio was rising on day 7. A further decrease in BIC and a sharp fall in the B/K ratio on day 8 led to initiation to high dose methylprednisolone therapy. There was a mild increase in BUN but no changes in Cr or urinary output.

Case 8. D. J., a 26-year-old woman, received a CD first transplant functioned satisfactorily with adequate urine output and a lowering of BUN and Cr levels (Fig. 8). The BIC fell as the B/K ratio was rising on the seventh day. A decrease in the B/K ratio and a further fall in the BIC on the eighth day were managed by methylprednisolone therapy (2 Gm. per day for 3 days) with improvement in B/K ratios and BIC. There was a mild temporary increase in BUN and no change in Cr or urine output during this period. Six months after transplant her BUN was 42 and her Cr was 1.0.

BIC AND B/K RATIO FALL TOGETHER

Case 9. R. M., a 23-year-old man, received a renal transplant from his father. The transplant functioned immediately with a good output of urine and a fall in the BUN and Cr levels (Fig. 9). On the seventh post-transplant day, he developed a temperature elevation to 103.4° F. and wound tenderness. There were no isotope studies on this day. Studies on the next day showed a fall in both the B/K ratio and the BIC. On this and the next day, the BUN and Cr and the urinary output remained essentially unchanged. Rapid failure of the transplant occurred. Heparin administration (20,000 units per day) was started on the thirteenth post-transplant day and was continued for 8 days. Allograft function improved slowly. He received hemodialysis five times during this period. Two years after transplant his BUN is 23 mg. percent and his Cr is 1.7 mg. percent.

Case 10. W. J., a 34-year-old woman with malignant hypertension, received a renal transplant from her brother. The transplant functioned im-

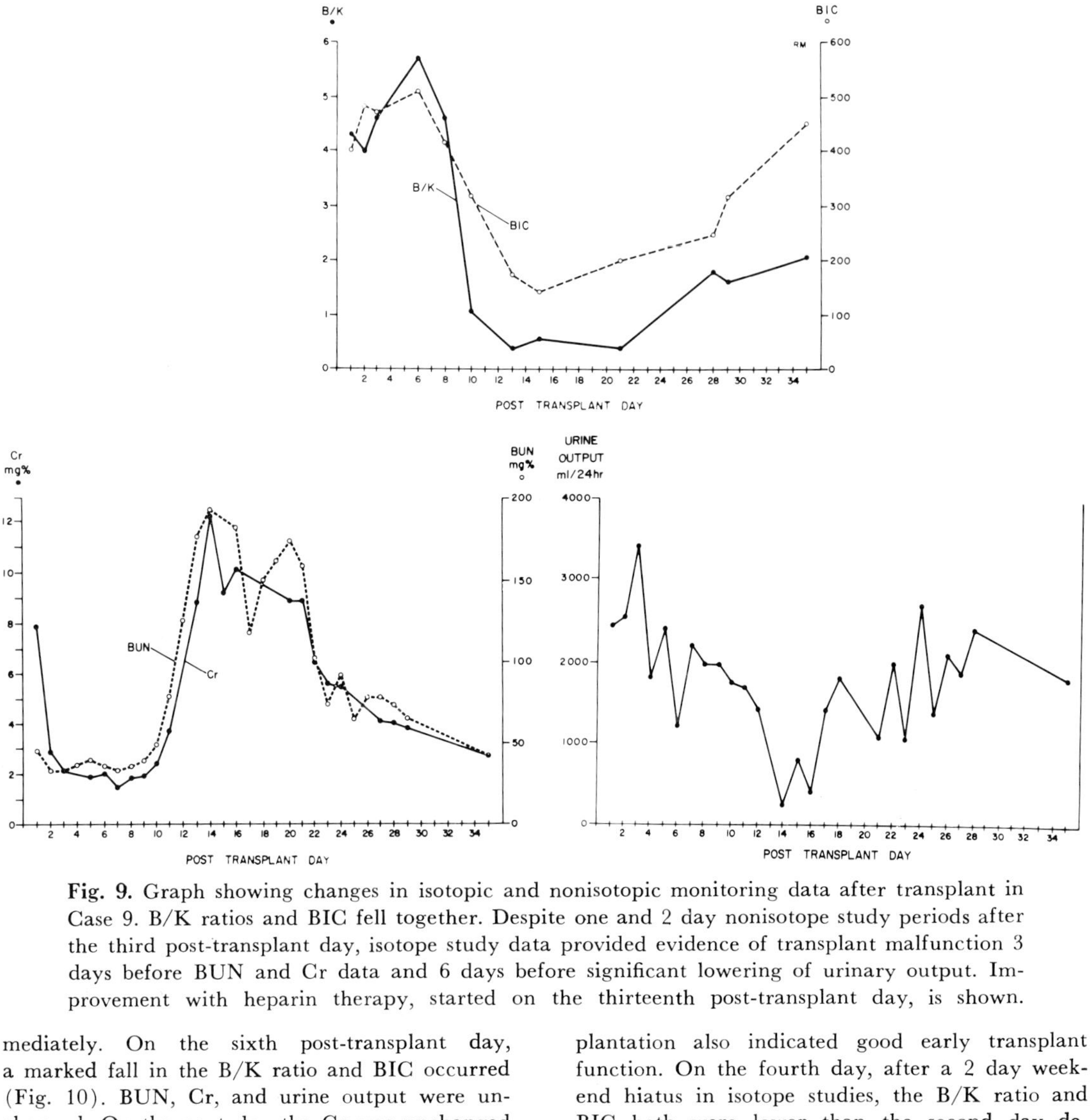

Fig. 9. Graph showing changes in isotopic and nonisotopic monitoring data after transplant in Case 9. B/K ratios and BIC fell together. Despite one and 2 day nonisotope study periods after the third post-transplant day, isotope study data provided evidence of transplant malfunction 3 days before BUN and Cr data and 6 days before significant lowering of urinary output. Improvement with heparin therapy, started on the thirteenth post-transplant day, is shown.

mediately. On the sixth post-transplant day, a marked fall in the B/K ratio and BIC occurred (Fig. 10). BUN, Cr, and urine output were unchanged. On the next day the Cr was unchanged while the BUN was elevated and the urinary output fell. Heparin administration (20,000 units per day) was started and was continued for 4 days. It was discontinued at the end of the tenth day when the patient experienced a massive cerebrovascular accident with vomiting and aspiration. Hemodialysis was started on the eleventh day and was employed five times. The aspiration pneumonitis proved rapidly fatal with death from respiratory insufficiency on the twenty-second post-transplant day. Transplant function improved during this terminal period with a return of urinary output to normal levels and a fall in BUN to 48.

Case 11. H. R., a 44-year-old man, received a CD first transplant. The transplant functioned immediately with a good urinary output and a prompt fall in BUN and Cr levels (Fig. 11). The B/K ratio and BIC on the first day after transplantation also indicated good early transplant function. On the fourth day, after a 2 day weekend hiatus in isotope studies, the B/K ratio and BIC both were lower than the second day determinations. Urinary output fell to one half prior levels on the fifth day, with a stable Cr and a rising BUN, and fell preciptiously the next day with a rise in BUN. Isotope study data also revealed marked deterioration in function. The transplant was removed on the twentieth post-transplant day.

DISCUSSION

Two of these 11 transplant recipients of kidneys which were affected by early post-transplant accelerated rejection had isotope studies every other day following transplantation, four had daily studies excluding weekends, and five had daily studies including weekends. As the study progressed, the information, which originally was reviewed as

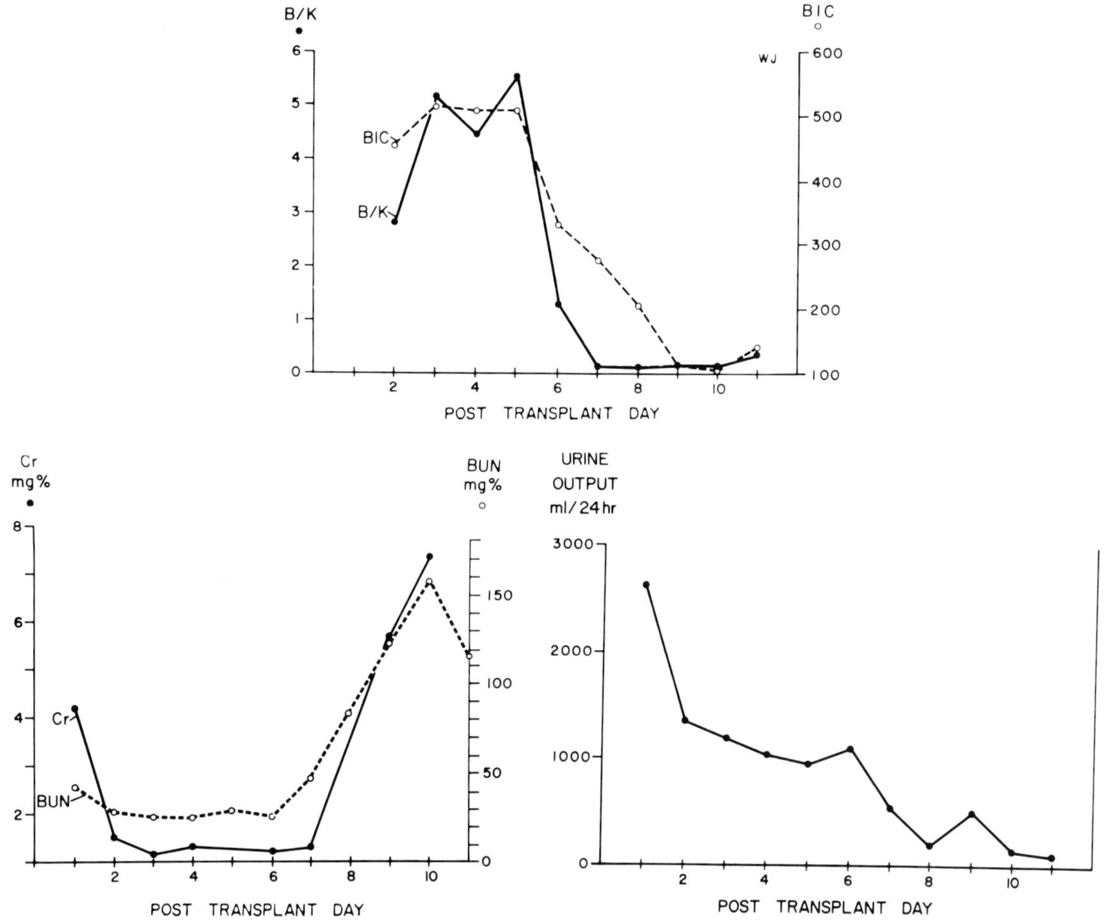

Fig. 10. Graph showing isotope study and nonisotope study monitoring data after renal transplant during the initial 11 post-transplant days in Case 10. B/K ratios and BIC fell together. Sharp falls in B/K ratio and BIC occurred one day prior to BUN and urinary output changes and 3 days prior to an elevation in Cr.

retrospective investigative data, proved to be so valuable that it was obtained with increasing frequency and recorded daily on the flow sheets. The information was obtained by phone as soon as it was available and was considered the most valuable and sensitive single type of information available for the early post-transplant monitoring of the function of the transplant. The isotope study data were employed both for the early detection of transplant malfunction and for the evaluation of the transplant response to malfunction therapeutic efforts as well as for the classification of the type of rejection and as an indication for the prompt initiation of antirejection therapy.

Data from the combined use of ^{131}I hippurate BIC and B/K ratio information provided highly sensitive and reliable information concerning the early onset of accelerated rejection. Despite the every-other-day isotope studies in two recipients and the weekend hiatuses of information in four (at 2 to 3, 4 to 5, 5 to 6, and 2 to 4 days after transplant), B/K ratio and BIC data gave advance indication of malfunction prior to BUN, Cr, and urine output information in all instances. A holiday-long weekend produced a 4 day hiatus of information in one case. Despite the limitations related to the infrequency and the missed periods of isotope studies, these data provided earlier information of transplant malfunction than that obtained from Cr data by one day in two cases, by 2 days in four cases and by 3, 4, and 5 days in one case each. The isotope

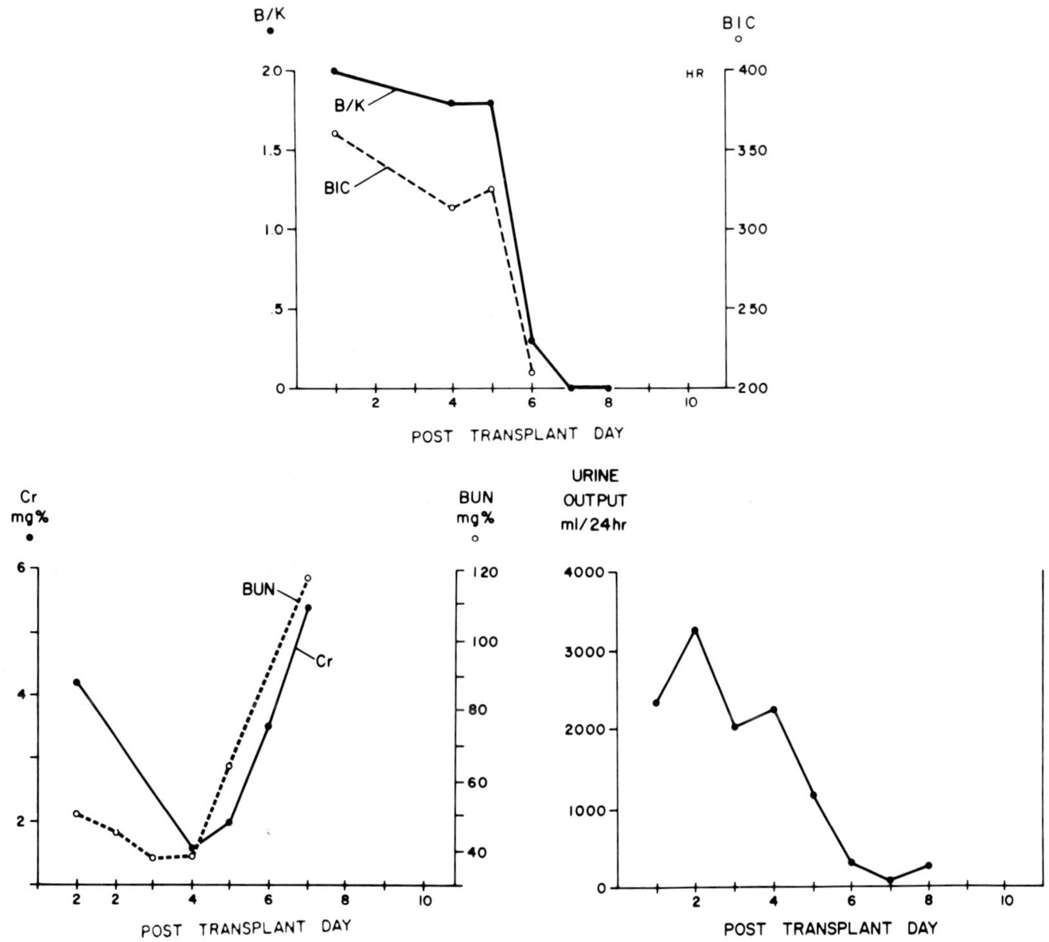

Fig. 11. Graph showing isotope study and nonisotope study after transplant monitoring data in Case 11. After a 2 day nonisotope study period, the B/K ratio and BIC fell together on day 4 from the second day post-transplant levels. This was one day before BUN rise and 2 days before Cr increase.

study data also provided earlier evidence of transplant malfunction than the BUN data by one day in four cases, by 2 days in three cases and by 3 days in two cases. In addition, these data provided earlier information of malfunction than urine output data by one day in four cases, by 2 days in three cases, by 3 days in one case, and by 6 days in one case. The isotope study data proved to be quite helpful, as additional information, in the evaluation of other indices of allograft function (BUN, Cr, and urine output) when these indices were equivocal, conflicting, or of questionable accuracy.

Evidence to suggest that accelerated rejection is due to recipient presensitization to donor transplant antigens has accumulated from radioimmunoassay studies[7] and from early post-transplant function data of machine-preserved cadaveric kidneys of good quality (from perfusion data) correlated with pre-transplant duration of hemodialysis and antibody-against-the-panel information.[12] This presensitization appears to be of intermediate titer with respect to antidonor transplant antigen antibody levels. Second-set cellular response also may play some role in accelerated rejection. The relative roles and magnitude of action of the humoral and cellular components of accelerated rejection may, at least theoretically, be dissected and studied from data of the type provided by the combined use of BIC and B/K ratio patterns of response and from their temporal relationships and the rapidity and degree of their respective daily alterations.

From the findings of this study, it appears that the type of accelerated rejection may be classified by the pattern of daily change in the BIC and B/K ratio data. Three major types of change were observed: (1) a rise in BIC while the B/K ratio was falling, (2) a fall in BIC while the B/K ratio was rising, and (3) a simultaneous fall in both BIC and B/K ratios. In five cases in this study, the B/K ratio fell as the BIC was rising (or was stable in one case), in three the BIC decreased initially as the B/K ratio was rising, and in three the BIC and B/K ratio fell together.

Razzak and associates[14] have found that BIC of ^{131}I hippurate provides a highly accurate index of renal blood flow in the presence of normal renal function. A rapid fall in allograft blood flow has been observed as a part of hyperacute renal allograft rejection, a type of rejection presumed to be due to high titers of antitransplant antibody. A fall in BIC while the B/K ratio is rising may suggest, theoretically, a predominant humoral antibody component in the accelerated rejection. The simultaneous fall in BIC and B/K ratio may also reflect this type of response. A rise in BIC at the time the B/K ratio is falling suggests a combination of allograft-increased blood flow and hyperemia in association with an increase in vascular permeability and immunoinflammatory edema fluid accumulation with a decreased passage of isotope into the urinary bladder. This type of pattern may be related to a predominantly cellular component of the accelerated rejection. This was the type of response which was observed consistently in the bilaterally nephrectomized, nonpresensitized, and nonimmunosuppressed dogs which received renal allografts. We recently have observed highly significant increases in ^{131}I hippurate accumulation (both per organ and per gram of tissue) in heterotopic heart allografts in nonpresensitized and nonimmuosuppressed rats in comparison to the isotope levels in the "native" (autologous) hearts at 6 and 7 days after grafting.[13]

With the passage of time and an increasing awareness of the significance and sensitivity of information from the combined used of daily BIC and B/K ratio studies as early indicators of the onset of accelerated rejection transplant malfunction, prompt antirejection treatment was initiated on the basis of these data alone and prior to the appearance of evidence of allograft malfunction as mirrored by changes in urine output or in BUN and Cr levels. Two of the recipients, whose isotope study changes led to prompt therapy with high-dose methylprednisolone, did not experience BUN, or urinary output alterations suggestive of transplant malfunction. Those recipients whose isotope-study evidence of transplant malfunction did not lead to prompt therapeutic efforts all experienced other (BUN, Cr, and urine output) evidence of malfunction.

Six of the recipients in this study lost their renal transplants by uncontrolled, early accelerated rejection or later recurrent acute and chronic rejection episodes and operative removal. Three of these recipients who had experienced short-term improvement in function had been given antirejection therapy in the form of high-dose methylprednisolone or antihistamine and antiserotonin drugs. The three patients who experienced rapid and uncontrolled accelerated rejection had not received heparin or high-dose methylprednisolone therapy. Two recipients died of cerebrovascular accidents and related complications at times when allograft function was improving. Both had prior histories of malignant hypertension and the cerebrosvascular accidents occurred during accelerated rejection malfunction of the transplants. One of them was on heparin and the other was on high-dose methylprednisolone therapy at the time of the cerebrovascular accident. Three recipients had reversal of the rejection malfunction and long-term (7 months and 1½ and 2 years) excellent transplant function. Two of these recipients had received heparin therapy for the malfunction. One of these recipients (Case 7) was found to have a reduction in blood histamine levels to one tenth of normal during the period of heparin therapy.[10]

CONCLUSION

Three types of BIC and B/K ratio alterations were observed: (1) a rise in BIC while B/K ratio was falling, (2) a fall in BIC while B/K ratio was rising, and (2) a simultaneous fall in BIC and B/K ratios. These changes may reflect the relative predominance of a sudden decrease in allograft blood flow and of allograft hyperemia and increased vascular permeability with immunoinflammatory edema fluid accumulation and, possibly, of the relative roles of humoral and second-set cellular immune responses in these events in these presumably presensitized recipients. Prompt antirejection therapy solely on the basis of isotopes study data in two cases appeared to have aborted the appearance of other clinical and laboratory changes associated with accelerated rejection malfunction (decreased urinary output and increase in BUN and Cr levels). We have found information from the combined use of ^{131}I hippurate BIC and B/K ratio studies to be the most valuable and sensitive type of data available for the daily, routine monitoring of post-transplant function of human renal allografts in recipients whose transplants function with reasonable adequacy in the immediate and early post-transplant period.

REFERENCES

1. Awad, W., Bennett, L. R., Martin, D. C.: Detection of renal homograft rejection with a single dose of radiohippuran, J. Urol. **100:** 233, 1969.
2. Egelston, T. A., Acchiardo, S., Rodriguez-Antunez, A., et al.: ^{131}I hippuran in the elevation of transplanted kidneys, Radiology **93:** 1145, 1969.
3. Figueroa, J. E., Rodriguez-Antunez, A., Nakamoto, A., et al.: The scintigram after renal transplantation in man, N. Engl. J. Med. **273:** 1406, 1965.
4. Hayes, M., and Moore, T. C.: Early detection and classification of renal transplant rejection by B/K scan ratio and blood isotope clearance data, Transplantation **12:** 139, 1971.
5. Hayes, M., and Moore, T. C.: Early detection of canine renal allograft rejection by reduction in the scan badder/kidney isotope intensity ratio, SURGERY **70:** 60, 1972.
6. Kountz, S. L., Laub, D. R., and Cohn, R.: Detecting and treating early renal homotransplant rejection, J. A. M. A. **191:** 997, 1965.
7. Lucas, Z. J., Coplon, N., Kempson, R., and Cohn, R.: Early transplant failure associated with subliminal sensitization, Transplantation **10:** 521, 1970.
8. Lubin, E., Levitus, Z., and Shimeoni, A.: Rapid sequential kidney scanning with ^{131}I hippuran, J. Nucl. Med. **9:** 567, 1968.
9. Magnusson, G., Collste, L., Franksson, C., et al.: Radiorenography in clinical transplantation, *in* Franksson, C., editor, Kidney transplantation, Stockholm, 1968, Almqvist and Wiksell, p. 60.
10. Moore, T. C., and Lemmi, C. A. E.: Effects of heparin and ALG with antiplatelet activity on blood and urinary histamine levels of human renal transplant recipients, Am. Surg. In press.
11. Moore, T. C., Thompson, D. P., and Hayes, M.: Correlation of renal bloodflow indices and histamine metabolism after canine renal allografting, Arch. Surg. **101:** 45, 1970.
12. Moore, T. C., Berne, T. V., and English, T. S.: Accelerated rejection of 36 immediate posttransplant functioning machine-preserved human cadaveric kidneys, SURGERY **75:** 357, 1974.
13. Moore, T. C., Vigran, T. S., and Lemmi, C. A. E.: ^{131}I hippurate isotope entrapment in rejecting heterotopic rat heart allografts, J. Thorac. Cardiovasc. Surg. Submitted for publication.
14. Razzak, M. A., Botti, R. E., MacIntire, W. J., and Pritchard, W. H.: External monitoring of ^{131}I hippuran disappearance as a measure of renal blood flow, Int. J. Appl. Radiat. Isot. **18:** 825, 1967.
15. Sharpe, A. R., Jr., King, E. R., Hume, D. M., et al.: Sequential response of the idodine-131 hippuran renogram in renal homotransplantation, J. Nucl. Med. **7:** 556, 1966.
16. Staab, E. V., Kelly, W. D., and Loken, M. K.: Prognostic value of radioisotope renograms in kidney transplantation, J. Nucl. Med., **10:** 133, 1969.
17. Weiss, E. R., Blahd, W. H., Winston, M. A., et al.: Scintillation camera in the evaluation of renal transplant, J. Nucl. Med., **11:** 69, 1970.

Transhepatic metabolism after end-to-side portacaval shunt in the young pig

Rosemary Hickman, M.D., Ch.M., James H. Crosier, M.B., Ch.B., Stuart J. Saunders, M.D., F.R.C.P., *and* **John Terblanche, Ch.M., F.C.S.(SA),** *Cape Town, South Africa*

End-to-side portacaval shunt was created in eight young pigs and metabolic changes were studied by transhepatic sampling techniques and lumbar puncture. The animals survived a mean of 25 days, with no obvious cause of death but failure to gain weight and inanition. Arterial ammonia levels rose despite maintained hepatic clearance. Cerebrospinal fluid (CSF) glutamine levels also rose for the first two weeks after shunt and there was significant correlation with arterial ammonia levels. Mean serum levels of cholesterol, alkaline phosphatase, amylase, and albumin fell after the procedure, but no changes were noted in acid-base status, osmolality, plasma potassium, glucose, aminotransferase (AAT), or urea.

From the Department of Surgery and Medicine, and the Medical Research Council Liver Research Group, University of Cape Town, and the Liver Clinic, Groote Schuur Hospital, Cape Town, South Africa.

PORTACAVAL SHUNTING for the relief of portal hypertension in patients with cirrhosis has undergone various phases of popularity.[19, 32, 53] Recently the operation has been recommended for children with hyperlipidemia[47] or with glycogen storage disease[49] because of related metabolic changes which have been noted to accompany diversion of portal blood from livers of normal rats,[1, 22] dogs,[6, 45] and monkeys.[21] Many other metabolic changes also occur with, as yet, ill-defined interrelationships.[15, 36, 37]

During a study of heterotopic liver transplantation in the pig, animals with portacaval shunts served as some controls.[8] A rapid rise in peripheral venous ammonia and cerebrospinal fluid (CSF) glutamine was noted and the present work was undertaken to evaluate this further. As no previous studies have been reported of transhepatic metabolism following portacaval shunt, recently described techniques of sampling[16] were used to evaluate the metabolic effect of acute portal diversion in the normal young pig.

Accepted for publication June 27, 1974.

This study was supported in part by the Medical Research Council of South Africa, the Harry Crossley Foundation, and the Herman and Caporn bequests to the University of Cape Town.

Reprint requests: Dr. Rosemary Hickman, Department of Surgery, Medical School, Observatory, Cape Town, South Africa.

MATERIALS AND METHODS

Eight young pigs aged 40 to 60 days and weighing between 16 and 32 kilograms (mean weight 21.3 kilograms) were starved for 24 hours and then anesthetized with sodium Pentothal (15 to 20 mg. per kilogram), given into an ear vein to allow passage of an endotracheal tube and a wide-bore gastric tube. Anesthesia was maintained with nitrous oxide and oxygen; the intravenous infusion solution was 10 percent invert sugar in Ringer's lactate.

Catheters (No. 8 Fr.) were introduced

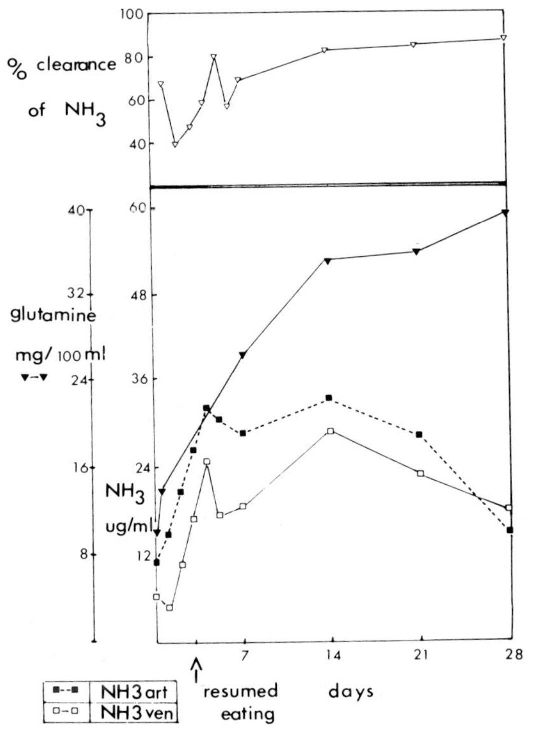

Fig. 1. The mean levels of arterial and venous ammonia and cerebrospinal fluid glutamine during the month of study, with the mean percentage hepatic clearance of ammonia.

into the right carotid artery and the external jugular vein. The latter was advanced through the superior vena cava and the suprahepatic vena cava into the left hepatic vein as previously described.[16] Through a midline abdominal incision, the portal vein was dissected free in the porta hepatis. Great care was taken to preserve the pancreaticoduodenal vein which drains into the portal vein high in the porta hepatis, in an attempt to maintain full insulin and glucagon supply to the circulation.[48] A portion of the intrahepatic cava proximal to the renal veins was dissected. End-to-side portacaval shunt was made with 5-0 silk and as this required less than 10 minutes, no portosystemic bypass was needed.[2] An anterior gastroenterostomy was made in an attempt to prevent gastric ulceration[9, 42] and the abdominal wound was closed in layers. Both neck catheters were left in situ for subsequent sampling and were sewn to the skin and the neck. The control clamp from an intravenous infusion set was threaded along the arterial catheter to prevent accidental hemorrhage.

Intravenous infusion was continued for 2 days and then the animals were returned to normal diet. Crystalline penicillin (600 mg.) and chloromycetin (1.0 Gm.) were given intravenously for 5 days. Blood samples were taken preoperatively and 15 minutes after opening of the shunt; lumbar puncture was repeated at the end of the operation. Blood was taken daily for 5 days and then at weekly intervals when animals were weighed and subjected to percutaneous liver biopsy and lumbar puncture[51] under light anesthesia with thiopentone sodium. At death, a complete autopsy was performed and specimens taken from liver, spleen, pancreas, kidneys, and any other organs which were obviously diseased. In addition, the portal vein and inferior vena cava were dissected out and patency of the shunt was ascertained. The position of the hepatic venous catheter was confirmed and collaterals searched for but never demonstrated.

Biochemical methods. Methods used for acid-base analysis and determination of aspartate aminotransferase (AAT), alkaline phosphatase, total protein and albumin, cholesterol, potassium, calcium, and osmolality have been previously described.[17] Ammonia was measured by the ion-exchange method of Kingsley and Tager,[20] amylase according to Pimstone.[34] CSF glutamine was determined by the method of Whitehead and Whitaker.[54]

RESULTS

Survival and weight. The mean survival time of these animals was 25 ± 1 days with a range of 15 to 31 days. Two animals had pneumonia at autopsy but there was no evidence of gastric ulceration in any. No other cause of death was obvious and animals apparently died of inanition. During life, the level of consciousness did not appear to be depressed, although in the third and fourth weeks animals responded less vociferously to handling, and in two, the change in squeal as described by McCance[25] was noted. The mean preoperative weight was 21.3 kilograms, and during the postoperative month of survival all animals failed to gain weight, especially when this was compared to the expected increase of 15 percent body weight per week for animals of this size.[25]

Ammonia and glutamine. During the month of study, the mean arterial and venous levels of ammonia tripled; liver ammonia clearance was impaired to 40 percent at the fifth day but this gradually improved (Fig. 1). Changes in blood ammonia level could not be attributed to changes in pH, nor was there profound respiratory alkalosis which promotes transfer of ammonia into the brain.[46]

The increase in levels of ammonia and glutamine immediately after creation of the shunt (Fig. 1) probably resulted from stasis in the mesenteric system during clamping, with subsequent release of ammonia into the circulation.

Mean CSF glutamine levels tripled within the first week and thereafter continued to increase slowly (Fig. 1). A significant correlation between CSF glutamine and plasma ammonia was noted during the first weeks (Fig. 2) ($p < 0.05$, $r = 0.91$), and lack of correlation at 3 and 4 weeks resulted from the plateau in glutamine levels. In five animals additional to this study, lumbar puncture was performed on days 2 and 4 post-shunt and the increase in CSF glutamine was found to have occurred within the first 2 days. These animals died within the first week and as repeated starvation and anesthesia were incriminated, subsequent samples were collected weekly.

Cholesterol, alkaline phosphatase, amylase, and serum protein. There were progressive falls in levels of cholesterol, alkaline phosphatase, and amylase in this study (Fig. 3). The fall in alkaline phosphatase was significant from the second day ($p < 0.001$) and isoenzyme studies demonstrated that the change was due to the bone and gut components. Mean levels of amylase and cholesterol were significantly different from preoperative values after the fifth day. The normal amylase value in pigs has been found to be 600 units and intraoperative values to be elevated to

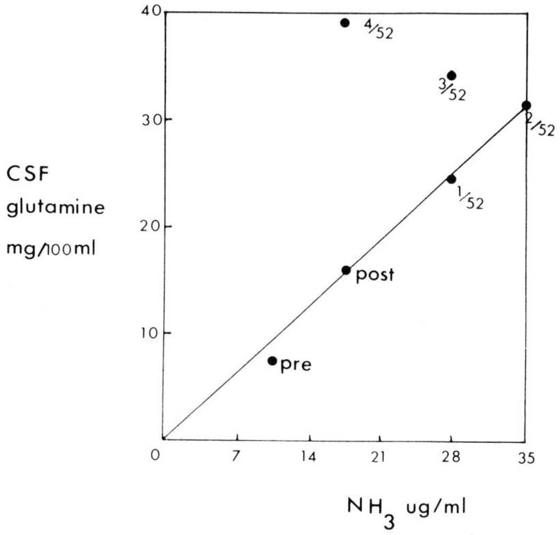

Fig. 2. The correlation between mean arterial ammonia and cerebrospinal fluid glutamine levels after portacaval shunt ($r = 0.091$, $P < 0.05$).

1,000 units (M. W. Waterworth, unpublished observation). Serum cholesterol fell during intravenous infusion and then rose with initial feeding, but the level was not sustained. A rise in serum protein was noted (Fig. 4) with a fall in albumin and a rise in globulin. Electrophoresis showed this to be in the α_1-, α_2-, and γ-globulin fractions ($p < 0.005$).

Other values. There were no significant changes during the period of study or in transhepatic samples in measurements of acid-base status, glucose, potassium, calcium, AAT, urea, or osmolality.

Histology. There were no outstanding features on light microscopy. A few sections showed isolated areas of fat infiltration but there was no necrosis. Lobules were not measured.

DISCUSSION

When a portacaval shunt is performed, the patients often have liver disease and almost always have hypertension of whatever etiology. Under these circumstances, natural portosystemic shunts have opened slowly[26] and liver function may have adjusted to increasing portal diversion.[40] When portacaval shunt is performed in normal animals, no such compensation can occur before diversion.

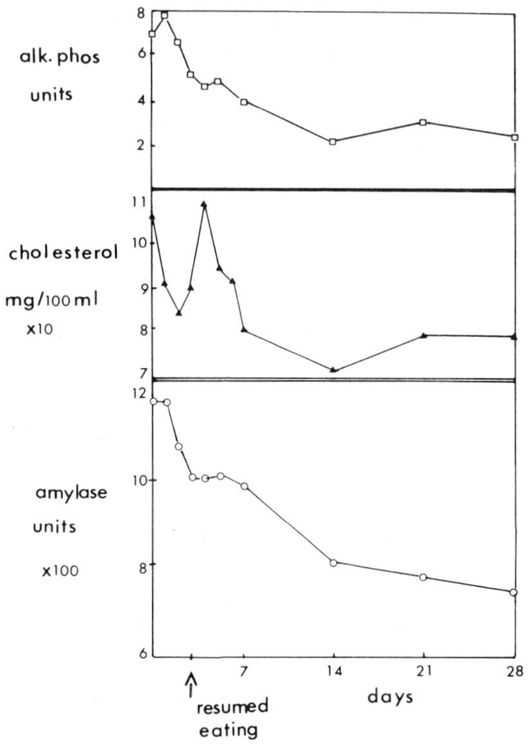

Fig. 3. The mean arterial levels of cholesterol, alkaline phosphatase, and amylase after portacaval shunt.

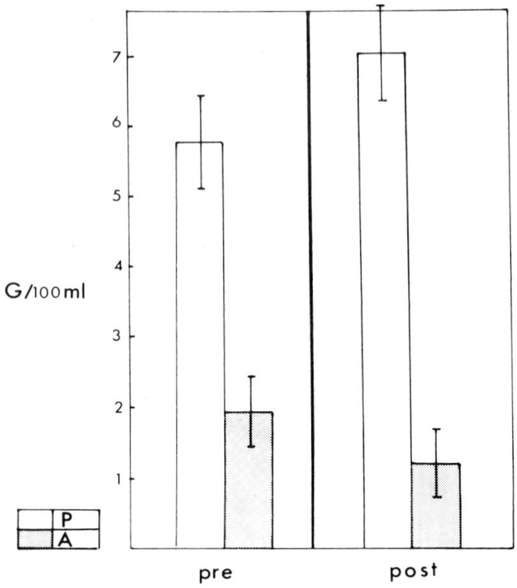

Fig. 4. The mean arterial levels (with standard error of the mean) of total serum protein and albumin (grams per 100 ml.) before and after portacaval shunt.

Observations made in this study confirmed those made in rats and dogs but the survival time was shorter and there was no obvious cause of death. The duration of survival was similar to that noted in small rats and might also be lengthened by administration of neomycin.[27] The failure to gain weight in growing animals has previously been noted in dogs[45] and rats,[22, 24] and it has been shown that the latter animals may eat one third less after operation when compared with sham-operated controls.[22] The food intake in these pigs was not measured but was apparently less than normal. In dogs an average weight loss of 20 percent is quoted, whether germ free or normal,[29] and some animals died within one month and 6 weeks postoperatively, manifesting emaciation and encephalopathy.[1, 4] In children with glycogen storage disease, however, a growth spurt was noted after portacaval shunt.[49]

Inadequate intake could be implicated in the changes in cholesterol, albumin, and alkaline phosphatase levels. Cholesterol values were not as low as noted in the previous series[8] in which no gastroenterostomy was performed and in which a high incidence of gastric ulceration was noted. The presence of such ulcers might have reduced food intake still further. A fall in serum cholesterol was first noted to follow Eck fistula by Winter and associates[56] in 1941. In these studies there was no impairment in intestinal absorption. This metabolic alteration has resulted in the recent proposal of portacaval shunt treatment for children with hyperlipoproteinemia.[47]

Reduction of alkaline phosphatase levels in young pigs following portacaval shunt resulted from decrease in the bone and gut components. In adult men[33] or monkeys,[21] no changes were noted in levels of alkaline phosphatase. Following partial hepatectomy in rats, the rise in alkaline phosphatase was interpreted as a response to liver regeneration.[31] The observed fall in alkaline phosphatase following portacaval shunt might be related to the role of portal blood in liver regeneration.[7, 12, 47]

The changes in serum proteins are similar to those noted in rats.[27] Decreased levels of serum albumin have also been noted in dogs after 6 weeks[40] and a lesser rate of protein synthesis has been proposed.[33, 45] In rats the rise in serum immunoglobulins following portacaval shunt has recently been shown to be due to circulation of bacterial lipopolysaccharides from the gut which were usually filtered in the liver.[27] Such circulating endotoxemia could also contribute to undernutrition in the pigs which are particularly susceptible to *E. coli* bowel infections.[28]

Recent studies by Olcay and associates[30] have shown reticuloendothelial dysfunction following acute portal vein occlusion, with endotoxemia.

The cause of failure to eat has not been clarified. A recent publication suggests the presence of receptors in the portal system which inter-react with the feeding and satiety centers in the hypothalamus.[37] The precise situation of these receptors is uncertain, but portal diversion might interfere with hypothalamic response.

Protein intoxication has been recorded since the first creation of the Eck fistula in dogs.[4, 29] In the pigs in this study, as in dogs,[10] the liver rapidly regained the capacity to clear ammonia. It is possible that the continued rise in arterial ammonia levels could be due to reduced delivery through the hepatic artery only. There is also clearance of ammonia in the eviscerated state,[40] suggesting a contributory mechanism by extrahepatic tissues in the presence of defective liver function. Preliminary studies of portal venous ammonia in portacaval shunted animals show high levels which must be cleared in extrahepatic tissues. Both ammonia and uric acid rise in the absence of sufficient oxygen,[32] an increase which could occur following portacaval shunt.

Cerebrospinal fluid glutamine has not often been measured following experimental portacaval shunt but there is well-recorded elevation in hepatic encephalopathy.[18] The pigs showed depressed responsiveness while glutamine levels rose rapidly within the first 2 days but improved to near normal thereafter. In previous studies attempting to induce hepatic necrosis in pigs, coma developed terminally for a few hours despite extensive liver damage and elevated CSF glutamine levels.[51] (The cerebral state of the pigs during most of the month of study would be graded as "minimal encephalopathy" according to Voorhees and associates.[53]) Ammonia may not be as toxic to pigs as it is claimed to be in human beings[3, 13] and dogs.[5, 11] In monkeys[21] there was no evidence of rise in blood ammonia or encephalopathy after portacaval shunt, and in children cerebral complications have not been noted.[49] Despite intensive investigation, the role of ammonia and glutamine in hepatic coma is only partly clarified[3, 35] and octopamine (a false neurotransmitter), ketoglutaramate, and fatty acids with mercaptans have recently been implicated.[23, 50, 57]

The lack of change in some measurements was of interest. AAT is a more sensitive index of liver damage in the pig than alanine aminotransferase,[55] the levels of which are low even in hepatic necrosis. Nevertheless, a rise in AAT has been noted after side-to-side shunt in monkeys[21] but not after Eck fistula.[14] In rats a five- to fifteen-fold increase in AAT occurred within the first 24 hours of shunt, but the rise is less in man or rabbits.[33] Mitochondrial[42] and microsomal[52] enzymes have been shown to be elevated in plasma. Acute ischemia of 30 minutes' duration in the pig has been shown to cause minimal change in AAT,[2] but it was anticipated that prolonged diversion might cause higher plasma levels.

Despite the importance of the liver in urea metabolism,[55] no change was noted in serum urea levels. However, for completeness, urinary clearance and urea synthesis and catabolism should also be studied.

There was no evidence of disturbed glucose metabolism despite prolonged inanition. In dogs glucose has been shown to be released from the liver after Eck fistula[14] and in man[3, 35] and dogs[54] it has been proposed that reduced metabolism of ammonia results from deficient glucose supplies, especially in the brain. Glucose tolerance has been reported to be abnormal in the dog.[14] Diversion of blood from portal receptors described previously might interfere with hormonal balance, especially of glucagon and insulin.[6, 48]

We wish to acknowledge the continued support and enthusiasm of Professor J. H. Louw, Head of the Division of Surgery. Expert technical assistance was rendered by Ms. J. Green, J. Fourie, C. Rose-Innes, and P. van Heerden. Histological specimens were prepared by Ms. S. Carstens and Mr. S. E. Abbott. The surgery was performed with the assistance of the staff of the J. S. Marais Surgical Laboratory.

REFERENCES

1. Assal, J. P., Levrat, R., Cahn, T., and Renold, A. E.: Metabolic consequences of portacaval shunting in the rat, Z. Ges. Exp. Med. **154:** 87, 1971.
2. Battersby, C., Hickman, R., Saunders, S. J., and Terblanche, J.: Liver function in the pig. I. The effect of 30 minutes' normothermic ischaemia, Br. J. Surg. **61:** 27, 1974.
3. Bessman, J. P., and Bessman, A. N.: The cerebral and peripheral uptake of ammonia in liver disease—a hypothesis for the mechanism of hepatic coma, J. Clin. Invest. **34:** 622, 1955.
4. Bollman, J.: The animal with an Eck fistula, Physiol. Rev. **41:** 607, 1961.
5. Brown, H., Brown, J., and Yashruti, S.: Hepatic coma and ammonia metabolism in dogs, J. A. M. A. **183:** 335, 1963.
6. Brown, H., Covelli, V. H., and Brown, M.: Insulin, ammonia, and glucose after portacaval shunting, SURGERY **66:** 383, 1969.
7. Bucher, N. L. R., and Swaffield, M. N.: Regeneration of liver in rats in the absence of portal splanchnic organs and a portal blood supply, Cancer Res. **33:** 3189, 1973.
8. Crosier, J., Immelman, E. J., Hickman, R., and Terblanche, J.: Unpublished observations, 1974.
9. Day, S. B., Skoryna, S. C., Webster, D. R., and MacLean, L. D.: Gastric hypersecretion and histamine levels in liver, stomach, duodenum, and blood following portacaval shunt in rats, SURGERY **54:** 764, 1963.
10. Drapanas, T., Kluge, D. N., Schreiber, H., and Stewart, J. T.: The direct removal of portal blood ammonia by the liver, Surg. Gynecol. Obstet. **111:** 58, 1960.
11. Eiseman, B., and Clarke, G. M.: Studies in ammonia metabolism. III. Experimental production of coma by carotid artery infusion of ammonium salts, SURGERY **43:** 476, 1958.
12. Fischer, J., Myers, A., and James, H.: Ornithine decarboxylase—a defect in liver regeneration following portacaval shunt, SURGERY **70:** 182, 1971.
13. Gips, C. H., Hindfelt, B., Holmin, T., and Kardel, T.: Some concepts in ammonia, portacaval shunts, and encephalopathy, Scand. J. Gastroenterol. **8:** 385, 1973.
14. Hallett, E. B., Hoton, G. W., Paterson, J. C. S., and Schilling, J. A.: Liver blood flow, hepatic glucose production, and splanchnic oxygen consumption in normal dogs following Eck fistula; liver blood flow before and after splenectomy, Surg. Gynecol. Obstet. **95:** 401, 1952.
15. Herz, R., Sautter, V., and Bircher, J.: Fortuitous discovery of urate nephrolithiasis in rats subjected to portacaval anastomosis, Experientia **28:** 27, 1972.
16. Hickman, R., Saunders, S. J., and Terblanche, J.: Liver function in the pig. II. Total hepatic and portal flow, S. Afr. J. Lab. Clin. Med. **48:** 1197, 1974.
17. Hickman, R., Simson, E., Saunders, S. J., and Terblanche, J.: Biochemical values in normal anaesthetized South African pigs, S. Afr. J. Lab. Clin. Med. **44:** 531, 1970.
18. Hourani, B. T., Hamlin, E. M., and Reynolds, T. B.: CSF glutamine as a measure of hepatic encephalopathy, Arch. Intern. Med. **127:** 1033, 1971.
19. Hourigan, K., Sherlock, S., George, P., and Mindel, S.: Elective end-to-side portacaval shunt—results in 64 cases, Br. Med. J. **4:** 473, 1971.
20. Kingsley, G. R., and Tager, H. S.: Ion exchange method of plasma ammonia nitrogen determination with Berthelot reaction, Stand. Meth. Clin. Chem. **6:** 115, 1970.
21. Kline, D. G., Cook, J. N., and Nance, F. C.: Eck fistula encephalopathy, Ann. Surg. **173:** 97, 1971.
22. Kyu, M. H., and Cavanagh, J. B.: Some effects of portacaval anastomosis in the male rat, Br. J. Exp. Pathol. **51:** 217, 1970.
23. Lam, K. C., Tall, A. R., Goldstein, G. B., and Mistilis, S. P.: False neurotransmitter—the role of octopamine in the pathogenesis of hepatic and renal encephalopathy, Scand. J. Gastroenterol. **8:** 465, 1973.
24. Masland, W. S.: Inter-relationships between diet and weight gain in rats with portacaval shunt, Am. J. Physiol. **206:** 304, 1964.
25. McCance, R. A.: Severe undernutrition in growing and adult animals, Br. J. Nutr. **14:** 59, 1960.
26. Mellemgaard, K., Winkler, K., Tygstrup, N., and Georg, J.: Sources of veno-arterial admixture in portal hypertension, J. Clin. Invest. **42:** 1399, 1963.
27. Meyers, O. L., Keraan, M., Engelbrecht, G. H. C., Hickman, R., Saunders, S. J., and Terblanche, J.: Gut, 1974. In press.
28. Moon, H. W., Whipp, S. C., and Baetz, A. L.: Comparative effects of enterotoxins from *E. coli* and *Vibrio cholerae* on rabbit and swine small intestine, Lab. Invest. **25:** 133, 1971.
29. Nance, F. C., and Kline, D. G.: Eck fistula

encephalopathy in germ-free dogs, Ann. Surg. **174:** 856, 1971.
30. Olcay, I., Kitahama, A., Miller, R. H., Drapanas, T., Trejo, R. A., and Di Luzio, N. R.: Reticulo-endothelial dysfunction and endotoxaemia following portal occlusion, SURGERY **75:** 64, 1974.
31. Oppenheimer, M. J.: *In* Hoffbauer, F. W., editor: Plasma alkaline phosphatase levels following partial hepatectomy, Trans. Josiah Macy Foundation, 5th meeting, New York, 1946, p. 36.
32. Orloff, M. J.: Current progress and problems in portal hypertension, *in* Saunders, S. J., and Terblanche, J., editors: Liver, Sir Isaac Pitman & Sons, Ltd., London, 1973, p. 273.
33. Ozawa, K., Kitamura, O., Yamaoka, Y., Kamano, T., Mizukami, T., Takeda, H., Takasan, H., and Honja, I.: Metabolic response of the liver of human beings and other mammals to deprivation of portal blood supply, Surg. Gynecol. Obstet. **137:** 623, 1973.
34. Pimstone, N. R.: A study of the starch-iodine complex: A modified colorimetric microdetermination of amylase in biologic fluids, Clin. Chem. **10:** 891, 1964.
35. Porro, G. B., Maiolo, A. T., and Della Porta, P.: Cerebral blood flow and metabolism in hepatic cirrhosis before and after portacaval shunt, Gut **10:** 894, 1969.
36. Reichle, F. A., Brigham, M. P., Reichle, R. M., Reilly, R. M., Tyson, R. R., and Rosemond, G. P.: Effect of portacaval shunt on tyrosine metabolism, Arch. Surg. **105:** 363, 1972.
37. Reichle, F. A., Brigham, M. P., Tyson, R. R., Reichle, R. M., Reilly, R. M., and Rosemond, G. P.: Serine metabolism after portacaval shunt, Arch. Surg. **100:** 163, 1970.
38. Schmitt, M.: Influences of hepatic portal receptors on hypothalamic feeding and satiety centers, Am. J. Physiol. **225:** 1089, 1973.
39. Sherlock, S.: Diseases of the liver, Oxford, 1968, Blackwell Scientific Publications.
40. Shorr, E.: *In* Hoffbauer, F. W., editor: Discussion, Trans. Josiah Macy Foundation, New York, 1949.
41. Smith, G. W., and Mouzas, G.: The metabolic response of the liver to portacaval shunt, SURGERY **68:** 341, 1973.
42. Spilg, H., Hickman, R., and Terblanche, J.: Unpublished observations, 1974.
43. Silen, W., Maudsley, D. L., Weinrich, W. L., and Harpur, H. A.: Studies of hepatic function in dogs with Eck fistula or portacaval transposition, Arch. Surg. **74:** 964, 1957.
44. Stabenau, J. C., Warren, K. S., and Rall, D. P.: The role of pH gradient in the distribution of ammonia between blood and CSF, brain, and muscle, J. Clin. Invest. **38:** 373, 1959.
45. Starzl, T. E., Chase, H. P., Putnam, C. W., and Porter, K. A.: Portacaval shunt for the treatment of hyperlipoproteinaemia, Lancet **940:** 944, 1973.
46. Starzl, T. E., Francavilla, A., Halgrimson, C. G., Francavilla, F. R., Porter, K. A., and Brown, T. H.: The origin, hormonal nature, and action of hepatotrophic substances in portal venous blood, Surg. Gynecol. Obstet. **137:** 179, 1973.
47. Starzl, T. E., Putnam, C. W., Porter, K. A., Halgrimson, C. G., Corman, J., Brown, B. I., Gatlin, R. W., Rodgerson, D. O., and Green, H. L.: Portal diversion for the treatment of glycogen storage disease in humans, Ann. Surg. **178:** 525, 1973.
48. Van Leenhoff, J. W., Hickman, R., Saunders, S. J., and Terblanche, J.: Massive liver cell necrosis in the pig induced with carbon tetrachloride, S. Afr. J. Lab. Clin. Med. **48:** 1201, 1974.
49. Vasanelli, P., and Chie Sara, E.: Microsomal drug metabolising enzymes—activity and induction in the rat liver after portacaval shunt, Arch. Int. Pharmacodyn. Ther. 158, 196, 1972. (Suppl.)
50. Vergara, F., Plum, F., and Duffy, T. E.: α-Ketoglutaramate: Increased concentrations in the CSF of patients in hepatic coma, Science **183:** 81, 1974.
51. Voorhees, A. B., Price, J. B., and Britton, R. C.: Portacaval shunt procedures for portal hypertension, Arch. Surg. **119:** 501, 1970.
52. Walker, C. O., and Schenker, S.: Pathogenesis of hepatic encephalopathy with special reference to the role of ammonia, Am. J. Clin. Nutr. **23:** 619, 1970.
53. Walser, M., and Bodenlos, T.: Urea metabolism in man, J. Clin. Invest. **38:** 1617, 1959.
54. Whitehead, T. B., and Whitaker, S. R. F.: A method for the determination of glutamine in CSF and the results in hepatic coma, J. Clin. Pathol. **8:** 81, 1955.
55. Wilson, G. D. A., Harvey, D. G., and Snook, C. R.: A review of factors affecting blood biochemistry in the pig, Br. Vet. J. **128:** 596, 1972.
56. Winter, I. C., Van Dolah, H. E., and Crandell, L. A.: Lowered serum lipid levels in the Eck fistula dog, Am. J. Physiol. **133:** 566, 1941.
57. Zieve, L., Doizaki, W. M., and Zieve, F. J.: Synergism between mercaptans and ammonia or fatty acids in the production of coma: A possible role for mercaptans in the pathogenesis of hepatic coma, J. Lab. Clin. Med. **83:** 16, 1973.

Removal of 5-hydroxytryptamine and norepinephrine from the pulmonary vascular space of man: Influence of cardiopulmonary bypass and pulmonary arterial pressure on these processes

C. N. Gillis, Ph.D., L. H. Cronau, M.D., Ph.D., N. M. Greene, M.D., *and*
G. L. Hammond, M.D., *New Haven, Conn.*

Pulmonary extraction of ^{14}C-5-hydroxytryptamine and ^{3}H-norepinephrine was measured in 23 anesthetized patients prior to and following cardiopulmonary bypass for aortocoronary saphenous vein grafts and/or valve replacement. Prior to cardiopulmonary bypass, lungs of patients with evidence of pulmonary hypertension, secondary to valvular disease, removed significantly ($P < 0.025$) more 5-hydroxytryptamine (5-HT) and norepinephrine (NE) from the pulmonary blood (78 ± 6 and 59 ± 11 percent, respectively) than did patients with normal pulmonary artery pressures (55 ± 6 and 22 ± 7 percent, respectively). In patients with preoperative pulmonary hypertension, percent extraction of 5-HT and norepinephrine following cardiopulmonary bypass was significantly ($P < 0.02$) lower (67 ± 6 and 38 ± 8 percent, respectively) than corresponding values for extraction of each substance before bypass. In contrast, pulmonary extraction of 5-HT and NE (76 ± 4 and 49 ± 10 percent, respectively) increased significantly ($P < 0.02$) in patients whose preoperative pulmonary artery pressures were within normal limits. There was no statistically significant difference between postbypass pulmonary extraction of either NE or 5-HT when values for patients with or without pulmonary hypertension were compared. It is apparent, therefore, that pulmonary hypertension is associated with increased biogenic amine extraction by lung; return of pulmonary arterial pressure toward normal tends to reverse this abnormality in amine removal by the lungs.

From the Departments of Anesthesiology, Pharmacology, and Surgery, Yale University School of Medicine, New Haven, Conn.

THE LUNG is a potentially important site for metabolism of certain vasoactive hormones.[7, 17] It is recognized that lungs of several species, including those of dog,[18, 20] cat,[6] rat,[1, 11] guinea pig,[10] and rabbit[12] remove both 5-HT and NE from blood in the pulmonary vascular space. Removal occurs in vivo as well as in isolated lungs perfused with either blood[6] or physiological medium.[1, 10-12] Recently we studied extraction of 5-HT and NE by lungs of seven anesthetized patients undergoing cardiopulmonary bypass for coronary revascularization by aortocoronary saphenous vein bypass grafting.[8] None had overt pulmonary disease or elevated left ventricular end-diastolic pressure (LVEDP). Prior to institution of cardiopulmonary bypass, 65 ± 4 percent (S.E.) of ^{14}C-5-HT and 23 ± 5 percent of ^{3}H-NE in blood sampled at the pulmonary artery, after rapid in-

Accepted for publication June 27, 1974.

This work was supported in part by United States Public Health Service Grant HL 13315 and Grants 473 and 435 from the Connecticut Heart Association.

Reprint requests: G. L. Hammond, M. D., Department of Surgery, Yale University School of Medicine, 333 Cedar St., New Haven, Conn. 06510.

Table I. *Pulmonary removal of NE and 5-HT before and after cardiopulmonary bypass*

No.*	Patient	Pulmonary arterial pressure	% extraction: ^{3}H-NE Prebypass	% extraction: ^{3}H-NE Postbypass	% extraction: 5-HT Prebypass	% extraction: 5-HT Postbypass
Patients with coronary artery disease:						
3	E. R.	28/10	38.8	82.1	68.8	89.0
4	A. P.	18/10	8.6	19.6	49.6	73.1
6	R. H.	22/9	24.4	76.5	47.5	87.2
7	J. P.	(10)‡	14.1	92.6	45.1	90.1
11	M. A.	(8)‡	16.1	19.0	73.3	73.0
12	H. H.	24/12	2.2	21.5	57.6	77.6
13§	M. L.	34/15	17.8	8.9	58.2	70.4
14	H. W.	(18)‡	23.7	11.1	78.0	64.9
15	D. F.	20/9	2.5	(−5.8)	50.1	59.7
28	J. G.	65/40	60.0	35.3	75.2	54.9
29	E. G.	(19)‡	1.3	29.3	13.5	47.1
31	J. M.	18/5	23.3	77.7	51.4	86.9
33	W. M.	26/8	29.7	95.4	30.7	93.3
		Mean	20.2	43.8	53.8	74.4
		±S.E.	±4.6	±9.8	±5.1	±4.1
Patients with valvular disease:						
18	J. M.	34/15	26.3	13.0	51.4	39.6
19	J. B.	36/16	94.9	64.9	95.7	81.3
21	W. H.	70/45	53.6	31.0	75.6	49.0
22§	J. G.	40/26	68.1	73.7	93.4	92.2
26§	L. C.	25/8	93.8	72.3	94.3	72.2
27§	C. T.	88/37	94.4	67.8	99.1	92.8
30	J. Y.	(20)†	6.4	33.2	58.4	76.2
32	J. T.	110/40	80.9	48.6	77.9	70.9
34§	H. R.	60/30	5.8	8.2	54.2	42.2
35	W. B.	120/50	92.6	30.6	97.6	71.6
		Mean	61.7	44.3	79.8	68.9
		±S.E.	±11.6	±7.8	±6.0	±6.0

*In some cases the study could not be completed, either for technical reasons or because the patient's condition did not permit it; thus numbering of cases is not consecutive.
†Only mean value of pulmonary artery pressure available.
‡Only LVEDP available.
§Female patients.

travenous injection of the amine into the median antecubital vein, was removed by the lungs of these patients. Immediately after cardiopulmonary bypass, percent removal of ^{14}C-5-HT and ^{3}H-NE was 81 ± 3 and 50 ± 12 percent, respectively. These data therefore demonstrated that both amines are removed from the pulmonary circulation of man and also suggested that cardiopulmonary bypass alters the process.

Both NE and 5-HT are potent vasoactive substances and therefore may alter vascular diameter and thus blood perfusion patterns within the lung. Accordingly, it is appropriate to question whether uptake of these amines by lungs of patients with evidence of pulmonary vascular change differs from that in normal lungs. We therefore studied removal of NE and 5-HT by lungs of patients with established cardiac valvular disease associated with pulmonary hypertension.

METHODS

Techniques used for isotope preparation and administration, as well as for anesthetic management of patients, were similar to those previously described in detail.[8] Two groups of patients, from whom informed consent had been obtained, were studied (Table I). Ten patients had mitral or aortic

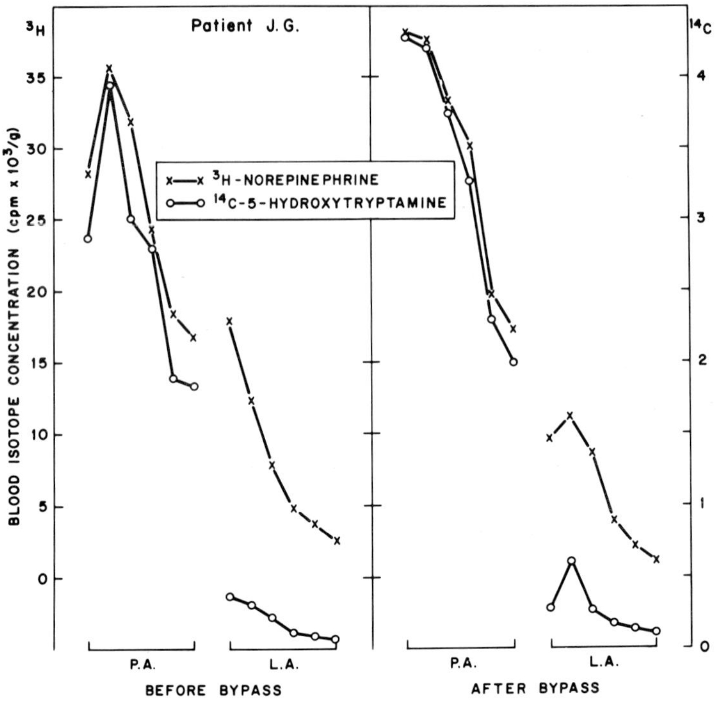

Fig. 1. Isotope concentrations in blood withdrawn continuously for approximately 30 seconds from the pulmonary artery *(P.A.)* and the left atrium *(L.A.)* both before and after cardiopulmonary bypass in a representative patient with pulmonary hypertension (mean P.A. pressure = 31 mm. Hg). At the start of injection of a mixture of ^{3}H-NE and ^{14}C-5-HT, withdrawal of blood was begun. In each isotope concentration profile illustrated, the first point on the left represents isotope concentration in the first blood fraction withdrawn; the last point on the right reflects isotope concentration in the sixth and last sample withdrawn.

valvular disease and most had pulmonary hypertension demonstrated during right heart catheterization. The second group of six patients (Nos. 14, 15, 28, 31, and 33 in Table I) were undergoing aortocoronary saphenous vein bypass grafting; data from these studies were added to those previously obtained in patients undergoing similar operations.[8]

All patients were anesthetized with oxygen–nitrous oxide and morphine sulfate and, in addition, received curare as an adjunct. Total doses of morphine administered during operation varied from 2 to 3 mg. per kilogram. Cardiopulmonary bypass was achieved by means of a Bentley bubble oxygenator aerated with 100 percent oxygen. Intraoperative measurements of pulmonary artery pressure were recorded by means of a Statham pressure transducer and appropriate polygraph.

Approximately 5 minutes after heparinization of the patient prior to cardiopulmonary bypass, and again about 10 minutes after bypass, 9 to 10 ml. of a solution of ^{14}C-5-HT and ^{3}H-NE was injected into a peripheral, intravenous, indwelling catheter, which was then flushed with whole blood under pressure. At the beginning of this injection, which took approximately 3 seconds, withdrawal of two 6 ml. samples of blood—one from the pulmonary artery, the other from the left atrium—was begun. Withdrawal of blood samples into plastic tubes attached to a Harvard withdrawal pump was continued at a constant rate until blood just filled the tubing (which took between 28 and 31 seconds). Tubes were then clamped at both ends and were rapidly transported to the laboratory where, approximately 20 minutes after withdrawal, blood was flushed out of each tube with 15 ml. of 0.6N perchloric acid and precipitated protein was sedimented by centrifugation at 10,000 g for 15 minutes. Total radioactivity (^3H and ^{14}C) in the resulting supernatant fluid was determined in a Packard model 3320 liquid scintillation spectrometer. In four experiments, each tube was segmented between clamps to give six fractions after which ^3H and ^{14}C in each were determined as described previously.[8] When tubes were fractioned in this manner, isotope in each fraction (i.e., counts per minute per Gm. of blood) was plotted sequentially to yield a "profile" of ^3H and ^{14}C concentration in blood during the period of withdrawal (Fig. 1). In these four cases total isotope collected at both sampling sites was calculated by adding the total amount of each isotope in the six segments obtained from the pulmonary artery and left atrium, respectively.[8] The difference between total isotope entering and leaving the lung during the 30 second sampling period provided a direct measure of pulmonary extraction of each amine. Percent amine extraction was calculated according to the formula,

$$\{1 - (I_{LA}/I_{PA})\} \times 100,$$

where I_{LA} and I_{PA} are total ^3H or ^{14}C in blood sampled at the left atrium and pulmonary artery, respectively.

In some experiments radioactivity associated with unchanged NE or 5-HT in blood samples was determined. For this purpose, blood from the plastic tubes was flushed in the operating room, by rapid passage of 15 ml. of chilled 0.6N perchloric acid through the tubes, as soon as possible after sampling blood from the pulmonary artery and left atrium of the patient. The resulting mixture of blood and perchloric acid was shaken thoroughly and kept chilled. After centrifugation, as before, the ^{14}C or ^3H associated with unchanged 5-HT or NE, respectively, was determined in samples of the supernatant fluid after passage over Biorex cation-exchange resin columns, which permit separation of each amine from its respective acid metabolites.[16]

Isotopes were prepared for injection and sterilized by Millipore (0.22 μ) filtration, as described previously.[8] Each injection contained 25 μc (6 to 8 μg NE base) of ^3H and 10 μc (7 to 9 μg 5-HT base) of ^{14}C in a lactate buffer/saline mixture, whose final pH was 4 to 5. ^3H-*dl*-norepinephrine (specific activity, 5 to 7 c. per millimole) or ^{14}C-5-hydroxytryptamine (as creatinine sulfate, specific activity, 55 or 57 mc. per millimole) were obtained from the New England Nuclear Corporation and the Amersham Searle Corporation, respectively. The significance of data was evaluated by the t test for paired data where appropriate, or by Student's t test.[2]

RESULTS

After Biorex column chromatography of suitably prepared (see Methods) blood samples from the pulmonary artery or left atrium, it was found that over 90 percent of the total ^3H or ^{14}C in these samples was associated with unchanged NE or 5-HT, respectively. The same results were obtained whether blood was taken from patients with normal or elevated pulmonary arterial pressure.

Examination of a representative isotope profile (i.e., concentrations of ^3H or ^{14}C in sequential fractions of segmented blood samples—see Methods) in a patient with pulmonary hypertension (Fig. 1) revealed that, as reported previously,[8] pulmonary arterial isotope, both before and after bypass, declined rapidly to background levels well within the 30 second withdrawal period used. Left atrial isotope concentrations before bypass declined also, although usually somewhat more slowly. There was no evidence of recirculation of isotope. Isotope profiles in patients with pulmonary hypertension were, therefore, essentially the same as those described previously for patients who had no demonstrated pulmonary hypertension.[8] This fact, coupled with the evidence that over 90 percent of the isotope in blood was associated with unchanged amine, supports our previous contention that the technique used gives a valid measure of amine extraction by lung.[8]

Table II. *Intraoperative pulmonary artery pressure and pulmonary extraction of ^{3}H-NE and ^{14}C-5-HT*

		Pulmonary arterial pressure*		% extraction			
				NE		5-HT	
No.	Patient	Prebypass	Postbypass	Prebypass	Postbypass	Prebypass	Postbypass
30	J. Y.	37/13	38/25	6.4	33.2	58.4	76.2
31	J. M.	26/11	23/7	23.3	77.7	51.4	86.9
32	J. T.	75/35	55/30	80.9	48.6	77.9	70.9
34	H. R.	55/25	45/15	5.8	8.2	54.2	42.2
35	W. B.	70/55	35/15	92.6	30.6	97.6	71.6

*Intraoperative measurements.

Table III. *Percent extraction of NE and 5-HT by lungs of patients with normal and elevated pulmonary artery (P.A.) pressures*

	^{3}H-NE			^{14}C-5-HT		
	Prebypass	Postbypass	P*	Prebypass	Postbypass	P*
Normal P.A. pressures (n = 13)	21.9 ± 6.8	48.5 ± 9.6	< 0.02	55.3 ± 5.8	76.2 ± 3.7	< 0.01
	P < 0.025†			P < 0.025†		
High P.A. pressures (n = 10)	59.4 ± 10.5	38.2 ± 7.8	< 0.01	77.9 ± 5.8	66.6 ± 6.1	< 0.02

*Pair t test: Significance of mean difference between pre- and postbypass amine extraction was calculated.

†Student's t test: Significance of differences between mean prebypass amine extraction by lungs of patients with normal or high P.A. pressures was calculated.

Table I shows percent extraction of both ^{3}H-NE and ^{14}C-5-HT in 23 patients; data from seven studies (patients 3, 4, 6, 7, 11, 12, and 13) were reported in our earlier study.[8] Patients were divided initially on the basis of pathology present, primarily coronary artery disease or valvular disease, with or without the simultaneous presence of coronary artery disease requiring one or more bypass grafts. Pulmonary artery pressures are listed for all subjects except for four of the coronary artery bypass graft patients (Nos. 7, 11, 14, and 29) for whom only LVEDP's were available. In one patient with valvular disease (No. 30) only mean pulmonary artery pressure was reported as part of the catheterization report. Initial examination of data for mean percent extraction of ^{3}H-NE and ^{14}C-5-HT (Table I) suggests that division of patients on the basis of pathology is appropriate since they seem to be representative of different experimental populations. Thus mean initial extraction values for both NE and 5-HT were higher in patients with valvular disease than in those with coronary arterial disease; also extraction of these amines by lungs of the former patients decreased after cardiopulmonary bypass while that of the coronary graft patients increased. The latter observation extends those described in our earlier report.[8]

However, closer inspection reveals certain inconsistencies in this classification. In one of the valve patients (No. 34) who had marked pulmonary hypertension, extraction of NE was low initially and essentially unchanged after bypass. It is also of considerable interest that in two patients with valvular disease (Nos. 22 and 30), who had mild elevations of pulmonary artery pressure, there was an increased NE extraction after bypass; the qualitative nature of this change is identical with that seen in coronary artery graft patients. In contrast, two of the patients with coronary artery disease (Nos. 13 and 28) showed decreased percent extraction of NE after cardiopulmonary bypass; this was associated with mild-to-moderately severe pulmonary hypertension. Thus it appears the presence or absence of pulmonary hypertension, rather than the presenting pathology, should form the basis for patient classification, at least with respect to pulmonary extraction of NE or 5-HT. The presence of pulmonary hypertension generally is associated both with higher initial (i.e., prebypass) percent extraction of both NE and 5-HT, as compared to patients with normal pulmonary artery pressures, and also with decreased amine extraction after cardiopulmonary bypass. In contrast, those patients with normal or near-normal pulmonary artery pressures show the opposite qualitative change in amine removal from the pulmonary vascular space following cardiopulmonary bypass.

In the majority of patients with pulmonary artery hypertension, correction of the hemodynamic defect was provided by surgery. Therefore, it might be proposed that the magnitude of initial (prebypass) amine extraction is related to the presence or absence of pulmonary hypertension while the qualitative change in extraction after bypass is related to the change in pulmonary artery pressure, brought about by the corrective surgery. Five patients in whom pulmonary artery pressures were measured intraoperatively provided an opportunity to test this hypothesis (Table II). In patient W. B. (No. 35) in whom a pronounced decrease in pulmonary arterial pressure occurred after valvular surgery, prebypass extraction of both amines was high and fell after bypass; to a lesser degree the same correlation was noted in patient J. T. (No. 32). In contrast, patient H. R. (No. 34), who had a smaller decline in pulmonary artery pressure after surgery, showed little change in amine extraction after cardiopulmonary bypass. Two other patients (Nos. 30 and 31, Table II) had no change in pulmonary artery pressure after surgery and showed an increase in percent extraction of both ^{3}H-NE and ^{14}C-5-HT after bypass.

Table III presents data for mean ^{3}H-NE and ^{14}C-5-HT extraction calculated from the individual values given in Table I. For these calculations patients were classified on the basis of the presence or absence of pulmonary hypertension, regardless of cardiac pathology. For the purpose of this classification, pulmonary hypertension was defined as present if *mean* pulmonary artery pressure was 22 mm. Hg or above. It can be seen (Table III) that patients with elevated pulmonary artery pressures had significantly elevated extraction of ^{14}C-5-HT ($P < 0.025$) and ^{3}H-NE ($P < 0.025$) as compared to those with normal pressures. Table III also shows that in both groups of patients extraction of amines immediately after cardiopulmonary bypass is not significantly different.

DISCUSSION

When precautions are taken to limit degradation of radioactive amines in blood (see Methods), Biorex column chromatography indicates that at least 90 percent of ^{3}H or ^{14}C in blood sampled at the pulmonary artery and left atrium after injection of ^{3}H-NE and ^{14}C-5-HT is associated with unchanged amine. Furthermore, this is true whether patients have normal or elevated pulmonary arterial pressure. Accordingly, measurement of total isotope in blood is an accurate reflection of unchanged amine. In our previous study, in which about 20 minutes elapsed between withdrawal and its deproteinization by perchloric acid, unchanged NE constituted only 24 to 29 percent of total ^{3}H, while the corresponding figure for unchanged 5-HT was 51 to 64 percent.[8] Thus it is apparent that rapid deproteinization of blood in the present study (carried out in the operating room immediately after withdrawal of blood) effectively limits metabolic or spontaneous degradation of these amines in blood. There is no difference in the percent of total radioactivity associated with metabolite (approximately 10 percent) in either left atrial or pulmonary arterial blood. Accordingly, these data confirm our previous suggestion that any metabolites of ^{3}H-NE or ^{14}C-5-HT formed in the lung are not released into the venous blood within the 30 second period between injection of the amines and withdrawal of blood, as prescribed in our technique.[8]

Patients undergoing aortocoronary saphenous vein bypass graft, for whom data were not previously presented (Nos. 14, 15, 28, 29, 31, and 33, Table I) were similar to the first such group studied.[8] Accordingly it seems justified to combine our information on all patients studied who were undergoing coronary bypass surgery. Data presented in this paper concerning 13 such patients confirm and expand those reported in our earlier study.[8] That is, prior to cardiopulmonary bypass, the lungs extract both NE and 5-HT from the blood during one circulation. The lung consistently removes 5-HT from the pulmonary circulation more effectively than it does NE; similar observations have been reported in rabbit[12] and dog[9, 20] lung. Furthermore, in patients in whom catheterization data indicated the presence of a normal or near normal pulmonary vascular pressure, removal of amine was enhanced following cardiopulmonary bypass. However, in patients with definite elevation of pulmonary artery pressure, secondary to cardiac valvular disease, extraction of both amines fell after cardiopulmonary bypass to levels that might be predicted had pulmonary hypertension not been present (Table I). Thus in terms of postcardiopulminary bypass amine extraction by lung, the two groups of patients were statistically indistinguishable. Previously we found no correlation between the change in amine extraction and the decrease in right ventricular outflow after bypass.[8] Similarly, there was no correlation between these variables in patients either with or without pulmonary hypertension in the present study. Accordingly, it is unlikely that altered cardiac output is related in any obvious manner to the quantitative change in amine extraction that follows a period of cardiopulmonary bypass.

Factors that might be linked to increased removal of amine by lungs of patients with pulmonary hypertension include (1) presence of a larger volume of pulmonary extravascular fluid (PEF) into which amine can pass; (2) availability of increased surface area within the pulmonary microvascular bed across which amines can be transported from the blood; (3) stimulation of the process responsible for NE and 5-HT removal by lung; and (4) the presence of a circulating hormone, present in unusually high concentrations in patients with pulmonary hypertension, which is capable of accelerating the "normal" rate of amine extraction by lung vasculature. The fact that angiotensin enhances NE uptake by perfused guinea pig lung suggests that a similar action could occur in man.[5] We are unaware of evidence that would allow definitive rejection of this possibility. However, it seems unlikely that such a hormonally induced effect could be reversed as rapidly as is apparent for the amine uptake process when the valvular defect causing pulmonary hypertension is corrected surgically (Table II). With regard to the first possibility mentioned above, data published by Luepker and associates[14] show that in nine of 11 patients with mean pulmonary arterial pressures above 22 mm. Hg, PEF volumes were increased above control values. If increased amine extraction by lungs of patients with pulmonary hypertension were due only to an increased volume of extravascular fluid accessible to amines, this implies that amine diffuses passively across vascular capillaries. Such a possibility is at variance with data from studies with a variety of experimental animals which suggest an energy-dependent and drug-sensitive process of amine removal, probably located at the capillary endothelial membrane.[1, 10-12, 19] The latter observations admittedly, however, do not rule out passive diffusion as at least a partial explanation for the mechanism in man. Within the context of proposal (2), above, the observations of Maloney, Roohalamini, and Wexler[15] concerning pressure diameter relationships of small vessels in isolated dog lung are relevant. These authors reported that the percent change in diameter per unit of pressure increase (i.e., vascular distensibility) ranged from 3.8 percent per centimeter of water for the smallest arteries to 0.5 percent for the largest veins. If in human lung the change in distensibility were of the order of 2 percent per centimeter of water pressure at the site of the amine uptake, a change of 25 cm. of water in mean pulmonary artery pressure could be associated with as much as a 50 percent change in surface area that is available for uptake of amines.

Our studies offer no clear explanation of the quantitative changes in NE or 5-HT extraction after cardiopulmonary bypass. Release of certain kinins and other substances from the blood,[3] particularly during cardiopulmonary bypass, may increase capillary permeability and thus enhance a normally small amount of passive amine movement out of the vascular space. Yet such a proposal is at variance with our previous study[8] which showed that pulmonary "extraction" of ^{3}H-water decreased after bypass, while percent removal of ^{14}C-5-HT administered simultaneously was increased. We recently observed a similar decrease in percent removal of ^{3}H-water after bypass in three patients with pulmonary hypertension (unpublished studies). Increased 5-HT extraction by lung, therefore, seems to be not simply a reflection of its passive diffusion into a larger extravascular water volume.

Reduced amine extraction by lung after correction of cardiac valvular defects may reflect a decreased "functional" surface area for amine uptake. This could occur as a result of surgical removal of a marked outflow resistance in the left heart. Data in Table II offer evidence suggestive of a direct correlation between acute decrease in pulmonary arterial pressure following valvular surgery and restoration (i.e., decline) in amine extraction toward "normal" post-bypass levels (patients 32 and 35, Table II). However, this conclusion must be tempered by the consideration that long-standing pulmonary hypertension may be associated with medial hypertrophy of small arteries and arterioles, with consequent reduction of vascular diameter and, therefore, a decreased effective capillary perfusion. The fact that two patients (Nos. 32 and 35, Table II) showed a rapid reduction in their intraoperative pulmonary artery pressure may argue against the presence of a permanent change in vascular structure in these patients, but others (e.g., Nos. 30 and 34, Table II) show evidence of some change which maintained the pulmonary hypertension immediately after bypass.

This study has extended our earlier observations, concerning removal of NE and 5-HT by human lung, by indicating that the magnitude of amine extraction generally is increased by the presence of pulmonary hypertension.[8] Although we cannot, at this point, offer more than highly speculative proposals to explain these data, their demonstration in man merits further study of the phenomenon, particularly in view of the potential for drug, as well as disease-induced changes in pulmonary biogenic amine extraction.[7]

REFERENCES

1. Alabaster, V. A., and Bakhle, Y. S.: Removal of 5-hydroxytryptamine in the pulmonary circulation of rat isolated lungs, Br. J. Pharmacol. **40:** 468, 1970.
2. Bernstein, L., and Weatherall, M.: Statistics for medical and other biological students, London, 1952, E. S. Livingstone, Ltd., p. 81.
3. Crosby, W. A., Snowden, S., and Parsons, V.: Changes in lung capillary permeability in renal failure, Br. Med. J. **4:** 388, 1972.
4. Davies, R. B., and Wang, Y.: Rapid pulmonary removal of 5-hydroxytryptamine in the intact dog, Proc. Soc. Exp. Biol. Med. **118:** 799, 1965.
5. Davilla, D., and Khairallah, P.A.: Effect of ions on inhibition of norepinephrine uptake by angiotensin, Arch. Int. Pharmacodyn. Ther. **185:** 357, 1970.
6. Gaddum, J. H., Hebb, C. O., Silver, A., and Swan, A. A. B.: 5-Hydroxytryptamine: Pharmacological action and destruction in perfused lungs, Q. J. Exp. Physiol. **38:** 255, 1952.
7. Gillis, C. N.: Metabolism of vasoactive hormones by lung, Anesthesiology **39:** 626, 1973.
8. Gillis, C. N., Greene, N. M., Cronau, L. H., and Hammond, G. L.: Pulmonary extraction of 5-hydroxytryptamine and norepinephrine before and after cardiopulmonary bypass in man, Circ. Res. **30:** 666, 1972.
9. Ginn, R., and Vane, J. R.: Disappearance of catecholamines from the circulation, Nature (Lond.) **219:** 740, 1968.
10. Gruby, L. A., Rowlands, C., Varley, B. Q., and Wyllie, J. H.: Fate of 5-hydroxytryptamine in the lungs, Br. J. Surg. **58:** 525, 1971.
11. Hughes, J. C., Gillis, C. N., and Bloom, F. E.: Uptake and disposition of norepinephrine in perfused rat lung, J. Pharmacol. Exp. Ther. **169:** 237, 1969.
12. Iwasawa, Y., Gillis, C. N., and Aghajanian, G.: Hypothermic inhibition of five-hydroxytryptamine and norepinephrine uptake by

lung: Cellular location of amines after uptake, J. Pharmacol. Exp. Ther. **186:** 498, 1973.
13. Lammerant, J., and de Herdt, P.: Catecholamine plasma levels in the pulmonary artery, the pulmonary vein, and the arterial tree of open-chest dogs during ambient air breathing and during acute anoxia, Arch. Int. Physiol. Biochim. **73:** 81, 1965.
14. Luepker, R., Liander, B., Korsgren, M., and Varnauskas, E.: Pulmonary intravascular and extravascular fluid volumes in exercising cardiac patients, Circulation **44:** 626, 1971.
15. Maloney, J. E., Roohalamini, S. A., and Wexler, L.: Pressure-diameter relations of small blood vessels in isolated dog lung, Microvasc. Res. **2:** 1, 1970.
16. Minard, F. N., and Grant, D. S.: A convenient method for chromatographic analysis of norepinephrine, dopamine, and serotonin, Biochem. Med. **6:** 46, 1972.
17. Said, S. I.: The lung as a metabolic organ, N. Engl. J. Med. **279:** 1330, 1968.
18. Starling, E. H., and Vereney, E. B.: Secretion of urine as studied on the isolated kidney, Proc. R. Soc. Lond. [Biol.] **97:** 321, 1925.
19. Strum, J. M., and Junod, A. F.: Radioautographic demonstration of 5-hydroxytryptamine-^{3}H uptake by pulmonary endothelial cells, J. Cell Biol. **54:** 456, 1972.
20. Thomas, D. P., and Vane, J. R.: 5-Hydroxytryptamine in the circulation of the dog, Nature (Lond.) **216:** 335, 1967.

Another look at rejection in pig liver homografts

C. Battersby, M.S., F.R.C.S., W. S. Egerton, M.S., F.R.A.C.S., Glenda Balderson, B.Sc., J. F. Kerr, Ph.D., F.R.C.P.A., *and* W. Burnett, Ch.M., F.R.C.S., *Brisbane, Australia*

Orthotopic liver homografting in 59 pigs was successful in producing survival beyond the immediate operative period in 29 animals. Survivors without immunosuppression were subjected to serial biopsy from 3 days to more than one year after transplantation. A composite picture of progressive histological changes in the group as well as in individuals has been built up. About 3 days after transplantation, there appeared in homografts (but not in autografts) progressive infiltration of the portal tracts by round cells, which was well established by the second postoperative week, and which was accompanied in severely affected animals by round-cell infiltration of the parenchyma, extensive death of hepatocytes by apoptosis, and canalicular bile stasis. The heavy round-cell infiltration coincided with the appearance of jaundice in about half the animals, and subsided spontaneously with the jaundice. By 4 weeks the lymphocytic infiltration was much less marked, but there developed a progressive fibrosis with disruption of the lobules and the appearance of regenerative nodules. This appeared to vary in speed of development and severity from animal to animal, but was present in most long-term survivors, despite apparent clinical and biochemical evidence of well being. Two long-term survivors died with biochemical and pathological evidence of progressive hepatocellular insufficiency. While acute rejection rarely causes death in this species, changes suggestive of chronic rejection occur in most animals and may cause death from liver failure.

From the Departments of Surgery and Pathology, University of Queensland, Brisbane, Australia

THE PIG has been widely used as an experimental animal in the study of orthotopic liver transplantation, and there appears little doubt that rejection of liver grafts in this animal is remarkably mild.[2, 3, 8, 12-14, 18, 20] However, experience from various laboratories has not been consistent, and it is not clear, for example, how commonly death occurs from acute rejection within the first 14 days after operation. The severity of progressive liver damage in long-term survivors has also not been studied systematically. Calne and associates[3] reported 36 pig liver transplants from which 20 animals survived beyond 3 days. Nine of these died between 7 and 81 days, and a variable degree of cholangitis was found in seven. No biopsies were reported, but tissues obtained at autopsy showed slight round-cell infiltration of portal tracts and interlobular septa, with an increase in fibrous tissue in the livers of only some long-term survivors. Terblanche and associates[20] also found it difficult to ascribe early death to any one factor. Only two of 25 animals surviving the operation died at the expected time of rejection (at 8 and 10 days, respectively). Dent and associates[7] reported death in three of 20 animals at 7 to

Accepted for publication June 27, 1974.

Reprint requests: C. Battersby, M.S., F.R.C.S., Department of Surgery, Clinical Sciences Building, Royal Brisbane Hospital, Brisbane, Queensland 4029 Australia.

Table I. *Survival times, maximum plasma bilirubin levels at the end of the first week, and blood compatibility data in three groups of liver transplants in pigs*

	*Group I**	*Group II†*	*Group III‡*
No.	16	25	18
Survivors beyond 24 hr.	7	13	9
Max. early bilirubin (mg./100 ml.) (mean ± S.D.)	Full data not available	3.6 ± 3.2	3.4 ± 2.61§
Average survival time (days) (mean ± S.D.) (eliminating deaths from misadventure)	112 ± 84	67 ± 71	62 ± 80§
Blood compatibility (donor cells to recipient serum)	Not available	All compatible	13/18

*Transplants within a colony of Large White Landrace cross breeds (not litter mates).
†Landrace to Large White Landrace cross breeds (unrelated colonies).
‡Berkshire to Large White Landrace.
§Not significant.

Table II. *Causes and times of death in pigs dying after immediate operative period*

Cause of death	*No.*	*Survival**		
		< 14 days	*14 to 370 days*	*Still alive**
Intestinal obstruction	5	7 (5), 15 (10), 17 (3)	6 (172), 10 (270)	5 (737), 12 (561), 20 (415), 27 (201)
Gastric ulcer	3	21 (10)	8 (63), 25 (41)	
Pulmonary abscesses	2	—	2 (63), 14 (36)	
Experimental causes	5	22 (5), 23 (8), 24 (7), 28 (5)	19 (60)	
Bile peritonitis	3	3 (7), 18 (6), 29 (1)	—	
Cholangitis	2	—	9 (14), 26 (20)	
Bile duct stricture	1	—	1 (224)	
Rejection	2	—	4 (370), 13 (55)	
Unknown cause	2	11 (7), 16 (10)	—	

*Experimental number is followed by survival time in days within parentheses. Pigs 1 to 7 belong to Group I, pigs 8 to 20 to Group II, and pigs 21 to 29 to Group III in Table I.

10 days after operation, and two of these had evidence of cholangitis.

In Starzl's laboratory there appeared to be more evidence of rejection than had been apparent in other centers.[14, 15] Ten animals out of 18 were reported to have died with the typical histological picture of rejection between 8 and 37 days after transplant, but, in six of these, other possible causes of death, such as bleeding from peptic ulceration, cholangitis, and pulmonary complications, were also present. It may be significant, however, that the Denver experiments were carried out on outbred animals of different color and breed, which was not consistently so in the reports from other centers.

Long-term biopsy material has been obtained only sporadically and the livers have been described either as normal or as showing only slight fibrosis.[3, 14, 18]

The objectives of the present study were (1) to evaluate the histological evidence of rejection seen in all animals at the end of the first week, and to define how often death at this time is a result of rejection, and (2) to clarify the long-term structural changes in a group of animals. Therefore, pigs were subjected to serial liver biopsy from 3 days to more than one year after transplantation and a composite picture of progressive histological changes was constructed.

METHODS

The animals used weighed 15 to 20 kilograms. The first 15 transplants were between animals obtained from a disease-free colony of Large White Landrace crossbred pigs. However, it became apparent that severe rejection was unusual within this colony and the question of a close genetic relationship between donor and recipient animals was raised; donors were therefore obtained for the next 26 experiments from an unrelated colony of Landrace pigs. Finally, in the last

18 transplants, the donor animals were black (Berkshire) and the recipients white (Landrace).

The technique used followed closely that of earlier workers.[4, 5, 19] Anesthesia was induced by thiopentone (20 mg. per kilogram), and maintained by a mixture of nitrous oxide, oxygen, and halothane. Systemic arterial blood pressure and central venous pressure were monitored, and blood, glucose, saline, and sodium bicarbonate were infused into the jugular vein of the recipient as judged necessary by serial estimations of hemoglobin, plasma electrolytes, and acid-base status. The liver was excised from the donor after being cooled in situ with heparinized Hartmann's solution to which sodium bicarbonate had been added (to bring the pH to 7.4) as well as 10 ml. of 10 percent procaine hydrochloride per liter. The organ was then placed in iced saline slush. The donor animal was heparinized and bled out, and the blood was used for transfusion of the recipient if there had been no aggregation of donor red cells by the recipient serum. Portal venous decompression in the recipient, which had been undergoing simultaneous hepatectomy, was by portajugular shunt, eliminating the need for splenectomy.

A similar protocol was followed in four animals in which an autograft rather than a homograft was done. Liver biopsies were taken from these animals at intervals from 3 to 38 days after transplant.

RESULTS

There appeared to be no difference in the results in the three groups (Table I). About 50 percent of the animals survived the operative period, and of these 60 percent in all groups developed a transient jaundice at the end of the first week. Precise bilirubin levels at this time and direct cross-match compatibility data are not available for Group I, as the possible significance was not appreciated at this time. Over-all survival times were similar for the three groups. Histological evidence of rejection is difficult to assess quantitatively, but the degree of lymphocyte infiltration in the first 4 weeks appeared to be the same in all groups. It was, therefore, decided to report the 59 transplants together.

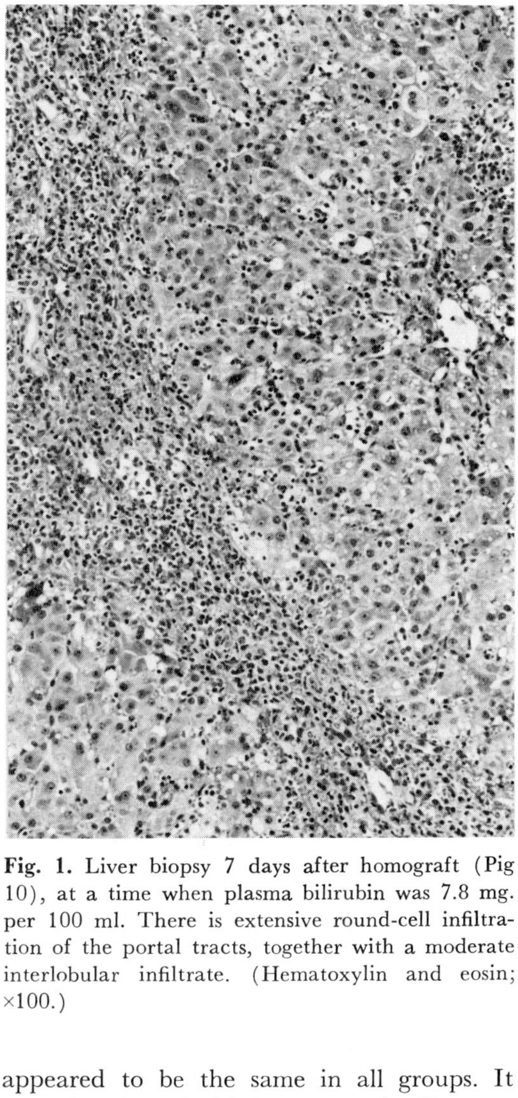

Fig. 1. Liver biopsy 7 days after homograft (Pig 10), at a time when plasma bilirubin was 7.8 mg. per 100 ml. There is extensive round-cell infiltration of the portal tracts, together with a moderate interlobular infiltrate. (Hematoxylin and eosin; ×100.)

When the operation had been technically satisfactory the pigs awoke rapidly and walked around the laboratory. Sometimes at this stage, however, animals developed an irreversible metabolic acidosis, which was eventually fatal. In those surviving more than a few hours, there was progressive coagulative necrosis in the liver, which was probably due to ischemia. The exact pathogenesis of this hepatic lesion is in doubt, and has been discussed in detail elsewhere.[1]

Twenty-nine animals survived the immediate postoperative period after homografting. The causes of death in 25 of them are

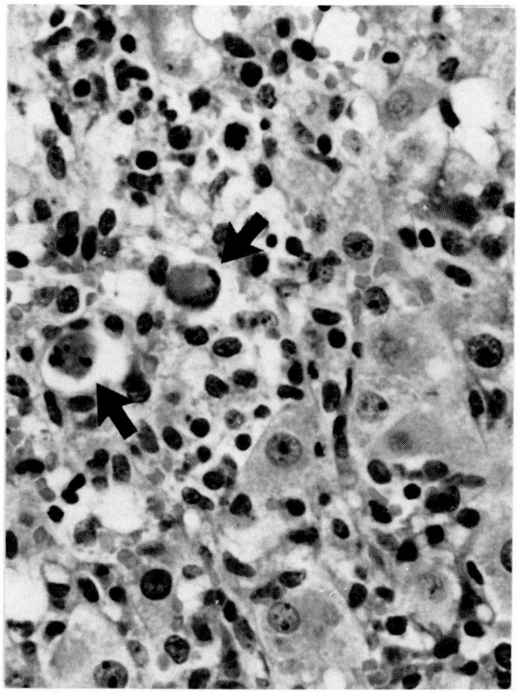

Fig. 2. Councilman bodies (arrowed) and round-cell infiltration of parenchyma in same biopsy as is illustrated in Fig. 1. (Hematoxylin and eosin; ×400.)

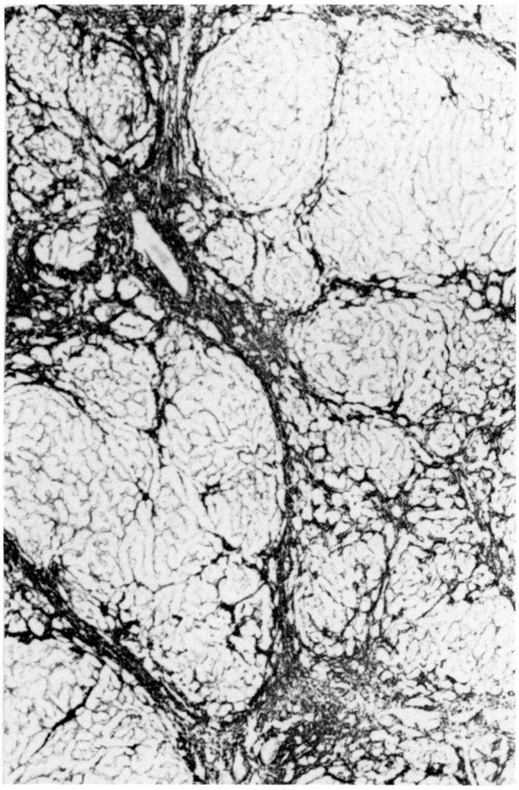

Fig. 3. Reticulin stain of liver biopsy 370 days after homograft (Pig 5) showing increase in connective tissue and loss of normal lobular architecture. (This animal is still alive and well 737 days after transplant.) (×40.)

given in Table II. In two animals it was difficult to be sure of the cause of death, and these will be discussed in detail later. After the first 14 days, rejection appeared the likely cause of death in only two animals, at 55 days and 370 days after transplant. Four animals are presently alive between 201 and 737 days postoperatively.

Serial biopsy supplemented by autopsy examination indicated that in all pigs there was a progressive round-cell infiltration of variable degree in the portal tracts beginning about 3 days after transplant, and being well established by 7 days. In the more severely affected animals, there was also a moderate degree of round-cell infiltration of the parenchyma (Fig. 1), and the presence of numerous Councilman bodies (Fig. 2) indicated extensive death of scattered single hepatocytes by shrinkage necrosis[10] or apoptosis.[11] This interpretation of the mode of cell death was confirmed by electron microscopy in five cases and will be illustrated in another paper. In such animals small arteries of the portal tracts sometimes showed endothelial swelling and round-cell infiltration of the intima.

Neither lymphoid infiltration of the portal tracts and parenchyma nor increased apoptosis were observed in the autograft material. While there was depletion of glycogen in the hepatocytes in the earlier biopsies, later biopsies in autografts were completely normal.

In 18 of the 29 animals these histological changes were accompanied by biochemical evidence of cholestasis, the plasma bilirubin sometimes reaching 8 mg. per 100 ml. Cholangiography on six animals while this jaundice was at its zenith failed to reveal extrahepatic obstruction in five cases and the jaundice faded rapidly.

In most homografts the round-cell infiltration seen at the end of the first week

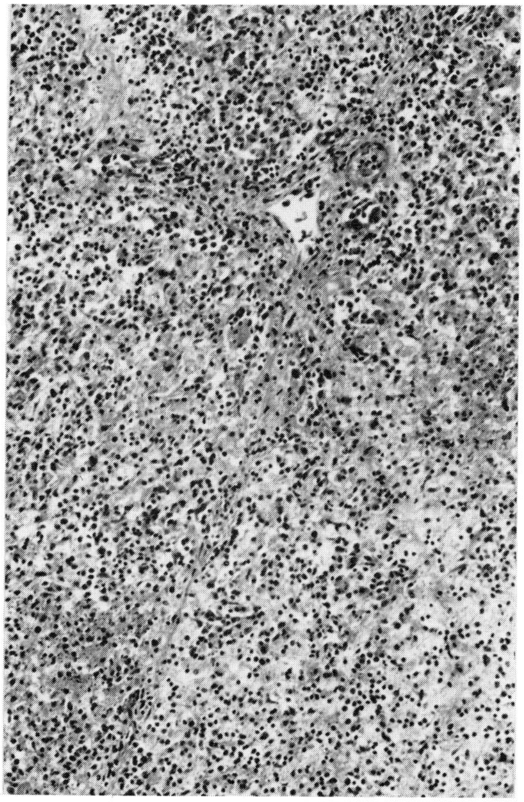

Fig. 4. Histological appearance at autopsy (Pig 11), 7 days after transplant when plasma bilirubin was 8.4 mg. per 100 ml. Parenchymal cells have completely disappeared, and there is massive round-cell infiltration throughout the lobules (compared with Fig. 1.). (Hematoxylin and eosin; ×100.)

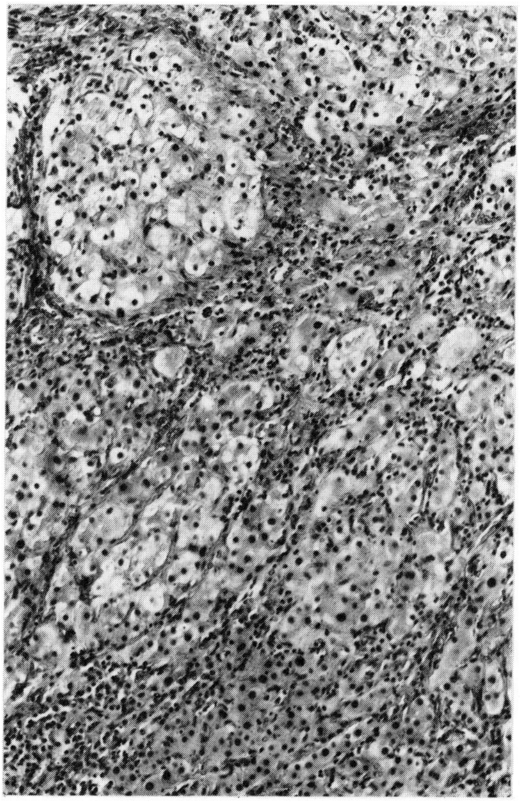

Fig. 5. Liver biopsy at 211 days after transplant (Pig 4). Note intense round-cell infiltration, dissection of parenchyma by fibrous septa, and nodules of hepatocytes. (Hematoxylin and eosin; ×100.)

slowly decreased and at 28 days was much less obvious. There was, however, in most of our long-term survivors, an increase in fibrous tissue which was best seen with a reticulin stain (Fig. 3). Despite apparent clinical and biochemical well being, the lobules were progressively broken up by fibrous tissues, and regenerative nodules appeared.

Detailed results of the leukocyte migration test[17] will be reported elsewhere, but inhibition of migration was inconstant, and did not correlate in time with maximal histological and biochemical evidence of rejection. There appeared to be no significant difference in results using this test between groups of pigs subjected to autograft, homograft, or bile duct ligation.

DISCUSSION

The difficulty of diagnosing liver rejection clinically or biochemically, or indeed, assessing its severity has been recognized previously.[7, 18] It is difficult to ascribe death in an animal to rejection on the basis of a histological appearance when biopsies from animals destined to survive for long periods show no less evidence of the rejection process. This is particularly so in death occurring in the first 4 weeks after transplantation, when a number of other factors such as gastric ulceration, cholangitis, biliary leak, and intra-abdominal sepsis take such a heavy toll of surviving animals. Often there are several factors occurring together to produce death —any one of which may do so on its own.

Two animals (Pigs 9 and 26) died 14 and

20 days postoperatively with raised plasma bilirubin and a high white cell count (WCC). Superficially rejection may have been blamed but both had a biliary collection in the subhepatic space, and one grew *E. coli* and *Klebsiella sp.* from the bile. Some minor histological features of rejection were seen in both, but there were many pus cells in the intrahepatic biliary radicles, and cholangitis seems a far more likely cause of death in these animals than does rejection.

Possible acute rejection. Two other animals died at 7 days (Pig 11) and 10 days (Pig 16), at a time when acute rejection might have been expected to be the cause.

A. Pig 11. This animal was jaundiced at death with a high WCC and mild elevations only of plasma alkaline phosphatase and aspartate amino transferase. At autopsy, there was no bile duct obstruction. Histological examination of the liver disclosed very heavy round-cell infiltration of both portal tracts and parenchyma, and massive loss of hepatocytes, most lobules being largely occupied by dilated sinusoids engorged with blood (Fig. 4). These appearances were not typical of those usually ascribed to rejection, but careful study failed to reveal any other cause of death, and similar, although rare, cases have previously been described.[6, 20]

B. Pig 16. This animal was not jaundiced. Enzyme levels were normal, but the WCC was markedly elevated. Histologically the hepatocytes appeared healthy and there was only a mild round-cell infiltration of the portal tracts. However, some of the radicles of the portal vein were acutely inflamed and there was an occasional microscopic abscess in the parenchyma. The cause of death may have been portal pyemia, although no obvious intra-abdominal sepsis was found at autopsy.

Thus of 59 animals, we have been able to find only two dying in the first 4 weeks after transplantation where there was no macroscopic cause of death, and one of these showed very mild changes of rejection only.

Chronic rejection. But what of chronic rejection? In longer surviving animals, we have found progressive hepatocellular loss and fibrosis, which has culminated in death consistent with that from hepatic insufficiency in two animals (Pigs 13 and 4) at 55 and 370 days, respectively, after transplantation.

A. Pig 13. This animal underwent cholangiography and biopsy at 41 days after transplant. There was no biliary obstruction. Histologically the liver showed extensive fibrosis with lobular dissection and isolation of small clumps of hepatocytes, continuing Councilman body formation, moderate round-cell infiltration of parenchyma, and a fairly severe canalicular bile stasis. These findings were confirmed at autopsy 14 days later.

B. Pig 4. This animal lived 370 days after transplant, but was noted to be losing weight and strength progressively in the last few months. There were mild jaundice, raised plasma enzyme levels, a very low plasma albumin, and a marked eosinophilia in the peripheral blood. Biopsies at 91, 211, and 333 days showed a progressive increase in fibrosis with lobular dissection, loss of hepatocytes, and persistent round-cell infiltration of both connective tissues and parenchyma (Fig. 5). At autopsy the liver showed fully developed cirrhosis. The bile duct was dilated below the anastomosis and contained an oval gallstone 1.5 cm. in length. There was no narrowing of the anastomosis and no dilatation above.

It is possible that this stone may have been responsible for some of the histological changes. Similar changes, however, were seen at one year in an animal (Pig 5) which is still alive and not jaundiced more than 2 years after transplantation. In addition, the obstruction in Pig 4 was not complete and the hepatic changes seem too gross to have been caused purely by this degree of organic obstruction. Functional bile duct obstruction remains a possibility, but no functional holdup at the bile duct anastomosis has been shown cholangiographically in the absence of organic narrowing.

At autopsy and at laparotomy in long-term survivors, evidence has been found of portal hypertension with dilated portal-systemic anastomotic veins, and dense vascular adhesions between the upper abdominal viscera, especially between the liver and the diaphragm. There is thus evidence of chronic liver disease, and we conclude that there is continuing slow rejection, which may eventually result in hepatocellular failure, but which is variable in its speed and severity from animal to animal.

Finally, the mode of hepatocyte loss in the livers showing evidence of rejection is of interest. Previous studies have drawn attention to the presence of numerous Councilman bodies in the parenchyma of hepatic transplants, and the ultrastructural changes have been interpreted as indicative of coagulative necrosis.[16] It is now known, however, that Councilman body formation is a manifestation of a distinct type of cellular death, which is fundamentally different from coagulative necrosis.[10] Unlike coagulative necrosis, it can be detected in the tissues of perfectly healthy animals, and evidence has recently accumulated that it complements mitosis in regulating the size of animal organs. The term apoptosis has been suggested to emphasize this kinetic role.[11] The results of the present study suggest that the type of cell death engendered by cellular-immune mechanisms might be apoptosis rather than coagulative necrosis; if substantiated, this conclusion would have important general biological implications.

REFERENCES

1. Battersby, C., Egerton, W. S., Balderson, G., Kerr, J. F., and Burnett, W.: Prediction of immediate survival after porcine hepatic transplantation, Aust. N. Z. J. Surg. Nov., 1974. In press.
2. Calne, R. Y., White, H. J. O., Yoffa, D. E., Maginn, R. R., Binns, R. M., Samuel, J. R., and Molina, V. P.: Observations on orthotopic liver transplantation in the pig, Br. Med. J. **2:** 478, 1967.
3. Calne, R. Y., White, H. J. O., Yoffa, D. E., Binns, R. M., Maginn, R. R., Herbertson, R. M., Millard, P. R., Molina, V. P., and Davis, D. R.: Prolonged survival of liver transplants in the pig, Br. Med. J. **4:** 645, 1967.
4. Calne, R. Y., Yoffa, D. E., White, H. J. O., and Maginn, R. R.: A technique of orthotopic liver transplantation in the pig, Br. J. Surg. **55:** 203, 1968.
5. Chalstrey, L. J., Parbhoo, S. P., Tappin, A., Baker, G. J., Gracey, J. R. H., Mullen, P. A., and Lester, R.: Technique of orthotopic liver transplantation in the pig, Br. J. Surg. **58:** 585, 1971.
6. Chomette, G., Garnier, H., Clot, J. P., Pinaudeau, Y., Auriol, M., and Brocheriou, C.: Etude microscopique de transplantations hepatique allogeniques chez le porc, Virchows Arch. Path. Anat. **347:** 176, 1969.
7. Dent, D. M., Hickman, R., Uys, C. J., Saunders, S., and Terblanche, J.: The natural history of liver allo and auto transplantation in the pig, Br. J. Surg. **58:** 407, 1971.
8. Garnier, H., Clot, J. P., and Chomette, G.: Orthotopic transplantation of the porcine liver, Surg. Gynecol. Obstet. **130:** 105, 1970.
9. Hunt, A. C.: Pathology of liver transplantation in the pig, *in* Read, A. E., editor: The liver, London, 1967, Butterworth & Co., Ltd.
10. Kerr, J. F. R.: Shrinkage necrosis; a distinct mode of cellular death, J. Pathol. **105:** 13, 1971.
11. Kerr, J. F. R., Wyllie, A. H., and Currie, A. R.: Apoptosis: A basic biological phenomenon with wide-ranging implications in tissue kinetics, Br. J. Cancer **26:** 239, 1972.
12. Lempinen, M., Salmenkivi, K., and Sivula, A.: Orthotopic liver transplantation in the pig, Acta Chir. Scand. **137:** 265, 1971.
13. Mieny, C. J., Moore, A. R., Homatas, J., and Eiseman, B.: Homotransplantation of the liver in pigs, S. Afr. J. Surg. **5:** 109, 1967.
14. Porter, K. A.: Pathology of liver transplantation, Transplant. Rev. **2:** 129, 1969.
15. Porter, K. A.: Pathology of the orthotopic homograft and heterograft, *in* Starzl, T. E., editor: Experience in hepatic transplantation, Philadelphia, 1969, W. B. Saunders Co.
16. Roessner, A., Lie, T. S., Schulz, D., v. Bassewitz, D. B., and Themann, H.: Zur feinstruktur der orthotop transplantierten, allogenen hundeleber, Virchows Arch. [Zellpathol.] **9:** 354, 1971.
17. Søborg, M., and Bendixen, G.: Human leukocyte migration as a parameter of hypersensitivity, Acta Med. Scand. **181:** 247, 1967.
18. Starzl, T. E.: Experience in hepatic transplantation, Philadelphia, 1969, W. B. Saunders Co.
19. Terblanche, J., Peacock, H. J. H., Bowes, J., and Hobbs, K. E. F.: The technique of orthotopic liver homotransplantation in the pig, J. Surg. Res. **8:** 151, 1968.
20. Terblanche, J., Peacock, J. H., Hobbs, K. E. F., Hunt, A. C., Bowes, J., Tierris, E. J., Palmer, D. B., and Blecher, T. E.: Orthotopic liver homotransplantation: An experimental study in the unmodified pig, S. Afr. Med. J. **42:** 486, 1968.

Alveolar morphometrics: Effects of positive end-expiratory pressure

Benedict D. T. Daly,* M.D., David A. Hughes, M.D.,** *and* **John C. Norman, M.D.,**
Houston, Texas

The effects of positive end-expiratory pressure (PEEP) on alveolar sac dimensions of the rat lung were investigated utilizing in vivo videomicroscopy. As PEEP was increased, alveolar sac volume at peak inspiration (alveolar capacity), alveolar sac volume at end expiration (alveolar functional residual capacity), and alveolar sac tidal volume increased linearly until a plateau was reached between 10 to 15 cm. H_2O PEEP. Monitored peak inspiratory pressure (PIP) increased by a factor of 2:1 with increasing levels of PEEP. Alveolar sac volumes plotted parametrically against PEEP resulted in pressure-volume curves which were similar to those obtained by plotting alveolar sac volumes against the PIP recorded at each volume. Alveolar sac volumes plotted against both PEEP and the mean PIP at each level of PEEP using three-dimensional isometric projections demonstrated that alveolar sac volumes could be related equally well to both applied levels of PEEP and the resultant increases in PIP.

From the Cardiovascular Surgical Research Laboratories of Texas Heart Institute, St. Luke's Episcopal and Texas Children's Hospitals, Houston, Texas

POSITIVE END-EXPIRATORY pressure (PEEP) is currently utilized in the ventilatory management of patients with acute respiratory failure characterized by large alveolar-arterial oxygen differences and decreased compliance.[3, 20] These abnormalities result from perfusion of partially or totally collapsed alveoli or terminal airways and increased pulmonary extravascular water with interstitial edema.[13, 14] The higher peak and mean airway pressures resulting from PEEP re-expand these terminal respiratory units and may retard water loss into the alveolar spaces and the interstitium.[4] Preliminary results of direct observations of the effects of PEEP at the alveolar level have only recently been reported.[16]

We have previously quantitated morphologic changes in alveolar sacs and alveoli during positive pressure respiration with an in vivo cinemicroscopy system which permits the visualization of terminal lung units during respiration.[17, 18] Subsequent attempts to characterize the effects of varying airway pressures were impeded by lung movement. The addition of a videotape system to the microscopy unit has permitted measurement of changing alveolar sac dimensions by analysis of recorded tapes viewed in slow motion. The purpose of this report is to describe the effects of PEEP on dynamic alveolar morphology utilizing these techniques.

Accepted for publication June 27, 1974.

This work was supported in part by United States Public Health Service Grant HL-14294-02 and Contract No. 4173-19G-4999-701.

Reprint requests: Benedict D. T. Daly, M.D., P.O. Box 20269, Houston, Texas 77025.

*Sylvia R. Herring, Scholar in Academic Thoracic and Cardiovascular Surgery.

**Mary A. Fraley, Fellow in Cardiovascular Surgical Research.

MATERIALS AND METHODS

Sprague-Dawley rats weighing 250 Gm. were anesthetized and tracheostomy was performed. Ventilation was maintained with a Harvard rodent respirator and the tidal volume (4 to 6 ml.) was adjusted to produce a peak inspiratory pressure of 15 to 20 cm. of water at a respiratory rate of 50 per minute, corresponding to the respiratory rate of these animals at rest. The end-expiratory pressure was controlled by immersing the outlet from the respirator in varying depths (0 to 20 cm.) of water (applied pressure). The anterior-inferior margin of the left upper lobe was exposed by thoracotomy and stabilized by affixing pipe cleaners to the lung surface with medical adhesive. The minimal traction and frictional resistance provided by these pipe cleaners kept the lung in contact with the coverslip above the microscope objectives but did not inhibit its normal expansion and contraction. In fact, the area of lung studied was gently supported so that compression at the lung surface was minimized. The microscope system consisted of a Wild-Heerbrug inverted metallurgical microscope with epiobjective lenses, a side-arm telescope, and a xenon arc light source. A black and white television camera with 2:1 interlace and automatic light control was attached to the side-arm telescope. Video signals from the television camera were initially channeled to an image enhancer and then to a 16 in. video television monitor and time-lapse videotape recorder with stepped slow motion and stop action. The animals were placed on a stand above the microscope and the stabilized lung margin apposed to a coverslip. The microscope was focused on alveolar sacs 1.5 mm. below the lung surface (Fig. 1). Vertical movement of the $\times$ 30 objective lens by 75 μ brought alveolar sacs and alveoli completely in and out of focus. Further vertical movement of the objective allowed focusing on deeper or more superficial alveolar units. The focus was varied during these recordings so that the maximum alveolar sac diameters of the units under study were recorded despite their movement in or out of a single plane of focus. Thus alveolar sac diameters were measured at peak inspiration and end expiration in several planes of focus so that the maximum diameter at each point in a respiratory cycle could be identified.

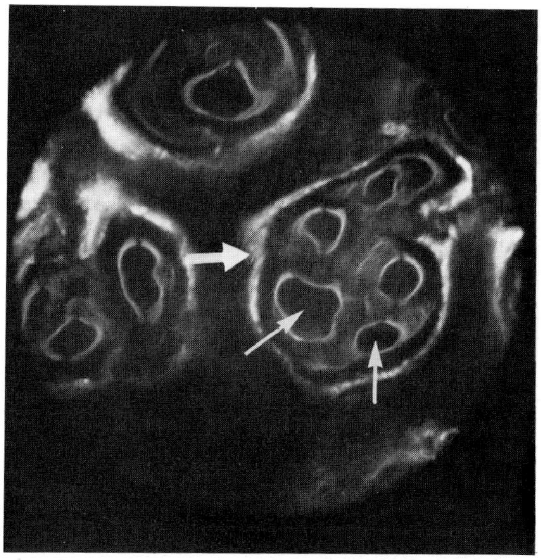

Fig. 1. A photomicrograph demonstrating the terminal respiratory units in the rat lung at peak inspiration (×174). The large arrow points to the wall of an alveolar sac and the small arrows point to alveoli.

Video recordings of control alveolar ventilation were made. Increasing levels of PEEP, i.e., 2.5, 5, 7.5, 10, 15, and 20 cm. H_2O were then applied sequentially and dynamic alveolar morphology recorded after stabilization of alveolar ventilation. The tidal volume from the respirator was maintained at the control level. The video tapes were reviewed in slow motion in steps up to $\frac{1}{61}$ of normal speed or video frames were individually advanced. The stereoscopic effect produced by the incident light-dark field illumination and the varying foci permitted determination of maximum alveolar sac diameters at peak inspiration and end expiration. These diameters were measured on the monitor at each level of PEEP from 0 to 20 cm. H_2O. Magnification was determined by viewing a calibrated grid through the microscope and measuring the grid lines (48 μ) on the television monitor. Mean alveolar sac diameters (S.E. ± 10 percent)

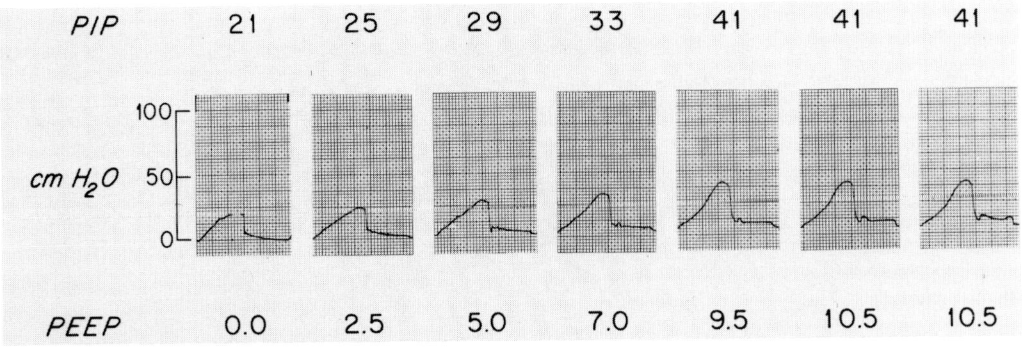

Fig. 2. A representative alveolar morphometrics airway pressure recording with a tidal volume of 4 ml. at a respiratory rate of 50. PIP increases by a factor of approximately 2:1 for each increment of PEEP until the elastic limits of the lung are reached at a recorded end-expiratory pressure of 10.5 cm. H_2O and a peak inspiratory pressure of 41 cm. H_2O.

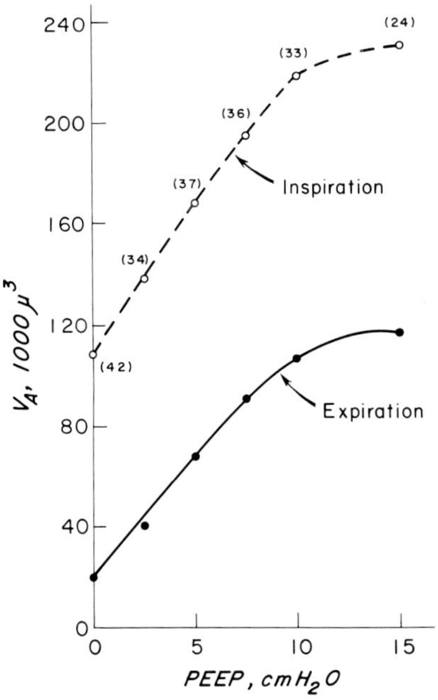

Fig. 3. Mean alveolar sac volumes at peak inspiration and end expiration at each level of applied PEEP. There is a nearly linear increase in alveolar sac volumes as PEEP is increased until the elastic limits of the lung are reached. The numbers of diameters measured for each point are enclosed by parentheses. As alveolar sac volume increased, the number of measurable alveolar sacs visualized on the television monitor decreased.

were converted to alveolar sac volumes (AV) by assuming a spherical shape of the sacs and using the formula $AV = \pi D^3/6$.

As measured increments of PEEP were applied without a change in tidal volume, the PIP increased by a factor of 2:1 (PIP:PEEP), and the recorded PEEP approximated the applied PEEP (Fig. 2). However, between 10 and 15 cm. H_2O of applied PEEP, expiration through the respiratory outflow valve ceased. This pressure varied from one animal to another due to differences in the elastic recoil of their lungs. Because of this variation in the level of PEEP at which expiration ceased, alveolar sac volumes were compared at levels of applied PEEP and recorded PIP.

RESULTS

Alveolar sacs were observed to increase in size in all dimensions with PEEP. Mean alveolar sac capacity (alveolar volume at peak inspiration), mean alveolar sac functional residual capacity (alveolar volume at end expiration), and alveolar sac tidal volume (alveolar volume at peak inspiration minus alveolar volume at end expiration), increased linearly with each increment of PEEP from 0 to 10 cm. H_2O (Fig. 3). At 15 cm. H_2O PEEP, a plateau was reached and no further increase in alveolar sac volumes could be attained. Control alveolar sac capacity increased 113 percent, alveolar sac functional residual capacity increased 499 percent, and alveolar sac tidal volume increased 32 percent. Because PIP increased nearly linearly as PEEP was applied, alveolar sac capacity, alveolar sac functional residual capacity, and alveolar sac tidal volume were determined according to grouped levels of recorded PIP, i.e., 15 to 24, 25 to 34, 35 to 44, 45 to 54, and 55 to 65 cm. H_2O

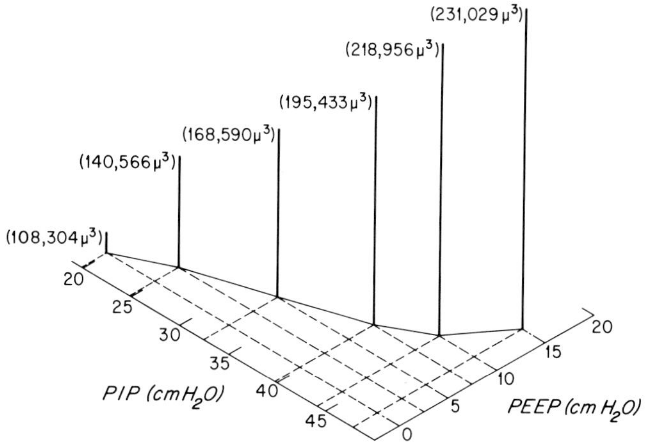

Fig. 4. An isometric projection showing the relationship between alveolar capacity and mean resultant PIP at each level of applied PEEP. Note the nearly linear relationship between alveolar capacity and both PEEP and PIP until the elastic limits of the lung are reached between 10 and 15 cm. H_2O.

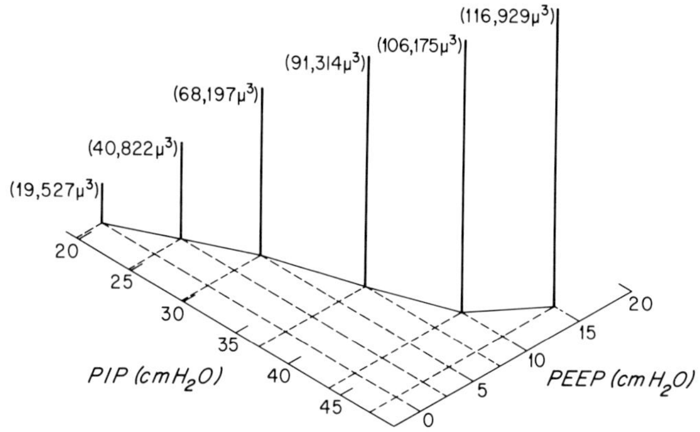

Fig. 5. An isometric projection showing the relationship between alveolar functional residual capacity and mean resultant PIP at each level of applied PEEP. Note the nearly linear relationship between alveolar functional residual capacity and both PIP and PEEP until the elastic limits of the lung are reached between 10 and 15 cm. H_2O.

(Fig. 4). Alveolar sac capacity determined in this fashion increased 87 percent, alveolar sac functional residual capacity increased 417 percent, and alveolar sac tidal volume increased 10 percent.

Since the recorded PIP at each level of PEEP varied from experiment to experiment, the mean PIP was determined for each level of PEEP from 0 to 15 cm. H_2O. Mean alveolar sac capacity, alveolar sac functional residual capacity, and alveolar sac tidal volume at each increment of PEEP were then compared simultaneously to both applied PEEP and the mean PIP at each level of PEEP. These results are illustrated as isometric projections in Fig. 5. There is a nearly linear relationship between PEEP and PIP from 0 to 10 cm. H_2O; alveolar sac capacity, alveolar sac functional residual capacity, and, consequently, alveolar sac tidal volumes correlate equally well with PEEP or PIP at any point along the base of the projections.

DISCUSSION

PEEP was first introduced in 1938 for treatment of pulmonary edema secondary to congestive heart failure.[5] Subsequently, it was employed as a method for increasing the partial pressure of oxygen for pilots during high-altitude flight.[7] However, because it increased the work of spontaneous breathing in these circumstances and decreased venous return and cardiac output, it was discontinued as a method of respiratory support in aviation medicine.[6] In 1967, PEEP was reintroduced as a method of treatment for acute respiratory failure.[2] Since that time its value in this syndrome has been established.

PEEP increases pulmonary functional residual capacity, lung compliance, and P_{AO_2}, and improvement in these factors parallels the levels of applied PEEP.[12] On the other hand, its effects on cardiac output are variable, although decreased pulmonary capillary transit time associated with increased intra-alveolar pressure has been cited as a possible mechanism to explain decreased alveolar-arterial oxygen gradients.[9, 15]

More specific means by which PEEP relieves hypoxemia at the alveolar level, however, remain to be established. The development of in vivo cinemicroscopy has permitted study of viable lung at the alveolar level. While other investigators have focused on the pulmonary microcirculation, we have studied dynamic alveolar morphology. Initial investigations detailed the microscopic anatomy of the terminal respiratory units in the rat lung.[17, 18] In observing lung under dark-field illumination with incident light, two distinctive terminal respiratory units are visualized. The first of these areas, which we define as alveolar sacs, maintains a stable morphologic appearance and is not deformed by respiration. The second structure, which we have termed alveoli, appears as out-pockets of the alveolar sac wall and is variably deformed by respiration. Measurements of alveolar sac diameters, therefore, included the alveoli which form the greater part of the alveolar sac wall viewed in three dimensions with varying focus. For this reason, quantitative measurements of alveolar sac diameters have been used for volume analyses. The recent addition of a videotape system to the microscopy unit has permitted these analyses to be extended to conditions of varying airway pressures.

In a previous report we noted that alveolar sac diameters at peak inspiration and end expiration increased with PEEP.[10] However, the difference between alveolar sac diameters at peak inspiration and end expiration decreased as PEEP was applied. When alveolar sac diameters are converted to alveolar sac volumes, it is apparent that alveolar sac tidal volume, or the difference between alveolar sac volumes at peak inspiration and end expiration, increases (Fig. 3). Thus, as alveolar sac capacity and alveolar sac functional residual capacity increase, alveolar sacs are ventilated at higher volumes, with an increased alveolar surface area during both inspiration and expiration. In addition, ventilation at the alveolar level increases despite the fact that the tidal volume from the respirator remains constant. These studies confirm the work of Dunnill[11] and Storey and Staub,[19] who demonstrated a proportionately greater increase in alveolar size relative to other lung structures with increased inflation.

Whether the observed changes in alveolar sac volumes are the result of increases in PEEP or resultant increases in PIP is open to question. In an animal model of pulmonary edema, other authors have demonstrated that optimal P_{AO_2}'s, achieved by PEEP or by raising the tidal volume to high levels (increased PIP), correlate with the mean airway pressure.[8] In the present study, the PIP increased by a factor of two times the PEEP, and the observed changes in alveolar sac volumes correlated with both PEEP and PIP. This latter relationship was demonstrated first by measuring alveolar sac volumes independently according to PEEP and then PIP. The resultant pressure volume relationships were similar. Second, alveolar sac volumes were compared simultaneously to the mean PIP and to the PEEP. Figs. 4 and 5 show a linear relationship between these volumes and both PEEP and PIP.

Since PEEP and PIP bear a nearly constant relationship, PEEP could be responsible for alveolar sac functional residual capacity and PIP for alveolar sac capacity without affecting the pressure volume curves in Fig. 3. This possibility is supported by the observation that alveolar sac functional residual capacity at 15 cm. H_2O PEEP is nearly the same as alveolar sac capacity at 15 to 20 cm. H_2O PIP (0 PEEP).

These studies have demonstrated the pressure-volume relationships in the terminal respiratory units of the lung that result from the utilization of PEEP. As PEEP is applied, the PIP increases by a factor of two times the applied PEEP. Transmission of these higher peak and end-expiratory pressures to the terminal respiratory units re-expands partially or totally collapsed alveoli. In addition, the resultant increase in alveolar sac dimensions in both inspiration and expiration and the increase in alveolar sac tidal gas exchange may contribute to decreased alveolar-arterial oxygen gradients. These changes in alveolar sac dimensions are linearly related to the PEEP until the elastic limits of the lung are approached.

REFERENCES

1. Anthonisen, N. R.: Effect of volume and volume history of the lungs on pulmonary shunt flow, Am. J. Physiol. **207:** 235, 1964.
2. Ashbaugh, D. C., Bigelow, D. B., Petty, T. L., and Levine, B. E.: Acute respiratory distress in adults, Lancet **2:** 319, 1967.
3. Ashbaugh, D. G., Petty, T. L., Bigelow, D. B., and Harris, T. M.: Continuous positive-pressure breathing (CPPB) in adult respiratory distress syndrome, J. Thorac. Cardiovasc. Surg. **57:** 31, 1969.
4. Barach, A. L.: Principles and practices of inhalation therapy, Philadelphia, 1944, J. B. Lippincott Company, pp. 52-57.
5. Barach, A. L., Martin, J., Echman, M.: Positive pressure respiration and its application to the treatment of acute pulmonary edema, Arch. Intern. Med. **12:** 754, 1938.
6. Barach, A. L., Eckman, M., Ginsburg, E., and Rumsey, C., Jr.: Studies on positive pressure respiration. III. Effect of continuous positive pressure breathing on arterial blood gases at high altitude, J. Aviation Med. **18:** 139, 1947.
7. Barach, A. L., Fenn, W. O., Ferris, E. B., and Schmidt, C. F.: The physiology of pressure breathing, J. Aviation Med. **18:** 73, 1947.
8. Cheney, F. W., and Martin, W. E.: Effects of continuous positive pressure ventilation on gas exchange in acute pulmonary edema, J. Appl. Physiol. **30:** 378, 1971.
9. Colgan, F. J., and Marocco, P. P.: The cardiorespiratory effects of constant and intermittent positive-pressure breathing, Anesthesiology **36:** 444, 1972.
10. Daly, B. D. T., Edmonds, C. H., and Norman, J. C.: In vivo alveolar morphometrics with positive end expiratory pressure, Surg. Forum **24:** 217, 1973.
11. Dunnill, M. S.: Effect of lung inflation on alveolar surface area in the dog, Nature **214:** 1013, 1967.
12. Falke, K. J., Pontoppidon, H., Kumar, A., Leith, D. E., Geffin, B., and Laver, M. B.: Ventilation with end-expiratory pressure in acute lung disease, J. Clin. Invest. **51:** 2315, 1972.
13. Gump, F. E., Mashima, Y., Jorgensen, S., and Kinney, J. M.: Simultaneous use of three indicators to evaluate pulmonary capillary damage in man, Surgery **70:** 262, 1971.
14. Hedley-Whyte, J., Laver, M. B., and Bendixen, H. H.: Effects of changes in tidal ventilation on physiologic shunting, Am. J. Physiol. **206:** 891, 1964.
15. Lutch, J. S., and Murray, J. F.: Continuous positive-pressure ventilation: Effects on systemic oxygen transport and tissue oxygenation, Ann. Intern. Med. **76:** 193, 1972.
16. McNary, W. F., Berman, H. S., Daly, B., and Norman, J. C.: The use of videotape to record and review data obtained by incident light dark-field microscopy of the living lung, Bibl. Anat. **11:** 44, 1973.
17. Moreci, A. P., and Norman, J. C.: Quantitative and qualitative changes in morphology of alveolar sacs with positive-pressure respiration, Proc. Soc. Exp. Biol. Med. **141:** 318, 1972.
18. Moreci, A. P., and Norman, J. C.: Measurements of alveolar sac diameters by incident-light photomicrography, Ann. Thorac. Surg. **15:** 179, 1973.
19. Storey, W. F., and Staub, N. C.: Ventilation of terminal air units, J. Appl. Physiol. **17:** 391, 1962.
20. Sugerman, H. J., Rogers, R. M., and Miller, L. D.: Positive end-expiratory pressure (PEEP); indications and physiologic considerations, Chest **62:** 86S, 1972.
21. Teplitz, C.: The ultrastructural basis for pulmonary pathophysiology following trauma, J. Trauma **8:** 700, 1968.

Allograft tolerance in the absence of circulating antibodies

R. Nowygrod, M.D., D. E. R. Sutherland, M.D., R. J. Howard, M.D., *and* **J. S. Najarian, M.D.,** *Minneapolis, Minn.*

Tolerance to skin allografts between chickens of different major histocompatibility genotypes was induced by intraembryonic injection of recipient animals with donor-strain spleen cells. To test the hypothesis that in vivo tolerance results from immunologic enhancement of the allograft by serum antibodies, tolerant animals were made agammaglobulinemic by neonatal excision of the bursa of Fabricius. Agammaglobulinemia was confirmed by the inability of bursectomized animals to produce agglutinating antibody to Brucella abortus and sheep red blood cells (SRBC) and by the absence of serum IgG and IgM by immunodiffusion assay. Skin graft survival times were the same in tolerant agammaglobulinemic and nonagammaglobulinemic animals, suggesting that in the chicken, in vivo skin allograft tolerance is not due to enhancing antibodies.

From the University of Minnesota, Department of Surgery, Minneapolis, Minn.

TOLERANCE, classically thought to result from the clonal elimination or paralysis of specifically activated T lymphocytes, is currently being re-examined as a possible manifestation of immunological enhancement.[5, 15] This phenomenon, originally described in experimental tumor systems,[9] can be defined as the failure to react against tumor antigens or histocompatibility alloantigens, which results from neutralization of normally functioning T lymphocytes by specific antitumor or antigraft antibodies. Much of the evidence in support of immunologic enhancement as the mechanism underlying tolerance derives from in vitro systems, demonstrating that washed lymphocytes from tolerant animals will respond normally against donor-strain target cells and that such reactivity can be specifically blocked by the addition of serum or antibody fraction from the tolerant host.[7] In the chicken it has been possible to eliminate circulating antibodies and humoral immune responsiveness without affecting T cell function by appropriate extirpation of the bursa of Fabricius, the primary avian lymphoid organ responsible for B cell maturation.[3] Failure to localize a bursal-equivalent organ in mammals prevents similar B cell ablation in nonavian species. The chicken, therefore, affords an excellent in vivo model for studying the role of antibodies in allograft tolerance. In addition, the availability of strains selected for uniformity with respect to major histocompatibility genotype facilitates evaluation of transplant results. In this study we have examined the effects of agammaglobulinemia on skin allograft tolerance to test, in

Supported by the Minnesota Medical Foundation, Grant SMF-115-73, and Health, Education, and Welfare Grant 5 P02 AM 13083-04.

Accepted for publication July 26, 1974.

Reprint requests: R. Nowygrod, M.D., Department of Surgery, Columbia-Presbyterian Medical Center, New York, N. Y. 10032.

vivo, the hypothesis that tolerance is an induced state of specific immunologic unresponsiveness rather than the result of an antibody-mediated inhibition of cellular allograft rejection. The results demonstrate that, in the chicken, tolerance induced by embryonic injection of donor strain spleen cells can be maintained in the absence of circulating IgG or IgM.

MATERIALS AND METHODS

Animals. Fertile hatching eggs, strains WC(B2/B2) and FS(B15/B21), defined at the major histocompatibility B locus, were purchased from Hy-line Laboratories (Johnston, Iowa) and incubated until hatching (days 20 to 22). Newborn chicks were kept in heated brooders for 2 weeks and then transferred to cages. All animals were fed Purina Startena chicken feed and tetracycline-supplemented tap water.

Agammaglobulinemia. Agammaglobulinemia was effected by bursectomy and irradiation in the newborn period as follows.

Bursectomy. Within 12 hours of hatching, the bursa of Fabricius was excised through an incision between the tail and cloaca. The degree of B cell ablation was assessed by (1) gross and microscopic examination of the hindgut for bursal remnants and microscopic examination of the spleen for presence of germinal centers; (2) agglutinin production following immunization with sheep red blood cells (SRBC) and *Brucella abortus;* and (3) serum assay for immunoglobulin by immunoelectrophoresis and Ouchterlony double diffusion in agar.

Irradiation. Irradiation was administered within 24 hours of hatching; 675 r were delivered at 35 r per minute by a Maximar 220 kv. machine, 15 Ma., with 0.25 mm. copper and one mm. aluminum filters.

Skin grafts. Skin grafting was performed as described by Cannon and Longmire.[2] A 2 cm. square piece of skin was rotated 180° on the graft bed. The grafts were held in place with several drops of collodion until day 10, at which time any remaining collodion was peeled off and inspection of the grafts begun. The grafts were checked every 2 days for 4 weeks and biweekly thereafter. All healthy grafts bore feathers or follicles and demonstrated microscopic epithelial and vascular continuity with host skin. Rejection was manifested by shrinkage, ulceration, and ultimate replacement of donor skin with scar tissue. The homozygous B2/B2 WC strain was used as the donor group and the heterozygous B15/B21 FS strain was used as the recipient group. Preliminary experiments revealed that tolerance was easier to induce with this combination than with the FS donor–WC recipient combination. All skin grafts were performed within the newborn period—donors and recipients were less than 2 days old. A specificity control group of 10 tolerant FS recipients bearing healthy WC skin grafts received thirty-party Ghostley strain newborn skin grafts at 4 to 8 weeks after initial WC skin grafting.

Immunization. The bursectomized and irradiated animals were given a primary immunization at age 4 weeks, which consisted of a 2×10^9 intraperitoneal injection of washed SRBC and 2×10^9 intramuscular injection of killed *B. abortus* organisms in complete Freund's adjuvant. The animals were given a single intraperitoneal injection of 2×10^9 Brucella organisms and 2×10^9 SRBC 3 weeks later. SRBC and *B. abortus* agglutinin titers were determined one week after the secondary immunization. Age-matched, sham-operated and irradiated, and untreated animals similarly immunized served as positive control groups.

Serum gamma globulin. Assay for chicken IgM and IgG was performed by serum immunoelectrophoresis (IEP) and for IgM by Ouchterlony double diffusion in agar. IgG and IgM standards were obtained by Sephadex G-200 fractionation of pooled normal chicken gamma globulins. Rabbit antichicken serum was prepared by injecting normal adult chicken serum in complete Freund's adjuvant into each rabbit's four footpads and four subcutaneous sites, followed by a similar secondary immunization 3 weeks later. Test serum was analyzed by IEP and Ouchterlony immunodiffusion 2 to 3 weeks after completion of Brucella and SRBC immunization.

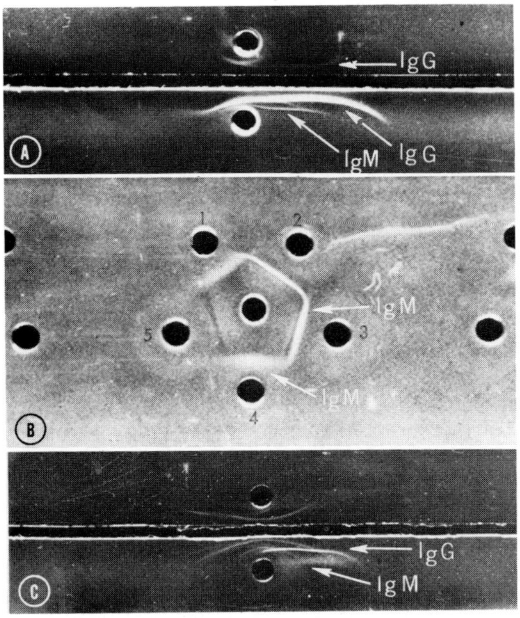

Fig. 1. Analysis of serum samples from bursectomized chickens by immunoelectrophoresis (*A* and *C*) and Ouchterlony double diffusion in agar (*B*). The same antisera were used in all three determinations. *A*, The lower well contains IgG and IgM isolated on Sephadex G-200. The upper well is a bursectomized serum sample which shows diminished but present IgG. *B*, Wells *2* and *3* contain the IgM standard. Lines of identity with bursectomized serum samples in *1* and *4* establish the presence of IgM. The sample in well *5* contains no detectable IgM. *C*, Two bursectomized serum samples from animals with negative antibody response to *Brucella abortus* and SRBC immunization are seen. The serum of the upper, but not the lower well contains no IgG or IgM.

Both IgM and IgG were detectable down to a protein concentration of 0.05 mg. per milliliter.

Tolerance induction. Tolerance was induced by the intravenous injection of embryonic donor spleen cells into the recipient embryo, as described by Rouse and Warner.[13] Fifty to 75 16-day-old WC embryo spleens were pooled and single cell suspensions were prepared by gentle grinding of the tissue through a No. 100 wire mesh screen. Cells were washed twice in Hanks Balanced Salt Solution and viability was determined by Trypan blue dye exclusion. Recipient FS embryos aged 15 to 16 days were injected with 2×10^6 viable WC spleen cells into a chorialIantoic vein and WC skin grafts were applied within 2 days after hatching.

RESULTS

Serum gamma globulins. The combined use of IEP analysis and Ouchterlony double diffusion in agar were successful in establishing the presence or absence of IgG and IgM in serum. A bursectomized serum sample with diminished, but present IgG is seen in the upper well of Fig. 1, *A*. Fig. 1, *B* shows three samples, two with IgM present and one with IgM absent. Fig. 1, *C* shows the immunoelectrophoretic patterns of two animals with no detectable agglutinin titers to either Brucella or SRBC. Only the sample in the upper well reveals no IgG or IgM.

Antibody production. Brucella agglutinin titers less than one and SRBC titers 2 or less were considered negative responses after preliminary testing of unimmunized age-matched animals revealed titers no higher than these. Fig. 2 shows the results for the bursectomized-irradiated animals and the sham-operated, irradiated animals. All irradiated and nonirradiated controls (nonbursectomized animals) developed agglutinin titers to one or both antigens. Of the 31 bursectomized-irradiated animals, 15 (48 percent) had no response to both antigens. Of these 15 antibody nonresponders, five (38 percent) had circulating serum immunoglobulin by IEP and Ouchterlony assay. Thus only 10 of the original 31 (32 percent) were truly bursectomized by both antibody production and immunodiffusion criteria.

B cell ablation. Gross examination of the hindgut was an inadequate parameter of B cell ablation; three of five bursectomized animals with positive antibody titers had no gross bursal remnant but did have at least one mature lymphoid follicle on microscopic examination of the hindgut. Serial microscopic sectioning of the hindgut also proved to be an inadequate parameter; three animals without antibody response to Brucella or SRBC, but with detectable circulating immunoglobulin, had no visible bursal follicles on serial microscopic sections, despite the presence of germinal centers in the spleen.

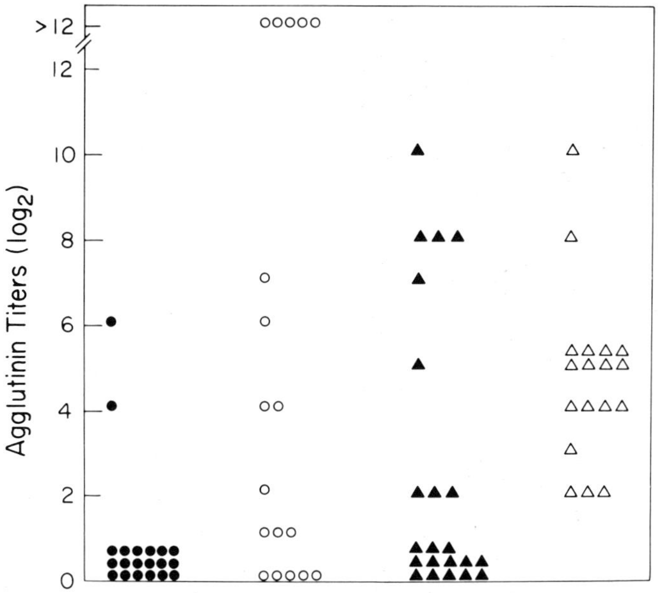

Fig. 2. Agglutinin titers are shown for bursectomized-irradiated animals and sham-operated irradiated controls. None of the controls but 48 percent of the bursectomized group had negative titers to both antigens. *Brucella abortus:* ● bursectomized, ○ control; sheep red blood cells: ▲ bursectomized, △ control.

Animals proved to be agammaglobulinemic by immunoelectrophoresis and Ouchterlony assay had no germinal centers and no positive antibody titers. Assessment of bursectomy results by antibody production and histologic examination thus proved to be inadequate, and only animals with undetectable serum immunoglobulins by immunodiffusion were considered truly bursectomized.

Skin graft survival. Fig. 3 depicts skin allograft survival for both spleen-cell–injected groups and control groups. The control animals consist of three groups that were not pretreated by intraembryonic injection of donor spleen cells: (1) bursectomized, irradiated (eight animals); (2) nonbursectomized, nonirradiated (33 animals); and (3) nonbursectomized, irradiated (21 animals). The only group of animals with significantly prolonged mean allograft survival time, by Student's t test, was the group pretreated with the donor strain spleen cells ($p < 0.001$). Of the 31 animals in this group, 24 (77 percent) maintained healthy grafts for 100 days. Of the seven animals that rejected their grafts, five did so after day 20 and two after day 60. In 10 FS recipients bearing healthy WC grafts for 4 to 8 weeks, third-party, Ghostley strain skin grafts were rejected within 3 weeks. Eight of the animals rejected the Ghostley skin allografts by 14 days after grafting and the remaining two rejected by day 20. The original WC skin grafts remained healthy throughout this period.

Agammaglobulinemia and graft survival. Fig. 4 illustrates the allograft survival of the 31 bursectomized animals pretreated by intraembryonic injection of donor spleen cells. The group is divided into (1) those which were agammaglobulinemic (10 animals), and (2) those which had positive antibody titers and/or detectable serum immunoglobulin (21 animals). Mean and median skin allograft survival times were 97 and 100 days, respectively, for the agammaglobulinemic group and 87 and 100 days for the nonagammaglobulinemic group. Nine of the 10 animals in the former group, and 17 of the 21 animals in the latter group maintained healthy allografts for the entire 100 days of observation. The difference in mean survival time is not significant by Student's t test ($p = 0.87$). Thus tolerance induction was equally successful in both agammaglobuline-

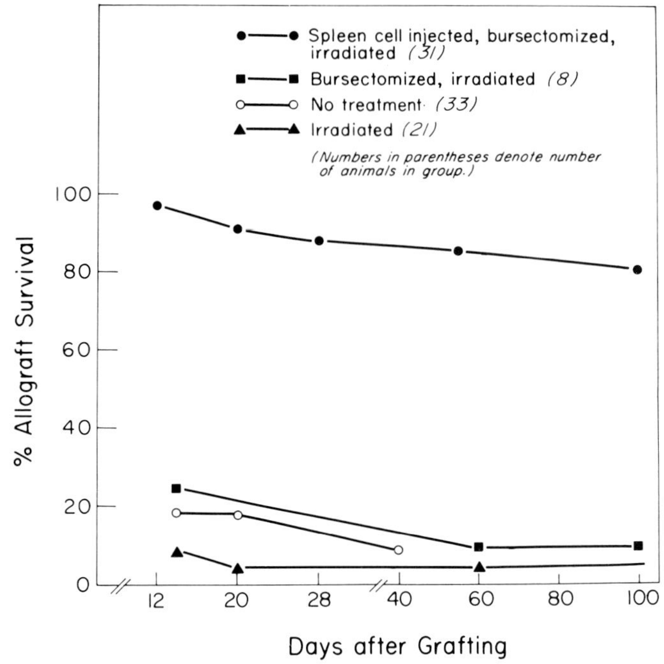

Fig. 3. Four groups of skin-allografted animals are depicted. Significant prolongation is seen only in the group pretreated by intraembryonic injection of donor spleen cells. The three control groups consist of untreated, irradiated, and bursectomized-irradiated animals.

mic animals and nonagammaglobulinemic animals.

DISCUSSION

The bursectomized chicken affords an excellent model to examine tolerance systems for their dependence on the presence of antibodies. Precaution must be exercised to assure that adequate bursal ablation has been effected since histologic criteria and the failure to produce detectable antibody activity do not assure agammaglobulinemia. In this study, only 10 of the 15 animals with a negative response to immunization with SRBC and Brucella were agammaglobulinemic at age 8 weeks, a time by which circulating maternal gamma globulins have disappeared.

Embryonic rather than adult donor spleen cells were used for tolerance induction to assure that these cells, when injected into embryos bursectomized at hatching, would not themselves produce antibody of donor strain origin and to preclude the complication of graft-vs.-host (GVH) reactions.[10, 14] Cooper and associates[3] have previously shown that to produce complete agammaglobulinemia, surgical bursectomy in the newborn period must be supplemented by x-irradiation to destroy peripheralized B cells. In Cooper and associates' experiments and in this study, possible T cell immunosuppression resulting from such treatment is discounted by the normal rejection of skin allografts in irradiated controls.

Our findings are in agreement with those of Rouse and Warner[13] and Crone,[4] who have reported that putative T cell tolerance, as measured by skin allograft prolongation and depression of GVH activity, can be induced equally well in bursectomized and nonbursectomized animals. In both studies intraembryonic injection of testosterone was used to induce bursal ablation and skin grafts were examined for a period of 3 to 4 weeks. While the absence of serum antibodies was supported by failure of spleen fragments to synthesize immunoglobulins in vitro[13] and failure to inhibit GVH response after preincubation of injected cells with sera from bursectomized animals,[4] neither study demonstrated conclusively that tolerant chickens

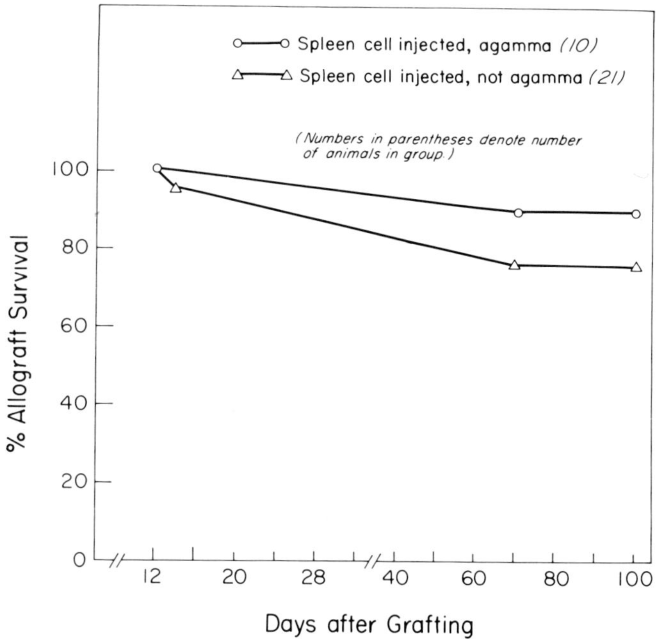

Fig. 4. The spleen-cell–pretreated animals are compared with respect to skin allograft survival times in agammaglobulinemic and nonagammaglobulinemic animals. Survival time is not significantly different between these two groups, suggesting that the lack of antibody is not affecting rejection times.

were agammaglobulinemic. We have attempted to counter this objection by using immunodiffusion criteria to establish absence of circulating IgG and IgM.

Yamanouchi and associates[18] have reported that in neonatally bursectomized quails, regression of virally induced Rouse sarcoma tumors is not augmented. In their study there was no difference in the tumor growth patterns between bursectomized and nonbursectomized animals, suggesting that in vivo enhancement was not a factor in the growth of this sarcoma. Bursectomy results were assessed only by antibody response to viral antigen and SRBC, and serum immunoglobulin determinations were not reported. Preliminary results in our laboratory utilizing nephroblastomas induced by tumor cell transplantation confirms the absence of in vivo enhancement in chickens, as assayed by tumor growth patterns in bursectomized and nonbursectomized hosts.

Hellstrom and associates[8] have shown that in mice rendered tolerant by neonatal injection of donor spleen cells, recipient lymphocytes were cytotoxic to donor fibroblasts in culture. This cytotoxicity could be significantly reduced by preincubation of the fibroblasts with recipient serum. They therefore suggested that the tolerance was the result of enhancing or blocking factors in the serum, presumably antibody or antibody-antigen complex. Attempts by Brent and associates[1] to reproduce these results in vivo in mice, using an identical tolerance induction protocol, failed. However, the critical experiments to test this hypothesis in vivo could not be done since, in the mouse, an ablatable bursal equivalent has not yet been defined, and, therefore, the means for inducing agammaglobulinemia did not exist.

Our findings that agammaglobulinemic chickens treated by a standard tolerogenic technique maintained skin allografts as well as did nonbursectomized animals demonstrate that conventional antibodies do not play an enhancing or blocking role in skin allograft tolerance as induced by the embryonic injection of donor cells. This view is in contrast to the interpretation placed on in vitro studies in rodents, dogs, and man by the Hellstroms[8] and others.[6, 11, 12, 17] In the chicken cellular tolerance appears to be a distinct phenomenon separate from enhancement.

REFERENCES

1. Brent, L., Brooks, C., Lubling, N., and Thomas, A. V.: Attempts to demonstrate an in vivo role for serum blocking factors in tolerant mice, Transplantation **14:** 382, 1972.
2. Cannon, J. A., and Longmire, W. P.: Studies of successful skin homografts in the chicken, Ann. Surg. **134:** 60, 1952.
3. Cooper, M. D., Peterson, R. D. A., South, M. A., and Good, R. A.: The functions of the thymus system and the bursa system in the chicken, J. Exp. Med. **123:** 75, 1966.
4. Crone, M.: Tolerance to allogeneic cells induced in bursectomized chickens, Scand. J. Immunol. **2:** 349, 1973.
5. Feldman, J. D.: Immunologic enhancement: A study of blocking antibodies, Adv. Immunol. **15:** 167, 1972.
6. Hattler, B. G., Davis, M., Soehnler, B., and Miller, J.: Prospective in vitro prediction of enhancement of canine renal allografts, SURGERY **74:** 163, 1973.
7. Hellstrom, K. E., and Hellstrom, I.: Immunological enhancement as studied by cell culture techniques, Ann. Rev. Microbiol. **24:** 373, 1970.
8. Hellstrom, I., Hellstrom, K. E., and Allison, A. C.: Neonatally induced allograft tolerance mediated by serum-borne factors, Nature **230:** 48, 1971.
9. Kalis, N.: Immunologic enhancement of tumor homografts in mice. A review, Cancer Res. **18:** 992, 1958.
10. Khattab, M. S., and Craig, J. V.: Allotype synthesis by adult donors' leukocytes and spleen cells injected into newly hatched chicks, Transplantation **10:** 33, 1970.
11. Phillips, S. M., Martin, J. W., Shaw, R. A., and Wegmann, T. G.: Serum mediated immunological nonreactivity between histoincompatible cells in tetra parental mice, Nature **234:** 146, 1971.
12. Pierce, G. E., Quadracci, L. J., Tremann, J. A., Moe, R. E., Striker, G. E., Hellstrom, I., Hellstrom, K. E., and Marchioro, M. D.: Studies on cellular and humoral immune factors in human renal transplantation, Ann. Surg. **174:** 609, 1971.
13. Rouse, B. T., and Warner, N. L.: Induction of T cell tolerance in agammaglobulinemic chickens, Eur. J. Immunol. **2:** 102, 1972.
14. Solomon, J. B.: The onset of immunological competence in the chicken, Folia Biol. **10:** 268, 1964.
15. Voisin, G. A.: Immunologic facilitation, a broadening of the concept of the enhancement phenomenon, Progr. Allergy **15:** 328, 1971.
16. Warner, N. L., and Szenberg, A.: Immunologic studies on hormonally bursectomized and surgically thymectomized chickens, *in* Good, R. A., and Gabrielson, A. E., editors: The thymus in immunobiology, New York, 1964, Paul B. Hoeber, Inc., Medical Book Division of Harper & Row, Publishers, p. 395.
17. Wegman, T. G., Hellstrom, I., and Hellstrom, K. E.: Immunological tolerance: "Forbidden clones" allowed in tetra parental mice, Proc. Natl. Acad. Sci. **68:** 1644, 1971.
18. Yamanouchi, K., Hayami, M., Satoshi, M., Fukuda, A., and Kobune, F.: Cellular immunity induced by Rous sarcoma virus in Japanese quail, Jap. J. Med. Sci. Biol. **24:** 1, 1971.

Pulmonary hypertension in acute hemorrhagic pancreatitis

Denis F. J. Halmagyi, M.D., D.Sc., J. H. Karis, M.D., *New York, N. Y.,*
F. G. Stenning, M.B., B.S., *Melbourne, Australia, and* **D. Varga, B.Sc.,** *Sydney, Australia*

Acute hemorrhagic pancreatitis was induced in eight greyhounds with a surgical technique, and the results were compared to changes in five sham-operated greyhounds. Pulmonary and femoral blood flows, systemic and pulmonary arterial blood pressures, blood gases, plasma levels of lactate, catecholamines, amylase, and glucose were measured prior to and for 24 hours following the interventions. Induction of pancreatitis was followed by gradual hypotension and six of eight dogs were dead after 24 hours; all sham-operated dogs remained alive the next day. Neither hypovolemia nor activation of vasodilator agents could be identified as the cause of circulatory failure. In the pancreatitis group mean pulmonary arterial pressure was 26 ± 5 and in the sham-operated group 15 ± 4 mm. Hg; pulmonary "wedge" pressure was 6 ± 5 mm. Hg, cardiac index 2.2 ± 0.3 L., and arterial blood gases were normal in both groups. In three patients admitted for acute hemorrhagic pancreatitis, Swan-Ganz catheters were inserted and pulmonary arterial mean pressures were found to be 36, 22, and 32 mm. Hg, respectively, with normal (8 to 10 mm. Hg) pulmonary "wedge" pressure and normal cardiac outputs. The similarity of these experimental findings with clinical results suggests that pulmonary hypertension is a hitherto unrecognized consequence of acute pancreatitis and that it is likely to be related to pulmonary arteriolar constriction secondary to the release of some vasoactive material from the injured pancreas.

From the Gordon Craig Research Laboratory, Department of Surgery, University of Sydney, Sydney, Australia, and the Departments of Surgery and Anesthesiology, College of Physicians and Surgeons, Columbia University, New York, N. Y.

THE MECHANISM of shock in acute hemorrhagic pancreatitis is controversial and the few circulatory studies reported fail to reveal any specific feature that would distinguish this type of circulatory failure from other types of shock.

Blood volume, as determined by a single isotope, is reduced,[3, 16] and this has been attributed to either blood loss into the peritoneal cavity,[8] or to plasma loss across the damaged capillaries in the pancreas,[1, 3] or to both. It has also been stated that in experimental acute pancreatitis hypotension develops rapidly, probably preceding the loss of plasma, suggesting that the fall in blood pressure may be related to the release of vasoactive substances.[1, 16] Indeed, the pancreas contains trypsinogen and kallikreinogen, and these, when activated, release plasma kinins from precursors. Plasma kinins are powerful vasodilators and could conceivably contribute to the genesis of shock.[10, 11, 16]

This study was supported by the National Heart Foundation of Australia.

Accepted for publication July 23, 1974.

Reprint requests: D. F. J. Halmagyi, M.D., Department of Surgery, PH-12-124, College of Physicians and Surgeons, Columbia University, 630 W. 168th St., New York, N. Y. 10032.

In most previous studies pancreatitis was induced by injection of bile or enzymes into the pancreatic duct. We utilized the technique described by Pfeffer, Stasior, and Hinton[13] and used by McCutcheon and Race.[9] Our first aim was to study the immediate circulatory, respiratory, and metabolic response to experimentally induced acute pancreatitis and to try to define its characteristic pattern. We then searched for the same pattern in three patients suffering from acute hemorrhagic pancreatitis.

METHODS

Animal studies. Thirteen greyhounds weighing 22 to 31 kilograms were studied. We have been using this breed over many years for their convenient size, excellent physical condition, and gentle nature. They are particularly well suited for experiments involving circulation of the limb.

The fasting supine animals were anesthetized with 15 mg. per kilogram of thiopentone intravenously. Anesthesia was maintained by a continuous intravenous infusion of 0.2 mg. per kilogram per minute of thiopentone, but later this dose could be reduced without having the animals regain consciousness. The trachea was intubated with a cuffed Magill tube.

A midline abdominal incision was made with standard surgical technique and the duodenum was divided just distal to the pylorus and, in addition, immediately distal to the major pancreatic duct. In eight dogs (experimental group) the ends of the isolated segment of the duodenum were closed by a double row of sutures and gastrointestinal continuity was established by end-to-end duodenostomy. Bile was excluded from the duodenal loop by ligation of the common bile duct. In five dogs (sham-operated group) the duodenum was divided proximally and distally in the same manner but anastomosed in situ to the divided ends and the bile duct was not ligated. The abdomen was then closed.

Both femoral arteries and veins were exposed 2 hours later, the animals were heparinized, and a double-lumen cardiac catheter was passed via the femoral vein under fluoroscopic guidance into the pulmonary artery with its distal opening in the wedge position. A cannulating flowmeter probe was inserted into the right femoral artery and a catheter built into the flowmeter probe was used for measurement of femoral artery pressure. Femoral arterial blood flow was measured with a squarewave electromagnetic flowmeter.[4] A nonoccluding polyethylene catheter was inserted into the right femoral vein. Details of this technique have been described elsewhere.[5]

Oxygen saturation of the arterial and mixed venous blood was measured with a Haemoreflector (Kipp and Zonen, Delft, Holland). Hemoglobin content of the arterial blood was measured spectrophotometrically and duplicate samples were spun in capillary tubes for 5 minutes in an Adams Autocrit for hematocrit measurements. Expired air was collected in Douglas bags; their contents were measured in a model E-40 wet test gas meter (Parkinson-Cowan, London) and analyzed for O_2 concentration in a Beckman model E-2 paramagnetic O_2 analyzer and for CO_2 concentration in a Beckman model LB-1 infra-red CO_2 analyzer. Femoral arterial and venous, pulmonary arterial, and pulmonary arterial wedge pressures were measured with Sanborn transducers and recorded on a direct-writing, multichannel Sanborn oscillograph. Details of these techniques have been previously described.[6, 7]

Arterial blood was taken anaerobically and analyzed immediately after collection at 38° C. for O_2 and CO_2 tensions and pH with Radiometer microelectrodes operating through a model 22 pH meter (Radiometer, Copenhagen).

Blood glucose was measured using the Gluco-Pak reagent set (Unitech Company, Panorama City, Calif.) based on the *o*-toluidine reaction and lactic acid was measured enzymatically.[12] Plasma amylase levels were measured[2] and were expressed in Street-Close units. The plasma level of catecholamines was measured fluorometrically, as described in detail elsewhere.[7]

A thermistor probe was introduced into the inferior vena cava, and blood temperature was continuously monitored on an elec-

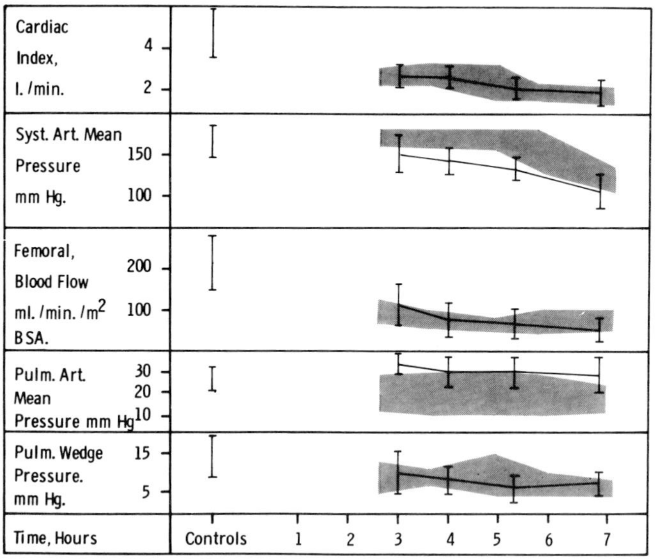

Fig. 1A. Immediate consequences of acute induced pancreatitis: circulatory changes. Shaded area: sham-operated animals, mean values ± standard deviations. Lines and vertical bars: pancreatitis dogs, mean values, and standard deviations.

tric thermometer (Type TE3, Electrolaboratoriet, Copenhagen).

The Fick principle was used to calculate cardiac output. Total systemic, pulmonary, and femoral arterial conductances were obtained by dividing blood flow (milliliter per minute per square meter of body surface area) by the arteriovenous pressure gradient (in millimeters of mercury) and were expressed in arbitrary units. Standard statistical methods were used for the evaluation of the results.

Gross postmortem examination was carried out in all animals.

Patient studies. Three patients admitted to the surgery-anesthesiology intensive-care unit of the Columbia-Presbyterian Medical Center with the diagnosis of acute pancreatitis were studied; all three had grossly elevated serum amylase levels. Cardiac output was measured by dye dilution, blood volume by RISA using a Volumetron, and pulmonary arterial and pulmonary arterial wedge pressures via a Swan-Ganz catheter.

RESULTS

Animal studies. These are summarized in Figs. 1 and 2.

To avoid excessive postoperative blood loss, heparin was withheld for 2 hours after

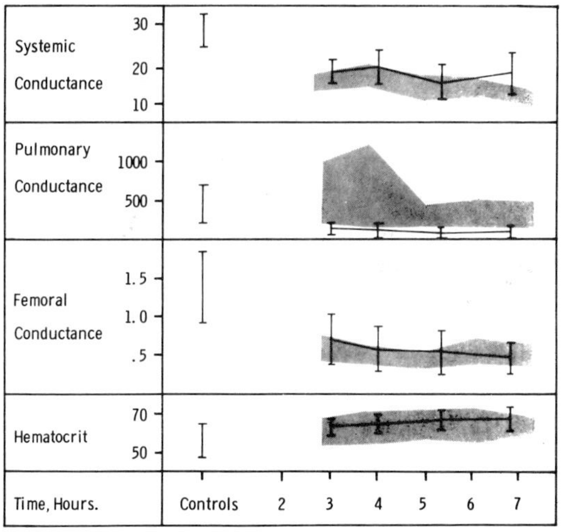

Fig. 1B. Conductance in acute induced pancreatitis. Legend as in Fig. 1*A*.

operation, and, accordingly, no preoperative circulatory measurements could be obtained. However, we did collect preoperative blood samples for catecholamine, lactate, amylase, and glucose measurements. The immediate circulatory response was assessed by comparing the results of the postoperative measurements with the normal values obtained in this laboratory over several years in a large number of greyhounds.[5-7]

Immediate changes. In both the experi-

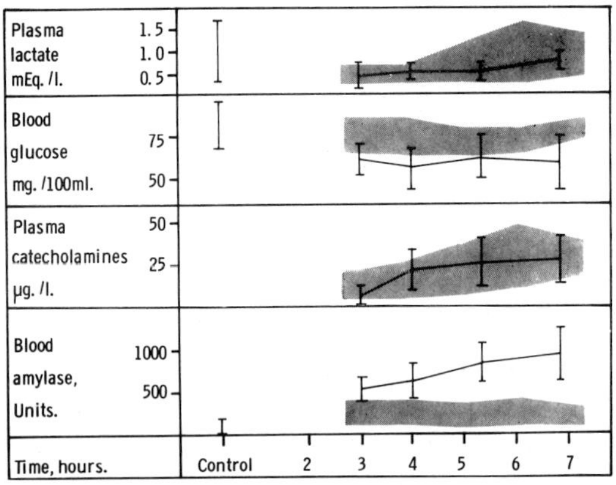

Fig. 2. Immediate consequences of acute induced pancreatitis: humoral changes. Shaded area: sham-operated animals mean values and standard deviations. Lines: pancreatitis dogs with standard deviations (vertical bars).

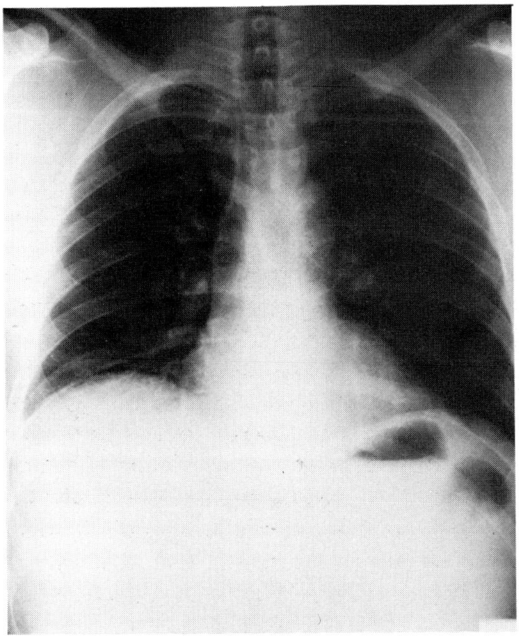

Fig. 3. Chest roentgenogram of Patient 3 at admission.

mental and the sham-operated groups, cardiac output ($P < 0.02$) and femoral arterial blood flow ($P < 0.02$) were reduced and blood pressure remained normal. Both systemic ($P < 0.01$) and femoral arterial ($P < 0.01$) conductances were low. Pulmonary arterial pressure was higher ($P < 0.01$) and pulmonary arterial conductance was lower ($P < 0.01$) in the experimental group

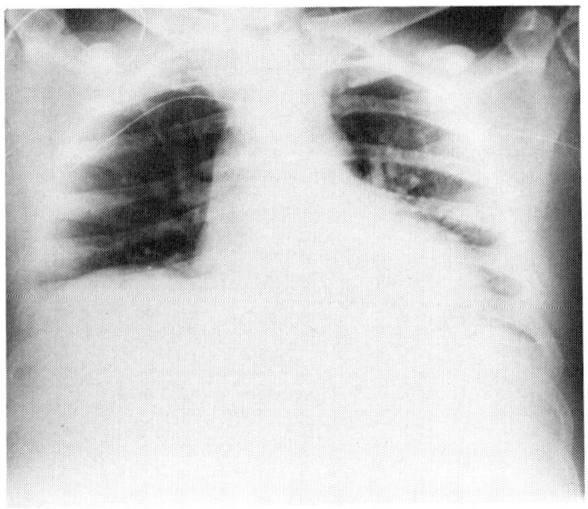

Fig. 4. Chest roentgenogram of Patient 3 on the fourth day. Note widespread opacities.

than in the sham-operated animals. In the experimental group blood glucose was lower ($P < 0.05$) and blood amylase was higher ($P < 0.01$) than in the sham-operated dogs. Plasma catecholamine level was in both groups many times higher than the normal value; plasma lactate, arterial blood gases, and pH were normal in both groups.

Further course. In the experimental group, systemic blood pressure fell to a lower level ($P < 0.02$), pulmonary artery pressure increased to a higher level ($P < 0.01$), pulmonary vascular conductance remained lower ($P < 0.01$) than in the sham-operated animals, and serum amylase continued to rise. Other parameters changed in a similar fashion in both groups, and arterial blood gases and pH remained normal in all animals.

After the last measurement the animals were laid on their side and restrained with wide canvas belts. Since at this stage vomiting was common in the experimental group, the Magill tube was not removed. A continuous intravenous infusion of 2 to 4 ml. per minute of 3.5 percent gelatin polymer in isotonic NaCl, K, and Ca (Haemaccell, Hoechst) was commenced and maintained overnight. All sham-operated dogs were alive the next morning. Of the experimental group, six dogs died within 14 hours after operation and two were alive the next day. Both these survivors were hypotensive (60 to 85 mm. Hg), their cardiac output was

Table I. *Circulatory parameters in acute hemorrhagic pancreatitis*

	Patient		
	1	2	3
Pulmonary arterial pressure (mm. Hg)	60/24 = 36	30/12 = 22	50/20 = 32
Pulmonary arterial wedge pressure (mm. Hg)	10	8	10
Cardiac output (L./min.)	5.50	5.40	9.00
Systemic arterial pressure (mm. Hg)	105/65	80/55	100/60
Blood volume (L.)	—	5.20	5.10

reduced (2.51 per minute per square meter of body surface area), and serum amylase levels were excessively elevated (1,720 and 1,280 U., respectively).

Postmortem findings. In the experimental group the pancreas was severely hemorrhagic and in the peritoneal cavity 300 to 1,500 ml. (mean 760 ml.) blood was found. In sham-operated animals (who were all killed on the second day), the pancreas appeared normal and the peritoneal cavity contained 500 to 900 ml. (mean 700 ml.) of blood. This was probably related to heparin.

Patient studies. Results of the first measurements obtained shortly after admission to the intensive-care unit are shown in Table I. In Patient 1 both blood flow and blood pressure were normal; Patient 2 was hypotensive with normal blood flow and blood volume; in Patient 3 cardiac output was high, blood pressure and blood volume were normal. In all three pulmonary arterial wedge pressure was normal but pulmonary arterial pressure was elevated.

In Patient 1 pulmonary arterial pressure decreased 3 days later to 40/20 (mean 26) mm. Hg, pulmonary arterial wedge pressure remained unchanged, and cardiac output was 6.0 L.; on the fourth day the Swan-Ganz catheter was removed and the patient was returned to the ward, where he eventually recovered. In Patient 2 pulmonary artery pressure was unchanged on the second day; the Swan-Ganz catheter was removed and she was returned to the ward, where she made an uneventful recovery. In Patient 3 pulmonary artery pressure remained elevated for the next 3 days; on the fourth day the patient died and the diagnosis of acute hemorrhagic pancreatitis was confirmed at autopsy.

Radiologic appearance of the lung and arterial blood gases were normal in Patients 1 and 2 and these were also normal at admission in Patient 3 (Fig. 3). However, on the second day Patient 3 developed respiratory distress, was intubated, and commenced on assisted ventilation. One day prior to his death he required 70 percent inspired O_2 concentration in order to maintain normal (93 mm. Hg) arterial Po_2. Chest roentgenogram, taken on that day, is shown in Fig. 4.

DISCUSSION

Contrary to previous descriptions, induction of pancreatitis in these dogs was not followed by rapid and dramatic deterioration of various physiological parameters. Instead, circulation showed a slow and progressive decline in both the sham-operated and experimental groups, accompanied by a reduction in vascular conductance (i.e., increased vascular resistance) in the total systemic and femoral arterial circuits, consistent with the high level of circulating catecholamines found in both groups of animals. Increased systemic arterial resistance in both sham-operated and pancreatic dogs was at variance with the hypothesis that activation of vasodilator agents contribute to pancreatitis-induced circulatory failure.

Postoperative blood loss was also a common feature in both sham-operated and pancreatitis dogs. The volume of the gelatin polymer administered was equal to, or in excess of, the amounts of blood recovered from the peritoneal cavities and, as indicated by the absence of lactic acidosis, the replacement of the blood loss was not grossly inadequate. Despite comparative blood loss and rate of replacement, circulatory failure and death occurred only in the pancreatitis group, suggesting that hypovolemia was not the principal cause of death.

In our three patients, blood volume was well maintained and this may have been a factor in preventing an increase in systemic arterial resistance. In addition, a septic component present in these patients could have also been responsible for the decreased vascular tone. The subordinate role played by hypovolemia and by the reduction in cardiac output is supported by findings in Patient 3: at 3 hours prior to death his blood volume was 5.3 L. and his cardiac output 8.5 L.

Clinical and radiological evidence of pulmonary complications are frequently seen in acute pancreatitis.[15] More recently, the early occurrence of arterial hypoxemia and hypocapnia was reported,[14] but we are unaware of any previous observation concerning the involvement of the pulmonary circulation.

At the onset of the disease, when pulmonary arterial pressure was already elevated, the chest x-ray and arterial blood gases were invariably normal in all dogs and in all patients, suggesting that respiratory failure is not prerequisite to the development of pulmonary hypertension or, in other words, hypoxia is not likely to represent its cause.

In both dogs and patients, pulmonary hypertension was accompanied by normal pulmonary artery wedge pressure; cardiac output was somewhat reduced in dogs and was normal or elevated in patients. We suggest that this hitherto unrecognized form of pulmonary hypertension is secondary to pulmonary arteriolar constriction and is probably related to the release of a pulmonary vasoactive agent from the damaged pancreas.

The skillful technical assistance of John Frazer and Margaret Horvat is gratefully acknowledged. Haemaccell was generously supplied by Hoechst Pty., Ltd.

REFERENCES

1. Anderson, M. C., Schoenfeld, F. B., Iams, W. B., and Suwa, M.: Circulatory changes in acute pancreatitis, Med. Clin. North Am. **47:** 127, 1967.
2. Bergmeyer, H. U.: Methods of enzymatic analysis, Weinheim, 1963, Verlag Chemie, p. 854.
3. Carey, L. C., and Rodgers, R. E.: Pathophysiologic alterations in experimental pancreatitis, SURGERY **60:** 171, 1966.
4. Goodman, A. H.: A transistorized squarewave electromagnetic flowmeter. I, II, Med. Biol. Eng. **7:** 115, 133, 1969.
5. Halmagyi, D. F. J., Goodman, A. H., and Neering, I. R.: Hindlimb blood flow and oxygen usage in hemorrhagic shock, J. Appl. Physiol. **27:** 508, 1969.
6. Halmagyi, D. F. J., Kennedy, M., and Goodman, A. H.: Response to dextran in posthemorrhagic shock after combined adrenergic receptor blockade, J. Appl. Physiol. **30:** 186, 1971.
7. Halmagyi, D. F. J., Kennedy, M., and Varga, D.: Combined adrenergic receptor blockade and circulating catecholamines in hemorrhagic shock, Eur. Surg. Res. **3:** 378, 1971.
8. Karmody, A. M., and Galloway, J. M. D.: Hemorrhagic shock in early acute pancreatitis, Br. J. Surg. **58:** 519, 1971.
9. McCutcheon, A. D., and Race, D.: Experimental pancreatitis: A possible etiology of postoperative pancreatitis, Ann. Surg. **155:** 523, 1962.
10. Nugent, F. W., Zubert, S., and Bulan, M. D.: Kinin precursors in experimental pancreatitis, Proc. Soc. Exp. Biol. Med. **130:** 566, 1969.
11. Ofstad, E.: Formation and destruction of plasma kinins during experimental acute hemorrhagic pancreatitis in dogs, Scand. J. Gastroenterol. **5** (Suppl. 5): 1970.
12. Olson, G. F.: Optimal conditions for the enzymatic determination of *l*-lactic acid, Clin. Chem. **1:** 8, 1962.
13. Pfeffer, R. B., Stasior, O., and Hinton, J. W.: The clinical picture of the sequential development of acute hemorrhagic pancreatitis in the dog, Surg. Forum **8:** 248, 1957.
14. Ranson, J. H. C., Roses, D. F., and Fink, S. D.: Early respiratory insufficiency in acute pancreatitis, Ann. Surg. **178:** 75, 1973.
15. Roseman, D. M., Kowlessar, O. D., and Sleisinger, M. H.: Pulmonary manifestations of pancreatitis, N. Engl. J. Med. **263:** 294, 1960.
16. Ryan, J. W., Moffat, J. G., and Thompson, A. G.: Role of bradykinin system in acute hemorrhagic pancreatitis, Arch. Surg. **91:** 14, 1965.
17. Schiller, W. R., Duprez, A., Iams, W. B., Suwa, M., and Anderson, M. C.: Experimental pancreatitis, Arch. Surg. **98:** 698, 1969.

Reticuloendothelial function: Determinant for survival following hepatic ischemia in the baboon

Isik Olcay, M.D., Klaus Holper, M.D., Akio Kitahama, M.D., Robert H. Miller, M.D., Theodore Drapanas, M.D., Rafael A. Trejo, M.D., Ph.D., *and* **Nicholas R. Di Luzio, Ph.D.,** *New Orleans, La.*

The influence of hepatic ischemia on reticuloendothelial (RE) function and on the development of systemic endotoxemia was evaluated and related to subsequent mortality patterns of Papio papio baboons. Of baboons undergoing 60 minutes of complete hepatic vascular occlusion, 60 percent manifested endotoxemia in both portal venous and femoral arterial plasma. All animals undergoing 90 minutes of hepatic ischemia developed systemic endotoxemia. Blood samples obtained from sham-operated and experimental animals prior to occlusion were endotoxin negative. The degree and persistence of endotoxemia did not appear to correlate with the ultimate fate of the animal. In contrast, RE dysfunction, as reflected by the impairment in the clearance of the ^{131}I-triolein RE test-lipid emulsion correlated with ultimate mortality patterns. Baboons which developed phagocytic depression 24 hours after hepatic insult ultimately died, while those which manifested minor modifications of RE function survived. These studies reveal that RE dysfunction may be contributory to fatal outcome in shock due to hepatic ischemia.

From the Departments of Surgery and Physiology, Tulane University School of Medicine, New Orleans, La.

Liver ischemia in the *Papio papio* baboon, induced by total normothermic hepatic occlusion, was associated with hepatic parenchymal and reticuloendothelial (RE) dysfunction.[10] In a retrospective analysis it was found that the degree of impairment of RE function significantly distinguished survivors from nonsurviving animals. Survival was associated with relatively normal phagocytic function, whereas the nonsurviving group manifested pronounced impairment of phagocytic activity. In contrast to these findings, alterations in hepatic parenchymal cell function did not distinguish the survivors from the nonsurviving group. Thus RE status rather than hepatic parenchymal function appeared to be of greater prognostic value following hepatic ischemia.

The reticuloendothelial system (RES), of which the Kupffer cells are the major functional component,[2] has been postulated to play an important role in systemic cardiovascular homeostasis.[8, 9, 15] Fine[7] proposed that bacterial endotoxins of intestinal origin are the final denominator in a variety of terminal shock forms. This possibility is, in part, based upon the previous observations that host defense against bacterial endotoxins depends upon the functional status of the RES.[1, 3, 17] The RES participates to a major

This study was supported in part by the American Heart Association, the Louisiana Heart Association, and National Institutes of Health Grant AM 13935.

Accepted for publication July 18, 1974.

Reprint requests: N. R. Di Luzio, Ph.D., Department of Physiology, Tulane University School of Medicine, New Orleans, La. 70112.

Table I. *The presence of endotoxin in various vascular components prior to, during, and following ischemia induced by total normothermic hepatic occlusion without venous decompression*

Animal No.	Ischemic interval (min.)	Endotoxin: Preocclusion: Portal vein and femoral artery	Endotoxin: During occlusion: Portal vein	Endotoxin: During occlusion: Femoral artery	Endotoxin: Postocclusion: Femoral artery
1	60	†	‡	‡	‡
2	60	†	‡	†	‡
3	60	†	†	†	†
4	60	†	‡	‡	‡
5	60	†	†	†	†
6	90	†	‡	†	‡
7	90	†	‡	†	‡
8	90	†	‡	†	§
9*	0	†	†	†	†

*Sham operated.
†Negative endotoxin concentrations.
‡Low (0.01 to 0.1 μg per milliliter) endotoxin concentrations.
§High (1.0 to 3.0 μg per milliliter) endotoxin concentrations.

Table II. *The presence of endotoxin in femoral arterial plasma prior to, during, and following ischemia induced by total normothermic hepatic vascular occlusion with venous decompression*

Animal No.	Ischemic interval (min.)	Endotoxin: Prior to operation	Endotoxin: During hepatic ischemia	Endotoxin: Following hepatic ischemia
10	90	†	†	†
11	90	†	‡	§
12	90	†	†	§
13	90	†	‡	‡
14*	0	†	‡	‡
15*	0	†	‡	§

*Sham occlusion.
†Negative endotoxin concentrations.
‡Low (0.01 to 0.1 μg per milliliter) endotoxin concentrations.
§Medium (0.1 to 1.0 μg per milliliter) endotoxin concentrations.

extent in the vascular clearance of endotoxin. Furthermore, since endotoxin detoxification is an exclusive property of the RES,[6, 11, 16] ischemic insult to Kupffer cells might result in their failure to detoxify endotoxin.

In view of the predicated importance of systemic endotoxemia in the development and progression of shock states and our previous observations of RE dysfunction in ischemic shock,[10] studies were undertaken to evaluate whether endotoxemia developed in portal and arterial blood following hepatic ischemia in the subhuman primate. An effort was made to correlate the occurrence and degree of endotoxemia and reticuloendothelial dysfunction with the development of shock and lethality following hepatic ischemia.

MATERIALS AND METHODS

Fifteen healthy *Papio papio* baboons of either sex and weighing between 9 and 16 kilograms were anesthetized and prepared for experimental procedures as previously described.[10] Since the method employed to determine phagocytic function was identical to that previously outlined,[10] it is not described herein.

The animals were divided into two main groups. One group of eight animals was subjected to 60 or 90 minutes of liver ischemia induced by total normothermic hepatic vascular occlusion without portacaval decompression. A sham operation was done on one animal for control purposes.

In a second group, six baboons underwent portacaval shunting by interposition of a Dacron graft. An end-to-side anastomosis was performed at each end of the graft to the inferior vena cava and to the portal vein. This procedure required a temporary interruption of portal vein flow for a period of approximately 20 to 25 minutes during insertion of the graft. Upon completion of the shunt, a normalization period of approxi-

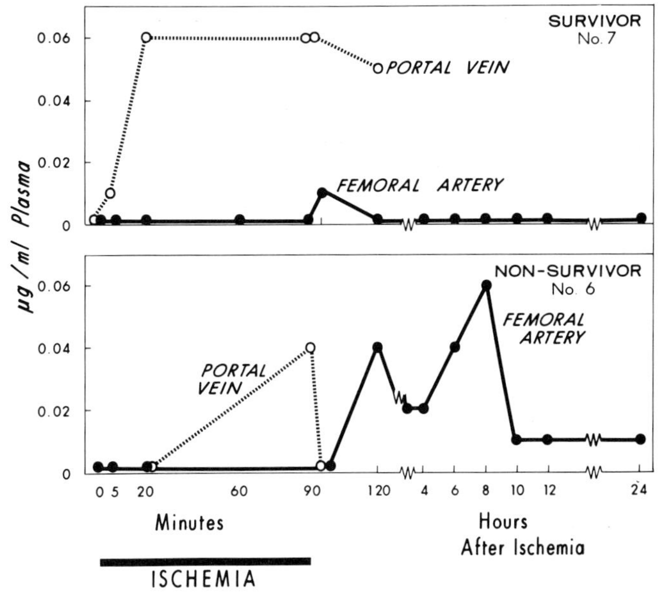

Fig. 1. The appearance of circulating endotoxin in portal vein and femoral artery in two representative experiments during and following 90 minutes of total hepatic ischemia without venous decompression. Peak levels occur either shortly after onset or in the final phase of the occlusion.

mately 15 minutes followed. Normothermic hepatic ischemia (90 minutes) was then produced in four of these animals. Following release of the occlusion and restoration of hepatic blood flow, the portacaval shunt which was left in place was ligated near both anastomoses and sectioned. Two animals with portacaval shunts, which did not undergo occlusion, served as sham controls. Portal vein samples were not obtained in this group in order to maintain the patency of the shunt. The portacaval shunt experiments were undertaken to determine the importance of stasis of the splanchnic vascular bed in the development of systemic endotoxemia following the induction of hepatic ischemia.

Endotoxin determinations[13, 14] were performed prior to, during, and at varying intervals following hepatic ischemia. Since the method to produce ischemia also included occlusion of the infrahepatic vena cava, caval blood as well as femoral arterial and portal venous blood were also tested for endotoxin.

RESULTS

In order to convey the response of the experimental baboons relative to the presence or absence of endotoxin in various vessels, a summary of the data is presented in Tables I and II. Plasma samples obtained from either portal vein (Table I) and the femoral artery (Tables I and II) prior to any initiation of experimental procedures were consistently negative for endotoxin. In 40 percent of the animals subjected to 60 minutes of ischemia, endotoxin was not detected in either portal vein, femoral artery, or inferior vena cava at any time during or following the occlusive episode. However, in the remaining 60 percent of the animals, endotoxin was detected both in portal vein and femoral artery blood (Table I).

In three baboons in which all preocclusive determinations for endotoxin were negative and which were subjected to 30 additional minutes of ischemia, i.e., 90 minutes without venous decompression, the plasma from the portal vein and femoral artery was endotoxin positive (Table I). The sham-operated animal was endotoxin free at all times throughout the experimental procedure.

The presence of a portacaval shunt in baboons subjected to 90 minutes of hepatic ischemia did not materially modify systemic endotoxemia (Table II). It appeared that in certain instances (baboons 14 and 15) the

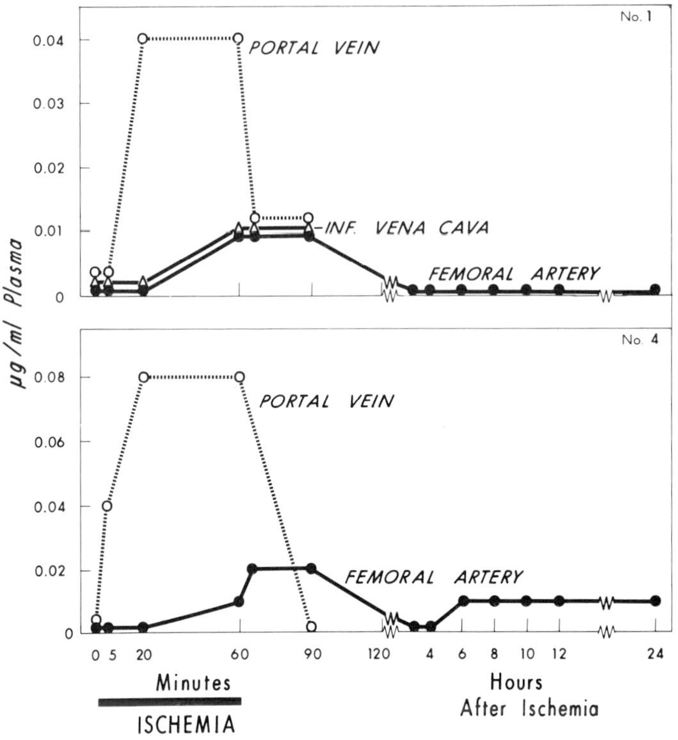

Fig. 2. Two representative experiments of endotoxin concentration of portal vein, femoral artery, and inferior vena caval plasma during and following 60 minutes of total hepatic ischemia without venous decompression. Endotoxin appeared in femoral arterial and inferior vena caval plasma prior to release of the occlusion.

insertion of the portacaval shunt alone resulted in transient periods of endotoxemia as denoted by the presence of endotoxin in femoral plasma.

In view of the diversity of the endotoxin response in different vessels, representative results are portrayed in the various figures (Figs. 1 to 8). Endotoxin was invariably first detected in the portal blood at early stages during the occlusive interval (Fig. 1). In three of the animals undergoing either 60 or 90 minutes of hepatic ischemia, endotoxin was detectable in portal venous blood almost immediately following the occlusion (as demonstrated in Fig. 1, baboon 7). In the other three baboons portal vein blood was positive for endotoxin 20 minutes following the onset of the occlusion (Fig. 1, baboon 6). Two of the animals did not show any endotoxin either in the portal or in the systemic blood during the occlusive interval. In 50 percent of the animals which were endotoxin positive, the peak portal endotoxin concentration occurred 20 minutes after onset of occlusion (Fig. 1, baboon 7). No further increase in concentration was demonstrated during the remainder of the occlusive period. In contrast, in the remaining 50 percent the highest endotoxin concentration was detected in the final phase of the occlusion (Fig. 1, baboon 6).

The initial appearance of endotoxin in femoral arterial blood in 66 percent of the baboons was shortly after release of the occlusion and restoration of hepatic blood flow (Fig. 1). The remaining population of baboons were endotoxin positive prior to release of occlusion (Fig. 2). During the occlusive period the endotoxin concentration was consistently higher in portal plasma than in the arterial blood. In all animals except one (Fig. 1, baboon 7) portal endotoxin concentration decreased immediately following release of the occlusion and re-establishment of portal

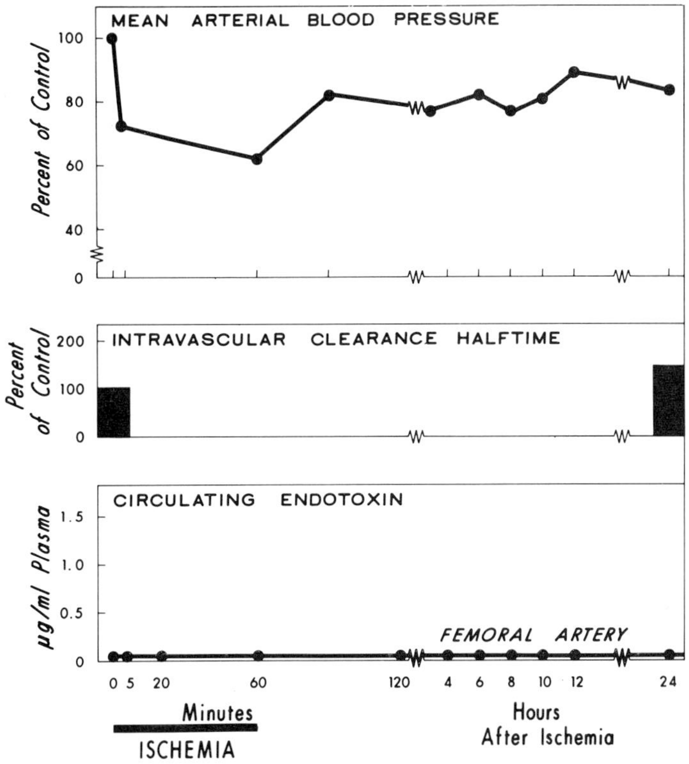

Fig. 3. The data derived from three animals which underwent 60 minutes of total hepatic occlusion denote that relatively normal phagocytic activity and the absence of circulating endotoxin were associated with early recovery and survival. The hypotension which occurred during occlusion of the hepatic vascular bed is also apparent.

vein and hepatic artery flow (Figs. 1 and 2). The magnitude and duration of portal endotoxemia during the occlusion did not correlate with the degree of subsequent endotoxemia in the systemic circulation following revascularization. The endotoxin concentration of infrahepatic plasma obtained from the vena cava was identical to that found in the arterial blood (Fig. 2).

The incidence and magnitude of endotoxemia was compared to the ultimate fate of the animal in an effort to establish a possible relationship between the events. Initial portal as well as postocclusive systemic endotoxin concentrations were not different in surviving and nonsurviving animals. The mean endotoxin concentration during the first 24 hour interval as determined by integrating the area under the endotoxin concentration curve, likewise denoted lack of correlation between the degree of endotoxemia and the ultimate outcome.

The results of experiments where endotoxin determinations and RE function were performed simultaneously were analyzed and grouped on the basis of survival time. Mean values of three animals (baboons 3, 4, and 5) are depicted in Fig. 3. The control intravascular clearance half time ($t_{1/2}$) of the RE test lipid emulsion was 18.7 ± 2.3 minutes. The assessment of RE function following 60 minutes of total hepatic ischemia without venous decompression indicated only slight prolongation of the half time to 145 percent of control values at the 24 hour interval. The mean systemic endotoxin concentration in these animals was essentially zero. In these three baboons the initial hypotensive episode during occlusion of hepatic blood flow was followed by recovery of arterial blood pressure to 83 percent of control values at 24 hours and subsequent survival of all three animals (Fig. 3).

In agreement with previous observations,

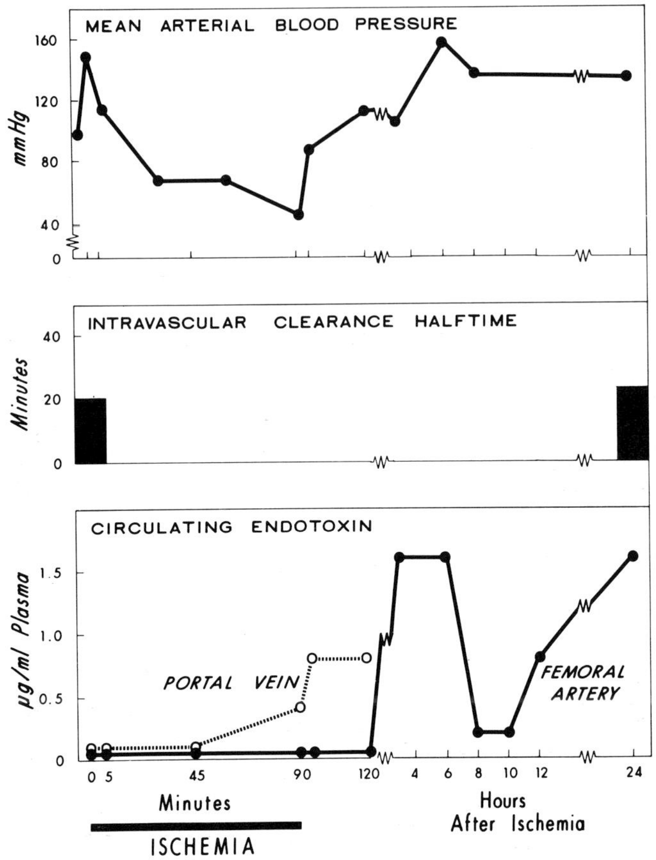

Fig. 4. The persistent endotoxemia in the presence of normal phagocytic activity was compatible with subsequent survival of this baboon which underwent 90 minutes of total hepatic occlusion.

persistent endotoxemia occurred in one of the baboons undergoing 90 minutes of ischemia over a period of 24 hours (Fig. 4). The persistence of endotoxemia was not associated with RE dysfunction, as reflected by normal vascular clearance of the lipid emulsion. During the occlusive interval, as generally observed, mean arterial blood pressure declined to a hypotensive state. Normalization of blood pressure and survival of the animal occurred in the obvious presence of sustained endotoxemia. An evaluation of RE function data of the 4 baboons (Figs. 3 and 4) which survived either 60 and 90 minutes of total hepatic ischemia indicated that phagocytic function was essentially unaltered.

The data relative to mean arterial blood pressure, phagocytic function, and systemic endotoxemia in three portacaval shunted animals which underwent 90 minutes of hepatic ischemia and died are presented in Fig. 5. The mean arterial blood pressure declined 25 percent within 5 minutes following the ischemic insult. Blood pressure continued to decrease to 47 percent of control at the end of the ischemic interval. The decrease of blood pressure occurred despite the presence of a patent portacaval shunt and the degree of hypotension was similar to that observed in nonshunted baboons.

Persistent endotoxemia was also observed in these three portacaval-shunted animals. The first positive interval of systemic endotoxemia occurred at the end of the hepatic ischemia when plasma endotoxin concentrations ranged from 0.1 to 0.8 μg per milliliter (Fig. 5). Peak endotoxin levels appeared in the three animals between 6 and 12 hours

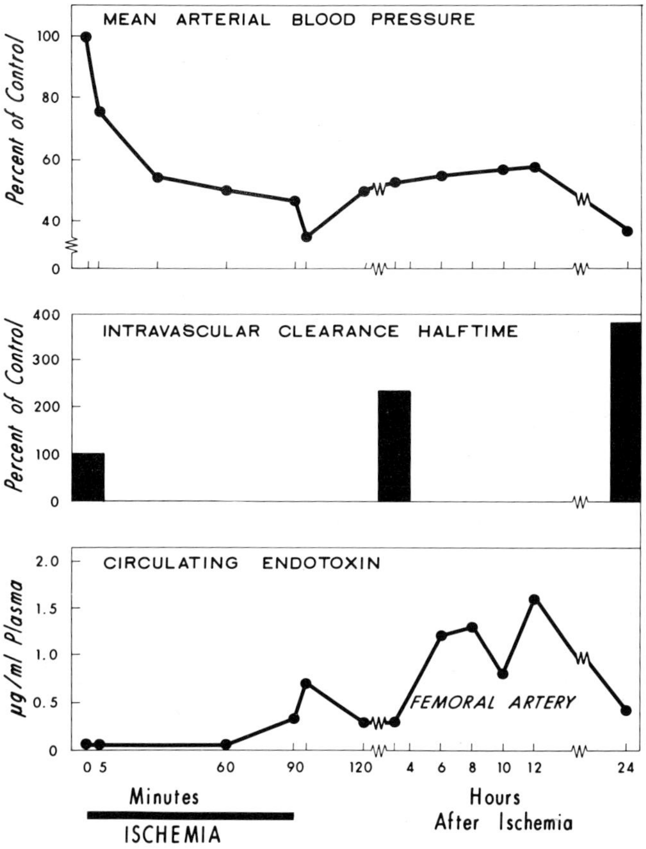

Fig. 5. Mean data relative to plasma endotoxin concentration, phagocytic function, and arterial blood pressure of three baboons which underwent 90 minutes of hepatic ischemia with portacaval shunting. Persistent endotoxemia in the presence of impaired RE function characterized the fatal outcome of these three baboons.

after ischemia and ranged from 1.6 to 3.2 μg per milliliter. A decline in circulating endotoxin was observed in all animals to a mean of 0.4 μg per milliliter at the 24 hour interval.

Phagocytic activity, as indicated by the intravascular clearance half time of the RE test lipid emulsion, was markedly depressed in these animals (Fig. 5). Compared to their mean control values of 19.1 $\pm$ 4.2 minutes, the half time periods at 3 and 24 hours were prolonged 2.4 and 3.8 fold, respectively. Pronounced depression of RE function and persistent endotoxemia was associated with the subsequent death of all animals. In contrast, no impairment of RE function was observed in the one animal which survived the 90 minute ischemic interval, as denoted by the unaltered intravascular clearance rate (Fig. 6). In this animal circulating endotoxin was not detected during the experiment. The mean arterial blood pressure was normalized at early postischemic intervals.

The course of two sham-operated baboons undergoing only portacaval shunting is depicted in Figs. 7 and 8. In one animal which survived (Fig. 7), phagocytic activity was not altered at the 3 and 24 hour intervals. Blood pressure was normalized in the presence of circulating endotoxin. In contrast, in the second sham-operated baboon a pronounced depression of phagocytic activity, as indicated by the prolongation of the half time from the initial value of 24 to 58 minutes occurred 24 hours after surgery (Fig. 8). Although endotoxin was initially present in the systemic circulation during the period of sham occlusion, endotoxin was not detectable

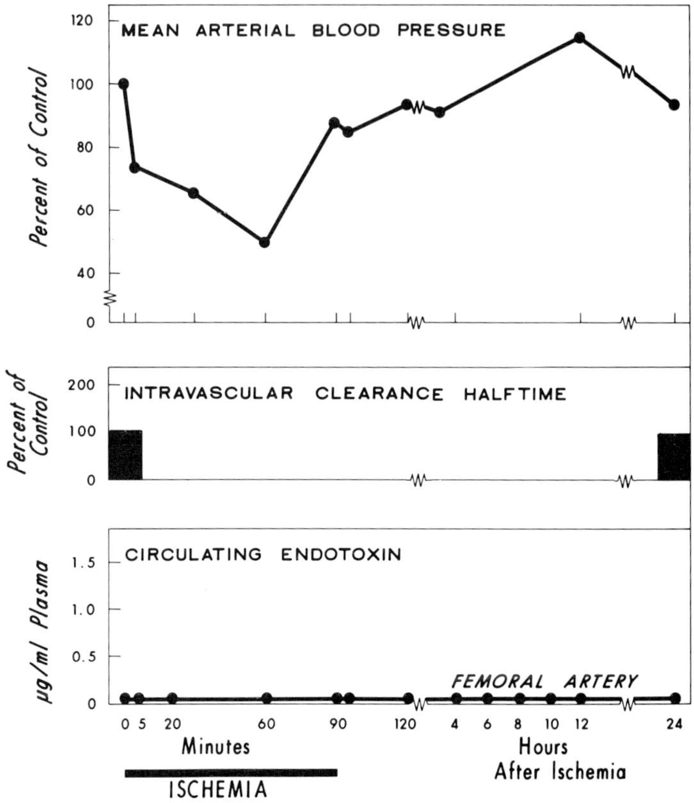

Fig. 6. Normal phagocytic activity, absence of endotoxemia and normalization of blood pressure is observed in one baboon surviving 90 minutes of hepatic ischemia with portacaval shunting.

in plasma at early intervals following restoration of hepatic blood flow. However, at the 6 hour interval endotoxin was again detectable. The endotoxin concentration continued to increase until the tenth hour and remained at this elevated level. A mild hypotensive response was observed in this baboon. The occurrence of RE dysfunction in this sham-operated baboon, which succumbed at 36 hours, supports the possible relationship between RE dysfunction and death.

DISCUSSION

These results confirm our previous findings of a suggested correlation between the status of RE function and the ultimate outcome of baboons subjected to hepatic ischemia.[10] Survival was consistently associated with normal RE function, while in contrast, death occurred in the presence of impairment of phagocytic activity. It appears that the degree of insult to the RES is an important factor which may determine the postischemic status of the baboon and its ability to resist shock.

In view of the hypotensive status induced following hepatic ischemia in certain, but not all of the baboons which subsequently died, consideration has to be made relative to the possibility that impaired phagocytic function could be mediated by reduced blood pressure and a resulting decrease in liver blood flow. This possibility appears unlikely since it was observed in previous studies[10] that liver blood flow was not altered in baboons when phagocytic function was significantly depressed.

Employing the Limulus test for assay of endotoxins, it was possible to determine the incidence, magnitude, and duration of endotoxemia and relate these changes to RE function and final outcome. Although Elin and

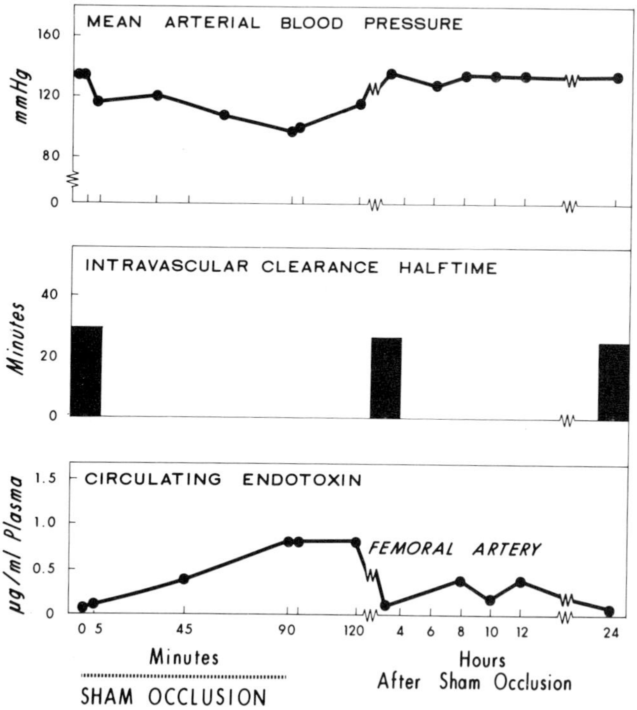

Fig. 7. Transient endotoxemia in the presence of normal phagocytic activity and blood pressure is denoted in one baboon following sham portacaval shunting. This animal recovered spontaneously.

Wolff[5] have reported the nonspecificity of the Limulus lysate test for endotoxins, their conclusions were based upon the positive reaction of the lysate with polynucleotides and certain coagulation factors, i.e., thrombin and thromboplastin. Our previous studies denoted that a negative Limulus lysate test was manifested in germ-free rats undergoing portal vein occlusion, an event which in conventional rats was associated with pronounced portal vein and systemic endotoxemia.[13] These findings would appear to indicate that gram-negative bacteria, present in the gastrointestinal tract, are the source of the endotoxins following restriction of hepatic flow. It therefore appears that nonspecific factors, as denoted by Elin and Wolff,[5] are not of importance in the hepatic ischemia model.

By simultaneous determinations of the concentrations of endotoxin in portal, caval, and arterial plasma, conclusions on the origin of endotoxin can be drawn. The consistent finding of higher endotoxin concentrations in portal plasma during the occlusion, as compared to endotoxin levels determined simultaneously in the systemic plasma, supports previous reports that the circulating endotoxin is of intestinal origin.[6, 7, 13] The appearance of detectable endotoxin in the arterial circulation prior to release of the occlusion suggests that the endotoxin travels either via direct portasystemic pathways in primates, as demonstrated by Milnes and associates,[12] or via lymphatic vessels. The endotoxin concentration determined in the infrahepatic vena cava plasma was uniformly equal to that found in arterial plasma, denoting the relative absence of extraction of endotoxin by peripheral tissues.

The role of circulating endotoxin in the induction of RE dysfunction appears to be minimal. The coexistence of endotoxemia and normal phagocytic activity appears to exclude a deleterious effect of endotoxin on the Kupffer cells insofar as phagocytic function is concerned. Circulating levels of endotoxin were, on occasion, well tolerated, as reflected

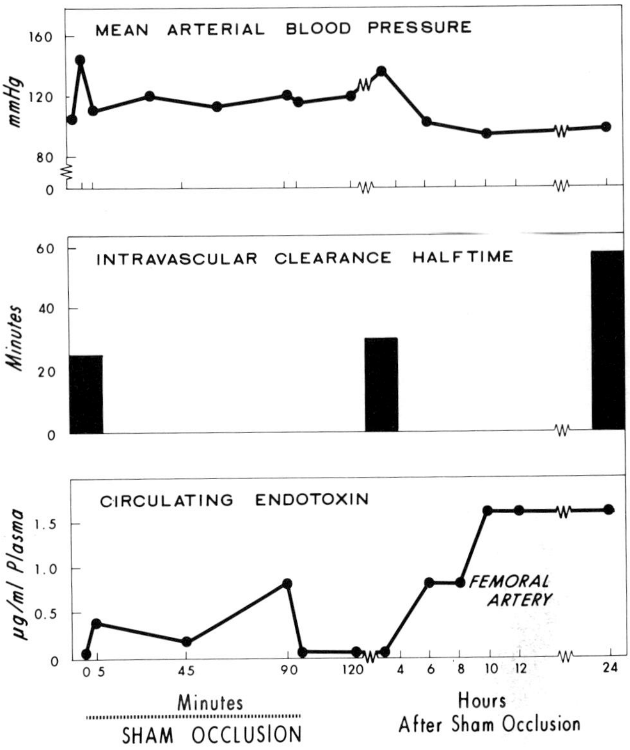

Fig. 8. Data obtained from one baboon which underwent portacaval shunting for control purposes. The transient endotoxemia was replaced by persistent endotoxemia and deteriorating of phagocytic activity. The baboon died 36 hours following the initiation of the sham operation.

in the normalization of blood pressure as well as the absence of lethality in the presence of normal phagocytic function. In contrast, lethality following ischemic insult was manifested only under circumstances where phagocytic function was markedly depressed. The impairment in phagocytic function may well reflect other functional alterations of macrophages, such as detoxification or other metabolic events, which may be of equal or greater significance in the response of the host to an ischemic insult. The present data support our previous observations[10] that the RE function test is of apparent value in the assessment of final outcome of the baboon following hepatic ischemia. Normal RE function 24 hours after ischemia was consistently associated with recovery of the animals, even in the presence of endotoxemia. In contrast, RE dysfunction was invariably associated with endotoxemia and subsequent death. These findings denote that measurement of the functional activity of Kupffer cells may be of significant value in the assessment of, as well as the prognosis of, hepatic ischemic injury.

REFERENCES

1. Beeson, P. B.: Effect of reticuloendothelial blockade on immunity to the Schwartzman phenomenon, Proc. Soc. Exp. Biol. Med. **64:** 146, 1947.
2. Biozzi, G., and Stiffel, C.: The pathophysiology of the reticuloendothelial cells of the liver and the spleen, *in* Popper, H., and Schaffner, F., editors: Progress in liver disease, New York, 1965, Grune & Stratton, Inc., p. 166.
3. Crafton, C. G., and Di Luzio, N. R.: Relationship of reticuloendothelial function activity to endotoxin lethality, Am. J. Physiol. **217:** 736, 1969.
4. Cuevas, P., and Fine, J.: Route of absorption of endotoxin from the intestine in nonseptic shock, J. Reticuloendothel. Soc. **11:** 538, 1972.
5. Elin, R. S., and Wolff, S. M.: Nonspecificity of the Limulus amebocyte lysate test: Positive

reactions with polynucleotides and proteins, J. Infect. Dis. **128:** 349, 1973.
6. Filkins, J. P.: Hepatic lysosomes and the inactivation of endotoxin, J. Reticuloendothel. Soc. **9:** 480, 1971.
7. Fine, J.: The intestinal circulation in shock, Gastroenterology, **52:** 454, 1967.
8. Gans, H.: Preservation of vascular patency as a function of reticuloendothelial clearance, SURGERY **60:** 1216, 1966.
9. Glass, K., Palmerio, C., and Fine, J.: Further evidence of the role of the reticuloendothelial system in the maintenance of vascular integrity, SURGERY **66:** 709, 1969.
10. Holper, K., Olcay, I., Trejo, R. A., Miller, R., Kitahama, A., Di Luzio, N. R., Brettschneider, L., and Drapanas, T.: Effects of ischemia on hepatic parenchymal and reticuloendothelial function in the baboon, SURGERY **76:** 423, 1974.
11. Levin, J., Poore, T. E., Zauber, N. P., and Oser, R. S.: Detection of endotoxin in the blood of patients with sepsis due to gram-negative bacteria, N. Engl. J. Med. **383:** 1313, 1970.
12. Milnes, R. F., and Child, C. G.: Acute occlusion by ligature of the portal vein in the *Macacus rhesus* monkey, Proc. Soc. Exp. Biol. Med. **70:** 332, 1949.
13. Olcay, I., Kitahama, A., Miller, R. H., Drapanas, T., Trejo, R. A., and Di Luzio, N. R.: Reticuloendothelial dysfunction and endotoxemia following portal vein occlusion, SURGERY **75:** 64, 1974.
14. Rojas-Corona, R. R., Skarnes, R., Tamakuma, S., and Fine, J.: The Limulus coagulation test for endotoxin. A comparison with other assay methods, Proc. Soc. Exp. Biol. Med. **132:** 599, 1969.
15. Selkurt, E. E.: Intestinal ischemic shock and the protective role of the liver, Am. J. Physiol. **197:** 281, 1959.
16. Starzecki, B., Reddin, J. L., Gran, A., and Spink, W. W.: Distribution of endotoxin-^{51}Cr in normal and endotoxin-resistant dogs, Am. J. Physiol. **213:** 1065, 1967.
17. Zweifach, B. W., Benacerraf, B., and Thomas, L.: The relationship between the vascular manifestation of shock produced by endotoxin, trauma, and hemorrhage. II. The possible role of the reticuloendothelial system in resistance to each type of shock, J. Exp. Med. **106:** 403, 1957.

Clinical review

The use of lymphangiography in melanoma

Irving M. Ariel, M.D., F.A.C.S., F.A.C.N.M., *New York, N. Y.*

Lymphography was used to locate metastases in the lymph nodes, thereby aiding in planning the policies for treatment of the cancer. The over-all diagnostic error was 30 percent, both false positive and false negative.

From the Department of Surgery, New York Medical College, and the Pack Medical Foundation, New York, N. Y.

PRINCIPLES of cancer treatment depend upon the local anatomic setting of the cancer and its method of spread. Many cancers spread via the lymphatic vessels to regional lymph nodes. Some knowledge regarding the logistics of lymphatic spread has been obtained by the institution of in vivo lymphography.

Living lymphography (lymphangioadenography) is defined as the roentgenography of the lymphatic channels (lymphangiography) and the lymph nodes (lymphadenography), following the injection of a radiopaque material into a lymphatic vessel. Accordingly, we have been provided with a new dimension in the visualization of the lymphatic dynamic state when cancerous metastases are transferred via a lymphatic vessel to a lymph node, as well as a means for the study of the sequence of events which follow such a transmission. The administration of a canceroidal agent, a radioactive isotope, permits the internal irradiation of not only cancerous deposits within a lymph node, but also of in-transit metastases.

Accepted for publication June 13, 1974.

This work was assisted by Grants in Aid from the Mr. and Mrs. Arnold Rosen Cancer Research Fund, and the Foundation of Clinical Research, New York, N. Y.

Reprint requests: Irving M. Ariel, M.D., F.A.C.S., Pack Medical Foundation, 139 E. 36th St., New York, N. Y. 10016.

LYMPHOGRAPHY IN THE DIAGNOSIS OF MALIGNANT NEOPLASMS

The diagnosis of metastases within a lymph node depends upon the fact that metastases do not concentrate the injected contrast medium, Ethiodol. The normal lymph nodes will concentrate the Ethiodol; when a metastasis of a given size is present, a vacuole remains.

Appearance of normal lymph nodes. The normal lymph node is usually ovoid with a regular contour. However, the normal node may also be "V" or "J" shaped, and frequently there is a small notch in the margin hilum, which is the point of entry of the lymphatic trunk. The opacified, normal lymph node presents a homogeneous and granular appearance. Sometimes a normal lymph node may be partially replaced by fat and/or fibrous tissue lending an appearance similar to that of a cancerous metastasis and a false-positive diagnosis is made. Fischer and Thornbury[6] call attention to another defect in normal lymphography that may lead to a false-positive diagnosis, that is, when two nodes lie closely adjacent, they give the radiographic appearance of a single node with a small space between, suggesting a metastasis. Special studies and oblique views help to delineate these defects.

Appearance of metastases. Metastases appear as a clear area, or vacuole, in an otherwise homogeneously filled lymph node. The observed patterns of metastases are numerous and varied. Frequently, lymph nodes containing metastases demonstrate marginal filling defects due to the presence of small metastases in the subcapsular region presenting a "moth-eaten" appearance. Usually these nodes are of normal size and do not become enlarged until extensive metastases are present.

A study by Koehler, Wohl, and Schaeffer[8] demonstrated that a metastasis must be a minimum of 5 to 10 mm. in diameter before it can be visualized roentgenographically. Numerous examples have been observed of completely normal-appearing lymph nodes containing microscopic deposits of cancer.

When a lymph node is completely replaced by cancer, the flow of the injected Ethiodol completely circumvents this node and it is not visualized roentogenographically. Therefore, the absence of opacification may give the surgeon a false sense of security.

The entire replacement of the node by cancer produces a stoppage in the flow of Ethiodol. Further testament to complete nodal replacement by cancer is the appearance of a pattern of fine, reticular, collateral lymphatic channels branching off from the area of abrupt obstruction.

The accuracy of diagnosing lymph-node metastases by lymphography averages about 30 percent. Errors may be made on two points: false negatives, in which no metastases are observed in a lymph node that appears roentgenographically normal, and false positives, in which defects that are not the result of metastases are observed within a node.

Additional benefits may be derived from lymphography: (1) It permits the oncologist to study both normal and abnormal lymphatic dynamics and to learn more about cancer spread. (2) Since the lymph nodes will retain the radiopaque medium for a period of 6 to 9 months, any change within the lymph node, such as a response to therapy or an increase in size due to cancerous growth, can be observed. (3) It offers the radiotherapist a landmark for the placement of radiotherapeutic portals. (4) One can study the response to x-ray therapy by observing any change in the size of the lymph node, particularly a decrease in size. (5) A repeat lymphogram will provide an assessment as to the status of the malignant process. (6) When chlorophyll is combined with Ethiodol, all the opacified lymph nodes are stained light green. Therefore, preoperative lymphography aids the surgeon, especially the surgical resident, in the visualization of the lymph nodes during the performance of a lymphadenectomy for cancer. (The Federal Drug Administration now prohibits the use of chlorophyll in this instance.) (7) It demonstrates to the surgeon the adequacy of his lymph-node dissection. A preoperative lymphogram is performed, and upon completion of a lymphadenectomy, a repeat roentgenogram taken on the operating table will demonstrate the presence of any retained lymph nodes. It must be borne in mind that a lymph node completely replaced by cancer (unopacified) will not be exhibited on x-ray. However, such cancerous nodes are usually markedly enlarged and are readily visible to the surgeon at the time of operation. (8) It demonstrates abnormalities of the mediastinum by any alteration in the anatomy of the thoracic duct.

COMPLICATIONS

Fischer and Thornbury,[6] in a review of 100 consecutive lymphograms, cite the following complications: (1) fever in 24 patients; (2) roentgenographically demonstrable contrast embolization in (a) lung (asymptomatic) in six patients and (b) liver (asymptomatic) in two patients; (3) extremity edema, worsened in three patients; (4) penile edema in two patients; (5) lymphangitis in two patients; (6) superficial thrombophlebitis in two patients; (7) aseptic incision separation in two patients; (8)

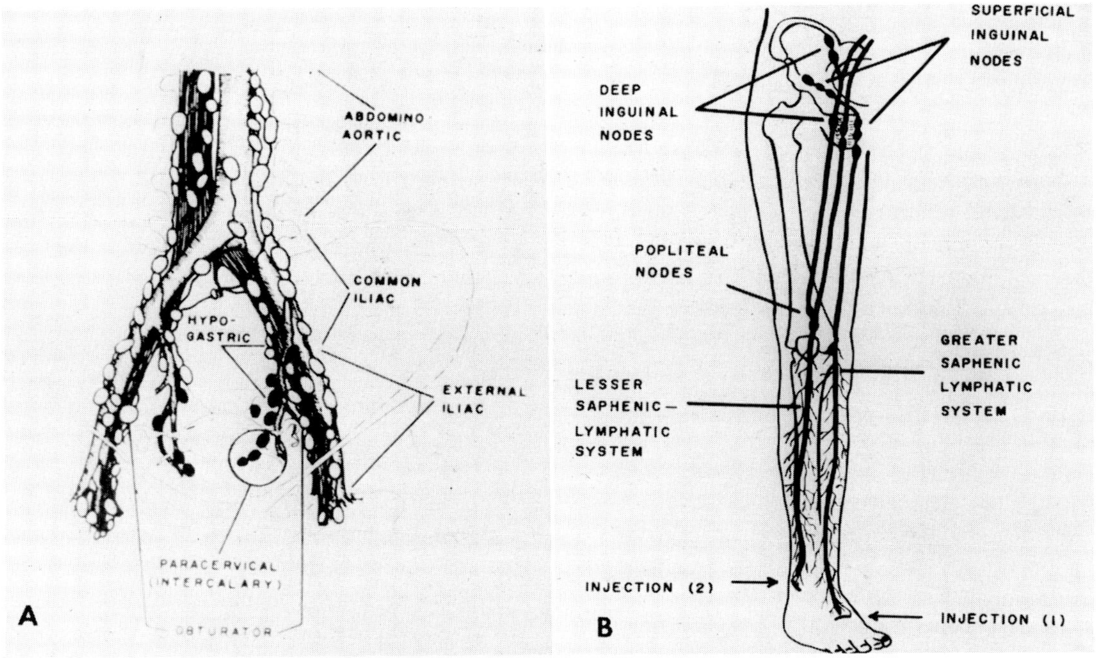

Fig. 1. *A,* Anatomy of lower abdominal lymph nodes; *B,* lymphatic vessels of lower extremity. Injection site 1, on dorsum of foot, drains into greater saphenous lymphatic system. Injection site 2, lateral aspect of ankle, drains into lesser saphenous system, into popliteal lymph nodes, and then to inguinal lymph nodes. (From Ariel and Resnick: Arch. Surg. **94:** 117, 1967.)

allergy to patent blue violet in two patients; (9) postconization parametritis exacerbation in one patient.

In our series of 300 lymphograms, we encountered no significant complications. Ten patients complained of a transient sense of ill-feeling which they could not pinpoint; five of these patients complained of transient mild nausea. The only reaction we have observed was that of slow healing of the incision at the injection site. Inasmuch as many of our patients reecived radioactive isotopes endolymphatically administered with the Ethiodol, we believe the slow healing to be the result of leakage at the site of incision. The simple procedure of pouring one liter of normal saline solution over the wound before it was suture closed obviated this difficulty in the last 100 patients treated.

Spillage of the contrast medium into the lung parenchyma via the thoracic duct is inherent in the technique. As a result, although symptoms are not produced in a patient with normal pulmonary function, a few serious sequelae have been described in patients with extensive pulmonary disease, and two fatal fat embolizations have been reported.[5, 7] This complication has been averted in our patients by means of limiting the amount of contrast medium injected. We inject no more than 6 ml. into each lower-extremity and 4 ml. into each upper-extremity lymphatic vessel.

An occasional patient may show a sensitivity to the dye. Rarely is a patient sensitive to the iodine; however, we had one such patient who developed a macular dermatitis, which responded readily to treatment.

LYMPHATIC DYNAMICS

A knowledge of the normal lymphatic anatomy and physiology provides us with a better understanding of the changes which may occur as a result of both metastasis and the performance of certain surgical and radiological procedures; this understanding will act as a guide to the best possible course of treatment.

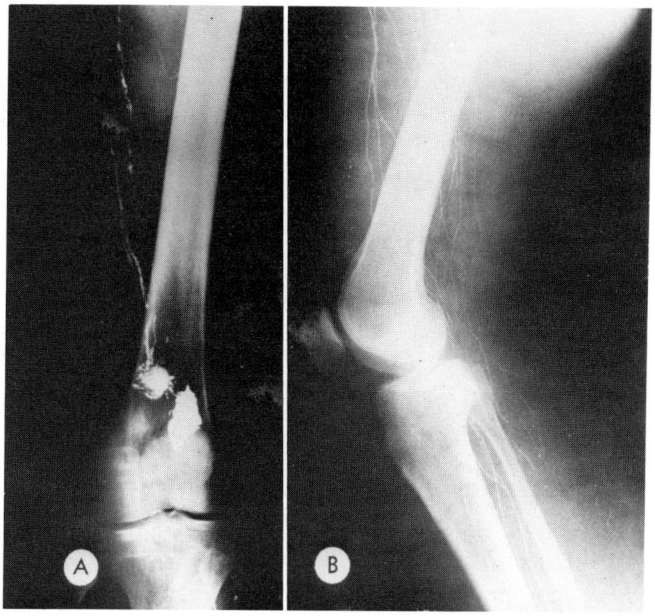

Fig. 2. *A,* Lymphogram of normal man demonstrating two popliteal lymph nodes. Injection made posterior to internal malleolus (courtesy of H. W. Fischer, M.D.). *B,* Lymphogram of a patient with melanoma, performed as in *A,* demonstrating well-developed chain of lymphatic vessels coursing popliteal space; no lymph nodes present. Dissection revealed one popliteal lymph node completely replaced by fat. (Reprinted by permission from the New York State Journal of Medicine, copyright by the Medical Society of the State of New York, Ariel, I. M.: Lymphography and endolymphatic administration of radioactive isotopes for treating cancer, N. Y. State J. Med. **68:** 1252, 1968.) (From Fisher, H. W., and Thornbury, J. R.: Lymphography in the diagnosis of malignant neoplasms, *in* Ariel, I. M., editor: Progress in clinical cancer, vol. 1, New York, 1965, Grune & Stratton, Inc., p. 118, by permission.)

NORMAL LYMPHATIC DYNAMICS

Normally, when Ethiodol is injected into a lymphatic vessel, the medium is transported throughout the lymphatic network with only a slight delay before deposition in the lymph nodes draining the region. The radiopaque material remains within the lymphatic vessels for 3 to 6 hours, and drains within 24 hours in almost every instance. In contrast to blood flow, lymphatic flow is either extremely slow or stagnant when the extremity is in the dependent position. With the patient in a horizontal position, it may take from one to 2 hours to inject 6 ml. of Ethiodol using a pressure pump. Following the intralymphatic injection of Ethiodol, serial roentgenograms will provide an index of the lymphatic distribution pattern.

Lower extremity lymphatic vessels. The lymphatic trunks of the lower extremity usually follow the course of the greater saphenous vein (saphena magna system). The lymphatic vessels vary from 0.25 to 1.0 mm. in diameter, usually retaining their caliber as they ascend toward the inguinal region and usually following a straight course to end abruptly (Fig. 1). When a contrast medium is injected into a lymphatic vessel on the dorsum of the foot (injection site *1,* Fig. 1, *B*), the lymphatic vessels are visualized as one or more trunks coursing proximally along the anteromedial aspect of the leg, converging toward the knee, then ascending and dividing into 12 to 16 divisions as they enter the superficial inguinal lymph nodes. If the opaque material is injected into a lymphatic vessel along the lateral aspect of the foot (injection site *2,* Fig. 1, *B*), the lymphatic vessels are seen to course proximally toward the popliteal fossa (saphena parva system), where one or two popliteal nodes are usually found. Popliteal nodes are found routinely in dogs, whereas in man they are absent in a significant number of patients (Fig. 2). The lymphatic vessels continue to course proximally to the deep lymphatic chain and terminate in the superficial inguinal vessels which course to the thigh and extend medially to enter the groin in juxtaposition to the femoral vessels. Somewhere along the course of the lymphatic vessels, valves are usually found which tend to prevent backflow. The lymph nodes of the saphena parva system (draining the back of the leg and following the course of the lesser saphenous vein) are said to lie deeper and more craniad than those draining the trunk of the greater saphenous system.

Inguinal and iliac lymph nodes (Fig. 1). There are from four to 10 inguinal nodes normally, both superficial and deep, presenting a variable pattern. Efforts to divide this group into subgroups based on a relationship to the greater saphenous vein are believed to be of no practical use in clinical roentgenographic diagnoses.

As originally described by Rouvier,[11] the efferent lymphatic vessels from the inguinal nodes continue proximally to the external iliac chain of nodes to divide into three chains: a lateral chain located lateral to the external iliac artery (one to four nodes), a middle group which lies on the posterior surface of the external iliac vein (two to four nodes), and a medial group (three to four nodes) posterior to the external iliac vein, usually in juxtaposition to the lateral pelvic wall. The obturator node is considered a part of the medial group of the external iliac chain of nodes and is found roentgenographically related; it may lie either in direct continuity with the remainder of the medial chain, or it may be somewhat distant, as a solitary node within the obturator fossa, usually between the external iliac vein and the obturator nerve and vessels.

Continuing proximally, the common iliac chain (four to 12 nodes lying in close relationship to the common iliac artery and vein) subdivides into the hypogastric nodes (two to eight in number) and courses along the hypogastric artery; from the common iliac nodes, several trunks course craniad along the aorta and inferior vena cava to form the abdominoaortic lymph node group (25 to 45 nodes). The abdominoaortic nodes are divided into four groups: (1) right lateral aortic, (2) left lateral aortic, (3) preaortic, and (4) retroaortic. Efferent lymphatic vessels from the abdominoaortic chain empty into the cisterna chyli usually at the level of the second lumbar vertebra. Rarely can lymph nodes be visualized in the posterior mediastinum, but not infrequently supraclavicular nodes may be seen in the region of the termination of the thoracic duct.

Upper extremity lymphatics. There are usually two groups of lymphatic vessels in the upper extremity, a lateral and a medial, which join above the elbow and usually follow the basilic vein along the inner aspect of the arm to the axillary chain of lymph nodes. The axillary nodes vary in number, are interconnected by many trunks, and their efferents may drain either directly into the subclavian vein or may lead to the supraclavicular nodes and then empty into the subclavian vein. Inconsistently, one or two small lymph nodes may be visualized in the epitrochlear region along the medial aspect.

Lymphatic-vascular communications. A communication normally exists between the lymphatic and venous systems. Rusznyak, Foldi, and Szabo[12, 13] have demonstrated anastomoses between the lymphatic vessels and the veins, especially in the thyroid, kidney, and liver. Blalock and associates[3] demonstrated the presence of numerous connections between the lymphatic vessels and the inferior vena cava, the azygous, and other veins, especially after ligation of the thoracic duct. Pressman and associates[10] demonstrated a communication between the lymph nodes and the blood vessels by injecting air into the lymph nodes of animals; the air was seen in

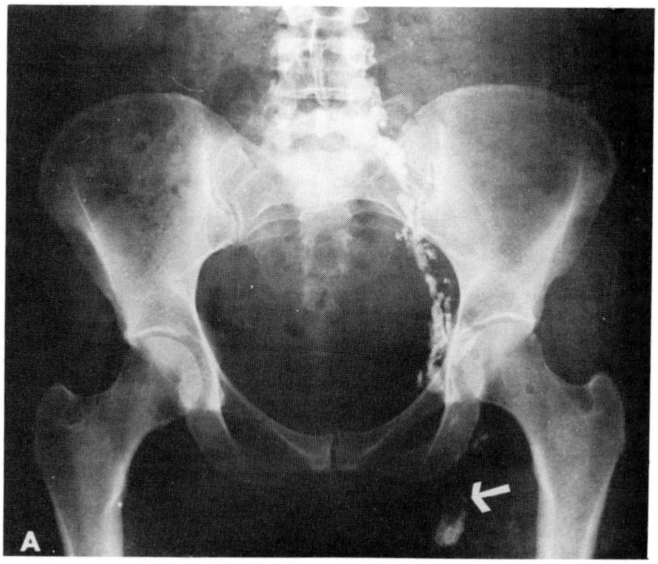

Fig. 3. Lymphogram of a patient with metastatic melanoma to left inguinal region, taken 5 days after injection of ethiodized oil. Note stagnation of lymphatic vessels and development of collateral circulation where presacral lymph nodes are visualized in midline. Note space-occupying lesions in the inguinal lymph nodes, a characteristic of metastases. (Reprinted by permission from the New York State Journal of Medicine, copyright by the Medical Society of the State of New York, Ariel, I. M.: Lymphography and endolymphatic administration of radioactive isotopes for treating cancer, N. Y. State J. Med. **68:** 1254, 1968.)

both the lymphatic vessels and the veins. Wallace and associates[17] demonstrated direct lymphatic-venous communications in the normal individual, found most frequently in the cervical region and to a lesser extent in the upper extremity. The communications were more abundant in individuals with lymphatic obstruction.

It is not surprising to note these connections between the lymphatic and venous systems, inasmuch as embryologically the lymphatic sacs are formed by a process of "budding" from the blood-vascular endothelium. Budding sacs from the anterior cardinal veins give rise to the lymphatic vessels of the head and neck. Sprouts from the mesonephric vein develop paired sacs which become the precursors of the skeletal lymphatics; two additional sacs are derived from the mesonephric vein—one later becomes the cisterna chyli and the lower thoracic duct and the other forms the lymphatic vessels of the abdominal viscera.

EFFECTS OF METASTASES—ALTERED LYMPHATIC DYNAMICS

Metastases in lymphatic vessels. Tumor implants lodged within either the lymphatic vessels or the lymph nodes may alter the normal lymphatic dynamics. The alteration is often determined by the implant's location and the degree of obstruction it causes. The blockage of a lymphatic vessel in either the leg or the arm may produce one or a combination of the following alterations in collateral lymphatic flow: (1) The anterior compartment may be completely blocked, shunting the lymphatic flow into the posterior compartment. (2) The anterior chain may be incompletely blocked, producing a partial shunt into the posterior compartment; function of both compartments remains. (3) Both compartments may be functional without evidence of block.

Accordingly, a cancer located on the dorsum of the foot may spread to the popliteal lymph nodes as a result of either an anatomic shunt to the posterior lymphatic chain or an obstruction in the anterior lymphatic chain.

Popliteal lymph nodes. When present, the popliteal nodes drain the lesser saphenous lymphatic system and may drain the greater saphenous system as well. Therefore, cancer cells may and do lodge in these nodes. Accordingly, when a malignant neoplasm is located in this area of drainage into the popliteal nodes (i.e., directly inferior to the popliteal space, the lateral aspect of the foot, the heel), the nodes should be included in the therapeutic plan.

It has been stated that "metastasis to the popliteal nodes is so rare that the possibility of its occurrence should not enter into the discussion of the management of melanoma of the lower extremity inferior to the condyles."[9] We disagree with this premise, for we have seen many instances of metastases of melanoma and other cancers (epidermoid carcinoma and sarcoma) to the popliteal and epitrochlear lymph nodes. Although the popliteal lymph nodes are absent in a certain percentage of people, they are present in others. The probability exists that these nodes undergo attrition with advancing age, as do many lymph nodes, and they are present in older individuals in a nonfunctioning, atrophic form.

Our data further suggest that if the lymphogram demonstrates a collateral route from the greater saphenous to the lesser saphenous system, the popliteal nodes should definitely be considered in the therapeutic plan. If lymphograms are not performed, at least a clinical search should be made in the popliteal and epitrochlear regions in all patients presenting either primary or secondary cancers distal to these sites.

Metastases in lymph nodes. When metastases in the lymph nodes have reached sufficient size, the resultant blockage shunts the lymph into alternate channels in order to maintain the integrity of lymphatic flow. A vast network of potential, not normally functioning lymphatic vessels is enlisted into service, and those in the immediate vicinity of the obstruction first become functional. In the lymphogram of a patient with metastatic melanoma to the left inguinal region taken 5 days after the injection of the contrast medium, stagnation of the lymphatic vessels was present and collateral circulation developed via the presacral chain of nodes (Fig. 3). Eventually, metastases were demonstrated in the lymph nodes of the opposite groin. Should this adjacent network prove insufficient, new groups of lymphatic vessels become functional in an effort to re-establish lymphatic flow. Often an unpredictable and bizarre form of lymphatic network will assume the function of lymph transportation (and, presumably, cancer cells) for great distances uninterrupted by lymph nodes.

The nature of the collateral lymphatic vessels is often determined by the level or location of an obstruction. Obstruction in the para-aortic lymphatic vessels may produce an atypical collateral network that may extend into the visceral lymphatics. Obstruction at the level of the porta hepatis may produce such stagnation of the lymphatic system distal to the blockage that the lymph nodes may be compressed and destroyed by the back pressure. Wallace and associates[17] demonstrated that obstruction at the thoracic duct produced by posterior mediastinal lesions hindered the normal flow of lymph and induced retrograde filling of the gastrointestinal trunk as well as the intercostal lymphatics.

Those collaterals called into play after an obstruction has become extensive are so eccentric and unpredictable that they defy any effort at interpretation, and the application of therapeutic modalities is nearly impossible. This was demonstrated in an obstruction in the iliac nodes secondary to a carcinoma of the cervix which produced a lymphatic collateral chain in the anterior abdominal wall to the axilla where a metastatic cancer was encountered.[15]

Perivascular lymphatics. The existence of potential spaces in perivascular locations was recently described by Wallace and his colleagues.[17] These spaces were successfully demonstrated by the investigators as an additional collateral route for the transport of lymph and tumor cells. They likened these perivascular spaces to the perineural or endoneural spaces which have been amply demonstrated to play a major role in the dissemination of tumor emboli. Although they have observed these perivascular spaces, they have been unable to establish their exact anatomy. Are they actual potential spaces between the vessel wall and its surrounding membrane, or do they constitute an integral part of the lymphatic system? However, these authors have shown conclusively the existence of a direct connection between the lymphatic system and these potential spaces to which lymph is transported and which offer a possible route for the unopposed transport of tumor cells. These spaces, located within the perivascular sheath, have been seen in patients with and without edema.

Stagnation of lymph. Radiopaque material injected into a lymphatic vessel normally empties from the lymphatics in from 4 to 24 hours. In the presence of obstruction, stagnation ensues and the injected material remains within the lymphatics for longer periods, as long as 2½ months and perhaps longer, as determined by the authors, but measurements have not been made.

Clinically, a stagnant lymphatic state may be manifest by the appearance of edema. An impediment to the free flow of lymph causes an increase in lymphatic pressure with the resultant deposition of lymph within the interstitial spaces of the extremities producing edema; however, stagnation of lymphatic flow has been observed without resultant edema. We interpret stagnant lymphatic flow as presumptive evidence of the existence of an obstruction in either the proximal chain of lymph nodes or within the proximal lymphatic vessels.

Fig. 4 is the lymphogram of a patient with metastases in the axilla from a primary melanoma of the left lateral chest wall. This patient manifested a direct lymphatic connection between the axillary and supraclavicular lymph nodes, illustrating a route for the passage of tumor emboli from the axilla into the supraclavicular region. The lymphogram showed the presence of metastases within the lymph nodes of the axilla; it demonstrated the retention of dye within the lymphatic vessels 3 days after the performance of the lymphogram, indicating stagnation in the lymphatic flow. In some instances, metastases within the lymph nodes may be so small as to go undetected lymphographically. For example, the stagnant state of the distal lymphatics in one patient prompted the excision of a groin lymph node for histologic study, which revealed the presence of metastases.

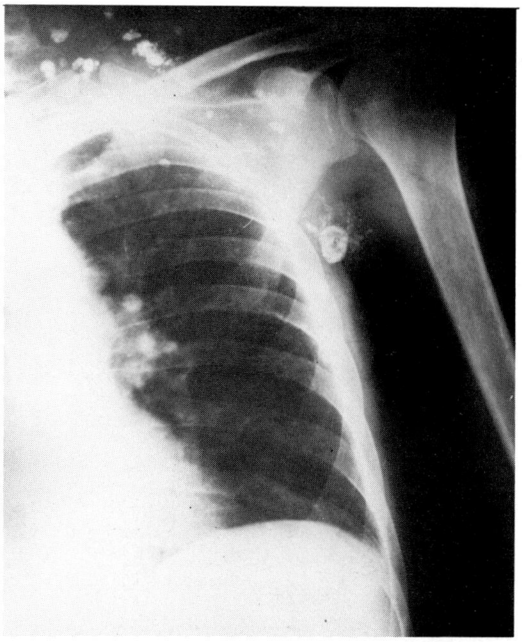

Fig. 4. Lymphogram demonstrating reconstituted lymphatic circulation. Regenerated lymphatic vessels communicate freely with supraclavicular lymph nodes; new collateral circulation developed with internal mammary chain of lymph nodes. Note residual lymph nodes in axilla harboring metastatic melanoma. Left radical axillary·dissection for melanoma performed elsewhere 2 years previously. (Reprinted by permission from the New York State Journal of Medicine, copyright by the Medical Society of the State of New York, Ariel, I. M.: Lymphography and endolymphatic administration of radioactive isotopes for treating cancer, N. Y. State J. Med. **68:** 1255, 1968.)

Lymphatic stagnation with ensuing edema may be only temporary, providing the development of collateral circulation is adequate.

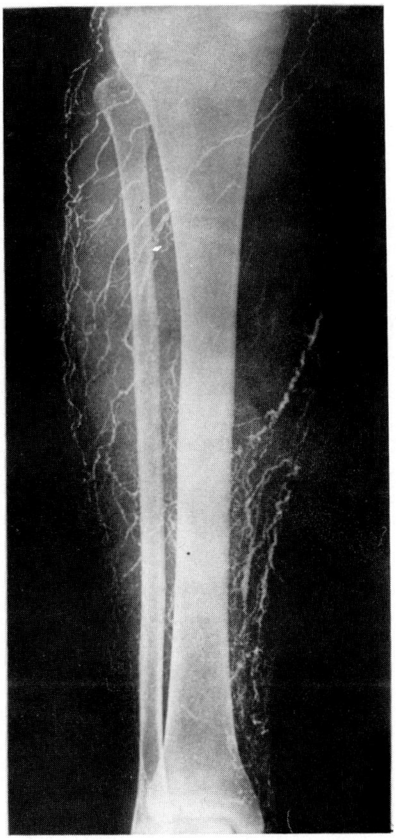

Fig. 5. Patient with marked lymphedema following radical groin dissection for melanoma with development of extensive network of cutaneous lymphatic vessels. (Reprinted by permission from the New York State Journal of Medicine, copyright by the Medical Society of the State of New York, Ariel, I. M.: Lymphography and endolymphatic administration of radioactive isotopes for treating cancer, N. Y. State J. Med. **68:** 1256, 1968.)

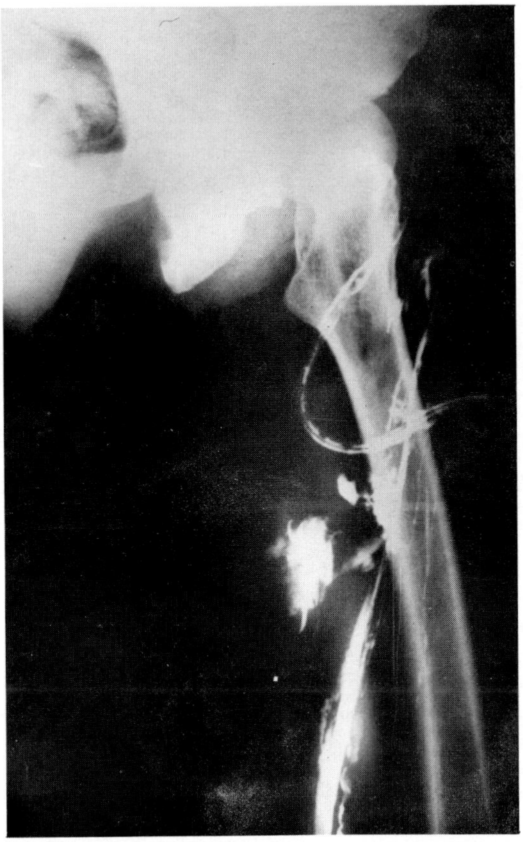

Fig. 6. Lymphogram taken 3 days after performance of radical groin dissection for melanoma. Note injected ethiodized oil removed by means of a hemovac within wound site. Note lymphocele. (Reprinted by permission from the New York State Journal of Medicine, copyright by the Medical Society of the State of New York, Ariel, I. M.: Lymphography and endolymphatic administration of radioactive isotopes for treating cancer, N. Y. State J. Med. **68:** 1257, 1968.)

Should this occur, the free flow of lymph within the lymphatics will be re-established and the edema will subside. However, if an adequate collateral circulation has not developed, the edema will become more pronounced as the lymphatic pressure increases.

Blocker and colleagues[4] have demonstrated that the normal intralymphatic pressures are subatmospheric in the lower extremity (0 to –16 mm. H_2O) with a decreasing gradient upward to the thoracic duct. With blockage, the intralymphatic pressure in the lower extremity is positive, going as high as 60 to 80 mm. H_2O. One patient with an inferior vena cava syndrome due to a mediastinal tumor had generalized edema from the nipple inferiorly and the extremely high intralymphatic pressure of 400 mm. H_2O in the lower extremity.

Reversal of flow. After a period of failure to establish satisfactory collateral circulation, a reversal in lymphatic flow occurs with the development of a functional superficial chain of dermal lymphatic vessels. In such instances, subsequent regurgitation of lymph occurs distally into a network of dermal lymphatic vessels (Fig. 5).

Lymphaticovenous anastomosis. Previous

comments have been made regarding the normal existence of lymphaticovenous anastomoses. In the presence of obstruction, potential, nonfunctioning lymphaticovenous openings become functional due to metabolic necessity, and certain new communications develop in the need to mobilize a collateral circulation for the stagnant lymph, present under an increased head of pressure resulting from obstruction.[6, 11, 17] Under such circumstances, the transport of tumor cells from the lymphatic into the vascular circulation is probably facilitated.

Lymphatic circulation time. We have observed, as have Stehlin and associates,[16] that in the presence of obstruction there is a delay in the time it takes for the dye to reach the inguinal lymph nodes. To ascertain the lymphatic circulation time from foot to groin, a Geiger counter is placed over the groin as the endolymphatic administration of ^{131}I-Ethiodol is begun into a foot lymphatic vessel, and the first recording is taken as the isotope reaches the groin. In 16 patients without evidence of obstruction, the time averaged 5 minutes and varied from 3 to 8 minutes. In the presence of clinically detectable metastases in the lymph nodes, the time averaged 10 minutes and varied from 5 to 20 minutes.

EFFECTS OF DISCONTINUOUS LYMPH-NODE DISSECTION ON LYMPHATIC DYNAMICS

Hazards of the operation. The performance of a discontinuous operation for melanoma is not without hazard.[1, 2] The following sequence of events occurs after a groin dissection.

1. There is an extensive escape of lymph through the severed lymphatic vessels resulting in the formation of a lymphocele. A lymphogram was performed 3 days after the radical groin dissection for a malignant melanoma (Fig. 6); a drain was left in situ. Salient in this instance is the observed escape of lymph and Ethiodol from the lymphatic system into the free tissue spaces of the dissection site, because the innumerable lymphatic vessels severed during the course of the dissection were not patent and therefore permitted the leakage; the drain functions as a suction apparatus for the lymph and Ethiodol. When the drainage tube is removed, the Ethiodol is retained within the free tissue spaces with the formation of a tract along the course of the tube.

Cancer cells in transit within the lymphatic vessels are deposited into the free tissue spaces where they may seed and grow, presenting as metastases.

2. A sealing off of the lymphatic vessels occurs at the incisional site. As a result, one or all of the following mechanisms can occur: (a) the lymphatic vessels may seal off and block the incisional region with the resultant retention of lymph in lymphatic vessels distal to the operative site; (b) re-establishment in continuity may take place by regrowth of the severed lymphatic vessels; (c) the blocked lymphatic vessels may form collateral channels with adjacent lymphatic vessels with the subsequent re-establishment of lymphatic flow; (d) due to lymphatic blockage and in the presence of an inadequate development of collateral circulation, a regurgitation of lymph occurs within the subsequently functional superficial or dermal lymphatic channels. As a result, edema of the extremity may occur (Fig. 5).

SATELLITOSIS OF MELANOMA

It is not uncommon to find dermal satellite metastases involving the skin of the leg after extensive metastases to the lymph nodes of the groin or subsequent to the surgical excision of these nodes. Satellite cancers have been noted in regions of expansive dermal lymphatic development secondary to an obstruction. It is believed that tumor emboli become implanted within the subcutaneous tissue and/or dermis via these dermal lymphatic vessels.

Malignant melanoma may spread either by direct infiltration or via lymphatic channels into the adjacent tissues, with the resultant deposition of cancer cells in the regional lymph nodes. Stehlin and associates[16] have applied the epigraph "in-transit metastases" to those cancer cells within the lymphatic vessels. This term emphasizes the fact that "cancer cells are conveyed via the lymphatic vessels to the regional lymph nodes." Stagnation of lymphatic flow, possibly attributable to proximal obstruction, hinders transportation and the stalled cancer cells implant and multiply to become a fixed metastatic deposit. The latter should be differentiated from the "floating cell" in transit within the lymphatics. Metastases may be found within the deep lymphatic vessels as well as in the newly developed dermal and subcutaneous lymphatic network. Accordingly, satellitoses may be considered the result of cancer cells presumably traveling in a retrograde manner within the tiny dermal lymhpatic vessels, developed in consequence of lymphatic obstruction with failure to promote adequate routes of collateral lymphatic flow; at least this is one mechanism in their development.

Metastases within the lymphatic vessels of the extremity may be present at any depth, and this should be considered in any planned attack upon malignant melanoma of an extremity. Consequently, melanoma cells may be found within the lymphatic vessels as (1) floating cells en route to the regional lymph nodes, (2) fixed within the deeper lymphatic vessels where they remain and grow, or (3) within the dermal lymphatic vessels transported in retrograde fashion and coming to a standstill to grow as satellitoses.

CONCLUSIONS

Since the lymph nodes retain the radiopaque medium for a period of 6 to 9 months, any change within the lymph node can be observed, such as a response to therapy, particularly a decrease in size, or an increase in size due to cancerous growth. A repeat lymphogram, especially in patients with lymphoma who must be followed for prolonged periods, provides an assessment as to the status of the malignant process.

Lymphography offers the radiotherapist a landmark for the placement of radiotherapeutic portals.

When chlorophyll is combined with Ethiodol, all the opacified lymph nodes are stained light green. Therefore, preoperative lymphography aids the surgeon, especially the surgical resident, in the visualization of the lymph nodes during the performance of a lymphadenectomy for cancer.

Lymphography demonstrates to the surgeon the adequacy of his lymph-node dissection. It demonstrates abnormalities of the mediastinum by any alteration in the anatomy of the thoracic duct.

Metastases in the lymph nodes produce the following alterations in lymphatic dynamics.

1. Stagnation of lymphatic flow which may produce edema. The "take" of cancer cells in transit is facilitated, as is the transport of cancer cells into the vascular compartment via lymphatic-vascular communications due to an increased head of lymphatic pressure.
2. Collateral lymphatic channels become so extensive and erratic as to defy interpretation of routes of cancer spread. Cancer cells may be conveyed uninterruptedly for great distances and to almost any region in the body.
3. If the collateral lymphatic circulation is inadequate, a reversal of lymphatic flow occurs via a group of newly developed, functional dermal lymphatic vessels. This is one modus operandi in the formation of dermal metastases (satellitosis of melanoma).

A discontinuous operation for melanoma, that is, the removal of the primary melanoma plus a groin or axillary dissection while completely ignoring the intervening lymphatics, not only aggravates the situation described above, but also permits the escape of cancer cells via the severed lymphatic vessels into the free tissue spaces where they may seed and grow.

REFERENCES

1. Ariel, I. M., and Resnick, M. I.: Altered lymphatic dynamics following groin and axillary dissection: Its relationship to treatment policies for malignant melanoma, SURGERY **61:** 210, 1967.
2. Ariel, I. M., and Resnick, M. I.: Altered lymphatic dynamics caused by cancer metastases, Arch. Surg. **94:** 117, 1967.
3. Blalock, A., Robinson, C. S., Cunningham,

R. S., et al.: Experimental studies on lymphatic blockage, Arch. Surg. **34:** 1049, 1937.
4. Blocker, T. G., Jr., Lewis, S. R., Smith, J. R., et al.: Lymphodynamics, Plast. Reconstr. Surg. **25:** 337, 1960.
5. Bron, K. M., Baum, S., and Abrams, H. L.: Oil embolism in lymphangiography: Incidence, manifestations and mechanisms, Radiology **80:** 194, 1963.
6. Fischer, H. W., and Thornbury, J. R.: Lymphography in the diagnosis of malignant neoplasms, *in* Ariel, I. M., editor: Progress in clinical cancer, vol. 1, New York, 1965, Grune & Stratton, Inc., p. 213.
7. Fuchs, W. A., and Book-Hederstrom, G.: Inguinal and pelvic lymphography, Acta Radiol. [Diag.] (Stockh.) **56:** 340, 1961.
8. Koehler, P. R., Wohl, G. T., and Schaeffer, B.: Lymphangiography—a survey of its current status. Am. J. Roentgenol. Radium Ther. Nucl. Med. **91:** 1216, 1964.
9. McNeer, G., and Das Gupta, T.: Routes of lymphatic spread of malignant melanoma, Cancer **15:** 168, 1965.
10. Pressman, J. J., Simon, M. B., Hand, K., et al.: Passage of fluids, cells and bacteria via direct communication between lymph nodes and veins, Surg. Gynecol. Obstet. **115:** 207, 1962.
11. Rouvier, H.: *In* Anatomy of the human lymphatic system, translated by Tobias, M. J., Ann Arbor, 1938, Edwards Brothers, Inc.
12. Rusznyak, I., Foldi, M., and Szabo, G.: *In* Lymphatic system, translated by Tobias, M. J., Ann Arbor, 1938, Edwards Brothers, Inc., p. 318.
13. Rusznyak, I., Foldi, M., and Szabo, G.: Lymphatics and lymph circulation, physiology and pathology, New York, 1960, Pergamon Press, Inc., p. 150.
14. Stehlin, J. S., Jr., Clark, R. L., Smith, J. L., Jr., et al.: Malignant melanoma of the extremities: experience with conventional therapy; a new surgical and chemotherapeutic approach to regional perfusion, Cancer **13:** 55, 1960.
15. Stehlin, J. R., Smith, J. L., Jr., and Clark, R. L.: Malignant melanoma, diagnosis and current treatment, Surg. Clin. North Am. **42:** 455, 1962.
16. Stehlin, J. S., Jr., Smith, J. L., Jr., Jing, Bao-Shan, et al.: Melanoma of the extremities complicated by in-transit metastases, Surg. Gynecol. Obstet. **122:** 3, 1966.
17. Wallace, S., Jackson, L., Dodd, G. D., et al.: Lymphatic dynamics in certain abnormal states, Am. J. Roentgenol. Radium Ther. Nucl. Med. **91:** 1187, 1964.

Brief clinical reports

Post-traumatic renovascular hypertension

M. N. Sechas, M.D., S. N. Plessas, M.D., *and* G. D. Skalkeas, M.D., *Athens, Greece*

An unusual case of post-traumatic arteriovenous communication between the right renal artery and the inferior vena cava is presented. Arterial hypertension and congestive heart failure were the prominent clinical features. Ligation of the renal artery and nephrectomy resulted in cure of the patient.

From the Second Department of Propedeutic Surgery, Athens University School of Medicine, Athens, Greece

THE WIDE propagation of renal angiography in recent years has resulted in a progressive increase in the number of diagnosed cases of arteriovenous (A-V) communications of the renal circulation.

The fistulas, being extremely rare, are divided into two types: congenital and acquired. The congenital ones, in which multiple points of communication between artery and vein exist, are also called varicose aneurysms. The acquired fistulas usually have only one point of communication and may be due to one of the following causes, listed in the order of their frequency: transcutaneous kidney biopsy, nephrectomy, renal carcinoma, renal injury, polycystic kidney, and ruptured renal artery aneurysm.

Only eight such acquired post-traumatic fistulas have been reported in the international literature.[2, 6, 9, 17]

We present a rare case of traumatic fistula between the right renal artery and the inferior vena cava (IVC), in which arterial hypertension was the prominent clinical feature.

Accepted for publication June 27, 1974.

Reprint requests: M. N. Sechas, M.D., Second Department of Propedeutic Surgery, Athens University School of Medicine, King Paul's Hospital, Athens 609, Greece.

CASE REPORT

A 37-year-old man was admitted to the hospital for investigation of arterial hypertension of 2 years' duration. The past history revealed a splenectomy performed 16 years earlier for a ruptured spleen following a car accident, and a repair of an incisional hernia 13 years earlier.

Two years prior to admission, the patient sustained a stab wound in the lower abdomen, for which an exploratory laparotomy was performed. Seven months later he started complaining of headache and intermittent diffuse abdominal pain extending to the right flank. He was admitted to another hospital, and hypertension and left ventricular hypertrophy were diagnosed.

Physical examination revealed a water-hammer pulse at a rate of 100 per minute and an arterial blood pressure of 250/130 mm. Hg. The jugular veins were normal. The liver was palpable three fingerbreadths below the costal margin. A thrill was palpated over the right paraumbilical area, extending to the right flank. A loud systolodiastolic murmur was heard over the same areas and could be traced along the vertebral column up to the thorax. The arterial pulses in the lower extremities were more prominent than normal.

The routine laboratory tests were within normal limits. Blood urea was 50 mg. percent, and creatinine 1 mg. percent and creatinine clearance 71 ml. per minute. The phonocardiogram recorded the characteristic murmur of A-V communication over the right renal region.

The plain chest film showed dilatation of all heart chambers (Fig. 1). X-ray of the kidneys, ureter, and bladder showed considerable diminution of the size of the right kidney and hypertrophy of the left kidney could be seen. Intravenous pyelogram failed to demonstrate excretion from this kidney.

Selective catheterization of the ureters was performed in order to perform split renal function tests, but there was no urine production from the right kidney. Retrograde pyelogram showed complete distortion of its pyelocalyceal system (Fig. 2). The functional disturbance of this kidney was further confirmed by the renogram (Fig. 3) and renal scan with ^{203}Hg.

Retrograde abdominal aortography revealed a simultaneous visualization of the aorta and the IVC, which was almost twice as wide as normal. The origin of the right renal artery was also markedly dilated subsequently forming two aneurysmal sacs and leading to communication with the IVC. There was failure of visualization of both the distal and intrarenal portions of the renal artery (Fig. 4). The above findings were confirmed by selective arteriogram of the right renal artery (Fig. 5).

The patient was started on antihypertensive treatment with little reduction of his blood pressure. On the contrary, he developed two episodes of congestive heart failure. For this reason surgical correction was decided upon.

At the operation the arteriographic findings were confirmed. The absence of any function from the right kidney, as revealed by the preoperative tests and the macroscopic appearance of the kidney, precluded any attempt for revascularization. The right renal artery was double ligated at its origin and the kidney was removed. The A-V communication was left intact.

The removed kidney weighed 30 grams and microscopically presented hypoplasia of the parenchyma with marked sclerosis of all vessels as well as inflammatory changes.

A dramatic fall in blood pressure (150/100 mm. Hg) was observed as early as the first postoperative day and 2 weeks later there was a considerable decrease in the size of the heart on the chest film (Fig. 6).

DISCUSSION

Since 1923, when Varela[18] described the first case, over 100 cases of A-V communications of the renal circulation have been reported.[8, 10, 11, 13, 17] These communications are either congenital are acquired[8] and may be intra- or extrarenal.

The congenital fistulas, usually being multiple, are mostly intrarenal and represent one third of the cases.[4]

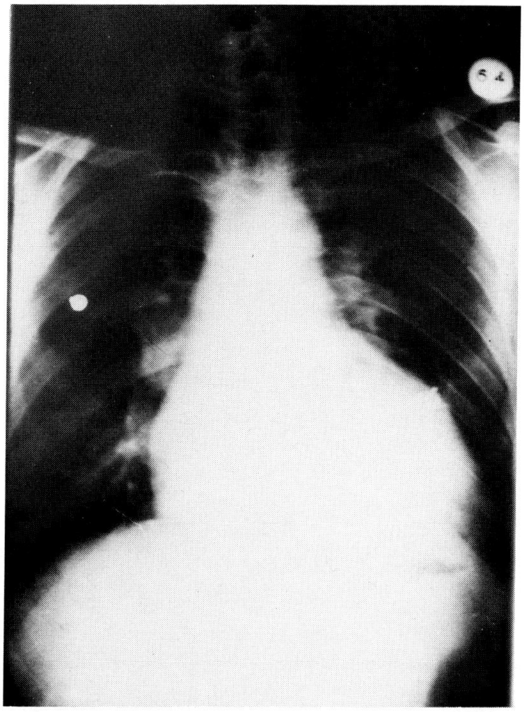

Fig. 1. Plain chest film showing cardiac enlargement and left ventricular hypertrophy.

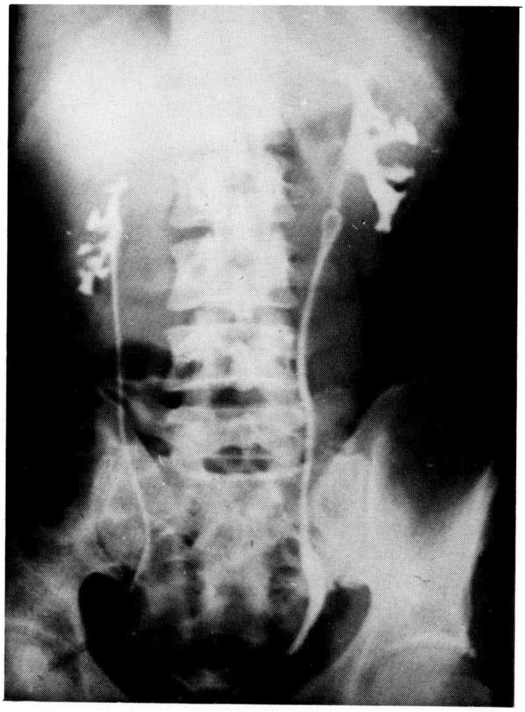

Fig. 2. Bilateral retrograde pyelogram with distortion of the right pyelocalyceal system.

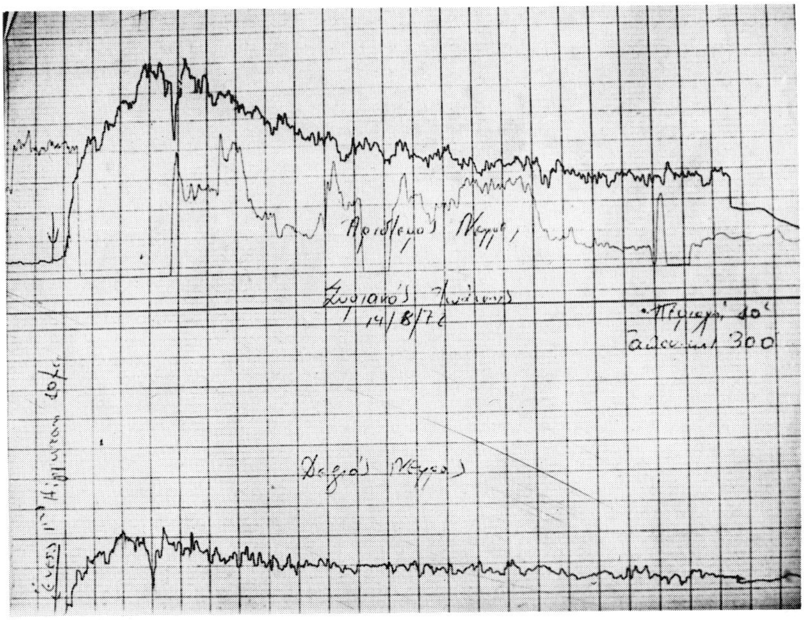

Fig. 3. Abnormal right kidney curve in the radioactive hippuran renogram (below) as compared to a normal curve of the left kidney (above).

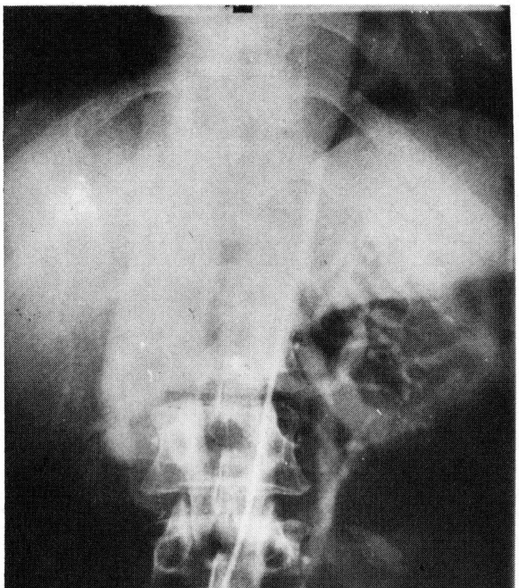

Fig. 4. Retrograde transfemoral aortogram. Simultaneous visualization of the aorta and of the dilated IVC, through an A-V fistula between the right renal artery and the IVC. The distal portion of the renal artery is not visualized.

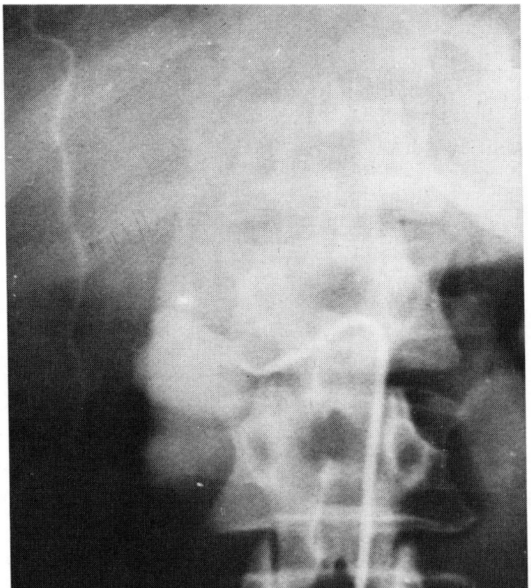

Fig. 5. Selective right renal angiogram showing two saccular aneurysms of the renal artery and communication to the IVC.

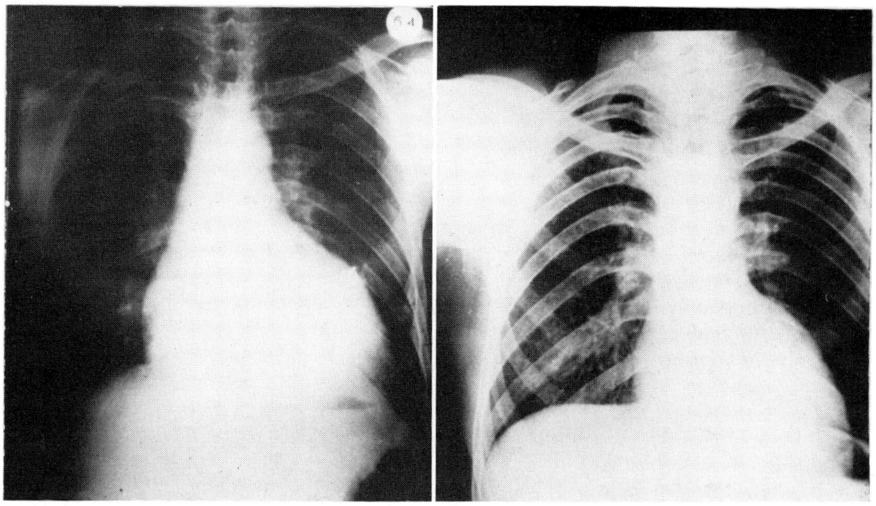

Fig. 6. The preoperative (left) chest film is compared to one taken 2 weeks after operation (right). The considerable decrease of the size of the heart is obvious.

In about 75 percent of the acquired variety, the communication is due to trauma (trauma to the flank or abdomen, renal needle biopsy, renal operations, etc.),[1, 5, 11, 17] other causes being tumors (hypernephroma),[15] inflammation, or atherosclerosis. Maldonado,[8] reviewing the international literature, found nine cases in which no primary cause could be incriminated and termed them idiopathic. Tynes and associates[17] reported one case of bilateral fistulas without history of trauma or previous disease.

As a result of the wide utilization of transcutaneous needle biopsy of the kidney in the study of renal disease, this method has tended to become the most common cause of acquired renal A-V fistulas.[9, 12, 16] The communications which develop following nephrectomy are apparently due to en bloc clamping and ligating of the renal pedicle with resultant necrosis of the vessels. In the case of renal cell carcinoma, the renal vessels become infiltrated by the neoplasm which undergoes necrosis with resultant A-V communication.

Most A-V fistulas are small and hemodynamically insignificant. Postbiopsy fistulas close spontaneously in about 50 to 70 percent of the cases.[3, 7] Others, causing marked shunting of arterial blood, need surgical correction. The hemodynamic disturbance in these cases consists of increased cardiac output and decreased peripheral resistance with systolic hypertension and a wide pulse pressure. Cardiac dilatation and hypertrophy with resultant heart failure are common.[4, 14] This sequence of events takes place only following nephrectomy. If the kidney is in its place, as was the case with our patient, it becomes ischemic due to reduction of flow distal to the communication, and diastolic hypertension is added to the clinical picture.

Nilsson and Ross,[12] however, reported the case of a hypertensive patient, who, following bilateral needle biopsies, showed a marked decrease in the blood pressure due to formation of bilateral A-V fistulas.

The most common symptoms of renal A-V fistulas are dyspnea, tachycardia (37 percent), light headedness (11 percent) and abdominal pain of undetermined mechanism (34 percent). Thrill, high-pitched continuous bruit with systolic accentutaion heard over the renal region (69 percent), increase of the size of the heart (57 percent), and hypertension (43 percent) are the usual physical findings.

In addition to the routine laboratory studies and the special tests for evaluation of renal function, aortography and selective renal arteriography may prove helpful in establishing the diagnosis and the indications for treatment.

Surgery is the treatment of choice, as these patients respond poorly to medical treatment, congestive heart failure being the fatal outcome.

Nephrectomy has been until recently the procedure most favored for management of renal A-V communications.[5, 9] However, the utilization of angiography and the refinement of surgical technique have resulted in a progressively increasing number of salvaged kidneys, provided that irreversible damage has not supervened.[11, 17]

The best approach seems to be exposing the communication through the veins, the artery being extremely friable, and ligation of all afferent and efferent branches. The aneurysm is then opened and the communication closed from inside.[10, 17]

The results are usually most satisfactory. The congestive heart failure, if present preoperatively, disappears and the size of the heart decreases. Hypertension is corrected in about 53 percent of the cases.[8]

REFERENCES

1. Aravanis, C., Michaelides, G., Alivisatos, C., and Lazarides, D.: Renal arteriovenous fistula following nephrectomy, Ann. Surg. **156:** 751, 1962.
2. Goldstein, A., Delaurentis, D., and Schwartz, A.: Post-nephrectomy arteriovenous fistula, J. Urol. **98:** 44, 1967.
3. Guilleumin, P., Parietti, R., and L'Hermite, J.: Guerison spontanée d'une fistule arterioveineuse après ponction biopsie du rein, J. Urol. Nephrol. (Paris) **78:** 871, 1972.
4. Holman, E.: The physiology of an arteriovenous fistula, Arch. Surg. **7:** 64, 1923.
5. Hutch, J., and Chisholm, E.: Intrarenal arteriovenous fistula, J. Urol. **88:** 150, 1962.
6. Kelly, D.: Renal arteriovenous fistula. A report of four cases and review of the literature, Br. J. Urol. **39:** 162, 1967.
7. Lindgardh, G., Lindqvist, B., and Lindström, B.: Renal arteriovenous fistula following puncture biopsy: A hemodynamic and functional study in four cases, Scand. J. Urol. Nephrol. **5:** 181, 1971.
8. Maldonado, J., Sheldon, S., Bernatz, P., Deweerd, J., and Harrison, E.: Renal arteriovenous fistula. A reversible cause of hypertension and heart failure, Am. J. Med. **37:** 499, 1964.
9. Malloy, T., Leberman, P., and Murphy, J.: Renal arteriovenous fistula, J. Urol. **98:** 40, 1967.
10. Merkel, F., and Sako, Y.: Surgical treatment for traumatic renal arteriovenous fistulas, Arch. Surg. **101:** 438, 1970.
11. Mguyen-Huu, Ngo-Gia-Hy, and Bui-Monz-Hung: Anevrysmes arterioveineux des vaisseaux rénaux, rein en place. Leur rôle dans l'hypertension arterielle d'origine rénale, Presse Med. **67:** 1680, 1959.
12. Nilsson, C., and Ross, R.: Bilateral renal arteriovenous fistulas and decreased blood pressure following renal biopsies, J. Urol. **97:** 176, 1967.
13. Poutasse, E.: Renal artery aneurysm: Report of 12 cases, two treated by excision of the aneurysm and repair of renal artery, J. Urol. **77:** 697, 1957.
14. Reid, M. R.: The effect of arteriovenous aneurysms upon the heart: With the report of a case studied by Professor Rudolph Matas, Dr. Georger Herrmann, and the author, Ann. Surg. **95:** 578, 1932.
15. Sontag, T. J., Patel, S. K., Petasnik, J. P., and Chambliss, J.: Hypernephromas with massive arteriovenous fistulas, Am. J. Roentgenol. Radium Ther. Nucl. Med. **117:** 97, 1973.
16. Smith, G. H., Reymero, A. R., and Dickey, B. M.: Intrarenal arteriovenous fistula and systemic hypertension following percutaneous renal biopsy, Nephron **5:** 24, 1968.
17. Tynes, W., Devine, C., Devine, P., and Poutasse, E.: Surgical treatment of renal arteriovenous fistulas: Report of 5 cases, J. Urol. **103:** 692, 1970.
18. Varela, M. E.: Aneurisma arteriovenoso de los vaso renales y asustolia consecutiva, Rev. Med. Lat. Am. **14:** 3244, 1923.

Staged palliative resection of recurrent carcinoma of the neck using an extra anatomic carotid bypass

Clyde O. Hagood, Jr., M.D., F.A.C.S., Colonel, USAF(MC), David J. Mozersky, M.D., Major, USAF(MC), *and* **Fulton W. Fite, M.D., F.A.C.S., Colonel, USAF(MC),**
Lackland Air Force Base, Texas

Recurrent carcinoma at the carotid bifurcation presents a therapeutic dilemma. Nonoperative treatment inevitably leads to exsanguinating hemorrhage and rapid death. Operative treatment (excision with or without vascular reconstruction) is fraught with the dangers of cerebral ischemia, secondary infection, and hemorrhage. Vascular reconstruction with delayed resection as described here is a unique solution to this difficult problem which may provide palliation in selected patients. We have been unable to find a previous report of a similar procedure.

From the Wilford Hall USAF Medical Center, Lackland Air Force Base, Texas.

RECURRENT squamous-cell carcinoma at the carotid bifurcation following radical cervical lymphadenectomy is a dreaded event that frequently leads to fatal exsanguinating hemorrhage. Palliative resection of the carotid without vascular reconstruction is fraught with prohibitive morbidity and mortality rates. Previously reported reconstructive efforts involved common carotid–internal carotid bypass either at the time of initial resection of the tumor or following radical lymphadenectomy.

This report outlines a procedure for patients developing recurrence at the carotid bifurcation following radical node dissection. It consists of a staged, extra-anatomic, distal subclavian–internal carotid–autogenous saphenous vein bypass procedure, followed in 3 weeks by an en bloc resection of the tumor and involved vessels.

Accepted for publication June 13, 1974.

Reprint requests: Clyde O. Hagood, Jr., Col, USAF (MC), CMR No. 8, Box 369501, Lackland AFB, Texas 78236.

REPORT OF A PATIENT

A 55-year-old Caucasian male patient had a laryngectomy for a squamous-cell carcinoma in 1969. He developed cervical nodal metastases in 1970, which were treated by irradiation and bilateral radical cervical lymphadenectomy. He did well until 1971 when he developed a mass over the bifurcation of the left carotid. Biopsy revealed recurrent squamous-cell carcinoma, and he was referred to Wilford Hall USAF Medical Center for treatment. Examination revealed a 5 by 5 cm. ulcerated mass fixed to the bifurcation of the left carotid artery. There was no evidence of other local recurrences or distant metastasis. The lesion seemed well localized to the area of the carotid bifurcation and a palliative resection seemed feasible if left cerebral circulation could be preserved.

Surgical procedure. The patient was given a volatile anesthetic agent and positioned supine with his head turned to the right. A 10 cm. incision was made slightly cephalad and

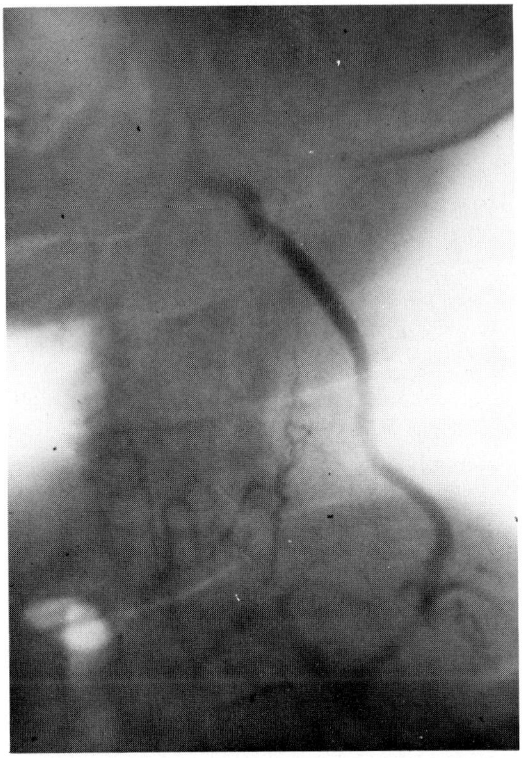

Fig. 1. Subtraction arteriogram taken 3 weeks following operation showing the lateral and posterior position of the graft. Both anastomoses are widely patent.

parallel to the middle third of the clavicle. The middle third of the clavicle was then resected exposing the distal subclavian artery and the proximal axillary artery. These vessels were isolated and prepared for anastomosis. The internal carotid was dissected through a 5 cm. incision extending from the tip of the mastoid to the angle of mandible. A tunnel was then created and directed under the anterior border of the trapezius as advocated by Loré.[2] An appropriate length of saphenous vein was harvested from the thigh and prepared for use as an arterial substitute. The distal subclavian artery was cross clamped proximally and distally following administration of 0.5 mg. aqueous heparin per kilogram of body weight. A 1.5 cm. incision was made in the cephalad aspect of the distal subclavian artery. The vein was reversed, the end was trimmed to the appropriate shape, and the anastomosis was done using running 5-0 synthetic suture. The vein was flushed, then cross clamped, and circulation was reinstituted to the arm. The vein was passed through the tunnel to the upper incision and divided at the appropriate level. The internal carotid was cross clamped proximally and distally and divided. Anastomosis without using a shunt was carried out with 5-0 synthetic suture material. Prior to completion of the anastomosis, flushing was carried out proximally to prevent air embolization. On completion, the proximal internal carotid was ligated and transfixed. The wound was closed in a routine fashion. The postoperative course was uneventful.

Three weeks following operation, arteriography demonstrated patency of the graft (Fig. 1). The patient was returned to the operating room and an en bloc resection of the tumor and carotid artery was performed using a Delto-Pectoral flap for reconstruction. Final modification of the flap was carried out several weeks later.

Following discharge from the hospital, the patient was returned to gainful employment and remained symptom free for one year. The patency of the graft was monitored during this interval using the Doppler Ultrasonic Flow Velocity Detector. He then developed metastasis in the base of the skull and died after a rapid downhill course.

DISCUSSION

Recurrent carcinoma of the carotid bifurcation has presented a most complex surgical problem. Expectant treatment has been unsatisfactory and has invariably led to rapid death from exsanguination. Early attempts at palliative treatment involved surgical excision of the carotid artery. Martin and his associates,[3] Watson and Silverstone,[6] and McComb[4] have, however, reported nearly a 50 percent mortality rate associated with these procedures. Most of the deaths were related to cerebral ischemia. Later efforts reported by Moore and Baker[5] have indicated that the mortality rate might be reduced to 11 percent. This figure is still unacceptable for a palliative operation.

Efforts to combine palliative resection with simultaneous vascular reconstruction were reported as early as 1952 by Conley.[1] Although this approach offered the theoretical advantage of preservation of carotid blood flow, the results were not spectacular. Of the 11 patients in his series, five died within 2 weeks of operation, four of complications related to sepsis. Loré[2] has suggested the concept of directing the bypass in such a way as to avoid the operative field and has reported two cases in which a circuitous Teflon (polytetrafluorethylene) common–internal carotid bypass graft has been used to re-establish continuity. In one of these cases, however, subsequent infection necessitated removal of the graft.

The procedure reported in the present communication, we believe, is a significant advance over previously reported operations. At the initial vascular reconstructive procedure the graft is directed well out of the proposed margins of the tumor resection. This is facilitated by using the distal subclavian artery as the source of the bypass graft. In addition, by using the distal subclavian instead of the common carotid, total cerebral ischemia time may be reduced. This may be important if one elects to perform the bypass without using a shunt.

After establishing vascular continuity, excision of the metastasis and adjacent artery may be completed and the resection need not be compromised by neurologic or vascular surgical considerations. The importance of the late problems which have plagued other attempts at vascular reconstruction under these circumstances (flap breakdown infection, delayed hemorrhage, or thrombosis) should be greatly reduced by this procedure.

Although it will be necessary to gain wider experience with this technique before questions relating to the reduction in morbidity and mortality rates can be answered, the results in our patient are encouraging. Staged subclavian–internal carotid artery bypass followed by wide en bloc resection of the tumor metastasis provides a method of treatment which adheres to the strictest principles of both vascular and oncologic surgery.

REFERENCES

1. Conley, J. J.: Carotid artery surgery in the treatment of tumors on the neck, Arch. Otolaryngol. **65:** 437, 1957.
2. Loré, J. M., Jr.: Vascular surgery in head and neck tumors, Arch. Otolaryngol. **83:** 109, 1966.
3. Martin, H. M., Del Valle, B. H., Ehrlich, H. W., and Cahan, W.: Neck dissection, Cancer **4:** 441, 1951.
4. McComb, W. S.: Carotid body tumors, Ann. Surg. **127:** 269, 1948.
5. Moore, O., and Baker, H. W.: Carotid artery ligation in surgery of the head and neck, Cancer **8:** 712, 1955.
6. Watson, W. L., and Silverstone, S. M.: Ligature of common carotid arteries in cancer of the head and neck, Ann. Surg. **109:** 1, 1939.

Spontaneous (pathologic) rupture of spleen in malignancies

C. P. Karakousis, M.D., *and* **E. G. Elias, M.D.,** *Buffalo, N. Y.*

Spontaneous (pathologic) rupture of the spleen is a rare clinical condition. Three cases are presented in association with three different malignancies, namely, metastatic malignant malanoma, acute monocytic leukemia, and Waldenstrom's macroglobulinemia. The clinical picture may be insidious and often obscured by how widespread the disease is or by the effects of therapy. A high clinical index of suspicion is required for early recognition. The presence of splenomegaly, thrombocytopenia, and/or a drop in the level of hemoglobin associated with these diseases, even in the absence of severe abdominal signs, should prompt surgical intervention.

From the Department of General Surgery, Roswell Park Memorial Institute, New York State Department of Health, Buffalo, N. Y.

SPONTANEOUS RUPTURE of the spleen is a well-recognized but rare clinical entity that occurs in abnormal spleens. It has been reported often with a variety of pathologic conditions, e.g., infectious mononucleosis, malaria, typhoid, splenic cysts, and leukemias. Several authors have supported the view that since minor physiologic trauma, such as coughing, straining, and other similar conditions, cannot be ruled out usually as a provocative factor in the rupture of the diseased organ, the term "spontaneous," denoting no external forces, should be abandoned in favor of "pathologic."[3-5] However, there is a fairly good concept of what constitutes trauma, and if there is no such history, the case should be classified as spontaneous. Though etiologic terms are generally preferable to descriptive ones, it is elected to retain the old terminology because it is well established and, more significantly, it stresses the clinical feature of absence of appreciable trauma which is important in the diagnosis of these cases.

The purpose of this report is to present three cases of spontaneous rupture of the spleen in three different malignancies.

CASE REPORTS

Case 1. S. L., a 71-year-old man, had malignant melanoma of the left preauricular region that was excised in May, 1966. He did well until 1970, when he developed a solitary metastasis in the left lung for which he underwent a left upper lobectomy. Subsequently he developed widespread metastases and in February, 1971, he was treated with chemotherapy that consisted of imidazol carboxamide and actinomycin D, but the disease progressed and he developed hepatosplenomegaly. On June 12, 1971, while at home, he developed left upper quadrant abdominal pain. The pain persisted and it became associated with nausea and vomiting. He was readmitted to our Institute with no history of trauma. Physical examination revealed hepatosplenomegaly. The liver measured 4 fingerbreadths below the costal margin. The spleen was palpable and tender. Pulse was 90 per

Accepted for publication June 27, 1974.

Reprint requests: C. P. Karakousis, Department of General Surgery, Roswell Park Memorial Hospital, 666 Elm, St., Buffalo, N. Y. 14203.

minute; blood pressure (B.P.), 190/100 mm. Hg; and temperature, 98.4° F. The bowel sounds were present. On admission the hemoglobin (Hgb.) was 9.1 Gm. percent and the hematocrit (Hct.) was 27 percent. The plain x-ray of the abdomen revealed a mass in the left upper quadrant displacing the splenic flexure of the colon; otherwise it was unremarkable. This was interpreted to be due to splenomegaly. He was put under observation and approximately 48 hours after admission the pulse rose to 136 per minute and the B.P. to 190/110; the temperature fell to 97.8° F., and, in the meantime, the Hgb. dropped to 6.6 Gm. percent, the Hct. to 21 percent, the white blood cell count (WBC) to 11,600, and the platelet count to 155,000. He was transfused with two units of whole blood and the Hgb. rose to 9.5 Gm. percent, the pulse to 100 per minute, the B.P. to 220/100, and the temperature to 99.4° F. The following day, two more units of whole blood were given but he suddenly became dyspneic and diaphoretic following a Fleet enema in preparation for barium enema. Chest x-ray revealed left pleural effusion and a left thoracentesis yielded 1,200 ml. of sanguineous fluid, after which there was some improvement of the dyspnea. The Hgb. was 9.5 Gm. percent, the WBC was 10,600, and the platelet count was 130,000. The patient died, however, on the morning of the fifth hospital day. The autopsy revealed metastatic melanoma to liver, intestines, left lung, and tongue, and a ruptured spleen that weighed 1,900 Gm., with hemoperitoneum of 1,800 ml. Ninety percent of the spleen was replaced by metastatic melanoma with cystic degeneration. The posterior surface of the lower splenic pole was the site of rupture and hematoma.

Case 2. H. D., a 69 year old man who was known to have severe emphysema, presented to a local hospital on July 4, 1972, with a 2 day history of persistent nausea and vomiting. A routine blood count revealed a Hgb. of 7.8 Gm. percent, a Hct. of 22.6 percent, and a WBC of 65,000, with the following differentials: 7 percent lymphocytes, 13 percent neutrophils, and 67 percent abnormal monocytes. Bone marrow biopsy and aspiration were consistent with acute myelomonocytic leukemia. On the second hospital day the patient began having tarry stools and vomiting coffee-ground material. The Hct. dropped to 18 percent and, following four units of whole blood transfusion, it rose to 33 percent. He was transferred to our Institute on July 12, 1972, for treatment of his leukemia and, on admission, he presented with severe respiratory distress. He was semicomatose; the pulse was 124 per minute, the B.P. was 120/60, the temperature was 101° F., the Hgb. was 9.6, the WBC was 98,000, and the platelet count was 32,500. An emergency tracheostomy was performed but the B.P. dropped to 70/40, the pulse to 128 per minute, and, in spite of supportive measures with digitalization, diuretics, and platelet transfusion, as well as with steroids and antibiotics, he remained hypotensive and oliguric overnight. On the following morning, the Hgb. dropped to 7.7 Gm. percent. The abdomen was soft and lax, and no signs of internal hemorrhage were suspected, but he died shortly afterward. It should be pointed out that, other than the respiratory distress, there was no history of trauma and no cardiac massage was attempted.

At autopsy there were moderate pulmonary congestion and a rupture of the spleen, which weighed 950 Gm., with massive intraperitoneal bleeding estimated to be over 1 L. Sections of the spleen showed a markedly thickened capsule with leukemic infiltration throughout the organ, areas of hemorrhage, old infarcts, hematomas, and parenchymal cell degeneration with necrosis.

Case 3. D. Y., a 45 year old woman, was admitted to our Institute on May 9, 1973, with a history of bleeding tendency, mainly menorrhagia, and anemia since November, 1972. On admission the liver and spleen were palpable 2 cm. below the costal margin. The Hgb. was 11.3 Gm. percent, the WBC was 3,850, with the following differential: neutrophils 31, stabs 24, lymphocytes 44, myelocytes 1. Platelets were in the range of 2,500 to 5,000 on three occasions. Total serum protein was 8.2 Gm. percent, with albumin 4.5 Gm. percent. Serum electrophoresis contained a gamma spike which appeared to be an immunoglobulin M (IgM). Immunoelectrophoresis confirmed the presence of monoclonal IgM peak (KLY) compatible with macroglobulinemia. The bone marrow was infiltrated with lymphocytes. On May 15, 1973, she developed a sudden dizzy spell and collapsed next to her bed but held onto it and slowly slid to the floor, so that there was no appreciable trauma. She complained of epigastric pain. On examination she looked pale; the pulse was 120 per minute, the B.P. was not obtainable, and the abdomen felt soft and lax, with slight tenderness over the epigastric area. An immediate blood count revealed a Hgb. of 6.9 Gm. percent and a Hct. of 18 percent. A few minutes later it became evident that she had an acute abdominal emergency. Intravenous infusion was started and she received whole blood and platelet transfusions. She was taken to the operating room where exploratory laparotomy revealed approximately 2,000 ml. of free blood in the peritoneal cavity, due to ruptured spleen. Splenectomy was performed. There was also slight oozing from two hematomas on the liver surface, easily controlled with Gelfoam packing. The spleen weighed 240 Gm. and there was subcapsular hematoma at the site of rupture. The postoperative course was benign, and the platelet count ranged from 5,000 to 20,000, yet there was no recurrence of bleeding. She was treated with chemotherapy that consisted of cytoxan and prednisone. Two months later she was readmitted with fever, developed respiratory insufficiency requiring tracheostomy, and finally died despite supportive measures. The autopsy revealed malignant lymphoproliferative disorder with Waldenstrom macroglobulinemia involving the lymph nodes and bone marrow.

DISCUSSION

Spontaneous rupture of the spleen has been reported in a variety of pathologic conditions that can be divided into (1) infections, (a) viral, as infectious mononucleosis, (b) parasitic, e.g., malaria, and (c) bacterial, as in typhoid and splenic abscess; (2) congenital anomalies of the spleen, as splenic cysts; (3) metabolic disorders, as Gaucher's disease; (4) degenerative conditions, as amyloidoses; and (5) malignancies, mainly leukemia (acute or chronic).[3] With regard to spontaneous rupture of the spleen in malignancies, most of the cases reported were in patients with leukemia. Although it is rare, by 1972 32 cases had been reported—18 of them in patients with acute leukemia[3, 4, 9, 10] and 14 in chronic leukemia.[6, 11] The etiologic factors of this phenomenon have been attributed to (1) neoplastic invasion of splenic capsule, (2) splenic infarctions followed by subcapsular hematomas, and (3) coagulation disorders that may lead to thrombosis or coagulation defects.[2] Hypercoagulability and thrombocytosis may lead to thrombosis and/or embolism with secondary splenic infarcts. On the other hand, fibrinolysis and hypocoagulable states as low plasma clotting factors or secondary to disseminated intravascular coagulopathy (DIC) may lead to bleeding incidents in the spleen. It should be pointed out that spontaneous rupture of the spleen always occurred in patients with splenomegaly.

All three of our patients had palpable spleens and two had thrombocytopenia. The one patient who had normal platelet count had metastatic melanoma, which is known to undergo cystic degeneration and is also known to be very vascular. The cystic degeneration and the vascular nature of such tumor may be the contributing factors in this case. It is clear from these three cases that the onset was insidious in the first two patients and acute in the third. The acute onset can be recognized easily, whereas the obscure clinical onset and course in patients receiving chemotherapeutic agents can be very puzzling to the clinician, who may attribute the anemia to bone marrow depression from the drug rather than to ruptured spleen, especially in the absence of abdominal signs.

Diagnostic paracentesis could be useful in establishing the diagnosis[12] but should be approached with great care in thrombocytopenic patients. Plain films of the abdomen, as reported by Pratt and associates,[8] are of no value, particularly in patients who have splenomegaly.

Scintiscanning may prove to be valuable in the diagnosis of obscure cases with delayed rupture,[7] and angiography is important in the syndrome of occult rupture of the spleen described by Drapanas and associates,[1] but most important is that the possibility of rupture of the spleen should be considered in the differential diagnosis.

Although most of the patients who had ruptured spleen succumbed in the postoperative period[2] as a result of their primary diseases, with the recent advances in hemostases and the control of fibrinolytic mechanisms in malignancies, some of these conditions could be palliated by splenectomy. The availability of platelet and leukocyte transfusions and epsilon-aminocaproic acid would enable the surgeon to carry out splenectomy and control the bleeding.

In conclusion, though the prognosis in patients with malignancy complicated with pathologic rupture of the spleen is usually grave, operative intervention is indicated to avert an immediate fatal outcome.

REFERENCES

1. Drapanas, T., Yates, A., Brickman, R., and Wholey, M.: The syndrome of occult rupture of the spleen, Arch. Surg. **99:** 298, 1969.
2. Hynes, E. H., Silverstein, N. M., and Fawcett, J. F.: Spontaneous rupture of the spleen in acute leukemia, Cancer **17:** 1356, 1964.
3. Hyun, H. B., Varga, F. C., and Rubin, J. R.:

Spontaneous and pathologic rupture of the spleen, Arch. Surg. **104:** 652, 1972.
4. Kaschub, W. R.: Pathological rupture of the spleen in acute leukemia, J. Maine Med. Assoc. **62:** 274, 1971.
5. Knoblich, R.: Pathologic (so-called spontaneous) rupture of the spleen in leukemia and lymphoma, Mich. Med. **65:** 105, 1966.
6. Leuridan, B., Sigam, M., Callens, J., and Langeron, P.: Spontaneous rupture of the spleen as a presenting sign of chronic myeloblastic leukemia, J. Sci. Med. Lille **88:** 537, 1970.
7. O'Mara, E. R., Hall, C. R., and Dombroski, L. D.: Scintiscanning in the diagnosis of rupture of the spleen, Surg. Gynecol. Obstet. **131:** 1077, 1970.
8. Pratt, D. B., et al.: Splenic rupture. A review of 114 cases, Minn. Med. **54:** 177, 1971.
9. Ravich, M. R., Reed, S. C., Stephaens, O. F., Vincent, C. P., and Gurnz, W. F.: Spontaneous rupture of the spleen in acute myeloid leukemia, Med. J. Aust. **1:** 90, 1971.
10. Schellmann, W. D., and Eckel, H.: Spontaneous splenic rupture in acute leukemia, Med. Welt **32:** 1733, 1969.
11. Stites, B. T., and Ultmann, E. J.: Spontaneous rupture of the spleen in chronic lymphocytic leukemia, Cancer **10:** 1587, 1966.
12. Tartaglia, A. P., et al.: Splenic rupture in leukemia, N. Engl. J. Med. **267:** 31, 1962.

Probable salmonella endocarditis treated with prosthetic valve replacement: A case report

Noriaki Yamamoto, M.D., Oscar Magidson, M.D., Christian Posner, M.D., A. Michael Mendez, M.D., Pablo Zubiate, M.D., *and* **Jerome Harold Kay, M.D.,** *Los Angeles, Calif.*

A case history of a 50-year-old woman with **Salmonella enteritidis** endocarditis, cured by mitral prosthetic valve replacement, is reported. The patient continues to do well without evidence of further infection 6 months after the operation.

From the Department of Thoracic and Cardiac Surgery and the Department of Medicine of the Saint Vincent's Hospital and the Los Angeles County–University of Southern California Medical Center, Los Angeles, Calif.

THE SALMONELLAE are primarily intestinal pathogens and, although salmonella endocarditis is an unusual occurrence, it is associated with a high mortality rate. The patient described in this paper was operated on in 1970, at which time her mitral valve was replaced with a mitral prosthesis. She developed salmonella endocarditis and congestive failure. The prosthesis was replaced with another identical mitral prosthesis and the patient appears to be cured of the endocarditis.

CASE REPORT

A 50-year-old woman was transferred from another hospital to the Saint Vincent's Hospital on April 6, 1973, with a high fever and chills of 4 weeks' duration. She had a past history of rheumatic fever at the age of 13 and a heart murmur discovered at the age of 20. At 38 years of age she noted shortness of breath, and a diagnosis of mitral stenosis was confirmed. In January, 1970, mitral valve replacement was performed with significant improvement.

The present illness was noted on March 5, 1973, when the patient was hospitalized with sudden onset of nausea, vomiting, high fever (105° F.), chills, and diarrhea. A blood culture was drawn on admission and was positive for salmonella group D. The blood cultures remained positive for 10 consecutive days. She was treated with ampicillin (3 Gm. intravenously daily) and tetracycline, (2 Gm. orally daily) with some improvement.

The patient was discharged on March 31, 1973, only to be readmitted on April 2, 1973, with recurrence of fever and chills. Blood cultures were again positive for the same organism. She was transferred to the Saint Vincent's Hospital for further evaluation and therapy on April 6, 1973.

Physical examination revealed that the patient had atrial fibrillation with a ventricular response of about 80 per minute. The blood pressure was 105/70 and her temperature was 98° F. on admission. Her temperature rose to 103° F. in the evening. The patient was a normally nourished, well-developed woman in no acute distress. She appeared markedly pale. There was no evidence of embolic phenomena. On auscultation of the lungs, râles were heard. The abdomen was soft

Supported in part by a grant from The Children's Heart Foundation.

Accepted for publication June 6, 1974.

Reprint requests: Jerome Harold Kay, M.D., University of Southern California, 2025 Zonal Ave., Los Angeles, Calif. 90033.

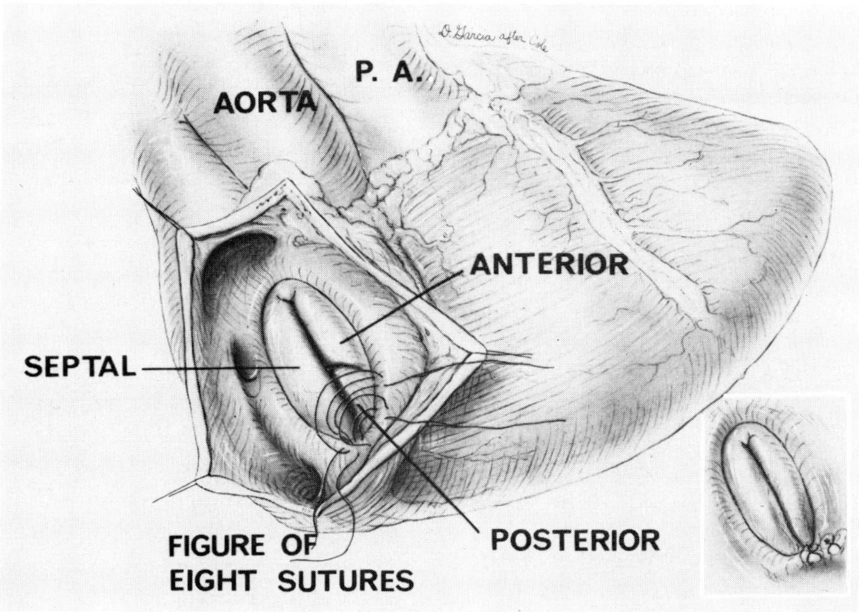

Fig. 1. Tricuspid annuloplasty.

and not tender. The liver was palpable 5 cm. below the right costal margin and there was no peripheral edema.

Laboratory findings were as follows: hemoglobin 9.6 Gm., hematocrit 29 percent, red blood cell count 3,270,000 per cubic millimeter; white blood cell count 13,900 per cubic millimeter, with 74 polymorphonuclear leukocytes, 15 percent lymphocytes, 5 percent monocytes, 5 percent band cells, and 1 percent eosinophils. Urinalysis was negative. Serum bilirubin values were normal. Serum protein electrophoresis revealed 6.2 Gm. of total protein with 2.0 Gm. of albumin and 0.5 Gm. of albumin-globulin ratio. Blood urea nitrogen value was 17 mg. per 100 ml. and creatinine was 1.4 mg. per 100 ml. Serum sodium was 129 mEq. per liter and serum potassium 4.6 mEq. per liter. Serum glutamic oxaloacetic transaminase activity was 82 U. Stool cultures were positive for salmonella type D. Three blood cultures were taken and were negative.

Chest roentgenogram revealed grade 4/5 cardiac enlargement on a scale of 6. The hilar and upper zone vessels remained slightly distended. The lungs were clear. There was a slight amount of pleural fluid in the costophrenic area. The liver scan demonstrated hepatomegaly. An electrocardiogram revealed atrial fibrillation with a ventricular response of about 80 per minute and nonspecific ST-T abnormalities.

The diagnosis on admission was salmonella endocarditis with congestive heart failure and she was on digoxin and lanoxin. Antibiotic therapy was started on April 6, with intravenous ampicillin, 9 Gm. the first day. The ampicillin was increased to 12 Gm. daily for a duration of 8 days and to 20 Gm. on and after April 15. There was no clinical improvement despite the therapy. Signs and symptoms of tricuspid insufficiency were detected on April 14; moreover, she complained of severe headache and double vision on April 19. This was diagnosed as septic cerebral emboli. At this time surgery with replacement of the mitral prosthesis was strongly urged. Although salmonella localization had not been found, it was considered probable that the site was on the mitral prosthesis. She continued to look acutely ill and continued in marked congestive failure. Her daily temperature continued as high as 103° F.

An operation was performed on April 27, 1973. The right atrium was grade 5/6 enlarged and there was a grade 5/6 systolic thrill in the right atrium. The systolic pulmonary artery pressure was thought to be about 70 mm. Hg. The left atrium was opened and examination revealed about 30 c.c. of vegetation between the disc and the flange of the prosthetic valve. This was piled up on the atrial side. There were a number of pockets of fluid in the wall along the cuff of the prosthetic valve. The vegetation, prosthetic valve, and a large cuff of mitral annulus were removed. The abscess areas were opened and all tissue removed was sent to the laboratory for culture. The mitral prosthesis, a No. 8 Kay-Shiley disc valve with a muscle guard, was replaced with an identical type prosthetic valve. The right atrium was opened and examination revealed a greatly dilated tricuspid annulus. The annulus would easily accommodate a tennis ball. A tricuspid annuloplasty was performed by eliminating the posterior leaflet by placing figure-of-eight sutures of No. 2 silk in the annulus of the tricuspid valve (Fig. 1).[4] This made for a very competent 2½ fingerbreadth valve. The total duration of aortic cross-clamping was 56 minutes.

The postoperative course was unremarkable. Streptomycin (1.0 Gm. intramuscularly) was given for 5 days as a standard postoperative antibiotic treatment. Daily ampicillin therapy was continued (20 Gm. intravenously). Although the vegetation removed at operation did not grow out any organisms and the smear was negative for organisms, it was felt this was the source of the infection and the ampicillin was, therefore, continued for 40 days postoperatively. After five days in the intensive-care unit the patient was transferred to the ward. The following day, her temperature rose to above 100° F. She continued to have temperature spikes to as high as 102° F. Stool culture on May 3 revealed the salmonella organism. After a week, the patient's temperature dropped and she felt far better than before the operation. All stool cultures were negative after May 7. She was discharged from the hospital on June 7, 1973, on ampicillin (2 Gm. orally daily). This was discontinued on Sept. 10, 1973, when she developed a rash. She continues to do well without evidence of infection 6 months postoperatively.

DISCUSSION

Saphra and Winter[7] reported on 7,779 human salmonella infections in 1957; 572 patients had focal manifestations, and bacterial endocarditis was noted in 20. Of the 20 cases, 13 were due to *Salmonella paratyphi* C and *S. choleraesuis;* one was due to *S. enteritidis.* All 20 cases had a rapidly fatal outcome. The organism in our patient was identified as *S. enteritidis.* Infection with this organism carries a very high mortality rate. Shulman[8] reviewed the literature of 15 cases of salmonella endocarditis. Only one of the 15 patients recovered and this was the first case report of salmonella endocarditis. Many cases of cardiac complications of salmonella infection have been reported, including acute paroxysmal auricular tachycardia,[8] pericarditis,[2] myocardial abscess,[3] and myocarditis.[6] Weinstein and Kaplan[9] reported on a 44-year-old man, who had an aortic prosthetic valve and developed salmonella aortitis and died due to rupture of the infected aorta just below the aortic prosthesis. They suggested that the appearance of bacteremia was especially ominous when such a prosthesis was present. A similar case was reported by Kleinman,[5] but the offending organism was *Staphylococcus aureus.* Bayer and associates[1] presented 14 postmortem cases of valve ring abscesses of the heart associated with atypical bacterial endocarditis, which included one instance of *S. choleraesuis* abscess.

Our case is unique in that this patient had a prosthetic mitral valve in place. Although the focus of salmonella was not detected prior to operation and the cultures of the vegetations removed during operation were sterile, the patient improved dramatically after replacement of the prosthetic mitral valve. The authors believe this to be the first case reported as a cure of *S. enteritidis* endocarditis with mitral prosthetic valve replacement.

The authors wish to thank Albert Attyah, M.D., for the referral and subsequent follow-up of this patient.

REFERENCES

1. Bayer, P. M., Pridun, N., and Wuketich, S.: Atypishe bakterielle endokarditis und klappenringabscess, Virchows Arch. [Zellpathol.] **352:** 182, 1971.
2. Bird, T.: *Salmonella typhimurium* pericarditis, Br. Heart J. **31:** 659, 1969.
3. Doraiswami, S., Friedman, S. A., and Kagan, A.: Salmonella endocarditis complicated by a myocardial abscess, Am. J. Cardiol. **26:** 102, 1970.
4. Kay, J. H., Masselli-Campagna, G., and Tsuji, H. K.: Surgical treatment of tricuspid insufficiency, Ann. Surg. **162:** 53, 1965.
5. Kleinman, L. A.: Recurrent bacterial endocarditis and aortitis with rupture of aorta: Report of a case with death four years after insertion of a Hufnagel valve, J. A. M. A. 173: 38, 1960.
6. Sanders, V., and Misanik, L. F.: Salmonella

myocarditis: Report of a case with ventricular rupture, Am. Heart J. **68:** 682, 1964.
7. Saphra, I., and Winter, J. W.: Clinical manifestations of salmonellosis in man: An evaluation of 7,779 human infections identified at the New York Salmonella Center, N. Engl. J. Med. **256:** 1128, 1957.
8. Shulman, B. H.: Cardiac complications in salmonella infections, Am. J. Dis. Child. **73:** 688, 1947.
9. Weinstein, L., and Kaplan, K.: Salmonella aortitis in a patient with a Hufnagel valve, Circulation **31:** 755, 1965.

Letters to the editors

Disseminated intravascular coagulation

To the Editors:

The syndrome now generally recognized by the name disseminated intravascular coagulation (DIC) was first noted many years ago by obstetricians who were confronted by uncontrollable bleeding associated with pregnancy. It was noted that in many cases fibrinogen was low or completely absent and the syndrome was thought to be only a consumption of fibrinogen. We now know that fibrinogen is the least affected of all clotting elements and that the syndrome has a very wide incidence involving all medical and surgical specialties.

However, as our knowledge of the syndrome has grown, controversies as to its incidence, importance, nature, and mechanism have multiplied and there is at present a great state of disagreement on almost every aspect of DIC.

The first two sentences in the 1973 *Year Book of Surgery* state, "Disseminated intravascular coagulation remains a concern in a variety of disorders of interest to surgeons. It is now appreciated that heparin is no longer to be regarded as primary therapy and correction of the initiating disorder should be emphasized."[1]

On page 21 of the same book, it is stated, "The major champion of the use of heparin, Dr. Hardaway, has recently tempered his enthusiasm." On page 51 of the same book, a study reports that coagulation changes were not seen in hemorrhagic shock in baboons. On page 59 of the same book, a study reports that while coagulation changes do not occur in hemorrhagic shock in baboons, they do occur in baboons as a result of bacteremia.

While it is gratifying to hear that DIC is now recognized as "a concern in a variety of disorders of interest to surgeons," it is disheartening to realize the great misunderstanding of DIC and its relationship to shock and other conditions.

DIC was first incriminated as a cause of tissue damage in 1954.[9]

DIC was first documented to be a factor in the etiology of shock in 1959.[7]

DIC was first promulgated to be the basic mechanism of a large number of clinical syndromes in 1961[2] and more completely in 1963.[8] In a monograph on DIC in 1966,[3] experimental and clinical treatment of shock and DIC was recommended. It stated (page 241): "Treatment is designed to restore normal condition and prevent DIC. The clinically most effective way of preventing DIC is preventing the stagnant, acid capillary flow which is necessary for the production of DIC. The first and most important step in this is producing an adequate blood volume." Heparin was not recommended for the treatment of DIC because (page 219): "it had to be administered before the onset of shock. It is inactivated in the presence of acidosis which occurs in shock. It does not prevent platelet agglutination which is the trigger mechanism of septic or endotoxin shock. It will not prevent coagulation produced by coagulase of staphylococci." In addition, it complicated the coagulation defect of DIC and is frequently dangerous. This opinion was expressed in numerous publications and many oral presentations given in the U. S. A., Canada, Mexico, South America, and many countries in Europe. In a book entitled *Clinical Management of Shock,* published in 1968,[4] it was stated on page 126: "The most effective method of preventing death . . . is by prevention of capillary stasis by means of volume addition and vasodilation." On page 87, it was stated: "Maintenance of a normal capillary blood flow is probably the best way to prevent DIC for two reasons: (1) it corrects the original primary deficiency

Vol. 76, No. 4, pp. 682-684

in such condition as shock, and (2) it is very hard for any of the many other causes for DIC to produce DIC in the presence of a normal capillary flow." Heparin was *not* recommended.

The opinions expressed above were based on considerable research work. It had been found in 1956 that, while infusion of incompatible blood in dogs would produce DIC if the dogs were first vasoconstricted by administering a surgical procedure, the DIC was not produced by incompatible blood alone.[10] It was found that the production of DIC required two separate factors—neither alone was adequate. These were (1) a stagnant, acid capillary flow, and (2) the presence of a thromboplastic agent in the blood stream.

These basic facts somehow have never been understood. Many medical and surgical authors have concluded that they could find no evidence of DIC in acute hemorrhagic shock in dogs, primates, or human beings. They found no evidence of pulmonary dysfunction or shock lung in acute hemorrhagic shock. Of course, this is prefectly true. Simple uncomplicated hemorrhage will not produce DIC even though severe and prolonged. It produces only one of the two requirements for DIC, namely a stagnant, acid capillary flow.[3, 4] Dogs do not die of pure hemorrhagic shock even though they are kept at 40 mm. Hg arterial pressure for 5 or more hours. However, if this shock is carried out by the usual Wiggers reservoir technique, almost all will die.[14] This is because the tubing and reservoir activate the coagulation mechanism completing the two requirements for production of DIC.[14] However, it is well documented that in refractory shock of any type DIC is present,[6, 15] and may be the cause of a bleeding tendency, acute respiratory failure, and other organ failure.

Hemorrhagic shock is always easily reversible until the point of death. It is only with the addition of a thromboplastic agent in the blood that DIC and refractoriness are produced. Common factors able to produce a thromboplastic agent are sepsis, tissue damage, and hemolysis.[3, 4] The best way to prevent or treat DIC is to promote capillary blood flow. Then even the abundance of a thromboplastic agent in the blood will not produce DIC. It has been shown that, even with large amounts of thromboplastic agents such as thrombin, hemolysis, or tissue damage, DIC will not be produced without a deficient capillary flow.[11] The massive liberation of thromboplastic agent resulting from intravenous infusion of distilled water or from injection of hemolyzed blood is harmless in the absence of a deficient capillary flow.[11] This is true in human beings as well as in animals. It was shown that the restoration of adequate capillary flow by means of volume administration and vasodilation would immediately stop DIC.[12] It was also shown that heparin could not act in the extremely low capillary and tissue pH that is present in shock.[13] It is inactivated in the very area that it is needed, namely the capillary.

To summarize, DIC is a common cause of refractory shock and a consumptive coagulopathy. Its treatment is by promoting capillary flow. Heparin is probably useless and may be dangerous.

Robert M. Hardaway, III, M.D.
Brigadier General, MC
Office of the Commander
William Beaumont Army Medical Center
El Paso, Texas 79920

REFERENCES

1. Schwartz, S. I., et al.: Year book of surgery, Chicago, 1973, Year Book Medical Publishers, Inc.
2. Hardaway, R. M.: Disseminated intravascular coagulation syndromes, Arch. Surg. **83:** 842, 1961.
3. Hardaway, R. M.: Syndromes of disseminated intravascular coagulation, Springfield, Ill., 1966, Charles C Thomas, Publisher.
4. Hardaway, R. M.: Clinical management of shock, Springfield, Ill., 1968, Charles C Thomas, Publisher.
5. Hardaway, R. M.: The fallacy of hemorrhagic shock models in dogs, *in* Microcirculatory approaches to current therapeutic problems symposia, Sixth European conference on microcirculation, Aalborg, 1970, p. 24.
6. Hardaway, R. M.: Disseminated intravascular coagulation as a possible cause of acute

respiratory failure, Surg. Gynecol. Obstet. **137:** 1, 1973.
7. Hardaway, R. M., and McKay, D. G.: Disseminated intravascular coagulation: A cause of shock, Ann. Surg. **149:** 462, 1959.
8. Hardaway, R. M., and McKay, D. G.: The syndromes of disseminated intravascular coagulation, Rev. Surg. **20:** 297, 1963.
9. Hardaway, R. M., McKay, D. G., and Williams, J. H.: Lower nephron nephrosis (ischemic nephrosis), Am. J. Surg. **87:** 41, 1954.
10. Hardaway, R. M., McKay, D. G., and Wahle, G. H.: Pathologic study of intravascular coagulation following incompatible blood transfusion in dogs, Am. J. Surg. **91:** 24, 1956.
11. Hardaway, R. M., et al.: Influence of trauma and hemolysis on hemorrhagic shock in dogs, J. Trauma **4:** 624, 1964.
12. Hardaway, R. M., et al.: Influence of vasoconstriction and vasodilation on disseminated intravascular coagulation in irreversible hemmorhagic shock, Surg. Gynecol. Obstet. **119:** 1053, 1964.
13. Hardaway, R. M., et al.: Clotting time of heparinized blood, Arch. Surg. **89:** 701, 1964.
14. Hardaway, R. M., et al.: The influence of extracorporeal handling of blood on hemorrhagic shock in dogs, Exp. Med. Surg. **23:** 28, 1965.
15. Hardaway, R. M., et al.: Intensive study and treatment of shock in man, J. A. M. A. **199:** 779, 1967.

Reply

To the Editors:

It appears that Dr. Hardaway's letter implies an inappropriate consideration by me regarding him as a past champion of the use of heparin. These comments were made personally by me in reference to an article which was being discussed and abstracted in the *Year Book of Surgery, 1973.* It is certainly possible that Dr. Hardaway's initial enthusiasm for heparin was overassessed by this editor, but I do feel obliged to indicate the statements appearing in Dr. Hardaway's monograph* which prompted the conclusion.

*Hardaway, R. M.: Syndrome of disseminated intravascular coagulation, Springfield, Ill., 1966, Charles C Thomas, Publisher.

1. Page 193: "Heparin will prevent death in irreversible hemorrhagic shock and ameliorate the toxic effects of surface-activated blood in dogs."

2. Page 219: "Heparin was found to be significantly effective in protecting dogs against death and DIC in irreversible hemorrhagic shock,[28*] and somewhat protective against endotoxin shock."[22*] However, it had to be administered before the onset of shock.

3. Page 239: "Any treatment must therefore begin at the start of endotoxin shock. Heparin and fibrinolysin are also successful if used early."

4. Page 269: There is a case report of a patient at the Walter Reed Hospital after open-heart surgery with a combination of afibrinogenemia and fibrinolysis *successfully* treated with fibrinogen, EACA, and heparin.

5. Page 346: Clotting abnormalities due to cancer are being discussed. "By injection of heparin in clinical cases, clotting factor differences could be alleviated. This is strong evidence that the bleeding tendency in these cases was due to an episode of DIC."

6. Page 363: "The etiologic mechanism in pseudomembraneous enterocolitis is intravascular coagulation. Heparin will prevent these changes to a large extent."

This editor does apologize if he has misrepresented so distinguished an investigator as Dr. Hardaway, but he feels that the above-mentioned statements were highly suggestive of an advocate of heparin.

Seymour I. Schwartz, M.D.
Strong Memorial Hospital
260 Crittenden Blvd.
Rochester, N. Y. 14620

*28. Hardaway, R. M., et al.: Ann. Surg. 155: 241, 1962.
22. Hardaway, R. M., et al.: Ann. Surg. 154: 791, 1961.

Volume 76 Number 5 SURGERY

NOVEMBER, 1974

Original communications

The choice of treatment for operable carcinoma of the breast

C. D. Haagensen, M.D., *New York, N. Y.*

This is a detailed report of the methods used to select patients from a personal series of 1,063 radical mastectomies performed over a period of 39 years and a presentation of the 10 year results. These results of radical mastectomy are compared with the results of other methods of treatment for operable breast carcinoma. The clinical and statistical requirements for a valid comparison of this kind are stated.

From the Columbia–Presbyterian Medical Center, New York, N. Y.

THIRTY-NINE YEARS AGO, in 1935, I began to perform the Halsted radical mastectomy. I believed then, as I still do, that it was the most thorough surgical method of eradicating breast carcinoma that was reasonable within the limitations of the regional anatomy and the pathology of the disease. I described my technique for the operation[16] in the pages of SURGERY in 1948. I and my residents have performed this same operation for 1,063 patients since 1935.

During recent years radical mastectomy has been increasingly challenged by a variety of less aggressive methods of treatment. It seems appropriate to review my experience with the operation in my personal series of patients and to compare my results with those obtained with other methods of treatment.

Accepted for publication March 19, 1974.

Reprint requests: C. D. Haagensen, M.D., Department of Surgery, Columbia University, 630 W. 168th St., New York, N. Y. 10032.

THE CLINICAL CLASSIFICATION OF BREAST CARCINOMA

Valid comparison of the results achieved with different methods of treatment of breast carcinoma depends primarily upon how the patients have been selected in the different trial series. Breast carcinoma is a slowly progressive disease and it is much more amenable to treatment in its earlier stages of advancement than later on in the course of the disease. For a fair comparison of methods of treatment, the clinical stage of advancement of the disease must be carefully de-

Table I. *The Columbia Clinical Classification*

Stage	*Clinical criteria*
A	No skin edema, ulceration, or solid fixation of tumor to chest wall; axillary nodes not clinically involved
B	No skin edema, ulceration, or solid fixation of tumor to chest wall; clinically involved axillary nodes, but less than 2.5 cm. in transverse diameter and not fixed to overlying skin or deeper structures of axilla
C	Any one of five grave signs of advanced breast carcinoma 1. Edema of skin of limited extent (involving less than one third of the skin over the breast) 2. Skin ulceration 3. Solid fixation of tumor to chest wall 4. Massive involvement of axillary lymph nodes: a single node, or group of fused nodes, measuring 2.5 cm. or more in transverse diameter 5. Fixation of the axillary nodes to overlying skin or deeper structures of the axilla
D	More advanced breast carcinoma, including 1. A combination of any two or more of the five grave signs listed above in Stage C 2. Extensive edema of skin (involving more than one third of the skin over the breast) 3. Satellite skin nodules 4. The inflammatory type of carcinoma 5. Clinically involved supraclavicular lymph nodes 6. Internal mammary metastases as evidenced by a parasternal tumor 7. Edema of the arm 8. Distant metastases

termined in each patient. This is based solely upon the *clinical* findings and is necessarily determined *before* treatment. Once the clinical stage of the disease is decided upon, it is of course never changed, no matter what the pathological findings following operation may be. Clinical staging makes it possible to compare the results of different methods of treatment in each stage separately. Otherwise such comparisons are like a race without a starting line.

Clinical staging is a new discipline in which most surgeons have not as yet had much experience. Its acceptance has been handicapped by the fact that the most widely used classification, the TNM plan of the International Union Against Cancer, first drafted in 1954, is so complex that it is not practical. Moreover, some of the clinical criteria used in it are poorly defined, while other important criteria are omitted.

At Columbia we have long been aware of the basic importance of clinical criteria to guide us in the selection of treatment for breast carcinoma. In 1943, just 31 years ago, we presented our criteria of operability. They were derived from close correlation of the clinical features of breast carcinoma with the results of treatment as recorded in a complete 10 year follow-up. The validity of our criteria of operability has been evidenced by their wide acceptance as a guide to the selection of patients for radical mastectomy.

From our experience with these criteria of operability we came to appreciate the great need for a practical plan for clinical classification. It must be simple enough to be kept clearly in mind by those who use it only infrequently in studying new patients with breast carcinoma. The criteria upon which it is based must be carefully chosen, and they must be so precisely defined that there is never confusion as to their meaning.

Our Columbia Clinical Classification for breast carcinoma, as it evolved from our experience with the disease more than 20 years ago, is shown in Table I. It has been used in our own clinic and in a number of other clinics long enough to convince us that it is practical and surprisingly accurate. It would be possible to improve its accuracy somewhat by adding certain other significant clinical factors, such as the size of the primary tumor, but our classification would then become too complex to be practical.

The greater accuracy of the Columbia Clinical Classification as compared with other clinical classifications is illustrated in the interpretation of the findings of axillary palpation. This is much the most important part of any clinical classification designed to define the stage of advancement of breast carcinoma. The palpation of the axilla is also the most difficult part of the clinical examination.

In the two most widely used clinical classifications, the TNM and the Manchester classifications, the patients are divided into

Table II. *Carcinoma of the breast: Clinical examination of the axilla correlated with pathological status of axillary nodes; radical mastectomy, 1935 to July, 1973*

Clinical findings in axilla	Number of patients	Axillary metastases: Number of patients	Axillary metastases: Percent	1 to 3 nodes involved: Number of patients	1 to 3 nodes involved: Percent	4 to 7 nodes involved: Number of patients	4 to 7 nodes involved: Percent	8 or more nodes involved: Number of patients	8 or more nodes involved: Percent
No palpable nodes	703	203	29	134	19	35	5	34	5
Palpable nodes not clinically involved	76	31	40	21	27	4	5	6	8
Clinically involved nodes less than 2.5 cm. in diameter and movable	240	179	74	75	31	41	17	63	26
Clinically involved nodes 2.5 cm. or more in diameter or fixed in axilla	44	41	93	13	30	11	25	17	38
Total number of patients	1,063	454	43						

two groups as regards the axillary findings—those who have no palpable axillary nodes and those in whom nodes are palpated. No matter what the characteristics of the palpable nodes in the latter group may be, it is assumed that they contain metastases. This is much too simplistic an interpretation of the axillary findings.

Good clinicians know that in many women small soft axillary nodes are palpated which represent only chronic lymphadenitis due to minor infections. We long ago learned that it is possible and useful to distinguish between these innocuous, smaller, softer nodes and the larger, firmer nodes which usually do contain metastases. We also learned from measuring the transverse diameter of larger axillary nodes that there is a critical size limit beyond which the possibility of surgical cure diminishes sharply. This limit is approximately 2.5 cm. The prognosis is even worse when these larger axillary nodes are fixed to the superficial or deep axillary structures.

These facts led us to classify our patients with breast carcinoma into four rather than two groups as regards the clinical findings in the axilla, as follows:

1—those with no palpable nodes,
2—those with smaller, softer nodes which are classed as not clinically involved,
3—those with larger, firmer nodes which are classed as clinically involved but which measure less than 2.5 cm. in transverse diameter,
4—those with clinically involved nodes which measure 2.5 cm. or more in transverse diameter or which are fixed.

The authors of the TNM and Manchester classifications did not think it worthwhile to attempt to categorize the axillary findings so precisely. McWhirter's[36] 1967 statement regarding the significance of axillary metastases is typical of their point of view. He stated, "Only the axillary group of nodes is removed in the conventional radical mastectomy. The long-term results show that when these nodes are involved the operation is rarely successful."

As evidence of the value of classifying patients with breast carcinoma into four clinical categories on the basis of axillary palpation, I can present data from my own series of radical mastectomies. In Table II the clinical findings in the axilla in 1,063 patients who subsequently underwent radical mastectomy are correlated with the pathological findings in the axillary nodes. There is a progressive increase in the percentage of axillary metastases through the four clinical categories—from 29 to 93 percent. Equally important is the fact that the percentage of patients with eight or more involved axillary nodes—an exceedingly grave degree of axillary involvement—increases from 5 to 38 percent through the four clinical categories.

In Table III the degree of axillary involvement found at radical mastectomy in my series of patients classified according to the

Table III. *Radical mastectomy for breast carcinoma: Extent of axillary metastasis correlated with 10 year survival—Personal series of cases, 1935 to July, 1963*

Columbia Clinical Classification	Number of axillary nodes with metastases	Number of patients	10 year survival: Number	10 year survival: Percent
Stage A	None	418	320	76.5
	1 to 3	131	89	68
	4 to 7	30	10	33
	8 or more	29	6	20
	Total	608	425	70
Stage B	None	48	34	70
	1 to 3	61	27	44
	4 to 7	37	14	38
	8 or more	40	5	12
	Total	186	80	43
Stage C	None	17	8	47
	1 to 3	21	6	29
	4 to 7	9	4	44
	8 or more	29	3	10
	Total	76	21	30
Stage D	None	1	0	
	1 to 3	2	1	
	4 to 7	1	0	
	8 or more	8	1	
	Total	12	2	17
Total		882		

Table IV. *Radical mastectomy for mammary carcinoma and frequency of microscopic axillary metastases*

Columbia Clinical Classification	Butcher, St. Louis, 1950-1955: Number of cases	Butcher, St. Louis, 1950-1955: Percent ax. met.	Miller, Detroit, 1951-1960: Number of cases	Miller, Detroit, 1951-1960: Percent ax. met.	Dahl-Iversen and Tobiassen, Copenhagen, 1950-1955: Number of cases	Dahl-Iversen and Tobiassen, Copenhagen, 1950-1955: Percent ax. met.	Haagensen, Columbia, New York, 1935-1955: Number of cases	Haagensen, Columbia, New York, 1935-1955: Percent ax. met.
Stage A	214	32.2	315	29.5	317	28.7	344	32.2
Stage B	135	75.5	90	84.4	69	76.8	138	76.0
Stage C	48	89.5	60	76.7	26*	46.2	63	76.2
All stages	397		465		412		545	

*This number of cases is too small to have any statistical significance.

Columbia Clinical Classification is correlated with 10 year survival. As the number of involved nodes increases, the survival rate falls in each of the advancing stages of the disease. Contradicting the pessimism of McWhirter, I can point out that, while the 10 year survival rate was 76.5 percent when no axillary nodes were found to be involved in my Stage A patients, 68 percent of those who had from one to three nodes involved survived for 10 years. The very grave prognostic significance of involvement of eight or more nodes in all of the clinical stages is also evident from this table.

The data shown in Table III provide the most accurate prognostic information available for patients who have been treated by radical mastectomy. Its accuracy is due to our classifying the clinical findings in the axilla in four different categories, which are

Table V. *Significance of edema of the breast skin as a prognostic sign: Radical mastectomy, 1935 to July, 1963*

Clinical group	Number of patients	10 year survival: Number	10 year survival: Percent
No edema of the skin; no clinically involved axillary nodes	608	425	70
Edema of limited extent; no clinically involved axillary nodes	10	6	60
No edema of the skin; clinically involved axillary nodes less than 2.5 cm. in diameter	186	80	43
Edema of limited extent and clinically involved axillary nodes less than 2.5 cm. in diameter	25	1	4

Table VI. *Conservative radical mastectomy for mammary carcinoma and crude survival rates in 250 cases—Handley, comparison of Columbia and TNM clinical staging*

Stage	Number of patients	10 year survival: Number	10 year survival: Percent
Columbia:			
A	127	69	54.3
B	98	41	41.8
C	21	4	18.0
D	4	0	0
Total	250	114	45.6
TNM:			
1	93	48	51.6
2	103	52	50.5
3	52	14	26.9
4	2	0	0
Total	250	114	45.6

a part of our Columbia Clinical Classification, as well as to our careful pathological studies of the extent of axillary node involvement in our radical mastectomy specimens.

Another indication of the accuracy of the Columbia Clinical Classification in terms of axillary involvement is seen in Table IV. In it the frequency of microscopical axillary metastases found at radical mastectomy is reported for each clinical stage in four different clinics. The findings were strikingly similar. It is remarkable that any clinical classification can be so accurate.

Another defect of the TNM clinical classification is the omission of edema of the skin as a clinical criterion. In the latest—1969—version of the TNM classification edema was not mentioned. Yet skin edema is one of the most important signs of an advanced stage of breast carcinoma. It results from blockage of the subdermal lymphatics by emboli of carcinoma cells. In order to assess as accurately as possible the significance of skin edema we classify these patients with edema in two groups—those in whom the edema involves less than one third of the skin over the breast, and those in whom the edema is more extensive. None of my patients who had extensive skin edema before treatment has been cured by any form of therapy. I learned this early enough to avoid ever performing radical mastectomy on such a patient. But my case series includes 35 patients who had skin edema involving less than one third of the skin over the breast. These patients were operated upon during the years when I was learning to assess the significance of this clinical phenomenon. The end results in these 35 patients are shown in Table V, in which the presence of limited skin edema is correlated with the clinical status of the axillary nodes. When skin edema of limited extent was present in patients who did not have clinically involved axillary nodes, the 10 year survival of 60 percent justified radical mastectomy. But when skin edema of even limited extent was present in patients with clinically involved axillary nodes, the survival rate of only 4 percent leaves no doubt as to the inoperability of these patients.

The best comparison of the practical value of the Columbia and TNM methods of clinical classification of breast carcinoma has been made by Handley. He classified the patients in his own series of 250 conservative radical mastectomies according to both the Columbia and the TNM clinical classification and correlated the clinical stages with the 10 year survival rates. His findings are shown in

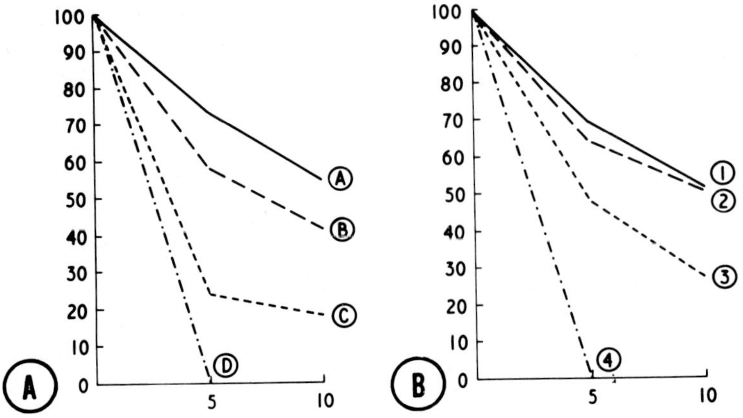

Fig. 1. Handley's crude survival rate in 250 patients on whom conservative radical mastectomies had been performed for mammary carcinoma; *A,* Columbia Clinical Classification; *B,* TNM Clinical Classification.

Table VI and Fig. 1. There was no real difference in the survival rates for stages 1 and 2 of the TNM classification, while there was a considerable spread between the survival rates for Stages A and B of the Columbia Classification. This fact makes the Columbia Classification much more useful than the TNM classification for distinguishing between the earlier stages of the disease. Another important advantage of the Columbia Classification is that it has been used in a number of carefully studied case series as a guide to the selection of patients for radical mastectomy. In our own clinic we perform the operation only for patients whose disease is classified as Stages A or B. The Stage C and D patients are treated by less drastic measures, such as irradiation, because the likelihood of cure by radical mastectomy is so poor that other methods will do as well or better. The TNM classification has not been much used as a guide for the selection of patients for radical mastectomy and its value in this regard remains untested.

Another clincal phenomenon which signifies incurability of breast carcinoma by surgery (except for certain inframammary carcinomas) is solid fixation of the tumor to the underlying chest wall. In our Columbia Classification we specify *solid* fixation and we mean just that. The tumor cannot be moved at all over the underlying chest wall. The Manchester classification also describes this phenomenon well with the statement, "complete fixation of the tumour to the chest wall." But in the TNM classification a confusing terminology regarding fixation is used. "Muscle fixation" signifies a T3 category, and "chest wall involved" signifies a T4 category. Neither of these terms refers to clearly recognizable clinical phenomena. They refer to pathological findings of doubtful clinical significance.

Carcinomas of the inframammary fold form a special group as regards fixation to the chest wall. The inframammary fold is a transverse ridge of abnormally dense mammary tissue across the caudad edge of the breast. Here the edge of the breast is bound down tightly to the deep fascial planes of the chest wall. Carcinomas sometimes develop in the inframammary ridge, and they are apt to be abnormally fixed to the underlying chest wall as compared with carcinomas occurring elsewhere in the breast. My series of radical mastectomies includes 23 patients with inframammary carcinomas. In 18 there was an abnormal degree of fixation. In nine, the abnormal fixation was only *relative*—that is, the tumor could be moved somewhat over the chest wall. This relative fixation has not, in my experience, been a contraindication to operation, and it is not a criterion in our Columbia Clinical Classification. In my other nine patients with inframammary carcinoma, the tumor was *solidly* fixed to the underlying chest wall. Yet four of the nine survived 10 years or more after radical mastectomy. Although the number of cases is small, my experience suggests that solid fixation of an inframammary carcinoma is not a contraindication to radical mastectomy provided the disease is otherwise classified as Stage A or B.

PERSONAL RESULTS WITH THE HALSTED RADICAL MASTECTOMY

Since 1935, when I began to perform the Halsted radical mastectomy in the Presbyterian Hospital, I have selected patients for the operation on the basis of careful study of the clinical features of their disease. The selection is defined in terms of the Columbia Clinical Classification, which I have discussed above. As I have learned more regarding the significance of the clinical features of breast carcinoma through the years, I have come to the conclusion that radical mastectomy, although it is the most successful of all surgical methods of attacking the disease, should be performed only on patients whose disease is classified as Columbia Stage A or B. The Stage C and D patients shown in my data who were treated by radical mastectomy are mostly from earlier years, before I became convinced that irradiation alone succeeds better with these patients whose disease is more advanced. My aim has always been to perform the best possible operation and to do it only on patients for whom it offers a better hope of cure than any other method of treatment.

Although the Columbia Clinical Classification has been the basis for my selection of patients for radical mastectomy, an additional method of selection was used between the years 1951 to 1966, inclusive. We had been aware that the clinical features alone upon which we relied for the selection of patients betrayed us into operating upon some patients whose disease was incurable by surgery. These were for the most part patients who had occult metastases at the periphery of the regional lymph node filter for the breast—the lymph nodes at the apex of the axilla and in the internal mammary chain. The frequency and the grave significance of internal mammary metastases had been demonstrated by Richard Handley. He learned to biopsy these nodes before performing radical mastectomy. Following his lead we began, in 1951, to perform preliminary biopsy of these internal mammary nodes to sharpen our selection of patients for radical mastectomy. In this separate preliminary biopsy procedure we combined biopsy of the primary tumor in the breast, excision of the lymph nodes at the apex of the axilla, and excision of the internal mammary nodes in the upper three interspaces. In general, we performed this preliminary triple biopsy only on patients whose disease, on clinical grounds, appeared to be somewhat more advanced. Between 1951 and 1966, inclusive, these biopsies were done upon a total of 1,007 patients.[19] When we found metastases in the apical or internal mammary nodes we did no further surgery, treating these patients with irradiation only. The 10 year survival rate in a total of 117 patients who were shown to have internal mammary metastases and who were treated by irradiation alone was 17 percent, which is statistically not different from the results of extended radical mastectomy with parasternal chest wall resection, including the internal mammary nodes.

In 1967 we terminated this triple biopsy clinical experiment, having learned all that we could hope to learn from it, and reported our results. Our conclusion was that all methods of treatment had failed disastrously and equally when metastases had reached these lymph nodes at the periphery of the regional lymph node filter at the apex of the axilla and in the internal mammary chain. We reverted to performing radical mastectomy straight off upon all patients whose breast carcinomas are classified as Columbia Stage A or B. Since we know that approximately 20 percent of these patients have occult internal mammary metastases, we regularly add postoperative prophylactic irradiation to the internal mammary nodes, excepting patients whose primary tumors are

Table VII. *Ten-year survival rates by clinical stage for radical mastectomy, and also for patients with metastases to subclavicular or internal mammary nodes treated only by irradiation: Personal series of cases, 1935 to July, 1963*

Columbia Clinical Stage	*Number of patients*	*10 year survival**	
		Number	*Percent*
Radical mastectomy:			
A	608	425	70
B	186	80	43
C	76	21	30
D	12	2	17
Total	882		
Positive subclavicular or internal mammary nodes—irradiation only:			
A	33	7	21
B	53	10	18
C	34	1	3
D	74	4	5
Total	194		
Entire series of patients including those treated by radical mastectomy as well as those with subclavicular or internal mammary metastases treated only with irradiation:			
A	641	432	67
B	239	90	38
C	110	22	20
D	86	6	7
Total	1,076		

*Two patients who died postoperatively and one lost to follow-up after 5½ years are counted as having died of breast carcinoma.

less than 3 cm. in diameter and are situated in the outer half of the breast. We know that in this group the frequency of internal mammary metastases is much less—probably only about 5 percent. When axillary nodes are found to be involved, this prophylactic internal mammary irradiation is always given. We can only hope that this will lessen, to some degree, the threat which internal mammary metastases impose.

During the years 1951 to July, 1963, these preliminary biopsies of the apical and internal mammary nodes were done in 194 patients with breast carcinoma in my personal series of cases. These 194 patients are, of course, included in my total series of personal cases for whom I herewith report 10 year results, so that my method of selection of patients is fully described.

In Table VII the 10 year results are presented for my entire series of 1,076 patients with breast carcinoma, including those treated by radical mastectomy as well as those excluded from the operation because of metastases in the apical or internal mammary nodes. This table gives complete information as to how my patients were selected for radical mastectomy. Those who wish to compare my results with the operation with the results of other methods of treatment need only select their patients in the same way that I have selected mine and use the same method of reporting end results.

A feature of the results in this personal series of radical mastectomies which I should like to emphasize is that they are the same in the ward patients where I served as first assistant to my pupil, the resident surgeon who did the operation, as they are in my private patients on whom I operated myself. The numbers of patients in the two groups are about equal. These data are shown in Table VIII. They substantiate the point which I have repeatedly made, namely, that the operation can be successfully taught to resident surgeons by sufficiently dedicated attending surgeons without penalizing the patients.

FREQUENCY AND EXTENT OF AXILLARY METASTASES

In this long personal series of radical mastectomies the frequency of axillary metastases has been 45.5 percent. This is somewhat lower than the frequency in some carefully documented modern series of radical mastectomies as shown in Table IX. This overall figure means very little. What is important is the frequency of axillary metastases in each of the advancing clinical stages of the disease.

This information, as well as the extent of axillary metastasis in terms of the numbers of involved nodes for each clinical stage, is correlated with 10 year survival rates in Table III. It is clear from this table that the status of the axillary nodes is overwhelmingly important in determining prognosis following radical mastectomy. Pathologists can make an essential contribution by studying the axillary specimens with the clearing technique and accurately determining the numbers of involved nodes as well as their exact position in the axillary node filter. When no more than three nodes contain metastases in patients whose disease is classified as Stage A, the survival rate is nearly as good as when there are no metastases. Involvement of eight or more nodes is, on the other hand, a very grave finding. These details are of critical importance in determining the further treatment in the individual patient.

LOCAL RECURRENCE

Local recurrence is a considerable threat following the usual type of radical mastectomy. It may be of three types. The first and least frequent type is local recurrence in the axilla. It signifies failure of the axillary dissection.

The second type is the parasternal moundlike tumor that is the outward manifestation of metastases to internal mammary nodes. These metastases are not chargeable to the surgeon in the sense of his having implanted them.

The third and by far the most frequent type of local recurrence is the development of nodules in the skin flaps on the chest wall. In general, such nodules must result from the implantation in the wound of carcinoma emboli that have escaped from blood vessels or lymphatics cut during the operation, from the implantation of carcinoma cells by instruments or sponges from a focus of carcinoma into which the surgeon has unwittingly carried his dissection, or from small unrecognized foci of carcinoma in breast tissue left by the operator on his thick skin flaps.

Whatever the explanation for local recurrence on the chest wall may be, the surgeon is certainly responsible for it. Either his operative technique has been faulty, or he has erred in choosing to operate upon carcinoma so far advanced that it is impossible to get it all out. This same criticism applies when there is recurrence in the axilla.

Although most recurrent nodules on the chest wall are distressingly genuine, the possibility of pseudorecurrence must always be kept in mind. Foreign-body cysts around suture material sometimes simulate true recurrence. Another form of pseudorecurrence is the bony, hard, fixed nodule that develops on a rib or costal cartilage where the surgeon's knife has nicked it. These prove to be merely proliferation of periosteum or perichondrium.

The frequency and site of local recurrence within 10 years in my personal series of radical mastectomies are shown in Table X. The most striking feature of these data is the infrequency of recurrence in the axilla; among a total of 328 patients whose disease was classified as clinical Stage A or B, constituting what we today regard as the operable group, and who were found to have axil-

Table VIII. *Ten-year survival of ward and private patients: Personal series of radical mastectomies, 1935 to July, 1963*

Columbia Clinical Classification	Private patients (Haagensen surgeon)		Ward patients (resident surgeon; Haagensen assistant)	
	Number of patients	Percent 10 year survival	Number of patients	Percent 10 year survival
Stage A	320	70	288	67
Stage B	72	42	114	43

Table IX. *Frequency of axillary metastases in radical mastectomy*

Author	Number of radical mastectomies	Percent with axillary metastases
Spratt and Donegan, Ellis Fischel Hospital, 1940-1958	704	56.7
Lewison, The Johns Hopkins Hospital, 1946-1950	253	54.5
Butcher, Barnes Hospital, 1950-1955	397	54.2
Miller, Grace Hospital, 1951-1960	465	48.6
Haagensen, Columbia-Presbyterian Medical Center, 1935–July, 1963	882	45.5
Dahl-Iversen and Tobiassen, Rigshospitalet, 1950-1955	425	41.1
Handley, Middlesex Hospital, 1946-1969	804	54.4

Table X. *Local recurrence within 10 years following radical mastectomy correlated with clinical stage and pathologically verified axillary metastases: Personal series of cases, 1935 to July, 1963*

Columbia Clinical Classification	*Status of axillary nodes*	*Parasternal recurrence*	*Chest-wall recurrence*	*Axillary recurrence*	*Total percent*
Stage A	No metastases, 418 cases	8	7	0	6.5
	Metastases, 190 cases	8	16	0	
Stage B	No metastases, 48 cases	1	0	0	18
	Metastases, 138 cases	5	26	2	
Stage C	No metastases, 17 cases	0	0	0	29
	Metastases, 59 cases	5	12	5	
Stage D	No metastases, 1 case	0	1	0	75
	Metastases, 11 cases	0	7	1	

lary metastases, only two developed axillary recurrence.

Of these 328 patients, 268 received no postoperative prophylactic irradiation; the only treatment to the axilla was a meticulous dissection. The two patients who had axillary recurrence were in this group; one had five of 18 nodes involved and the other had 11 of 21 nodes involved. These facts are a very strong argument for meticulous axillary dissection in operable carcinoma of the breast.

Postoperative prophylactic irradiation was given to the axilla in 64 of these 328 patients —to those who had a considerable number of nodes involved. Those who received it had an average of 11.5 involved nodes. None of these 64 patients had axillary recurrence. The prophylactic irradiation must, of course, receive a good deal of credit for this achievement. This experience has led us to recommend irradiation to the axilla when a total of eight or more nodes are involved.

The parasternal local recurrences representing internal mammary metastases have occurred in my patients who did not have preliminary internal mammary biopsy, which we began to perform in 1951. When biopsy revealed metastasis, we did not do radical mastectomy. These parasternal recurrences developed within 10 years in 22 of my clinical Stage A and B patients. None had had the prophylactic postoperative irradiation to the internal mammary region which we now give.

The chest-wall recurrences are much the most frequent type of local recurrence following radical mastectomy. In Table XI chest-wall recurrence within 10 years is correlated with the extent of axillary metastasis in my personal series of cases. Chest-wall recurrence was rare when there were no axillary metastases. It was distressingly frequent, however, when a total of eight or more axillary nodes were involved; 24 percent of these patients whose disease was classified as clinical Stage A and 45 percent of those whose disease was clinical Stage B developed chest-wall recurrence. The 25 patients in these two groups who developed chest-wall recurrence had an average of 16 axillary nodes involved by the disease.

These local recurrences on the chest wall when many axillary nodes are involved are understandable. Even the most meticulous surgeon often fails to get the disease all out of the axilla under these circumstances. Since the chest-wall dissection is part of the same operative field as the axillary dissection, he will probably leave foci of carcinoma beneath the skin flaps.

I did not, in my earlier experience with breast carcinoma, fully realize the danger of chest-wall recurrence when there was extensive axillary involvement. Moreover, I was hesitant to give prophylactic postoperative irradiation to the chest wall for fear of irradiation damage to my thin skin flaps and my skin graft. Thus very few of my patients were given chest-wall irradiation, even when a good many nodes contained metastases. I have come to realize that this was a mistake. My skin flaps and skin grafts tolerate irradiation very well, provided that

Table XI. *Radical mastectomy for breast carcinoma: Extent of axillary metastases correlated with frequency of chest-wall local recurrence within 10 years: Personal series of cases, 1935 to July, 1963*

Columbia Clinical Classification	Extent of axillary metastasis	Number of patients	Local chest-wall recurrence within 10 years: Number of patients	Local chest-wall recurrence within 10 years: Percent
Stage A	No nodes involved	418	7	2
	1 to 3 nodes involved	131	6	4
	4 to 7 nodes involved	30	3	10
	8 or more nodes involved	29	7	24
	Total	608	23	4
Stage B	No nodes involved	48	0	0
	1 to 3 nodes involved	61	3	5
	4 to 7 nodes involved	37	5	13
	8 or more nodes involved	40	18	45
	Total	186	26	14
Stage C	No nodes involved	17	0	0
	1 to 3 nodes involved	21	4	19
	4 to 7 nodes involved	9	1	11
	8 or more nodes involved	29	7	24
	Total	76	12	16
Stage D	No nodes involved	1	1	
	1 to 3 nodes involved	2	0	
	4 to 7 nodes involved	1	1	
	8 or more nodes involved	8	6	
	Total	12	8	66
Total number of patients		882		

Table XII. *Average interval between radical mastectomy and local recurrence and average length of survival after local recurrence in 73 patients: Personal series of cases, clinical stages A and B, 1935 to July, 1963*

Columbia Clinical Classification	Parasternal recurrence: Average interval between operation and recurrence (mo.)	Parasternal recurrence: Average survival after recurrence (mo.)	Chest-wall recurrence: Average interval between operation and recurrence (mo.)	Chest-wall recurrence: Average survival after recurrence (mo.)	Axillary recurrence: Average interval between operation and recurrence (mo.)	Axillary recurrence: Average survival after recurrence (mo.)
Stage A	59	67.5	58.5	27.5	—	—
Stage B	69	21.5	27	18	21	31

it is given slowly over a period of 6 weeks or more. I now advise that all patients found to have eight or more axillary nodes involved receive prophylactic irradiation to the chest wall as well as to the axilla and the supraclavicular region.

One of the controversial questions regarding the technique of radical mastectomy continues to be whether or not skin grafting will decrease the likelihood of local recurrence. Halsted, in his 1912 paper, described the method of skin grafting which he had employed for 16 years and concluded, "It is better to remove too much skin than too little, for the mistake of excising an insufficient quantity is quite fatal to the patient's chance of recovery."

The opposite view was held by Sampson Handley, who wrote in 1906, "The area of skin taken away in the operation should ob-

Table XIII. *Site of first distant metastases within 10 years following radical mastectomy correlat*
July, 1963

Columbia Clinical Classification	*Status of axillary nodes*	*Supraclavicular*	*Opposite axilla*	*Distant skin*
Stage A	No metastases, 418 cases	2	0	3
	Metastases, 190 cases	4	0	2
Stage B	No metastases, 48 cases	0	0	0
	Metastases, 138 cases	9	1	3
Stage C	No metastases, 17 cases	0	0	0
	Metastases, 59 cases	5	1	1
Stage D	No metastases, 1 case	0	0	0
	Metastases, 11 cases	1	0	0
Total	No metastases, 484 cases	2	0	3
	Metastases, 398 cases	19	2	6

viously be no larger than necessary, and no healthy skin should be removed."

It is Sampson Handley's point of view which has won out since these two distinguished students of breast carcinoma disagreed. In the standard radical mastectomy today so little skin is sacrificed that the skin flaps can be brought together, albeit with some tension.

Early in my experience with breast carcinoma I saw so many patients in whom entirely inadequate so-called radical mastectomy with thick skin flaps and no skin graft was followed by early local recurrence in the operative field that I was convinced of the wisdom of sacrificing almost all of the skin over the protuberant breast and also dissecting really thin flaps of the remaining skin back to the midline medially and to the edge of the latissimus muscle laterally. This has been my practice with few exceptions and I believe that it is responsible for the fact that local recurrence on the chest wall has developed within 10 years in only 6.2 percent of my patients with Columbia Stage A and B carcinoma.

Donegan and his associates,[12] in their study of local recurrence in their series of 704 patients treated by radical mastectomy, reported a 5 year cumulative local recurrence rate of 17.5 percent. Skin grafting was done in only 289 of the 704 patients. There was no significant difference in the local recurrence rate in those whose wounds were grafted.

Unfortunately, it is a fact that skin recurrences often appear later than 5 years after operation. In order to provide a fair test of the value of skin grafting as regards avoidance of local recurrence, we should compare the 10 year results in case series carefully classified as to clinical stage of advancement, all treated by radical mastectomy, but some series of cases grafted and the others not.

Richard Handley has provided comparable data of this kind. He has used the Columbia Clinical Classification to stage his patients and has used a skin graft in about one half of them. Local recurrence on the chest wall within 10 years in his Stage A and B patients was approximately twice as frequent as it was in my series of radical mastectomies, in which almost all patients had skin grafts.

A second reason why I intend to continue skin grafting is that I am convinced that it is a kindness to the patient, quite apart from the matter of local recurrence. One advantage of skin grafting is that it saves the patient discomfort. It is amazing to me how painless radical mastectomy usually is if the skin flaps are not sutured with tension. My patients often tell me they have had no pain at all postoperatively. On the other hand, I see many patients whose skin flaps have been pulled together with tension sutures and who have had a good deal of pain as a consequence. The sensation of constriction of the chest that all patients have to some degree for a considerable time after *th clinical stage and pathologically verified axillary metastases: Personal series of cases, 1935 to*

Lung	Bone	Liver	Other abdominal	Brain	Other	Total number	Percent
18	27	4	0	3	2	59	14
18	27	5	5	2	1	64	33
2	1	0	0	0	0	3	6
9	26	4	2	1	5	60	43
0	2	0	0	0	0	2	12
19	13	0	0	2	3	44	75
0	1	0	0	0	0	1	100
4	4	0	0	0	2	11	100
20	31	4	0	3	2	65	
50	70	9	7	5	11	179	

radical mastectomy is much more marked in patients whose skin flaps have been sutured under tension.

A third reason that impels me to suture the skin flaps without tension and to graft skin is that I know that this is the way to make certain of perfect wound healing and to avoid edema of the arm. Necrosis, infection, and fibrosis are the triad that lead to edema of the arm, and they are, unfortunately, frequent when the skin flaps are pulled together under tension.

Donegan emphasized the grave significance of local recurrence after radical mastectomy. Forty-six percent of his 146 patients who developed local recurrence died of their disease within one year after the local recurrence, and only four percent lived more than 5 years.

My own experience with local recurrence has not been so unfortunate. Thirty percent of the 73 patients who developed local recurrence in my personal series of 794 radical mastectomies performed for patients whose disease was classified as Stage A or B died within a year after their local recurrence. Twelve percent lived more than 5 years, and two of these patients still survive 22.4 and 29.3 years, respectively, after parasternal recurrence which was treated by irradiation.

In studying the time at which local recurrence occurs, the clinical stage of the disease as well as the type of local recurrence should be considered. Table XII shows the average length of time elapsing between operation and local recurrence, as well as the length of survival after local recurrence, in the 73 patients in my personal series of cases who developed local recurrence. These patients are classified by clinical stage, and their recurrences are classified in the three usual types—parasternal, chest walls, and axilla. It will be seen from this table that in the clinical Stage A patients local recurrences developed later, and the patients survived somewhat longer than the Stage B patients. It is also apparent that the patients with parasternal recurrence do better than those with chest-wall recurrence.

Our experience has taught us that all three types of local recurrence—parasternal, axillary, and skin-flap and skin-graft recurrences—are better treated by irradiation than by surgery. Most surgeons have enough common sense not to attempt to excise the parasternal and axillary recurrences, but many cannot resist the temptation to excise small solitary recurrences in the skin flaps. In so doing they spread the recurrent disease around and make the radiotherapist's task of controlling it more difficult. Radiotherapy usually succeeds in controlling solitary skin recurrences, and when new ones develop in adjacent areas they too can be successfully dealt with by irradiation. This is not true of the surgical attack; the surgeon is soon hopelessly defeated in his effort to control successive local recurrences. It is, therefore, my practice to treat local recurrence with irradiation.

Table XIV. *Numbers of patients with first recurrence within 10 years, by site and year following radical mastectomy in clinical stage A and B cases: Personal series, 1935 to July, 1963*

Site of recurrence	Postoperative year 1	2	3	4	5	6	7	8	9	10	After 10 years	Total
Bone	19	20	10	15	5	2	3	3	3	1	6	87
Lung	2	13	7	12	2	2	3	4	2	0	5	52
Parasternal	1	7	4	4	2	0	1	1	1	0	4	25
Chest wall	8	21	5	3	3	1	0	2	2	0	3	48
Axilla	1	0	1	0	0	0	0	0	0	0	0	2
Liver	4	5	1	0	2	0	1	0	0	0	1	14
Other abdominal	2	2	0	2	0	1	0	0	0	0	0	7
Supraclavicular	7	6	0	1	1	0	0	0	0	0	1	16
Contralateral axilla	1	0	0	0	0	0	0	0	0	0	0	1
Distant skin	3	1	3	1	0	0	0	0	0	0	1	9
Brain	1	1	2	1	1	0	0	0	0	0	0	6
Other	2	1	0	0	1	2	2	0	0	0	1	9
Total	51	77	33	39	17	8	10	10	8	1	22	276

DISTANT METASTASIS

Distant metastasis is, of course, the sword of Damocles that hangs over the patient who has had a locally successful radical mastectomy.

In my personal series of 882 radical mastectomies, distant metastases (excluding local recurrence on the chest wall and parasternal and axillary recurrence) developed in a total of 244 patients within 10 years. The sites of first distant metastasis in these patients are shown in Table XIII.

The striking prognostic significance of axillary metastases again emerges from these data regarding distant metastases. Distant metastases were 3½ times more frequent in patients with axillary metastases than in those whose axillae were not involved.

Osseous and pulmonary metastases were much the most frequent types of distant metastasis in my patients.

THE TIME OF LOCAL RECURRENCE AND DISTANT METASTASIS AFTER RADICAL MASTECTOMY

It is important to study the time of local recurrence and metastasis because it gives us a better concept of the natural history of the disease and how its course is influenced by different types of treatment.

There have been a good many individual case reports of the very late development of local recurrence and distant metastasis. These reports have been tabulated by the Mortons[38] and, more recently, by Danckers, Hamann, and Savage.[10] Pawlias, Dockerty, and Ellis[40] reported a series of 45 cases of late local recurrence. In general, it can be said that the more complete and the longer the follow-up, the more late recurrences will be found, although they are still comparatively infrequent after 10 years.

It is important to look critically into the genuineness of presumed late "recurrence." Many of the case reports are so incomplete that no definite conclusion can be drawn from them. It is more than likely that, rather than being examples of true late recurrence, they represent one of three other phenomena, as follows.

1. **The persistence rather than recurrence of carcinoma.** Patients whose carcinoma has been locked up by irradiation fibrosis until it finally begins to grow again belong in this category. Since these patients are never free from disease, it is not proper to classify them as having late recurrence.

2. **Metastasis from a different primary carcinoma.** In patients who develop metastasis after a long period of freedom from evidence of their disease, it is often not certain that the source is the original breast carcinoma. It may be a different and occult

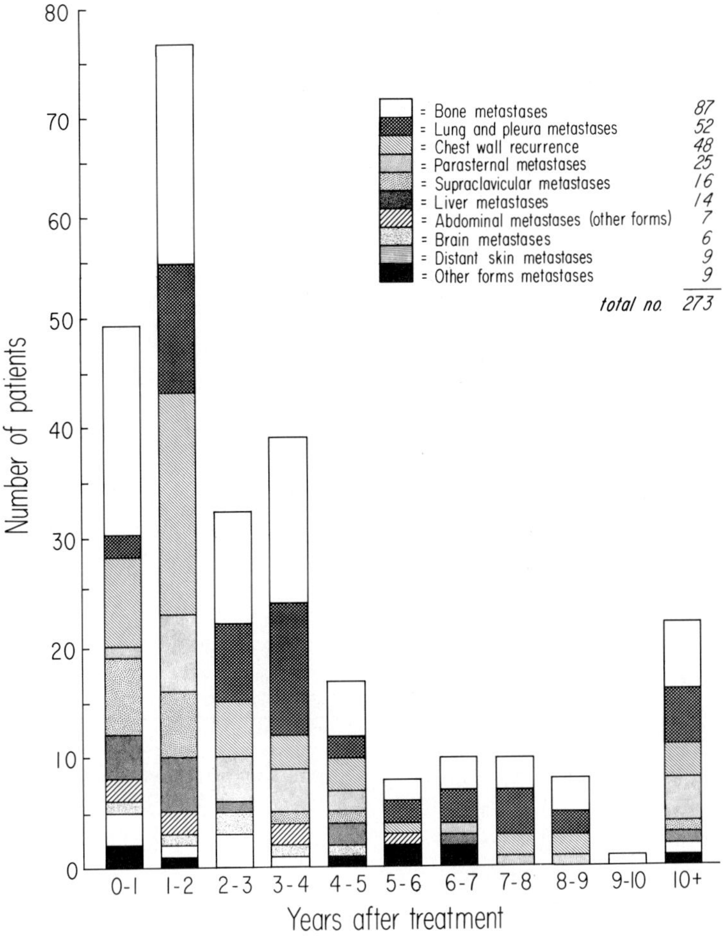

Fig. 2. Time and site of first recurrences of carcinoma in 273 patients in the Haagensen series.

primary carcinoma. Small primary carcinomas from the lung and pancreas are particularly likely to be missed clinically, and they may closely resemble breast carcinoma microscopically. The possibility of metastasis from a small occult primary carcinoma of the opposite breast must also be kept in mind. These possibilities can be ruled out only by autopsy.

3. **New primary mammary carcinoma developing from mammary tissue left on thick skin flaps.** As I have already pointed out, the skin flaps of the standard American radical mastectomy are so thick that they often include a good deal of mammary tissue. It is likely that carcinoma reappearing in the flaps a long time after operation is sometimes a new primary lesion, arising in the residual mammary tissue. Wawro[49] has described a convincing example of this phenomenon. In his patient the new primary carcinoma developed in breast tissue left on a skin flap from 2 to 4 cm. thick, 17 years after the original operation.

In studying the time of recurrence in my personal series of radical mastectomies, I have focused upon the 794 patients whose disease was classified as Clinical Stages A and B because they are the ones in whom we now perform radical mastectomies. After their initial recurrence, patients often develop recurrences in other sites. Their actual extent cannot be known without complete autopsy studies, which we do not have.

We do, however, know the time and site of the first recurrence in almost all of the

Table XV. *First recurrence of breast carcinoma more than 10 years after radical mastecton*

Case number	Patient	Age	Date of operation	Clinical stage	Size of primary tumor (cm.)	Status of axillary nodes	Microscopi type of tum
1	H. T.	59	Oct., 1948	B	2.0	2 positive in 24	Grade I
2	C. S.	55	Apr., 1945	A	2.0	No metastasis in 18	Intraducta
3	L. K.	65	Feb., 1941	A	2.0	No metastasis in 14	Grade I
4	H. B.	55	June, 1939	A	4.5	No metastasis in 36	Grade I
5	M. H.	49	July, 1945	A	4.0	1 positive in 30	Grade II
6	H. B.	45	Mar., 1942	B	4.5	7 positive in 14	Grade I
7	L. L.	32	Feb., 1942	A	4.0	8 positive in 17	Grade I
8	M. M.	47	Oct., 1949	B	3.5	4 positive in 20	Grade I
9	A. L. B.	63	Apr., 1950	A	3.0	2 positive in 34	Grade II
10	H. M.	47	July, 1940	B	6.5	6 positive in 19	Grade I
11	N. P.	50	Jan., 1942	B	8.0	3 positive in 10	Grade I
12	L. B.	63	Sep., 1944	A	3.5	No metastasis in 18	Grade I
13	L. C.	49	Jan., 1948	B	5.0	6 positive in 14	Grade III
14	L. B.	47	June, 1937	B	10.0	15 positive in 18	Mucoid
15	M. V.	55	Oct., 1942	A	6.0	No metastasis in 10	Intraductal
16	M. T.	51	Dec., 1947	A	3.0	1 positive in 11	Small cell
17	M. H.	53	June, 1941	A	4.0	1 positive in 18	Small cell
18	L. C.	63	June, 1947	A	2.0	3 positive in 30	Intraductal
19	C. N.	72	Sep., 1939	B	5.0	1 positive in 28	Grade III
20	L. L.	64	Oct., 1961	B	10.0	4 positive in 17	Mucoid
21	E. C.	40	Mar., 1958	B	8.0	No metastasis in 36	Grade I
22	A. A.	43	June, 1959	A	Small	3 positive in 30	Grade III

patients in my personal series. The number of first recurrences is, of course, considerably smaller than the total number of recurrences, but the data regarding first recurrence are comparatively accurate and useful. The first recurrences within 10 years are shown in Table XIV and in Fig. 2. From these data it is seen that recurrence develops most often within the first 4 years after operation and decreases in frequency thereafter.

Occasionally recurrence appears after 10 years. At the present writing, recurrence has developed more than 10 years after operation in a total of 22, or 3 percent, of my 794 Clinical Stage A and B patients. I have summarized the pertinent details of these patients with very late recurrence in Table XV. Their recurrences were spread over a long period of years. In two patients (Cases 7 and 4) recurrence developed more than 20 years after operation.

The details of the course of the disease in these two patients are summarized below.

CASE REPORTS

Case 7. Mrs. L. L., 32 years of age, discovered a small tumor in her left breast but did not consult us for a year because it did not seem to change much. When admitted in February, 1942, she had a typical 4 cm. carcinoma of the upper inner sector of the breast without any clinically involved axillary nodes. Her disease was classified as clinical stage A. Radical mastectomy was done. Eight of a total of 14 axillary nodes contained metastases. The primary tumor was a well-differentiated Grade I carcinoma. No postoperative irradiation was given.

In November, 1962, 20 years and 9 months after operation, induration was noted at the base of the right side of her neck. Shortly thereafter a right Horner's syndrome developed and chest films showed slight indentation of the trachea on the right side and elevation of the right diaphragm. A biopsy of the right supraclavicular mass confirmed the diagnosis of metastases of her original breast carcinoma.

Irradiation was given to the right mediastinum and the right infraclavicular and supraclavicular regions.

Within a year the patient developed metastases to the brain, as well as to the dorsal spine, pelvic bones, and humerus. She died in August, 1964.

There was no autopsy, but it seems likely that she originally had metastases to her right internal mammary nodes, and after slowly growing over a period of many years in these nodes, her disease reached the nodes in the lymphatic terminus at the base of her right neck, and there generalized through the blood stream. Prophylactic irradiation *rsonal series, 1935 to July, 1963*

First recurrence	*Interval from operation to recurrence (yr.)*	*Subsequent recurrence elsewhere*	*End result*	*Autopsy*
edial skin flap, March, 1959	10.4	Scalp, Oct., 1961	Died May, 1962	No
rasternal—3rd, Feb., 1958	13.3	Liver, lungs, bones, ovary	Died Aug., 1968	Yes
in graft, March, 1960	19.1	Supraclavicular + pleural, 1963	Died Sep., 1968	Yes
ge skin graft, April, 1967	27.8	None	Died Dec., 1969	No
rasternal—2nd, Feb., 1958	12.7	Bones, pleura, Dec., 1959	Died July, 1961	No
rasternal—3rd, Nov., 1966	14.7	Lung, bones, June, 1967	Died June, 1968	No
praclavicular nodes, Nov., 1962	20.7	Brain, bones, Nov., 1963	Died Aug., 1964	No
ura, Dec., 1965	14.1	—	Died May, 1969	Yes
ura, March, 1964	13.9	—	Died Sep., 1966	No
ura, Feb., 1955	14.3	Spine and liver	Died Feb., 1956	Yes
ura, Jan., 1954	12.0	—	Died Dec., 1954	No
nes, June, 1958	13.6	—	Died Feb., 1959	No
nes, Aug., 1958	10.6	Lung, Sep., 1958	Died Aug., 1959	No
mur, April, 1949	11.8	—	Died Oct., 1953	No
ver, May, 1956	13.5	Ovary, omentum	Died July, 1956	Yes
stant skin, March, 1959	11.6	Bones, April, 1959	Died Dec., 1959	Yes
bcutaneous neck, Oct., 1959	18.3	Pleura, Nov., 1965	Died Feb., 1966	No
rtebrae, Aug., 1963	16.0	Lung, Aug., 1963	Died Apr., 1964	Yes
rasternal—2nd, Dec., 1949	10.2	—	Died Aug., 1951	No
lvic bones, Dec., 1972	11.1	—	Living Oct., 1973	—
mbar spine, Dec., 1972	14.9	—	Living Mar., 1973	—
ura, July, 1970	11.0	—	Living Apr., 1972	—

to her internal mammary region might have saved her.

Case 4. Miss H. B., 55 years of age, noticed dimpling of the skin just above the areola of her right breast and on palpation felt a lump beneath the area of skin retraction. The tumor measured 4.5 cm. in diameter and had the clinical characteristics of a carcinoma. There were no clinically involved axillary nodes and the disease was classified as a Clinical Stage A carcinoma. Radical mastectomy was performed in June, 1939. A total of 36 axillary nodes were free of metastases. The primary tumor was a well-differentiated Grade I carcinoma. The individual tumor cells were comparatively regular in size and shape, and were often arranged in tubules.

No postoperative irradiation was given.

In April, 1967, 27 years and 10 months later, I noted an 8 mm. erosion at the edge of the skin graft along its inner upper border. It was so characteristic of local recurrence that it was treated by irradiation. The erosion healed satisfactorily.

In October, 1969, however, the irradiated area broke down, and biopsy of the area was done. The sections showed carcinoma similar to the original breast carcinoma removed more than 30 years previously. A limited excision of the chest wall was done and the defect was closed with a flap mobilized from the opposite breast. She died in December, 1969.

These late skin recurrences in the skin graft and in the skin flaps in three of my patients, 10, 19, and 27 years postoperatively, can be explained theoretically by the fact that my very thin flaps as well as the skin grafts provide a poorly vascularized site in which a minute focus of well-differentiated carcinoma may remain locked up in scar tissue for a very long time.

These late recurrences usually occurred with well-differentiated carcinomas. Seventeen of my 22 cases were of this type. These lesions lack the growth vigor of less well-differentiated carcinomas and grow slowly.

EDEMA OF THE ARM AFTER RADICAL MASTECTOMY

The complications of shock and infection which were formerly a hazard, to some degree, of radical mastectomy, have been solved, and edema of the arm is the only postoperative complication of any consequence. It remains, however, the greatest penalty that women have to face after the average standard radical mastectomy.

It is necessary first of all to define what we mean by edema. A good many patients have transitory slight increase in the diameter of the arm following radical mastectomy. This might be defined as an increase of less than 3 cm. in the diameter of the arm. This amount of edema usually shortly disappears with the restoration of arm function. An exception must be made for the baggy enlargement of the ventral aspect of the upper arm. This is seen in obese patients with relaxed tissues, and results from severing the axillary fascia. It cannot be avoided. The edema to which I refer as a formidable complication affects the whole arm or the entire upper arm. This kind of edema, which makes the patient socially unpresentable and which gives her a feeling of tension in the tissues of the arm, varies greatly in degree.

When the diameter of the patient's forearm, a month or so after operation, is increased by more than 3 cm., but is not strikingly edematous, she may be said to have moderate arm edema. A marked degree of edema may develop in patients who had poor wound healing, who are obese, or who have had postoperative irradiation to the axilla and supraclavicular regions.

Britton and Nelson,[4] who have written one of the best papers dealing with postmastectomy lymphedema of the arm, tabulated its frequency as reported in 14 different case series. It varied between 6.7 and 62.5 percent. Daland's[9] experience was typical: 27.8 percent of his patients had moderate or severe arm edema.

In tabulating the frequency of arm edema, the patients in whom edema develops as the result of local recurrence of the carcinoma in the axillary and supraclavicular regions should be set apart or excluded. This type of edema is not directly related to the surgery that has been performed. What might be called *surgical* edema, that developing in patients who have been treated surgically but remain free of clinical evidence of axillary or supraclavicular recurrence, should be further classified into two types. *Postoperative* surgical edema is the type that occurs immediately following operation. It must be regarded as the consequence of some sort of fault in surgical technique. *Secondary* surgical edema is the type that develops many months or years after operation as the result of a new infection in the arm through a portal of entry on the hand or arm. The surgeon cannot be held responsible for secondary edema, except to the extent that he may have failed to warn his patient that any minor wound or infection on the hand or arm subsequent to radical mastectomy is a serious matter.

It is sometimes difficult to distinguish true postoperative edema from the edema developing as a result of later infection. For instance, the patient may go home after operation and shortly thereafter burn her forearm while cooking, with the result that she develops edema, for which her surgeon is truly not responsible.

In my personal series of patients, postoperative edema has been infrequent. Only about 5 percent have developed it. Secondary edema, resulting from infection gaining entry through the skin of the hand or arm, has been more frequent. Approximately 8 percent of my patients have had secondary episodes of cellulitis of the arm which have left some degree of permanent edema.

Following the extirpation of the axillary lymph nodes into which the arm lymphatics empty, adequate collateral lymphatic circulation usually develops within a month if wound healing is normal. It is true that the reserve capacity of the lymphatic circulation is encroached upon. In most patients, however, no edema results. Edema, then, must be due to some other factor that causes a further encroachment upon the lymphatic drainage of the arm. The evidence indicates that this is *infection.*

Halsted, with his wonderful facility for discovering the essential truth of every problem that he put his mind to, was the first to describe the clinical picture of edema of the arm following mastectomy. He called it "elephantiasis chirurgica." He correctly described the two types which I have mentioned—that which follows shortly after operation and that which may develop any time subsequent to operation, sometimes years later, following an episode of infection. He observed that when a skin graft was used to cover the defect on the chest wall and the skin flaps were not sutured under tension, marginal necrosis of the flaps and consequent infection and inflammation were avoided. "Swollen arms of dimensions sufficient to distress or annoy the patient were no longer observed . . . ," he stated.

My experience with arm edema duplicates Halsted's. I have long been convinced that fibrosis following infection in radical mastectomy wounds which have healed badly is its underlying cause. Surgeons who handle the skin flaps too roughly and bring them together under tension invite necrosis of the skin margins as well as the formation of a dead space in the axilla in which fluid accumulates and infection develops. Arm edema often follows.

I believe that postoperative arm edema has not been a serious problem for me because I have learned how to achieve perfect wound healing. I handle the skin flaps gently and take great care not to suture them so tightly that I compromise their circulation. I use a generous skin graft. I dress my wounds myself. Even with ward patients, for whom I act as first assistant while my resident surgeon operates, I supervise the postoperative care of the wound.

Postoperative irradiation to the axilla certainly increases the frequency and degree of edema of the arm. Several experienced clinicians have emphasized this relationship (Lobb and Harkins;[33] Holman, McSwain, and Beal[29]; Daland[9]; and Hollenbach[28]).

The radiodermatitis with moist desquamation of the skin, which was formerly observed following intensive 250 kv. radiotherapy, provided an ideal portal of entry for infection. Today, with carefully supervised cobalt therapy, this kind of radiodermatitis is not seen and the hazard of infection in the arm no longer exists. Nevertheless, my experience has convinced me that irradiation to the axillary region, no matter how skillfully given, adds somewhat to the degree of postoperative edema of the arm, probably because it increases the amount of fibrosis in the axilla and, therefore, adds to the obstruction of lymphatic channels. For this reason, postoperative axillary irradiation should be avoided unless there are definite indications for it.

The patient who escapes edema of the arm immediately following radical mastectomy should be told by her surgeon that she is vulnerable to *secondary* edema for the rest of her life. She must be made to realize that any trauma to the hand or arm which provides a portal of entry for bacteria may lead to infection and edema. Burns, cuts, abrasions, and paronychia are the most frequent sources of infection. Patients should be urged to avoid manicurists, because manicurists invariably push the cuticle back and in this way induce a minor degree of infection.

OPERATIONS OTHER THAN THE HALSTED RADICAL MASTECTOMY

When Halsted visited Billroth's clinic in Vienna in 1879 he found the leader of German surgery treating breast carcinoma with what we would today describe as simple mastectomy and in some patients also with limited axillary dissection. Billroth's local recurrence rate was 82 percent, and his 3 year cure rate only 4.7 percent. There was, of course, no radiotherapy or hormonal treatment in those days. Even patients with very advanced disease were treated by surgery.

Halsted had a much more imaginative concept of surgery than did Billroth and after he returned to Roosevelt Hospital and the College of Physicians and Surgeons in New York he began, in 1882, to perform the first true radical mastectomy. By 1894 he was able to report, "In 50 cases operated upon by the complete method we have been able to trace only three local recurrences."

Surgeons the world over quickly adopted the Halsted operation, or the similar operation devised by Willy-Meyer about the same time, and proved that radical mastectomy cured many patients in whom the disease had not extended beyond the limits of the dissection. My own 10 year results with the Halsted operation detailed above illustrate what can be achieved with it in patients whose disease is carefully classified as to its

Table XVI. *Results of treatment in mammary carcinoma—10 year survival, Columbia Clini*

Stages of Columbia Clinical Classification	*Miller, simple mastectomy*		*Handley & Thackray, conservative radical mastectomy*		*Butcher, radical mastectomy*	
	Number of patients	*10 yr. survival %*	*Number of patients*	*10 yr. survival %*	*Number of patients*	*10 yr. survival %*
A	105	40	77	61	216	56
B	34	26	58	25	135	30
C	18	22	8	14	48	31
D	45	9	0	—	26	0
Total	202		143		425	

*From Haagensen, C. D., et al.: Treatment of early mammary carcinoma: Cooperative international study, Ann. Surg. 170:

clinical stage of advancement on the basis of the Columbia Clinical Classification.

Despite such data, surgeons have recently begun to abandon radical mastectomy. Their disillusionment is, I believe, explained by two factors. First of all, surgeons have not learned how to select patients for radical mastectomy on the basis of an accurate and practical clinical classification. As long ago as 1943, Stout and I worked out criteria of operability[18] based on the careful assessment of the clinical features of breast carcinoma. But many surgeons continue to ignore them. Radical mastectomy for inoperable breast carcinoma (Clinical Stages C and D in our Columbia Clinical Classification) not only punishes the patient with a futile operation when irradiation alone would have done just as well or better, but it destroys the confidence of the surgeon in the superiority of radical mastectomy for patients whose disease is operable.

The second reason for the loss of confidence in radical mastectomy is that many surgeons are unwilling to devote the time and patience required to do the operation well. They perform it indifferently, using a great variety of techniques which are not meticulous and thorough and which give inferior results.

Radical mastectomy has been attacked recently in both the lay and the medical press, by lay women as well as physicians. A wide variety of less aggressive methods of treatment have been advocated in its place. These include irradiation alone, local excision of the primary tumor, or simple mastectomy, as well as curtailed modifications of radical mastectomy—all used alone or supplemented by irradiation. The question of how to treat breast carcinoma has been debated on public television programs—a ridiculously inadequate forum for the discussion of so complex a problem. Crile, an advocate of very limited surgery, has presented his argument in book form for the laity.

Support for this attack on radical mastectomy within the medical profession comes from dissident surgeons and radiotherapists who ignore the facts of pathology and disparage the reports of results of treatment already available. Their attack is summed up by Bernard Fisher[14] in Pittsburgh and Sir Hedley Atkins[3] in London, who have stated that we do not know how best to treat carcinoma of the breast and that we can only find out from clinical trials which include such limited methods as lumpectomy and simple mastectomy. They ignore the reports of the results of radical mastectomy by surgeons of the preceding generation, such as Taylor and Wallace[44] from the Massachusetts General Hospital and Finney, Merkel, and Miller[13] from the Johns Hopkins Hospital, which were based on data which were just as good as any we have today with the exception that their patients were not selected for operation on the basis of any formal clinical classification. They were expert clinicians, however, and had learned fairly well how to distinguish between operable and inoperable cases.

The formal clinical classifications for breast carcinoma which are available today make *assification**

Haagensen & Cooley, radical mastectomy		Dahl-Iversen & Tobiassen, extended mastectomy		Williams & Stone, total mastectomy + axillary dissec. + irrad.		Kaae & Johansen, McWhirter method	
umber of patients	*10 yr. survival %*	*Number of patients*	*10 yr. survival %*	*Number of patients*	*10 yr. survival %*	*Number of patients*	*10 yr. survival %*
344	70	352	57	68	59	159	50
138	40	75	24	57	46	28	32
63	27	34	35	16	19	9	0
11	18	15	7	1	0	3	0
556		476		142		199	

).

it much easier to compare different methods of treatment because end results may now be compared in each of the advancing clinical stages of the disease. This was the purpose of a cooperative international study, "Treatment of early mammary carcinoma,"[20] based on the Columbia Clinical Classification in which the results of seven different methods of treatment were compared. It was published in 1969. Local recurrence and survival rates at 10 years were reported. Anglem and Leber,[1] in their admirable recent review, "The dubious case for conservative operation in operable cancer of the breast," have endorsed this study. The 10 year survival rates for the seven different methods of treatment are presented in Table XVI.

In a recent editorial in the *Journal of the American Medical Association,* I discussed our "Great leap backward in the treatment of carcinoma of the breast,"[17] and reviewed the results of several of the less aggressive methods of treatment currently being advocated as a substitute for radical mastectomy. I will discuss these methods more thoroughly here. Their value should be viewed critically from three points of view. First, are they reasonable in terms of our present knowledge of the natural history and pathology of breast carcinoma? Second, what is their penalty for the patient? Third, what are their results in terms of local recurrence and survival at 10 years?

LOCAL EXCISION

There is no reason to believe that mere local excision of a palpable primary breast carcinoma, even when a few centimeters of the surrounding breast tissue are included in the excision, will be any more successful today than in Paget's time when there were no 10 year survivors. We know today that in more than half of the patients there are multiple impalpable foci of the disease in the breast which the local excision will not remove, and that in an equal proportion of the patients there will be axillary metastases which will also be left untreated. In the light of these facts mere local excision must be regarded as an entirely unacceptable method of treatment. There are no significant modern data as to the results of local excision alone. No conscientious surgeon can justify treating breast carcinoma in an operable stage with this method.

LOCAL EXCISION PLUS IRRADIATION

When local excision of the primary tumor is supplemented with irradiation to the breast and the axilla, there will be some survivors. Peters[41] has treated in this way a series of 129 patients whose carcinomas were classified as Stage I by the International TNM Clinical Classification. In order to make an exact comparison of her results with mine achieved with radical mastectomy I have reclassified my cases according to the TNM classification. This comparison is shown in Table XVII.

Local excision supplemented by irradiation, of course, avoids sacrifice of the breast, but the likelihood of cure is so much less than after a good radical mastectomy that

Table XVII. *Results of treatment in mammary carcinoma—10 year survival International TNM Clinical Classification—Stage I wedge resection plus irradiation compared with radical mastectomy*

Peters, 1935 to 1962		*Haagensen, consecutive patients, 1935 to July, 1963*					
Wedge resection plus irradiation		*Radical mastectomy*		*Irradiation only, biopsy-proved metastases internal mammary or subclavicular nodes*		*Combined series of patients*	
Number of patients	*10 yr. survival (%)*	*Number of patients*	*10 yr. survival (%)*	*Number of patients*	*10 yr. survival (%)*	*Number of patients*	*10 yr. survival (%)*
129	44.5	450	74.5	16	33	466	73

patients who are told the facts and convinced of their truth will usually choose radical mastectomy.

SIMPLE MASTECTOMY

A generation ago a group of surgeons, exemplified by Hartmann,[27] Fitzwilliams,[15] Deaton,[11] and Case,[7] began to advocate simple removal of the breast as a substitute for radical mastectomy. This trend received support from a comparison of the results of simple and radical mastectomy in Rockford, Ill., made by Smith and Meyer[43] in 1959. They concluded that they "... could demonstrate no reason for performing more than simple mastectomy." Two years later Shimkin, Koppel, Connelly, and Cutler[42] of the National Cancer Institute restudied the Rockford data and reaffirmed the finding that the survival rates "... were practically identical whether radical or simple mastectomy was used as the primary treatment." The truth about the Rockford studies is that patients in these trial series were not accurately classified as to the clinical extent of their disease, making valid comparison of results impossible.

In the light of our modern knowledge of the pathology of breast carcinoma, simple mastectomy alone is an inadequate method of treatment both locally and in the axilla. The local extent of the sacrifice of skin and subcutaneous tissue is usually much more limited in simple than in radical mastectomy. Indeed, in simple mastectomy breast tissue is usually left on the thick flaps. Since carcinoma is often more widespread in the breast than the surgeon suspects, limited local surgery results in a higher local recurrence rate.

When simple mastectomy is the sole method of treatment for patients with operable carcinoma of the breast (Stages A and B in the Columbia Clinical Classification) more than one half of them will have axillary metastases which are left untreated. The excuse often given is that breast carcinoma is incurable when the axillary nodes are involved. The fact is that axillary dissection, which is part of radical mastectomy, succeeds surprisingly well. My Table III shows that in Stage A patients with from one to three involved axillary nodes the 10 year survival rate was 68 percent, while it was 44 percent in Stage B patients. None of these 192 patients developed axillary recurrence.

From the patient's point of view, the penalty in mutilation is not much greater for a skillfully done radical mastectomy than for simple mastectomy. In both operations she loses her breast. With perfect wound healing after radical mastectomy, edema of the arm is rare and arm function is almost normal. There should be no operative mortality from either type of operation.

Fortunately, Miller[37] has reported the results in a carefully classified and followed series of patients in whom the treatment was only mastectomy, without significant supplemental irradiation or hormonal treatment. The 10 year local recurrence and survival rates in Miller's case series are compared with

Table XVIII. *Results of treatment in mammary carcinoma, Columbia Clinical Classification, simple mastectomy only compared with radical mastectomy*

	Miller, 1927 to 1956			*Haagensen, consecutive patients, 1935 to July, 1963*						
	Simple mastectomy only			*Radical mastectomy*			*Irradiation only, biopsy-proved metastases internal mammary or subclavicular nodes*		*Combined series of patients*	
		10 yr. results			*10 yr. results*					
Stage	*Number of patients*	*Local recurrence (%)*	*Survival (%)*	*Number of patients*	*Local recurrence (%)*	*Survival (%)*	*Number of patients*	*10 yr. survival (%)*	*Number of patients*	*10 yr. survival (%)*
A	115	37	40	608	6.8	70	33	21	641	67
B	34	50	26	186	18	43	53	18	239	38

Table XIX. *Results of treatment in mammary carcinoma in patients under 65 years of age, International TNM Clinical Classification, simple mastectomy plus irradiation compared with radical mastectomy*

	McWhirter, 1941 to 1956		*Haagensen, 1935 to July, 1963*					
	Simple mastectomy followed by irradiation		*Radical mastectomy*		*Irradiation only, biopsy-proved metastases, internal mammary or subclavicular nodes*		*Combined series, radical mastectomy, irradiation only*	
Clinical stage	*Number of patients*	*10 yr. survival (%)*	*Number of patients*	*10 yr. survival (%)*	*Number of patients*	*10 yr. survival (%)*	*Number of patients*	*10 yr. survival (%)*
I	600	54	360	78	16	33	376	76
II	491	43	137	55	12	16	149	52
III	690	24	185	45	47	15	232	40

those in my series of radical mastectomies in Table XVIII. The much higher local recurrence rate and the far lower survival rate after simple mastectomy should convince anyone that it is an inferior method of treatment.

In patients whose carcinoma is clearly inoperable, simple mastectomy has often been used as a palliative procedure to rid the patient of her large or ulcerated tumor. As the efficacy of irradiation in controlling the primary tumor temporarily has improved, the need for palliative simple mastectomy has decreased. I have long since abandoned it because I have learned that radiotherapy alone works better.

Another use of simple mastectomy which I must strongly condemn is when a surgeon, unable to make a definite pathological diagnosis, compromises by performing simple mastectomy, with the intention of proceeding with radical mastectomy when a definite diagnosis becomes available. In so doing he is very apt to sacrifice the patient's only chance of cure because his initial limited dissection cuts into carcinoma and implants it widely. Lockhart and Ackerman[34] reviewed a series of cases in which simple mastectomy had been done preceding radical mastectomy and found the results disastrous.

SIMPLE MASTECTOMY PLUS IRRADIATION

In 1941 McWhirter[36] in Edinburgh introduced the method of treatment for breast carcinoma which is named for him. It consists of simple mastectomy followed by a course of irradiation to the chest wall, axilla, and supraclavicular region given over a 3 week period. The tumor dose approximates 4,000 rads. McWhirter's method is probably the one most used in Britain, and it is widely used everywhere.

It should be understood that in McWhirter's method the main reliance is upon irradiation. It cannot be assumed that the limited surgery removes the primary breast carcinoma in its entirety; and there is no surgical attack upon the axillary nodes. If the primary tumor is of considerable size, its removal by simple mastectomy may facilitate the effort of the radiotherapist to control it, but in general the same factors which limit the effectiveness of irradiation when it is used alone as a method of treatment for breast carcinoma also apply to the McWhirter treatment.

In his most recent report of his results, McWhirter excluded patients 65 years of age and over. He used the TNM Clinical Classification. I have reclassified my patients treated by radical mastectomy in the same manner. The results of the two methods of treatment are compared in Table XIX. In all three clinical stages radical mastectomy gives a decidedly superior 10 year survival rate.

McWhirter refrains from giving a local recurrence rate following his method of treatment. After intensive irradiation it is sometimes difficult to differentiate between induration due to fibrosis and true local recurrence. However, Kaae and Johansen,[30] in Copenhagen, tested McWhirter's method in a trial series in which they followed his technique carefully, and in their report they included local recurrence rates. Since they used the Columbia Clinical Classification, these local recurrence rates in their patients treated by McWhirter's method can be compared with my local recurrence rates following radical mastectomy. In Kaae and Johansen's Stage A patients the 10 year local recurrence rate was 19 percent, and in Stage B patients 29 percent. In my Stage A patients treated by radical mastectomy the local recurrence rate was 6.5 percent and in Stage B patients 18 percent.

In patients treated by McWhirter's method the chest wall is not as much disfigured as after a radical mastectomy with a skin graft. However, they are penalized to some degree by the irradiation they receive. And the McWhirter method is clearly a bad bargain in terms of both local recurrence and survival.

MASTECTOMY PLUS AXILLARY DISSECTION

The method of treatment which today provides the sharpest competition for radical mastectomy is a compromise procedure which is best called mastectomy plus axillary dissection. This operation is usually called "modified" radical mastectomy, a name which implies that it is much more extensive than it really is. The procedure is certainly not a radical mastectomy in the sense in which both Halsted and Willy-Meyer used the term. In the Halsted radical mastectomy, which I perform, the skin over most of the protuberant breast is sacrificed, necessitating a skin graft. The skin flaps are thin and do not include any mammary tissue. Both pectoral muscles are removed. With sharp dissection I get an average of 30 nodes out of the axilla.

The "modified" radical mastectomy which has recently become fashionable is a much less radical procedure. The breast is removed through a transverse incision, with so little sacrifice of skin that the wound can be closed without a skin graft. The skin flaps are cut so thick that mammary tissue remains on them. The pectoralis major muscle is left intact and retracted medially, providing only limited access to the axilla. A blunt axillary dissection with scissors removes only the more lateral axillary nodes. The entire procedure is completed in between an hour and an hour and a half. Mastectomy plus axillary dissection is the most accurate name for this operation. Techniques for it have been described by Patey and Dyson,[39] by Handley, by Madden,[35] and by many other surgeons. In actual practice the thoroughness of the operation varies greatly.

There are perfectly good reasons why the results of this limited operation should be expected to be somewhat inferior to those of the radical mastectomy which I have described. (1) When the excision of the skin and subcutaneous tissues over the breast is so limited that a skin graft is not required, the surgeon in his dissection will occasionally get too close to the carcinoma, which may extend more widely in the breast than he thinks, and local recurrence will follow. If breast tissue left on the skin flaps contains carcinoma, or if the disease has penetrated to the deep aspect of the breast, local recurrence is also inevitable. (2) When the pectoral muscles are not removed the interpectoral nodes are not excised, and if there is carcinoma in them, the patient is doomed. (3) The axillary dissection which is done in this limited operation is usually more brutal and less complete than in the Halsted radical mastectomy. In the "modified" operation strong traction medially on the pectoralis major will expose the axillary structures for only about two thirds of the distance from the lateral edge of the operative field where the axillary vein crosses the white tendon of the latissimus dorsi, to the point where the vein passes, medially, beneath the subclavius muscle.

Patey devised a technique which makes it possible to perform a more complete axillary dissection. The patient's arm is held vertically by an assistant so that the elbow points toward the ceiling. This relaxes the pectoralis major and makes it possible to retract it further medially, while preserving its nerve and arterial supply. The pectoralis minor is divided. With this technique Patey states that he is able to dissect the axilla up to the lateral border of the first rib.

Handley has adopted the Patey technique and performs what is probably the most thorough and meticulous mastectomy with axillary dissection. He prefers to call his operation a "conservative" radical mastectomy. He sacrifices so much skin that in more than one half of his patients he has to use a skin graft. His skin flaps are thinner than those of most surgeons. He takes from 2 to 3 hours to perform his operation. Handley emphasizes the cosmetic advantage of his operation. The transverse incision disfigures the chest wall less than the vertical Halsted incision, and when the pectoralis major is preserved it forms a bridge across the anterior axilla and maintains the contour of the anterior axillary fold. My answer is that these cosmetic advantages are less important than the local recurrence and survival rates.

Handley has classified his patients according to our Columbia Clinical Classification. He has biopsied the internal mammary nodes before deciding as to treatment; when he finds them involved he does not perform his complete operation but merely removes the breast and irradiates the axilla and internal mammary region. The results in these patients are reported in a separate category in his data. Like Handley I have refrained from radical mastectomy in my patients in whom internal mammary metastases were demonstrated by preliminary biopsy and treated with irradiation alone. These patients are also reported in a separate category in my data. Thus Handley's results with his operation and mine with the Halsted radical mastectomy are strictly comparable. They are shown in Table XX.

In Handley's Stage A patients treated by "conservative" radical mastectomy the local recurrence rate at 10 years was 12 percent, and in Stage B patients 24 percent. In my Stage A patients treated by the Halsted radical mastectomy the local recurrence rate was 6.5 percent, and in Stage B patients 18 percent.

These data show that the Halsted radical mastectomy has the advantage of a lower local recurrence and a higher survival rate. These differences are small, but, I believe, real. I have now performed more than 1,000 radical mastectomies, and these results lead me to conclude that I will have obtained 10 year survival in some 67 patients who would not have reached it if I had done the Handley operation. This has been achieved at the cost of approximately 3,500 more hours of operating time than I would have needed if I had done Handley's operation. Looking back I must say that as a physician dedicated to the ideal of giving my patients the best chance for survival I am duty bound to make this extra effort. I have failed often enough to cure breast carcinoma to be con-

Table XX. *Results of treatment of mammary carcinoma, Columbia Clinical Classificati*

	Handley, 1946 to 1962					
	"Conservative" radical mastectomy		*Simple mastectomy plus irradiation, biopsy-proved metastases, internal mammary nodes*		*Combined series of patien*	
Clinical stage	*Number of patients*	*10 yr. survival (%)*	*Number of patients*	*10 yr. survival (%)*	*Number of patients*	*10 yr. survival (%)*
A	160	63	11	9	171	60
B	91	37.5	21	9.5	112	32

vinced that no reasonable effort is too great in dealing with this formidable disease.

MORE EXTENDED OPERATIONS

None of the operations which I have discussed above, including the Halsted mastectomy, attempts to remove any but the axillary lymph nodes. They are therefore all inadequate in terms of our modern knowledge of the occurrence of metastases in other regional lymph node groups—the internal mammary and the supraclavicular nodes. In an attempt to meet this challenge surgically, a variety of new operations have recently been devised which combine some type of mastectomy and axillary dissection with removal of either the internal mammary or the supraclavicular nodes, or both.

RADICAL MASTECTOMY COMBINED WITH SUPRACLAVICULAR DISSECTION AND INTERNAL MAMMARY AND MEDIASTINAL LYMPH NODE DISSECTION

Wangensteeen and Lewis at the University of Minnesota devised the most radical surgical attack upon breast carcinoma. It included not only the conventional radical mastectomy but also supraclavicular dissection as well as dissection of the internal mammary and mediastinal lymph nodes. To achieve this, the chest was opened widely by splitting the sternum and detaching the first rib and elevating the clavicle. The operation was done in two stages. Lewis[31] reported a 13 percent operative mortality rate in a series of 50 patients. In something over 40 percent of the patients, no lymph node metastases were found in any of the dissected areas.

I cannot conceive of any justification for this operation. It had a high morbidity, a considerable mortality rate, and in a high percentage of the patients in whom it was done it was unnecessary.

RADICAL MASTECTOMY PLUS SUPRACLAVICULAR DISSECTION PLUS EXTRAPLEURAL EXCISION OF THE INTERNAL MAMMARY LYMPH NODE CHAIN

Dahl-Iversen and Tobiassen[8] in Copenhagen began, in 1948, to dissect the supraclavicular nodes as part of their radical mastectomy. In 1950 they extended their surgical attack to the internal mammary nodes. They evolved a conservative method of removing them extrapleurally, by cutting the second, third, and fourth costal cartilages 1 to 1.5 cm. from the sternal border. The costal cartilages were then raised with gauze strips so that the internal mammary vessels and all accompanying lymphatic and fatty tissue were removed in this way from the upper four interspaces.

As reported in our cooperative international study, "Treatment of early mammary carcinoma," this operation had a considerable morbidity, and the results were not as good as those of the Halsted radical mastectomy. Dahl-Iversen and his associates abandoned their operation some time ago.

nservative" radical mastectomy compared with radical mastectomy

Haagensen 1935 to July, 1963					
Radical mastectomy		Irradiation only, biopsy-proved metastases, internal mammary or subclavicular nodes		Combined series of patients	
'umber of patients	10 yr. survival (%)	Number of patients	10 yr. survival (%)	Number of patients	10 yr. survival (%)
608	70	33	21	641	67
186	43	53	18	239	38

RADICAL MASTECTOMY COMBINED WITH EN BLOC RESECTION OF THE CHEST WALL IN THE INTERNAL MAMMARY AREA

More radical surgical methods of combining radical mastectomy with *en bloc* resection of the full thickness of the chest wall in the internal mammary area have been devised by Urban[47] and by Ariel[2] in New York. In the Urban operation the sternum is split and the second, third, fourth, and fifth ribs are cut just lateral to their costochondral junctions. This leaves a defect of considerable size in the chest wall, which Urban closes with a fascia lata graft.

This operation has been more widely done than any of the other surgical procedures which include excision of the internal mammary nodes. The largest unselected case series is that of Bucalossi and associates[5]; the 10 year survival rate in 64 patients with proven internal mammary metastases was 20 percent.

I do not believe that these results justify a continuation of surgical attempts to deal with internal mammary metastases. It is my hope that prophylactic irradiation of these nodes, following the Halsted radical mastectomy, will give us better results.

REQUIREMENTS FOR THE VALID COMPARISON OF DIFFERENT METHODS OF TREATMENT

The main reason for the confusion regarding the best treatment for breast carcinoma is that the methods of studying case series and reporting results have not met reasonable standards. For example, in a recent report by Wise, Mason, and Ackerman,[50] no actual 10 year survival data were included; hypothetical long-term results were extrapolated from short-term results. This misleads the gullible reader.

It has recently become fashionable to regard randomized prospective trials as the only valid method of comparing results. My statistician consultants agree that there is no magic in the terms *prospective* or *randomized.* At Columbia we began in 1935 a prospective study of the treatment of breast carcinoma, and we have carried it forward ever since. Our clinical and pathological findings have been recorded in great detail, as illustrated in this paper. The stage of advancement of the disease has been carefully determined in all patients on the basis of the Columbia Clinical Classification. The results of radical mastectomy have been studied by our statisticians and reported in unequalled detail. What makes our study significant is its completeness, not when it was begun.

The fact that in so-called random studies several different forms of treatment are carried out simultaneously and their results compared in the same clinic is also inconsequential. There is no reason why the results of different methods of treatment carried out in different clinics cannot be compared provided that they meet the same standards. We suggest the following minimal requirements for the comparison of methods of treatment for carcinoma of the breast.

1. The unit case records must contain all essential clinical data—preferably recorded on a diagram as well as in a written description.

2. The clinical stage of advancement of the disease must be accurately determined for every patient, so that the results of different methods of treatment can be compared in each of the different clinical stages. The Columbia Clinical Classification is the most accurate one and the easiest to use.

3. Case series should consist of consecutive patients of all ages with breast carcinomas of all sizes, situated in all sectors of the breast, treated by the method being studied.

4. The technique of treatment being tested must be fully described and strictly followed in every patient. There are great differences in surgical and radiotherapeutic techniques and results differ accordingly.

5. Only carcinomas of accepted pathological types should be included in the trial series. Lobular carcinoma in situ (so called) is not true carcinoma. We prefer to call it *lobular neoplasia* and we do not include it among our breast carcinomas.

6. Results of treatment should be expressed in terms of the actual numerical frequency of local recurrence and the survival after 10 years. Patients dying of intercurrent disease and those lost track of are counted as dying of breast carcinoma.

There are already at hand enough valid data, as I have reviewed them in the preceding pages, to demonstrate beyond doubt that certain methods of treatment give such inferior results in operable carcinoma of the breast that no informed and conscientious surgeon can justify their use. Local excision of the primary tumor supplemented by irradiation, and simple mastectomy alone, are in this class. I believe that it is morally wrong to condemn patients to be treated with these methods in random studies without explaining to them the advantages and disadvantages of other methods of treatment. Physicians who do so should recall that Rabelais long ago said, "Science without conscience is but ruination of the soul."

McWhirter's simple mastectomy supplemented by irradiation gives somewhat better results which are, however, distinctly inferior to those of radical mastectomy. Patients should be told these facts before they decide how they wish to be treated.

Mastectomy plus axillary dissection, when very well done, gives results which approach but do not equal those of the Halsted radical mastectomy. With regard to this choice we need to decide whether cosmetic advantages take precedence over survival to some degree. We, of course, need more and better data to help make this choice. Until it is available my data as to the results of the Halsted radical mastectomy set a standard for comparison and suggest that this operation is the best method yet found for controlling this dangerous disease.

REFERENCES

1. Anglem, T. J., and Leber, R. E.: The dubious case for conservative operation in operable cancer of the breast; Ann. Surg. **176:** 625, 1972.
2. Ariel, I. M.: A conservative method of resecting the internal mammary lymph nodes en bloc with radical mastectomy, Surg. Gynecol. Obstet. **100:** 623, 1955.
3. Atkins, H., Hayward, J. L., et al.: Treatment of early breast cancer: A report after ten years of a clinical trial, Br. Med. J. **2:** 423, 1972.
4. Britton, R. C., and Nelson, P. A.: Causes and treatment of postmastectomy lymphedema of the arm, J. A. M. A. **180:** 95, 1962.
5. Bucalossi, P., Veronesi, U., et al.: Enlarged mastectomy for breast cancer, Am. J. Roentgenol. Radium Ther. Nucl. Med. **111:** 119, 1971.
6. Butcher, H. R.: Radical mastectomy for mammary carcinoma, Ann. Surg. **170:** 883, 1969.
7. Case, T. C.: Extended simple mastectomy for carcinoma of the breast, J. Int. Coll. Surg. **18:** 26, 1952.
8. Dahl-Iversen, E., and Tobiassen, T.: Radical mastectomy with parasternal and supraclavicular dissection for mammary carcinoma, Ann. Surg. **170:** 889, 1969.
9. Daland, E. M.: The incidence of swollen arms

after radical mastectomy and suggestions for prevention, N. Engl. J. Med. **242:** 497, 1950.
10. Danckers, U. F., Hamann, A., and Savage, J. L.: Postoperative recurrence of breast cancer after 32 years, SURGERY **47:** 656, 1960.
11. Deaton, W. R., Jr.: Simple mastectomy for carcinoma of the breast, SURGERY **37:** 720, 1955.
12. Donegan, W. L., et al.: A biostatistical study of locally recurrent breast carcinoma, Surg. Gynecol. Obstet. **122:** 529, 1966.
13. Finney, G. G., Merkel, W. C., and Miller, D. B.: Carcinoma of the breast; study of 298 consecutive cases, Ann. Surg. **125:** 673, 1947.
14. Fisher, B.: Status of adjuvant therapy: Results of The Surgical Adjuvant Breast Project studies on oophorectomy, postoperative radiation therapy, and chemotherapy. Other comments concerning clinical trials, Cancer **28:** 1654, 1971.
15. Fitzwilliams, D. C. L.: A plea for a more local operation in really early breast carcinoma, Br. Med. J. **2:** 405, 1940.
16. Haagensen, C. D.: A technique for radical mastectomy, SURGERY **19:** 100, 1946.
17. Haagensen, C. D.: A great leap backward in the treatment of carcinoma of the breast, J. A. M. A. **224:** 1181, 1973.
18. Haagensen, C. D., and Stout, A. P.: Carcinoma of the breast. Criteria of operability, Ann. Surg. **118:** 1032, 1943.
19. Haagensen, C. D., et al.: Metastasis of carcinoma of the breast to the periphery of the regional lymph node filter, Ann. Surg. **169:** 174, 1969.
20. Haagensen, C. D., Cooley, E., et al.: Treatment of early mammary carcinoma: A cooperative international study, Ann. Surg. **170:** 875, 1969.
21. Halsted, W. S.: The results of treatment for the cure of cancer of the breast performed at the Johns Hopkins Hospital from June, 1889, to January, 1894, Johns Hopkins Hosp. Rep. **4:** 297, 1894-95.
22. Halsted, W. S.: The swelling of the arm after operations for cancer of the breast—*elephantiasis chirurgica*—its cause and prevention, Bull. Johns Hopkins Hosp. **32:** 309, 1921.
23. Handley, R. S.: The technic and results of conservative radical mastectomy (Patey's operation), *in* Ariel, I. M., editor: Progress in clinical cancer, New York, 1965, Grune & Stratton, Inc., p. 462.
24. Handley, R. S.: Personal communication, 1970.
25. Handley, R. S.: Personal communication, 1973.
26. Handley, R. S., and Thackray, A. C.: The internal mammary lymph chain in carcinoma of the breast, Lancet **2:** 276, 1949.
27. Hartmann, H.: Résultats des opérations limitées dans le cancer du sein, Int. Union Against Cancer **8:** 161, 1952.
28. Hollenbach, F.: Vermeidung des Armödems nach Mamma-Amputation, Chirurg **20:** 374, 1949.
29. Holman, C., McSwain, B., and Beal, J. M.: Swelling of the upper extremity following radical mastectomy, SURGERY **15:** 757, 1944.
30. Kaae, S., and Johansen, H.: Simple mastectomy plus postoperative irradiation by the method of McWhirter for mammary carcinoma, Ann. Surg **170:** 895, 1969.
31. Lewis, F. J.: Extended or super-radical mastectomy for cancer of the breast, Minnesota Med. **36:** 763, 1953.
32. Lewison, E. F., and Smith, R. I.: Results of breast cancer treatment at Johns Hopkins Hospital, 1946-1950, SURGERY **53:** 644, 1963.
33. Lobb, A. W., and Harkins, H. N.: Postmastectomy swelling of the arm, West. J. Surg. **57:** 550, 1949.
34 Lockhart, C. E., and Ackerman, L. V.: The implications of local excision or simple mastectomy prior to radical mastectomy for carcinoma of the breast, SURGERY **26:** 577, 1949.
35. Madden, J. L.: Modified radical mastectomy, Surg. Gynecol. Obstet. **121:** 1221, 1965.
36. McWhirter, R.: Cancer of the breast, J. Radiol. Electr. **48:** 768, 1967.
37. Miller, E.: Simple mastectomy for mammary carcinoma, Ann. Surg. **170:** 879, 1969.
38. Morton, J. J., Jr., and Morton, J. H.: Cancer as a chronic disease, Ann. Surg. **137:** 683, 1953.
39. Patey, D. H., and Dyson, W. H.: The prognosis of carcinoma of the breast in relation to the type of operation performed, Br. J. Cancer **2:** 7, 1948.
40. Pawlias, W. T., Dockerty, M. B., and Ellis, F. H., Jr.: Late recurrence of carcinoma of the breast, Ann. Surg. **148:** 192, 1958.
41. Peters, M. V.: Personal communication, 1972.
42. Shimkin, M. B., et al.: Simple and radical mastectomy for breast cancer; a re-analysis of Smith and Meyer's report from Rockford, Illinois, J. Natl. Cancer Inst. **27:** 1197, 1961.
43. Smith, S. S., and Meyer, A. C.: Cancer of the breast in Rockford, Illinois, Am. J. Surg. **98:** 653, 1959.
44. Taylor, G. W., and Wallace, R. H.: Carcinoma of the breast; fifty years experience at the Massachusetts General Hospital, Ann. Surg. **132:** 833, 1950.
45. Spratt, J. S., Jr., and Donegan, W. L.: Can-

cer of the breast, Philadelphia, 1967, W. B. Saunders Co.

46. TNM. General Rules. Geneva, Int. Union Against Cancer, 1969.
47. Urban, J. A.: Radical excision of the chest wall for mammary cancer, Cancer **4:** 1263, 1951.
48. Urban, J. A., and Castro, E. B.: Selecting variations of surgical procedure for breast cancer, Cancer **28:** 1615, 1971.
49. Wawro, N. W.: The case for de novo origin of late recurrence of cancer of the female breast, SURGERY **35:** 470, 1954.
50. Wise, L., Mason, A. Y., and Ackerman, L. V.: Local excision and irradiation; an alternative method of treatment for early mammary cancer, Ann. Surg. **174:** 392, 1971.

Penetrating vascular injuries of the thoracic outlet

Robert L. Hewitt, M.D., Arnett D. Smith, M.D., Mathis L. Becker, M.D., Edward S. Lindsey, M.D., James B. Dowling, M.D., *and* **Theodore Drapanas, M.D.,** *New Orleans, La.*

Penetrating vascular injuries involving vessels of the base of the neck, supraclavicular area, and upper chest regions require a precise plan for prompt exposure of the injured vessels. Seventy-four patients with major vessel injury resulting from wounds of the cervicothoracic region were operated on. Bleeding, hematoma, signs of ischemia, or arteriovenous fistula were the frequent indications for operation, but location of the injury was also important. Arteriography was usually indicative of the site of arterial injury and, therefore, was helpful in the operative approach. Thirty-seven patients required thoracotomy and 37 were operated on through cervical, supraclavicular, or infraclavicular approaches without thoracotomy. Seven patients in the series died; all deaths were related to consequences of blood loss and shock. An increasing trend toward use of a thoracic approach for management of patients with major vascular injuries of the thoracic outlet has been observed, and these approaches have been described.

From the Department of Surgery, Tulane University School of Medicine, New Orleans, La.

PENETRATING INJURIES involving major blood vessels of the base of the neck, supraclavicular area, and upper chest represent a demanding problem. Arterial injuries in these areas along with wounds to the aorta result in the highest mortality rate of all arterial injuries.[2, 3] These injuries represent a special problem in operative approach because of frequent difficulty in gaining prompt access to the wounded vessels. The decision for use of either thoracotomy, an extrathoracic approach, or a combination of those approaches is sometimes complex. Unnecessary thoracotomy and sternotomy are not desirable, yet adequate exposure should be the dominant consideration. Furthermore, the site of vascular injury is often not apparent until operative exposure is accomplished. Management of patients with such injuries requires a precise plan for prompt exposure of the aortic arch, innominate, carotid, subclavian, and axillary arteries. Steenberg and Ravitch[5] directed attention to the important features in operative approach to injuries of the cervicothoracic region and, subsequently, others have reported extensive application of those principles.[1, 3] The operative approaches to these vascular injuries and the indications for them are presented in the following report, which is based on experiences with 74 patients.

Accepted for publication July 16, 1974.

Reprint requests: Robert L. Hewitt, M.D., Department of Surgery, Tulane University School of Medicine, 1430 Tulane Ave., New Orleans, La. 70112.

CLINICAL EXPERIENCE

Seventy-four consecutive patients with major vessel injury resulting from wounds of the cervicothoracic region treated on the Tulane University Surgical Service, Charity Hospital of Louisiana, from 1960 through

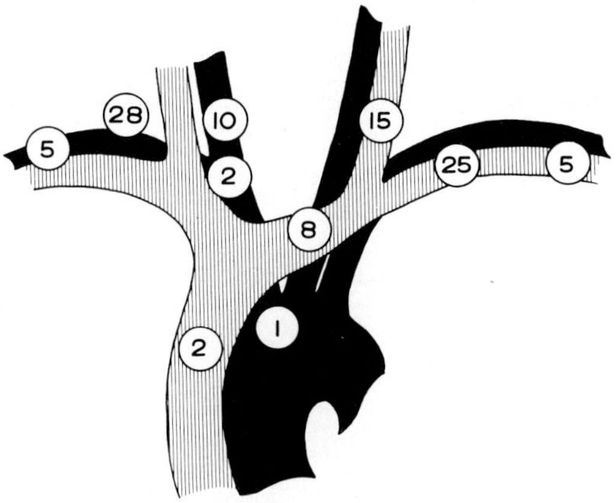

Fig. 1. Distribution of vascular injuries of the upper chest and base of neck in 53 patients.

Table I. *Vessels injured and results*

Major vessel	*No. of patients**	*No. of deaths*
Carotid artery	10 (4)	0
Subclavian artery	28 (18)	6
Innominate artery	2 (2)	1
Axillary artery	5 (2)	0
Aortic arch	1 (1)	0
Superior vena cava	2	0
Internal jugular vein	11	0
Subclavian vein	7	0
Innominate vein	5	0
Axillary vein	3	0
	74	7

*Numbers in parentheses indicate associated vein injury.

1973, comprise the basis of this report. The patients ranged from 9 to 63 years of age, with an average age of 29 years. Forty-eight patients sustained stab wounds, and 26 had low-velocity gunshot wounds. Carotid artery and jugular vein injuries, other than those resulting from wounds at the base of the neck, were excluded from this review. Findings in each patient suggested injury to a major blood vessel of the thoracic outlet. Twenty-seven patients sustained combined arterial and venous injuries, nine sustained arterial injuries only, and 28 had venous injuries only. The distribution of the 46 arterial and 55 venous injuries among the 74 patients is demonstrated in Fig. 1.

More than half of the patients were markedly hypotensive on admission, with systolic blood pressure of 80 mm. Hg or less. Most patients had extensive hematoma of the lower neck, supraclavicular area, or upper chest, and more than half had roentgenographic evidence of hemothorax or obvious hematoma in the mediastinum. A summary of the injuries and results is presented in Table I.

Subclavian artery. The frequent findings for the 28 patients with subclavian arterial injuries included: hypotension, associated subclavian vein injury, and hemothorax. Approximately half of the patients had no palpable distal pulse. Phrenic nerve injury was observed in four patients, brachial plexus or ulnar nerve injury in three, spinal cord injury in one, and injury to the thoracic duct in two. Nineteen of these patients had direct repair of the artery, eight had repair with either a vein graft or Dacron graft, and one was treated by ligation. The six deaths among patients with subclavian arterial injury were related to blood loss. Three of those deaths were in patients over 50 years of age, and two of the three required immediate thoracotomy in the emergency room to control bleeding. Four of the six deaths were related to prolonged and profound hypotension prior to operation; the fifth patient died as a result of air embolism during autotransfusion, and the sixth died of complications resulting from stress ulceration and gastric bleeding following operation. Among patients who survived, none developed ischemia of the upper extremity, although one patient's subclavian artery was ligated and two others were known to develop thrombosis following repair. One of these patients has arteriographic evidence of retrograde vertebral flow distal to thrombosed graft but is asymptomatic. One patient required late amputation because of brachial plexus injury.

Common carotid artery. Among the 10 patients with common carotid injuries, six were hypotensive (systolic pressure $<$ 80 mm. Hg), four of whom were either comatose or semicomatose. All of the 10 patients had primary suture repair. None died, but two of the hypotensive patients who were comatose experienced permanent hemiplegia.

Axillary artery. The five patients with

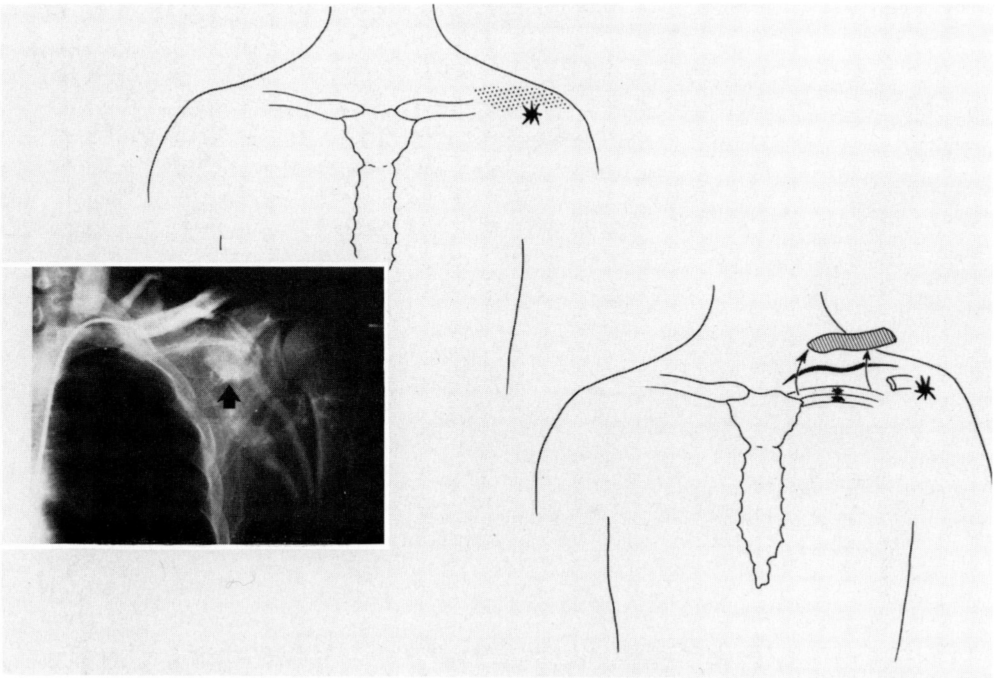

Fig. 2. Selective subclavian arteriogram demonstrating rapid runoff of contrast material through an arteriovenous fistula (Patient 1).

axillary artery injuries presented with hematoma extending above the clavicle, and one of these also had hemothorax. Peripheral pulses were detected in one. Four had repair by direct suture and one required a vein graft; all had a satisfactory result.

Aorta: Innominate artery. The one patient with aortic injury and one of the two patients with innominate artery injury are presented as brief case reports. The patient with aortic injury and the patient with innominate artery injury survived; one patient with innominate artery injury died as a result of delay in recognition of the injury.

Venous injuries. Among the 28 patients with venous injuries only, there were no deaths. One patient sustained cardiac arrest but was resuscitated. The injured vein was repaired by direct suture in 18 patients and was ligated in 10. Among the 27 patients with combined arterial and venous injuries, 11 had repair of the injured vein and 16 were treated by ligation. Three patients who required ligation of their subclavian veins experienced moderate edema of the upper extremity, but the edema was not permanent. No other complications directly attributable to venous repair or ligation were observed.

MANAGEMENT

The complexity in management of patients with injuries to the cervicothoracic region and the decisions regarding the type of approach are well demonstrated in the following four case presentations:

Patient 1. A 24-year-old man was admitted with a hematoma of the left supraclavicular area following a stab wound located inferior to the lateral part of the clavicle. Exploration of the axillary artery through an infraclavicular incision, with division of the pectoralis minor tendon, did not disclose an arterial injury. Eight days later, the patient was observed to have an arteriovenous fistula of the subclavian artery and vein which was repaired electively, and his course following the operation was uncomplicated. Fig. 2 illustrates the selective subclavian arteriogram in this patient and demonstrates the difficulty in visualization of the exact site of the fistula due to rapid shunting of contrast material into the vein.

Comment. The inadequacy of an infraclavicular approach to evaluate a possible wound of the

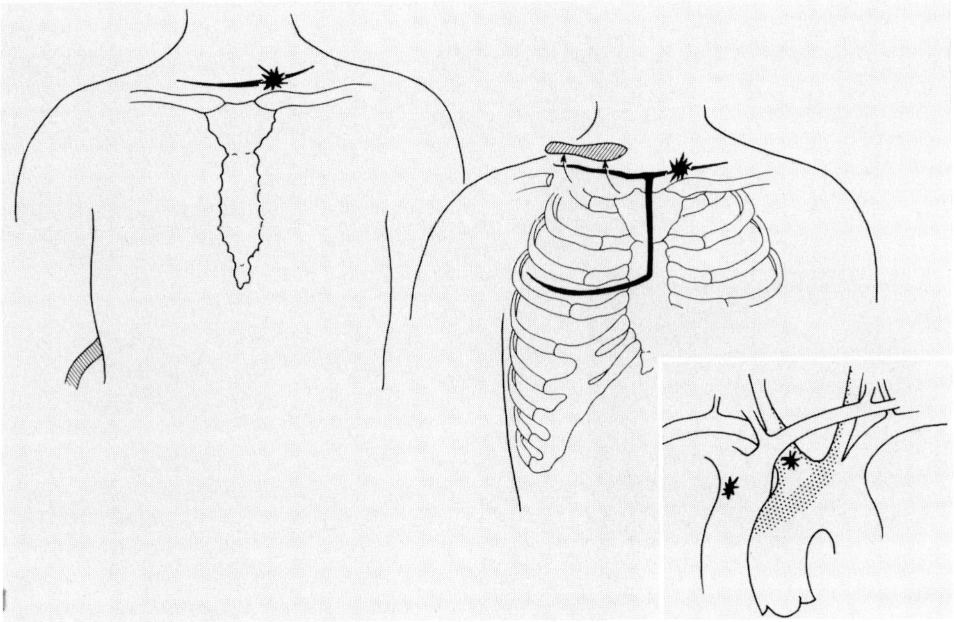

Fig. 3. Diagram of injury and management (Patient 2).

subclavian artery is apparent. Adequate exploration would have included a supraclavicular approach with resection of the clavicle, as was required at the second operation.

Patient 2. A 26-year-old man sustained a stab wound of the base of the neck just above the left sternoclavicular joint (Fig. 3). On chest roentgenogram the superior mediastinum was widened slightly, and there was evidence of a small amount of blood in the right chest. A right tube thoracotomy was performed, and the neck was explored. Although a trace of hematoma was noted in each carotid sheath, no arterial injury was identified. Five hours later, while the patient was still in the recovery room, a massive hematoma developed in the neck and resulted in tracheal compression and cardiac arrest. The patient was intubated and resuscitated, and the mediastinum was explored through a median sternotomy combined with a right third interspace incision. Perforating injuries of the innominate artery and vein were repaired, but the patient remained decerebrate following the operation and died.

Comment. The inadequacy of the initial exploration was obvious. The presence of hematoma in the carotid sheaths should have prompted exploration to the origin of the hematoma, which, in this case, would have lead to sternotomy and exposure of the innominate artery and aortic arch, as was performed during the second operation.

An example of the appropriate management of a similar case is presented with the next patient.

Patient 3. A 26-year-old man sustained a stab wound of the base of the neck near the left sternoclavicular junction. The patient was completely stable and had minimal neck hematoma. The superior mediastinum was widened on roentgenogram, but an arch aortogram was within normal limits (Fig. 4). Exploration through a median sternotomy disclosed hematoma along the left carotid and subclavian arteries. A perforating injury to the left innominate vein and penetrating injury to the aortic arch were discovered and repaired. The patient's course following operation was uneventful.

Comment. The normal arch arteriogram is not surprising since many arterial injuries are not readily apparent by arteriography. Even without evidence of widened mediastinum on roentgenogram, the presence of hematoma along the course of major arteries would have led to the discovery of the injury.

A critical decision is the selection of the appropriate incision for proximal control, yet, reserving the use of thoracotomy or sternotomy for instances where it is required. The use of multiple incisions is often required and is exemplified in the following case.

Patient 4. A 34-year-old man sustained a gunshot wound of the left supraclavicular area and was admitted with tachycardia and a systolic blood pressure of 80 mm. Hg. A left tube thora-

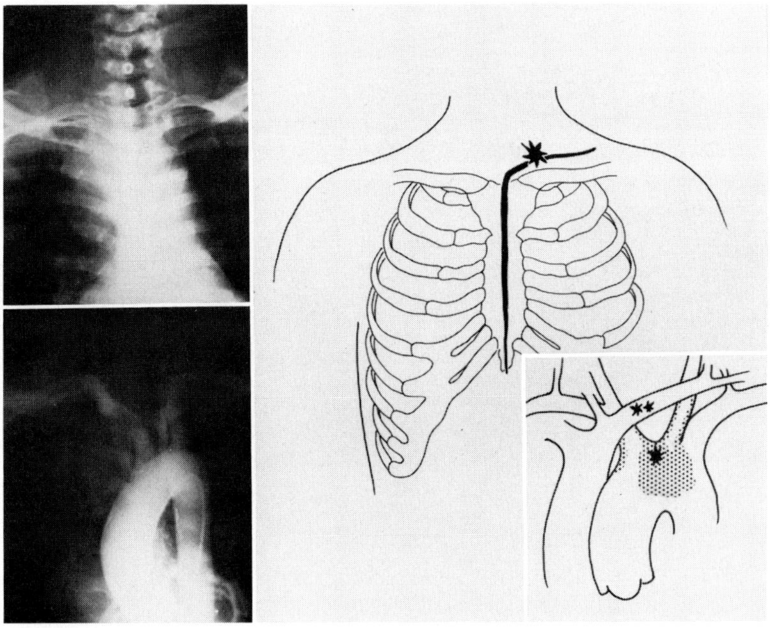

Fig. 4. Roentgenogram demonstrating a widened superior mediastinum and normal arch aortogram in patient with aortic arch injury (Patient 3).

cotomy yielded approximately 100 ml. of blood. During blood transfusion the patient remained stable; chest roentgenogram demonstrated a widened mediastinum and a missle in the right hilar region (Fig. 5). All pulses were palpable. Injury to the left subclavian artery was suspected and through a left anterior third interspace incision a large hematoma was noted to surround the subclavian artery and to extend over the aortic arch. While the hematoma was tamponaded by an assistant, a median sternotomy was performed and extended to meet the third interspace incision. This exposure disclosed hematoma beneath the adventitia of the aortic arch and left subclavian artery. Following proximal control of the left subclavian artery, dissection was continued distally to near the exit of the artery from the thorax, where the injury appeared to be located. A left supraclavicular incision with division of both heads of the sternocleidomastoid muscle, division of the strap muscles and anterior scalene muscle, and resection of the medial two thirds of the clavicle allowed control of the distal subclavian artery and its branches. A perforating injury to the subclavian artery was then repaired by resection of a small segment of artery and interposition of a Dacron graft. The patient had an uncomplicated recovery.

Comment. The approach used in this patient was emphasized by Steenberg and Ravitch,[5] who emphasized initial control of the bleeding intrathoracic vessel by an anterior third interspace incision; while the vessel is controlled by pressure or clamp, a median sternotomy is performed to gain control and provide exposure for repair. Control of the distal subclavian artery requires a supraclavicular approach as described in this case.

During the period of this study a more aggressive approach to the management of patients with suspected injury to vessels of the thoracic outlet has evolved. Bleeding, as evidenced by hemothorax, mediastinal hematoma, and hematoma over the upper thorax, supraclavicular area, or neck, was observed to be the most reliable sign of vascular injury. The combination of bleeding and location of the penetrating wound is sometimes more reliable than arteriography. Fig. 6 demonstrates an arteriogram and a venogram performed in a patient with a gunshot wound of the supraclavicular area and minimal chest wall hematoma. The arteriogram did not demonstrate injury, but venogram confirmed a massive hematoma about the vessels. Exploration confirmed an extensive injury of the first portion of the axillary artery. Despite the inaccuracy of arteriography in the above patient and in the patient with an aortic injury (Patient 3), arteriography is frequently helpful in precisely localizing the injury. Arteriography is now used routinely in patients who are stable and when time permits.

An increasing trend toward the use of a

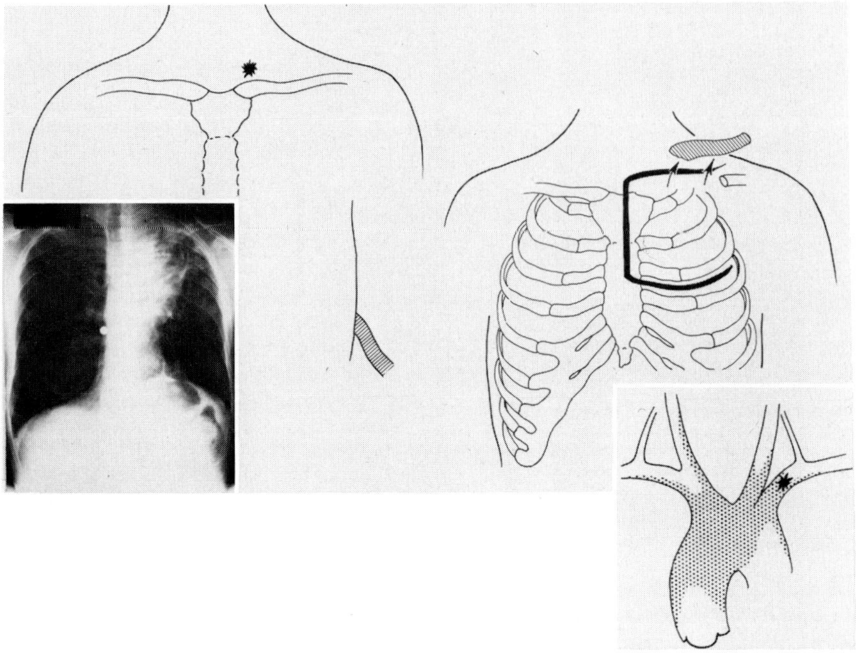

Fig. 5. Roentgenogram demonstrating widened superior mediastinum, left hemothorax, and missile in right hilum; an anterior third interspace incision offered exposure for proximal control of the injured left subclavian artery prior to definitive exposure through a "trap door" incision.

thoracic approach for achieving more central exposure of vascular injuries in this area is apparent from this study (Fig. 7). Thoracotomy, sternotomy, or a "trap door" approach was used in 37 of the 74 patients in this series. A thoracic approach was used in 18 of the initial 50 patients and in 19 of the subsequent 24 patients.

DISCUSSION

Penetrating injuries involving major blood vessels of the base of the neck, supraclavicular area, or upper chest often present difficulty in the choice of operative management. The indications for operation are usually apparent: bleeding, hematoma, signs of ischemia, arteriovenous fistula, or location of the wound. The approach and extent of operation require additional planning. Aortography may be especially helpful in precisely localizing injuries of the innominate, subclavian, or proximal carotid arteries. Aortography should be done routinely when circumstances permit, and retrograde femoral aortography is preferable in most instances. The presence of active arterial bleeding is a contraindication to the delay imposed by arteriography; even when time does permit arteriography, a surgeon should be at the patient's side.

The possible need for extensive exposure as accomplished with thoracotomy, sternotomy, or resection of the clavicle makes consideration of proximal control more complex for these vascular injuries as compared to most other peripheral vascular injuries. Several important principles of approach for injuries to vessels of the thoracic outlet and upper chest are demonstrated in Fig. 8. Although an infraclavicular approach is often adequate for injuries to the axillary vessels (Fig. 8, *A*), proximal control of the subclavian artery through a supraclavicular approach may be desirable for injuries to the first portion of the axillary artery (Fig. 8, *B*). Subclavian injuries may often be repaired through such an incision with resection of the medial part of the clavicle if necessary. More extensive exposure is afforded by using both incisions or by combining the two as a

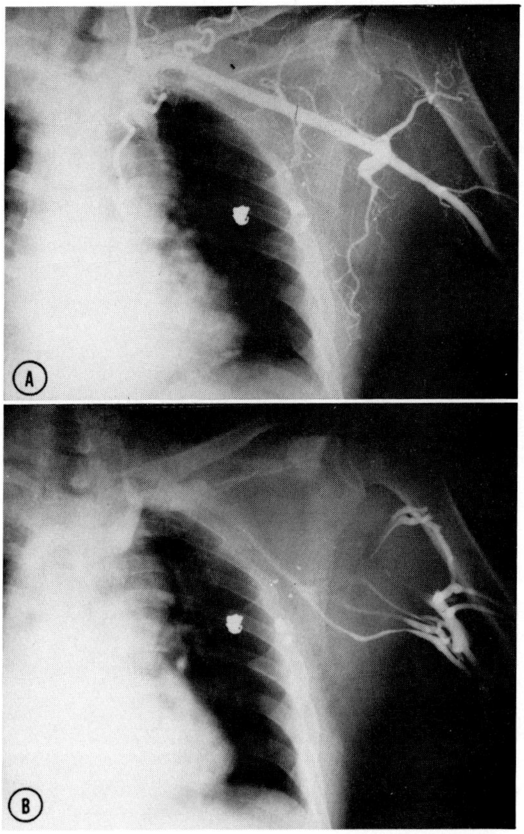

Fig. 6. *A,* Arteriogram demonstrating no evidence of injury in patient with severe subclavian arterial injury; *B,* venogram demonstrating massive hematoma about vessels which was the indication for exploration.

continuous incision. More proximal control may be afforded through a third interspace and sternotomy combined with a supraclavicular approach with resection of the medial part of the clavicle, the "trap door" incision (Fig. 8, *C*). Extensive exposure of the aortic arch and central great vessels may be afforded through a sternotomy, and the incision may be extended longitudinally into the cervical area or transversely over the supraclavicular area for more distal exposure (Fig. 8, *D*). The decision for the type of approach often is complicated by the concept that most or all penetrating injuries of the neck are explored while uncomplicated penetrating injuries of the chest are usually not.[4] The relative merits of proximal control and adequate exposure outweigh the possible morbidity from sternotomy or thoracotomy

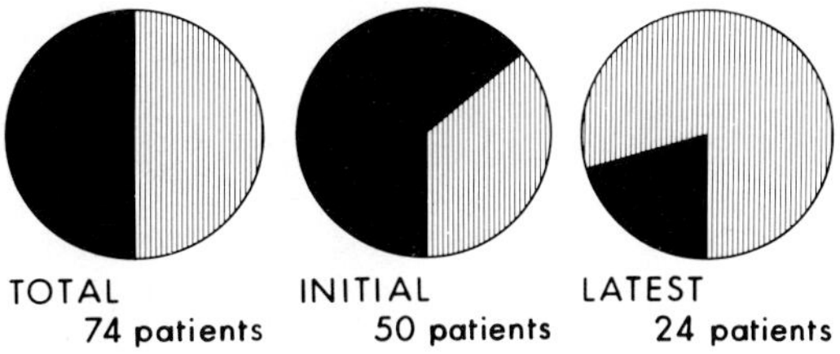

Fig. 7. Trend in more frequent use of thoracic approach in management of patients with penetrating injuries of the thoracic outlet. Black area, extrathoracic approach; striped area, thoracic approach (thoracotomy, sternotomy, or "trap door").

in management of suspected injuries of the proximal vessels.

The present experience confirms that the presence of hematoma is the most constant sign alerting to major vascular injury. Exploration should, therefore, include inspection of the vessels proximal to the hematoma. Application of this principle would have avoided the overlooking of an arterial injury, as described in Patients 1 and 2, in whom hematoma beneath the adventitia of the artery was apparent. The presence of mediastinal hematoma following penetrating injury is indication for exploration of the mediastinum even in absence of signs of blood loss or when aortography is negative, as illustrated in Patient 3. The combination of hematoma and the site and trajectory of the injury may be even more compelling indications for exploration than either finding alone.

The possibility of concurrent injury to the mediastinum or intrathoracic vessels must always be considered in patients with injuries to the neck. Otherwise, neck exploration alone may even be misleading if considered negative. The possibility of the sudden onset of bleeding into the thorax or neck from an unrecognized vessel injury occurring following exploration of the neck may be catastrophic (Patient 2).

An interesting observation in the present series was that most patients operated on for venous injury had repair rather than ligation of the vein, while most patients operated on for arterial and venous injury were treated by ligation of the vein. This observation reflects largely the more extensive

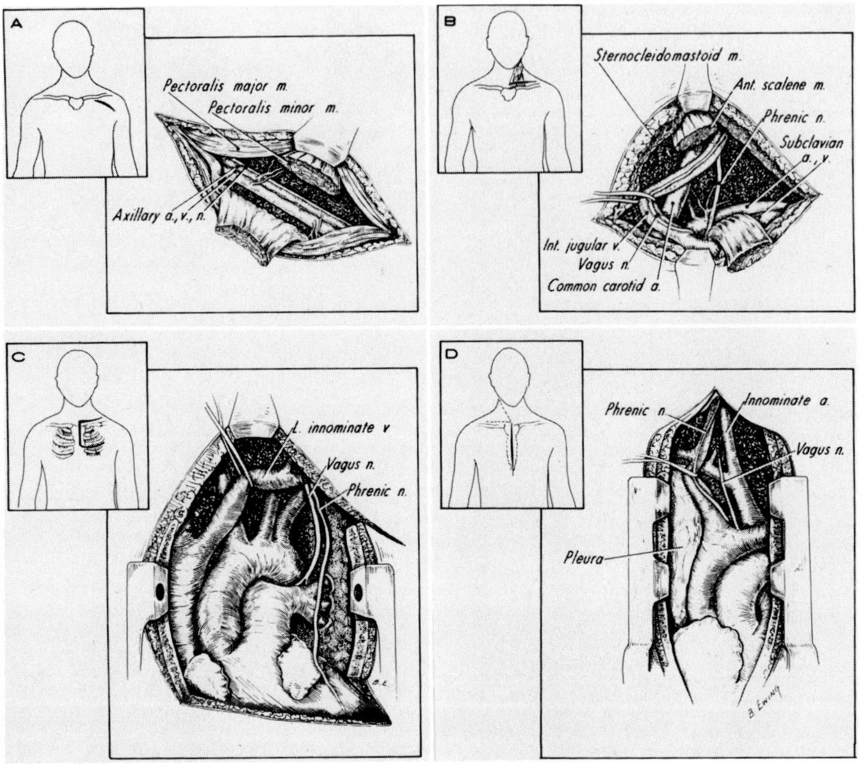

Fig. 8. *A,* Injuries to the axillary vessels may be exposed through an infraclavicular approach. *B,* If injury involves the first portion of the axillary artery or the subclavian artery a supraclavicular approach is required. A supraclavicular approach may be used to control the subclavian artery while an infraclavicular incision is used to approach an injured axillary artery. More extensive exposure is afforded by utilizing a continuous incision or by resection of the medial portion of the clavicle. *C,* More proximal injuries of the subclavian, innominate, or carotid arteries may be exposed using a third interspace incision combined with a supraclavicular incision, resection of the medial part of the clavicle and sternotomy, the "trap door" incision. *D,* Exposure through median sternotomy. Incision may be extended as shown.

injuries in the latter group, and also that concern with arterial repair accounts for less attention to the venous injury than in situations of isolated venous injury. Permanent edema of the upper extremity was not observed as a consequence of repair or ligation of injured innominate, subclavian, or axillary veins, and this observation would appear to support the safety of ligation of these veins when collateral venous supply is known to be adequate. Even so, we have preferred repair to ligation whenever possible and would strongly advise repair if collateral venous supply is in question.

REFERENCES

1. Brawley, R. K., Murray, G. F., Crisler, C., and Cameron, J. L.: Management of wounds of the innominate, subclavian, and axillary blood vessels, Surg. Gynecol. Obstet. **131:** 1130, 1970.
2. Bricker, D. L., Noon, G. P., Beall, A. C., Jr., and De Bakey, M. E.: Vascular injuries of the thoracic outlet, J. Trauma **10:** 1, 1970.
3. Drapanas, T., Hewitt, R. L., Weichert, R. F., and Smith, A. D.: Civilian vascular injuries: A critical appraisal of three decades of management, Ann. Surg. **172:** 351, 1970.
4. Hunt, T. K., Blaisdell, F. W., and Okimoto, J.: Vascular injuries of the base of the neck, Arch. Surg. **98:** 586, 1969.
5. Steenberg, R. W., and Ravitch, M. M.: Cervico-thoracic approach for subclavian vessel injury from compound fracture of the clavicle: Considerations of subclavian-axillary exposures, Ann. Surg. **157:** 839, 1963.

Directional Doppler studies of supraorbital artery flow in internal carotid stenosis and occlusion

Frank W. LoGerfo, M.D., *and* **G. Robert Mason, M.D.,** *Baltimore, Md.*

A directional Doppler flowmeter was used to determine the direction of supraorbital artery flow in 13 patients with disease of the internal carotid arteries and in 10 controls. Supraorbital artery flow is antegrade in normal subjects and with internal carotid stenosis of up to 75 percent by diameter. Flow is retrograde with complete occlusion or extreme stenosis. The test is of clinical value in screening stroke patients and in the evaluation of patients undergoing carotid endarterectomy. However, retrograde flow is not an index of the clinical significance of a carotid stenosis.

From the Department of Surgery, University of Maryland Hospital, Baltimore, Md.

THE DOPPLER FLOWMETER determines the frequency shift in an ultrasound beam as it is reflected from moving blood cells. This Doppler shift is converted to a voltage output which is directly proportional to the velocity of blood flow. Recently a directional Doppler flowmeter has become available which utilizes a phase analyzer to determine the direction as well as the velocity of flow.* There are separate output channels for flow toward the probe and for flow away from the probe.

The supraorbital artery is a branch of the ophthalmic artery and derives its blood flow from the circle of Willis. The vessel traverses the roof of the orbit, crossing the rim at the easily palpable supraorbital notch. Normally the direction of supraorbital artery flow is from the orbit to the forehead (Fig. 1). However, if there is occlusion of the internal carotid artery, flow in the supraorbital is reversed as it receives blood from the external carotid system (Fig. 2). Under these circumstances the primary source of collateral flow is the superficial temporal artery.

This reversal of supraorbital flow with internal carotid occlusion has been demonstrated previously.[5] The purpose of the present study was to determine the relationship between reversal of supraorbital flow and the degree of internal carotid stenosis.

TECHNIQUE OF SUPRAORBITAL ARTERY STUDY

The supraorbital notch is palpated at the rim of the orbit and the probe is placed over the artery, just inside the rim. The probe is then angled posteriorly so that the beam will be directed against the normal flow of blood (Fig. 1). With some practice the artery is easily identifiable. It is important to maintain the probe crystals perpendicular to the vessel and not to stray medially with the beam, as the lateral nasal artery and other collaterals

Accepted for publication July 26, 1974.

Reprint requests: Frank W. LoGerfo, M.D., Assistant Professor of Surgery, University Hospital, Boston University Medical Center, Boston, Mass. 02118.

*Parks Electronics Model 806.

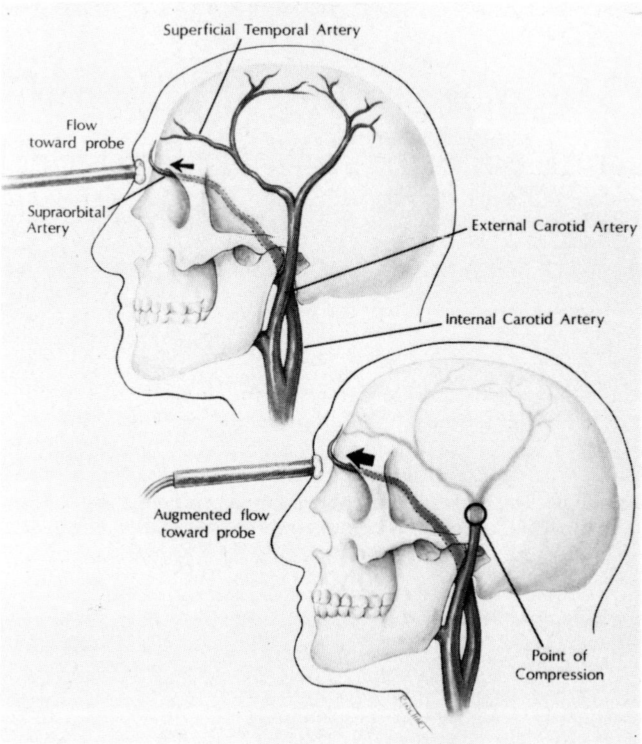

Fig. 1. The normal direction of blood flow in the supraorbital carotid artery is toward the probe (top). With compression of the superficial temporal artery this flow is augmented (bottom).

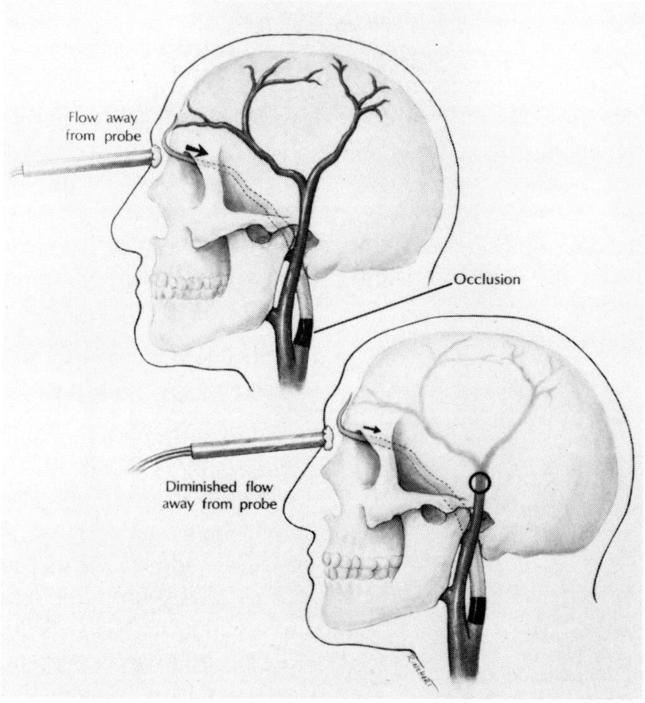

Fig. 2. With occlusion of the internal carotid artery flow in the supraorbital artery is away from the probe (top). This flow is diminished by compression of the superficial temporal artery (bottom).

Table I. *Results of Doppler supraorbital study*

Case No.	Clinical symptoms	Supraorbital flow Right	Supraorbital flow Left	Angiography: Diameter reduction internal carotid (%) Right	Angiography: Diameter reduction internal carotid (%) Left	Other findings
Internal carotid occlusion:						
1.	Left hemiparesis	Retro	Retro	100	100	
2.	Ligation left internal carotid for cav. sinus fistula	Ante	Retro	0	100	
3.	Aorto-iliac disease, bilateral carotid bruits	Retro	Ante	100	50	
Internal carotid stenosis:						
4.	Dizziness, ataxia, left carotid bruit	Ante	Ante	0	60	Left subclavian steal
5.	Buzzing in left ear, bilateral carotid bruits	Ante	Ante	60	70	
6.	Transient weakness left arm, systolic and diastolic right carotid bruit	Retro	Ante	95	0	
7.	Transient left facial weakness, dizziness, bilateral carotid bruits	Ante	Ante	70	60	
8.	Dizziness, ataxia, no bruit	Ante	Ante	60	0	Left subclavian steal
9.	Dizziness, bilateral carotid bruits	Ante	Ante	60	60	
10.	Transient aphasia, previous minor stroke, no bruit	Ante	Ante	50	50	
11.	Transient aphasia and monocular blindness, bilateral carotid bruits	Ante	Ante	75	70	
12.	Abdominal aneurysm, bilateral carotid bruits	Ante	Ante	60	60	
13.	Aorto-iliac disease, bilateral carotid bruits	Ante	Ante	60	60	
Controls:						
10 patients	Average age, 62 years; no bruits	Ante	Ante	0 (3 patients)	0 (3 patients)	

are in the area. Also no pressure should be applied as it is very easy to inadvertently compress the supraorbital artery.

Having found the artery, the examiner may then use the panel meters or the recorder output to determine direction of flow. In some cases flow may be so low that an accurate determination cannot be made on this basis. As a confirmatory test, the ipsilateral superficial temporal artery is compressed while listening to the supraorbital flow. Normally this produces an increase in flow as the supraorbital supplies additional blood to the forehead (Figs. 1 and 3). However, if the supraorbital flow is reversed and is originating from the external carotid system, this maneuver will markedly diminish supraorbital flow (Figs. 2 and 4).

RESULTS

Twenty-three patients were studied by the above technique, the results of which are summarized in Tables I and II. Angiography was performed where it was clinically indicated; no patient was subjected to angiography specifically for the purpose of this investigation. Three of the patients who underwent angiography were found to have essentially normal extracranial vessels and are included among 10 controls. The remainder of the 10 controls were presumed to have normal vessels on clinical grounds alone.

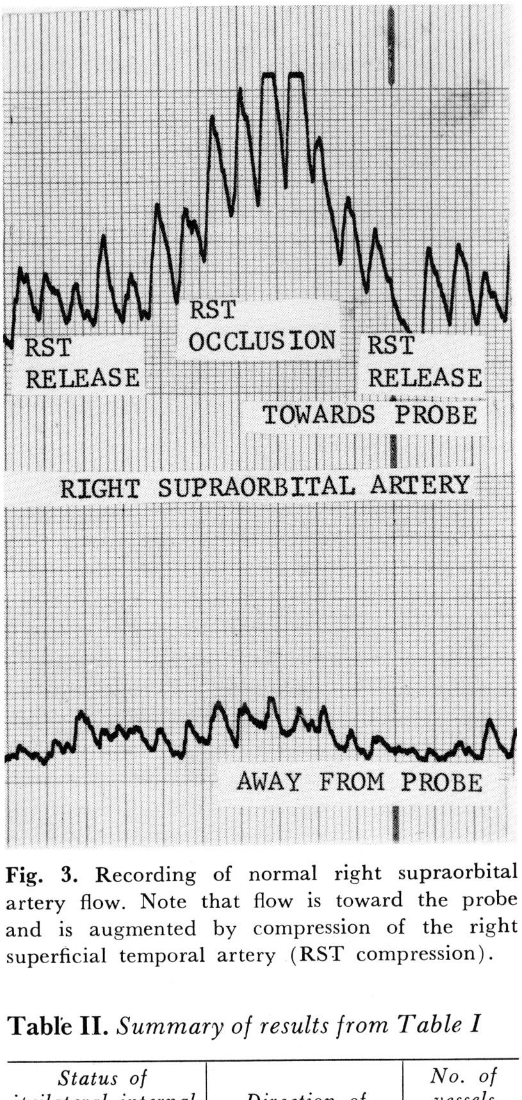

Fig. 3. Recording of normal right supraorbital artery flow. Note that flow is toward the probe and is augmented by compression of the right superficial temporal artery (RST compression).

Table II. *Summary of results from Table I*

Status of ipsilateral internal carotid artery	*Direction of supraorbital flow*	*No. of vessels studied*
Normal	Antegrade	23
Stenosis of 50 to 75%	Antegrade	16
Stenosis of 95%	Retrograde	1
Complete occlusion	Retrograde	4

Of the total group of 46 internal carotid arteries, 25 were normal, 17 were stenotic, and four were completely occluded. Supraorbital flow was antegrade in 25 of 25 instances of a normal ipsilateral internal carotid artery and in 16 of 17 instances of internal carotid stenosis. Flow was retrograde in four of four cases of complete occlusion of the ipsilateral internal carotid and in one case of extreme stenosis.

The degree of stenosis was between 50 and 75 percent diameter reduction in 16 cases, all of which were associated with antegrade supraorbital flow. The one instance of stenosis associated with retrograde flow was so extreme that it was initially interpreted as complete occlusion. However, on a subtraction study and at the subsequent operation the vessel was shown to be patent, with a stenosis estimated to be 95 percent of the diameter.

DISCUSSION

Antegrade supraorbital flow means that pressure in the internal carotid system is higher than in the external carotid–superficial temporal system. If a pulse is palpable in the superficial temporal artery, it is reasonable to assume that an equivalent pulsatile flow is present in the ophthalmic artery. Otherwise, supraorbital flow would be retrograde and would not be augmented by superficial temporal compression. In all of our cases of internal carotid stenosis, a pulse was easily palpated in the superficial temporal artery. Nonetheless, we found supraorbital flow to be antegrade even in the face of marked internal carotid stenosis, as exemplified by Case 11 (Fig. 5). In this instance there was stenosis of 75 percent of the diameter or 94 percent of the cross-sectional area of the internal carotid. At first glance it may be surprising that this degree of stenosis did not cause reversal of supraorbital flow. However, Brisman, Grossman, and Correll,[3] using an electromagnetic flowmeter, found no decrease in internal carotid flow with 75 percent stenosis. In experimental studies of stenosis of the dog aorta[6] and iliac artery[7] no decrease in flow was noted until more than 70 percent of the diameter was compromised. Baker and associates[1] showed that decrease in flow and mean pressure distal to an experimental aortic stenosis did not occur until 97 percent of the diameter was compromised. This flow decrease was heralded by the appearance of a diastolic bruit. Our own results concur with these experimental findings in that reversal

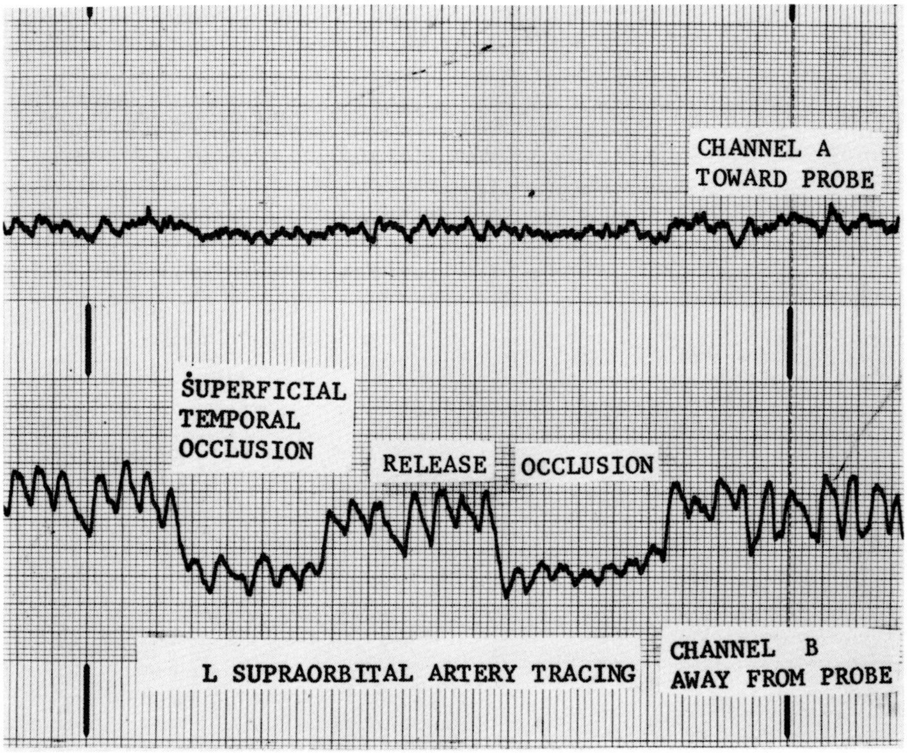

Fig. 4. Recording of left supraorbital artery flow in Case 1 with internal carotid occlusion. Note that flow is away from probe and is diminished but not obliterated by compression of the left superficial temporal artery. There is marked diastolic flow especially apparent just prior to compression.

of supraorbital flow did not occur with stenotic lesions known to be hemodynamically insignificant. Flow reversal did occur with complete occlusion and with extreme (95 percent) internal carotid stenosis where a diastolic bruit was present. We believe, therefore, that supraorbital flow correlates with flow in the ipsilateral carotid territory and that antegrade flow indicates adequate flow distal to an internal carotid stenosis.

While antegrade supraorbital flow demonstrates that an internal carotid stenosis is not hemodynamically significant, it does not rule out its clinical significance. In fact, six of our 10 patients with internal carotid stenosis had transient ischemic attacks in the carotid territory in the face of antegrade supraorbital flow (Table I). This finding supports the contention[4] that transient ischemic attacks in the carotid territory frequently represent an embolic rather than flow phenomenon.

Retrograde supraorbital flow indicates complete occlusion of the ipsilateral internal carotid. It was present in all four instances of occlusion in our series. In addition, Machleder and Barker[5] found retrograde supraorbital flow in 10 cases of internal carotid occlusion with one false positive. Early in our study we found what was thought to be retrograde flow in a patient who proved to have only 50 percent stenosis. However, upon restudying the patient, antegrade flow was demonstrated. This false positive was probably a result of listening to a collateral vessel, such as the lateral nasal artery, rather than the supraorbital. As mentioned earlier, such errors can be avoided by strict attention to the orientation of the probe and crystals. We have also noticed that when retrograde flow is present, there is usually a diastolic component and the flow is markedly diminished, but not obliterated, by superficial temporal

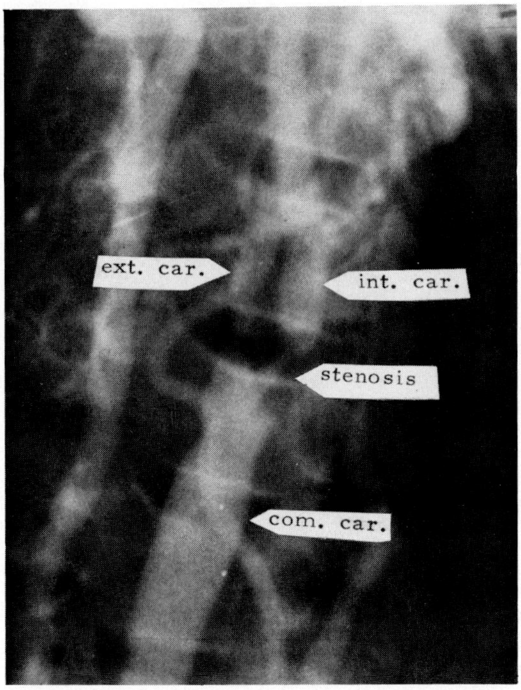

Fig. 5. This patient (Case 11) had transient ischemic attacks in the carotid territory and stenosis of 75 percent of the diameter of the internal carotid artery. However, flow in the ipsilateral supraorbital artery was antegrade.

compression (Fig. 4). If the examiner encounters flow which is heard in systole only and which is obliterated by superficial temporal occlusion, he is probably listening to a collateral of the external carotid system and should check the probe orientation.

Doppler supraorbital artery studies are of value in patients undergoing carotid endarterectomy. In particular the presence of antegrade flow following operation will confirm patency of the internal carotid. Should neurologic signs and retrograde flow subsequently develop, the surgeon can quickly and reliably make diagnosis of internal carotid occlusion. The test is also useful in determining the patency of the internal carotid arteries in acute stroke patients. It does not appear to be of value in determining the clinical significance of a stenosis of the internal carotid artery.

REFERENCES

1. Baker, J. D., Del Banco, T. L., Price, J. B., et al.: Experimental study of murmurs in stenotic arteries, SURGERY **59:** 88, 1966.
2. Bergentz, S. E., Haggendal, E., and Iyilsson, N. Y.: Pre and postoperative cerebral blood flow in patients with carotid artery stenosis, *in* Brock, M., editor: Cerebral blood flow, New York, 1969, Springer-Verlag, pp. 161-162.
3. Brisman, R., Grossman, B. L., and Correll, J. W.: Accuracy of transcutaneous Doppler ultrasonics in evaluating extracranial vascular disease, J. Neurosurg. **32:** 529, 1970.
4. Crawford, E. S., De Bakey, M. E., Blaisdell, F. W., et al.: Hemodynamic alterations in patients with arterial insufficiency before and after operation, SURGERY **48:** 76, 1960.
5. Machleder, H. I., and Barker W. F.: Stroke on the wrong side: Use of the Doppler ophthalmic test in cerebral vascular screening, Arch. Surg. **105:** 943, 1972.
6. May, A. G., DeWeese, J. A., and Rob, C. G.: Hemodynamic effects of arterial stenosis, SURGERY **33:** 513, 1963.
7. Schenk, W. G., Menno, A. D., and Martin, J. W.: Hemodynamics of experimental coarctation of the aorta, Ann. Surg. **153:** 163, 1961.

A comparison of gastric emptying before and after vagotomy with antrectomy and vagotomy with pyloroplasty

I. A. Donovan, F.R.C.S., I. F. Gunn, F.R.A.C.S., Anne Brown,
J. Alexander-Williams, M.D., Ch.M., F.R.C.S., *Birmingham, England, and*
R. J. Clarke, M.D., F.R.C.S., *Somerset, England*

The rate of gastric emptying of a 750 ml. 10 percent dextrose meal was studied by a double-dye dilution technique in 23 patients with duodenal ulcer. Fourteen were restudied 3 months after vagotomy with pyloroplasty (V+P) and nine 3 months after vagotomy with antrectomy (V+A). Two points in the emptying were taken to express the results: (1) the volume emptied by 10 minutes after ingestion of the meal as a measurement of initial gastric incontinence or cascading, and (2) the time taken for complete emptying of the stomach as a measurement of active muscular gastric emptying. Statistical comparison of the preoperative and postoperative results by Student's t test showed that both operations significantly shortened the time taken for complete emptying of the stomach ($p < 0.025$ for V+P and $p < 0.05$ for V+A). However, only after V+P was there a significant increase above preoperative levels in the volume of early emptying ($p < 0.001$). After V+A two groups were identifiable: five of the nine patients emptied rapidly, whereas four behaved similarly to the way they did before operation. Rapid early emptying of the meal after either operation correlated with the clinical symptoms of dumping ($p < 0.01$).

From The General Hospital, Birmingham, England

One of the suggested advantages of vagotomy with pyloroplasty (V+P) over vagotomy with antrectomy (V+A) is that V+A removes the antrum and, therefore, might be followed by more precipitous gastric emptying and, consequently, a higher incidence of dumping and diarrhea.

However, some published results of the relative incidence of postoperative symptoms do not support this hypothesis. Cox and his colleagues[3] found an incidence of episodic diarrhea of 20.9 percent following V+P, but of only 14.6 percent following V+A.

Goligher and his colleagues,[5] in a 5 to 8 year followup of V+P and V+A, found the incidence of diarrhea and dumping to be approximately the same after the two operations.

We have measured the rate of gastric emptying in patients before and after V+A and before and after V+P to see if there is any demonstrable difference and have related the results to symptoms of dumping 3 months after operation.

MATERIAL AND METHODS

Twenty-nine male patients with duodenal ulcers were studied before operation. Fourteen of these were studied 3 months after V+P and nine others 3 months after V+A.

A 750 ml. solution of 10 percent dextrose in water was used and the residual volume

Accepted for publication July 16, 1974.

Reprint requests: J. Alexander-Williams, M.D., The General Hospital, Steelhouse Lane, Birmingham, B4 6NH, England.

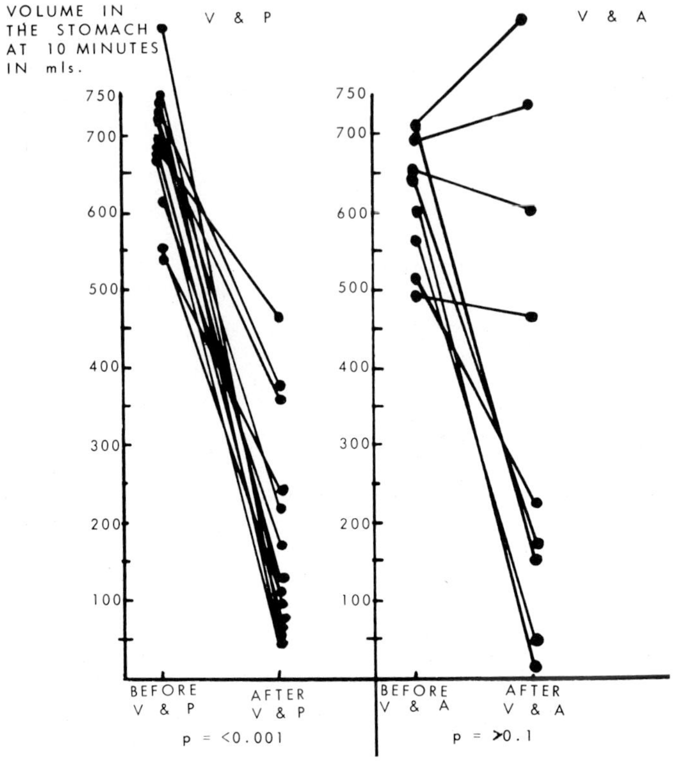

Fig. 1. The volume in the stomach 10 minutes after the meal, before and after either vagotomy and pyloroplasty or vagotomy and antrectomy.

in the stomach calculated using a double sampling dye dilution technique[4] with S^{35} phenol red as the indicator. All the tests were performed with the patient in the sitting position.[2]

Previous studies of gastric emptying after gastric surgery from our unit have shown that there is a great increase in early gastric emptying after operation.[2] This is best illustrated by the results at 10 minutes after the meal, and we therefore selected the volume remaining at this time as the first point for comparison of the emptying studies. The second point at which comparison was made was the time taken for complete emptying to occur. In practice this was said to have been achieved when the estimated volume fell below 20 ml.

The results were statistically analyzed with Student's t test. Because of the skewed distribution of the results, the original figures were converted to logarithms before being subjected to analysis and comparison. The chi-square test was applied when considering the incidence of dumping relative to rapid early emptying.

RESULTS

After V+P there was considerable alteration in the pattern of emptying, with a significantly reduced volume remaining in the stomach 10 minutes after the meal, as shown in Fig. 1 ($p < 0.001$). After V+A there were two reactions among patients, four of the nine behaved in a similar fashion to the V+P group and emptied rapidly, and the other five showed little alteration from the preoperative state.

Fig. 2 illustrates the alterations in final emptying times in the two groups of patients. In both, complete emptying was significantly faster after operation ($p < 0.025$ for V+P and $p < 0.05$ for V+A).

Early dumping symptoms only occurred in patients who had less than 300 ml. remaining in the stomach at 10 minutes (see Fig.

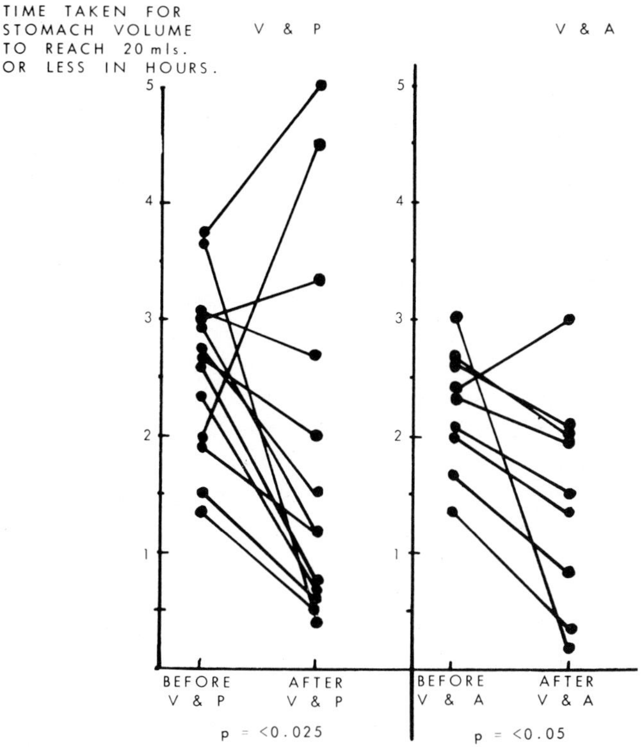

Fig. 2. The time taken for the stomach volume to reach 20 ml. or less, before and after either vagotomy and pyloroplasty or vagotomy and antrectomy.

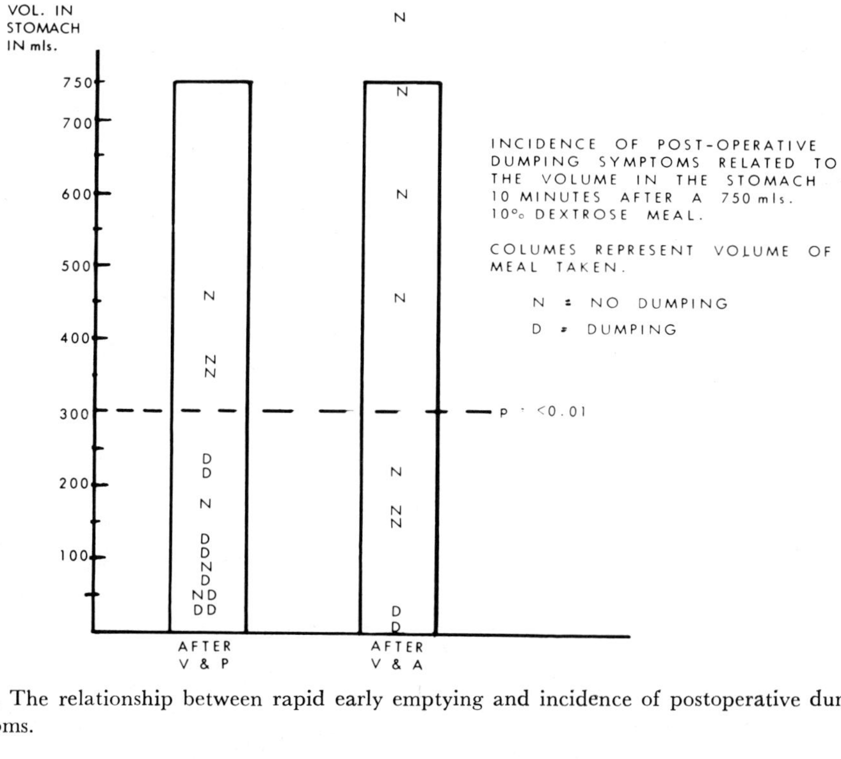

Fig. 3. The relationship between rapid early emptying and incidence of postoperative dumping symptoms.

3). This correlation is significant at the one percent level when analyzed by the chi-square test.

DISCUSSION

This study does not support the suggestion that gastric emptying is less affected by V+P than by V+A. On the contrary, it suggests that rapid early emptying is likely to be more common after V+P than after V+A.

This rapid early emptying has been aptly described as "gastric incontinence."[6] Two possible explanations for the phenomenon are disruption of the pyloroantral mechanisms and abolition of the receptive relaxation of the body of the stomach in response to an incoming meal.[1] Abolition of this faculty is the likely explanation for the increase in early emptying reported after proximal gastric vagotomy[2] where the pyloroantral mechanism has not been disturbed. After V+A and V+P presumably both destruction of the pyloroantral mechanism and abolition of receptive relaxation play a part in the genesis of gastric incontinence.

In the V+A group there were two patients who showed little change from the preoperative state and two patients who emptied less at 10 minutes after than before operation. Both of the latter suffered from fullness after meals, suggestive of early gastric retention, but their final emptying times were not prolonged.

The findings of Cox and his colleagues[3] and Goligher and his colleagues[5] are, to some extent, explained by the similar patterns of gastric emptying after V+P and V+A. Symptoms of diarrhea and dumping, which are related to the disturbance of gastric emptying caused by these operations, should be expected to have a similar incidence.

Clarke and Alexander-Wiliams[2] were able to relate gastric incontinence to the incidence of dumping symptoms. In this paper we have also found a relationship between rapid early emptying and the incidence of dumping.

Goligher and his colleagues[5] showed that the incidence of recurrent ulceration after V+A was significantly less than after V+P, with no difference in operative mortality rate. Such data indicate that V+A is the better operation, providing that it has no side effects. Our study supports the view that V+A will cause no more sequelae from rapid gastric emptying than will V+P.

REFERENCES

1. Cannon, W. B., and Lieb, E.: Receptive relaxation of the stomach, Am. J. Physiol. **29:** 250, 1911.
2. Clarke, R. J., and Alexander-Williams, J.: The effect of preserving antral innervation and of a pyloroplasty on gastric emptying after vagotomy in man, Gut **14:** 300, 1973.
3. Cox, A. G., Spencer, J., and Tinker, J.: *In* Williams, J. A., and Cox, A. G., editors: After vagotomy, London, 1969, Butterworth & Co., Ltd., pp. 119-130.
4. George, J. D.: New clinical method for measuring the rate of gastric emptying: The double sampling test meal, Gut **9:** 237, 1968.
5. Goligher, J. C., Pulvertaft, C. N., Irvin, T. T., Johnston, D., Walker, B., Hall, R. A., Willson-Pepper, J., and Matheson, T. S.: 5 to 8 year results of truncal vagotomy and pyloroplasty for duodenal ulcer, Br. Med. J. **1:** 7, 1972.
6. McKelvey, S. T. D.: Gastric incontinence and postvagotomy diarrhoea, Br. J. Surg. **57:** 741, 1970.

Effect of aging, organ allografting, and surgical stress on rat thymus histidine decarboxylase activity

Thomas C. Moore, M.D., Michael C. Sinclair, M.D., Columbus D. McAlpin, M.D., Griffith A. Weber, A.B., *and* **Carlos A. E. Lemmi, M.A.,** *Torrance, Calif.*

The normal or "resting" level of thymic histidine decarboxylase (HDC) enzyme activity in rats has been found to be quite high in comparison with the normal or "resting" levels observed in prior studies of other lymphoid organs. The resting level of activity is affected by age. It is higher in young rats and lower in old rats. The effect of organ allografting (heart and kidney) and of nonallografting surgical stress (renal isografting and simple laparotomy) on thymic HDC activity in the initial 10 days following operation was studied in 113 inbred Lewis rats. Both organ allografting and simple surgical stress produced a marked early (days 1 and 2) depression in thymic HDC activity. A significant later increase in thymic HDC activity above normal levels occurred after cardiac allografting. A mild decrease in thymic weights occurred. Lower thymic weights often were associated with high levels of thymic HDC activity. It is suggested that thymic HDC activity may play an important role in normal thymus function and in the thymic response to immunologic and nonimmunologic surgical stress. These changes may be involved in the release and recruitment of lymphoid cells to and from lymphoid organs and also may be related to changes in the metabolism of other vasoactive substances in thymic and other lymphoid tissues, to vasoactive substance receptors on lymphocytes, and to levels of lymphoid cellular cyclic adenosine monophosphate (AMP) activity.

From the Research Laboratory of the Division of Pediatric Surgery and Renal Transplantation, Harbor General Hospital, Campus, UCLA School of Medicine, Torrance, Calif.

EVIDENCE has been obtained in recent years to suggest a role of importance for vasoactive substances in both the afferent and efferent arcs of the immune response. Renal allografting in the rat has been found to be associated with an increase in plasma kallikrein activity which was not encountered following isografting.[20] An increase in prostaglandin E (PGE) activity has been demonstrated in the coronary sinus venous blood of heart allografts in nonimmunosuppressed rats.[3] Marked (33 fold) elevations in rat heart allograft levels of PGE activity have been found in the second 5 days after heart allografting. Significant increases in splenic and thymic PGE activity also have been found in the second 5 days after heart allografting in the rat.[15]

It is of interest that PGE and the kinins share many physiological and biochemical actions with histamine, including potent stimulation of cellular cyclic adenosine monophosphate (AMP) activity. It also is of interest that lymphocytes possess cell mem-

Supported by grants from National Institutes of Health (AM-10373), the Los Angeles County Heart Association, and the John A. Hartford Foundation.

Accepted for publication July 26, 1974.

Reprint requests: Thomas C. Moore, M.D., Chief, Pediatric Surgery and Renal Transplantation, Harbor General Hospital, 1000 W. Carson St., Torrance, Calif. 90509.

brane receptors for histamine and PGE, that these receptors may be exposed or expressed following an immune challenge, and that these changes are related to levels of antibody production and to lymphocytic cellular cytotoxic activity.[1, 8, 27]

Elevated levels for the urinary excretion of histamine have been observed following skin, kidney, and heart allografting in rats, dogs, and man.[11, 16, 17, 22, 28] Activity of histidine decarboxylase (HDC), the histamine-forming enzyme, has been found to be elevated in the spleens of rats following skin[14] and kidney[19] allografting and following sheep red blood cell (SRBC) immunization.[23] The major elevation in splenic HDC activity occurred in the initial 5 days following the immune challenge. A peak elevation in splenic HDC was found at 4 days after both renal allografting and SRBC immunization. There was a rapid fall in activity thereafter. The elevation in splenic HDC activity which followed SRBC immunization was correlated temporally with the level of hemolytic (19S) antibody formation as measured by the agar plaque assay. Splenic HDC activity following SRBC immunization peaked one day before the peak elevation in 19S antibody formation. Schayer[26] has reported an increase in lymph node HDC activity of mice following an immune challenge with complete Freund's adjuvant.

Skin[16] and renal parenchymal[19] allograft levels of HDC activity have been found to increase in the second 5 days following grafting. Peak elevations (33 and 25 fold) in HDC activity occurred at 10 days after grafting for both skin and kidney. There was a rapid decline in activity thereafter. The 10 day allograft peak elevation in HDC activity has been found to be the period of peak accumulation in numbers of stimulated, immunocompetent lymphocytes (medium and large size) in heterotopic heart allografts in rats.[2] This also was the period of the peak elevation in lymphotoxin (LT) lymphokine activity of lymphocytes extracted from cardiac allografts per 10^6 lymphocytes obtained.[2] Concanavalin A (Con A) and Con A–stimulated rat lymphocyte lymphokines administered in vivo by intrasplenic injection have produced an increase in splenic HDC activity 4 days after injection.[21] These substances, on incubation in vitro with rat spleen, have led to a release of histamine into the incubating fluid and to subcellular shifts in histamine levels with decrease in the nuclear and increases in the mitochondrial and microsomal percents of total cellular histamine.[21]

Inhibitors of HDC activity have been found to prolong first-set skin allograft survival in rats[9] and to suppress antibody formation following strong immunologic challenges with SRBC and salmonella flagellar antigen in rats and mice.[23] They also have been found to prolong second-set skin allograft survival in rats when given before both first- and second-set allografting but not when given only at the time of second-set skin allografting.[10]

These observations and the time sequence of elevations in activity have suggested a possible role for HDC activity in the recruitment and release of immunocompetent lymphocytes of the appropriate clone from reticulonendothelial organs and in their accumulation at the target organ or tissue site of immunologic effector response, such as an allograft. The work of Majno and associates[6, 7] is of interest in this regard. They have shown that the vascular site of action of histamine and of bradykinin is the postcapillary venule, an anatomic area of importance in the recirculation of small, immunocompetent lymphocytes.

Because of the recognized role of the thymus in cellular immunity, the present study was carried out to investigate in the rat the thymic HDC response to aging, to kidney and heart allografting, and to nonimmunological surgical stress in the form of renal isografting and simple laparotomy.

MATERIAL AND METHODS

Male inbred Lewis rats were used as allograft and isograft recipients and in simple surgical stress and aging studies. Male Brown Norway (BN) rats were employed as kidney and heart allografting donors. Recipient rats weighed approximately 350 grams.

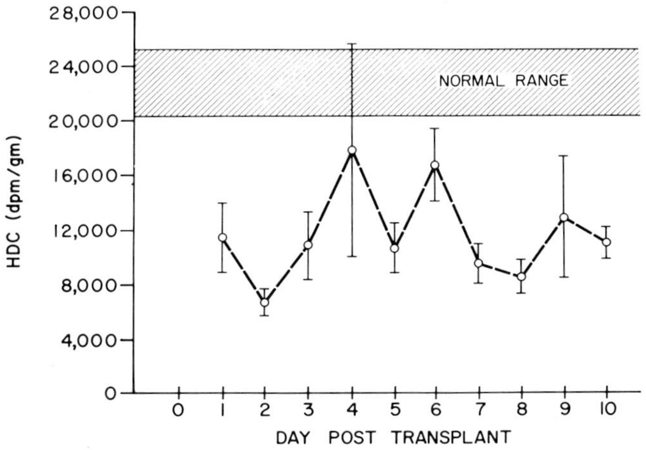

Fig. 1. Early postoperative depression in thymic histidine decarboxylase (HDC) activity following renal allografting in the rat.

Ether was used for anesthesia. Renal transplants were performed by the technique of Lee.[5] Both recipient kidneys were left intact in renal transplant studies. Heterotopic heart allografts were performed by the technique of Ono and Lindsey,[24] in which the donor-heart ascending aorta was anastomosed end to side to the recipient abdominal aorta and in which the donor heart pulmonary artery was anastomosed end to side into the recipient infrarenal inferior vena cava. Simple, nontransplant surgical stress was produced by laparotomy with mobilization and reattachment of one kidney. No antibiotics, immunosuppressives, or other drugs were used. Recipient rats were fed a standard rat pellet Purina Chow diet and were given water *ad libitum* following operation.

Rats from each group were killed on a daily basis during the initial 10 days following operation. The thymuses were removed and quick frozen in a dry ice–acetone mixture or in liquid nitrogen for storage at –87° C. in an ultradeep freezer for later HDC assay.

Just prior to HDC assay, the frozen thymuses were weighed. HDC activity was assayed by the ^{14}C radioisotope method of Schayer.[25] This method involved the incubation of ^{14}C histidine and pyridoxal phosphate with a known weight of tissue for a 3 hour period at 37° C. under nitrogen in a Dubnoff metabolic incubator. The ^{14}C histamine produced was converted to benzene-sulfonyl histamine (BSH). The BSH was purified by repeated recrystallizations over a period of 5 days. HDC activity, corrected for tissue blank, background activity, and recovery of BSH were calculated and expressed as disintegrations per minute (d.p.m.) per gram of tissue. All data are presented as the arithmetic mean ± the standard error of the mean (S.E.M.).

RESULTS

Frozen thymuses from 47 renal-allografted rats, from 11 renal-isografted rats, from 30 heart-allografted rats, and from 25 rats subjected only to the surgical stress of simple laparotomy were weighed and assayed for HDC activity.

Thymuses of normal, nonoperated Lewis rats in the approximate 350 gram weight range (350 ± 6 grams) were found to have an unusually high normal or "resting" level of HDC activity (22,675 ± 2,464 d.p.m. per gram of tissue) for lymphoid tissue. This normal level of activity was approximately 5 times higher than that of normal spleen[14, 19] and approximately 20 times higher than that of normal appendix[18] and of normal small intestinal Peyer's patches[14] lymphoid tissue.

During the course of this study, the effect of rat age and size on rat thymus HDC activity was considered. Thymuses from four small, young rats of a mean weight of 38

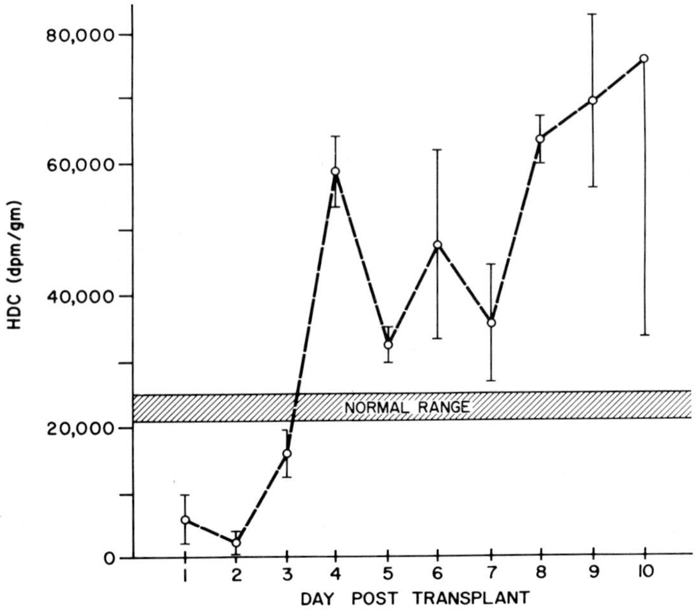

Fig. 2. Early postgrafting decrease in thymic HDC following heterotopic (abdominal) heart allografting in the rat followed by later increases in thymic HDC activity.

grams were removed and compared with those of four large, older rats of a mean weight of 422 grams for weight, for percent of total body weight, and for HDC activity. The thymuses of the young rats constituted a larger percentage of total body weight (0.21 vs. 0.04 percent). Thymic HDC activity per gram of thymus was greater in the young rats (66,033 ± 17,981 d.p.m. vs. 13,007 ± 2,514 d.p.m.), $p < 0.025$. HDC activity also was greater in the young rats per total thymus (4,424 ± 363 d.p.m. vs. 2,224 ± 275 d.p.m.), $p < 0.001$.

Thymic HDC activity in the early post-transplant period following renal allografting was substantially below normal values for rats of 350 ± 6 grams of weight (Fig. 1). The lowest reduction in HDC below normal values of 22,675 ± 2,464 d.p.m. per gram was found 2 days after allografting ($p < 0.0005$). Some early, mild reduction in thymic weights on days 3 and 4 (not statistically significant), followed by a mild gain in weight on day 10 (not statistically significant), occurred in this group of rats. Four or five rats in this group were killed on each day after transplant.

Heterotopic heart allografting also produced an early post-transplant reduction in thymic HDC activity with the maximum depression at days 1 and 2 (4,508 ± 2,441 d.p.m. per gram). This was significantly below that of normal values for rats of 360 ± 6 grams (22,675 ± 2,464 d.p.m. per gram), $p < 0.001$ (Fig. 2). As with renal allografting, the greatest reduction in thymic HDC activity occurred in the initial days after grafting. A progressive rise in HDC activity took place after the second day maximum depression. This increase in activity at days 8 and 9 (66,945 ± 7,705 d.p.m. per gram) resulted in values significantly above normal levels ($p < 0.00025$). A progressive reduction in thymus weights after transplant occurred in this group of animals (Fig. 3). The major reduction below thymus weights at day one occurred at days 3 and 4. This early post-allograft reduction in thymic weight was statistically significant ($p < 0.025$). There was no significant change in thymic weights thereafter. One heart-allografted rat was killed 24 days after allografting. At this time thymic HDC activity was 37,347 d.p.m. per gram and thymic weight was 220 milligrams. Two rats in this group were killed on post-transplant days 2 and 8. Three and four rats

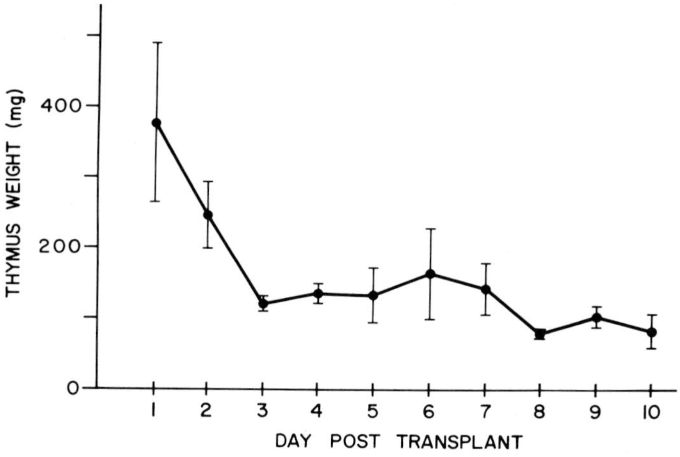

Fig. 3. Early reduction in thymus weights following heart allografting.

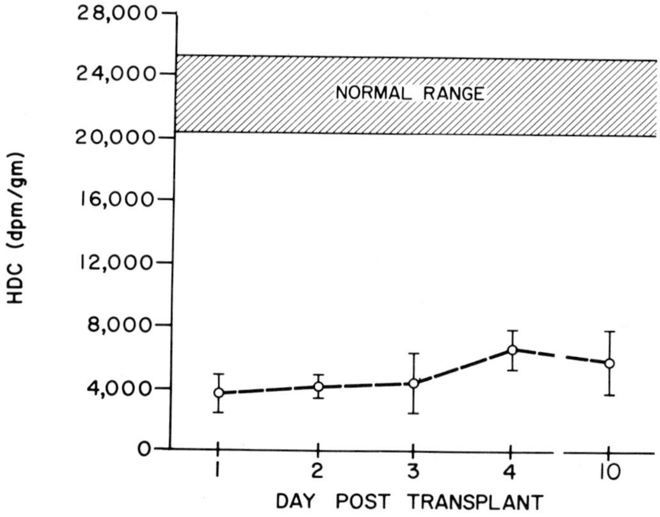

Fig. 4. The effect of nonimmunological surgical stress (simple laparotomy) on thymic HDC activity at intervals following operation.

were killed on all other of the initial 10 post-transplant days.

Three renal-isografted rats were killed on post-transplant days one, 5, and 8, and two were killed on day 10. On day one, HDC activity was 1,319 ± 254 d.p.m. per gram. This was significantly lower than normal levels ($p < 0.00025$). Thymic weights at day 10 were significantly lower than day 1 weights ($p < 0.005$). Five of the eight thymuses from animals killed at 5, 8, and 10 days had HDC activities in the 3,000 to 6,000 d.p.m. per gram range and weights in the 114 to 145 gram range. One animal on each of these 3 days had a smaller thymus (49, 60, and 42 milligrams) and a considerably higher HDC level (21,538, 15,788, and 36,131 d.p.m. per gram).

Five of the surgical stress–laparotomy animals were killed on each of 5 days following operation (days 1 through 4 and on day 10). Thymic HDC values on days 1 and 2 (3,552 ± 768 d.p.m. per gram) were reduced significantly below normal levels (Fig. 4) for rats of 350 ± 6 grams ($p < 0.000025$). Determinations were concentrated in the initial 5 days after operation because of the early allografted rat thymus changes in HDC ac-

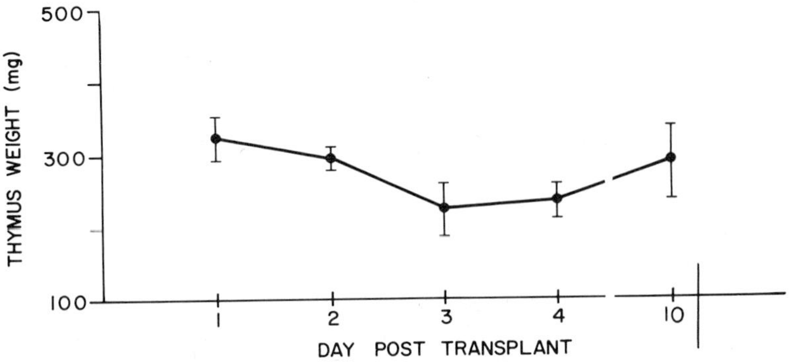

Fig. 5. Thymus weight changes following simple surgical stress (laparotomy) at intervals following operation.

tivity. The 10 day levels were still depressed ($p < 0.001$) below normal values. Some mild reduction in thymus weight below day 1 levels occurred at days 3 ($p < 0.05$), and 4 ($p < 0.025$), following simple surgical stress (Fig. 5). By day 10 mean thymic weights had returned to the day 1 postoperative levels.

DISCUSSION

The thymus is the principal source of immunologically competent, long-lived, circulating lymphocytes. It appears early in the phylogenetic development of the lymphoid system in vertebrates and is unique among lymphatic organs in that it is almost fully developed before birth. Thymic development is independent of immunologic stimulus, while the development and structure of the spleen and lymph nodes clearly are dependent upon antigenic stimulation.[29]

The short generation time of thymic lymphocytes (between 6.5 and 8.5 hours) is approximately 3 to 5 times shorter than the generation time of lymphocytes in the spleen or lymph nodes.[30] The high thymic mitotic index and the precocious development of the thymus, as compared with other lymphatic organs, have prompted the hypothesis that the thymus releases lymphocytes to seed other lymphatic organs.

Although other lymphatic organs decrease somewhat in size with puberty, the thymus undergoes a rather marked but gradual atrophy with aging (age involution). The thymus also may undergo sudden involution in illness and following trauma (stress involution).

In the study reported here, thymic HDC activity decreased promptly and markedly from normally high-resting levels following both immunologic and nonimmunologic stress. Thymic weights also decreased, most markedly after heart allografting. The major reductions in thymic HDC occurred at days 1 and 2, and the major reductions in thymic weights (when they occurred) were found at days 3 and 4 after allografting and after nonimmunological surgical stress. Low thymic weights were associated with high thymic HDC activity per gram of thymic tissue. In heart-allografted animals, a marked increase in thymic HDC activity occurred after the early postgrafting decrease.

The early postoperative fall in thymic HDC activity following both immunologic and nonimmunologic stress suggested an independence of thymic HDC response from pure immunologic stimulus. This differed from the splenic HDC response which, in a prior study, was found to be increased by tissue and organ allografting but not by isografting.[19] These findings were similar to those cited above in which thymic activity had been found to be independent of pure immunologic stimulus as compared with other lymphatic organs. Thymic weight decreased after both immunologic and nonimmunologic stress, most markedly after cardiac allografting. Splenic weights, in prior studies, were increased after renal allografting in rats but were decreased following renal isografting. HDC activity of Peyer's patches lymphoid tissue and of the appendix were unchanged by skin and renal allografting in rats.[14, 18]

The time sequence of changes in lymphoid organ and target allograft organ changes in HDC activity following allografting is of interest. The early one and 2 day maximum thymic decrease in HDC activity, the 4 day maximum increase in splenic HDC activity, and the 10 day allograft peak increase in HDC activity suggest a possible role for lymphatic organ HDC activity in the derecruitment (shedding) and recruitment (attraction) of immunocompetent lymphocytes to and from these lymphoid organs and for allograft organ HDC activity in the recruitment of these lymphocytes to the target organ of immunologic assault.

The second 5 day postallograft increases in thymic HDC activity following cardiac allografting suggest a possible immunologic-stimulated alteration in thymic activity as reflected in HDC activity. A significant ($p < 0.01$) increase in thymic PGE activity at 7, 8, and 9 days following heart allografting in rats (BN to Lewis) has been observed recently by one of us (T. C. M.) and by Jaffe.[15] This increase in thymic PGE activity was associated with a reduction in thymic weight. These findings suggest, in addition, that multiple vasoactive substance metabolic alterations may be involved in these thymic changes which occur in response to the cellular (T cell) immune response to organ allografting. Major vasoactive substances of similar physiologic and biochemical action (histamine, PGE, and the kinins) may release and be released by one another.[20] These observations also are of importance with respect to the findings by Melmon and associates[8] of lymphocyte receptors for histamine and PGE, which become exposed or expressed following an immune challenge, and to the potent stimulatory effect of histamine and PGE on cellular cyclic AMP activity.[1, 8, 27]

The reason for the difference in thymic HDC response to renal and cardiac allografting with respect to the later increases in activity is unclear. The small number of animals studied following renal isografting and the wide spread in some of the later period HDC activity data make this information difficult to interpret. Following simple laparotomy surgical stress, thymic HDC activity remained at depressed levels in the initial 10 days following operation.

The stimulation of lymphoid organ activity by organ allografting as manifested in HDC activity in this and in prior studies cited above appears to have a negative counterpart in a suppression of lymphoid (splenic) HDC activity in the immune depression situation of uncontrolled malignant tumor growth. In a recent study we have observed that uncontrolled growth, during a 5 week period, of syngenic transplanted SV-40 tumors in hamsters has been associated with a 10 fold depression in host splenic HDC activity below normal levels of activity.[4] Repeated injections of these tumors with a vasoactive substance (bradykinin) has slowed the growth of injected tumors, has resulted in marked mononuclear cell invasion of both injected tumors and of noninjected tumors as well in two tumor animals, and has been associated with a 5 fold increase in host splenic HDC activity above the 10 fold depression levels produced by uncontrolled tumor growth.[4]

REFERENCES

1. Bourne, H. R., Lichtenstein, L. M., Melmon, K. L., et al.: Modulation of inflammation and immunity by cyclic AMP; receptors for vasoactive hormones and mediators of inflammation regulate many leukocyte functions, Science **184:** 19, 1974.
2. Granger, G. A., and Moore, T. C.: Accumulation of lymphotoxin secreting lymphoid cells in rat heart allografts, Surgery **76:** 542, 1974.
3. Jaffe, B. M., and Moore, T. C.: Elevation in prostaglandin E activity of rat heart allograft coronary sinus venous blood, Int. Res. Comm. Sys. Med. Sci. **2:** 1417, 1974.
4. Koppleman, L., Moore, T. C., Lemmi, C. A. E., and Porter, D. D.: Effects of bradykinin injection into syngenic SV-40 hamster tumors on rate of tumor growth and splenic histidine decarboxylase activity, Int. Res. Comm. Sys. Med. Sci. **2:** 1272, 1974.
5. Lee, S.: An improved technique of renal allografting in the rat, Surgery **61:** 771, 1967.
6. Majno, G., Palade, G. E., and Schoefl, G. I.: Studies on inflammation: II. The site of action of histamine and serotonin along the

vascular tree; a topographical study, J. Biophys. Biochem. Cytol. **2:** 607, 1961.
7. Majno, G., Gilmore, V., and Leventhal, M.: On the mechanism of vascular leakage caused by histamine-type mediators, Circ. Res. **21:** 833, 1967.
8. Melmon, K. L., Weinstein, Y., Shearer, G. M., et al.: Separation of specific antibody-forming mouse cells by their adherence to insolubilized endogenous hormones, J. Clin. Invest. **53:** 22, 1974.
9. Moore, T. C.: Histidine decarboxylase inhibitors and the survival of skin homografts, Nature **215:** 871, 1967.
10. Moore, T. C.: Histidine decarboxylase inhibitors and second-set allograft survival, Arch. Surg. **99:** 470, 1969.
11. Moore, T. C., and Chang, J.: Urinary histamine excretion in the rat following skin homografting and autografting, Ann. Surg. **167:** 232, 1968.
12. Moore, T. C., and Schayer, R. W.: Histidine decarboxylase activity of autografted and allografted rat skin, Transplantation **7:** 99, 1969.
13. Moore, T. C., and Lawrence, W., Jr.: Suppression of antibody formation by histidine decarboxylase inhibitors, Transplantation **8:** 224, 1969.
14. Moore, T. C., and Schayer, R. W.: Histidine decarboxylase activity of the rat spleen following skin allografting, Ann. Surg. **171:** 609, 1970.
15. Moore, T. C., and Jaffe, B. M.: Prostaglandin E levels of heterotopic rat heart allografts and of host lymphoid tissues at intervals postgrafting, Transplantation. In press.
16. Moore, T. C., Thompson, D. P., and Hayes, M.: Correlation of renal blood flow indices and histamine metabolism data after canine renal allografting, Arch. Surg. **101:** 45, 1970.
17. Moore, T. C., Thompson, D. P., and Glassock, R. J.: Elevation in urinary and blood histamine following clinical renal transplantation, Ann. Surg. **173:** 381, 1971.
18. Moore, T. C., Sinclair, M. C., and Lemmi, C. A. E.: Effect of renal allografting on rat appendiceal histidine decarboxylase activity, Int. Res. Comm. Sys. Med. Sci. (73-5) **47:** 2, May 1973.
19. Moore, T. C., Sinclair, M. C., and Lemmi, C. A. E.: Elevation in host splenic and allograft parenchymal and capsular histidine decarboxylase activity and weights following renal allografting in rats, SURGERY **75:** 203, 1974.
20. Moore, T. C., Sinclair, M. C., and Lemmi, C. A. E.: Elevation in rat plasma kallikrein activity following renal allografting, Am. J. Surg. **127:** 287, 1974.
21. Moore, T. C., Granger, G. A., and Lemmi, C. A. E.: In vivo elevation in rat splenic histidine decarboxylase activity by intra-splenic injection of Con A and Con A activated lymphokines, Int. Res. Comm. Sys. Med. Sci. **2:** 1458, 1974.
22. Moore, T. C., Cleveland, R. J., Thompson, D. P., and Nelson, R. J.: Vasoactive amine metabolism following canine and human heart transplantation, Ann. Surg. **154:** 51, 1971.
23. Moore, T. C., Lemmi, C. A. E., Orlando, J. C., and Pinkerton, W.: Correlation of splenic histidine decarboxylase activity and antibody formation following SRBC immunization, Transplantation **11:** 347, 1971.
24. Ono, K., and Lindsey, E. S.: Improved technique of heart transplantation in rats, J. Thorac. Cardiovasc. Surg. **57:** 225, 1969.
25. Schayer, R. W.: Formation and binding of histamine by rat tissues in vitro, Am. J. Physiol. **187:** 63, 1956.
26. Schayer, R. W.: Role of histamine in Freund's adjuvant action, Fed. Proc. **29:** 617, 1970. (Abs.)
27. Shearer, G. M., Melmon, K. L., Weinstein, Y., and Sela, M.: Regulation of antibody response by cells expressing histamine receptors, J. Exp. Med. **136:** 1302, 1972.
28. Sinclair, M. C., Lemmi, C. A. E., and Moore, T. C.: Elevation in urinary excretion of histamine following renal allografting in rats, J. Surg. Res. In press.
29. Weiss, L.: The cells and tissues of the immune system, Englewood Cliffs, N. J., 1972, Prentice-Hall, Inc., p. 79.
30. Weiss, L.: The cells and tissues of the immune system, Englewood Cliffs, N. J., 1972, Prentice-Hall, Inc., p. 88.

Complications of related kidney donation

Panyiotis K. Spanos, M.D., Richard L. Simmons, M.D., Ernest Lampe, M.D., Luca C. Rattazzi, M.D., Carl M. Kjellstrand, M.D., Frederick C. Goetz, M.D., *and* John S. Najarian, M.D., *Minneapolis, Minn.*

The complications of nephrectomy in 287 healthy volunteers to relatives requiring kidney transplantation have been reviewed. A total complication rate of 28.2 percent included a 3.1 percent incidence of wound complications, an 8.7 percent incidence of lower urinary complications, and a 15 percent incidence of minor intrathoracic complications. There were no deaths and only four serious complications. Two serious late complications were related to development of glomerulonephritis and hemolytic-uremic syndrome in donors; both donors are currently well. One pulmonary embolus and one case of deep thrombophlebitis occurred but responded to anticoagulation. Kidney donation is a relatively safe procedure carrying important benefits for the recipient.

From the Departments of Surgery and Medicine, University of Minnesota, Minneapolis, Minn.

ALTHOUGH there is still controversy about the use of related volunteer donors for kidney transplantation, related transplants do function better than unrelated ones. For example, the Human Renal Transplant Registry[1] reports the 2 year functional survival of related transplants as approximately 70 percent compared to 47 percent for cadaver kidneys. These results have not improved over the past 5 years, despite the advent of newer immunosuppressive agents and the development of tissue typing techniques. It is likely that immunogenetic factors thus far undetectable by in vitro techniques facilitate the survival of kidneys from relatives.

Nevertheless, willingness to utilize living relatives as donors requires documentation of continued low morbidity of the donor nephrectomy and continuing attempts to further lower the complication rate. There are several reports demonstrating satisfactory renal function following kidney donation.[5, 15, 16] There are also long-term studies after nephrectomy showing that there is no increase in mortality rate in this group of patients.[2] The present study reviews the morbidity in 287 volunteer donors who gave kidneys to their relatives between 1963 and June, 1973. We paid particular attention to the length of hospitalization and compared the morbidity of donation in older to younger donors. We also compared the last 100 cases (1972 to 1973) to those done previously to see if modification in the donor management had lessened the complication rate.

This work was supported by Grant No. AM 13083 from the United States Public Health Service, and Grant No. RR-400 from the General Clinical Research Centers Program of the Division of Research Resources, National Institutes of Health.

Accepted for publication Aug. 27, 1974.

Reprint requests: Richard L. Simmons, M.D., Box No. 185, Mayo Memorial Bldg., University of Minnesota, Minneapolis, Minn. 55455.

MATERIALS AND METHODS

A total of 505 renal transplants were performed at the University of Minnesota be-

Table I. *Protocol for the study of a potential related donor*

1. History and physical examination
2. Hematology Hematocrit, leukocyte, differential, and platelet counts
3. Coagulation Prothrombin, partial thromboplastin, and thrombin times
4. Chemistry Serum Na^+, K^+, Cl^-, CO_2^-, SGOT, bilirubin, uric acid, Ca^{++}, P, BUN, creatinine, fasting blood sugar, glucose tolerance test
5. Urine Urinalysis, 24 hour urine for creatinine clearance
6. Microbiology Clean catch urine culture 2 times
7. Immunology Blood type (major and minor), tissue typing, leukocyte cross match for recipient anti-donor and leukocyte antibodies, Venereal Disease Research Laboratory, Australian antigen
8. X-ray Chest x-ray, posterior-anterior and lateral intravenous pyelogram, renal arteriograms
9. Isotope Bilateral renogram
10. Electrocardiogram

tween 1963 and June, 1973; 287 transplants were from living donors. Our donor selection criteria have been extensively described[17] but Table I briefly lists those procedures carried out to discover contraindications to donation. When the potential donor is from a family with a history of diabetes mellitus, he must be given the standard workup described in Table I, and, in addition, he must complete the protocol listed in Table II. The sequence of studies involves blood and tissue typing and a brief preadmission interview to discover major contraindications from the patient's previous medical history. After admission, a detailed history and physical examination, urinalysis, cultures, renography, and intravenous pyelography are carried out. Finally, all other studies being normal, renal arteriography is performed. Spanos and colleagues[20] have previously reported a 25 percent incidence of renal abnormalities in these relatives of patients with kidney failure which contraindicate donation.

The preoperative preparation and operative procedures currently utilized have been described in detail.[17] Certain procedural and operative alterations were undertaken in 1971 in order to minimize certain complications. These changes included the elimination of the twelfth rib resection, previously utilized to facilitate operative exposure, and the institution of the prophylactic use of sulfisoxazole for 5 days following nephrectomy in order to reduce the incidence of urinary infections. The introduction of these changes accounts for the division of our material into the first 187 cases vs. the last 100 cases (Table III).

Table II. *Additional protocol to study potential related donors for diabetic recipients*

Preparation: 300 Gm. carbohydrate diet, 3 days	
Days 1-3	Needle biopsy, right quadriceps muscle
Day 4	Cortisone-glucose tolerance test,[8] *Part I.* Eat at least 200 Gm. additional carbohydrate
Day 5	Cortisone-glucose tolerance test, *Part II*
Day 6	Rest day
Day 7	Intravenous glucose tolerance test[6]; Creatinine clearance (24 hr.), daily glucose and protein; Kidney biopsy (open) at time of transplant—for electron microscopy and immunofluorescent studies
Repeat all above studies three years after transplantation	

Intraoperative management. Two days prior to transplantation, the donor is readmitted to the hospital, and the creatinine clearance and urine cultures are repeated. The day before operation a central venous pressure (CVP) catheter is inserted via a brachial vein and the central position is confirmed radiographically. The CVP is monitored during and after operation, as a guide for fluid administration. At 6 A.M. on the day of operation, a rapid infusion of fluids is started, and the urine output is monitored; Najarian and his colleagues[14] have shown that an active diuresis in the donor organ at the time of renal artery occlusion will mean prompt function of the graft in the recipient. The CVP is measured again in the operating room before the patient is placed in the lateral decubitus position. A transverse flank incision starts at the rectus sheath 1 to 2 cm. above the umbilicus, passes just below the twelfth rib, and terminates behind the posterior axillary line. The rib is not resected to eliminate problems with postoperative pneumothorax. In all other respects, the donor nephrectomy follows the procedure previously described in detail.[13, 17]

RESULTS

No deaths occurred in our series of 287 related kidney donors, but there were one or more complications in 81 (28.2 percent) of these patients. These complications were observed during all phases of treatment, from the preoperative evaluation through long-term follow-up.

Complications during potential donor evaluation. Only two complications were seen during work-up of the prospective donor. Only one, a femoral thrombosis after arteriography, necessitated an operation. The only other complication was bacteremia after renal arteriogram. The patient developed chills and fever of 104°, which we treated with cephalothin systemically for 5 days. One week later the donor nephrectomy was performed without complication.

Intraoperative complications. The only complication in 287 operations was hypotension during anesthesia induction in one patient. The operation was postponed for a week to study the possibility of myocardial infarction. When that possibility was excluded, donor nephrectomy was carried out without complication.

Postoperative complications. A total of 78 of 287 donors developed complications after donation (27.1 percent). Most but not all of the complications were mild and easy to manage. Fever was a common occurrence in the first 24 hours after operation, but, with good pulmonary care, it usually disappeared by the end of the first day after operation.

Wound complications. Wound complications appeared in nine (3.1 percent) of our patients. Five consisted of subcutaneous seromas or hematomas and four of these (1.4 percent) were subcutaneous infections. There were no deep infections. The incidence of wound problems was higher in the older group of donors (Table IV). There have been no wound infections in the last 100 patients (Table III). We feel that this slight improvement is the result of more careful and conservative use of the electrocautery in the superficial tissues of the wound.

Table III. *Comparison of last 100 consecutive cases with the first 187 cases*

Complications	*First 187 cases* No.	%	*Last 100 consecutive cases* No.	%
Wound:				
Infection	4		—	
Hematoma	1		2	
Persistent pain	—		1	
Subcutaneous emphysema	1		—	
Total patients	6	3.2	3	3.0
Urinary tract:				
Infection	20		3	
Retention	—		1	
Proteinuria	2		—	
Dysuria	1		—	
Total patients	21	11.2	4	4.0
Pulmonary:				
Pneumomediastinum	8		8	
Pleural effusion	3		7	
Atelectasis	9		7	
Pneumothorax	5		—	
Pulmonary embolus	1		—	
Total patients	26	14.0	22	22.0
Other:				
Hemolytic uremic syndrome	—		1	
Thrombophlebitis	1		1	
Prolonged ileus	1		—	
Glomerulonephritis	1		—	
Femoral thrombosis	1		—	
Psychological stress	1		—	
Arrhythmia	1		—	
Hypotension during induction	1		—	
Radial nerve palsy	1		—	
Bacteremia after arteriogram	1		—	
Cytomegalovirus fever	—		1	
Total patients	9	5.0	3	3.0

Urinary tract complications. Urinary tract complications were relatively common. Urinary tract infections were the most frequent complication and occurred in 23 of 287 (8 percent) (Table IV). Most were asymptomatic and were discovered on routine culture.

Table IV. *Complications of kidney donors*

Complications	< 45 *yrs of age* No.	< 45 *yrs of age* %	> 45 *yrs of age* No.	> 45 *yrs of age* %	*Total* No.	*Total* %
Wound:						
Hematoma	1		2		3	
Infection	2		2		4	
Subcutaneous emphysema	1		—		1	
Chronic pain	1		—		1	
Total patients	5	2.2	4	6.3	9	3.1
Urinary tract:						
Infection	17		6		23	
Retention	1		—		1	
Dysuria	1		—		1	
Proteinuria	1		1		2	
Total patients	18	8.1	7	10.9	25	8.7
Pulmonary:						
Pneumomediastinum	13		3		16	
Atelectasis	7		9		16	
Pleural effusion	5		5		10	
Pneumothorax	4		1		5	
Pulmonary embolus	1		—		1	
Total patients	29	13.0	14	21.9	43	15.0
Other:						
Thrombophlebitis	2		—		2	
Late glomerulonephritis	1		—		1	
Late hemolytic uremic syndrome	1		—		1	
Psychological stress	1		—		1	
Predonation femoral thrombosis after arteriography	1		—		1	
Transient arrhythmia	—		1		1	
Radial nerve palsy	—		1		1	
Hypotension during induction	—		1		1	
Prolonged ileus	—		1		1	
Bacteremia after arteriogram	—		1		1	
Cytomegalovirus fever	—		1		1	
Total patients	6	2.7	6	9.5	12	4.2
Total patients with complications	54/223	24.2	27/64	42.2	81/287	28.2

No symptomatic cases of pyelonephritis occurred. Table V lists the organisms cultured in these patients. *E. coli* was the most frequently cultured. Table IV shows that there was no significant difference in the occurrence of urinary tract infections with age of donor. Table III demonstrates a decreased incidence in the last 100 patients. We have used a 5 day course of sulfisoxazole postoperatively in the last 100 donors and have, thereby, reduced this complication from 8 to 3 percent. All urinary tract infections have been treated with appropriate antibiotics, and we have had no late postoperative urinary tract problems. All of the other urinary tract complications were transient and self limited.

Pulmonary complications. Of 287 donors, 43 (15 percent) developed complications involving intrathoracic organs, and 16 (5.6 percent) were asymptomatic mediastinal problems (Table IV). Pneumomediastinum was a frequent and peculiar complication that is absolutely benign and needs no treatment. It was a purely roentgenologic finding, without concomitant clinical symptoms or signs, which always resolved spontaneously. Analysis of our data in Table IV shows that this complication is slightly more frequent in the younger group of donors and there is no predilection for right or left nephrectomies. Pneumomediastinum is probably the result of para-aortic dissection at the level of the renal artery. Air advances in between the tissue planes and appears around the intrathoracic aorta.

Pulmonary atelectasis and pleural effusion are the most frequent intrapleural complications and were of brief clinical importance in 16 of 287 (5.6 percent) and 10 of 287 (3.5 percent) patients, respectively, (Tables III and IV). Both complications occurred much more frequently in older donors and have not been eliminated by experience in the most recent patients. No patient had to undergo thoracentesis for the pleural effusion, and no patient's hospitalization was prolonged beyond 5 days after operation because of atelectasis. Atelectasis usually cleared on the second day, with coughing and occasional use of intermittent positive-pressure breathing.

Asymptomatic pneumothorax was a roentgenographic finding in five of 287 (1.7 percent) patients. The pneumothorax was usually small (< 10 percent) but was aspirated in one patient. We have not encountered a pneumothorax in our last 100 patients (Table III) since the twelfth rib tip is no longer resected.

A pulmonary embolus occurred on the tenth day after operation in a 26-year-old donor while at home. He was readmitted and was seriously ill for one week but responded to treatment with anticoagulants. There have been no long-term sequelae.

Other complications. We have 12 complications listed as "other" complications in Tables III and IV. One case of superficial thrombophlebitis required no treatment; a single case of deep thrombophlebitis required hospitalization and anticoagulation. The prolonged ileus occurred in an older donor who required nasogastric drainage, but the only consequence to the patient was a 5 day longer stay in the hospital.

Although psychological depression is not uncommon during the first 24 to 48 hours,[15] only one patient developed serious depression. This patient was seen by a psychiatrist and her hospitalization was prolonged for 3 days. Then, seen as an outpatient for regular checks at one month, 6 months, and one year postoperatively, there were no psychiatric problems and no further psychiatric consultation was needed.

The transient radial nerve palsy, probably due to pressure during anesthesia, and unknown fever were prolonged complications (Table V). The patient with radial nerve palsy required 6 weeks of physical therapy but recovered without sequelae. The patient who developed the fever of unknown origin was initially discharged on the fifth day after operation. One week later, he returned with low-grade fever and ileus. He was hospitalized for 3 weeks before the fever subsided. No source was found for the fever, but cytomegalovirus inclusion disease virus was isolated from his urine. The appearance of complement-fixing antibodies to the virus coincided with his recovery.

Table V. *Organisms cultured from donors with urinary tract infections after operation*

Infection	*No.*
Escherichia coli	17
Proteus mirabilis	3
Alpha-streptococcus	3
Klebsiella	3
Enterococci *(Streptococcus faecalis)*	2
Coliform bacilli	1
Candida albicans	1
Staphylococci, coagulase-negative	2
Total patients	23/287 (8%)

Late complications. Two complications developed late after the initial discharge from the hospital. Glomerulonephritis developed in a middle-aged man 8 months after nephrectomy. He developed a sore throat and acute fluid retention and elevation of his serum creatinine from 1.3 to 4.8 mg. per 100 ml. He made a spontaneous recovery and his current creatinine clearance is 72 ml. per minute.

Hemolytic uremic syndrome developed in a 21-year-old female donor, whose recipient sister had lost her own kidneys from hemolytic uremic syndrome.[4] The donor had a smooth postnephrectomy course with a serum creatinine of 1.2 mg. per 100 ml., but 3 weeks later she was readmitted with the serious hemolytic uremic syndrome proved by renal biopsy. She was treated successfully with streptokinase and heparin infusion, and dialysis was necessary for 2 months. Dialysis is no longer required but she has an elevated serum creatinine of 2.4 mg. per 100 ml. while her blood urea nitrogen is 50 mg. per 100 ml.[4] This patient is the only donor with impaired renal function.

Hospitalization. The mean stay after donor nephrectomy for the last 100 consecutive donors was 5.13 days (range, 4 to 10 days). Rarely is a donor kept in the hospital for more than 5 days. The patients have discomfort and pain for the first 48 hours, but by the third day after operation, they start asking when they can leave.

Postdonation renal function was evaluated in 100 random cases just before discharge at 5 days. The average predonation blood urea nitrogen rose from 12.7 to 15.8 mg. per 100 ml. The mean creatinine clearance at the time of discharge was 69 percent of the average prenephrectomy value.

DISCUSSION

There is no doubt that transplantation from a living related donor is far superior to transplantation with a cadaver kidney; the long-term results are twice as good. The patient awaiting a kidney does not need to be subjected to long periods of dialysis with its danger and psychological stress, and the incidence of acute renal failure after transplantation is only one third of that after cadaver transplantation.[9] It is comforting also to know that the survival after unilateral nephrectomy is no different from that of a normal population of a similar age distribution.[2]

Our own experience as well as that of others[16, 19] support the general finding that donor nephrectomy is a safe procedure. Although the total incidence of complications in our group was relatively high (28.2 percent), the incidence of serious complication was very low (4 of 287, 1.4 percent). Only one complication (femoral thrombosis) required an operation, but three complications were life threatening: pulmonary embolus, glomerulonephritis, and hemolytic uremic syndrome. However, when one reviews these complications, only one of these seems actually to be related to the donation itself (pulmonary embolus).

The appearance of the hemolytic uremic syndrome was particularly disturbing. This experience plus other evidence suggesting a familial tendency in this disease may contraindicate sibling donation in these cases.[3, 12]

Our experience with minor complications is similar to that of Smith and associates[19] and Penn and associates.[16] Wound infections, pulmonary problems, and urinary tract infections account for almost 90 percent of the complications seen. Four patients had wound infections (1.4 percent). Two of these wound infections were seen in patients over 45 years of age, accounting for our incidence of 3 percent in this age group. Smith and co-workers reported an over-all incidence of wound infection of 2.5 percent and the incidence of wound infection in Penn's series was 1.8 percent. We have not seen wound infections in the last 100 patients and we attribute this to the more conservative and careful use of the electrocautery.

Pulmonary problems account for 50 percent of our complications. The most often seen were pneumomediastinum, an absolutely benign problem, and atelectasis which uniformly cleared with coughing. Pneumothorax, which occurred in 10 percent of Penn's cases, has not been seen since rib resection was abandoned. The slightly higher incidence of pulmonary complications in donors older than 45 years of age would not seem to contraindicate donation from patients in this age group.

Urinary tract infections were present in 8 percent of our patients whereas Penn had a similar incidence of 10 percent. This problem has also been minimized in the last 100 cases by prophylactic treatment postoperatively with a 5 day course of sulfisoxazole after removal of the urinary catheter.

There are two groups of donors which deserve special consideration. Kidneys from living donors older than 45 years of age appear to function as well as younger kidneys.[20] Similarly, residual renal function in the donor is equivalent to that remaining in younger donors and the serious complications did not occur in this group. But inevitably such donors will not be utilized as often if care is taken to exclude donors with other illnesses.[21] Prospective donors from siblings of recipients with diabetic nephropathy should also be evaluated more thoroughly (Table II). Diabetes is transmitted by recessive genes of one or more loci according to Steinberg[22] and Simpson.[18] Consequently, though the incidence of diabetes in the general population is only 2 percent, the incidence of heterozygous carriers of diabetes may reach 24 percent.[11] Fajans and Conn[8] established the cortisone-glucose tolerance test in an effort to predict future development of diabetes. In follow-up studies,[5, 7, 8] they showed that 25 percent of subjects with "positive response" to the initial cortisone-glucose tolerance test had developed diabetes and another 10 percent "probable diabetes." On the other hand, in a control with subjects with negative initial response, only one developed diabetes. In addition to the Fajans and Conn test, we have employed a high-dose intravenous glucose tolerance test[6] for screening of potential donors from families with a history of diabetes mellitus. In a very rare case donors with "positive response" have been used and then the chances of development of diabetes in the future were always explained with all the possible consequences.

REFERENCES

1. Advisory Committee to the Renal Transplant Registry: The Eleventh Report of the Human Renal Transplant Registry, J. A. M. A. **226:** 1197, 1973.
2. Anderson, G., Hansen, J. B., and Jorgensen, S. J.: Survival after nephrectomy, Scand. J. Urol. Nephrol. **2:** 91, 1968.
3. Anthony, P. P., and Kaplan, A. B.: Fatal haemolytic-uremic syndrome in two sibs, Arch. Dis. Child. **43:** 316, 1968.
4. Bergstein, J., Michael, A. F., Kjellstrand, C. M., et al.: Hemolytic-uremic syndrome in adult sisters, Transplantation **17:** 487, 1974.
5. Conn, J. W.: The pre-diabetic state in man, Diabetes **7:** 347, 1958.
6. Dyck, D. R., and Moorhouse, J. A.: A high-dose intravenous glucose tolerance test, J. Clin. Endocrinol. Metab. **26:** 1032, 1966.
7. Fajans, S. S.: Diagnostic tests for diabetes mellitus, *in* Williams, R. H., editor: Diabetes, New York, 1960, Paul B. Hoeber, Inc., Medical Book Division of Harper & Row, Publishers, pp. 389-422.
8. Fajans, S. S., and Conn, J. W.: The approach to the prediction of diabetes mellitus by modification of the glucose tolerance test with cortisone, Diabetes **3:** 296, 1954.
9. Kjellstrand, C. M., Simmons, R. L., Shideman, J. R., et al.: Acute tubular necrosis after renal transplantation. Pathogenesis, prognosis and comparison to surgical disease, *in* Friedman, E. A., and Eliahou, H. E., editors: Proceedings of Acute Renal Failure Conference, Washington, D. C., 1974, Department of Health, Education, and Welfare Publication No. (NIH) 74-608, p. 329.
10. Krohn, G. A., Odgen, D. A., and Holmes, J. H.: Renal function in 29 healthy adults before and after nephrectomy, J. A. M. A. **196:** 322, 1966.
11. Lenz, W.: Medical genetics, Lanze, E. F., translator, Chicago, 1963, University of Chicago Press, p. 56.
12. Liebeman, E.: Hemolytic-uremic syndrome, J. Pediatr. **80:** 1, 1972.
13. Marchioro, T. L.: Donor nephrectomy, *in* Starzl, T. E., editor: Experience in renal transplantation, Philadelphia, 1964, W. B. Saunders Company, pp. 68-83.
14. Najarian, J. S., Gulyassy, P. P., Stoney, R. J., et al.: Protection of the donor kidney during homotransplantation, Ann. Surg. **164:** 398, 1966.
15. Ogden, D. M.: Donor and recipient function two to four years after renal homotransplantation. A paired study of 28 cases, Ann. Intern. Med. **67:** 998, 1967.
16. Penn, I., Halgrimson, C. G., Ogden, D., et al.: Use of living donors in kidney transplantation in man, Arch. Surg. **101:** 226, 1970.
17. Simmons, R. L., Kjellstrand, C. M., and Najarian, J. S.: Technique, complications and results, *in* Najarian, J. S., and Simmons, R. L., editors: Transplantation, Philadelphia, 1972, Lea & Febiger, Publishers, pp. 445-495.
18. Simpson, N. E.: Multifactoral inheritance: A possible hypothesis for diabetes, Diabetes **13:** 462, 1964.
19. Smith, R. B., Walton, K., Lewis, E. L., et al.: Operative morbidity among 40 living kidney donors, J. Surg. Res. **12:** 199, 1972.
20. Spanos, P. K., Simmons, R. L., Simmons, R. G., et al.: The aging related kidney donor: Prognosis for donor, recipient and kidney, Abstr. Sixth Ann. Meeting Am. Soc. Nephrol, 1973, p. 99.
21. Spanos, P. K., Simmons, R. L., Kjellstrand, C. M., et al.: Screening potential related transplant donors for renal disease, Lancet **1:** 645, 1974.
22. Steinberg, A. G.: The genetics of diabetes: A review, Ann. N. Y. Acad. Sci. **82:** 197, 1959.

New method of reconstruction of the alimentary canal after total gastrectomy

Józef Kalemba, M.D., *and* **Bogdan Lazarkiewicz, M.D.,** *Wroclaw, Poland*

We present a new technique of reconstruction of the alimentary tract after total gastrectomy that is based on a modified Hunt pouch. The esophagus is anastomosed into an opening in the upper end of the anterior pouch suture line, so placed that all of the intra-abdominal esophagus can be covered with portions of the pouch wrapped around it in a manner reminiscent of a gastric fundoplication. We have performed the operation on nine patients with three deaths, with no suture line leaks, and with no incidence of reflex or diarrhea.

From the Medical School, Wroclaw, Poland.

SINCE Schlatter's first total gastrectomy in 1897, more than 50 different methods of reconstruction of the alimentary canal after total gastrectomy have been reported. The mortality rate today, though substantially lower than in the past, remains relatively high and the complication rate significant.[4, 6-9, 13, 17] The poor nutritional status of patients with gastric cancer aggravates the problem of anastomosis to the serosa-free esophagus.

The search for a simple, easy, and safe method of reconstruction has led to two principal solutions:[5] (1) reconstruction of the alimentary route through the duodenum and (2) reconstruction bypassing the duodenum. If the duodenum is to be left in line, one employs an interposed segment of small or large intestine between the esophagus and duodenum. Whether the duodenum is bypassed or not, the intestinal segment anastomosed to the esophagus may be fashioned into a pouch or reservoir.

Direct anastomosis of the duodenum to the esophagus, without an interposed intestinal segment, is possible at times. The anastomosis is likely to be under dangerous tension. Duodenal reflux into the esophagus is an undesirable aftereffect of direct esophago-duodenal anastomosis. Interposition of an extrapolated intestinal loop between the esophagus and the duodenum tends to prevent the reflux and permits anastomoses without tension but substantially increases the magnitude of the operative procedure and the number of anastomoses.

It is substantially simpler and technically less demanding to restore the alimentary canal, bypassing the duodenum by some form of esophagojejunal anastomosis. The experiments of Scott and associates[18] demonstrate that such reconstructions after total gastrectomy are compatible with maintenance of adequate nutrition. It is our conviction that the best method of reconstruction after total gastrectomy involves the formation of a pouch as a replacement stomach to prevent

Accepted for publication August 5, 1974.

Reprint requests: Józef Kalemba, M.D., Clinical General Surgery II, Medical School, Wroclaw, Poland.

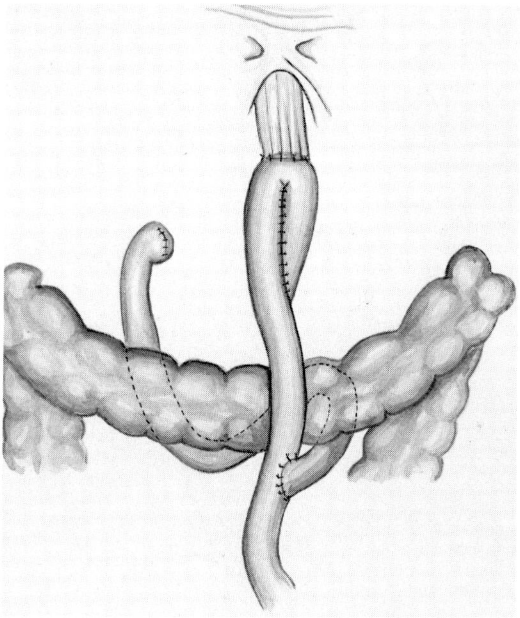

Fig. 1*A*. Hunt technique for gastric pouch reconstruction with jejunum.

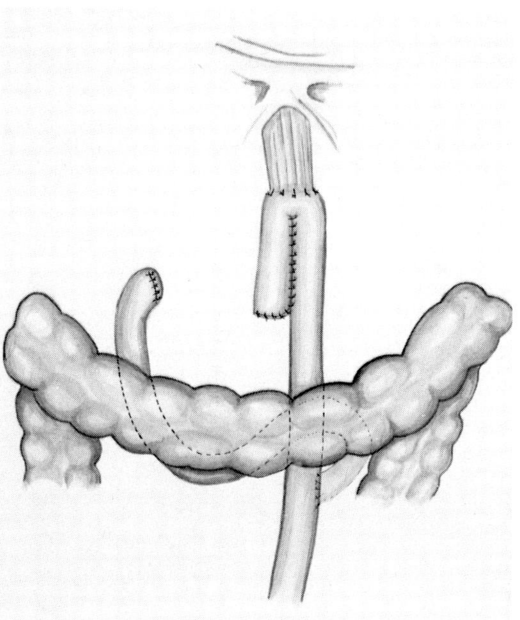

Fig. 1*B*. Lima-Basto technique for gastric pouch reconstruction with jejunum.

reflux and to avoid the rapid entrance of ingested food into the intestinal stream, which often leads to diarrhea.[2, 12, 16] The Roux-Y reconstructions with proximal pouches, re-

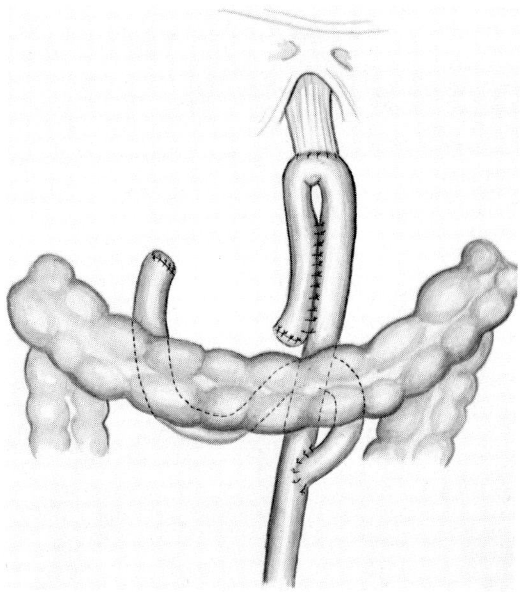

Fig. 1*C*. Rodino technique for gastric pouch reconstruction with jejunum.

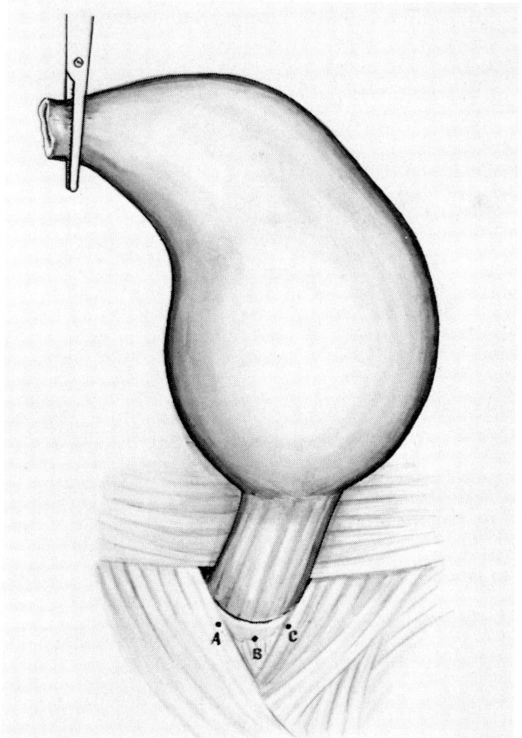

Fig. 2. The duodenum has been transected and the distal end closed. The esophagus is to be divided at the appropriate level. The points *A, B,* and *C* mark the sites to which the pouch will be tacked.

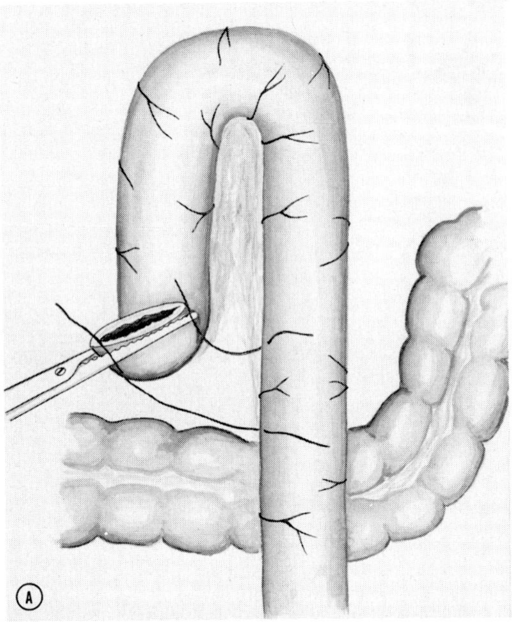

Fig. 3*A*. The Hunt-type pouch is created with limbs 12 to 15 cm. long. The proximal limb held by a noncrushing clamp is left open and limbs are approximated with interrupted sutures.

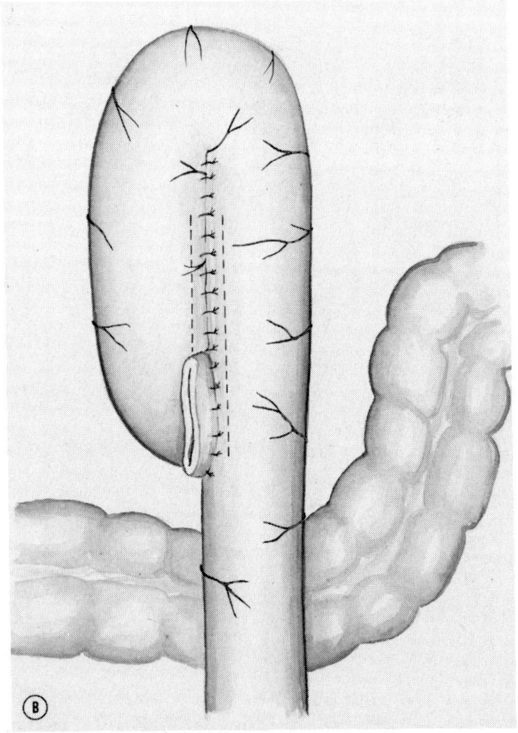

Fig. 3*B*. The two limbs are incised, the incision in the proximal limb being continuous with its open end. The incision is carried no further than 2½ cm. from the upper junction of the limbs.

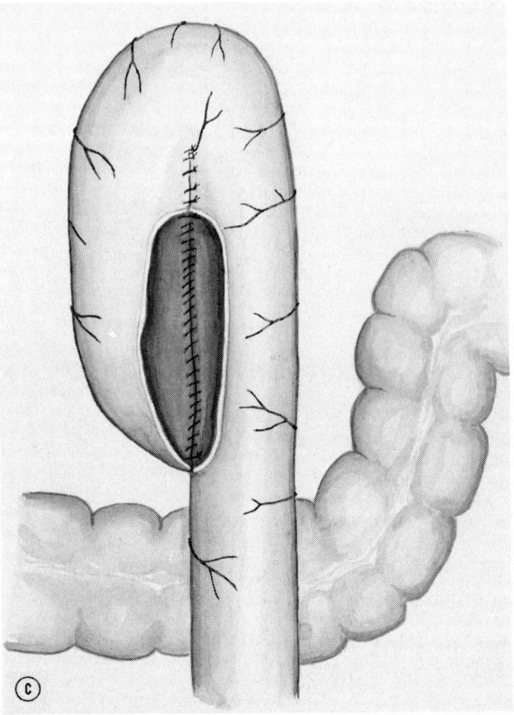

Fig. 3*C*. The appearance after completion of the continuous posterior suture line.

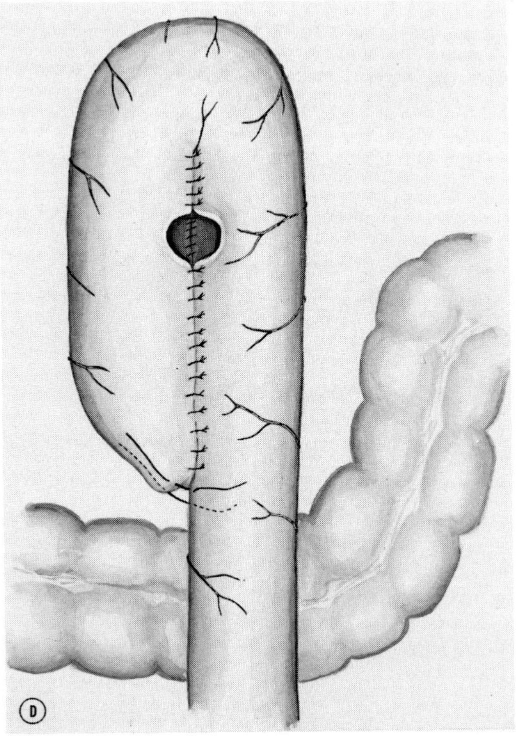

Fig. 3*D*. The completion of the anterior suture line with, an opening at the upper end for anastomosis with the esophagus.

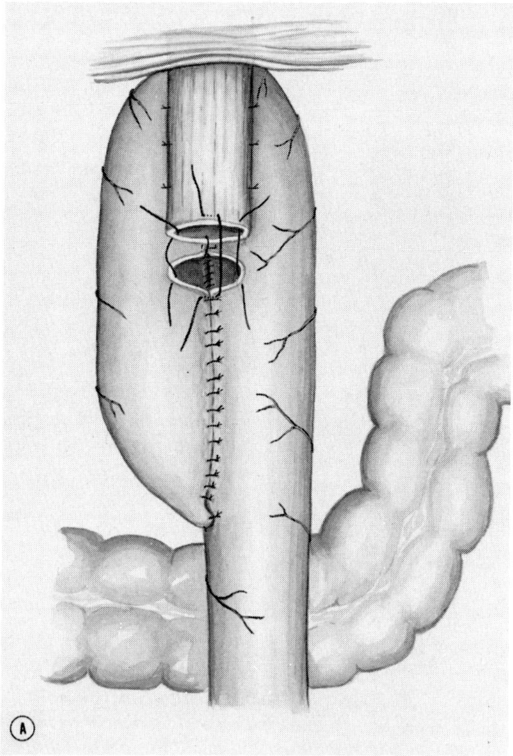

Fig. 4*A*. The esophageal anastomosis. The pouch has been tacked to the diaphragm and the preaortic tissues (at the points indicated in Fig. 2). The esophagus is tacked to the anterior surface of the pouch above the point of anastomosis with interrupted sutures on both sides, and then anastomosis is performed between the esophagus and the opening in the anterior pouch suture line with the usual interrupted suture technique.

ported by Hunt[4] in 1952 (Fig. 1*A*) and by Lima-Basto[7] in 1956 (Fig. 1*B*) and the technique described by Rodino[15] in 1952 (Fig. 1*C*) represent commonly used variations.

While reconstructions of this kind function satisfactorily, leaks of the esophagojejunostomy or the end of the jejunum have continued to be a problem. The technique of reconstruction after total gastrectomy, reported herewith, creates a pouch, prevents reflux, and provides a new and satisfactory technique for protecting the esophagojejunal suture line. As indicated in Figs. 2, 3, and 4, after the stomach has been removed, the duodenum is closed and a modified Hunt pouch is constructed with an opening remaining at the upper end of the anterior pouch suture line. The end of the esophagus

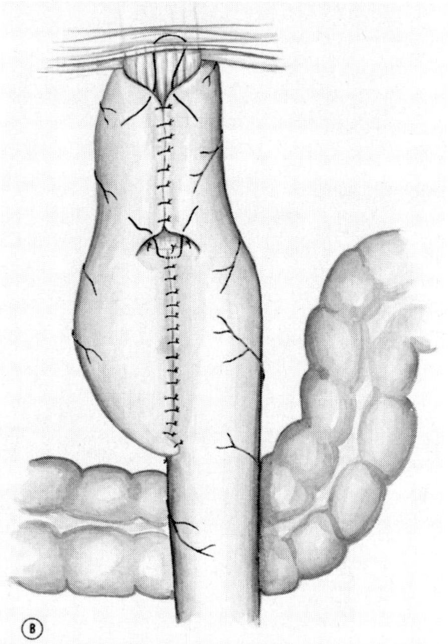

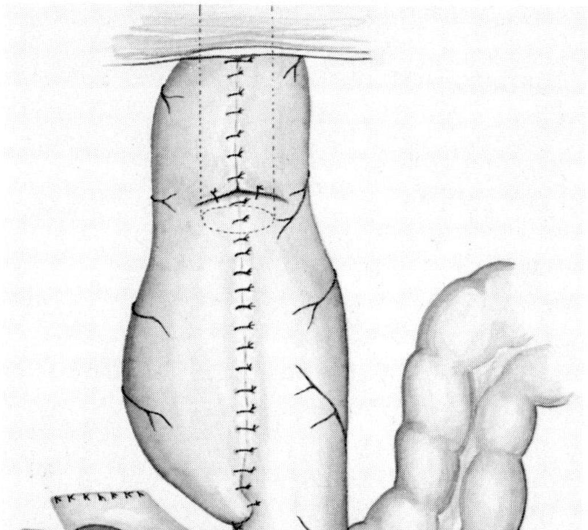

Fig. 4*B*. The pouch is wrapped around the intra-abdominal portion of the esophagus in the manner depicted and then suspended anteriorly from the diaphragm.

Fig. 4*C*. A Roux-Y anastomosis of the proximal jejunum to the efferent limb of the pouch completes the reconstruction.

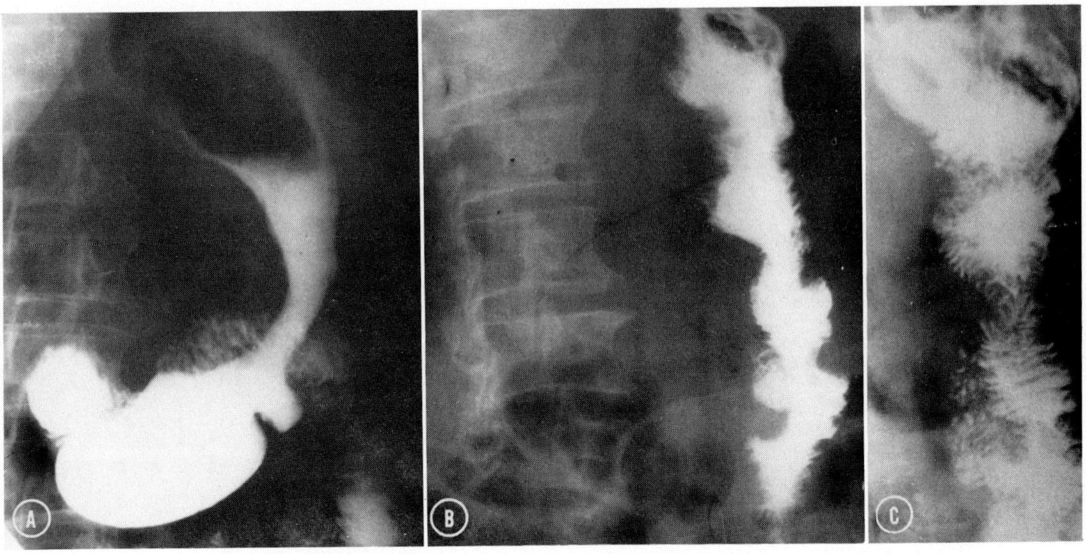

Fig. 5. *A,* Extensive adenocarcinoma of the stomach in a 63-year-old woman. *B,* Barium meal, day 16, demonstrating satisfactory retention in a pouch. *C,* Two months later there has been a gratifying enlargement of the pouch. The patient's general condition is satisfactory, without complications, sequelae, diarrhea, or symptons of flux.

is sutured into this opening. The pouch is tacked to the diaphragm and then wrapped around the esophagus very much in the fashion of a Nissen[12] fundoplication.

We have now performed this procedure on nine patients with three deaths. Despite our small experience and the novelty of the method, our satisfaction with the results, in terms of both mortality rate and function (Fig. 5), prompts us to present our technique.

REFFERENCES

1. Allen, W.: Cancer of the stomach, Surg. Gynecol. Obstet. **92:** 757, 1951.
2. Dzadek, J.: Erfahrurngen mit totaler abdominaler Gastrectomie und Ersatzmagen, Chirurg **25:** 170, 1954.
3. Herzog, K. H.: Operationen am Magen und Zwolffingerdarm. Bier-Braun-Kummell chirurgische Operationslehre, Leipzig, 1972, Johan Ambrosius Barth.
4. Hunt, C. J.: Construction of food pouch from segment of jejunum as substitute for stomach in total gastrectomy, Arch. Surg. **64:** 601, 1952.
5. Kock, N. G., Lewin, E., and Petterson, S.: Partial or total gastrectomy for adenocarcinoma of the cardia, Acta Chir. Scand. **135:** 340, 1969.
6. Largiader, F., and Sauberli, H.: Die totale Gastrectomie, Bruns Beitr, Klin. Chir. **7:** 601, 1972.
7. Lima-Basto, E.: Functional adaptation after total gastrectomy, *in* Proceedings of the World Congress of Gastroenterology, Washington, D. C., 1958, (Baltimore, 1959, The Williams & Wilkins Company), p. 1075.
8. Maden, J.: Atlas chirurgicznej techniki, P. Z. W. L., Warszawa, 1968.
9. Magill, T. G., and Simmons, R. L.: Resection of cardioesophageal carcinoma, Arch. Surg. **94:** 865, 1967.
10. Marshall, S., and Uram, H.: Total gastrectomy for gastric cancer—effects upon mortality, morbidity, and curability, Surg. Gynecol. Obstet. **99:** 657, 1954.
11. Nassehi, A. T.: Nahtinsuffizienz nach Cardiaresektion, Munchen, 1963, dissertation.
12. Nissen, R.: Der operierte Magen, Dtsch. Med. Wochenschr. **88:** 742, 1963.
13. Oszacki, J., Nowotwory, Z., Nielubowicz, J. et al.: Chirurgia kliniczna, P. Z. W. L. Warszawa, 1971.
14. Randall, H. T.: Alteration in gastrointestinal tract function following surgery. Nutrition and dumping syndrome after gastrectomy, Surg. Clin. North. Am. **36:** 585, 1958.
15. Rodino, D.: Contribution à la technique de l'anastomose oesophagojéjunale après gastrectomie totale, J. Chir. (Paris) **68:** 716, 1952.
16. Sanchez, R. E., and Gordon, H. E.: Com-

plications of total gastrectomy, Arch. Surg. **100:** 136, 1970.
17. Schlatter, C.: Oesophago-enterostomy after extirpation of the stomach, Lancet **1:** 141, 1898.
18. Scott, H. W., Law, D. H., Gobbel, W. G., et al.: Clinical and metabolic studies after total gastrectomy with Hunt-Lawrence food pouch, Am. J. Surg. **115:** 148, 1968.
19. Szabo, L. E., Karacsonyi, S., and Füredi, E.: Zur metastasebildung des Oesophagus und Kardiakarzinoms, Acta Chir. Acad. Sci. Hung. **8:** 301, 1967.

The need for pediatric surgeons as determined by the volume of work and the mode of delivery of surgical care

Mark M. Ravitch, M.D., *and* **Bruce A. Barton, M.S.,** *Pittsburgh, Pa.*

An analysis of the relative advantages and disadvantages of supplying pediatric surgeons according to a fixed population ratio or according to the capacity of appropriately distributed special centers for pediatric surgery to accommodate the volume of work in the United States suggests the following. (1) Distribution of pediatric surgeons by a fixed surgeon:population ratio might require 4 to 6 times as many general pediatric surgeons as would the delivery of specialized surgical care by general pediatric surgeons in centers. (2) The result of distribution of pediatric surgeons principally in relation to population would be to provide a minimal continuing experience in major pediatric surgery for most of the surgeons and so to decrease the volume in the training centers as to make it difficult or impossible to train future pediatric surgeons or to expand knowledge of pediatric surgery. (3) The centers in approximately 48 cities (with several centers in some of the largest cities) would appear to satisfy regional institutional and educational needs and to provide a well-distributed network.

From the Department of Surgery, Montefiore Hospital, and the Departments of Surgery and Biostatistics, University of Pittsburgh, Pittsburgh, Pa.

THE NEED for general pediatric surgeons in the United States in the coming decades depends on the manner in which pediatric surgical care is to be delivered. If pediatric surgeons are to be distributed strictly on a one surgeon per X hundred thousand population basis, the need could be enormous. By the same token, the requirement for general pediatric surgeons will differ if, on the one hand, we expect that *all* general surgery (including appendectomies, herniorrhaphies, various types of minor surgery, etc.) for children below, say, the age of 14, is to be done by pediatric surgeons, or if, on the other hand, we assume the special expertise of pediatric surgeons should be applied to the very special problems of pediatric surgery—essentially all surgery of the neonate, the surgery of major congenital anomalies, and the surgery of malignant tumors. Pediatric surgery in these special areas deals with conditions which occur in one in 5,000 to one in 10,000 to 20,000 live births, so that, if pediatric surgeons were distributed on a population ratio basis, it is entirely likely that a general pediatric surgeon, making an adequate living performing appendectomies and inguinal herniorrhaphies, might see one or two of these special conditions in a year. The predictable result would be a progressive decline in the operative, diagnostic, and therapeutic skills of the pediatric surgeon from the level at which he left his residency training, with an inevitable reflection in the results obtained in the treatment of these occasional patients. By the same token, the widespread scattering

Accepted for publication August 2, 1974.

Reprint requests: Mark M. Ravitch, M.D., Department of Surgery, University of Pittsburgh, Pittsburgh, Pa. 15213.

in every community in the country of cases of this sort would result in so small a patient load in the pediatric hospitals that the training programs from which future pediatric surgeons should be derived would be ineffective, and the opportunity to advance pediatric surgery from the study of significant series of cases would be lost.

There is the further feature that the surgery of congenital anomalies and of malignant tumors in children, and most surgery in the neonates, require for their successful performance a constellation of services and talents, which it is simply not feasible or economically sensible to provide, except in special centers. One is speaking of the neonatologist, the pediatric anesthesiologist, the pediatric radiologist, the pediatric pathologist, the pediatric oncologist and chemotherapist, and the special facilities of pediatric and neonatal intensive-care units, radiology departments, respiratory therapists, etc.

In the last quarter of the twentieth century in this country, transportation by ground and by air is such as to make it readily acceptable that, in almost any neonatal condition, the time required for transportation from anywhere in the country to a major center would be offset by the great advantages accruing to the child from treatment at a center. While the transportation of adults to centers for the treatment of special problems makes equally good sense, it does introduce the major problem of dislocating families, etc. In the case of children, particularly of infants, this is much less significant. The newborn, in particular, has not yet established himself in the family and his removal some distance from home has not the same significance as, let us say, the transportation of the father away from his children, from contact with his business, etc. The cost of transportation of newborn children, whether by ambulance or helicopter, would clearly be substantially less than the cost of establishing and maintaining hundreds of specially equipped and staffed centers around the country, apart from the obvious fact that qualified personnel for such centers are not available and, if they became available, would lose their expertise in installations with so predictably small a case load.

There is the additional factor that not only is there a declining birth rate in this country, but specifically a declining birth rate of babies born to very young mothers and to very mature mothers, i.e., the two groups in which there is special risk that babies with congenital anomalies will be produced. The pediatric surgeons of this country are under the very distinct impression that they are currently seeing fewer congenital anomalies in the major centers than they did only a few years ago. In the absence of reliable figures, it cannot be stated whether this represents a decline in the appearance of congenital anomalies or a dispersion throughout the country of surgeons who consider themselves competent to care for children with congenital anomalies, so that the infants have not been referred to centers on the same scale as previously.

It seems worthwhile to see whether the magnitude of the need for pediatric surgical services can be arrived at in terms of the frequency of occurrence of serious pediatric surgical conditions at present and at intervals in the future.

If we make our assumptions for the need of pediatric surgeons on the basis that a population of 100,000 or of 200,000 could "support" a pediatric surgeon, the projected population of the United States in 1975 of 215,588,000 would indicate a need for 2,156 to 1,078 pediatric surgeons, and in 1985 a need for 2,409 to 1,205 pediatric surgeons. If we assumed pediatric surgeons and their patients would not be well served in small communities, although with a peripheral and rural population that might nevertheless reach these numbers, and we restricted the siting of pediatric surgeons to communities of a minimum of 100,000 or 200,000 population, we would come up in 1975 with a need for 1,252 or 578 pediatric surgeons, and in 1985 with a need for 1,546 or 726. In any case, it seems unlikely that these surgeons could survive economically unless they did most of the general surgery in infants and children of whatever degree of simplicity or complexity. We have already alluded to the progressive diminution in the expertise of such surgeons and to the less than optimal support they and their patients would receive in terms of facilities and professional collaboration.

To arrive at an estimate of the number of pediatric surgeons functioning in centers and the number of centers that might be required, it was necessary to arrive at an estimate of the volume of special pediatric surgery which is required. There is no national statistical reservoir of the volume of pediatric surgery in general, nor of the number of cases of any one kind which are treated by surgeons. The very large statistical bank in Ann Arbor, CPHA, is not useful in this regard. An analysis of their data base shows that children's hospitals have been excluded almost systematically and only one or two university hospitals are included in which there is any recognized special interest in pediatric surgery. Furthermore, most diagnostic codes have been made without any special input from pediatric surgeons and it is not a simple matter to pluck from such a registry the kinds of cases in which we are interested, although the computer program could be directed to make an appropriate search and the results would at least give us the volume of special pediatric surgery which is being performed in this large group of nonspecialized hospitals. Discharge diagnoses from lying-in hospitals are frequently erroneous. The correct diagnosis is subsequently made in the pediatric hospital to which the infant has been transferred, or the infants are discharged before the presence of an anomaly is recognized.

One of the striking results of our inquiry has been the demonstration that there is not at hand a ready statistical base from which to draw conclusions as to the need for pediatric surgeons and/or pediatric surgical centers. Most articles on pediatric surgical problems list a figure for the incidence of the particular problem under discussion. When this is given as the number of cases seen in that hospital, or of the proportion to other conditions seen during the same period of time, it is of interest but not useful for the present study. These papers originate largely from pediatric surgical centers. Nowhere in the country do all pediatric surgical problems come to the recognized children's hospital center, so that over all a center's disease roster usually represents only part of the load in its drawing area and the figures would be low. By the same token, special conditions come to some individual surgeons or hospitals from all over the country and from abroad because of long-established special interest in a given problem, and for these conditions figures derived from these surgeons or hospitals would be high. Surprisingly enough, an inquiry addressed to most of the major pediatric surgical units disclosed the fact that many of them did not keep a running tabulation of their annual experience.

Since we are dealing with conditions of considerable rarity, it seemed reasonable to assume that, if we were able to secure reliable data from a number of sources which came to their estimates of incidence in several ways, and if these were all within a reasonable range and not dissimilar from those arrived at in the past by a variety of methods, these would be sufficiently accurate for the present purpose. Furthermore, the rarity of the conditions suggests that even a modest error in the accuracy of the projections would not result in a case load sufficiently different to suggest a totally different order of magnitude in the kind of support required.

Given the extraordinarily broad range of the special problems of pediatric surgery, it seemed impractical to attempt to secure a total picture of all the conditions which might fall into this grouping. Instead, we have attempted to gather figures for the following six groups of congenital anomalies and three tumors: (1) esophageal atresia and tracheoesophageal fistula; (2) omphalocele and gastroschisis; (3) imperforate anus; (4) intestinal atresia; (5) congenital diaphragmatic hernia; (6) Hirschsprung's disease; (7) rhabdomyosarcoma; (8) Wilms' tumor, and (9) neuroblastoma.

Our assumption has been that experienced

pediatric surgeons in major pediatric surgical clinics, understanding the ratio of these index cases to other major conditions and to the simpler problems dealt with daily, could come up with a valid estimate of the number of pediatric surgeons which would be required in a center which would be expected to treat a given number of these index conditions. Also, it might be reasonable to assume for the specialties within pediatric surgery, i.e., neurosurgery, urological surgery, orthopedic surgery, plastic surgery, and cardiac surgery, that if, for instance, in an extant center the volume of work in general pediatric surgery would increase by a predicted factor, it would increase by a similar factor in these specialties, modified by the degree to which more or less work in that specialty is being done now outside of centers than is the case for general pediatric surgery.

We had thought the incidence of these index conditions could be established readily enough from recorded data. This proved not to be the case. In general in this country, prospective studies on these conditions have not been done nor have we found thus far, in a search that still continues, the information available nationally from the United States Public Health Service, the Bureau of Census, or the Children's Bureau, nor from the health departments or other agencies of any of the 50 states.

Our basic calculations were from the raw data from the following sources:

1. The Hospital Utilization Project based in Monroeville, Penn., which collects abstracts of records from hospitals in several states, but for which we programmed a computer search for all the records from Allegheny County as containing a mix of general hospitals of all kinds as well as a major pediatric hospital.

2. The commonwealth of Pennsylvania's Department of Health Study of 1963 of the incidence of congenital anomalies in the state of Pennsylvania, which accounted for almost 96 percent of all births and, presumably, a similar percentage of anomalies. This covered the first four congenital anomalies, which would be expected to be recognized at birth.

3. The data from the National Center for Disease Control in Atlanta, Ga., covering a continuing surveillance of hospital records in the Atlanta area from October, 1967, to December, 1971. Again this study was concerned only with defects which became evident in the first 2 weeks of life and was useful, therefore, only with respect to the first four congenital malformations.

4. The Connecticut Cancer Registry had a well-defined base population so that it could provide data for inclusion in this study with respect to tumors.

5. The Third National Cancer Survey provided data on the incidence of the three childhood neoplasms for 4 years in the Pittsburgh SMSA (standard metropolitan survey area) and for 1969 for the entire survey.

The only two non-neoplastic conditions, studied in persons under 15 years of age, although congenital conditions—Hirschsprung's disease and diaphragmatic hernia—have only one data source, the Hospital Utilization Project (HUP). Other sources listed these conditions, but only for newborn infants, and a significant proportion of cases of Hirschsprung's disease and diaphragmatic hernia are not recognized in the newborn infant. It therefore required a study of a complete survey of hospital records, which was available to us from HUP.

Vital statistics are not useful because, in general, these malformations are not reportable by law, either separately or on birth certificates, and for surviving infants there would be no death certificate in any case. It has been demonstrated for Missouri[10] that, although that state requires by law the reporting of birth defects, crosschecking of birth certificates with hospital records shows that fewer than 50 percent of the defects are reported.

The statistical calculations required to relate the reported incidence to live births or population will be reported elsewhere and have been evaluated and accepted by biostatisticians at the School of Public Health at the University of Pittsburgh.

It is likely that our incidence rates are, in fact, higher than those suggested in the literature dealing with specific anomalies. The reason for this is that the codification of disease conditions is imprecise. Thus a good many conditions other than intestinal atresia may be lumped under its code number. For our purposes this still represents a valid indication of the workload of pediatric surgeons.

Here and there the literature does record what would appear to be valid figures for the occurrence of congenital anomalies in given populations, although most articles dealing with a surgical problem in pediatrics usually quote a secondary or tertiary source, which on further check may not be found to be based on an altogether valid study. Nevertheless, it is of interest to compare our figures with some of those reported.

For esophageal atresia and tracheoesophageal fistula, we calculated an incidence rate of one per 5,077 live births, with an upper limit of one per 4,486 and a lower limit of one per 5,847. Cameron Haight's[5] 30 year study of every newborn infant in Washtenaw County, Mich., gave an incidence of one in 4,425 live births, close to our upper figure. Rickham and Johnston,[16] between 1953 and 1968 in Liverpool, saw 223 cases or roughly one in 3,000 live births for the northwest portion of England and for north Wales, assuming they saw all the babies with this defect born in that area and that none of the babies with this defect went elsewhere. Anderson and Reed,[1] after a review of the literature, concluded that the incidence is approximately one in 6,000 live births, somewhat below our lower figure.

For imperforate anus and variants, we came to a figure of one per 2,523 live births, with an upper limit of one per 2,315 and a lower limit of one per 2,771. The British Perinatal Mortality Survey[3] found an incidence of one per 3,300 live births for the week they surveyed, a little below our lowest rate. Unsupported figures from other authors vary from one in 1,500 live births to one in 5,000 live births.[1, 22]

For omphalocele and gastroschisis, we found an incidence rate of one per 2,461 live births, with an upper limit of one per 2,287 and a lower limit of one per 2,663. Rickham and Johnston[17] found an incidence of one per 6,000 for omphalocele and one per 30,000 for gastroschisis. From Birmingham, England, McKeown, McMahon, and Record,[11] from 1941 to 1951, found the incidence of omphalocele to be about one in 3,200 live births. The incidence of omphalocele from Adelaide, Australia,[20] is given as one in 4,000 live births, from 1946 to 1969, and of gastroschisis as one in 40,000. Soper and Green,[21] in Iowa from 1951 to 1960, gave an incidence of one in 3,800 for omphalocele. O'Leary and Clymer[13] had one omphalocele in 5,000 deliveries at the University of Oklahoma, but Jarcho,[7] in 5,017 deliveries at Sydenham Hospital in New York, found an incidence of one in 2,455. Since our study included gastroschisis, our rates are found to be close to those reported.

For intestinal atresia and variants, we found an incidence rate of one per 2,710 live births, with an upper limit of one per 2,480 and a lower limit of one per 2,988. Rickham and Johnston[18] again, for the years 1956 to 1968, estimated an incidence of one per 5,000 live births. Moore and Stokes[12] report from Indiana an incidence of one in 6,000 live births. Evans,[4] after an exhaustive study of the literature, suggests that the incidence would be one in 1,500 births, including stillborns.

Our calculations of the incidence of congenital diaphragmatic hernia yield a figure of one per 4,776 live births. Rickham and Johnston[15] found a rate of one per 12,000 live births from Liverpool. Lister,[8] writing from Sheffield, suggested on the basis of indirect calculations an incidence of about one in 10,000 live births. The John Gaston Hospital in Memphis, from 1948 to 1966, reported an incidence of about one in 7,000 live births.[6] A 10 year review of the Evanston, Ill., hospital yielded an incidence of one per 1,200 deliveries.[2] Although the rates vary widely, and there may be some question in some studies of the accuracy of reporting or diagnosis, the rate from our study is within the range of the rates in the literature.

For Hirschsprung's disease, the incidence

in Allegheny County was one per 8,333 live births. Rickham and Johnston[19] calculated an incidence of one per 10,000 live births. Madsen[9] from Denmark reports an incidence of one per 4,700 births, from a total of 124,000 births. Our figure is roughly midway between the Birmingham and Copenhagen figures.

Actually, since diaphragmatic hernia and Hirschsprung's disease are recognized at all ages, it is the rate per population under age 15 which contributes to the workload of the pediatric surgeon. This rate is one per 12,100 children under age 15 for congenital diaphragmatic hernia and one per 12,569 children under 15 years of age for Hirschsprung's disease.

For the tumors, from Allegheny County, the Connecticut Cancer Registry, and two segments of the Third National Cancer Survey—which includes seven metropolitan areas, two entire states, and Puerto Rico—the figures are as follows:

For rhabdomyosarcoma, the average rate was one per 202,741 population under age 15, with an upper limit of one per 179,979 and a lower limit of one per 232,094. All the reported figures in the surgical literature which we found dealt with the number of cases admitted to a hospital or the proportion of all childhood cancer cases represented by rhabdomyosarcoma in a given hospital over a certain period of time. In the absence of any knowledge as to the population base for those periods, these figures are not useful for this study.

For Wilms' tumor, the average incidence rate was one per 101,370 population under 15 years of age, with an upper limit of one case per 93,728 and a lower limit of one case per 110,370 population.

For neuroblastoma, the average rate was one per 128,048 population under 15 years of age, with an upper limit of one per 116,290 and a lower limit of one case per 142,450. One valid study was found in the literature for 1943 to 1956, that of Pinkel, Dowd, and Bross[14] from Buffalo, which yielded an incidence of about one case of neuroblastoma per 100,000 population under 15 years of age, very close to our average rate of one per 128,000, with a variance of 116,000 to 142,000.

Now what does this mean in terms of the total load for pediatric surgeons? Converting all our figures to the incidence of anomalies in any one given year in the entire population of the United States under age 15, we find that, in 1970, there should have been 738 tracheoesophageal fistulas and variants, 1,474 imperforate anuses and variants, 1,511 omphaloceles and variants, 1,372 intestinal atresias, 4,785 diaphragmatic hernias, 4,607 cases of Hirschsprung's disease, 386 rhabdomyosarcomas, 571 Wilms' tumors, and 452 neuroblastomas. Fifteen years later in 1985, assuming a constant birthrate—which one might as well assume since biostatisticians and demographers are unable to make any valid predictions—the increase is to 774 tracheoesophageal fistulas, 1,558 imperforate anuses and variants, 1,598 omphaloceles, 1,451 intestinal atresia and its variants, 5,060 diaphragmatic hernias, 4,871 cases of Hirschsprung's disease, 302 rhabdomyosarcomas, 604 Wilms' tumors, and 478 neuroblastomas. The total number of these index problems of pediatric surgery would have been 15,790 in 1970 and can be expected to rise to 16,696 in 1985.

Now we have not included such obviously special lesions as sacrococcygeal teratoma, cervical hygroma, lung cysts, mediastinal tumors, biliary atresia, choledochal cysts, liver tumors, etc. We would consider that these require the special constellation of services and individual talents of pediatric surgical centers as much as do the nine conditions we have chosen as index conditions.

For the year from May 1, 1973, to April 30, 1974, at the Children's Hospital of Pittsburgh, a review of the operating room records shows 146 procedures done with diagnoses from the nine index conditions. Clearly some children with Hirschsprung's disease or imperforate anus had several procedures. There were 177 procedures in the operating room record in the same period done by general pediatric surgeons, which could be considered "special" under the following headings: necrotizing enterocolitis, pectus excavatum, pyloromyotomy, malrotation, clitorrhaphy, cystic hygroma, exstrophy of the bladder, splenectomy—including trauma—biliary atresia, vascular rings, hypospadias, other malignancy, and a variety of miscellaneous conditions. Herniorrhaphies, appendectomies, and major traumatic problems were excluded. It will be seen that the index conditions represented somewhat less than half the total number of operative procedures and a smaller proportion than this of individual patients. If one assumed that most children with pyloric stenosis would not be sent to a center and children with ruptured spleens would also not be transported to a center, the proportion of the index conditions to the major problems of general pediatric surgery comes pretty close to one to one.

Since all our incidence figures are, if anything, on the high side, and since the birthrate may continue to fall, it is not likely that our figures will underestimate the need for pediatric surgeons.

The required output of pediatric surgeons from training programs in the United States will obviously depend on whether the need for pediatric surgeons is calculated on some population basis or on the center concept. To arrive at some notion of the number of cities in which centers might have to be provided, we indicated, on a population map of the United States (Fig. 1), those major centers already functioning and obviously justifying their existence, accepting existing patterns, which in some cases might result in centers being placed in what might be considered to be competing areas. In addition, centers were postulated in rapidly growing centers of population which had not yet justified the creation of a center but obviously had or soon would have a population size and a distance from existing centers which would justify such a designation.

Clearly the volume of patients and the availability of institutions and established patterns would dictate, in a number of the larger cities, the presence of more than one center.

There is no need at this juncture to propose sites or finite numbers for centers or to indicate the number of residents required to be trained each year. The few existing training programs appear to be capable of maintaining the existing number of pediatric surgeons and it is not at all clear that any great increase will be required. Furthermore, if the need for pediatric surgeons turns out to be greater than predicted, the supply can be rapidly increased. For the graduates of general surgical residency programs it would be only 2 years "in the pipeline" before additional pediatric surgeons would be available. Well over half of the projected 48 or more centers would not have pediatric surgical residency programs. If additional output of pediatric surgeons proved to be required, several of these could institute such programs on relatively short notice.

The pediatric surgeons in those of the 48 or more centers which will not have training programs for pediatric surgeons will be aided by residents rotating through from the associated general surgical programs. This will ensure a very substantial supply of surgeons scattered about the country, who have more than an ordinary awareness of the problems of pediatric surgery, and who have the capacity to deal with the problems not requiring the facilities of a center, the ability to recognize the problems requiring transportation to a center, and the ability to prepare the children properly for such transportation.

Fig. 1. Population distribution map of 1970, with numerators for the number of index conditions and denominators for the number of millions in the circled areas. It will be noted that Hawaii is included (there is no circle) and that Alaska, like the other sparsely populated areas of the country, mainly the western and upper midwestern states, is not. The population concentrations in a number of the circled areas are such that obviously more than one center would be required. In almost all these areas, there are now pediatric facilities which function to some known degree as referral centers or could very easily be brought up to the standard required in terms of complexity of available services, etc.

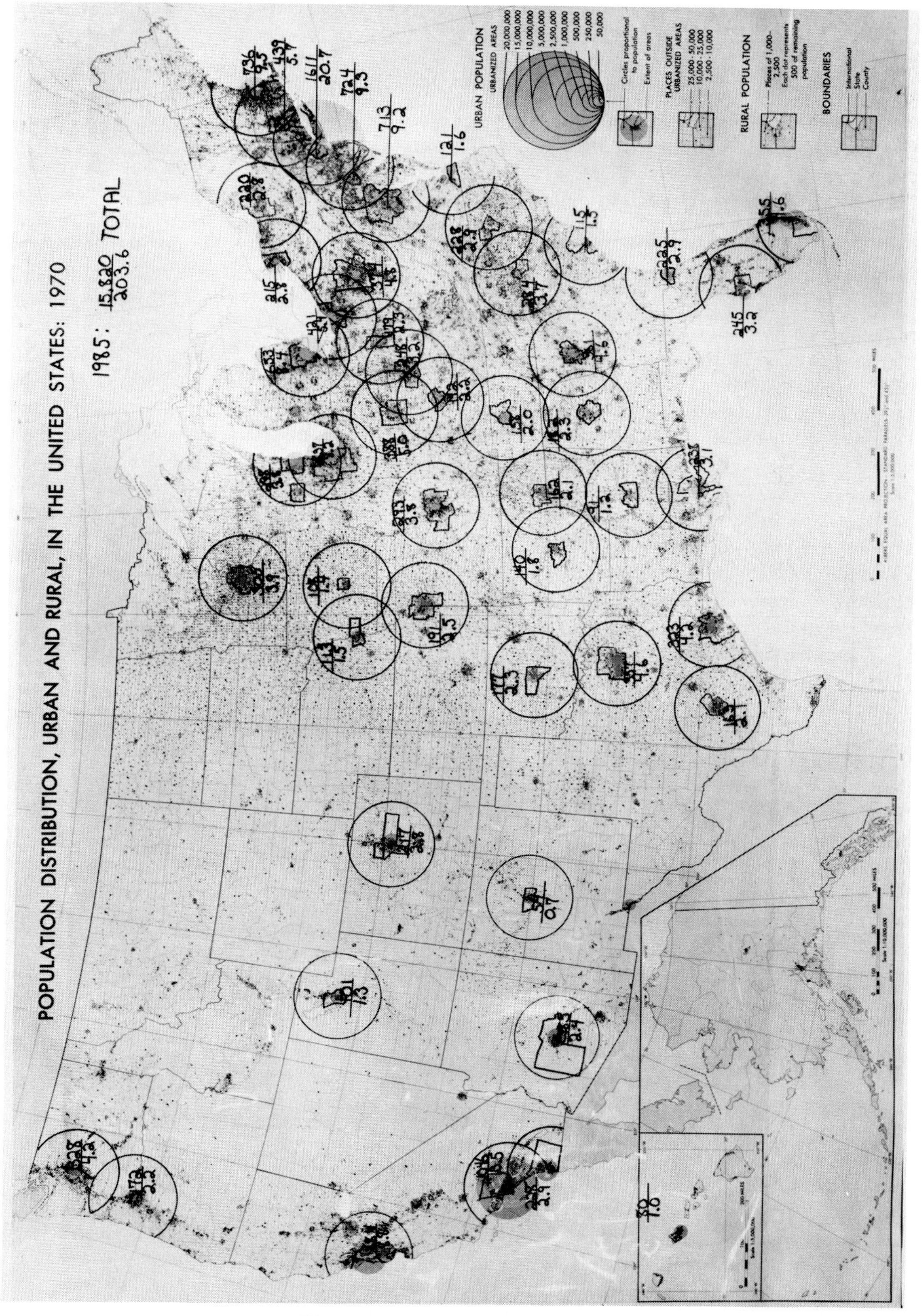

Fig. 1. For legend, see opposite page.

Currently we have under 300 pediatric surgeons. If pediatric surgeons were based solely according to population, one for each 100,000 or 200,000 population within a city, the number of pediatric surgeons required in 1985 would be 1,546 or 726. If we had that many pediatric surgeons and the surgery of these anomalies were evenly divided, then each man would see from 27 to 55 of these index anomalies per year and from 70 to 140 major problems of any kind. On the other hand, if all children with these problems were to be treated in centers—and let us assume the final plan accepted the 48 or more areas which we have indicated on our maps—the very smallest number in 1985 would be Salt Lake City with 101 of these index conditions and 202 major pediatric surgical problems. The New York metropolitan area, with 1,611 and 3,222, would obviously require several centers. The city of Pittsburgh, which now has five surgeons who devote themselves exclusively to general pediatric surgery, would have 374 index patients (748 total) in 1985, which would mean, if the patients were equally distributed and no new pediatric surgeons were added, each of these men would see about three index problems every 2 weeks or three "good" cases each week. If we had one pediatric surgeon for every 100,000 population in Pittsburgh and its drawing area (for convenience, assumed to be the area within 100 miles of the city), we would have 48 pediatric surgeons and, if it were one per 200,000, we would have 24 pediatric surgeons. Similar calculations can be made in any area of the country.

We are not yet prepared to make any prediction of the number of pediatric surgeons which might be required. If we were to have 300 surgeons limiting themselves to general pediatric surgery in the centers which would be receiving these patients, then, by 1985 over the entire country, were distribution to be precisely even, the 16,696 cases of the index conditions would mean 55 of these patients a year for each of the 300 surgeons, or 110 major pediatric surgical cases per man per year, roughly two per week. It can be seen that even allowing for some inequalities in various parts of the country and for considerable errors in our calculations, 300 general pediatric surgeons would quite easily carry the load. We are talking of scarcely more than one of these nine index conditions per week through the year. Even if we assume these index conditions represent only half the volume of serious and special problems for the pediatric surgeon, we would be talking about fewer than three cases per week, and if they represent only a quarter of the significant problems, we would be talking about only four or five major cases a week per man. The hours involved in the care of many of these infants apart from the operation, the numerous other duties and responsibilities which surgeons in institutions of this kind have, the certainty that there will and should continue to be a significant burden of everyday pediatric surgical problems in the "centers," all keep us from the obvious fallacy of assuming any vigorous surgeon can do three to five cases a day and that the number of surgeons needed is, therefore, substantially less than, let us say, the figure of 300 used in the example above.

If we assume either a 2:1 or 1:1 ratio (other special conditions: index conditions), we can calculate the following annual rates per 100,000 population:

2:1			
9 index	27.27	±	2.86
Other	54.54	±	5.67
Total	81.81	±	8.53
1:1			
9 index	27.27	±	2.86
Other	27.27	±	2.86
Total	54.54	±	5.72

From the total figures, we can thus determine that, for each 100,000 population, assuming a range from the highest possible to the lowest possible incidence, we can expect annually from approximately 90 to 50 index and other special cases, which is roughly one every 3 to 4 days to less than one a week.

It is perfectly clear that the surgeon who begins to do a considerable number of these major problems is not going to be able to do the large number of infant hernias, undescended testes, etc., which now constitute a very large portion of the practice and the principal source of income of a great many pediatric surgeons. Inevitably, as the special pediatric centers become filled with patients with the grave illnesses which require their special facilities, a considerable number of the less complicated problems will be treated in other hospitals by general surgeons. Very possibly these would be men whose general surgical training had been in programs with which pediatric surgical centers were associated and who had had at least some exposure to pediatric surgery. While the elegance of the operative technique employed by such men may not meet the standards of purist pediatric surgeons, it is not likely that the patients will suffer seriously.

REFERENCES

1. Anderson, R., and Reed, S.: The likelihood of recurrence of congenital malformation, Lancet **74:** 176, 1954.
2. Bowers, V. M., Jr., McElin, T., and Dorsey, J. M.: Diaphragmatic hernia in the newborn: Diagnostic responsibility of the obstetrician, Obstet. Gynecol. **6:** 262, 1955.
3. Butler, N., and Alberman, E., editors: Perinatal problems: The second report of 1958 British Perinatal Mortality Survey, London, 1969, The Williams & Wilkins Company, p. 309.
4. Evans, C.: Atresias of the gastrointestinal tract, Surg. Gynecol. Obstet. (Int. Abst. Surg.) **92:** 1, 1951.
5. Haight, C.: Congenital esophageal atresia and tracheoesophageal fistula, *in* Mustard, W. T., Ravitch, M. M., Snyder, W. H., Jr., Welch, K. J., and Benson, C. D., editors: Pediatric surgery, Chicago, 1969, Year Book Medical Publishers, Inc., p. 357.
6. Jackson, T.: Congenital diaphragmatic hernia, Arch. Surg. **95:** 102, 1967.
7. Jarcho, J.: Congenital umbilical hernia, Surg. Gynecol. Obstet. **65:** 593, 1937.
8. Lister, J.: Recent advances in the surgery of the diaphragm in the newborn, Prog. Pediatr. Surg. **2:** 30, 1970.
9. Madsen, C. M.: Hirschsprung's disease, translated by Harris, C. N., Springfield, Ill., 1964, Charles C Thomas, Publisher, p. 25.
10. Marienfeld, C. J.: Personal communication, May 21, 1973.
11. McKeown, T., McMahon, B., and Record, R. G.: An investigation of 69 cases of exomphalos, Am. J. Hum. Genet. **5:** 168, 1953.
12. Moore, T., and Stokes, G.: Congenital stenosis and atresia of the small intestine, Surg. Gynecol. Obstet. **97:** 719, 1953.
13. O'Leary, C., and Clymer, C.: Umbilical hernia, Am. J. Surg. **52:** 38, 1941.
14. Pinkel, D., Dowd, J., and Bross, I.: Some epidemiological features of malignant solid tumors of children in the Buffalo, New York, area, Cancer **16:** 29, 1963.
15. Rickham, P. P., and Johnston, J. H.: Neonatal surgery, London, 1969, Appleton-Century-Crofts, Inc. (Division of Meredith Pub. Co.), p. 179.
16. Rickham, P. P., and Johnston, J. H.: Neonatal surgery, London, 1969, Appleton-Century-Crofts, Inc. (Division of Meredith Pub. Co.), p. 203.
17. Rickham, P. P., and Johnston, J. H.: Neonatal surgery, London, 1969, Appleton-Century-Crofts, Inc. (Division of Meredith Pub. Co.), p. 257.
18. Rickham, P. P., and Johnston, J. H.: Neonatal surgery, London, 1969, Appleton-Century-Crofts, Inc. (Division of Meredith Pub. Co.), p. 320.
19. Rickham, P. P., and Johnston, J. H.: Neonatal surgery, London, 1969, Appleton-Century-Crofts, Inc. (Division of Meredith Pub. Co.), pp. 382-383.
20. Savage, J. P., and Davey, R. B.: The treatment of gastroschisis, J. Pediatr. Surg. **6:** 148, 1971.
21. Soper, R., and Green, E.: Omphalocele, Surg. Gynecol. Obstet. **113:** 501, 1961.
22. Stephens, F. D., and Smith, E. D.: Ano-rectal malformations in children, Chicago, 1971, Year Book Medical Publishers, Inc., p. 160.

The effect of sepsis on acute gastric ulcerations in the rat

R. Rasche, M.D., *and* **W. C. Butterfield, M.D.,** *Waterbury, Conn.*

Subcutaneous injections in the rat with **S. Aureus** and **E. coli** were compared with controls to determine the effect of infection on gastric secretion and on the formation of acute ulcerations in the pyloric-ligated and restraint models. A statistically significant decrease in ulcerations in the pyloric-ligated group and a decrease, although not statistically significant, in the restraint group occurred in the animals infected with **E. coli**. Gastric acidity was also inhibited in the **E. coli** group. The **E. coli** animals were febrile while the **S. aureus** animals were not. The inhibitory effect of temperature elevation on gastric secretion, which has been repeatedly documented in the literature, is believed to be the explanation for the observed results.

From the Division of Surgery, St. Mary's Hospital, Waterbury, Conn.

SEVERAL clinical studies report an association between stress ulcers and sepsis.[1, 11, 12, 15, 25] From 29 to 83 percent of patients with stress ulcers have concurrent sepsis.[5, 19] Little experimental work has been done in this area, however, and it is unclear whether sepsis is simply a coexistent phenomenon or an etiological agent.

The purpose of the following experiment was to test the effects of infection with *Escherichia coli* and *Staphylococcus aureus* on the incidence of acute gastric ulceration in the rat using the ulcerogenic models of pyloric ligation[29] and physical restraint.[9] *E. coli* and *S. aureus* were chosen for study because of their frequent association with stress ulceration and infection in man.[1, 13, 15, 16]

METHOD

1. Gastric ulcers—pyloric ligation model. Sixty male rats (COBS rats: Charles River, CD strain), weighing between 270 and 350 grams, were paired by weight and placed in wire mesh cages to minimize coprophagia. Food, but not water, was withheld from the animals for 72 hours prior to pyloric ligation. Forty-eight hours before pyloric ligation, the backs of 15 pairs of rats were shaved and injected. One member of each pair received a 1.0 ml. subcutaneous injection containing *S. aureus* (10^9 CFU) and 30 mg. of sterile talc. The remaining member, the control animal, received a 1.0 ml. subcutaneous injection of normal saline and 30 mg. of sterile talc.

Fourteen hours before pyloric ligation, the backs of the remaining 15 pairs of rats were shaved and injected. One member of each pair received a 1.0 ml. subcutaneous injection containing *E. coli* (10^9 CFU) and 30 mg. of sterile talc. The remaining member received a 1.0 ml. subcutaneous injection of normal saline and 30 mg. of sterile talc.

Each animal was lightly anesthetized with ether immediately before pyloric ligation. Rectal temperature was recorded with a

Accepted for publication August 12, 1974.

Reprint requests: W. C. Butterfield, M.D., Division of Surgery, St. Mary's Hospital, 56 Franklin St., Waterbury, Conn. 06702.

telethermometer. The abdomen was shaved and, through a midline abdominal incision, the pylorus was isolated and ligated with No. 4-0 silk. The abdomen was closed and the incision covered with collodion. Following operation, food and water were withheld from the rats.

The rats in all groups were killed ten hours after pyloric ligation. The skin was incised and examined for pus; the abdomens were opened and the stomachs removed. A second observer, unaware of the identity of the group, opened each stomach along the greater curvature and examined it under the dissecting microscope for the presence of ulcers. The number of stomachs with ulcers and the number of ulcers per stomach 1.0 mm. or greater in size were recorded.

2. Gastric acid—pyloric ligation model. Sixty male rats were paired by weight. The rats were initially treated as in the preceding experiment except that the *S. aureus* group was injected earlier (60 hours before ligation) in an effort to establish a more virulent infection.

The 30 pairs of rats were killed 4 hours after ligation. The skins were incised and examined for pus; the abdomens were opened and the esophagus ligated with No. 4-0 silk to prevent loss of gastric contents. The stomachs were removed, washed in normal saline, and carefully dried. A nick was made in the wall of each stomach along the greater curvature and the gastric contents were filtered through gauze to remove saliva and detritus. The volume of gastric juice from each stomach was measured and the pH determined with a Beckmann pH meter. The stomachs were then examined for the presence of ulcers and the number of ulcers greater than or equal to 1.0 mm. in diameter were recorded.

3. Gastric ulcers—restraint model. Fifty-one male rats were matched for weight and distributed equally in three groups. Food but not water was withheld from the animals 24 hours prior to restraint. The rats' backs were shaved and injected 22 hours prior to restraint. The control group received a 1.0 ml. subcutaneous injection of normal saline and 30 mg. of sterile talc. The two experimental groups received a subcutaneous injection of a 1.0 ml. solution containing either *S. aureus* (10^9 CFU) or *E. coli* (10^9 CFU) and 30 mg. of sterile talc.

The rats were restrained as follows: each rat was lightly anesthetized with ether. Rectal temperatures were determined with a telethermometer. Ties of heavy twine were placed on the rats' front and back extremities and the rats were inserted into wire mesh envelopes. The envelopes were tacked to the tabletop along the perimeter of the rats' bodies. Care was taken not to compromise respiration. The ties around the extremities were tacked to the tabletop with sufficient tension to immobilize the legs. Six hours later the rats were killed. The abdomens were opened and explored for evidence of perforation and the stomachs were removed. The skins were incised to check for pus. The stomachs were opened along the greater curvature and examined for ulcers by an examiner unaware of the identity of the group.

In a second experiment, 51 rats were matched for weight and distributed equally in three groups. This experiment was identical to the preceding experiment except that the group receiving *S. aureus* was injected 48 hours prior to restraint and the group receiving *E. coli* was injected 12 hours prior to restraint. In addition, the rats were restrained for 10 hours. The changes in time from injection to restraint were made to increase the infection in the *S. aureus* group which had not appeared to be very ill and to lessen the infection in the *E. coli* group which had appeared to be severely ill. The period of restraint was lengthened to increase the number of ulcers.

RESULTS

Pus was present in all animals on gross examination, with considerably greater quantities observed in the *S. aureus* group.

A statistically significant elevation in rectal temperature was observed in the *E. coli* experimental group when measured 18 hours following injection. However, no statistically

Table I. *Effect of* **E. coli** *on frequency of ulcers—pyloric ligation model*

Treatment	10 hours of pyloric ligation beginning 14 hours after injection		4 hours of pyloric ligation beginning 14 hours after injection	
	Stomachs with ulcers (%)	Mean number of ulcers ≥ 1.0 mm.	Stomachs with ulcers (%)	Mean number of ulcers ≥ 1.0 mm.
Control	66.6*	9.4†	73.3‡	3.2§
E. coli	14.4‖	0.78	13.3	0.13

$*\chi^2 = 8.19$, df = 1, p = 0.005.
†t = 2.75, df = 27, p = 0.01.
‡$\chi^2 = 10.6$, df = 1, p = 0.005.
§t = 2.34, df = 14, p = 0.05.
‖One animal died prior to pyloric ligation.

Table II. *Effect of* **S. aureus** *on frequency of ulcers—pyloric ligation model*

Treatment	10 hours of pyloric ligation beginning 48 hours after injection		4 hours of pyloric ligation beginning 60 hours after injection	
	Stomachs with ulcers (%)	Mean number of ulcers ≥ 1.0 mm.	Stomachs with ulcers (%)	Mean number of ulcers ≥ 1.0 mm.
Control	80.0	13.4	26.6*	0.13
S. aureus	80.0	19.1	40.0	1.46

*One animal died following pyloric ligation.

Table III. *The effect of* **E. coli** *on the pH and total acid of gastric juice*

Treatment	Mean pH	Mean total acid (moles)
Control	1.7	10.5×10^{-5}
E. coli	2.3*	1.93×10^{-5}†

*t = 4.7, df = 14, p = 0.001.
†t = 5.7, df = 14, p = 0.001.

Table IV. *The effect of* **S. aureus** *on the pH and total acid of gastric juice*

Treatment	Mean pH	Mean total acid (moles)
Control	1.7	11.07×10^{-5}
S. aureus	1.6	8.45×10^{-5}

significant difference in rectal temperatures was observed between the group receiving *S. aureus* and the controls.

1. Gastric ulcers—pyloric ligation model. Ulcers in the pyloric ligation model were confined to the forestomach. Statistically significant decreases in both the number of stomachs with ulcers and the mean number of ulcers equal to or greater than 1.0 mm. in length were observed in the experimental groups which received *E. coli* when compared with the control groups (Table I). No statistically significant differences were noted between the experimental groups which received *S. aureus* and the control groups (Table II).

2. Gastric acid—pyloric ligation model. Both a statistically significant increase in pH of the gastric juice and a statistically significant decrease in the total acid (hydrogen ion content), a value derived by multiplying the antilog of the pH by the volume of the gastric juice, was observed in the group which received *E. coli* when compared to the control group (Table III). No difference was observed in the pH of the gastric juice or the total acid between the control group and the group which received *S. aureus* (Table IV).

3. Gastric ulcers—restraint model. Perforation of the stomach was not observed in the restraint model. Gastric ulcers in this model were confined to the glandular region of the stomach. The number of stomachs with ulcers was less in the *E. coli* group, but the difference was not statistically significant. No statistically significant difference was observed in the number of stomachs with ulcers or in the mean number of ulcers greater than or equal to 1.0 mm. in diameter between control and experimental groups (Tables V and VI).

Table V. *Effect of* **E. coli** *on frequency of ulcers—restraint model*

Treatment	6 hours of restraint 22 hours after injection		8 hours of restraint 12 hours after injection	
	Stomachs with ulcers (%)	Mean number of ulcers ≥ 1.0 mm.	Stomachs with ulcers (%)	Mean number of ulcers ≥ 1.0 mm.
Control	41.2*	0.18	23.5‡	0.12
E. coli	26.6†	0.20	5.9	0.06

*One animal died during restraint.
†Two animals died prior to restraint, five animals died during restraint.
‡Two animals died during restraint.

Table VI. *Effect of* **S. aureus** *on frequency of ulcers—restraint model*

Treatment	6 hours of restraint beginning 22 hours after injection		8 hours of restraint beginning 48 hours after injection	
	Stomachs with ulcers (%)	Mean number of ulcers ≥ 1.0 mm.	Stomachs with ulcers (%)	Mean number of ulcers ≥ 1.0 mm.
Control	41.2*	0.18	23.5†	0.12
S. aureus	35.3‡	0.35	23.5	0.24

*One animal died during restraint.
†Two animals died during restraint.
‡One animal died during restraint.

DISCUSSION

Although many clinical series suggest an etiological role for sepsis in the formation of stress ulcerations, there are few experimental attempts to elucidate this apparent relationship, and many of the early experimental projects are poorly controlled and have other obvious defects. In 1857 Lebert[21] noted gastric ulceration in a dog after injecting pus intravenously. In 1916 Rosenow[26] caused gastric and duodenal ulcers in animals by the intravenous injection of streptococci cultured from the depths of human peptic ulcers but did not obtain results with cultures of other bacteria. An attempt by Saunders[28] to duplicate these studies was unsuccessful. More recently, Douglass, Falk, and La Veen[13] increased the incidence of perforated gastroduodenal ulceration in hypersecreting guinea pigs infected with coagulase-positive staphylococci. An *E. coli* group had no effect. Howe, Wigglesworth, and Porell[18] produced wound infections in dogs and noted a significant rise in gastric secretion compared to the controls with clean wounds. A disconcerting finding in this study was the continued hypersecretion of some of the dogs for weeks after the infections were healed. Hartman[17] produced ulcers in dogs with 50 to 60 percent burns and reported an incidence of 78 percent acute ulceration. Treatment with penicillin reduced the incidence of ulceration to 23 percent.

Two recent studies, though not dealing with sepsis, suggest a possible role for bacteria or bacterial products in the production of stress ulcers. Rosoff and Goldman,[27] using a restraint rat model, demonstrated a decrease in acute gastric ulcerations when the rats were pretreated with oral polymyxin B and the coliform flora in the feces was decreased. Nance, Kaufman, and Batson,[24] using a similar restraint rat model, found that germ-free rats had a marked reduction in the incidence and severity of gastric ulceration compared to either rats with a normal gastrointestinal flora or germ-free rats contaminated with normal fecal flora. Feeding neomycin to rats with a normal flora reduced the incidence of ulcerations. Neomycin had no effect on gastric ulceration in the germ-free animals. The authors concluded that bacterial factors appeared to play a significant role in the pathogenesis of stress ulcers. The observations of Einheber and associates[14] are opposite to the results of this study. They studied the incidence of stress ulcers in mice with 35 percent body surface burns and were unable to find any difference in the incidence of ulcerations between the germ-free and "conventionalized" (multicontaminated, formerly germ-free) mice. Since some of the germ-free animals died within a day of burning from ulcer complications, the authors felt that bacteria could not be implicated.

It was obvious from a review of the literature that only a few recent experiments deal directly with the association of sepsis and stress ulceration. The original purpose of our study was to confirm the observations of Douglass, Falk, and La Veen[13] that subcutaneous infection increased the incidence of ulcers. We did not feel, however, that the histamine-stimulated guinea pig was the best animal model to use. We chose the restraint rat model instead, since, as noted by Brodie,[8] this model appears to mimic the stress ulcerations seen in man. The ulcers are superficial, gastric, multiple, and lack an inflammatory component. The pyloric ligation model was used in order to study gastric secretion, since it is difficult to quantitate acid in the restraint model.

Our results differed from the Douglass study in two ways. First, the significant changes occurred with the *E. coli* group and not with the *S. aureus* group. Second, the changes were opposite to those observed by Douglass. The *E. coli* group had significantly *fewer* ulcers in the pylorus-ligated rats and fewer ulcers, although not of statistical significance, in the restraint rats. Total hydrogen ion content was also significantly decreased in the *E. coli* group. The decrease in acid secretion might explain the decrease in ulceration in the *E. coli* group.

The lack of a decrease in acid in the *S. aureus* group remains to be explained. Both groups were obviously infected, as judged by the presence of pus in the wounds at the time of death. The *E. coli* group was sicker than the *S. aureus* group and had loose stools, but the outstanding difference between the groups was the temperature response to the infection. The *E. coli* group was febrile and the *S. aureus* group was not. A review of the literature supplied a possible explanation. Indeed, as far back as 1833, William Beaumont[4] had written:

> "In febrile diathesis or predisposition from whatever cause . . . the villous coat becomes red and dry, at other times pale and moist and loses the smooth and healthy appearance; the secretions become greatly vitiated, greatly diminished, or entirely suppressed, and mucous coat scarcely perceptible, the follicles flat and placcid, with secretions insufficient to protect the nervous papillae . . . . When there are corresponding symptoms of disease, as dryness of the mouth, thirst, accelerated pulse, etc., no gastric juice can be extracted, not even in the application of alimentary stimulus . . . . "

Since Beaumont's observations, several other investigators have verified the inhibitory effect of fever on gastric secretion. Berglund and Chang[6] compared patients with fever caused by typhoid, paratyphoid, tuberculosis, bronchopneumonia, lung abscess, and cirrhosis of the liver with patients with intestinal diseases without fever. Achlorhydria was found in all the febrile cases and in none of the afebrile ones. In a similar study of 106 febrile patients tested by the histamine method of gastric analysis, Chang[10] found an average decrease of gastric acidity to one third of normal. A third of the patients, about eight times the normal incidence, showed achlorhydria. The decrease in gastric function was proportional to the height of the fever. Ninety percent of the patients recovered normal gastric function soon after the disappearance of the fever. In a clinical study of gastric analyses done on 325 patients with tuberculosis, Kruger,[20] reported that the incidence of achlorhydria rose with the increase in degree of fever. While only 17 percent of those with temperatures below 100.5° F. were achlorhydric, 50 percent of those over 102° F. were achlorhydric. It would appear that the temperature elevation and not the infection is important since gastric acidity has also been shown to be depressed by the administration of pyrogenic killed bacterial products as well.[3, 10, 22, 23, 30, 31] Indeed, an elevation of the temperature by physical means alone seems effective. Meyer, Cohen, and Carlson,[23] using Pavlov pouches in dogs, were able to depress gastric secretion by elevating the temperature 2 to 4° F. by enclosing them in a hot box. Bandes, Hollander, and Bierman[2] demonstrated similar results on man using a heating cabinet. In both experiments the effects were transitory and disappeared with the return of the temperature to normal. In our experiments the inhibitory effect of *E. coli* infection, which raised the temperature, and the lack of any effect with *S. aureus* infection, which did not elevate the temperature, fits well with these observations from the literature. It is suggested that the decrease in the aggressive factor of acidity is the explanation for the decrease in ulcerations in the rats infected with *E. coli.*

We would not wish these findings to be interpreted as evidence that sepsis has no role in the development of stress ulcers. Other factors associated with sepsis but not studied in our experiment may be ulcerogenic.

REFERENCES

1. Altemeier, W. A., Fuller, W. S., and Mc Donough, J. J.: Sepsis and gastrointestinal bleeding, Ann. Surg. **175:** 759, 1972.
2. Bandes, J., Hollander, F., and Bierman, W.: The effect of physically induced pyrexia on gastric acidity, Gastroenterology **10:** 697, 1948.
3. Baume, P. E., Nicholls, A., and Baxter, C. H.: Inhibitation of gastric secretion by purified bacterial lipopolysaccharide, Nature (Lond.) **215:** 59, 1967.
4. Beaumont, W.: Experiments and observations on the gastric juice and the physiology of digestion, Boston, 1929, Harvard University Press, p. 107.
5. Beil, A. R., Mannix, H., and Beal, J. M.: Massive upper gastrointestinal hemorrhage after operation, Am. J. Surg. **108:** 324, 1964.
6. Berglund, H., and Chang, H. C.: Transitory character of the achlorhydria during fever demonstrated by the histamine test, Proc. Soc. Exp. Biol. Med. **26:** 422, 1929.
7. Blickenstaff, D., and Grossman, M. I.: A quantitative study of the reduction of gastric secretion associated with pyrexia, Am. J. Physiol. **160:** 567, 1950.
8. Brodie, D. A.: Stress ulcer as an experimental model of peptic ulcer disease, *in* Pfeiffer, C. M., editor: Peptic ulcer, Philadelphia and Toronto, 1971, J. B. Lippincott Co., pp. 71-81.
9. Brodie, D. A., and Hanson, H. M.: A study of the factors involved in the production of gastric ulcers by the restraint technique, Gastroenterology **36:** 353, 1960.
10. Chang, H. C.: Gastric secretion in fever and infectious diseases, J. Clin. Invest. **12:** 155, 1933.
11. Crawford, F. A., Hammon, J. W., and Shingleton, W. W.: The stress ulcer syndrome: A clinical and pathologic review, Am. J. Surg. **121:** 344, 1971.
12. Douglass, H. W., Jr., and La Veen, H. H.: Stress ulcers: A clinical and experimental study showing the roles of mucosal susceptibility and hypersecretion, Arch. Surg. **100:** 178, 1970.
13. Douglass, H. W., Jr., Falk, G. A., and La Veen, H. H.: Infection: A cause of acute peptic ulceration in hypersecreting animals, SURGERY **68:** 827, 1970.
14. Einheber, A., Wren, R. E., Porro, R. F., et al.: Curling's ulcer in the germ free mouse, Nature **214:** 298, 1967.
15. Garvey, J. M., and Fogelman, M. J.: Septic peptic ulceration, J. Trauma **6:** 644, 1966.
16. Goodman, A. A., and Frey, C. F.: Massive upper gastrointestinal hemorrhage following surgical operation, Ann. Surg. **167:** 180, 1968.
17. Hartman, F. W.: Curling's ulcer in experimental burns. II. The effect of penicillin therapy, Ann. Surg. **121:** 54, 1945.
18. Howe, C. W., Wigglesworth, W. C., and Porell, W. J.: Gastric secretory responses to surgical stress and infection, Surg. Forum **2:** 34, 1952.
19. Kirtley, J., Scott, H. W., Sawyers, J., et al.: The surgical management of stress ulcers, Ann. Surg. **169:** 801, 1964.
20. Kruger, A. L.: Gastric acidity in pulmonary tuberculosis, Am. J. Dig. Dis. **10:** 111, 1943.
21. Lebert, H.: Traite d'anatomie pathologique générale et spéciale, Paris, 1857, J. B. Baillière et Fils, p. 537.
22. Mc Ginty, D. A., Wilson, M. L., and Rodney, G.: The ulcer inhibitory action of pyrogens, Proc. Soc. Exp. Biol. Med. **70:** 334, 1949.
23. Meyer, J., Cohen, S. J., and Carlson, A. J.: Contribution to the physiology of the stomach, XLVI. Gastric secretion during fever, Arch. Intern. Med. **21:** 354, 1918.
24. Nance, F. C., Kaufman, H. J., and Batson, R. C.: The role of the microbial flora in acute gastric stress ulceration, SURGERY **72:** 68, 1972.
25. Pruit, B. A., Jr., Foley, F. D., and Moncreif, J. A.: Curling's ulcer: A clinical-pathology study of 323 cases, Ann. Surg. **172:** 523, 1970.
26. Rosenow, E. C.: Causation of gastric and duodenal ulcer by streptococci, J. Infect. Dis. **19:** 333, 1916.
27. Rosoff, C. B., and Goldman, H.: Effect of the

intestinal flora on acute gastric stress ulceration, Gastroenterology **55:** 212, 1968.
28. Saunders, E. W.: The serologic and etiologic specificity of alpha streptococci of gastric ulcers: A bacteriologic study, Arch. Intern. Med. **45:** 347, 1930.
29. Shay, H., Komarov, S. A., Fels, S. S., et al.: A simple method for the uniform production of gastric ulceration in the rat, Gastroenterology **5:** 43, 1945.
30. Vanzant, F. R., and Snell, A. M.: The effect of injection of nonspecific protein on the pain of ulcer and on gastric secretion: A clinical and experimental study, J. Clin. Invest. **11:** 647, 1932.
31. Wyllie, J. H., Limbosch, J. M., and Nyhus, L. M.: Inhibition of gastric acid by bacterial lipopolysaccharide, Nature **215:** 879, 1967.

Uveitis and vitiligo associated with BCG treatment for malignant melanoma

Robert C. Donaldson, M.D., Samuel A. Canaan, Jr., M.D., Robert B. McLean, M.D., *and* **Lauren V. Ackerman, M.D.,** *St. Louis, Mo.*

Uveitis and vitiligo developed in two patients undergoing treatment with bacillus Calmette-Guerin (BCG) for malignant melanoma. Both patients are living and well after 33 and 32 months of nonspecific immunotherapy. To explain this unusual response, we propose that BCG (and possibly isoniazid) may be capable of augmenting a cytotoxic autoimmune reaction directed toward melanin-producing cells in certain patients with melanoma. Close parallels between the clinical course of our patients and two probable autoimmune diseases, the halo nevus and the Vogt-Koyanagi-Harada syndrome, are discussed in support of this theory.

From the Departments of Surgery, Ophthalmology, and Surgical Pathology, the Veterans Administration Hospital, and the Washington University School of Medicine, St. Louis, Mo.

Uveitis and vitiligo developed in two patients with metastatic melanoma treated postoperatively by multiple intradermal vaccinations with BCG* (bacillus Calmette-Guérin). Melanoma regressed in both patients, and they have maintained normal weight and activity during follow-up periods of 33 and 32 months, respectively.

Of great interest to us is the close parallel between the response of these patients and the clinical course of the halo nevus and the Vogt-Koyanagi-Harada syndrome. Both of the latter conditions are believed to be caused by activation of an autoimmune response.

METHODS

BCG was administered exclusively by intradermal injection in normal skin areas. A 0.1 c.c. aliquot of the standard dilution for tuberculosis vaccination, containing from 400,000 to 900,000 viable organisms, was given at each injection site in both patients. The number of injection sites used at any one time and the frequency of repeat vaccinations were decided on the basis of the growth status of the tumor and potential toxic complications from BCG in each individual patient. One patient received isoniazid, which may have played a role in his response.

CASE SUMMARIES AND RESULTS

Case 1. M. L., a 75-year-old Negro man, was admitted to the St. Louis Veterans Administration Hospital on July 23, 1969, for treatment of a black area beneath his right thumbnail, which had been increasing in size for several months. In addition, the patient complained of anorexia and a 30 pound weight loss developing in recent months. Biopsy of the mass beneath the right thumbnail revealed malignant melanoma, and on Aug. 18, 1969, the thumb was amputated. Gastrointestinal x-rays revealed a prepylôric gastric ulcer, which improved with conservative management. On Sept. 10, 1969, a right axillary dissec-

Accepted for publication August 12, 1974.

Reprint requests: Robert C. Donaldson, M.D., Surgical Service, Veterans Administration Hospital, St. Louis, Mo. 63125.

*Manufactured by Glaxo Laboratories, Ltd., Greenford, Middlesex, England; distributed by Eli Lilly & Co., Indianapolis, Ind.

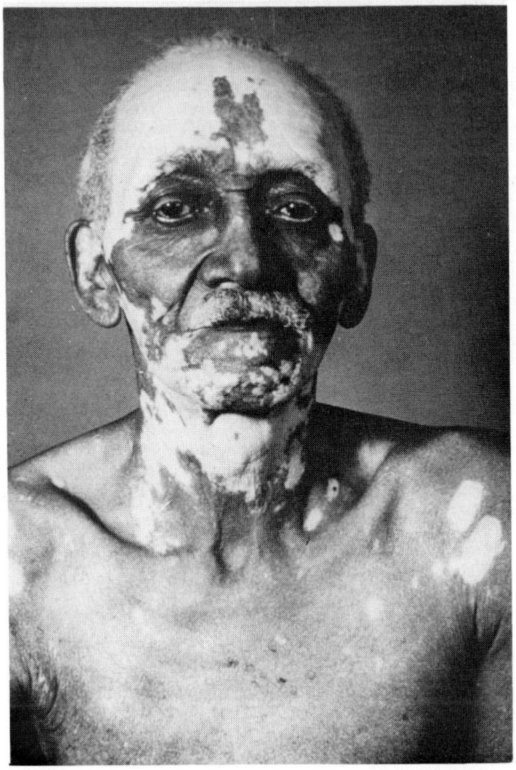

Fig. 1. Patient M. L. with vitiligo involving face and neck as well as circumscribed areas of otherwise normal skin surrounding each pair of BCG vaccination scars in both deltoid areas. Note a halo of depigmentation about an intradermal lesion in left supraclavicular area.

tion was done, revealing four lymph nodes containing malignant melanoma. The patient enjoyed good health until December, 1970, at which time he was readmitted with the complaint of a recurrent mass in the right axilla and progressive swelling of the right arm. Chest X-ray and laminograms revealed the development of multiple nodular densities in both lung fields compatible with metastatic melanoma.

Because of recent interest in isoniazid as a possible cancer chemotherapeutic adjuvant,[5, 6] a therapeutic trial was started on Jan. 8, 1971, at a dose of 400 mg. daily (6 mg. per kilogram). Examination of the patient 3 months later revealed more than a 90 percent decrease in edema of the right arm, a 50 percent decrease in size of the right axillary mass, and a definite decrease in size of the nodules in the lungs, documented by chest x-ray. On June 21, 1971, an intermediate-strength (5 TU) tuberculin test was read as mildly positive. A 0.1 c.c. aliquot of BCG was injected intradermally in each deltoid area. Within 7 days, both vaccination sites were necrotic and subsequently required 2½ months to heal. Isoniazid therapy has continued uninterrupted during the BCG vaccination periods and only recently has been discontinued (Nov. 18, 1973). At a follow-up examination on Sept. 27, 1971, all edema was noted to have disappeared from the right arm. The right axillary node mass had remained 50 percent smaller than at the onset of treatment and was estimated to be 2 cm. in greatest diameter. Chest x-ray revealed no increase in size or number of pulmonary nodules. In December of 1971, 6 months following vaccination with BCG, the patient noted the onset of small depigmented areas of the face and dorsum of the hands and the appearance of white patches of hair on his head. The depigmentation progressed until more than 50 percent of the facial skin was involved (Fig. 1). A one to 2 cm. halo of depigmentation developed in normal skin surrounding the scar of each BCG injection site in the skin over the anterior deltoid areas (Fig. 1). Also, clearly demonstrated in Fig. 1 is a halo nevus (? halo melanoma) in the left supraclavicular area. The patient was not checked for uveitis at this time because we were unaware of its possible association with the treatment schedule.

BCG vaccination was repeated in each deltoid area on March 3, 1972. At a follow-up on Jan. 2, 1973, the patient complained for the first time of progressively decreasing vision in both eyes and of the presence of floaters. He was referred to the Department of Ophthalmology. Visual acuity with maximum correction was 20/30 in the right eye and 20/25 in the left eye. Much of the hair of the scalp, eyebrows, and eyelashes was white (poliosis). The conjunctivae of both eyes were normal in appearance. A few pigmented keratic precipitates and a trace of cells (1+) and flare (haze) were present. The irides were normal except for moderate atrophy. Marked irregularity of the pupillary pigment fringe was noted. No synechiae were observed and the angles were normal. The lenses showed anterior pigment deposits and mild, posterior subcapsular opacities, and the vitreous was clear in both eyes. Mild pigment dispersion and clumping were present in both maculae, consistent with senile macular change. The remainder of the fundus was normal. The similarity between the clinical picture in this patient and the Vogt-Koyanagi-Harada syndrome was noted by the ophthalmologist at this time. No specific therapy was given; the patient's cells and flare cleared, and vision improved slowly over a 2 month period.

BCG vaccinations were repeated on April 17, 1973 (two sites). Six months later, in October, 1973, the patient again developed an acute flare-up of uveitis with marked impairment of vision. Funduscopic examination revealed multiple, small, yellow elevated hemispheric lesions of the choroid

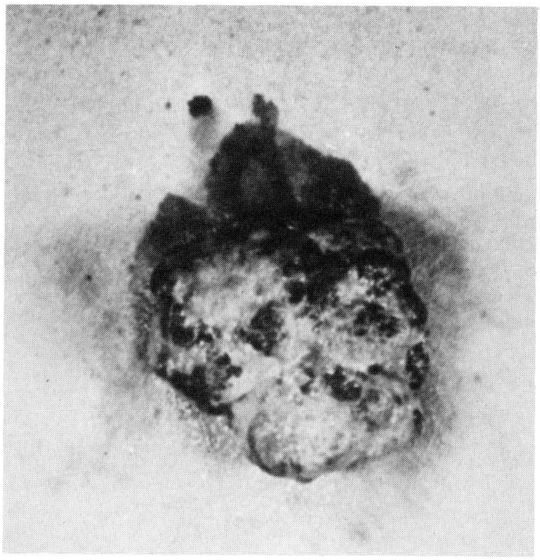

Fig. 2. Patient A. D. with exophytic primary lesion measuring 10 by 10 by 8 cm.

bilaterally. Fluorescein angiography of the fundus was compatible with the Vogt-Koyanagi-Harada syndrome. Isoniazid was discontinued for a period of 3 months, during which time visual acuity rapidly improved in contrast to the slow resolution encountered with first episode of uveitis.

Evidence of increase in size of pulmonary nodules and the right axillary mass was noted on March 7, 1974, and led to the decision to accept the risk of recurrence of uveitis and give a repeat vaccination with BCG.

Examination of the patient 6 weeks later on April 22, 1974, showed definite improvement. Chest x-ray revealed a decrease in size of some lesions and complete disappearance of others. The right axillary mass showed no progression, and the liver scan was negative. Vision was normal, but there was definite extension of vitiligo in several areas. The patient was asymptomatic and maintaining a normal weight of 142 pounds.

In summary, the patient was a Negro with postoperative recurrence of metastatic malignant melanoma, in whom the combination of uveitis and vitiligo, similar to that seen in the Vogt-Koyanagi-Harada syndrome, has been activated on two separate occasions, appearing each time approximately 6 to 9 months following vaccination with BCG. The melanoma was converted from an aggressive growth phase to partial regression, followed by a quiescent phase compatible with a normal life style for this patient, which continues after a 33 month follow-up.

Case 2. A. D., a 51-year-old Caucasian man was admitted to the St. Louis Veterans Administration Hospital on May 30, 1971, with a necrotic, exophytic mass, 10 cm. in diameter, at-

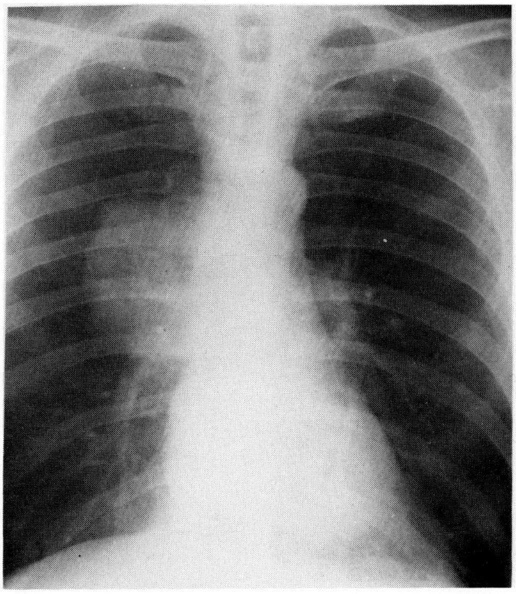

Fig. 3. Chest x-ray of patient A. D. showing large right hilar mass believed initially to be metastatic melanoma.

tached to the skin overlying the midportion of the right posterior rib cage (Fig. 2). It started as a small "black spot" one year prior to admission. Biopsy revealed malignant melanoma. Two enlarged nodes (2 by 3 cm.) were palpable in the right axilla. Chest x-ray was interpreted as showing a large right hilar mass (Fig. 3), believed to be metastatic melanoma, and the patient was considered incurable. An intermediate-strength (5 TU) tuberculin test was positive (12 mm.). Intradermal vaccination with BCG (four sites) was done on June 2, 1971. On June 4, 1971, the primary tumor mass was shaved off at the skin level by electrocautery excision as a palliative procedure, and the subsequent granulating wound was covered with a skin graft which took 100 percent. On July 20, 1971, a repeat chest x-ray was completely negative for hilar metastases (Fig. 4). Reevaluation of the chest x-rays indicated that the primary tumor mass itself had been responsible for casting the shadow in the area of the right hilum noted on the first chest x-ray. Consequently, a wide re-excision of the pigmented area surrounding the original mass (Fig. 5) was done on July 27, 1971. Histopathologic examination of the specimen (Fig. 6) revealed no microscopic evidence of melanoma, which was surprising in view of the large black deposits of pigment in the skin surrounding the primary site. A right axillary dissection was performed on Aug. 16, 1971, revealing the presence of metastatic melanoma in two lymph nodes (Fig. 7). Subsequent treatment was limited to periodic vaccinations with BCG on

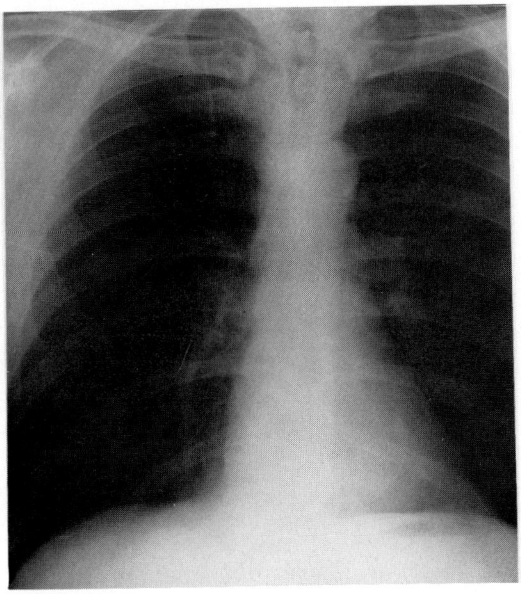

Fig. 4. Repeat chest x-ray of patient A. D. following palliative resection of the primary lesion showing the absence of the hilar shadow noted in Fig. 3.

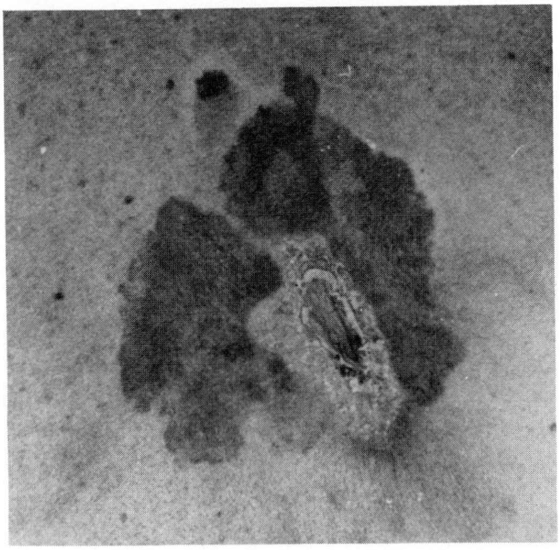

Fig. 5. Pigmented area surrounding the site of the primary lesion of patient A. D. Note healed skin graft in the center.

Oct. 27, 1971 (one site), June 14, 1972 (nine sites), Feb. 10, 1973 (two sites), July 18, 1973 (2 sites), and Jan. 16, 1974 (one site). A 0.1 c.c. aliquot of the standard dilution of BCG (Glaxo) was used at each site. No isoniazid has been given.

Vitiligo was first noted in July, 1972, after the patient had developed a deep suntan and was best visualized on the face and dorsum of the hands (Fig. 8). In January, 1973, approximately 6 months following the June 14, 1972, BCG vaccination at nine sites, the patient developed uveitis similar to that of patient M. L., but of less severity. For several weeks the patient had noticed floaters and gradually decreasing visual acuity. With correction, visual acuity was 20/20 in both eyes. A streak of white hair was noted in the right eyebrow, but the eyelashes remained normal. No conjunctival injection was present. A few pigmented keratic precipitates and cells (1+) and flare (haze) were present in both eyes, and both irides were atrophic. The pigmented pupillary fringe was irregular in the right eye and was completely replaced with a ring of white, diaphanous tissue in the left eye. One posterior synechia was present in the left eye and broke on dilatation. Iris nodules were not observed, and the angles were normal. Both lenses had coarse pigment deposits on their anterior surfaces. The vitreous, posterior pole, and periphery were normal bilaterally. The patient was given atropine and topical steroid therapy, which was followed by complete disappearance of his cells and flare within 3 weeks. Subsequent BCG vaccinations have not been associated with increased vitiligo or return of uveitis, as was true in Case 1. A possible explanation for the observance of uveitis on only one occasion may lie in the degree of stimulation with BCG. In this patient, it followed only the nine-site vaccination treatment. All other vaccinations were at one or two sites only. Also, the lesser degree of both uveitis and vitiligo in this patient, as compared to the previous patient, may reflect the absence of isoniazid in his treatment schedule.

Examination of the patient on April 18, 1974, approximately 32 months after the initial BCG vaccinations, revealed no palpable evidence of enlarged lymph nodes in the cervical, axillary, or inguinal area. Chest x-ray and liver scan were both negative. The patient weighed 184 pounds and was entirely asymptomatic.

DISCUSSION

Attempts to augment cell-mediated immune defense against human leukemia, melanoma, and squamous-cell carcinoma by BCG have been reported by Mathè and associates,[13] Morton and associates,[14] Gutterman and associates,[9] and Donaldson.[5, 6] Each group of workers has documented improvement in the status of certain cancer patients, and they emphasize the need for further investigation of BCG in the treatment of cancer.

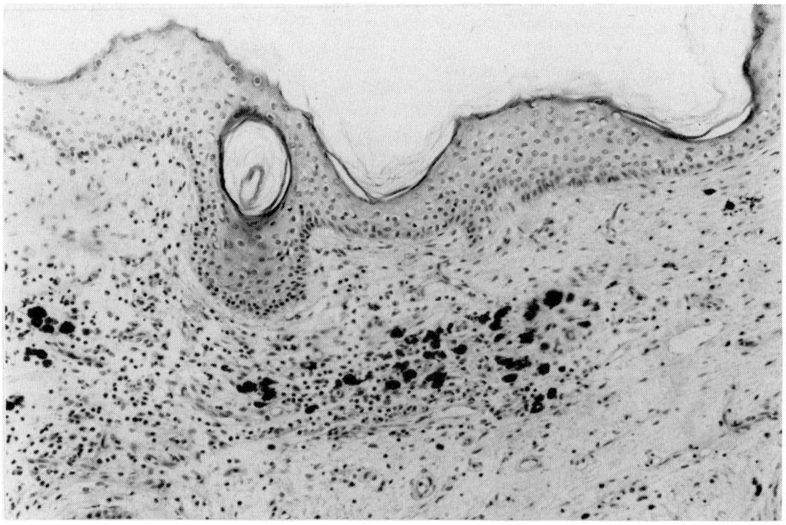

Fig. 6. Photomicrograph of the pigmented area of Fig. 5 following excision, showing no evidence of malignant melanoma. Small collections of melanin pigment are demonstrated by Fontana stain, and there is some evidence of lymphocytic infiltration. (Original magnification, ×120.)

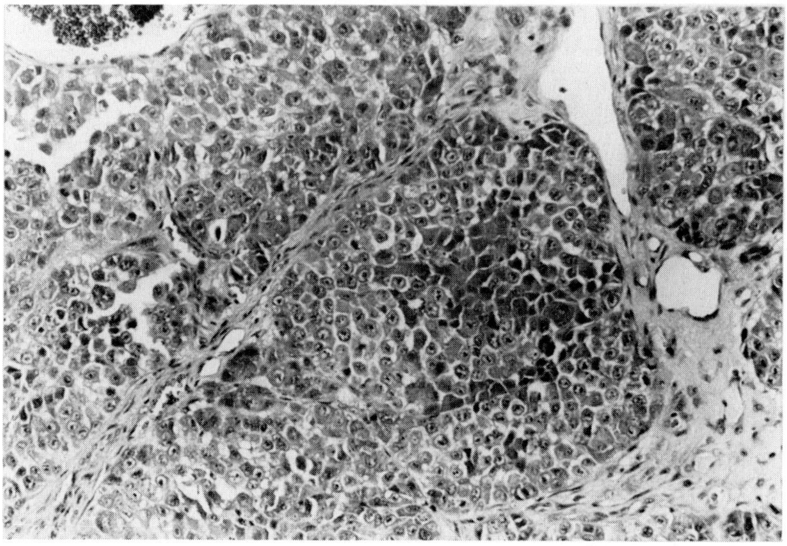

Fig. 7. Photomicrograph showing undifferentiated malignant melanoma in a lymph node from right axillary dissection, patient A. D. (Original magnification, ×300.)

The unique association of BCG with the development of uveitis and vitiligo, coupled with unexpected long-term survival which we have observed in two patients with malignant melanoma, has not, to our knowledge, been described previously. However, closely paralleling our observations in man is a report by Hornung and Krementz[10] demonstrating the development of vitiligo of the face in chimpanzees receiving immunizing doses of human melanoma. The authors conclude that the vitiligo is a manifestation of an autoimmune reaction. Of interest is the strikingly similar 6 to 8 month delay in appearance of vitiligo following initiation of BCG injections in man and melanoma injections in chimpanzees.

A uveitis-vitiligo syndrome has been re-

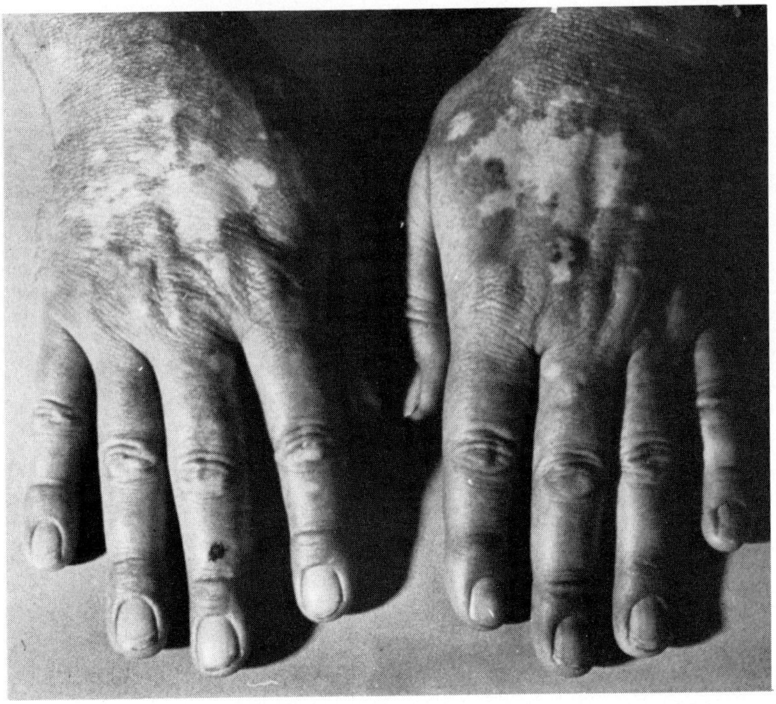

Fig. 8. Vitiligo on dorsum of hands of patient A. D.

ported in sympathetic ophthalmia, Harada's disease, and the Vogt-Koyanagi syndrome. Although signs of meningeal irritation and eighth nerve impairment have not been noted to date, the clinical courses of our patients do have several features in common with these clinical entities, suggesting that they may have similar etiologic mechanisms.

In 1949, Bruno and McPherson[1] reported four cases of Harada's disease and noted that the clinical picture overlaps that of the sympathetic ophthalmia and Vogt-Koyanagi syndrome. All three conditions may actually be variants of the same disease entity with hypersensitivity to uveal pigment playing a major role in the etiology. Woods and Little[16] and Friedenwald[8] demonstrated hypersensitivity to melanin in sympathetic ophthalmia. Coles[2] suggested that a hypersensitivity reaction rather than actual invasion by tubercle bacilli may be the cause of uveal tuberculosis. In favor of this theory is the work of Collins[3] wherein heat-killed tubercle bacilli were used as an adjuvant to uveal tissue to produce uveitis in guinea pigs. An infiltration of lymphocytes and epitheloid cells was noted, which resembles the histopathologic picture of sympathetic ophthalmia in man. In his controls, Collins was unable to demonstrate this reaction when guinea pig uvea or adjuvant was injected alone.

Depigmented halos about nevi and intradermal metastases of malignant melanoma, although rare in occurrence, do bear some resemblance to the clinical course of our patients. In 1965 Kopf, Morrill, and Silberberg[11] published their personal experience with leukoderma acquisitum centrifugum (halo nevus). The lesion consists of a sharply defined halo of total loss of pigment surrounding a densely pigmented nevus. Eventually the nevus disappears, leaving a disc-shaped area of depigmentation. More than one halo nevus may occur simultaneously while other nearby nevi may remain uninvolved. Two patients with malignant melanoma developed depigmented halos about intracutaneous deposits of tumor. The first patient developed a halo about the primary lesion. Subsequently, the disease progressed rapidly with death occurring 7 months after the initial observation. The second patient developed halos about cutaneous metastases of melanoma after 6 months of chemotherapy with actinomycin, mitomycin C, mephalan, vinblastine, mithramycin, and streptonigrin. The disease progressed more slowly, leading to death 3 years after onset. In 1968 Wayte and Helwig[15] gave a detailed clinicopathologic report on a series of 108 halo nevi. The nevi are usually compound and infiltrated with lymphocytes and histiocytes, and the halo area contains dopa-negative clear cells in the epidermis. By electron microscopy these cells are identified as Langerhans cells. In 1973 Epstein and associates[7] reported on the development of multiple halo nevi in five patients following the removal of primary malignant melanomas. They conclude that halo nevi are probably caused by an immune reaction to melanoma antigens. Lewis and Copeman[12] postulated that halo nevi may actually represent a stage of malignant melanoma undergoing immunologic rejection. Normally, in most individuals, the immunologic surveillance system rejects the melanoma before it becomes visible, thus accounting for the rarity of halo nevi.

In our experience, uveitis and vitiligo have been associated with BCG injections only with melanoma. Approximately 2,600 intradermal injections of BCG have been given over a period of 2½ years to 155 patients with a wide variety of cancers other than malignant melanoma. This group consisted of 129 Caucasian and 26 Negro patients, and, so far, none has complained of visual difficulties or developed vitiligo. Only one serious complication has been encountered in this series of patients receiving BCG. A patient developed a high fever 24 hours following a routine vaccination with BCG at four sites simultaneously. BCG septicemia, although unproved by blood culture, was suspected. The patient recovered rapidly following treatment with isoniazid at 5 mg. per kilogram for 10 days.

Since isoniazid is known on rare occasions to activate the autoimmune disease, systemic lupus erythematosus,[4] it is interesting to speculate on the possible effect of this drug on the clinical course of patient M. L. He received isoniazid as the only treatment for 5½ months prior to the first vaccination with BCG, during which time there was partial regression of the melanoma, well documented by physical examination and chest x-ray. Following the first vaccination with BCG, this patient developed more extensive uveitis and vitiligo than did patient. A. D., who had not received isoniazid. Six months following the second BCG vaccination, patient M. L. developed a second episode of severe uveitis which cleared within one week after discontinuance of isoniazid. Perhaps isoniazid deserves further study as a possible adjuvant to immunotherapy of malignant melanoma.

The foregoing observations suggest the possibility that uveitis and vitiligo, plus excellent long-term regression of malignant melanoma, occurring in our patients may represent a cytotoxic autoimmune reaction augmented by BCG (and ? isoniazid) and directed toward melanin-producing cells. As of April 22, 1974, both patients were living and well 33 and 32 months, respectively, after onset of treatment.

ADDENDUM

During the past year, isoniazid combined with multiple intradermal vaccinations with BCG (Glaxo) has been given to three additional patients with malignant melanoma. At the onset of treatment all had histologic proof of metastatic melanoma and clinical evidence of progressive disease either in the lungs, liver, or subcutaneous nodules. A 31-year-old woman continues to respond after 4½ months with complete regression of all measurable disease, relief of back pain, return of appetite, and a 10 pound gain in weight. Two men, 50 and 43 years of age, had partial or complete regressions of individual lesions lasting 9 and 3 months, respectively. Uveitis and vitiligo have not, as yet, been detected in these patients.

In all five of our patients, there is a definite correlation between intensity of local inflammatory response to BCG and the degree and duration of regression of melanoma. The best regressions are maintained in patients who continue to show intense local reactions to BCG at the intradermal vaccination site.

REFERENCES

1. Bruno, M. G., and McPherson, S. D., Jr.: Harada's disease, Am. J. Ophthalmol. **32:** 513, 1949.
2. Coles, R. S.: Uveitis associated with systemic diseases, Surv. Ophthalmol. **3:** 377, 1963.
3. Collins, R. C.: Experimental studies on sympathetic ophthalmia, Am. J. Ophthalmol. **32:** 1687, 1949.
4. Delepierre, F., Rullière, R., and Coury, C.: Systemic lupus erythematosus and lupus-like syndrome. A rare complication of prolonged treatment with isoniazid and other anti-tuberculosis agents concerning two new cases, Rev. Tuberc. Pneumol. (Paris) **35:** 397, 1971.
5. Donaldson, R. C.: Methotrexate plus bacillus Calmette-Guérin (BCG) and isoniazid in the treatment of cancer of the head and neck, Am. J. Surg. **124:** 527, 1972.
6. Donaldson, R. C.: Chemoimmunotherapy for cancer of the head and neck, Am. J. Surg. **126:** 507, 1973.
7. Epstein, W. L., Sagebeil, R., Spitler, L., et al.: Halo nevi and melanoma, J. A. M. A. **225:** 373, 1973.
8. Friedenwald, J. S.: Notes on allergy theory of sympathetic ophthalmia, Am. J. Ophthalmol. **17:** 1008, 1934.
9. Gutterman, J. U., Mavligit, G., McBride, C., et al.: Active immunotherapy with BCG for recurrent malignant melanoma, Lancet **1:** 1208, 1973.
10. Hornung, M. O., and Krementz, E. T.: Specific tissue and tumor responses of chimpanzees following immunization against human melanoma, SURGERY **75:** 477, 1974.
11. Kopf, A. W., Morrill, S. D., and Silberberg, I.: Broad spectrum of leukoderma acquisitum centrifugum, Arch. Dermatol. **92:** 14, 1965.
12. Lewis, M. G., and Copeman, P. W. M.: Halo nevus—a frustrated malignant melanoma? Br. Med. J. **1:** 47, 1972.
13. Mathé, G., Amiel, J. L., Schwarzenberg, L., et al.: Active immunotherapy for acute lymphoblastic leukemia, Lancet **1:** 697, 1969.
14. Morton, D. L., Eilber, F. R., Malmgren, R. A., et al.: Immunological factors which influence response to immunotherapy in malignant melanoma, SURGERY **68:** 158, 1970.
15. Wayte, D. M., and Helwig, E. B.: Halo nevi, Cancer **22:** 69, 1968.
16. Woods, A. C., and Little, M. F.: Uveal pigment—hypersensitivity and therapeusis, Arch. Ophthalmol. **9:** 200, 1933.

Effect of sera obtained from normal and partially hepatectomized rats and patients on the growth of cells in tissue culture

Achilles A. Demetriou, M.D., Eli Seifter, Ph.D., *and* **Stanley M. Levenson, M.D.,** *Bronx, N. Y.*

The effect of posthepatectomy and normal rat or human serum on cultured cells derived from rat hepatocytes was studied. Hepatectomies (70 percent), sham hepatectomies, and unilateral nephrectomies were performed in rats, and serum obtained 24 hours later was added to the culture medium. Addition of serum (5 and 10 percent) from hepatectomized rats caused considerable stimulation of cell growth; this effect was not altered when serum from rats which underwent hepatectomy and unilateral nephrectomy was added to the medium. Serum from normal, sham-hepatectomized or unilaterally nephrectomized rats produced no effect on cell growth. Similarly, serum from normal human beings or from a patient who had undergone a negative laporotomy following trauma produced no effect. In contrast, serum (5 and 10 percent) from a man 14 days following 75 percent hepatectomy done because of liver injury stimulated cell growth considerably. Initial attempts to isolate the stimulating factor revealed that the active compound(s) is entirely filtrable through cellophane membrane and has molecular weight (MW) of less than 12,000. We conclude: (1) normal serum does not contain an inhibitor of cell growth, (2) a factor stimulating cell growth in vitro is present in the serum of rats and man following partial hepatectomy, and (3) this stimulating factor has a MW of less than 12,000.

From the Departments of Surgery and Biochemistry, Albert Einstein College of Medicine, Bronx, N. Y.

LIVER REGENERATION is an important biological phenomenon. The specific regulatory stimulus for liver regeneration remains unknown. It has been proposed that (1) a factor appears in the serum of hepatectomized animals which stimulates liver regeneration; (2) a factor is present in the serum of normal rats which inhibits regeneration; following hepatectomy the concentration of this factor falls, permitting liver regeneration; and (3) both (1) and (2) are true. Further, the presence of certain modifying factors, i.e., factors which modify the rate of liver regeneration but are not in themselves fundamental to liver regeneration, have been implicated. The purpose of the experiment reported in this paper was to clarify some aspects of these matters.

Supported in part by Army Medical Research and Development Command Contract DADA-17-70-C to the Albert Einstein College of Medicine, and Research Career Award 5 K06 GM 14, 208 (S. M. Levenson) from the National Institutes of Health.

Accepted for publication August 12, 1974.

Reprint requests: Achilles A. Demetriou, M.D., Rm. 744, Forchheimer Bldg., Albert Einstein College of Medicine, 1300 Morris Park Ave., Bronx, N. Y. 10461.

MATERIALS AND METHODS

Male Long Evans rats (250 to 300 grams) obtained from the Charles River Breeding Laboratories, Wilmington, Mass., were used. Hepatectomies (70 percent) were performed according to the technique described by Higgins and Anderson[10] under light ether anesthesia. Sham hepatectomies consisted of an

Table I. *The effect of supplementation of Eagle's basal medium with several concentrations of fetal calf serum (FCS), normal rat serum, and normal human serum on the growth of cells in vitro**

Supplement to basal medium (%)	No. of flasks	Day 3	Day 4	Day 5	Day 6
No FCS	10	7.0† ± 0.1	9.5† ± 0.3	10.0† ± 0.3	24.0† ± 0.7
2.5 FCS	10	4.6† ± 0.2	12.0† ± 0.6	28.0† ± 1.3	33.0† ± 0.7
5.0 FCS	10	14.0† ± 1.4	19.0† ± 0.8	38.0† ± 1.0	64.0† ± 1.2
10 FCS	10	63.0 ± 1.1	160.0 ± 1.7	278.0 ± 4.8	244.0 ± 5.9
10 FCS 10 normal rat serum	10	70.0 ± 0.9	121.0 ± 1.7	205.0 ± 4.2	270.0 ± 6.5
10 FCS 5.0 normal rat serum	10	67.0 ± 1.3	135.0 ± 2.7	243.0 ± 6.5	269.0 ± 5.6
10 FCS 1.0 normal rat serum	10	45.0 ± 1.2	160.0 ± 4.2	249.0 ± 5.9	230.0 ± 4.9
10 FCS 10 normal human serum	10	52.0 ± 2.1	152.0 ± 6.4	176.0† ± 8.2	232.0 ± 7.7
10 FCS 5.0 normal human serum	10	48.0 ± 1.4	167.0 ± 5.6	249.0 ± 7.8	260.0 ± 6.4
10 FCS 1.0 normal human serum	10	55.0 ± 2.2	143.0 ± 4.0	224.0 ± 5.1	256.0 ± 5.9

*Results are expressed as number of cells $\times 10^3 \pm$ S.E.

†$p < 0.01$, calculated using Student's t test for two independent means (10-percent FCS vs. each other experimental group).

abdominal incision plus gentle palpation of the liver. Some rats underwent 70 percent hepatectomy plus unilateral nephrectomy or nephrectomy alone. All rats were anesthetized lightly with ether 24 hours following operation and were exsanguinated by closed cardiac puncture. The blood was collected in sterile tubes. The blood of five rats of each group was pooled aseptically, allowed to clot for 2 to 3 hours at room temperature, and then the serum was obtained by centrifugation. The serum was kept frozen at –20° C. until used; in no case was the serum kept frozen for longer than 10 days.

Venous blood was drawn from patients 14 days following operation and processed in a similar way, but not pooled. Serum was obtained from the following patients: (1) a previously healthy 26-year-old man who underwent 75 percent hepatectomy and right nephrectomy because of a gunshot wound to the abdomen; (2) a 27-year-old previously healthy man who underwent right hepatic lobectomy because of metastatic colonic carcinoma of the liver; (3) a 44-year-old man, previously healthy, who underwent a right nephrectomy because of a penetrating stab wound to the right flank; (4) a 22-year-old woman previously in good health who underwent a negative laparotomy following blunt abdominal trauma; and (5) a healthy young man about 26 years of age.

Cell culture assay. E_1 cells derived from rat hepatocytes were used. The cells were grown in 250 ml. flasks (Falcon Plastics, Oxnard, Calif.) Eagle's minimal essential medium* supplemented with nonessential amino acids,* antibiotics,* and various concentrations of fetal calf serum* were used. The serum to be studied was added to the medium just prior to cell inoculation. The total volume of medium in each flask was 10 ml. and the initial cell inoculum was 20,000 cells. The cultured cells were maintained at 37°

*Grand Island Biological Co., Grand Island, N. Y.

Table II. *The effect of supplementation of Eagle's basal medium with various concentrations of hepatectomized rat and human serum on the growth of cells in vitro**

Supplement to basal medium (%)	*No. of flasks*	*Day 3*	*Day 4*	*Day 5*	*Day 6*
10 FCS	10	63.0 ± 1.1	160.0 ± 4.6	278.0 ± 4.8	244.0 ± 5.9
10 FCS 10 hepatectomized rat serum	10	188.0† ± 2.3	347.0† ± 2.0	634.0† ± 1.7	1,327† ± 8.1
10 FCS 5.0 hepatectomized rat serum	10	170.0† ± 1.2	271.0† ± 3.7	608.0† ± 1.3	1,201† ± 9.8
10 FCS 2.5 hepatectomized rat serum	10	146.0† ± 1.2	226.0† ± 4.1	547.0† ± 4.7	923.0† ± 6.1
10 FCS 1.0 hepatectomized rat serum	10	67.0 ± 1.5	128.0 ± 1.9	187.0† ± 7.7	259.0 ± 2.9
10 FCS 10 hepatectomized human serum	10	134.0† ± 2.1	195.0 ± 2.8	424.0† ± 8.0	904.0† ± 9.8
10 FCS 5.0 hepatectomized human serum	10	136.0† ± 2.8	190.0 ± 3.2	380.0† ± 4.5	825.0† ± 9.1
10 FCS 2.5 hepatectomized human serum	10	160.0† ± 1.9	255.0† ± 4.0	533.0† ± 9.3	806.0† ± 9.2
10 FCS 1.0 hepatectomized human serum	10	61.0 ± 1.2	169.0 ± 2.6	270.0 ± 3.9	218.0 ± 4.7

*Results are expressed as number cells × 10^3 ± S.E.
†$p < 0.01$, calculated using Student's t test for two independent means (10 percent FCS vs. each other experimental group).

C., in 5 percent CO_2; the medium was changed every 48 hours. The same specific medium was used to feed the cultures. At 3, 4, 5, and 6 days the cells were harvested with trypsin* and counted in a hemocytometer (Improved Neubauer, 0.10 mm. deep). Replicate counts (four) were performed on each flask.

Ultrafiltration. An initial volume of 20 ml. of serum was used. All filtrations were carried out at 4° C. Serum from normal controls or experimental groups was passed sequentially through three Millipore filters (Millipore Filter Corp., Bedford, Mass.); the pore diameters were: 0.8μ, 0.45μ, and 0.22μ. The filtered serum was then passed through a dialysis membrane (Seamless Cellulose Dialyzer Tubing) for 1½ hours in an ultrafiltration chamber (Republic Seitz Filter Corp., Milldale, Conn.). About one ml. remained unfiltered through each of the Millipore filters, while 2 ml. remained unfiltered through the dialysis membrane.

*Grand Island Biological Co., Grand Island, N. Y.

RESULTS

Table I shows that when fetal calf serum is added to the basal medium in concentrations varying from 2.5 to 10 percent, there is a proportional increase in the rate of cell multiplication. Table I shows also that addition of serum from normal rats or man in concentrations of 1.0 to 10 percent to medium containing 10 percent fetal calf serum neither inhibits nor stimulates cell growth significantly. In contrast, the addition of serum from partially hepatectomized rats or human beings (Table II) results in significant ($p < 0.01$) stimulation of cell growth with serum concentrations of 2.5 to 10 percent and no stimulation with 1.0 percent serum concentration. Table III shows that addition of serum from sham-hepatectomized rats does not affect the growth of the cells. Similar results were obtained when serum

Table III. *The effect of supplementation of Eagle's basal medium with various concentrations of serum from sham-hepatectomized rats and a patient who underwent a negative laparotomy on the growth of cells in vitro**

Supplement to basal medium (%)	No. of flasks	Day 3	Day 4	Day 5	Day 6
10 FCS	10	63.0 ± 1.1	160.0 ± 4.6	278.0 ± 4.8	244.0 ± 5.9
10 FCS 10 sham-operated rat serum	10	62.0 ± 1.4	120.0 ± 1.8	224.0 ± 2.1	241.0 ± 7.4
10 FCS 5.0 sham-operated rat serum	10	69.0 ± 1.7	134.0 ± 2.0	233.0 ± 1.4	267.0 ± 1.5
10 FCS 1.0 sham-operated rat serum	10	65.0 ± 1.2	111.0 ± 1.4	202.0† ± 1.9	236.0 ± 1.5
10 FCS 10 negative laparotomy human serum	10	60.0 ± 1.0	133.0 ± 1.5	209.0† ± 3.2	238.0 ± 4.5
10 FCS 5.0 negative laparotomy human serum	10	55.0 ± 1.2	124.0 ± 1.4	235.0 ± 5.0	248.0 ± 6.1
10 FCS 1.0 negative laparotomy human serum	10	67.0 ± 1.2	131.0 ± 1.6	256.0 ± 3.3	223.0 ± 6.0

*Results are expressed as number of cells × 10^3 ± S.E.

†$p < 0.01$, calculated using Student's t test for two independent means (10 percent FCS vs. each other experimental group).

Table IV. *Effect of supplementation of Eagle's basal medium with serum from nephrectomized or nephrectomized and hepatectomized rats and humans**

Supplement to basal medium (%)	No. of flasks	Day 3	Day 4	Day 5	Day 6
10 FCS	10	63.0 ± 1.1	160.0 ± 4.6	278.0 ± 4.8	244.0 ± 5.9
10 FCS 10 nephrectomized rat serum	10	54.0 ± 1.1	126.0 ± 2.7	255.0 ± 4.8	314.0 ± 4.4
10 FCS 10 nephrectomized and hepatectomized rat serum	10	145.0†‡	228.0†‡	413.0†‡	995.0†‡
10 FCS 10 nephrectomized human serum	10	61.0 ± 1.5	130.0 ± 2.8	226.0 ± 4.0	240.0 ± 7.0
10 FCS 10 nephrectomized and hepatectomized human serum	10	127.0†‡ ± 2.3	236.0†‡ ± 6.1	488.0†‡ ± 8.1	1,042†‡ ± 20.6

*Results are expressed as number of cells × 10^3 ± S.E.

† or ‡ $p < 0.01$, calculated using Student's t test for two independent means († 10 percent FCS vs. each other experimental group. ‡ Nephrectomized vs. nephrectomized and hepatectomized rat or human serum.)

from a patient who underwent a negative laparotomy following blunt abdominal trauma was added to the medium (Table III). The addition of serum from a rat or a patient with unilateral nephrectomy to the medium (Table IV) also had no significant effect on cell growth, but serum from rats or a patient who underwent partial hepatectomy and unilateral nephrectomy (Table IV) stimulated growth to a significant degree ($p < 0.01$) and to about the same extent as did serum from rats and patients undergoing hepatectomy alone.

The results of the Millipore filtration and ultrafiltration experiments indicate that none of the normal rat or human serum filtrates or ultrafiltrates had any effect on cell growth (Table V). In contrast, Table VI shows that filtrates 1 to 4 of hepatectomized (rat or human) serum significantly stimulate cell

Table V. *Effect of supplementation of Eagle's basal medium with serum fractions from normal rats and humans**†

Experimental conditions‡	*No of flasks*	*Day 3*	*Day 4*	*Day 5*	*Day 6*
Normal rat serum:					
Filtrate 1	10	66.0 ± 1.3	115.0 ± 2.4	250.0 ± 6.0	402.0 ± 2.1
Filtrate 2	10	60.0 ± 1.2	118.0 ± 9.9	208.0 ± 1.1	340.0 ± 2.1
Filtrate 3	10	68.0 ± 1.4	126.0 ± 1.8	235.0 ± 3.7	400.0 ± 2.9
Filtrate 4	10	54.0 ± 1.1	110.0 ± 2.3	244.0 ± 4.0	408.0 ± 7.6
Fraction 4a	10	69.0 ± 2.3	170.0 ± 5.2	259.0 ± 7.1	313.0 ± 9.0
Fraction 5	10	55.0 ± 1.1	123.0 ± 2.6	261.0 ± 7.1	328.0 ± 8.8
No supplement	10	68.0 ± 1.2	117.0 ± 2.4	273.0 ± 4.6	300.0 ± 2.0
Normal human serum:					
Filtrate 1	10	72.0 ± 3.1	130.0 ± 4.2	240.0 ± 5.0	358.0 ± 7.0
Filtrate 2	10	65.0 ± 2.5	110.0 ± 2.3	205.0 ± 5.1	343.0 ± 1.8
Filtrate 3	10	58.0 ± 1.5	125.0 ± 3.6	241.0 ± 5.5	316.0 ± 2.3
Filtrate 4	10	60.0 ± 1.6	118.0 ± 2.5	235.0 ± 4.7	300.0 ± 7.6
Fraction 4a	10	68.0 ± 2.4	130.0 ± 4.1	261.0 ± 7.3	370.0 ± 8.2
Fraction 5	10	64.0 ± 2.5	120.0 ± 3.6	249.0 ± 5.7	325.0 ± 8.0
No supplement	10	62.0 ± 1.1	133.0 ± 3.9	247.0 ± 5.2	400.0 ± 7.7

*Results are expressed as number of cells $\times 10^3 \pm$ S.E.

†$p < 0.01$, calculated using Student's t test for two independent means (no supplement group vs. each other group).

‡Basal medium, 10 percent FCS, and supplement as noted; filtrate and fraction concentration is 5 percent.

growth ($p < 0.01$) as does fraction 5, the ultrafiltrate ($p < 0.01$), but fraction 4A (residue of Millipore filtrate 4 remaining unfiltered through the dialysis membrane) does not affect cell growth.

DISCUSSION

Evidence suggesting the presence of a "stimulating" factor in the serum of hepatectomized rats was provided by Bucher, Scott, and Aub[1] in experiments with parabiotic rats; when partial hepatectomy was performed on one member of a parabiotic pair or on two members of parabiotic triplets, increased numbers of mitoses were found in the intact liver of the parabiont that had not undergone partial hepatectomy. Although Weinbren[17] confirmed this observation, Rogers, Shaka, and Pechet[13] failed to do so. Studies by Moolten and Bucher[12] of carotid-to-jugular crosscirculation of blood between partially hepatectomized and normal rats produced further evidence in support of humoral control; deoxyribonucleic acid (DNA) synthesis was stimulated in the normal partner when measured 20 hours after the beginning of the exchange at a rate of flow of 2 ml. per hour. Friedrich-Freksa and Zaki[5] reported an increase in the mitotic rate in livers of normal rats following the injection of serum from hepatectomized rats. However, other investigators reported contradictory results.[17]

Glinos[8] suggested that an inhibitor is present in normal rat serum which decreases following partial hepatectomy. In experiments performed in vitro, Glinos and Gey[9] showed that normal rat serum inhibited the growth of fibroblasts, whereas hepatectomized rat serum had a stimulating effect on cell growth. Dilution of plasma, accomplished by repeated plasmapheresis in normal rats, stimulated mitotic activity in the livers of these animals;[7] this was attributed to the dilution of a factor(s) which is normally present in the serum of the intact animals and which inhibits liver regeneration. Fluid restriction of hepatectomized rats inhibited hepatic mitotic activity;[7] this was attributed by Glinos to an increase in the concentration of the inhibitor in the serum. Glinos suggested that albumin was the inhibitory serum factor. Tissue-specific mitotic inhibitors named "chalones" by Bullough and Lawrence[2] have been demonstrated in a number of tissues. The best studied is the epidermal chalone. The chalone inhibits DNA synthesis by acting on the presynthetic G_1 phase.[3] Verly and his associates[16] have recently succeeded in isolating from rabbit liver (using ethanol precipi-

Table VI. *Effect of supplementation of Eagle's basal medium with serum fractions from hepatectomized rats and humans**

Experimental conditions‡	*No. of flasks*	*Day 3*	*Day 4*	*Day 5*	*Day 6*
Hepatectomized rat serum:					
Filtrate 1	10	151.0 ± 5.0	248.0 ± 6.7	504.0 ± 9.0	1,064 ± 9.7
Filtrate 2	10	169.0 ± 5.3	303.0 ± 6.8	567.0 ± 7.0	1,222 ± 19.5
Filtrate 3	10	148.0 ± 5.0	286.0 ± 6.7	529.0 ± 9.8	1,010 ± 18.4
Filtrate 4	10	150.0 ± 5.2	308.0 ± 6.9	627.0 ± 10.9	1,120 ± 15.5
Fraction 4a	10	66.0† ± 1.3	115.0† ± 2.4	238.0† ± 4.9	340.0† ± 2.2
Fraction 5	10	130.0 ± 2.0	241.0 ± 6.3	508.0 ± 10.0	1,000 ± 15.5
No supplement	10	62.0 ± 1.1	133.0 ± 2.7	247.0 ± 5.1	334.0 ± 2.1
Hepatectomized human serum:					
Filtrate 1	10	136.0 ± 2.3	251.0 ± 6.7	518.0 ± 9.5	1,100 ± 18.7
Filtrate 2	10	150.0 ± 5.2	327.0 ± 7.0	610.0 ± 12.0	1,215 ± 20.5
Filtrate 3	10	164.0 ± 5.2	310.0 ± 7.0	624.0 ± 10.1	1,130 ± 16.0
Filtrate 4	10	151.0 ± 5.3	296.0 ± 6.8	577.0 ± 11.0	1,000 ± 17.0
Fraction 4a	10	62.0† ± 2.2	130.0† ± 2.5	245.0† ± 5.2	392.0† ± 6.0
Fraction 5	10	120.0 ± 4.4	249.0 ± 6.5	572.0 ± 10.9	1,064 ± 17.6
No supplement	10	65.0 ± 1.3	127.0 ± 2.5	251.0 ± 5.3	387.0 ± 6.1

*Results are expressed as number of cells $\times 10^3 \pm$ S.E.

†All filtrates and fractions are significantly ($p < 0.01$) greater than the control (no supplement) except fractions 4a.

‡Basal medium, 10 percent FCS, and supplement as noted; filtrate and fraction concentration is 5 percent.

tation, G-50 Sephadex chromatography, and ultrafiltration) and concentrating 450 fold a liver chalone. They have shown that the hepatic chalone is a polypeptide of low molecular weight. The chalone activity was measured by the inhibition of DNA synthesis in liver slices taken from the remaining lobe of a subtotally hepatectomized rat 24 hours following hepatectomy.

Investigators who found a factor stimulating liver regeneration have made few attempts to isolate and chemically define this factor. Gentile, Ali, and Grace,[6] on the basis of enzymatic inhibition studies, suggested that ribonucleic acid (RNA) may be the stimulating factor present in serum. Wrba and Volm[19] suggested that liver regeneration may be the result of increased catalase levels in the serum following hepatectomy. Recently several investigators have stressed the importance of insulin and glucagon as factors which may regulate liver regeneration. Several investigators[18] used a rat preparation devoid of portal organs to study the effect of glucagon on liver regeneration. Partial hepatectomy in this preparation was followed by a delay in the peak DNA response (in the liver); infusion of glucagon restored the peak DNA response in time nearly to that of the control rats. Fisher and associates[4] demonstrated by use of extracorporeal crosscirculation that a humoral factor regulating liver regeneration does not arise from the liver remnant but rather is present in the portal blood. Other investigators[15] have performed experiments in which partial hepatectomy and selective resection of splanchnic organs was undertaken. These studies suggested that the "hepatotrophic" factor originates from the pancreas and/or the duodenum. Levi and Zeppa[11] demonstrated a fourfold increase in DNA synthesis in isolated rat livers, which were perfused with a blood-simulating suspension that had been previously circulated through an isolated regenerating liver. They interpreted their results as indicating that the liver itself is the site of origin of the "hepatotrophic" factor. Other investigators, however, failed to reproduce this experiment.[14]

The data reported in this study support the hypothesis that a "stimulating" factor is present in the serum of man and rats following partial hepatectomy. Increasing concentrations of serum from hepatectomized rats or man resulted in stimulation of cell growth in vitro. The presence of an "inhibitory" factor in the serum of normal human subjects or rats is not supported by our experiments since increasing concentrations of normal serum failed to inhibit cell growth as would be expected were an inhibitor present. Our results are contradictory to those obtained by Glinos and Gey,[9] who found that addition of increasing concentrations of serum from normal rats inhibited cell growth. Glinos and Gey, in their experiments, used very high concentrations of both control and experimental serum (20 and 50 percent); in addition, the system for estimating cell growth used by them was different from ours (they estimated fibroblastic outgrowth on glass, whereas in our experiments the cells were harvested with trypsin and counted in a hemocytometer). Another important difference from our experiment is that the culture medium was not renewed during the 6 day experimental period in Glinos' study.

Serum from normal rats or human patients who underwent unilateral nephrectomy had no effect on cell growth, whereas serum from hepatectomized and nephrectomized (unilateral) rats or patients behaved identically to the serum of rats or patients who underwent hepatectomy alone, suggesting that nephrectomy does not alter the effect of serum from hepatectomized rats on human beings on the growth of cells in vitro.

The results of our fractionation experiments show clearly that the stimulating factor present in serum following partial hepatectomy is ultrafiltrable and has a molecular weight of 12,000 or less. Further studies are under way to elucidate the chemical nature of this factor(s).

REFERENCES

1. Bucher, N. L. R., Scott, J. F., and Aub, J. C.: Regeneration of the liver in parabiotic rats, Cancer Res. **11:** 457, 1951.
2. Bullough, W. S., and Lawrence, E. B.: The control of epidermal mitotic activity in the mouse, Proc. R. Soc. Br. **151:** 517, 1960.
3. Elgjo, K.: Epidermal cell proliferation during the first 24 hours after injection of an aqueous skin extract (chalone), Virchows Arch. [Zellpathol.] **4:** 119, 1969.
4. Fisher, B., Szuch, B., Levine, M., et al.: A portal blood factor as the humoral agent in liver regeneration, Science **171:** 575, 1971.
5. Friedrich-Freksa, H., and Zaki, F. G.: Spezifische Mitose-Auslosung in normaler Rattenleber durch Serum von partiell hepatektomierten Ratten, Z. Naturforsch. **98:** 394, 1954.
6. Gentile, J. M., Ali, E., and Grace, J. T.: Effects of posthepatectomized rat sera on cultured cells, J. Surg. Oncol. **1:** 3, 1969.
7. Glinos, A. D.: Environmental feedback control of cellular growth, *in* Teir, H., and Rytomaa, T., editors: Control of cellular growth in adult organisms, New York, 1967, Academic Press, Inc.
8. Glinos, A. D.: The mechanism of liver growth and regeneration, *in* McElroy, W. D., and Glass, B., editors: The chemical basis of development, Baltimore, 1958, Johns Hopkins Press.
9. Glinos, A. D., and Gey, G. O.: Humoral factors involved in the induction of liver regeneration in the rat, Proc. Soc. Exp. Biol. Med. **80:** 421, 1952.
10. Higgins, G. M., and Anderson, R. M.: Experimental pathology of the liver; restoration of the liver of the white rat following partial surgical removal, Arch. Pathol. **12:** 186, 1931.
11. Levi, J. U., and Zeppa, R.: Source of the humoral factor that initiates hepatic regeneration, Ann. Surg. **174:** 364, 1971.
12. Moolten, F. L., and Bucher, N. L. R.: Regeneration of rat liver; transfer of humoral agents by cross circulation, Science **158:** 272, 1968.
13. Rogers, A. E., Shaka, J. A., Pechet, G., et al: Absence of a "humoral factor" affecting hepatic regeneration in parabiotic rats, Am. J. Pathol. **39:** 561, 1961.
14. Sera, Y., Neustein, H., Nicholson, M. O., et al.: Failure of perfusate passed through regenerating liver to increase DNA synthesis in cells of isolated perfused normal liver, Surg. Forum **24:** 386, 1973.
15. Sgro, J. C., Charles, A. C., Chandler, J. G., et al.: Site of origin of the hepatotrophic portal blood factor involved in liver regeneration, Surg. Forum **24:** 377, 1973.
16. Verly, W. G., Deschamps, Y., Pushpathadam, J., et al.: The hepatic chalone. I. Assay method for the hormone and purification of the rabbit liver chalone, Can. J. Biochem. **49:** 1376, 1971.
17. Weinbren, K.: Regeneration of the liver, Gastroenterology **37:** 657, 1959.
18. Whittemore, A. D., Kasuya, M., Fodor, P. B., et al.: Hepatic regeneration in the rat without portal organs, Surg. Forum **24:** 384, 1973.
19. Wrba, H., and Volm, M.: Depressive action of serum of partially hepatectomized rats on tumor cells in vitro, Eur. J. Cancer **3:** 143, 1967.

The hemodynamic response to positive end-expiratory ventilation in hypovolemic patients

Alden H. Harken, M.D., Murray F. Brennan, M.D., Beverly Smith, R.N., *and*
Ernest M. Barsamian, M.D., *Roxbury and Boston, Mass.*

Acutely ill patients can little afford the depressed cardiac output (CO) frequently associated with positive end-expiratory pressure (PEEP) ventilation. PEEP has occasionally, however, been recognized as improving CO. The purpose of this study was to describe the hemodynamic response of acutely ill patients to PEEP. In addition, we hoped to identify some parameter that might correlate with a patient's ability not only to tolerate, but even to augment CO in response to increased airway pressure. Hemodynamic and ventilatory parameters with and without PEEP were evaluated in 27 patients following cardiac operation. Preoperative left ventricular end-diastolic pressure (LVEDP) was 12.9 ± 1.1 mm. Hg (mean ± S.E.) in patients with improved CO on PEEP. In patients whose CO decreased with PEEP, LVEDP was 7.6 ± 1.1 mm. Hg. These values were significantly different ($p < 0.01$). Increased intrathoracic pressure (with PEEP), relative to extrathoracic resistance, may boost a failing left ventricle and augment CO. On hemodynamic grounds, no absolute contraindications to PEEP exist. If a patient appears to warrant PEEP to improve gas exchange, a trial of ventilation with PEEP will rapidly determine hemodynamic tolerance. It is reasonable to foresee a day when PEEP will be used routinely not only to improve gas exchange but also, in selected patients, to augment CO.

From the Division of Surgery, Veterans Administration Hospital, West Roxbury, Mass., and the Peter Bent Brigham Hospital, Harvard Medical School, Boston, Mass.

POSITIVE-PRESSURE breathing was first successfully accomplished 200 million years ago by the frog.[7] It was not until 25 years ago, however, that Otis and associates[21] and Cournand and associates[3] demonstrated the potentially deleterious effect of positive-pressure ventilation on cardiac output (CO). Guyton[9] subsequently showed that compensatory increase in peripheral venous tone was necessary to re-establish the positive gradient between extra- and intrathoracic veins essential for a stable CO. Similarly, Sykes, Adams, and Finlay[25] noted that hypovolemic dogs could sustain their CO in the face of positive end-expiratory pressure (PEEP) ventilation, while hypovolemic animals could not compensate and CO fell. Multiple groups[13, 18, 19] have equated an increase in airway pressure (especially with PEEP) with a decrease in CO. Conversely, for years several groups have recognized and utilized positive-pressure ventilation for its salutory hemodynamic[11] and hemostatic[15] effects. PEEP may offer a dramatic reduction in pulmonary shunting in many acutely ill patients. These patients are frequently the ones, however, who can least tolerate any change in CO. The controversy

Accepted for publication August 12, 1974.

Reprint requests: Major Alden H. Harken, MC, Division of Surgery, Department of the Army, Walter Reed Army Institute of Research, Walter Reed Army Medical Center, Washington, D. C. 20012.

Table I. *Decreased cardiac output in response to PEEP—Group A**

Patient	*Operation*	Δ *cardiac index* %	Δ *cardiac index* Cardiac index	Δ *blood volume* (%)	*FRC/TLC* (%)	*LVEDP*
R. M.	VR	–18	2.8 /2.3	–8	63	5
K. C.	CABG	–40	1.8 /1.1	–31	70	5
W. S.	VR	–33	1.9 /1.3	–22	55	8
E. R.	VR	–26	2.8 /2.1	–14	55	7
D. C.	CABG	–16	2.5 /2.1	–14	55	15
W. M.	CABG	–8	2.5 /2.3	–13	43	7
J. R.	CABG	–10	3.4 /3.1	–12	56	5
H. F.	CABG	–9	1.6 /1.4	–3	58	6
H. F.†	CABG	–13	3.0 /2.5	0	58	6
V. R.	VR	–28	3.0 /2.2	–2	56	0
R. B.	CABG	–14	2.8 /2.4	+5	62	13
K. B.	CABG	–35	2.6 /1.7	–25	61	7
K. B.†	CABG	–25	2.3 /1.7	–13	61	7
E. N.	VR	–19	2.7 /2.2	–15	60	15
Mean		–21	2.55/2.03	–12	58	7.6
Standard error		±2.7	0.13/0.14	±2.7	±1.6	±1.1

*VR: valve replacement; CABG: coronary artery bypass graft; Δ cardiac index: percent change (liters per square meter per minute); Δ blood volume: percent change (liters); FRC/TLC: ratio of functional residual capacity to total lung capacity; LVEDP: left ventricular and diastolic pressure (mm. Hg).

†Studied on first postoperative day.

over the hemodynamic effects of PEEP remains. This led us to investigate the hemodynamic alterations associated with PEEP. We reasoned that hypovolemic patients with compromised myocardial function following cardiac operation would be most responsive to increased airway pressure. Immediately following cardiac operation, patients characteristically have an expanded extracellular compartment but low circulating blood volume.[2] The purpose of this study was to describe the hemodynamic response of "high-risk" patients to PEEP. In addition, we hoped to identify some parameter that might predict a patient's ability not only to tolerate, but even to augment CO in response to increased airway pressure.

METHODS

Twenty-seven patients were randomly selected for study prior to cardiac operation. Sixteen patients were scheduled for coronary artery bypass grafts and 11 were scheduled for valve replacement. In all patients blood volume, functional residual capacity (FRC), total lung capacity (TLC), and resting left ventricular end-diastolic pressure (LVEDP) were measured preoperatively. Blood volume was measured with radioiodinated serum albumin. FRC and TLC were measured with the standard helium dilution technique.[1] Left ventricular pressure was measured during cardiac catheterization. Intraoperatively, arterial and central venous catheters were inserted. On return to the intensive care unit (ICU), patients were ventilated via endotracheal tubes with a volume-regulated ventilator.

Within one hour of arrival in the ICU, with the patient hemodynamically stable, arterial blood gases, blood volume, and dye-dilution CO were obtained. The expiratory tube of the ventilator was then placed under 10 cm. of water (end-expiratory pressure 10 cm. H_2O). Following 30 minutes of equilibration on continuous positive pressure, arterial blood gases and CO were repeated. All CO's were performed in duplicate.

Fourteen of these patients were restudied in exactly the same manner 16 to 20 hours later.

Five of the initial 27 patients served as controls. They followed exactly the same protocol but were ventilated without end-expiratory pressure. Twelve sets of CO's were determined on these patients at 30 minute intervals in the postoperative period.

Throughout the study period, arterial oxy-

Table II. *Less than 5 percent change in cardiac output in response to PEEP—Group B**

Patient	Operation	Δ cardiac index %	Δ cardiac index Cardiac index	Δ blood volume (%)	FRC/TLC (%)	LVEDP
J. R.†	CABG	−5	2.62/2.50	−6	56	15
W. M.†	CABG	−4	3.34/3.22	+15	43	7
G. O.†	CABG	0	0.83/0.83	−21	50	10
P. B.	VR	0	3.0 /3.0	−13	56	0
C. C.	CABG	+5	1.60/1.68	−2	64	10
J. M.	CABG	−4	2.13/2.05	−15	54	8
Mean		−1.3	2.25/2.21	−7	54	8.3
Standard error		±1.5	.38/ .36	±5	±2.8	±2.0

*VR: valve replacement; CABG: coronary artery bypass graft; Δ cardiac index: percent change (liters per square meter per minute); Δ blood volume; percent change (liters); FRC/TLC: ratio of functional residual capacity to total lung capacity; LVEDP: left ventricular end diastolic pressure (mm. Hg).

†Studied on first postoperative day.

Table III. *Increased cardiac output in response to PEEP—Group C**

Patient	Operation	Δ cardiac index %	Δ cardiac index Cardiac index	Δ blood volume (%)	FRC/TLC (%)	LVEDP
P. H.	CABG	+7	1.7 /1.8	−21	57	10
P. H.†	CABG	+11	2.2 /2.5	−7	57	10
D. C.†	CABG	+16	2.8 /3.2	+2	55	15
A. B.	CABG	+17	1.8 /2.1	−18	54	12
A. B.†	CABG	+9	2.5 /2.8	−12	54	12
G. O.	CABG	+18	1.4 /1.7	−37	50	10
C. P.	VR	+32	0.51/0.67	−12	55	13
R. L.	VR	+13	2.3 /2.6	−29	52	22
R. L.†	VR	+11	2.3 /2.5	−27	52	22
J. M.†	CABG	+34	2.1 /2.8	−7	54	8
F. E.	VR	+19	2.1 /2.5	0	68	9
F. J.	CABG	+13	1.5 /1.7	−11	43	12
F. J.†	CABG	+13	2.2 /2.8	−2	43	12
R. B.†	CABG	+25	1.7 /2.2	+28	62	13
Mean		+17	1.94/2.28	−10.9	54	12.85
Standard error		±2.2	0.15/0.17	±4.3	±1.7	±1.1

*VR: valve replacement; CABG: coronary artery bypass graft; Δ cardiac index: percent change (liters per square meter per minute); Δ blood volume; percent change (liters); FRC/TLC: ratio of functional residual capacity to total lung capacity; LVEDP: left ventricular end diastolic pressure (mm. Hg).
†Studied on first postoperative day.

gen tensions remained above 100 torr at all times. Any study in which Pa_{CO_2} changed more than 4 torr was rejected.

RESULTS

In order to facilitate evaluation, the patients were arbitrarily divided into four groups: Group A, 14 patients (Table I) decreased CO more than 5 percent in response to 10 cm. H_2O PEEP; Group B, six patients (Table II), changed CO less than ± 5 percent in response to PEEP; Group C, 14 patients (Table III), increased CO more than 5 percent in response to PEEP; and Group D, six patients (Table IV), served as controls.

As anticipated,[2] all groups of patients displayed low circulating blood volume postoperatively due to a contracted vascular compartment: Group A (↓ CO) down 12 ± 2.7 percent (mean ± S.E.M.); Group C (↑ CO) down 10.9 ± 4.3 percent; and Group D (control) down 15 ± 3.9 percent. The patients, therefore, had uniformly low blood volumes and the groups did not differ significantly. In all of the 14 instances that patients were

Table IV. *Change in cardiac output per 30 minutes without PEEP—Control group**

Patient	Operation	Δ cardiac index %	Δ cardiac index Cardiac index	Δ blood volume (%)	FRC/TLC (%)	LVEDP
H. D.	CABG	+3	2.0 /2.14	−24	63	8
		0	2.14/2.14			
		0	2.14/2.14			
E. N.†	VR	0	3.8 /3.8	+2	60	15
L. P.	CABG	−3	1.8 /1.75	−20	58	11
M. T.	VR	+3.6	2.05/2.13	−20	52	11
		−3.6	2.13/2.05			
P. T.	CABG	0	2.25/2.25	−18	42	10
		−6	2.25/2.13			
P. T.†	CABG	0	2.5 /2.5	−10	42	10
		0	2.5 /2.5			
		+5	2.5 /2.63			
Mean		−0.1	2.34/2.34	−15	53	10.8
Standard error		±.9	0.15/0.15	±3.9	±3.7	±0.9

*VR: valve replacement; CABG: coronary artery bypass graft; Δ cardiac index: percent change (liters per square meter per minute); Δ blood volume; percent change (liters); FRC/TLC: ratio of functional residual capacity to total lung capacity; LVEDP: left ventricular end diastolic pressure (mm. Hg).

†Studied on first postoperative day.

restudied on the first postoperative day, blood volume increased over that measured on the day of operation. Cardiac index (mean ± S.E.M.) was 2.12 ± 0.26 L. per square meter per minute in these 14 patients prior to PEEP on the day of operation and increased to 2.47 ± 0.30 L. per square meter per minute on the first day after operation. Following PEEP, cardiac index was 2.06 ± 0.20 L. per square meter per minute and increased to 2.51 ± 0.30 L. per square meter per minute on the day following operation.

There was a relatively even mix of valve and coronary artery operations in Groups A, C, and control (D).

The FRC/TLC ratio was not significantly different in Groups A, C, and control (D). The mean scores ± standard error were 58 ± 1.6 percent, 54 ± 1.7 percent, and 53 ± 3.7 percent, respectively. Patients in Group C did show a tendency toward less hyperinflation ($p < 0.1$).

Resting LVEDP was significantly higher in Group C (↑ CO) than in Group A (↓ CO) ($p < 0.01$). Mean LVEDP in Group A was 7.6 ± 1.1 mm. Hg. Mean LVEDP in Group C was 12.85 ± 1.1 mm. Hg. In both groups end diastolic pressures were similar to the control group: Group A vs. D ($p > 0.1$); Group C vs. D ($p > 0.2$).

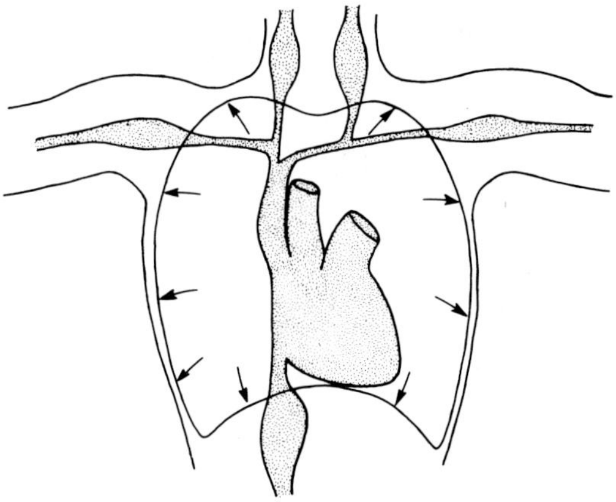

Fig. 1. Cardiac output falls with an increase in intrathoracic pressure and consequent decrease in venous return.

DISCUSSION

As previously noted, there is ample precedent[12, 17, 19] for a decrease in CO associated with PEEP breathing. The prevalent explanation is that the increase in intrathoracic pressure decreases venous return and thus diminishes CO (Fig. 1).

This reasoning very adequately explains why hypervolemic dogs can sustain their CO in the face of PEEP, while hypovolemic dogs

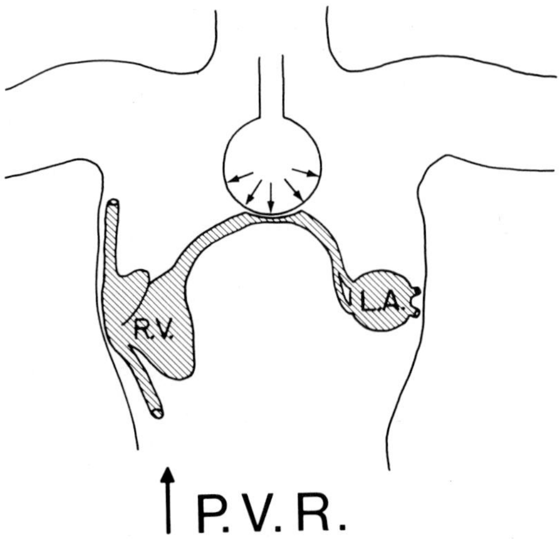

Fig. 2. Increased pulmonary vascular resistance leads to a decrease in cardiac output.

cannot.[24] This reasoning similarly explains why patients with "sympathetic dysfunction"[22] (cervical cord transection or ganglionic-blocking medication) cannot sufficiently increase venous tone to re-establish a positive extra- to intrathoracic venous pressure gradient. In these patients CO falls with PEEP.

It was anticipated that all patients would respond to PEEP with a fall in CO (Group A). The decreased venous return (Fig. 1) associated with increased intrathoracic pressure might decrease the preload on a failing heart. This redistribution of blood or autophlebotomy might also increase CO, however.

Patients exhibiting little or no change in CO in response to PEEP have previously been observed.[11, 16] Falke and associates[5] studied 10 patients with acute respiratory failure. They found an increase in CO associated with 5 cm. H_2O PEEP in three of the 10 patients. Little has been said about the mechanism of such an increase in CO associated with PEEP.

Two and a half centuries ago, Sir John Floyer[6] wrote:

> "An intermitting pulse depends on the stop of the circulation thro' the lungs: because the left ventricle of the heart, by that stop, wants sufficient blood to continue its constant pulsation, and this is plain in the asthma, where the pulse intermits, because of the constriction, which stops the circulation through the lungs."

Mead and Whittenberger,[20] continuing the work of Floyer, were able to show that pulmonary vascular resistance (PVR) increases in ex vivo dog lung with increasing lung volume. Vascular resistance, therefore, should be least at end expiration (FRC). Permutt, Bromberger-Barnes, and Bane[22] noted that interalveolar capillary resistance increased with increasing airway pressure. They termed the flow from these high-pressure pulmonary capillaries to the lower pressure left atrium a "vascular waterfall."[22] West,[26] however, has distinguished two varieties of intrapulmonary vessels. The small interalveolar vessels respond directly to airway pressure. They exhibit an increase in vascular resistance as lung volume increases. The larger extra-alveolar vessels respond primarily to changes in interstitial pressure and may actually exhibit a decrease in vascular resistance with increasing lung volume. Grenvik[8] has recognized this phenomenon clinically. He studied thoracic surgical patients after operation and noted a decrease in PVR associated with a change from spontaneous to controlled ventilation. An increase in PVR might well account for the decrease in CO associated with PEEP in Group A patients (Fig. 2); conversely, FRC probably varies with level of consciousness and certainly can be altered voluntarily. FRC changes with disease, obesity, smoking, and body position.[4, 13] If a patient's FRC were below "normal" on intermittent positive pressure ventilation, and PEEP increased it to "normal," PVR might well decrease and CO improve (Group C patients). However, if the patient's FRC were already above "normal" prior to the institution of PEEP, PVR should increase with the increased lung volume. Pulmonary elasticity must also be critically important, for this governs the degree to which airway pressure is transmitted to the intrapulmonary vessels. For these reasons we looked at the ratio of FRC to total lung capacity as a guide to hyperinflation. We expected the FRC/TLC ratio to be lower in Group C (↑ CO) patients, thus permitting PEEP to elevate FRC

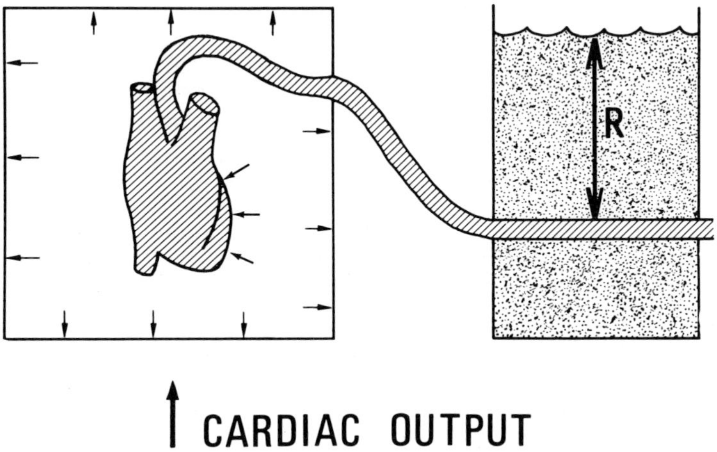

Fig. 3. With a fixed systemic vascular resistance, an increase in intrathoracic pressure (and thus left ventricular pressure) will relatively decrease the load on the left ventricle and cardiac output will increase.

toward "normal" with a concomitant decrease in PVR and increase in CO. The tendency in that direction (Tables I and III) is not statistically significant ($p < 0.1$).

The third mechanism by which PEEP might alter or increase CO is depicted in Fig. 3. With the exception of the coronary and bronchial circulations, all the vascular beds fed by the left ventricle are outside the thorax. Assuming the systemic vascular resistance remains constant, an increase in intrathoracic pressure by PEEP (and thus left ventricular pressure) should relatively decrease the load on the left ventricle. CO should increase. This mechanism has been evaluated in dogs by Harken and Giordano.[10] They demonstrated a parallel increase in pulmonary artery wedge and esophageal (pleural) pressures with PEEP. No increase in transmural ventricular pressure was noted, indicating an increase in ventricular pressure with PEEP relative to the systemic vascular bed (Fig. 3). CO increased 25 percent of the time with 10 cm. H_2O PEEP. In these dogs when pleural pressure was then rendered zero by opening the chest widely, CO fell. Indeed, Levine, McIntyre, and Glovsky[16] report the case of a 40-year-old trumpet player who was asked to participate in six one-mile parades. He had angina which developed repeatedly while marching the steady cadence of a parade. This patient noted, however, that when he began playing his trumpet his angina was relieved. Once during a parade, when the music had stopped, chest pain developed and he requested that the leader start the next song immediately. Levine collected three other patients who demonstrated the same phenomenon. In each angina was relieved without cardiac slowing, as would be necessary if relief were mediated via the carotid sinus.

In a group of patients in whom left ventricular function limits CO then, an increase in intrathoracic pressure (relative to peripheral resistance) with PEEP might reasonably be expected to increase CO (Fig. 3). In fact, the patients benefited by PEEP were the group with elevated LVEDP's before operation. Looking at all the groups, it is apparent that left ventricular function is not the whole solution. Evidently other factors, such as effective blood volume, peripheral venous tone, PVR, and, perhaps, degree of hyperinflation (FRC/TLC), are operative.

The purpose of this study was to evalute the hemodynamic effects of PEEP in acutely ill patients. We hoped to divorce the hemodynamic sequelae from the well-recognized influence of PEEP on gas exchange by requiring an arterial oxygen tension above 100 torr throughout the study period. In light of this oxygen surplus, we feel that changes in arterial oxygen tension (above 100 torr) had little influence on CO. Likewise, arterial carbon dioxide tension (Pa_{CO_2}) is recognized as influencing CO.[24] For this reason, we discarded any sets of observations in which Pa_{CO_2} changed more than 4 torr. By eliminating the bias of gas exchange in this manner, we feel that several conclusions are permissible concerning the pure hemodynamic effects of PEEP on CO.

PEEP ventilation does not invariably reduce CO. Hypovolemia and impaired peripheral venous tone are relative, but not absolute contraindications to PEEP. Not infrequently CO responds favorably to PEEP. In these instances it appears that left ventricular function is limiting CO prior to the institution of PEEP. The state of the intrapulmonary vessels must also be important. As has been discussed, PVR may either rise or fall with an increase in lung volume. Current evidence must be refined, but it suggests that PVR might correlate with some parameter of hyperinflation, such as FRC/TLC ratio.

It is currently safe to conclude that on hemodynamic grounds, no absolute contraindications to PEEP exist. If a patient appears to warrant PEEP to improve gas exchange, he should not be deprived of this valuable ventilatory adjunct. A trial of ventilation with PEEP should rapidly eliminate questions of any patient's hemodynamic tolerance. It is even reasonable to foresee a day when PEEP will be used routinely in selected patients to augment CO.

REFERENCES

1. Bates, D. V., and Christie, R. V.: Intrapulmonary mixing of helium in health and in emphysema, Clin. Sci. **9:** 17, 1950.
2. Breckenridge, I. M., Digerness, S. B., and Kirklin, J. W.: Increased extracellular fluid after open intracardiac operation, Surg. Gynecol. Obst. **131:** 53, 1970.
3. Cournand, A., Motley, H. L., Werko, L., et al.: Physiological studies of the effects of intermittent positive pressure breathing on cardiac output in man, Am. J. Physiol. **152:** 162, 1948.
4. Craig, D. B., Wahba, W. M., Don, H. F., et al.: Closing volume and its relationship to gas exchange in seated and supine positions, J. Appl. Physiol. **31:** 717, 1971.
5. Falke, K. J., Pontoppidan, H., Kumar, A., et al.: Ventilation with end expiratory pressure in acute lung disease, J. Clin. Invest. **51:** 2315, 1972.
6. Floyer, J.: Treatise of the asthma, London, 1717.
7. Gans, C., DeJongh, H. J., and Farger, J.: Bullfrog *(Rana catesbeinana)* ventilation: How does the frog breathe? Science **103:** 1223, 1968.
8. Grenvik, A.: Respiratory, circulatory and metabolic effects of respirator treatment: A clinical study in the post-operative thoracic surgical patients, Acta Anaesthesiol. Scand. [Suppl.] **19:** 1, 1966.
9. Guyton, A. C.: Circulatory physiology: Cardiac output and its regulation, Philadelphia, 1963, W. B. Saunders Company, p. 380.
10. Harken, A. H., and Giordano, J.: The hemodynamic effects of continuous positive pressure ventilation, Clin. Res. **22:** 505, 1974.
11. Harken, D. E., and Bjork, V.: Personal communication.
12. Hedley-Whyte, J., Pontoppidan, H., and Morris, M. J.: The response of patients with respiratory failure and cardiopulmonary disease to different levels of constant volume ventilation, J. Clin. Invest. **45:** 1543, 1966.
13. Kumar, A., Falke, K. J., Geffin, B., et al.: Continuous positive pressure ventilation in acute respiratory failure. N. Engl. J. Med. **283:** 1430, 1970.
14. Leblanc, P., Ruff, F., and Milic-Emili, J.: Effects of age and body position on 'airway closure' in man, J. Appl. Physiol. **28:** 448, 1970.
15. Lefemine, A. A., and Harken, D. E., Postoperative care following open-heart operations: Routine use of controlled ventilation, J. Thorac. Cardiovasc. Surg. **52:** 207, 1966.
16. Levine, J. J., McIntyre, K. M., and Glovsky, M. M.: Relief of angina pectoris by Valsalva maneuver, N. Engl. J. Med. **275:** 487, 1966.
17. McIntyre, R. W., Laws, A. K., and Ramachandran, P. R.: Positive expiratory pressure plateau: Improved gas exchange during mechanical ventilation, Can. Anaesth. Soc. J. **16:** 447, 1969.
18. McMahon, S. M., and Halprin, G. M.: Modification of intrapulmonary blood shunt by end expiratory pressure application in patients with acute respiratory failure, Chest **59:** 275, 1971.
19. McMahon, S. M., Hayrin, G. M., and Sieker, H. O.: Positive end-expiratory airway pressure in severe arterial hypoxemia, Am. Rev. Respir. Dis. **108:** 526, 1973.
20. Mead, J., and Whittenberger, J. L.: Lung

inflation and hemodynamics: A critical comprehensive presentation of physiological knowledge and concepts, *in* Penn, W. O., and Rahn, H., editors: Handbook of physiology, Washington, D. C., 1964, American Physiological Society, p. 477.

21. Otis, A. B., Rahn, H., Brontman, M., et al.: Ballistocardiographic study of changes in cardiac output due to respiration, J. Clin. Invest. **25:** 413, 1946.
22. Permutt, S., Bromberger-Barnes, B., and Bane, H. N.: Alveolar pressure, pulmonary venous pressure and the vascular waterfall, Med. Thorac. **19:** 47, 1962.
23. Pontoppidan, H., Geffin, B., and Lowenstein, E.: Acute respiratory failure in the adult, N. Engl. J. Med. **287:** 799, 1972.
24. Prys-Roberts, C., Kelman, G. R., Greenbaum, R., et al.: Circulatory influences of artificial ventilation during nitrous oxide anesthesia in man. II. Results: The relative influence of mean intrathoracic pressure and arterial carbon dioxide tension, Br. J. Anaesth. **39:** 533, 1967.
25. Sykes, M. K., Adams, A. O., and Finlay, W. E.: The effects of variations in end-expiratory inflation pressure on cardio-respiratory function in normo, hypo and hypervolemic dogs, Br. J. Anaesth. **42:** 669, 1970.
26. West, J. B.: Effects of interstitial pressure, *in* Fishman, A. P., and Hecht, H. H., editors: The pulmonary circulation and interstitial space, Chicago, 1969, University of Chicago Press, p. 43.

Lymphocyte output by the isolated perfused rabbit thymus

O. Ekwueme, M.D., F.R.C.S., *and* **A. P. M. Forrest, B.Sc., M.D., Ch.M., F.R.C.S.,**
Cardiff, Wales

The isolated thymic perfusion system has been used to re-examine the question of lymphocyte output from the thymus. In one experiment serial leukocyte and differential counts were performed on perfusate samples over a 6 hour perfusion period. In another, thymic cells were labeled in vivo by daily intravenous injections of tritium-labeled thymidine; the thymus was then excised and perfused, and a search was made in the perfusate for labeled cells. The findings confirm that a significant emigration of small and medium lymphocytes occurs from the thymus. It is suggested that the isolated perfused thymus preparation could make a significant contribution to the wider question of lymphopoiesis and lymphocyte transport in the body.

From the Surgical Unit, Welsh National School of Medicine, Cardiff, Wales

THE THYMUS is a well-known center of lymphocyte production. Evidence for this has accumulated from morphological observations,[5, 14] from mitotic counts[1, 27, 35, 53] and from studies of dioxyribonucleic acid (DNA) turnover.[2, 17, 41, 60] The production of such massive numbers of cells in the thymus raises the question as to what is the fate of these cells. As the thymus does not increase indefinitely in şize, a steady state must be present in which cell production is balanced by a cell elimination process. Theoretically this elimination process could be either by cell degeneration locally in the thymus or by export of cells from the organ. Considerable evidence has accumulated in support of the hypothesis that most, if not all, of these cells do not emigrate but degenerate in the thymus.[14, 31, 34] On the other hand, evidence in support of the suggestion that lymphocytes emigrate from the thymus has accumulated from several, largely indirect methods of study: from the ontogenetic development of the thymus and other lymphatic tissues,[4, 47] from thymectomy of both newborn[39, 40] and adult animals[33, 44] and man,[26] from cell population kinetics, as studied by the mitotic index,[28, 38] and from other morphological studies.[8, 24, 52, 55] Other methods include the use of chromosone markers and parabosis or thymus implants,[12, 24, 30, 40] the transfer of labelled cells,[19, 41, 50] and direct selective labeling of the thymus.[42, 45, 59] However, because of the limitations inherent in these various methods of study, other approaches to the problem are still required. We have developed a method of isolated thymic perfusion with a view to employing this in experimental tumor immunotherapy,[15] and the unique potentials of this system as an additional tool in studies of thymic function have become apparent, as it provides an experimental system that is rigidly controllable to a degree unattainable by other available

Accepted for publication August 12, 1974.

Reprint requests: O. Ekwueme, M.D., F.R.C.S., Department of Surgery, University of Nigeria Teaching Hospital, P.M.B. 1129, Enugu, Nigeria.

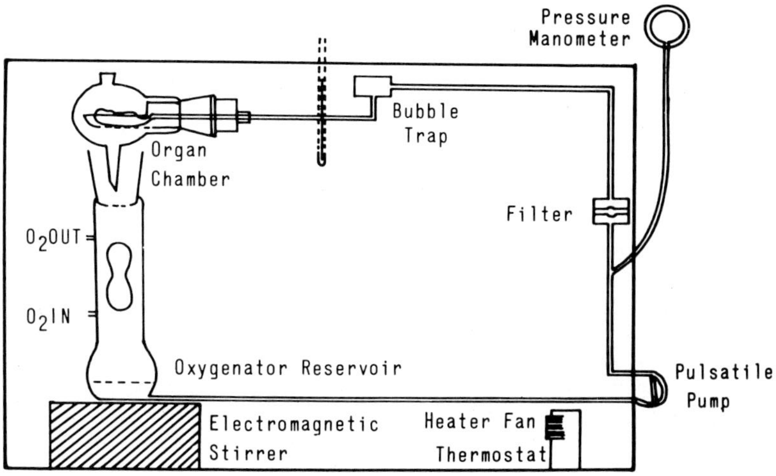

Fig. 1. Perfusion circuit.

methods of study. In this study, the isolated perfused thymus preparation has been used to re-examine the question of lymphocyte output by the thymus.

MATERIALS AND METHODS

The development of our method of isolated perfusion of the thymus and its evaluation has been described in detail elsewhere,[16] and is briefly summarized here.

The perfusion system. The thymuses were perfused in a pump oxygenator system which is schematically depicted in Fig. 1. The system, apart from the leads to the pump, was enclosed in a perspex chamber, the temperature inside which was maintained at 38° C. by means of a thermostatically regulated heater and fan. All tubing was of siliconized rubber of 1 mm. internal diameter. A humidified gas mixture of 95 percent oxygen and 5 percent carbon dioxide was passed through the oxygenator at a rate of about 200 ml. per minute. Open thymic venous return drained by gravity from the organ chamber into the oxygenator, and the arterialized blood was propelled to the thymus by a Watson-Marlow microperfusion pump.

Operative technique. Male and female New Zealand white rabbits, 4 months of age, were used for this experiment. Each animal was anesthetized by intravenous Nembutal (30 to 45 mg. per kilogram of body weight), followed by 3,000 I.U. of heparin. After 10 minutes, blood for perfusion was taken by arterial puncture. Using sterile instruments, the skin was incised in the midline from the jaw to the midabdomen. It was then dissected off and clipped aside, thus exposing the chest. This was then cleaned with Hibitane and sterile towels were applied. With a sterile technique, the abdomen was opened and the diaphragm was incised. The ribs were cut along the mid axillary line on both sides and the anterior chest wall was gently elevated. The left subclavian artery was exposed and the internal thoracic branch was identified. Through an incision at the base of the subclavian artery, a one-inch long fine nylon cannula was inserted into the internal thoracic artery and tied in place by a ligature placed just lateral to the anterior vena cava. A second ligature was placed at the base of the subclavian artery. The internal thoracic artery was then ligated distal to the thymic branch, and, if a sternal twig was present between the proximal and distal ligatures, this also was ligated (Fig. 2). The left lobe of the thymus was then separated from the right and from other mediastinal structures, and, by sectioning the other branches of the subclavian artery and the left anterior vena cava proximal and distal to the entrance of the thymic vein, the thymus could then be transferred to the organ chamber.

The anoxic interval was usually less than 20 minutes. Throughout the dissection the

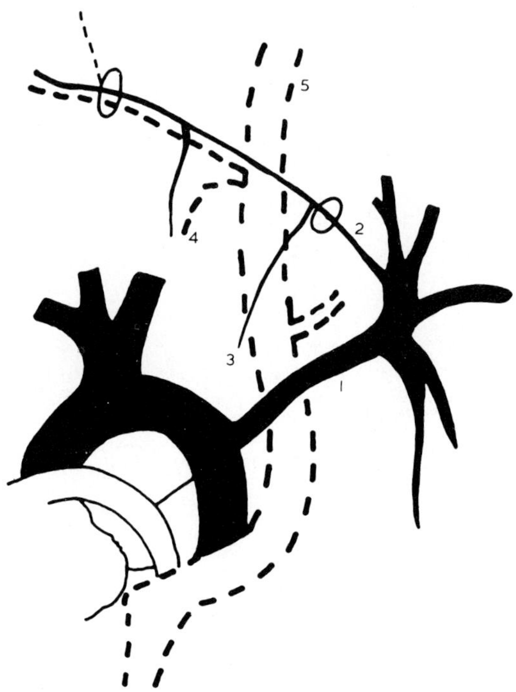

Fig. 2. Schematic representation of the dissection of the left lobe of the rabbit thymus for ex vivo perfusion: *(1)* subclavian artery; *(2)* internal thoracic artery; *(3)* pericardiacophrenic artery; *(4)* thymic artery and vein; *(5)* anterior vena cava.

thymus was handled as little as possible and kept moist with drops of saline.

Conduct of the perfusion. The perfusate was diluted autologous blood.[16] It had a normal osmolality, and the hematocrit varied between 15 and 20 percent. The reduction in viscosity associated with a low hematocrit has been shown to be an advantage in perfusing isolated organs.[6, 9] The circuit was primed with 20 ml. of the perfusate and the pump was run at a low setting during the thymic dissection. At the beginning of perfusion the pump was adjusted to produce an initial pressure of 30 mm. Hg and the system was then left to find its own level. The flow pressure and pH were recorded at hourly intervals throughout the perfusion. The pressure was recorded with an aneroid manometer; the flow rate was determined by the rate of drop formation at the exit of the organ chamber; the pH was determined by the Astrup microelectrode assembly.

Lymphocyte counts. Lymphocyte counts were performed in 20 thymic perfusions. Samples (0.5 ml.) were taken from the reservoir before and 15 minutes after the start and, subsequently, at hourly intervals throughout the 6 hour perfusion period. Quadruplicate estimations of total leukocyte count were made on each sample with standard hematological techniques.[11] Simultaneously, several blood smears were prepared and stained with Jenner-Giemsa. A differential lymphocyte count was performed for each sample of perfusate from counts of at least 500 leukocytes on each of two slides. Monocytes were grouped with lymphocytes, as they constitute only a small proportion of the mononuclear cells[54] and are not usually satisfactorily identifiable in routine smear preparations of rabbit blood.[27]

Control perfusions. The effect of the circuit on the white cell content of the perfusate was investigated in 10 control perfusions. In these, the normal circuit, but without a thymus, was set up concurrently with an experimental perfusion. Serial blood samples were then taken and the total leukocyte and lymphocyte contents determined.

In vivo labelling experiments. Four male New Zealand white rabbits, 4 months of age, were used for this study. Each animal received five daily intravenous injections of tritiated thymidine 0.25 μc per milligram of body weight (The Radiochemical Center, Amersham; specific activity, 5.0 Ci per millimole). Twenty-four hours after the last injection, a thymic lobe was excised and perfused. In these experiments, blood for perfusion was obtained from another rabbit that had not received radioactive material. Preperfusion and hourly samples were taken from the reservoir for total and differential leukocyte determinations in the usual way. In addition, at one, 3, and 6 hours a lymphocyte-rich suspension was prepared from each specimen by differential sedimentation according to the method of Brent and Medawar.[7] These were smeared on gelatin-coated slides and, when dry, were fixed in absolute ethyl alcohol for 15 minutes and subjected to autoradiography. A cell suspension from

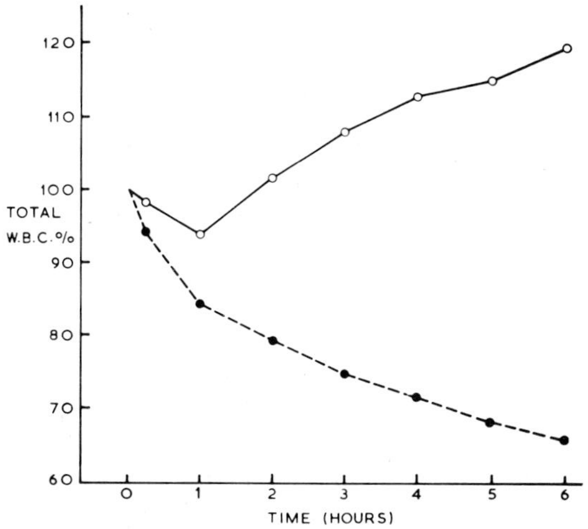

Fig. 3. Total leukocyte count during perfusion recorded as a percentage of the preperfusion count: ○ = thymic perfusion; ● = control perfusion.

the nonperfused lobe of the thymus was also prepared for autoradiography.

Autoradiography was performed by layering Kodak AR 10 autoradiographic stripping film onto the specimens. After drying, the slides were exposed for 6 weeks at 4° C. in airtight boxes with calcium chloride as desicant. They were developed for 4 minutes in Kodak D19 developer, rinsed in water, and fixed with Kodak Unifix. They were then washed in running water and dried by exposure. The specimens were stained with Giemsa according to the method of Gude, Upton, and Odell[22] and were examined at ×1,000 magnification.

RESULTS

1. Lymphocyte counts. The mean values of the total leukocyte and differential counts from 10 thymus perfusions are shown in Table I, and the mean values from five control perfusions in Table II. These are presented graphically in Figs. 3, 4, and 5.

In the control experiments (no thymus in the circuit), the mean total leukocyte count fell sharply in the first hour and then progressively at a reduced rate throughout the perfusion period. At the end of 6 hours, the total leukocyte count was 65.7 percent of the preperfusion value, falling from 5,926 per cubic millimeter to 3,893 per cubic millimeter. Thus there was a progressive destruction of leukocytes during perfusion (Fig. 3). That polymorphonuclear leukocytes and lymphocytes were not affected to the same degree is illustrated by Fig. 4, which shows a progressive increase in the percentage lymphocyte count above the preperfusion level during control perfusion. Consequently, although the mean total leukocyte count fell to 65.7 percent of the preperfusion value at 5 hours, the lymphocyte count fell only to 72.5 percent (Fig. 5).

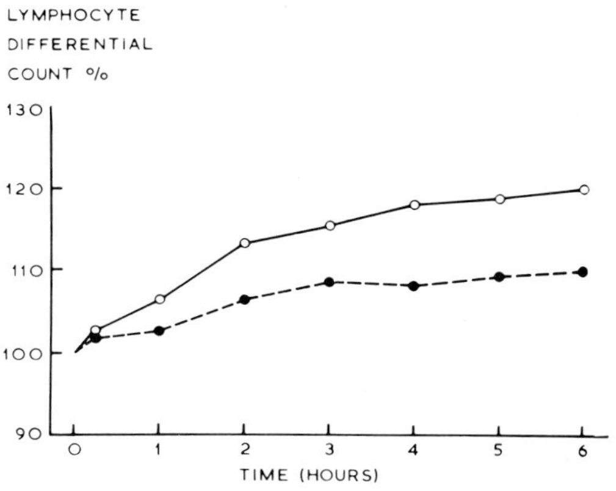

Fig. 4. Perfusion lymphocyte differential count during perfusion, recorded as a percentage of the preperfusion value: ○ = thymic perfusion; ● = control perfusion.

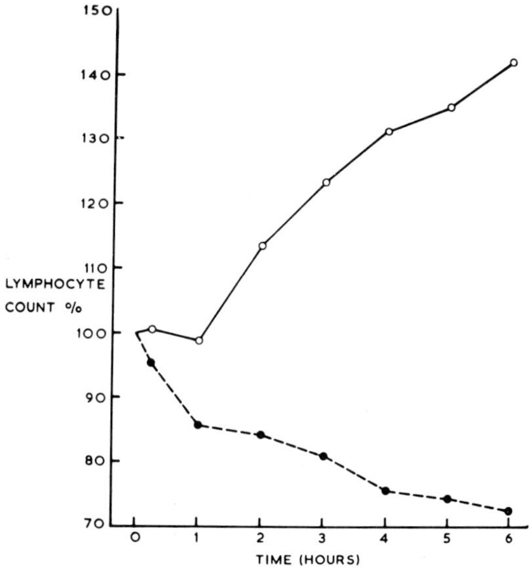

Fig. 5. Absolute lymphocyte count during perfusion recorded as a percentage of the preperfusion count: ○ = thymic perfusion; ● = control perfusion.

Table I. *Mean leukocyte counts in 10 thymic perfusions*

Time (hr.)	*Total leukocyte count per mm.³*	*Lymphocyte (%)*	*Lymphocyte count per mm.³*
0	4,627	77.8	3,635
¼	4,540	79.9	3,549
1	4,332	82.8	3,592
2	4,686	88.2	4,124
3	4,986	90.2	4,489
4	5,202	92.1	4,784
5	5,297	92.9	4,920
6	5,506	93.8	5,188

Table II. *Mean leukocyte counts in five "control" perfusions*

Time (hr.)	*Total leukocyte count per mm.³*	*Lymphocyte (%)*	*Lymphocyte count per mm.³*
0	5,926	76.7	4,571
¼	5,570	78.1	4,355
1	4,984	78.7	3,913
2	4,680	81.7	3,849
3	4,420	83.5	3,702
4	4,237	83.1	3,457
5	4,033	84.2	3,395
6	3,893	84.7	3,312

Table III. *Mean hourly lymphocyte output during thymic perfusion**

First hour	*Second hour*	*Third hour*	*Fourth hour*	*Fifth hour*	*Sixth hour*
13.2	16.1	13.2	13.5	5.1	9.1

*Output of cells at each hour is expressed as a percentage of the preperfusion lymphocyte count.

The result from the thymic perfusion experiments showed a different pattern from those of control experiments. The total leukocyte count after a slight fall in the first hour rose progressively throughout the perfusion period, and at 6 hours the total leukocyte count was 119 percent of the preperfusion value (Fig. 3). As the polymorphonuclear leukocyte count showed a fall of the same degree as in control experiments, the rise in total leukocyte count was due to a progressive increase in lymphocyte numbers. Thus although the total leukocyte count was 119 percent of the preperfusion level at the end of 6 hours perfusion, the lymphocyte count had risen to 142.7 percent (Fig. 5) from a preperfusion count of 3,635 per cubic millimeter to 5,188 per cubic millimeter.

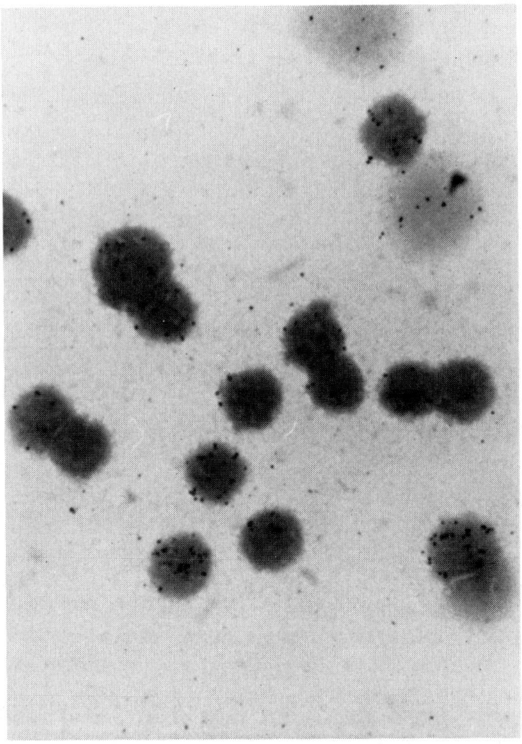

Fig. 6. Autoradiograph of a smear of thymus cell suspension from a rabbit following five daily intravenous injections of tritiated thymidine 0.25 μCi per kilogram. Thymus excised 24 hours after last dose. Exposure time, 6 weeks. (Original magnification ×1,000.)

In the presence of progressive leukocyte destruction, as demonstrated in the control experiments, the true lymphocyte output during thymic perfusion is clearly more than is suggested by the counts, as it can be assumed that the circuit on its own would effect cell destruction to the same extent in both the thymic and control perfusions. Thus in Fig. 5 the difference between the values for the thymic and control perfusions at each hour would represent the true lymphocyte output. From this the hourly cell output can be calculated (Table III). It will be seen that there was a steady output of lymphocytes in the first 4 hours, at an average

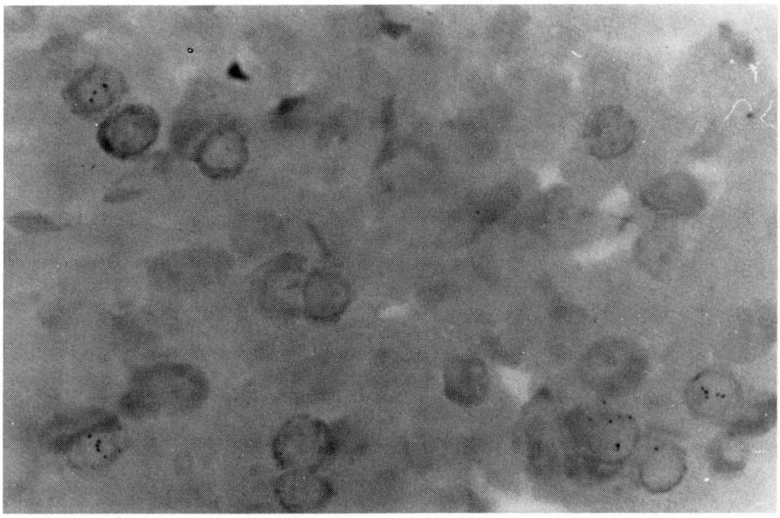

Fig. 7. Autoradiograph of a smear preparation of a lymphocyte-rich suspension prepared from thymic perfusate at the end of a 6 hour perfusion. The animal had received a 5 day course of tritiated thymidine prior to excision of the thymus for perfusion. Labeled lymphocytes are present in the perfusate. Agglutinated erythrocytes and polymorphonuclear leukocytes account for the dense background; some distorted polymorphonuclear leukocytes are also seen. Exposure time, 6 weeks. (Original magnification, ×1,000.)

hourly rate of 14 percent of the preperfusion value, and the initial fall in cell counts during the first hour was due to the marked leukocyte destruction at this time, which could not be completely made up by cell output. During the last 2 hours of perfusion, cell output was still occuring, but at a reduced rate.

2. In vivo labelling experiments. The mean proportion of labeled cells in the thymus before perfusion was 67.3 percent. The labeled cells included all classes of cells—small, medium, and large lymphocytes (Fig. 6).

Labeled cells were present in the perfusate after the first hour, with increasing numbers at 3 and 6 hours (Fig. 7). These cells included both small and medium, but not large lymphocytes and were largely lightly labeled cells. Even in these lymphocyte-rich preparations, a variable proportion of polymorphonuclear leukocytes was present, As these could not always be identified with certainty, differential counting of labeled lymphocytes was not possible. Consequently, quantitation of total lymphocyte output by this method could not be attempted. However, the identification of labeled cells in the perfusate in progressively increasing numbers confirms the results of the cell-counting experiments, that lymphocytes were donated to the perfusate during perfusion. It also means that at least some of the donated cells were produced within the 5 days prior to perfusion.

DISCUSSION

Several objections have been raised to the various methods that have hitherto been employed in the study of the emigration of cells from the thymus. The influence of thymectomy on the output of lymphocytes from the thoracic duct, the blood lymphocyte content, and the lymphoid tissues of animals have been taken to be indications that the thymus normally exports large numbers of lymphocytes.[33, 40, 44] However, the thymus is thought to exert a regulatory influence on lymphopoiesis in other lymphoid tissues. Saline extracts of human or mouse thymus produce a lymphocytosis in young mice.[32] In young thymectomized rodents, a restoration toward normal blood lymphocyte levels has been acheived with the use of various thymic extracts[3, 25] and, to a lesser extent, with thymus enclosed in Millipore diffusion chambers.[56] Consequently, the results obtained from these thymectomy experiments could also be due to the removal of a stimulator of lymphopoiesis.

Although histological studies are suggestive of cell migration from the thymus,[8, 24, 28, 38, 52, 55] an exact determination of the direction of cell movement is not possible from these static studies. There is evidence that lymphoid cells can seed to the thymus under certain conditions, for example, during the regeneration of the thymus after irradiation.[21, 49] Furthermore, during the regeneration of syngeneic thymus there is a gradual and complete replacement of the mitotic lymphoid cells of the graft by host-type cells.[13, 20, 24, 39] Therefore, the results of histological studies cannot be taken as evidence of the movement of cells from the thymus into the blood, any more than in the opposite direction.

Studies with thymus grafts[12, 24, 40] do not reproduce the state of affairs in the normal thymus. Some amount of tissue disruption must take place following grafting, and graft-derived cells might thus escape and seed the host tissues. Even if this possibility were discounted, as grafting results in the death of many of the cells in the graft, any migrating cells must be the survivors of the grafting process and are, therefore, a selective group of cells. Although thymus grafts bear a close histologic and cytologic resemblance to the normal thymus, functional and other differences have been demonstrated.[35, 37, 48]

Cell transfusion experiments[19, 41, 50] do not measure the migration of thymic lymphocytes but attempt to elucidate the fate of such migrated cells. Taken on their own, therefore (except, perhaps, cell injection directly into the thymus[50]), they constitute only a very indirect evidence for cell migration from the thymus.

The most direct evidence for the migration of thymic lymphocytes has come from studies in which thymic cells were selectively labeled radioactively.[42, 45, 59] However, this method also has certain limitations. The surgical procedure cannot be considered physiological, and there is the possibility that any migration of cells from the thymus is a stress-induced process. When parenchmal injections are used, the possibility has to be excluded either of emigration of cells along the needle track or of extrathymic cells entering the thymus along the track, becoming labeled, and then migrating to the periphery. Furthermore, as the presence of a "thymus-blood barrier" has been demonstrated electron microscopically,[8, 58] it is possible that direct introduction of radioactive label into the thymus may have stimulated the cells in an abnormal way. Finally, there is the possibility of reutilization of the label,[26, 51, 57] and, if all thymic lymphocytes died in situ, release of label to the general circulation with peripheral lymphocyte labeling might thereby result.

These critical remarks do not necessarily invalidate the results obtained using these methods of study. However, they do suggest that other approaches to the problem are still required. The use of the isolated ex vivo thymus perfusion preparation in the study of lymphocyte output by the thymus has the advantage that, with the use of an initial priming volume, all cell output can be harvested in the perfusate. The results of this experiment are in support of an emigration of lymphocytes from the thymus. Using 4-month-old rabbits and a 20 ml. priming volume, there was a steady increase in lymphocyte count in the first 4 hours of perfusion at an average rate of 14 percent of the preperfusion count, or 1×10^7 cells per hour. Assuming an equal output from both lobes of the thymus, this would amount to 2×10^7 cells per hour for the two lobes. Larsson,[29] by measuring thymic blood flow and arteriovenous cell difference, performed a similar quantitative estimation of the output of lymphocytes from the thymus of young guinea pigs and concluded that at least 6,000 lymphocytes leave the thymus every minute through the veins, that is 3.6×10^5 cells per hour. The larger estimate for the rabbit thymus in this study reflects not only its much larger size but also its greater cortex/medulla ratio.[23]

However, other factors may be involved.

Nagaya and Sieker[43] have suggested the possibility of a feedback mechanism controlling lymphocyte production and emigration. They found that the peripheral lymphocyte count of rats receiving daily injections of antilymphocyte serum was increased when the blood lymphocyte count was low, whereas it was decreased when the count returned toward normal. The amount of cell emigration could, therefore, be determined by the level of circulating lymphocytes or of a thymic humoral factor. As the perfusate used in this experiment was diluted blood, the resultant lymphopenia may have been a stimulus to a greater than normal emigration of cells, the rate of cell output tailing off as the circulating lymphocyte numbers approached the normal value.

Perfusion studies after prior labeling of thymic cells in vivo with tritiated thymidine have yeilded further evidence in support of thymic cell emigration in that labeled cells were identified in the perfusate during perfusion. With in vivo direct labeling of thymic cells, labeled cells have been identified in various peripheral lymphoid organs.[30, 42, 59] The method of ex vivo perfusion after total animal labeling avoids the limitations of the methods using direct labelling of thymic cells, although it gives no indication of the destination of the emigrating cells.

The findings of this experiment are in agreement with the suggestion that only small and medium lymphocytes, but not larger cells, emigrate from the thymus. The fact that the cells that migrated from the thymus tended to be the less densely labeled ones suggests that these were not cells that were primarily labeled but were the result of mitotic division of labeled cells, with consequent dilution of the label. Clearly these cells were produced during the 5 days prior to perfusion, but no further information on the intrathymic life span of the thymic lymphocyte is obtainable from the design of the present experiment. Craddock and coworkers[10] and Metcalf and Wiadrowski[36] have suggested that thymus small lymphocytes leave the organ after an intrathymic life span of 3 to 4 days. However, Nossal and Gorrie[46] identified labeled cells in the lymph nodes and spleen of 4-to-6-week-old guinea pigs as early as one hour after direct intrathymic labeling; and Everett, Reike, and Caffrey[18] have suggested that thymic cell migration occurred on a random basis.

The possibility has to be considered that the cell output during thymus perfusion is a passive washout phenomenon. If this were the case, the cell output would be expected to be maximal in the first hour, falling off to negligible values as perfusion progressed. On the contrary, active cell production has been shown to be continuous during perfusion,[16] and cell output continued at a constant rate during the first 4 hours of perfusion, suggesting that this was an active process. The possibility that the subsequent reduction in output in the latter stages of perfusion was due to a return toward normal of the perfusate lymphocyte count has been discussed, but it is also possible that this is a reflection of a reduction in the vitality of the organ preparation.

This initial study has been limited to the restricted question of lymphocyte emigration from the thymus. However, it is clear that by varying the design of the experiment a further range of information could become available. The controllable experimental conditions offered by the isolated thymic perfusion system should make a significant contribution to the wider question of lymphopoiesis and lymphocyte transport in the body.

We would like to acknowledge the technical assistance of Mr. Robert L. Davies.

REFERENCES

1. Andreasen, E., and Christensen, S.: The rate of mitotic activity in the lymphoid organs of the rat, Anat. Rec. **103:** 501, 1949.
2. Andreasen, E., and Ottesen, J.: Studies on the lymphocyte production: Investigations on nucleic acid turnover in the lymphoid organs, Acta Physiol. Scand. **10:** 258, 1945.
3. Asanuma, Y., Goldstein, A. L., and White, A.: Reduction of the incidence of wasting disease in neonatally thymectomized CBA-W mice by the injection of thymosin, Endocrinology **86:** 600, 1970.
4. Auerbach, R.: Genetic control of thymus lymphoid regeneration, Proc. Nat. Acad. Sci. **47:** 1175, 1961.

5. Beard, J.: The true function of the thymus, Lancet **1:** 114, 1899.
6. Brauer, R. W., Pessotti, R. L., and Pizzolato, P.: Isolated rat liver perfusion. Bile production and other properties, Proc. Soc. Exp. Biol. (N. Y.) **78:** 174, 1951.
7. Brent, L., and Medawar, P. S.: Tissue transplantation: A new approach to the "typing" problem, Br. Med. J. **2:** 269, 1963.
8. Clark, S. L., Jr.: The thymus in mice of strain 129/J, studied with the electron microscope, Am. J. Anat. **112:** 1, 1963.
9. Couch, N. P., Cassie, G. F., and Murray, J. E.: Survival of the excised dog kidney perfused in a pump oxygenator system, SURGERY **44:** 666, 1958.
10. Craddock, C. S., Nakai, G. S., Fukuta, H., et al.: Proliferative activity of the lymphatic tissues of rats as studied with tritium-labelled thymidine, J. Exp. Med. **120:** 389, 1964.
11. Dacie, J. V., and Lewis, S. M.: Practical haematology, ed. 4, London, 1968, J. & A. Churchill, Ltd., p. 60.
12. Davies, A. J. S., Festenstein, H., Leuchars, E., et al.: A thymic origin of some peripheral blood lymphocytes, Lancet **1:** 183, 1968.
13. Dukor, P., Miller, J. F. A. P., House, W., et al.: Regeneration of thymus grafts. I. Histological and cytological aspects, Transplantation **3:** 639, 1965.
14. Dustin, A. P.: Recherches d'histologie normale et expérimentale sur le thymus des amphibiens anoures, Arch. Biol. **30:** 601, 1920.
15. Ekwueme, C. O.: M.D. thesis, University of London, 1972.
16. Ekwueme, O.: A method of thymic perfusion and its evaluation, Clin. Exp. Immunol. **14:** 609, 1973.
17. Everett, N. B.: Caffrey, R. W., and Reike, W. O.: Recirculation of lymphocytes, Ann. N. Y. Acad. Sci. **112:** 887, 1964.
18. Everett, N. B., Reike, W. O., and Caffrey, R. W.: The kinetics of small lymphocytes in the rat, with special reference to those of thymic origin, *in* Good, R. A., and Gabrielson, A. E., editors: The thymus in immunobiology, New York, 1964, Harper and Row, publishers, p. 291.
19. Fichtelius, K. E.: The destination of thymus lymphocytes, *in* Wolstenholme, G. E. W., and O'Connor, M., editors: Ciba Foundation symposium on Haemopoiesis, London, 1960, J. & A. Churchill, Ltd., p. 204.
20. Ford, C. E.: Traffic of lymphoid cells in the body, *in* Wolstenholme, G. E. W., and Porter, R., editors: Ciba Foundation Symposium. Thymus: Experimental and clinical studies, London, 1966, J. & A. Churchill, Ltd., p. 131.
21. Gengozian, N., Urso, I. S., Congdon, C. C., et al.: Thymus specificity in lethally irradiated mice treated with rat marrow, Proc. Soc. Exp. Biol. Med. **96:** 714, 1957.
22. Gude, W. D., Upton, A. C., and Odell, F. T., Jr.: Giemsa staining of autoradiograms prepared with stripping film, Stain Technol. **30:** 151, 1965.
23. Hammar, J. A.: New views as to the morphology of the thymus gland and their bearing on the problem of the function of the thymus, Endocrinology **5:** 543, 1921.
24. Harris, J. E., and Ford, C. E.: Cellular traffic in thymus: Experiments with chromosome markers, Nature **201:** 884, 1964.
25. Jankovic, B. D., Isakovic, K., and Horvat, J.: Effect of a lipid fraction from rat thymus on delayed hypersensitivity reactions of neonatally thymectomized rats, Nature **208:** 356, 1965.
26. Joske, A. A.: The effects of thymectomy on the lymphocyte count in patients with myasthenia gravis, Med. J. Aust. **45:** 859, 1958.
27. Kellum, W. E., and Forkner, C. E.: The normal blood picture in the rabbit by the vital staining method, Anat. Rec. **25:** 109, 1923.
28. Kindred, J. E.: Quantitative studies on lymphoid tissues, Ann. N. Y. Acad. Sci. **59:** 746, 1955.
29. Larsson, B.: A quantitative estimation of the venous output of lymphocytes from the thymus in guinea pigs, Acta Pathol. Microbiol. Scand. **67:** 586, 1966.
30. Linna, J. J.: Cell migration from the thymus to other lymphoid organs in hamsters of different ages, Blood **31:** 727, 1968.
31. Matsuyama, M., Wiadrowski, M. B., and Metcalf, D.: Autoradiographic analysis of lymphopoiesis and lymphocyte migration in mice bearing multiple thymic grafts, J. Exp. Med. **123:** 559, 1966.
32. Metcalf, D.: Thymus origin of some plasma lymphocytosis simulating factor, Br. J. Cancer **10:** 442, 1956.
33. Metcalf, D.: The effect of thymectomy on the lymphoid tissues of the mouse, Br. J. Haematol. **6:** 324, 1960.
34. Metcalf, D.: The autonomous behaviour of normal thymus grafts, Aust. J. Exp. Biol. Med. Sci. **41:** (Suppl.): 437, 1963.
35. Metcalf, D.: The thymus and lymphopoiesis, *in* Good, R. A., and Gabrielson, A. E., editors: The thymus in immunobiology, New York, 1964, Harper and Row, Publishers, p. 150.
36. Metcalf, D., and Wiadrowski, M.: Autoradiographic analysis of lymphocyte proliferation in the thymus and in thymic lymphoma tissue, Cancer Res. **26:** 483, 1966.
37. Metcalf, D., Sparrow, N., Nakamura, K., et al.: The behaviour of thymus grafts in high

and low leukaemic strains of mice, Aust. J. Exp. Biol. Med. Sci. **39:** 441, 1961.

38. Michalke, W. D., Hess, M. W., Riedwyl, H., et al.: Thymic lymphopoiesis and cell loss in newborn mice, Blood **33:** 541, 1969.
39. Miller, J. F. A. P.: Role of the thymus in transplantation immunity, Ann. N. Y. Acad. Sci. **99:** 340, 1962.
40. Miller, J. F. A. P.: Effect of neonatal thymectomy on the immunological responsiveness of the mouse, Proc. R. Soc. (B) **156:** 415, 1962.
41. Mims, C. A.: Experiments on the origin and fate of lymphocytes, Br. J. Exp. Pathol. **43:** 639, 1962.
42. Murray, G. A., and Woods, P. A.: Studies on the fate of lymphocytes. The immigration and metamorphosis of *in situ* labelled thymic lymphocytes, Anat. Rec. **150:** 113, 1964.
43. Nagaya, H., and Sieker, H. D.: Feedback mechanisms of thymic lymphocyte production, Proc. Soc. Exp. Biol. Med. **126:** 131, 1967.
44. Nakamoto, A.: The influence of the thymus on the blood picture, especially on lymphocytes. I. Effects of thymectomy on the peripheral blood and lymph nodes, Acta Haematol. Jap. **20:** 179, 1957.
45. Nossal, G. J. V.: Studies on the rate of seeding of lymphocytes from the intact guinea pig thymus, Ann. N. Y. Acad. Sci. **120:** 171, 1964.
46. Nossal, G. J. V., and Gorrie, J.: Studies on the emigration of thymic cells in young guinea pigs, *in* Good, R. A., and Gabrielson, A. E., editors: The thymus in immunology, New York, 1964, Harper and Row, Publishers, p. 288.
47. Papermaster, B. W., Condie, R. M., Finstad, J., et al.: Significance of the thymus in the evolution of the lymphoid tissue and acquired immunity, *in* Good, R. A., and Gabrielson, A. E., editors, New York, 1964, Harper and Row, Publishers, p. 551.
48. Pepper, F. J.: Transplantation of thymic tissue in inbred strains of mice, J. Endocrinol. **22:** 349, 1961.
49. Popp, R. A.: Repopulation of thymus by immunologically competent cells derived from donor marrow, Proc. Soc. Exp. Biol. Med. **108:** 561, 1961.
50. Rankin, J. J.: Circulation of lymphocytes and thymocytes in the normal and leukaemic mouse, Acta Anat. **40:** 221, 1960.
51. Reike, W. O.: The in vivo re-utilization of lymphocytic and sarcoma DNA by cells growing in the peritoneal cavity, J. Cell Biol. **13:** 205, 1962.
52. Sainte-Marie, G., and Leblond, C. P.: Origin and fate of cells in the medulla of rat thymus, Proc. Soc. Exp. Biol. Med. **98:** 909, 1958.
53. Sainte-Marie, G., and Leblond, C. P.: Elaboration of a model for the formation of lymphocytes in the thymus cortex of young adult rats, Blood **26:** 765, 1965.
54. Shermer, S.: The blood morphology of laboratory Animals, ed. 3, Philadelphia, 1954, F. A. Davis Company, p. 54.
55. Toro, I., and Olah, I.: Penetration of thymocytes into the blood circulation, J. Ultrastruct. Res. **17:** 439, 1967.
56. Trench, C. A. H., Watson, J. W., Walker, F. C., et al.: Evidence for a humoral thymic factor in rabbits, Immunology **10:** 187, 1966.
57. Trowell, O. A.: Re-utilization of lymphocytes in lymphopoiesis, J. Biophys. Biochem. Cytol. **3:** 317, 1957.
58. Weiss, L.: Electron microscopic observations on the vascular barrier in the cortex of thymus of the mouse, Anat. Rec. **145:** 413, 1963.
59. Weissman, I. L.: Thymus cell migration, J. Exp. Med. **126:** 291, 1967.
60. Yoffey, J. M., Hanks, G. A., and Kelly, L.: Some problems of lymphocyte production, Ann. N. Y. Acad. Sci. **73:** 47, 1958.

The influence of glucose on gastrin and insulin release in the enteroinsular axis

Stanley R. Friesen, M. D., Robert E. Bolinger, M.D., *and* **Joseph L. Kyner, M.D.,**
Kansas City, Kan.

The plasma levels of immunoreactive gastrin (IRGA) and immunoreactive insulin (IRI) were studied in 21 subjects during the oral glucose tolerance test. There was a rise in the IRGA which reached peak levels later than that for IRI. IRI and IRGA levels were correlated in such a way that earlier high levels of IRGA were associated with more prolonged elevations in the IRI. Furthermore, the group of 11 subjects with some degree of glucose intolerance showed significantly higher IRGA levels than did the normal subjects. Likewise the obese group had significantly higher levels than did those with normal body weight. An intravenous glucose tolerance test carried out on seven subjects was accompanied by a similar rise in serum gastrin. The sequence of events suggests that the increased IRGA during the glucose tolerance test was of pancreatic rather than gastric origin. The data support the existence of an enteroinsular axis in normal and abnormal clinical states.

From the Departments of Surgery and Medicine, and the Clinical Research Center, University of Kansas Medical Center, Kansas City, Kan.

THE RELEASE of polypeptide hormones from the embryologically and cytochemically similar endocrine cells of the foregut is influenced by both exocrine and endocrine products which result in normal endocrine homeostasis during good health. In abnormal clinical states, such as the Zollinger-Ellison (Z-E) syndrome and other clinical manifestations of the multiple endocrine adenomatosis syndromes (MEA I and II), there is an imbalance in the homeostatic mechanisms, which produces a variety of clinical pictures. It is known, for instance, that calcium affects parathormone, calcitonin, and gastrin release[22]; hydrochloric acid affects gastrin[9] and secretin release[1]; glucose affects insulin,[3, 25] gastric-inhibiting polypeptide,[3, 25] and gastrin levels[6]; secretin, cholecystokinin (CCK), and glucagon affect serum gastrin levels[7, 10, 16, 20]; pentagastrin stimulates thyrocalcitonin secretion[14]; thyrocalcitonin inhibits gastrin release,[2, 23]—to name a few reported examples. These interrelationships probably account for the high incidence of multiple endocrinopathies when one of the foregut endocrine systems becomes imbalanced for genetic or other reasons; they also may contribute to the confusion regarding the pathogenesis of the Z-E and MEA syndromes (theories of pituitary instigation, "gastric factor" in the enteroinsular axis, genetic and nesidioblastosis)[5] and could, in addition, account for the occasional observation of ulcerogenic tumor regression after total gastrectomy.[4]

When the interactions within the entero-

Supported in part by Grant (RR-828) from the General Clinical Research Center's Program of the Division of Research Resources, National Institutes of Health.

Accepted for publication August 12, 1974.

Reprint requests: Stanley R. Friesen, M.D., The University of Kansas Medical Center, College of Health Sciences Hospital, Rainbow Blvd. at 39th, Kansas City, Kan. 66103.

insular axis are examined specifically, the ingestion of glucose is bound to induce a series of primary hormonal responses and homeostatic reactions extending over several hours. Several of the gastrointestinal hormones secreted after the ingestion of various foodstuffs are known to mediate insulin release by the islets.[27] The secretion of gastrin has not been shown to be a part of this response but is classically known to be stimulated by a decrease in gastric acidity and inhibited by increasing acidity.[9, 17, 26] Gastrin tetrapeptide, on the other hand, is known to evoke the release of insulin from the islets,[18] although the concentrations necessary to do this are above the physiologic range. Vance and associates[28] have noted an associated hypersecretion of glucagon and insulin in patients with nesidioblastosis and have postulated a hyperreactivity of the enteroinsular axis. Oral glucose has been demonstrated to stimulate immunoreactive gastric inhibitory polypeptides (GIP) in normal man[3] and in patients after vagotomy and pyloroplasty[25] as further evidence for an enteroinsular axis.

Since gastrin has been demonstrated to be present in the delta cell of the islets,[13, 21] the possibility of the participation of gastrin in the hypersecretory response of the islet cell to glucose should be examined. In this study the behavior of the serum gastrin during the oral glucose tolerance test will be examined. Any possible association between gastrin and insulin secretion will be sought by a study of the correlations between various parameters of the secretory curve of the two hormones.

METHODS

Clinical. The study was carried out on 21 healthy subjects, six of whom were over 120 percent of ideal body weight. All of the subjects had normal fasting plasma glucose levels, but 11 of the group showed either a one hour glucose greater than 180 or a 2 hour glucose greater than 140. An oral glucose tolerance test was carried out for 6 hours following the ingestion of 100 Gm. of glucose as Glucola. A group of six normal controls was tested in the same manner following the ingestion of 180 ml. of water and subsequent blood sampling for 4 hours. Plasma glucose was determined on the AutoAnalyzer.[11] Immunoreactive insulin (IRI) was determined by the method of Herbert and associates,[15] using dextran-coated charcoal.

Immunoreactive gastrin (IRGA). Antiserum to crude gastrin II was produced in guinea pigs by the method of Yalow and Berson.[29] Antiserum was used in a final dilution of 1:6,000. Antibody prepared by this method had no significant cross-reaction with insulin or pancreozymin. Pure synthetic gastrin 1 to 17* was iodinated with I^{125} by the method of Greenwood and Hunter.[12] Radioimmunoasay was carried out using 100 λ of standard gastrin in concentrations of 50, 100, 500, 1,000, 5,000, and 10,000 picograms (pg.) per milliliter. Unknown serum was used in a volume of 300 λ. Antiserum and labeled hormone were added each in a volume of 100 λ, giving about 500 counts per minute. Final volume was adjusted to 700 λ with barbiturate buffer 0.02M, pH 8.0, containing 0.02M ethylene diamine tetra-acetic acid, and 0.3 percent bovine serum Albumin (Armour). Control tubes were set up for each unknown serum, using all reagents except antiserum. Incubation at 4° C. was carried out for 48 hours. Separation of bound from free label was carried out by adding 0.5 ml. of Amberlite,[29] 20 mg. per milliliter, and centrifuging at 4° C. Supernatant solution was counted and gastrin concentrations calculated with a curve fitting program. Before calculation to correct for nonspecific binding, counts in the tubes containing no antiserum were subtracted from the counts in the tubes containing antiserum. Experimental error was ± 10 percent of the IRGA value.

RESULTS

Mean fasting plasma immunoreactive gastrin (IRGA) levels shown in Table I were 99 ± 15 pg. per milliliter and, 2 hours after

*Imperial Chemical Industries Limited, Mereside Alderly Park, Macclesfield Cheshire, England.

Table I. *Plasma levels during oral glucose tolerance test*

	Fasting	Hours ½	1	2	3	4	5	6
All cases, n = 21								
Glucose (milligrams per 100 ml.)								
Mean	91	149	179	134	86	75	73	74
S.E.*	3	11	14	12	7	4	3	4
IRI† (microunits per milliliter)								
Mean	25	134	204	193	103	40	22	20
S.E.	6	23	33	31	34	10	5	6
IRGA‡ (picograms per milliliter)								
Mean	99	119	156	250	152	140	113	95
S.E.	15	24	41	47	23	30	19	19
Cases with normal glucose tolerance, n = 10:								
Glucose (milligrams per 100 ml.)								
Mean	88	113	124	93	77	78	79	71
S.E.	4	8	9	8	11	5	6	8
IRI† (microunits per milliliter)								
Mean	27	106	146	121	44	22	14	12
S.E.	11	15	41	26	11	5	5	5
IRGA‡ (picograms per milliliter)								
Mean	80	73	99	161	123	123	102	65
S.E.	21	18	31	42	22	43	31	22
Cases with glucose intolerance, n = 11:								
Glucose (milligrams per 100 ml.)								
Mean	93	183	228	172	95	73	70	77
S.E.	3	14	15	14	9	6	4	4
IRI† (microunits per milliliter)								
Mean	22	159	256	259	157	55	29	28
S.E.	5	42	48	46	62	18	8	9
IRGA‡ (picograms per milliliter)								
Mean	116	161	208	330	177	156	124	122
S.E.	21	40	71	75	38	43	24	28

*Standard error of the mean.
†IRI: immunoreactive insulin.
‡IRGA: immunoreactive gastrin.

glucose ingestion, increased to a mean peak of 250 ± 47 pg. per milliliter (Fig. 1). Mean IRGA levels at 2 hours were significantly different from fasting levels ($P < 0.01$). Increases in IRGA levels were accompanied by similar increases in glucose and IRI, although the mean peaking times for glucose, IRI, and IRGA were at 77, 82, and 130 minutes, respectively.

Results of a blank test using 180 ml. of water are shown in Table II, where it is noted that extensive variability obtains in the gastrin levels at 30 minutes; however, the basal levels are maintained throughout the succeeding 4 hours. For that reason, no data from the 30 minute gastrin levels are included in the assessment of the effect of glucose ingestion on gastrin blood levels. Correlations are shown in Table III. Earlier IRI peaking was associated ($r = -0.567$) with later IRGA peaking. The peaking times for glucose and IRI were associated with one another but dissociated from that of IRGA, as shown by the chi-square test ($P < 0.005$). IRGA levels at one hour correlated well with IRI levels at 3 and 4 hours ($P < 0.001$), while the magnitude of later IRGA peaks was correlated with high 6 hour IRI levels ($P < 0.05$). The integral increase in IRGA between one and 2 hours

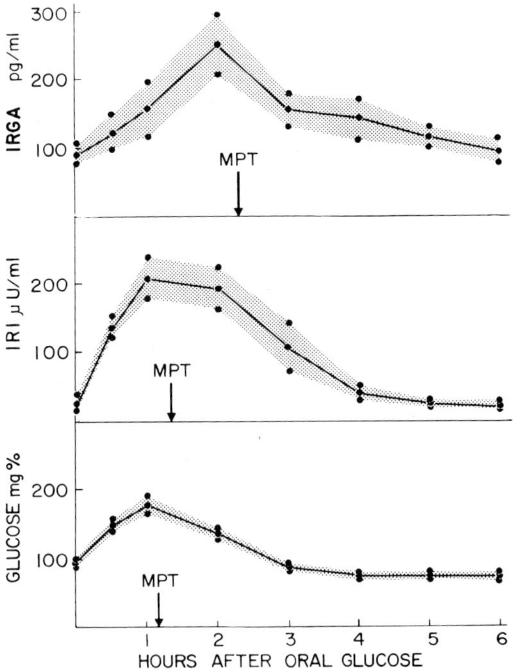

Fig. 1. Relation of plasma levels of IRGA, IRI, and glucose to the oral administration of glucose. Mean peaking time (MPT) is indicated by the arrow. Standard error of the mean is shown.

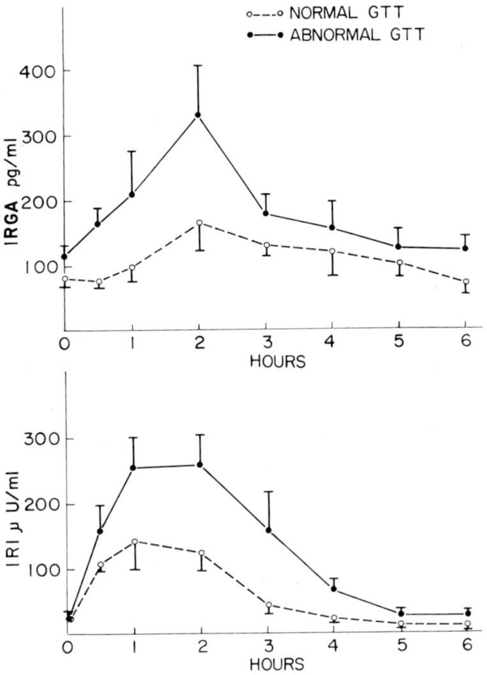

Fig. 2. Plasma IRI and IRGA response to oral glucose is shown for subjects with normal glucose tolerance (dotted line) and for those with abnormal glucose tolerance (solid line). Standard error of the mean is shown.

correlated ($P < 0.01$) with the level of IRI at 3 hours. The levels of IRGA and IRI at 3 hours showed a significant correlation with one another. In five cases a smaller secondary peak in IRGA occurred at 4 to 6 hours. Because of the variation in the peaking time of the curves for IRI and IRGA, the values at the apex of each curve were compared, excluding 30 minute values for aforementioned reasons. The one hour IRGA correlated with both the magnitude and time of the peak IRI ($P < 0.01$). Thus the greater the one hour IRGA, the later the insulin peak. The 4 hour ($P < 0.01$) and 6 hour ($P < 0.05$) IRGA levels were also correlated with the value for the peak IRI.

By analysis of variance, both the IRGA and IRI levels were significantly higher ($P < 0.001$) in the group showing decreased glucose tolerance (Fig. 2). When the subjects were grouped according to weight, those who were greater than 120 percent

Table II. *Plasma levels after ingestion of 180 ml. of water (n = 6)*

		Hours				
	F	*½*	*1*	*2*	*3*	*4*
Immunoreactive gastrin (picograms per milliliter):						
Mean	54	284	50	49	57	68
S.E.	20	195	21	7	24	19
Immunoreactive insulin (microunits per milliliter):						
Mean	26	20	22	22	22	23
S.E.	4	4	4	4	5	6

of their ideal body weight showed significantly higher IRGA levels ($P < 0.01$) and IRI levels than did the nonobese group. Differences between the groups were most marked at 4 hours ($P < 0.02$).

The IRGA levels following the intravenous injection of glucose are shown in Table IV for seven subjects. A similar increase in the IRGA is noted with peak values occurring at one to 2 hours which

Table III. *Correlations*

	Variable A (hr.)	Variables vs.	Variable B (hr.)	r	P
1	½	IRI*	3 IRG†	0.507	0.05
2	1	IRI	3 IRG	0.512	0.05
3	1	IRI	4 IRG	0.448	0.05
4	2	IRI	3 IRG	0.513	0.05
5	3	IRI	3 IRG	0.675	0.01
6	3	IRI	4 IRG	0.512	0.05
7	3	IRI	6 IRG	0.664	0.001
8	1	IRG	3 IRI	0.785	0.001
9	1	IRG	4 IRI	0.727	0.001
10	Fasting	IRG	Glucose nadir	0.496	0.05
11	1	IRG	IRI peak time	0.560	0.01
12	1	IRG	IRI peak	0.556	0.01
13	3	IRG	Glucose peak time	0.490	0.05
14	4	IRG	IRI peak	0.560	0.01
15	5	IRG	Glucose nadir	0.441	0.05
16	6	IRG	IRI peak	0.511	0.05
17	6	IRI	IRG peak time	0.501	0.05
18	IRG peak time		Insulin peak time	-0.567	0.01
19	IRG peak time		6 IRI	0.510	0.05
20	2 IRG area		3 IRI	0.572	0.01

*IRI: immunoreactive insulin.
†IRG: immunoreactive gastrin.

Table IV. *Serum gastrin during intravenous glucose tolerance test**

		Minutes				
	Fasting	15	30	45	60	120
Mean	136	212	240	224	316	319
S.E.	42	55	41	67	89	103

*Picograms per milliliter (n = 7).

are significantly higher ($P < 0.01$) than fasting values.

DISCUSSION

The studies described herein demonstrate a significant rise in the serum gastrin level during the oral glucose tolerance test and a peaking of the curves for glucose, insulin, and gastrin occurring in that order of time. Placebo oral tests carried out using an equal volume of water evoked erratic changes in the serum gastrin during the first 30 minutes, probably related to distension of the stomach,[24] but caused no significant changes thereafter. Since the more consistent peak in the serum gastrin followed that of the insulin peak, the possibility that gastrin might be triggering the release of insulin appears to be excluded. The correlations between peak values of gastrin and insulin neither support nor exclude any cause-and-effect relationship between the secretion of these two hormones but do suggest a communality in the secretory mechanism. The appearance of the gastrin peaks at a time after maximal mucosal stimulation of the stomach would probably have been completed suggests an extra-antral source for the gastrin. Moreover, the late appearance of the peak in proximity to that of the insulin is more consistent with the hypothesis that the islet is a source for the gastrin. The similarity of response during the intravenous glucose tolerance test tends to support this. A significant contribution to the peripheral venous level of gastrin from the pancreatic effluent in the dog following antral stimulation has been noted by Friesen and associates.[5] Further evidence of an extra gastric contribution to the serum gastrin level has been noted by Korman, Soveny, and Hansky[19] after gastrectomy. Vance and associates[28] have noted an associated exaggerated plasma insulin and glucagon response in patients with subtotal gastrectomy and multiple endocrine adenomatosis and have ascribed this to hyperactivity of the enteroinsular axis. The early increase in GIP levels slightly before or simultaneously with the increase of insulin in normal subjects as reported by Crockett and associates,[3] suggests an intestinal origin of GIP. Thomford and associates[25] have shown that the early GIP response to oral glucose in patients having had vagotomy and pyloroplasty is greater than in normal individuals; this augmented (GIP) response to glucose is presumably due to glucose intolerance in these operated patients, an observation which is similar to the enhanced insulin and gastrin response reported here with glucose intolerance. A similarly related hyper-response of insulin and gastrin is reported here in patients with glucose intolerance and insulin hypersecretion and suggests a common event related to islet cell activity as the source of the changes in the plasma level of both hormones during the glucose tolerance test.

REFERENCES

1. Bayliss, W. M., and Starling, E. H.: The mechanism of pancreatic secretion, J. Physiol. **28:** 325, 1902.
2. Becker, H. D., Reeder, D. D., Scurry, M. T., et al.: Inhibition of gastrin release and gastric secretion by calcitonin in patients with peptic ulcer, Am. J. Surg. **127:** 71, 1974.
3. Crockett, S. E., Cataland, S., Brown, J. C., et al.: Immunoreactive gastrin inhibitory polypeptide levels following oral glucose ingestion, Clin. Res. **22:** 465A, 1974.
4. Friesen, S. R.: A gastric factor in the pathogenesis of the Zollinger-Ellison syndrome, Ann. Surg. **168:** 483, 1968.
5. Friesen, S. R.: Zollinger-Ellison syndrome, Curr. Probl. Surg. April 1972.
6. Friesen, R. H., Friesen, S. R., and Bolinger, R. E.: Pancreatic gastrin response to intravenous glucose in the dog. Unpublished data.
7. Friesen, S. R., Hermreck, A. S., and Mantz, F. A., Jr.: Glucagon, gastrin and carcinoid tumors of the duodenum, pancreas and stomach: Polypeptide "apudomas" of the foregut, Am. J. Surg. **127:** 90, 1974.
8. Friesen, R. H., Frazier, R. L., Lukert, B. P., et al.: Antral influence on pancreatic islet function in dogs, Surg. Forum **23:** 367, 1972.
9. Friesen, S. R., Crosby, I., Boggan, M. D., et al.: An experimental study of the antral gastrin mechanism, SURGERY **75:** 517, 1974.
10. Gallagher, N. D., and Stening, G. F.: Effect of cholecystokinin and secretin on gastric hypersecretion in a patient with the Zollinger-Ellison syndrome, Aust. N. Z. J. Med. **4:** 393, 1972.
11. Grady, H. J., and Lamar, M. A.: Glucose determination by automatic chemical analysis, Clin. Chem. **5:** 542, 1959.
12. Greenwood, F. C., and Hunter, W. M.: The preparation of ^{131}I labeled human growth hormone of high specific radioactivity, Biochem. J. **89:** 114, 1963.
13. Greider, M. H., and McGuigan, J. E.: Cellular localization of gastrin in the human pancreas, Diabetes **20:** 389, 1971.
14. Hennessy, J. F., Gray, T. K., Cooper, C. W., et al.: Stimulation of thyrocalcitonin secretion by pentagastrin and calcium in two patients with medullary carcinoma of the thyroid, J. Clin. Endocrinol. Metab. **36:** 200, 1973.
15. Herbert, V., Lau, K. S., Gottlieb, C. W., et al.: Coated charcoal assay for insulin, J. Clin. Endocrinol. Metab. **25:** 1375, 1965.
16. Isenberg, J. I., Walsh, J. H., Passaro, E., Jr., et al.: Unusual effect of secretin on serum gastrin, serum calcium and gastric acid secretion in the patient with suspected Zollinger-Ellison syndrome, Gastroenterology **62:** 626, 1972.
17. Jackson, B. M., Reeder, D. D., and Thompson, J. C.: Dynamic characteristics of gastrin release, Am. J. Surg. **123:** 137, 1972.
18. Kikuchi, M., Tokeshi, K., and Ide, T.: Plasma insulin response to intravenous administration of tetragastrin (C-terminal tetrapeptide amide of gastrin in man), Metabolism **20:** 433, 1971.
19. Korman, M. G., Soveny, C., and Hansky, J.: Extragastric gastrin, Gut **13:** 346, 1972.
20. Korman, M. G., Soveny, C., and Hansky, J.: The effect of glucagon on serum gastrin. II. Studies in pernicious anemia and the Zollinger-Ellison syndrome, Gut **14:** 459, 1973.
21. Lomsky, R., Langr, F., and Vortel, V.: Immunochemical demonstration of gastrin in mammalian islets of Langerhans, Nature (Lond.) **223:** 618, 1969.
22. Passaro, E., Jr., Basso, N., and Walsh, J. H.: Calcium challenge in the Zollinger-Ellison syndrome, SURGERY **72:** 60, 1972.
23. Sizemore, G. W., Go., V. L. W., Kaplan, E. L., et al.: Relations of calcitonin and gastrin in the Zollinger-Ellison syndrome and medullary carcinoma of the thyroid, N. Engl. J. Med. **288:** 641, 1973.
24. Sugawara, K., Isaza, J., Curt, J. R., et al.: Distension of the pyloric antrum as a stimulus for gastrin release, Br. J. Surg. **100:** 201, 1970.
25. Thomford, N. R., Sirinek, K. R., Crockett, S. E., et al.: Augmented gastric inhibitory polypeptide response to oral glucose after vago-

tomy and pyloroplasty, Presented at meeting of Cent. Surg. Assoc. Feb. 1974.

26. Trudeau, W. L., and McGuigan, J. E.: Relations between serum gastrin levels and rates of gastric hydrochloric acid secretion, N. Engl. J. Med. **284:** 408, 1971.
27. Unger, R. H., and Eisentraut, A. M.: Enteroinsular axis, Arch. Intern. Med. (Chicago) **123:** 261, 1969.
28. Vance, J. E., Stoll, R. W., Fariss, B. L., et al.: Exaggerated intestinal glucagon and insulin responses in human subjects, Metabolism **21:** 405, 1972.
29. Yalow, R. S., and Berson, S. A.: Radioimmunoassay of gastrin, Gastroenterology **58:** 1, 1970.

Clinical review

The elective surgical treatment of chronic duodenal ulcer: A critical review

Leslie Wise, M.D., *and* **Walter F. Ballinger, M.D.,** *St. Louis, Mo.*

The few controlled, prospective studies suggest that the results for elective, duodenal ulcer surgery following vagotomy with pyloroplasty, vagotomy with gastroenterostomy, vagotomy with antrectomy and simple Billroth II type partial gastrectomy are not very different. There is no one "best" operation because each of these procedures seems to have some advantages and some disadvantages. Depending on the preference of the individual surgeon, he may perform any of these procedures, with the proviso that the mortality rate from the procedure should be under 1 percent; if he can achieve this with resection, this is probably slightly preferable to the simple procedures. If truncal or selective vagotomy is used, then gastrojejunostomy is probably slightly preferable to pyloroplasty as the drainage procedure. In the future, all studies should be prospective, randomized, and of at least five and, preferably more, years' duration. Cases excluded from the study must be followed as carefully as those included.

From the Department of Surgery, Washington University School of Medicine, St. Louis, Mo.

DURING the last three decades numerous claims have been made as to the "best" operation for chronic duodenal ulcer. During the 1930's, bypassing the ulcers by gastrojejunostomy was quite commonly performed, but it was soon realized that the operation was followed by a high incidence of marginal ulceration.[30] The next operation which gained favor was partial gastrectomy, but this was also abandoned to a large extent because of its supposed side effects (weight loss, dumping, nutritional disabilities, etc.) and, in the 1950's, truncal vagotomy with drainage was popularized. This was superseded by selective vagotomy with or without drainage and, quite recently, highly selective vagotomy without drainage has become the latest fashion in duodenal ulcer surgery. The purpose of this review is to analyze critically the results of these various procedures.

Accepted for publication April 4, 1974.

Reprint requests: Leslie Wise, M.D., Department of Surgery, Washington University School of Medicine, St. Louis, Mo. 63110.

SOURCES OF VARIABILITY

There are literally hundreds of papers published on the various operations for duodenal ulcer and the results vary considerably. The sources of this variability may be discussed under four headings.

1. Selection of patients. Among other factors age, sex, and the indications for operation may all influence prognosis. It has been shown that the death rates due to peptic ulcer in men per 100,000 population are low under the age of 30 years, become higher after age 60, and achieve a rate of 80 per 100,000 by age 80.[1] It has also been shown that the results of ulcer operations are significantly worse in females than in males.[10] The indications for operation, of course, may

Table I. *Clinical material (Cox series)*

	Vagotomy with gastrojejunostomy	*Billroth II partial gastrectomy*
Number of patients in study	81	79
Not available for follow-up	30	24
Available for follow-up	51 (84%)	55 (82%)
Reasons for unavailability:		
Postoperative death	1*	1†
Reoperation for recurrence	4	2
Carcinoma of stomach (died)	1	—
Unrelated late deaths	8	4
Unrelated, miscellaneous reasons	16	17

*Pulmonary edema.
†Enterocolitis.

Table II. *General evaluation of symptomatic outcome (Cox series): Patient's evaluation**

Symptoms	*No. of patients* — *Vagotomy with gastrojejunostomy*	*Billroth II partial gastrectomy*
None	30	25
Mild	14	18
Moderate	6	9
Severe	1	3
Total	51	55

*After Cox, A. G.: Br. Med. J. 1: 288, 1968.

also have a major effect on the results; emergency operations, especially those for hemorrhage, may result in higher mortality and morbidity rates than elective procedures. This obvious point is mentioned since such heterogeneous groups have been included in many "prospective, controlled series."

2. Selection of operation. Many surgeons tend to perform a "lesser" operation, such as vagotomy and drainage, for high-risk subjects. In addition, the surgical procedure is often modified according to the technical difficulties experienced at laparotomy, e.g., a "difficult" duodenum may influence a surgeon toward vagotomy and gastroenterostomy rather than partial gastrectomy. Obviously such selection may influence the results.

3. Operations not standarized. Such factors as size and shape of gastric remnant, size of stoma, type of pyloroplasty (e.g., Finney, Heineke-Mikulicz, Jaboulay, etc.), type of gastrojejunostomy (antecolic vs. retrocolic, isoperistaltic vs. antiperistaltic), and completeness of vagotomy are often not defined clearly in many articles.

4. Follow-up assessment. The main factors which should be considered are: (1) Who collected and assessed the results? The operating surgeon's assessment may well be biased. Ideally the results should be graded "blindly" by an independent observer. (2) What criteria were taken into account in the assessment (e.g., mortality rate, diarrhea, dumping, metabolic sequelae, etc.)? (3) Definition of terms (e.g., diarrhea, dumping). (4) Completeness of follow-up. (5) Duration of follow-up.

It should be obvious therefore that only controlled, prospective, randomized, clinical trials will help us answer the question as to which is the "best" elective operation for chronic duodenal ulcer. The results of the published trials will be reviewed. If cases are excluded from study series it is just as important to follow these cases as those included in the study.

GLASGOW TRIAL (NO. 1)

This trial was first set up in Glasgow by Sir Charles Illingworth in the middle 1950's.[7] The aim was to compare the results of three operations: (1) partial gastrectomy with gastroenterostomy (i.e., Billroth II type gastrectomy), (2) truncal vagotomy with gastrojejunostomy, and (3) gastroenterostomy alone. It soon became obvious that gastroenterostomy alone was frequently followed by marginal ulceration and therefore this procedure was soon eliminated from the study. In 1968 Cox[5] reported the results of this series. Only male patients admitted for elective duodenal ulcer surgery were included in the study. The choice of operation was determined by random selection after exploration of the abdomen had confirmed the diagnosis and shown that either operation could be performed with safety. The minimum follow-up period was 8 years and

Table III. *Allocation and subsequent fate of 568 male duodenal ulcer patients treated by different elective operations**

	Operative methods used			
	In Leeds/York trial, 1959-1962			In study, 1963-1965
	Vagotomy and gastroenterostomy	Vagotomy and antrectomy	Subtotal gastrectomy	Vagotomy and pyloroplasty
Number in each group	126	132	117	192
Operative deaths	0	0	0	1
Subsequent deaths	4	11	3	10
Untraced cases	3	5	7	17
Traced cases 5 to 8 years after operation	119	116	107	164

*After Goligher, J.C., et al.: Br. Med. J. 1: 7, 1972.

83 percent of the original patients were available for review (Table I). The vagotomy and gastrectomy groups of patients were similar when age, height, weight, and time since operation were compared. Although the over-all number of alimentary symptoms in each group was approximately the same, sensation of fullness after meals was significantly ($p < 0.001$) more common after partial gastrectomy. This was also accompanied by inability to eat large meals and a 20 percent incidence of postcibal sweating and faintness as opposed to a 10 percent incidence following vagotomy with gastroenterostomy. The over-all general evaluation of the symptomatic outcome is shown in Table II. The differences are not significant.

This study indicates that the differences between the symptomatic results of vagotomy with gastrojejunostomy vs. partial gastrectomy are insignificant, except for recurrent ulceration which is less common after gastrectomy, and postcibal fullness which is less common after vagotomy with gastroenterostomy.

THE LEEDS/YORK TRIAL

In this trial the results of three operations were compared:[10, 12] (1) truncal vagotomy with posterior, dependent gastrojejunostomy, (2) truncal vagotomy with antrectomy (Billroth II type reconstruction), and (3) standard partial gastrectomy (i.e., two thirds to three fourths distal resection) with Billroth II type reconstruction. The trial was open for the acceptance of new patients from 1959 to 1962 in the participating institutions at Leeds and York; there were nine surgeons who contributed to the trial. During that period 634 patients (507 men and 127 women) were admitted for the elective ("cold") surgical treatment of chronic duodenal ulcer.

It was decided to allow the surgeons to reject some of their cases from the trial either before laparotomy or in the light of the operative findings. Thus many surgeons excluded from the trial patients with a history of pulmonary tuberculosis or who were very thin because they felt that gastrectomy should be avoided in these subjects. On the other hand, for patients with a history of fairly recent hemorrhage, some surgeons considered, rightly or wrongly, that partial gastrectomy was the best treatment. Again at laparotomy with very adherent posterior wall ulcers it was sometimes considered that resection was too hazardous and so vagotomy with gastroenterostomy was performed. Once the decision was made to include the case in the trial, the choice of operation was out of the surgeon's control. Out of the 507 male patients, 132 (26 percent) were rejected from the trial and were mostly treated by vagotomy with gastroenterostomy. These patients were also followed and the results were very similar to those of the vagotomy with gastroenterostomy group in the trial except for a higher Visick IV group grading of the functional results (17 vs. 11 percent). The assessment of the results was made by a small panel of clinicians who were not al-

Table IV. *Frequency of symptoms due to disturbance of alimentary function 5 to 8 years after operation*

	Operations used			
Symptoms	*Vagotomy and gastroenterostomy (% of about 119 cases)**	*Vagotomy and antrectomy (% of about 116 cases)**	*Subtotal gastrectomy (% of about 107 cases)**	*Vagotomy and pyloroplasty (% of about 161 cases)**
Epigastric fullness	40.2	36.3	36.5	37.1
Early dumping	17.9	8.6	21.5	11.9
Late dumping	6.0	4.3	0.9	1.9
Nausea	12.8	17.2	23.4	17.6
Food vomiting	4.3	9.6	5.6	4.4
Bile vomiting	14.5	13.8	13.1	10.1
Heartburn	19.9	15.7	8.4	12.6
Flatulence	17.9	22.8	19.8	20.1
Dysphagia	1.1	0.0	0.0	0.6
Diarrhea	26.3	23.2	6.5	21.7

*The percentages relate to the total number of cases in which the particular symptom was elicited, which in some instances were a few less than the numbers indicated. Reprinted with permission from Goligher, J. C., et al.: Br. Med. J. 1: 7, 1972.

Table V. *Bowel habit 5 to 8 years after operation**

	Operations used			
Bowel habit	*Vagotomy and gastroenterostomy (% of 118 cases)*	*Vagotomy and antrectomy (% of 112 cases)*	*Subtotal gastrectomy (% of 107 cases)*	*Vagotomy and pyloroplasty (% of 161 cases)*
No change	42.3	39.3	57.0	50.4
Improved†	31.4	37.5	36.5	27.9
Diarrhea (all forms)	26.3	23.2	6.5	21.7
Severe diarrhea	5.1	2.7	0.9	4.3

*Modified after Goligher, J. C., et al.: Br. Med. J. 1: 7, 1972.

†"Improved" means that the stools have become somewhat looser and possibly a little more frequent; and regarded by the patient as an agreeable effect of the operation. The "diarrhea" ranged from 3 to 10 or more stools per day and it was usually mild.

lowed to know which operation had been performed until after they had recorded their findings, thus avoiding any bias from preconceived ideas of the relative advantages and disadvantages of the different operative methods.

From 1963 to 1965, inclusive, the co-operating surgeons in a second Leeds/York trial treated, in addition, 192 men with chronic duodenal ulcer by elective truncal vagotomy and Heineke-Mikulicz pyloroplasty.[11] The five to eight year results of this study have been compared with the results obtained in the first Leeds/York trial. Such a comparison is open to criticism; however, all the patients were derived from the same hospital areas and the methods of assessment were identical.

As seen in Table III, there were no operative deaths in the Leeds/York trial; there was, however, one postoperative death in the vagotomy-pyloroplasty series which was due to bronchopneumonia. Twenty-eight patients died subsequent to discharge from hospital; all these deaths were from unrelated causes. All patients in this series were followed for a minimum of 5 to 8 years. The results are discussed under three headings.[8]

1. Symptoms due to alimentary dysfunction. Contrary to popular belief, most of these symptoms occurred with approximately equal frequency after all these operations (Table IV). Diarrhea, however, was relatively rare after partial gastrectomy. The alterations in bowel habit were further analyzed as shown in Table V. It is quite clear that in this respect partial gastrectomy gave better results than the three vagotomy

Table VI. *Recurrence of ulcer 5 to 8 years after operation**

Degree of certainty of diagnosis of recurrence	Operations used: Vagotomy and gastroenterostomy (119 cases)	Vagotomy and antrectomy (116 cases)	Subtotal gastrectomy (107 cases)	Vagotomy and pyloroplasty (164 cases)
Proved at laparotomy	3	0	1	11
Highly suspected	4	2	1	7
Total	7	2	2	18

*Modified after Goligher, J. C., et al.: Br. Med. J. 1: 7, 1972.

Table VII. *Visick grading 5 to 8 years after operation**

Category	Operations used: Vagotomy and gastroenterostomy† (% of 119 cases)		Vagotomy and antrectomy† (% of 116 cases)		Subtotal gastrectomy† (% of 117 cases)		Vagotomy and pyloroplasty‡ (% of 164 cases)	
I. Excellent	44	70	50	78	49	77	45	68
II. Very good	26		28		28		23	
III. Satisfactory	19		14		17		18	
IV. Unsatisfactory	11		8		6		14	

*After Goligher, J. C., et al.: Br. Med. J. 1: 7, 1972.
†Leeds/York trial.
‡Not in the trial.

operations. In any discussion on diarrhea it is most important to have a clear definition of the term. Lack of such a definition accounts for some of the variations reported in the incidence of diarrhea.

Gastric resection (whether in the form of the classical partial gastrectomy or as antrectomy-vagotomy) was followed by a significantly greater weight loss (approximately 10 pounds) than vagotomy-gastroenterostomy, where there was no significant change in weight. The weight changes following vagotomy-pyloroplasty were not published.[11]

2. Recurrent ulcerations. Proved or highly suspected ulcers were less frequent after gastric resection procedures than after vagotomy with simple drainage (Table VI). The incidence was highest after vagotomy-pyloroplasty. The incidences of proved and highly suspected recurrent ulcers were 6.7 and 4.3 percent, respectively, after vagotomy-pyloroplasty, 2.5 and 3.3 percent after vagotomy-gastroenterostomy, 0 and 1.7 percent after vagotomy-antrectomy, and 0.9 and 0.9 percent after partial gastrectomy. The differences between vagotomy-pyloroplasty vs. vagotomy-antrectomy or standard partial gastrectomy are statistically significant, but those between vagotomy-pyloroplasty vs. vagotomy-gastroenterostomy are not.

3. Visick grading (over-all assessment). The results have been graded by a modification of the Visick classification[35] and are shown in Table VII. It can be seen that the over-all results after vagotomy-pyloroplasty are worse than after the other operations: 14 percent of patients unhappy after vagotomy-pyloroplasty, 11 percent after vagotomy-gastroenterostomy, 8 percent after vagotomy-antrectomy, and only 6 percent after partial gastrectomy. In the light of these findings, Goligher and co-workers[11] suggested that truncal vagotomy with pyloroplasty has not lived up to its expectations and its place as the currently most popular procedure in the elective surgical treatment of duodenal ulcer should be reconsidered.

Only 127 female patients were eligible for inclusion in the Leeds/York trial. Of these, 50 were rejected because several of the surgeons were unhappy about the alleged poor results of partial gastrectomy in female patients.[10] There were no operative deaths among the remaining 77 patients, but the number available for follow-up in the three subgroups was not sufficient to allow mean-

Table VIII. *Comparison of incidence of postgastric operation syndromes 5 to 8 years after vagotomy and gastroenterostomy in male and female patients**

Symptoms	*Males (% of 215 cases)*	*Females (% of 66 cases)*	*P*
Bile vomiting	13.7	35.4	< 0.001†
Nausea	15.7	38.5	< 0.001†
Epigastric fullness	39.0	56.9	< 0.001†
Early dumping	16.2	16.9	> 0.95
Late dumping	5.7	1.6	> 0.2
Flatulence	18.7	25.8	> 0.3
Heartburn	18.3	23.8	> 0.5
Reflux	6.7	11.1	> 0.3
Food vomiting	4.3	15.6	< 0.01†
Dysphagia	1.1	4.2	Not stated

*Reprinted with permission from Goligher, J. C., et al.: Br. Med. J. 2: 781, 1968.
†Statistically significant.

Table IX. *Comparison of percentage of Visick grading in all male and female patients at latest follow-up 5 to 8 years after vagotomy and gastroenterostomy**

Category	*Males (% of 215 patients)*		*Females (% of 66 patients)*	
I	45	71	28	58
II	26		30	
III	15		20	
IV	14		22	

*Reprinted with permission from Goligher, J. C., et al.: Br. Med. J. 2: 781, 1968.

ingful conclusions. A comparison, however, could be made between the results of all the male and female patients who had vagotomy-gastroenterostomy (this included not only patients in the trial, but also those rejected patients who had vagotomy-gastroenterostomy). Table VIII provides a comparison of the incidence of gastrointestinal symptoms in men and women. Bilious vomiting, nausea, epigastric fullness, and food vomiting were significantly more common in females. The recurrent ulceration rate was 5 percent for men and 9 percent for women. The differences in Visick grading are shown in Table IX. It should be noted that the number of Category IV cases among the women was 8 percent higher than in men, while the proportion of combined Categories I and II

Table X. *Distribution of the patients in the four groups**

Group	*Operation*	*No. of patients*
1	Random vagotomy and pyloroplasty	204
2	Random vagotomy and gastrojejunostomy	200
3	Pyloroplasty with vagotomy added (excluded from random trial)	42 (8%)
4	Gastrojejunostomy chosen as drainage and vagotomy added (excluded from random trial)	101 (18%)
	Total	547

*Reprinted with permission from Kennedy, F., et al.: Br. Med. J. 2: 71, 1973.

cases in women was 13 percent lower than in men.

GLASGOW TRIAL (NO. 2)

Kennedy and associates[24] reviewed their results of a controlled clinical trial on 547 patients who underwent truncal vagotomy combined with either gastrojejunostomy or pyloroplasty for the elective surgical treatment of chronic duodenal ulcer in the University Department of Surgery at the Western Infirmary, Glasgow, between 1965 and 1971. Excluded from the study were patients with combined gastric and duodenal ulcers and all patients undergoing emergency operations for the complications of duodenal ulcerations. When the diagnosis was confirmed at laparotomy, the surgeon first decided that either gastrojejunostomy or pyloroplasty would be equally safe and then the patient was randomly allocated to one of these two groups. If the diagnosis was in doubt then the pylorus was opened to confirm the presence of duodenal ulcer and closed as a pyloroplasty; truncal vagotomy was then added and this group of patients was excluded from the trial and categorized as Group 3. When pyloroplasty was regarded as technically unsafe, the patient received a gastrojejunostomy and truncal vagotomy and was allocated to Group 4 (Table X). All pyloroplasties were of the Heineke-Mikulicz type. There were no statistically significant differences between Groups 1 and 2 regarding sex, age, length of history, body weight, severity of symptoms, or acid output. The over-all operative mortality rate, including the rejected cases, was 0.5 percent; for the patients in the trial it was 0.25 percent (Table XI).

Of the 404 patients in the trial, 331 (82 percent) were assessed at least 2 years after operation, the mean length of follow-up being just over 4 years. Proved recurrent ulceration and dumping symptoms occurred more commonly after vagotomy-pyloroplasty, whereas bilious vomiting was more frequent after vagotomy-gastroenterostomy (Table XII). The over-all incidence of severe diarrhea was 1.1 percent, with no significant difference between the groups. These results indicate that almost 90 percent of the patients undergoing vagotomy and simple drainage had a good result. The final Visick grading is somewhat in favor of gastroenterostomy as the drainage procedure of choice (Table XII).

Table XI. *Period in hospital and major early complications**

	Group 1 (N = 204)	*Group 2 (N = 200)*
Time in hospital (days)	11.9 ± 0.3	12.2 ± 0.3
Deaths	None	1 Superior mesenteric arterial occlusion
Reoperation	2 Bleeding pyloroplasty 1 Subphrenic abscess	2 Stomal delay 2 Subphrenic abscess 2 Wound dehiscence
Cardiovascular complications	3 Deep vein thrombosis 3 Pulmonary embolism 1 Myocardial infarction 1 Atrial fibrillation	5 Deep vein thrombosis 2 Pulmonary embolism 1 Pericarditis

*Reprinted with permission from Kennedy, F., et al.: Br. Med. J. 2: 71, 1973.

Table XII. *Late results of Glasgow trial**

	Group 1 (N = 166)	*Group 2 (N = 165)*
Proved recurrent ulcer	4.8%	3.0%
Bilious vomiting	6%	16%
Dumping symptoms	27%	16%
Visick I and II†	150	152
Visick III†	12	12
Visick IV†	4	1

*Compiled from Kennedy, F., et al.: Br. Med. J. 2: 71, 1973.

†Final clinical assessment after reoperation for recurrent ulcer or bilious vomiting.

TRUNCAL VS. SELECTIVE VAGOTOMY

It has been suggested that the denervation of the small bowel and biliary tree may be responsible for the occasional diarrhea which follows truncal vagotomy. Truncal vagotomy has also been implicated in the pathogenesis of cholelithiasis.[25] Therefore selective gastric vagotomy is a theoretically more attractive procedure. There are five published "controlled" trials of truncal vs. selective vagotomy: (1) Kraft and associates (1967), (2) Mason and associates (1968), (3) Sawyers and associates (1968), (4) Kennedy and Connell (1969), and (5) Kronberg and associates (1970).

Kraft and co-workers[28] found no significant difference between the results of selective and truncal vagotomy in a 4 year follow-up. The trial entry, however, was not randomized, the drainage procedure was not standardized, the operation was performed for conditions other than duodenal ulcer, and the follow-up was incomplete.

Mason and co-workers[31] also attempted to compare the results of total vs. selective vagotomy. With the early selective cases, however, they had a very high incidence of incomplete vagotomies due to technical inexperience. Even after they obtained more experience, the incidence of incomplete vagotomies was 50 percent higher with the selective than with the truncal technique. The follow-up in this series was only 3 months. At that stage, the incidence of diarrhea was somewhat less after selective vagotomy. Unfortunately, again in this series, the drainage procedure was not standardized.

In a trial on 145 patients, Sawyers and associates[35] compared the clinical effects of truncal vs. selective vagotomies. Unfortu-

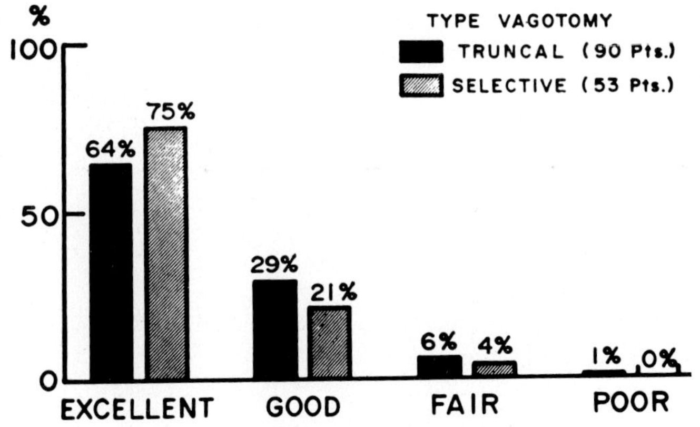

Fig. 1. Comparison of the clinical results of truncal vagotomy and selective vagotomy in 143 patients. (From Sawyers, J. L., et al.: Am. J. Surg. **115:** 165, 1968.)

nately, in only 67 percent of the cases was duodenal ulcer the primary indication for operation and the case material included emergency operations. Furthermore, in approximately 15 percent of cases, truncal vagotomy was performed because of technical difficulties or because the patient was a poor risk even though the randomized card indicated selective vagotomy and so the truncal technique was used in 63 percent of the patients, while selective gastric vagotomy was performed in only 37 percent. The drainage procedure was again not standardized and it included antral resection, pyloroplasty, and, in one case, gastrojejunostomy. The follow-up period ranged from 6 to 30 months. There were three differences found in the results: (1) there was a higher incidence of diarrhea in the truncal group (21 vs. 12 percent); (2) there was a higher incidence of positive Hollander tests in the truncal group (19 vs. 2 percent); (3) there was one recurrent ulcer in the truncal group and no recurrent ulcer in the selective group. The over-all clinical results, however, were the same in the two groups (Fig. 1).

In a randomized, controlled trial by Kennedy and Connell and their colleagues[25, 26] from Belfast, the 5 year follow-up results of selective and truncal vagotomy, each combined with pyloroplasty, were compared. The two groups were comparable as far as age, sex, and preoperative maximal acid output were concerned. There was no significant difference in the incidence of dumping, but there was a higher incidence of incomplete vagotomy, recurrent ulceration, and diarrhea in the truncal group. Two of 45 Hollander tests in the selective group and nine of 43 Hollander tests in the truncal group were positive in the immediate postoperative period. In three patients there was a proved recurrent ulcer; all three occurred in the truncal group. No patient died in either group and there were no significant differences in the postoperative complications. Furthermore, there was no significant difference in the 5 year over-all clinical grading between the two groups (Table XIII).

Kronberg and associates[29] reported on a controlled, randomized trial of truncal vs. selective vagotomy. The series included 81 patients with chronic duodenal ulcer. The drainage operation was a Heineke-Mikulicz pyloroplasty in 72 patients; four patients with selective and five with truncal vagotomy had a gastrojejunostomy because of severe pyloric scarring. Seventy-six patients were re-examined 5 years later. Although no difference in histamine- or insulin-activated gastric acid secretion could be demonstrated 10 days after the operation, 5 years later the insulin-activated secretion was higher after selective than after truncal vagotomy. This suggests a higher incidence of incomplete vagotomies with the selective than with the truncal procedure. At the 5 year follow-up no difference was found in the recurrent ulcer rate, but diarrhea was more frequent after truncal than after selective vagotomy; one patient with the truncal procedure was incapacitated due to diarrhea. Dumping symptoms and weight changes were equal in the two groups.

SAWYERS AND SCOTT TRIAL

Sawyers and Scott,[34] in a randomized study, compared the results of selective vagotomy with pyloroplasty (Finney or Jaboulay) vs. selective vagotomy with antrectomy (BI or BII). Only patients undergoing elective operations for duodenal ulcer were included. The 79 patients admitted to this study have been followed for 12 to 45 months, with an average follow-up of 30 months. There were 57 men and 22 women in the series with an age range from 16 to 76 years. There was no significant difference in the incidence of dumping or diarrhea between the two groups. Only one patient developed a recurrent ulcer (following selective vagotomy and Billroth I antrectomy); at reoperation an incomplete vagotomy was demonstrated. There was no significant difference in the postoperative insulin tests between the two groups: approximately 10 to 15 percent had incomplete vagotomies. There has been no operative death and the over-all clinical results are shown in Table XIV. The study suggests that selective gastric vagotomy with pyloroplasty produces just as good a clinical result as selective vagotomy with antrectomy. This is contrary to the past clinical experience of Scott and Sawyers and their colleagues[36] of the superior clinical benefits from truncal vagotomy-antrectomy compared to truncal vagotomy-pyloroplasty.

BELFAST TRIAL OF PYLOROPLASTY VS. GASTROJEJUNOSTOMY

Kennedy and associates[27] recently reported on the 2 to 5 year results (mean, 3½ years) of a double-blind, randomized, controlled trial comparing gastrojejunostomy and Finney pyloroplasty, each with selective vagotomy for the elective treatment of chronic duodenal ulceration. There were no operative deaths. The follow-up rate was 97 percent. There were two proved recurrences after pyloroplasty and one after gastrojejunostomy. The Visick grading was also marginally better for gastrojejunostomy. In addition, after gastrojejunostomy there was slightly less dumping, less increase of bowel frequency, and less flatulence; bilious vomiting, however, was less common after pyloroplasty. Although these differences were not statistically significant, the results of this trial suggest that with selective vagotomy gastrojejunostomy is a better drainage procedure than pyloroplasty.

Table XIII. *Clinical grading at 5 year follow-up, Belfast trial**

Grade	*Vagotomy*	
	Truncal (N = 49)	*Selective (N = 46)*
I	29	27
II	11	20
III	2	0
IV	4	2
Proved recurrent ulceration	3	0
Significant diarrhea	2	0

*Compiled from Kennedy, T., and Connell, A. M.: Lancet 1: 899, 1966.

Table XIV. *Critical appraisal of the over-all clinical results with selective vagotomy (Sawyers and Scott trial)**

	Antrectomy	*Pyloroplasty*
Excellent	27	22
Good	11	16
Fair	0	1
Poor	1	1

*Reprinted with permission from Sawyers, J. L., and Scott, W. H.: Ann. Surg. 174: 541, 1971.

JORDAN AND CONDON TRIAL

In the trial of Jordan and Condon,[23] 200 consecutive male, veteran patients requiring elective operation for duodenal ulcer were studied. The indications for operation were varied and included bleeding, obstruction, and perforation (Table XV). In two patients the primary indications for operation were not reported. Secondary operative procedures included aortofemoral bypasses in

Table XV. *Primary indications for operation (Jordan and Condon trial)**

Operation	Intractability No.	Intractability %	Bleeding No.	Bleeding %	Obstruction No.	Obstruction %	Perforation† No.	Perforation† %
Vagotomy and drainage	70	66	24	22	12	11	1	1
Vagotomy and resection	71	78	12	13	6	7	2	2

*Reprinted with permission from Jordan, P. H., and Condon, R. E.: Ann. Surg. 172: 547, 1970.

†Recent reperforation and continued intractability.

Table XVI. *Major complications associated with operative technique**

Complications	*V-P in 94*	*V-GE in 14*	*V-A-BI in 73*	*V-A-BII in 19*
Wound infection	7	1	5	3
Wound disruption	2	0	0	0
Stomal dysfunction	7	3	1	1
Reoperation for stomal dysfunction	2	2	0	1
Duodenal fistula	2	0	1	1
Reoperation for intestinal obstruction	1	0	0	0
Patients hospitalized postoperatively in excess of 10 days	29	7	18	12
Average postoperative hospitalization (days)	12	16	11	18
Operative deaths	2	0	0	0

*Reprinted with permission from Jordan, P. H., and Condon, R. E.: Ann. Surg. 172: 547, 1970.

Table XVII. *Jordan and Condon series*

Operation	*No.*	*Operative deaths*	*Incomplete vagotomy (%)*	*Recurrent ulcer*
Vagotomy and pyloroplasty	94	2	50	8 reoperated 3 under observation
Vagotomy and resection	92	0	13	None

Table XVIII. *Veterans Administration Cooperative Study Group: 5 year follow-up*

	Total No. of patients	*Operative deaths* (%)*	*No. of patients available for 5 yr. study for recurrent ulceration*	*Recurrent ulcers managed by operation†*	*No. of patients available for 5 yr. study for over-all grading*	*Over-all grading‡ Visick I and II (%)*	*Over-all grading‡ Visick IV (%)*
Vagotomy and drainage	337	0.6	226	7.3%— Pyloroplasty, 8.9% Gastroenterostomy, 5.7%	219	85.0	4.1
Vagotomy and antrectomy	331	0.9	236	0.8%— BI, 1.5% BII, 0.6%	223	86.6	3.1
Vagotomy and hemigastrectomy	343	0.6	273	1.1%— BI, 3.5% BII, 0.5%	266	88.0	2.3
Gastric resection only	346	1.8	242	4.5%— BI, 3.7%§ BII, 4.4%	234	90.6	2.1
Total	1,357		977		942		

*No significant difference between the four groups (Postlethwait).

†Recalculated from data in article.

‡Excludes deaths and patients with reoperation for any reason.

§There were only 27 BI gastric resections.

two patients and hiatal hernia repair in 11 patients. It should also be noted that at operation "the primary active ulcer or the residual scar was located in the duodenum in 194 and in the prepyloric area, at the pylorus or just proximal to the pylorus in 16 patients." This means that a small number of gastric ulcers were also apparently included in this series. Each patient was assigned preoperatively to either truncal vagotomy with Heineke-Mikulicz pyloroplasty (V-P) or truncal vagotomy with Billroth I antrectomy (V-BI). Surgeons were given the option to substitute gastroenterostomy (V-GE) for pyloroplasty or Billroth II type reconstruction for BI in case the duodenum was too scarred. In the original randomized study 98 patients were assigned V-P and 102 V-BI. In 10 patients the protocol was violated and a drainage operation was performed instead of resection. The operations actually performed were V-P in 94, V-GE in 14, V-BI in 73, and V-BII in 19. The operative complications are listed in Table XVI. The follow-up period ranged from 5 months to 5 years. There were no significant differences in the frequency of postoperative gastrointestinal symptoms between the two groups. The over-all results are shown in Table XVII. All the recurrent ulcers occurred in the vagotomy-pyloroplasty group. Again there was no significant difference in the over-all follow-up evaluations made by patients in the two groups; approximately 86 percent of patients in each group considered themselves much better as a result of the operation.

This trial suggests that truncal vagotomy with resection is superior to truncal vagotomy with simple drainage because of its lower recurrence rate without the association of increased morbidity and mortality rates. These results are similar to the nonrandomized findings of Sawyers and associates.[36] It should be noted that in the Jordan and Condon study a number of patients who randomly should have had resection did not have it because it was considered too hazardous. Therefore the statement that truncal vagotomy with resection is better than truncal vagotomy with simple drainage should be qualified insofar as that the higher recurrence rate after vagotomy and simple drainage is probably acceptable in those cases where the risk of resection is great.

Table XIX. *Comparison of effects of truncal and selective vagotomy* on incidence of postvagotomy diarrhea†*

	Truncal vagotomy		*Selective vagotomy*	
Ref. No.	*No. of patients*	*% with diarrhea*	*No. of patients*	*% with diarrhea*
3	100	26	100	12
6	131	2	44	2
13	60	68	52	29
14	30	50	44	6
39	43	9	22	0
26	50	37	50	27
28	42	33	40	20
32	90	21	53	12
15	300	23	100	9
17	81	36	101	12
34	118	7	100	9
27	35	46	36	11
25	50	30	48	8
Total	1,130	24.6	790	12.3

*With pyloroplasty, gastrojejunostomy, or antrectomy.
†Reprinted with permission from Johnston, D., et al.: Br. Med. J. 3: 788, 1972.

Table XX. *Bowel habit one year after truncal or selective vagotomy and pyloroplasty or highly selective vagotomy without drainage procedure**

	Truncal vagotomy and pyloroplasty (50 patients) (%)	*Selective vagotomy and pyloroplasty (50 patients) (%)*	*Highly selective vagotomy (50 patients) (%)*
No change	40	50	58
Improved	36	32	40
Diarrhea	24	18	2
Mild or moderate	18	16	2
Severe	6	2	0

*Reprinted with permission from Johnston, D., et al.: Br. Med. J. 3: 788, 1972.

VETERANS ADMINISTRATION COOPERATIVE TRIAL (POSTLETHWAIT)

In 1973 Postlethwait and Price and their colleagues[32, 33] reported the results of a

Table XXI. *Clinical incidence of early dumping one year after truncal or selective vagotomy and pyloroplasty or highly selective vagotomy without drainage procedure**

	Truncal vagotomy and pyloroplasty (50 patients) (%)	Selective vagotomy and pyloroplasty (50 patients) (%)	Highly selective vagotomy (50 patients) (%)	Controls (50 patients) (%)
Mild or moderate	20	32	6	4
Severe	0	2	0	0
Total	20	34	6	4

*Reprinted with permission from Humphrey, C. S., et al.: Br. Med. J. 3: 785, 1972.

Veterans Administration Cooperative Study Group. All patients were male veterans presenting for operation for chronic duodenal ulcer. Excluded from randomization were patients who had any previous operation altering gastric function but not simple closure of a perforated ulcer. Participants were advised to exclude all patients having emergency operation for hemorrhage or perforation and "this was almost totally observed." After abdominal exploration, the surgeon determined whether any one of the four trial operations could be performed without danger to the patient; the suitable subjects were then randomly assigned to one of four groups. A total of 1,357 patients were included in this trial in nearly equal groups: truncal vagotomy-drainage in 337, truncal vagotomy-antrectomy in 331, truncal vagotomy-hemigastrectomy in 343, and gastric resection only in 346. This represented 53 percent of all operations for duodenal ulcer in the 17 participating hospitals. The type of drainage as well as the reconstruction after resection was left to the judgment of the surgeon. Antrectomy indicated removal of 20 to 30 percent of the distal stomach, hemigastrectomy was an estimated 50 percent distal resection, and the gastrectomies without vagotomy were distal two thirds to three quarters resections. In all, 15.3 percent of the patients were lost to 5 year follow-up. The operative mortality rate for these procedures varied from 0.6 to 1.8 percent for gastric resection, but Postlethwait states that "the differences among these rates were not statistically significant" (Table XVIII).

The recurrence rates for vagotomy with simple drainage (i.e., pyloroplasty or gastroenterostomy) and for simple gastric resection were statistically higher than the recurrence rates for vagotomy-antrectomy and for vagotomy-hemigastrectomy. It is interesting to note that patient satisfaction was highest with simple gastric resection.

NEW PROCEDURES

The exact cause for the dumping syndrome and diarrhea which sometimes follow gastric surgery is not clear. The basic defect responsible for dumping seems to be the loss of pyloric control of gastric emptying; the main defect responsible for diarrhea is thought to be the extragastric vagal denervation associated with truncal vagotomy. The operation of highly selective vagotomy without a drainage procedure was introduced in the hope of minimizing dumping and diarrhea. In Table XIX[20] the effects of truncal and selective vagotomy on the incidence of diarrhea are compared. About 25 percent of patients experienced episodic diarrhea after truncal vagotomy and 12.5 percent after selective vagotomy, each with a drainage procedure. The diarrhea was usually mild, but in about 2 percent it was so severe that the operation had to be regarded as a failure. Burge and co-workers[2] suggested that in the absence of organic pyloric stenosis, selective vagotomy without drainage is an adequate procedure; others,[4, 39] however, have found that gastric stasis may occur without drainage and that in some cases this may be complicated by gastric ulcer.

Johnson and associates[20] reviewed the results in 150 patients who had undergone elective surgery for duodenal ulcer at least one year previously in the University Depart-

Table XXII. *Controlled trials for the elective surgical management of chronic duodenal ulcer*

Series	*Operation*	*Follow-up period*	*No. of patients and completeness of follow-up*	*Over-all evaluation*
1. Glasgow trial (Cox) No. 1	BII gastrectomy vs. vagotomy with gastrojejunostomy	Minimum of 8 yr.	Approx. 80 patients in each group, 83% follow-up	No significant difference (1) Recurrent ulcer, vagotomy > gastrectomy (2) Postcibal symptoms, gastrectomy > vagotomy
2. Leeds/York trial (Goligher et al.)	(a) Vagotomy with gastrojejunostomy (b) Vagotomy with BII antrectomy (c) BII gastrectomy	5-8 yr.	Approx. 120 patients in each group, 96% follow-up	No significant difference, except vagotomy and gastrojejunostomy had highest incidence of recurrence
3. Leeds/York supplementary trial	Vagotomy with pyloroplasty vs. operations in Leeds/York trial	5-8 yr.	192 patients, 88% follow-up	Vagotomy and pyloroplasty gave highest recurrence rate and poorest Visick grading
4. Glasgow trial (Kennedy et al.) No. 2	Vagotomy with pyloroplasty vs. vagotomy with gastrojejunostomy	At least 2 yr.; mean just over 4 yr.	Approx. 200 patients in each group, 83% follow-up	Results very similar, however (1) Visick grading gastrojejunostomy better than pyloroplasty (2) Recurrent ulcer, gastrojejunostomy < pyloroplasty (3) Bilious vomiting, gastrojejunostomy > pyloroplasty
5. Belfast trial for drainage procedure (Kennedy et al.—Ref. 27)	Selective vagotomy with Finney pyloroplasty vs. selective vagotomy with gastrojejunostomy	2-5 yr. (mean 3½yr.)	50 patients in each group, 94% follow-up	Over-all results slightly better with gastrojejunostomy
6. Belfast trial for type of vagotomy (Kennedy and Connell)	Selective vagotomy with pyloroplasty vs. truncal vagotomy with pyloroplasty	5 yr.	50 patients in each group, 95% follow-up	No significant difference except for higher incidence of diarrhea in truncal group
7. Copenhagen trial (Kronberg et al.)	Selective vagotomy with simple drainage vs. truncal vagotomy with simple drainage	5 yr.	Approx. 40 patients in each group, 97% follow-up	No significant difference except for higher incidence of diarrhea in truncal group
8. Sawyers et al. trial No. 1 (Sawyers et al.)	Truncal vagotomy with "drainage" vs. selective vagotomy with "drainage"	6 to 30 mo. after operation	145 patients in study group—63% had truncal and 37% had selective vagotomy, 100% follow-up	No significant difference in over-all clinical results, except for decrease in incidence of diarrhea and in percentage of incomplete vagotomies with selective procedure

Table XXII. *Cont'd*

Series	*Operation*	*Follow-up period*	*No. of patients and completeness of follow-up*	*Overall evaluation*
8. Sawyers et al. trial No. 1—Cont'd				Criticism of study: (a) Drainage procedure not standardized (b) In only 67% of cases was the primary indication for operation a chronic duodenal ulcer
9. Sawyers and Scott trial No. 2 (Sawyers and Scott)	Selective vagotomy with pyloroplasty vs. selective vagotomy with antrectomy	Average of 30 mo. with 12-45 mo. range	Approx. 40 patients in each group, 100% follow-up	No significant clinical difference; no operative death
10. Jordan and Condon trial	Truncal vagotomy with simple drainage vs. truncal vagotomy with antrectomy	5 mo. to 5 yr.	Approx. 100 patients in each group, approx. 90% follow-up	Truncal vagotomy with antrectomy gave better results than truncal vagotomy with simple drainage; V+A had a lower recurrence rate without association of increased mortality and morbidity
11. VA study	(1) Vagotomy and simple drainage (2) Vagotomy and antrectomy (3) Vagotomy and hemigastrectomy (4) Gastric resection only	5 yr.	Approx. 240 patients in each group, 72% follow-up	Vagotomy and simple drainage → high recurrence rate (7.3%); vagotomy and resection → approx. 1% recurrence rate (BI > BII); gastric resection only → almost 2% operative mortality and relatively high (4%) recurrence rate but good Visick grading
12. Wastell study	Highly selective vagotomy with pyloroplasty vs. highly selective vagotomy without drainage	3 to 12 mo.	16 patients without drainage and 20 with drainage	Two recurrent ulcers in group without drainage

ment of Surgery at the Leeds General Infirmary. The operative procedures used were: (1) truncal vagotomy-pyloroplasty, (2) selective vagotomy-pyloroplasty, and (3) highly selective vagotomy without a drainage procedure. This series was a retrospective review; the last 50 consecutive patients treated by each type of vagotomy and seen at least one year after operation (mean, 20 months) were chosen for analysis. The results are shown on Table XX. Seventy-five other patients with duodenal ulcer were also questioned before operation and three admitted to occasional attacks of diarrhea. These results suggest that, after highly selective vagotomy without a drainage procedure, the incidence of diarrhea is no higher than that in a control population. The incidence of dumping is shown in Table XXI[16]; it was significantly less frequent in patients who had undergone highly selective vagotomy without a drainage procedure than in patients who had undergone truncal or selective vagotomy with pyloroplasty ($P < 0.05$ and < 0.001, respectively). Up to date, in this series of highly selective vagotomies without drainage there has been no death and no proven recurrent ulceration.[9] Highly selective vagotomy without drainage reduces the secretion of gastric acid and pepsin as effectively as does truncal or selective vagotomy with a drainage procedure.[21, 22, 40] It has also been shown that highly selective vagotomy without drainage does not result in delayed gastric emptying.[41] In a 2 year follow-up of this series the over-all clinical results of highly selective vagotomy without drainage were much better than those of truncal or selective vagotomy with drainage.[9, 19]

The experience of Wastell and co-workers,[39] however, has been somewhat different. In 1972 they reviewed the results of a prospective, clinical trial comparing highly selective vagotomy with and without drainage. The follow-up period varied from 3 to 12 months. In the 16 patients without drainage there were two definite recurrent duodenal ulcers, causing them to advise caution in the adoption of highly selective vagotomy without drainage for the elective surgical treatment of duodenal ulceration.

The results of the controlled trials for the elective surgical treatment of chronic duodenal ulcer are summarized in Table XXII.

REFERENCES

1. Blumenthal, I. S.: Digestive disease as a national problem. III. Social cost of peptic ulcer, Gastroenterology **54:** 86, 1968.
2. Burge, H., MacLean, C., Stedeford, R., Pinn, G., and Hollanders, D.: Selective vagotomy without drainage. An interim report, Br. Med. J. **3:** 690, 1969.
3. Burge, H. W., Rizk, A. R., Tompkin, A. M. B., Barth, C. E., Hutchison, J. S. F., Longland, C. J., McLennan, I., and Miln, D. C.: Selective vagotomy in the prevention of post-vagotomy diarrhea, Lancet **2:** 897, 1961.
4. Clarke, R. J., McFarland, J. B., and Williams, J. A.: Gastric stasis and gastric ulcer after selective vagotomy without drainage procedure, Br. Med. J. **1:** 538, 1972.
5. Cox, A. G.: Comparison of symptoms after vagotomy with gastrojejunostomy and partial gastrectomy, Br. Med. J. **1:** 288, 1968.
6. Elliot-Smith, A., Painter, N. S., and Porter, R.: Selective vagotomy and post-vagotomy diarrhea, Lancet **2:** 1036, 1961.
7. Forrest, A. P. M.: The treatment of duodenal ulcer by gastroenterostomy, gastroenterostomy and vagotomy and partial gastrectomy, Gastroenterologia **89:** 307, 1958.
8. Goligher, J. C.: The comparative results of different operations in the elective treatment of duodenal ulcer, Br. J. Surg. **57:** 78, 1970.
9. Goligher, J. C.: Elective surgical treatment of duodenal ulcer, Br. Med. J. **2:** 420, 1973.
10. Goligher, J. C., Pulvertaft, C. N., DeDombal, F. T., Conyers, J. H., Duthie, H. L., Feather, D. B., Latchmore, A. J. C., Shoesmith, J. H., Smiddy, F. G., and Willson-Pepper, J.: Five- to eight-year results of Leeds/York controlled trial of elective surgery for duodenal ulcer, Br. Med. J. **2:** 781, 1968.
11. Goligher, J. C., Pulvertaft, C. N., Irvin, T. T., Johnston, D., Walker, B., Hall, R. A., Willson-Pepper, J., and Matheson, T. S.: Five- to eight-year results of truncal vagotomy and pyloroplasty for duodenal ulcer, Br. Med. J. **1:** 7, 1972.
12. Goligher, J. C., Pulvertaft, C. N., and Watkinson, G.: Controlled trial of vagotomy and gastroenterostomy, vagotomy and antrectomy and subtotal gastrectomy in elective treatment of duodenal ulcer: Interim report, Br Med. J. **1:** 455, 1964.
13. Harkins, H. N., Stavney, L. S., Griffith, C. A., Savage, L. E., Kato, T., and Nyhus, L. M.: Selective gastric vagotomy, Ann. Surg. **158:** 448, 1963.
14. Hedenstedt, S., and Lundquist, G.: Selective gastric vagotomy versus total abdominal vagotomy, Acta Chir. Scand. **131:** 448, 1966.
15. Hendry, W. G., and Abdulla, K. H.: Diarrhea after vagotomy. A comparative study of truncal and bilateral selective vagotomy, Br. J. Surg. **56:** 1, 1969.
16. Humphrey, C. S., Johnston, D., Walker, B. E., Pulvertaft, C. N., and Goligher, J. C.: Incidence of dumping after truncal and selective vagotomy with pyloroplasty and highly selective vagotomy without drainage procedure, Br. Med. J. **3:** 785, 1972.
17. Inberg, M. V.: Clinical experience with selective gastric and total abdominal vagotomy. Special reference to insulin test and post-vagotomy diarrhea, Ann. Chir. Gynaec. Fenn. 58 (Suppl. 165): 1969.
18. Jepson, K., Lari, J., Humphrey, C. S., Smith, R. B., Wilkinson, A. R., and Johnston, D.: A comparison of the effects of truncal, selective and highly selective vagotomy on max-

imal acid output in response to pentagastrin, Ann. Surg. **178:** 769, 1973.

19. Johnston, D., Goligher, J. C., Pulvertaft, C. N., Walker, B. E., Amdrup, E., and Jensen, H. E.: The two- to four-year clinical results of highly selective vagotomy (parietal-cell vagotomy) without drainage procedure for duodenal ulcer, Gut **13:** 842, 1972.
20. Johnston, D., Humphrey, C. S., Walker, B. E., Pulvertaft, C. N., and Goligher, J. C.: Vagotomy without diarrhea, Br. Med. J. **3:** 788, 1972.
21. Johnston, D., and Wilkinson, A. R.: Highly selective vagotomy without a drainage procedure in the treatment of duodenal ulcer, Br. J. Surg. **57:** 289, 1970.
22. Johnston, D., Wilkinson, A. R., Humphrey, C. S., Smith R. B., Goligher, J. C., Kragelund, E., and Amdrup, E.: Serial studies of gastric secretion in patients after highly selective (parietal-cell) vagotomy without a drainage procedure for duodenal ulcer. Part I. The effect of highly selective vagotomy on basal and pentagastrin-stimulated maximal acid output, Gastroenterology **64:** 1, 1973.
23. Jordan, P. H., and Condon, R. E.: A prospective evaluation of vagotomy-pyloroplasty and vagotomy-antrectomy for treatment of duodenal ulcer, Ann. Surg. **172:** 547, 1970.
24. Kennedy, F., MacKay, C., Bedi, B. S., and Kay, A. W.: Truncal vagotomy and drainage for chronic duodenal ulcer disease: A controlled trial, Br. Med. J. **2:** 71, 1973.
25. Kennedy, T., and Connell, A. M.: Selective or truncal vagotomy? A double blind randomized controlled trial, Lancet **1:** 899, 1966.
26. Kennedy, T., Connell, A. M., Love, A. H. G., MacRae, K. D., and Spencer, E. F. A.: Selective or truncal vagotomy? Five-year results of a double-blind, randomized, controlled trial, Br. J. Surg. **60:** 944, 1973.
27. Kennedy, T., Johnston, G. W., Love, A. H. G., Connell, A. M., and Spencer, E. F. A.: Pyloroplasty versus gastrojejunostomy. Results of a double-blind, randomized, controlled trial, Br. J. Surg. **60:** 949, 1973.
28. Kraft, R. O., Fry, W. J., Wilhelm, K. G., and Ransom, H. K.: Selective gastric vagotomy. A critical appraisal, Arch. Surg. **95:** 625, 1967.
29. Kronberg, O., Malstrom, J., and Christiansen, P. M.: A comparison between the results of truncal and selective vagotomy in patients with duodenal ulcer, Scand. J. Gastroenterol. (Suppl.) **5:** 519, 1970.
30. Lewisohn, R.: The frequency of gastro-jejunal ulcers, Surg. Gynecol. Obstet. **40:** 70, 1925.
31. Mason, M. C., Giles, G. R., Graham, N. G., Clark, C. G., and Goligher, J. C.: An early assessment of selective and total vagotomy, Br. J. Surg. **55:** 677, 1968.
32. Postlethwait, R. W.: Five year follow-up results of operations for duodenal ulcer, Surg. Gynecol. Obstet. **137:** 387, 1973.
33. Price, W. E., Grizzle, J. E., Postlethwait, R. W., Johnson, W. D., and Grabicki, P.: Results of operation for duodenal ulcer, Surg. Gynecol. Obstet. **131:** 233, 1970.
34. Sawyers, J. L., and Scott, W. H.: Selective gastric vagotomy with antrectomy or pyloroplasty, Ann. Surg. **174:** 541, 1971.
35. Sawyers, J. L., Scott, W. H. J., Edwards, W. H., Shull, H. J., and Law, D. H., IV: Comparative studies of the clinical effects of truncal and selective gastric vagotomy, Am. J. Surg. **115:** 165, 1968.
36. Scott, H. W., Jr., Sawyers, J. L., Gobbel, W. G., Herrington, J. L., Edwards, L. W., and Edwards, W. H.: Vagotomy and antrectomy in surgical treatment of duodenal ulcer, Surg. Clin. North Am. **46:** 349, 1966.
37. Tovey, F. I.: A comparison of polya gastrectomy, total and selective vagotomy, and of pyloroplasty and gastrojejunostomy, Br. J. Surg. **56:** 281, 1969.
38. Visick, A. H.: The study of the failures after gastrectomy, Ann. R. Coll. Surg. Eng. **3:** 266, 1948.
39. Wastell, C., Colin, J. F., MacNaughton, J. I., and Gleeson, J.: Selective proximal vagotomy with or without pyloroplasty, Br. Med. J. **1:** 28, 1972.
40. Wilkinson, A. R., Humphrey, C. S., Mason, M. C., Smith, R. B., and Johnston, D.: Serial gastric tests after highly selective vagotomy without drainage-comparison with truncal and selective vagotomy with drainage, Br. J. Surg. **58:** 295, 1971.
41. Wilkinson, A. R., and Johnston, D.: Effect of truncal, selective and highly selective vagotomy on gastric emptying and intestinal transit of food-barium meal in man, Ann. Surg. **178:** 190, 1973.
42. Williams, E. J., and Irvine, W. T.: Functional and metabolic effects of total and selective vagotomy, Lancet **1:** 1053, 1966.

Brief clinical reports

Aberrant pancreas causing pyloric obstruction

Yoichi Matsumoto, M.D., Yoshio Kawai, M.D., *and* **Ken Kimura, M.D.,** *Kobe, Japan*

A case of aberrant pancreas at the pylorus, which caused typical clinical features of hypertrophic pyloric stenosis, was reported. When an unusual appearance of the pyloric mass is noted in cases operated on as hypertrophic pyloric stenosis, biopsy should be done. If the aberrant pancreatic tissue is found, gastrectomy, including the pylorus, and gastroduodenostomy should be performed.

From the Department of Surgery, Kobe Children's Hospital, Kobe University School of Medicine, Kobe, Japan.

ABERRANT PANCREAS of the gastrointestinal tract is not uncommon and is usually asymptomatic. Once located at the pylorus, however, it causes pyloric obstruction and it is almost impossible to differentiate it from congenital hypertrophic pyloric stenosis. Even at operation, the diagnosis is very difficult to make because of the rarity of the condition. We considered it worthwhile to report a case of aberrant pancreas at the pylorus, incorrectly diagnosed as congenital hypertrophic pyloric stenosis.

CASE REPORT

A 5-day-old female infant was admitted with vomiting and melena. On admission she weighed 3,690 Gm., and she appeared to be icteric and cyanotic when she cried. Grade III systolic murmur was audible at the anterior chest but the breath sounds were normal. An olivelike mass was palpated in the right upper quadrant. The abdomen was moderately distended and the liver was palpable 2.5 cm. below the costal margin. Laboratory studies were within normal limits except for elevated serum bilirubin. The chest x-ray film was normal. The abdominal plain film showed a distended stomach with minimal gases in the intestines. Upper gastrointestinal series showed pyloric obstruction and barium enema was normal (Fig. 1). The preoperative diagnosis was hypertrophic pyloric stenosis and she was operated on with Ramstedt's procedure at the age of 7 days.

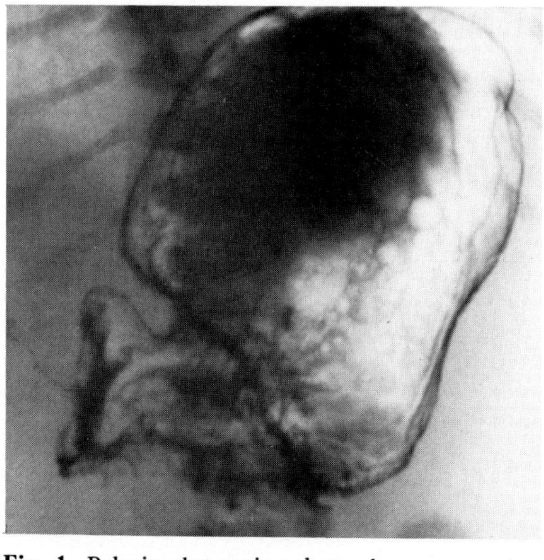

Fig. 1. Pyloric obstruction shown by upper gastrointestinal series.

A transverse incision was made in the right upper quadrant and the peritoneal cavity was

Accepted for publication July 16, 1974.

Reprint requests: Yoichi Matsumoto, M.D., Department of Surgery, Kobe Children's Hospital, Kobe, Japan.

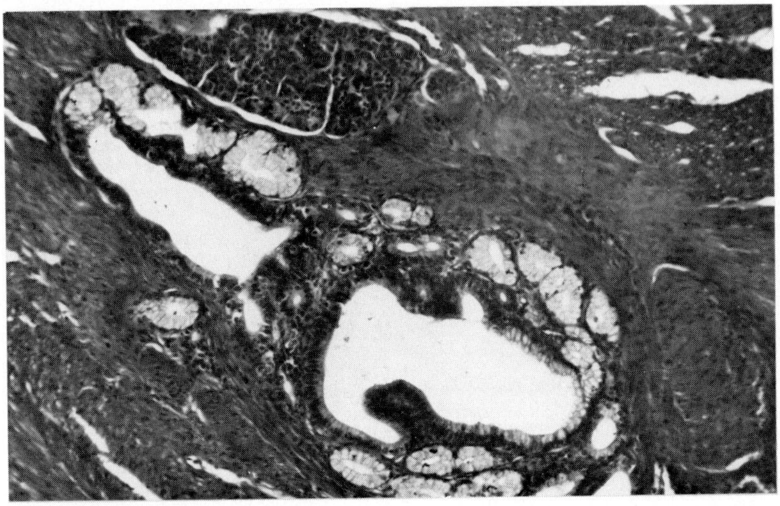

Fig. 2. The resected pyloric mass, showing pancreatic acini and ducts in the hypertrophied muscular structure with lymphocyte and histiocyte infiltration.

entered. A mass was noted at the pylorus but the serosal surface of this mass was rough and irregular, with yellowish tissue underneath the serosa. Its appearance was neoplastic and different from that of hypertrophic pyloric stenosis. Consistency of the mass was similar to hypertrophic pyloric stenosis. Ramstedt's procedure was then abandoned, and, after biopsy of the mass, a retrocolonic gastrojejunostomy was performed in antiperistaltic fashion.

The pathologist reported an absence of muscular hypertrophy and a remarkable fibrosis was noted in the biopsy specimen. The glandular structure was seen with the distended cavity lined by the glandular epithelium, similar to the pancreatic ducts, but there was no pancreatic parenchyma. At this point, the pathologic diagnosis was not definitely aberrant pancreas at the pylorus.

The patient did well after operation and subsequent cardiac catheterization revealed the interatrial septal defect. About 2 months after operation, she started vomiting again. The vomitus contained bile at this time.

She was initially managed conservatively, but after vomiting increased in frequency, she was readmitted to the hospital, 6 months after operation. On the second admission, she weighed 7,400 Gm. and still the pyloric olive was palpated. Upper gastrointestinal series showed delayed gastric emptying with stenosed gastrojejunal anastomosis, but minimal patency of the pylorus was noted.

A laparotomy was performed by an upper abdominal transverse incision. The firm pyloric mass was noted with a smooth serosal surface and its appearance was normal at this time. There was no yellowish tissue underneath the serosa. After detaching the gastrojejunal anastomosis, an antrectomy of the stomach, including the mass, was done, followed by gastroduodenostomy.

Pathologic study of the resected mass showed the pancreatic acini and ducts in the hypertrophied muscular structure with lymphocyte and histiocyte infiltration. The islet structure was not observed. There were no abnormal findings at the pyloric mucosa (Fig. 2).

Follow-up after the second operation showed normal development and growth.

COMMENT

Aberrant pancreas causing pyloric obstruction is extremely rare and only a few cases have been reported.[1, 2, 3] In the case reported here, vomiting and melena started soon after birth and our preoperative diagnosis was that of an unusual type of hypertrophic pyloric stenosis, even though the onset of symptoms of hypertrophic pyloric stenosis usually occurs after 2 weeks. A review of the literature showed no case reported with correct preoperative diagnosis. The case reported by Kernohan and Morison[2] was of a 17-day-old male infant admitted with typical clinical course of hypertrophic pyloric stenosis. Ramstedt's procedure was performed, followed by persistent vomiting, diarrhea, and tarry stool. He died 11 weeks later. At autopsy the cause of gastrointestinal hemorrhage could not be determined. Komi and associates[3] reported a case of a 2-month-old boy who started vomiting at 1 week of age. In this case, the upper gastrointestinal series was unusual as with hypertrophic pyloric stenosis, and the preoperative diagnosis was gastric tumor. Distal gastrectomy was done, including the pyloric mass, and the pathologic study revealed a mucosal lesion at the pylorus with a bleeding point.

We believe that diagnosis based on operative findings is not reliable and only pathologic or histologic study of the biopsy specimen allows an accurate diagnosis. In our case, the biopsy specimen did not contain the pancreatic parenchyma and only the adenogranular tissue was observed. The gastrojejunostomy was palliatively done and the postoperative course was closely followed. Gastrectomy in infants is a grave procedure, but we feel that distal gastrectomy with gastroduodenostomy is the treatment of choice.

REFERENCES

1. Collet, R. W.: Prepyloric polyps in stomach of childhood, Am. J. Dis. Child. **72:** 545, 1946.
2. Kernohan, R. J., and Morison, J. E.: Symptomatic pancreatic heterotopia of pylorus associated with bilateral renal necrosis in an infant, Arch. Dis. Child. **31:** 276, 1956.
3. Komi, N., Takahashi, K., and Suzuki, S.: A clinical study of aberrant pancreas causing pyloric obstruction with hemorrhage, Igaku-no-ayumi **70:** 265, 1969.

Solitary rectal ulcer: A cause of life-threatening hemorrhage

Herman Delancy, M.D., *and* **William Stroud Hitch, M.D.,** *Savannah, Ga.*

Three cases of massive hemorrhage from solitary ulcer of the rectum are presented. Each occurred in a patient seriously ill from causes unrelated to the gastrointestinal tract. The bleeding occurred suddenly and without prodromal symptoms and was life threatening in each patient. Treatment is directed toward local control of the bleeding point and diversion of the fecal stream. A combined abdominotransanal approach utilizing a low colotomy is a useful way of identifying and controlling this source of hemorrhage.

From the Department of Surgery, Memorial Medical Center, Savannah, Ga.

MASSIVE RECTAL BLEEDING presents a difficult challenge in diagnosis and treatment. This report deals with an unusual cause of rectal bleeding which has not previously been discussed in detail. Three case studies and comments on management are included.

CASE REPORTS

Case 1. E. H., a 54-year-old woman, underwent removal of a large meningioma from the left cerebellar fossa. On the thirteenth postoperative day she experienced a sudden onset of left hemiplegia, which was thought to be caused by a cerebral embolus. She recovered from this episode rather slowly and required frequent enemas for bowel evacuation. On the twenty-third hospital day she developed profuse rectal bleeding. Proctoscopic examination demonstrated a shallow bleeding ulcer on the anterior wall of the rectum 6 cm. from the dentate line. The ulcer was cauterized with good control of the bleeding. She again developed profuse rectal bleeding 2 days later and proctoscopic examination showed extension of the ulceration with an active arterial bleeder. This time bleeding was controlled by oversewing from below. After control of the bleeding, it was noted that the adjacent rectal mucosa was unremarkable. However, 2 days later she again had sudden onset of severe, bright red rectal bleeding. On this occasion she underwent a diverting colostomy and oversewing of the ulcer from below. At this time an ulcer was noted on the posterior midline 8 cm. from the dentate line. Multiple biopsies of the ulcer crater were taken and demonstrated only mild inflammation. Her colostomy was closed one month later and rectal bleeding never recurred for the remainder of her life.

Case 2. C. M., a 47-year-old woman, was admitted acutely ill with diabetic ketoacidosis. Appropriate treatment was instituted but the patient remained obtunded and incontinent of feces. On the sixth hospital day she suddenly passed an estimated liter of bright blood via the rectum. This was followed by a continuation of semiliquid stool and bright red blood. Coagulation studies were normal. Proctoscopic examination in bed was unsuccessful because of profuse bleeding, which completely obscured the field. Barium enema demonstrated multiple filling defects considered to be blood clots. At emergency laparotomy the entire left colon was found to be distended with blood. In the absence of obvious bleeding sites and with no radiographic evidence of diverticulosis, it was elected to do a low anterior colotomy to determine if the bleeding was coming from the rectum or from the colon. The rectum was cleared of blood by suction and immediately refilled, thus localizing

Accepted for publication July 26, 1974.

Reprint requests: Herman Delancy, M.D., 5102 Paulsen St., Savannah, Ga. 31405.

the site of bleeding to the rectal segment. The patient was placed in the lithotomy position while a sertile field was maintained above, and a proctoscope was introduced. By maintaining suction through the colotomy, it was possible to localize a vigorous arterial bleeder on the posterior lateral wall 10 cm. above the dentate line. The bleeder was contained within a small shallow ulcer. Multiple biopsies were taken from the wall of the ulcer and hemostasis was obtained by oversewing the bleeding artery. The colotomy was closed and a diverting transverse colostomy was constructed. The patient experienced no further bleeding but died one week later of uncontrollable diabetic ketoacidosis. Autopsy revealed pulmonary emphysema, intercapillary glomerulosclerosis, and acute and chronic pyelonephritis. The colonic mucosa was entirely normal aside from a small area of inflammation in the region of the colotomy. The biopsies of the ulcer crater showed only submucosal hemorrhage.

Case 3. R. L., a 57-year-old man, developed cardiac arrest while undergoing bone marrow aspiration. Resuscitative efforts resulted in sternal fracture. Tracheostomy with mechanical ventilation was required. He became septic 2 days later and had a moderate amount of diarrhea. On the seventh day he developed massive, painless rectal bleeding. Four units of whole blood were required during a one hour period to maintain systolic blood pressure at 100 mm. Hg. Proctoscopic examination was attempted, but bleeding was so profuse that successful examination could not be accomplished. While awaiting angiography, the patient became shocky, and it was elected to forego any further studies and to resort to operation. Emergency laparotomy revealed the colon to be filled with blood to the level of the mid ascending colon. No obvious site of bleeding was apparent and there was no gross evidence of diverticular disease. Because of our previous experience, a low sigmoid colotomy was performed, and it was determined that the bleeding point was in the rectum. The patient was placed in lithotomy position, and, by aspirating blood from above and below, it was possible to localize the site of bleeding to a shallow ulcer on the posterior rectal wall 6 cm. from the dentate line. A large artery in the base of the ulcer was suture ligated and a diverting colostomy was constructed. The patient experienced no further bleeding and made an uneventful recovery. Colostomy closure was performed 2 months later.

DISCUSSION

Solitary ulceration into a submucosal artery in an otherwise normal rectum caused life-threatening hemorrhage in three patients. The ulcers occurred in the rectal ampulla 6 to 10 cm. above the dentate line in patients seriously ill from other causes. Solitary ulcer of the rectum has previously been discussed,[2, 3] but we have not been able to document a previous report of this entity as a source of life-threatening hemorrhage. Microscopic examination of biopsy specimens has provided no clue as to the etiology of the ulcer. One of our patients (Case 1) had constipation requiring frequent enemas. It is possible that this ulcer resulted from pressure necrosis—a stercoraceous ulcer. The other two patients were not constipated but rather had other difficulty with bowel movement—bowel aberrations of fecal incontinence and moderate diarrhea. The management of these cases may be difficult. As noted in Cases 2 and 3, protoscopic examination is frequently unrewarding due to severity of the bleeding. Further, the diagnosis may easily be confused with other causes of massive colonic bleeding such as diverticular disease.[5] Angiography may be useful but also may be hazardous because of delay in controlling the severe bleeding that occurs. Obviously colectomy with ileoproctostomy, as performed for diverticular disease,[1, 4] will be useless in this situation. The presence of bright red arterial blood and clot may be clues that the bleeding is coming from erosion of an artery in the rectal ampulla. If this condition is suspected, it seems wise to do a colotomy above the peritoneal reflection to isolate the rectal pouch. If the blood is coming from the rectum, then the bleeding point can be quickly visualized from below with the help of colotomy and vigorous suction. Although exposure may be difficult, the bleeding point can usually be concontrolled by transfixing or oversewing from below. The construction of a diverting colostomy is advisable to prevent recurrent bleeding. It is probably unwise to re-establish intestinal continuity until the patient has regained a normal state of good health and is no longer prone to fecal impactions or other bowel dysfunction.

REFERENCES

1. Bruders, C. W.: Bleeding from diverticula of the colon, Surg. Clin. North Am. **52:** 317, 1972.

2. Haskell, B., and Rovner, H.: Solitary ulcer of the rectum, Dis. Colon. Rectum **8:** 333, 1965.
3. Madigan, M. R., and Morson, B. C.: Solitary ulcer of the rectum, Gut **10:** 871, 1969.
4. McGuire, H. H., Jr., and Haynes, B. W., Jr.: Massive hemorrhage from diverticulosis of the colon: Guidelines for therapy based on bleeding patterns in fifty cases, Ann. Surg. **175:** 852, 1972.
5. Noer, R. J., Hamilton, J. E., Williams, D. J., and Broughton, D. S.: Rectal hemorrhage: Moderate and severe, Am. Surg. **155:** 796, 1962.

Occlusion of popliteal artery caused by popliteal cysts

James D. Schlenker, M.D., Kent Johnston, M.D., *and* **Jerry S. Wolkoff, M.D.,**
Cleveland, Ohio

This is the first reported case of popliteal artery occlusion caused by popliteal cysts. The patient presented with acute ischemia of the foot and lower leg. The popliteal cysts were excised, the arteries were thrombectomized, and the blood flow was re-established.

From the Department of Surgery, Case Western Reserve University School of Medicine, and Cleveland Veterans Administration Hospital, Cleveland, Ohio.

POPLITEAL CYSTS can simulate different vascular abnormalities. When they are painful and tender, they can be confused with thrombophlebitis.[5, 12] When they transmit the pulsation of the popliteal artery, they may appear as popliteal aneurysms.[1, 12] Popliteal cysts have been reported to cause venous obstruction, but arterial obstruction has not been reported.[5, 12] It is the purpose of this paper to document a case of acute ischemia of the leg secondary to occlusion of the popliteal artery by popliteal cysts.

CASE REPORT

A 56-year-old man was admitted for evaluation of the sudden onset of pain and numbness in the left foot and ankle of 10 hours' duration, which had occurred while sitting, and which subsequently prevented ambulation. He denied pain or swelling of the left knee.

He had undergone a cup arthroplasty for severe osteoarthritis of the right hip 23 years previously and a meniscectomy of a torn medial meniscus of the right knee 22 years earlier. At the time of the hip and knee operations, multiple osteochondromatous loose bodies were found in the joints. A biopsy of the synovium of the hip joint was consistent with the diagnosis of synovial osteochondromatosis.[13] Except for occasional locking of the right hip in flexion, he had improved ability to ambulate. He smoked one pack of cigarettes per day and had chronic bronchitis with a productive cough and moderate exertional dyspnea, for which he was treated with bronchodilators.

On physical examination the left leg was cold and blue below midcalf. Capillary and venous filling were prolonged. Sensory and motor function of the left foot were diminished. The pulses in the right leg were normal. The left femoral pulse was normal and the left popliteal pulse was stronger and wider than usual. Dorsalis pedis and posterior tibial pulses on the left side were absent. There was no evidence of knee joint effusion.

The hematocrit was 60 percent and the white blood cell count was 15,300. The chest x-ray showed chronic fibrotic changes. A right femoral arteriogram revealed a complete occlusion of the popliteal artery with no delayed visualization of the posterior tibial, anterior tibial, or peroneal arteries (Fig. 1).

Under local anesthesia the left common femoral artery was explored. A Fogarty catheter could be passed to the level of the knee joint but no farther, and no thrombus was extracted. Under general anesthesia the popliteal space was explored through a medial longitudinal incision. After the deep fascia had been incised, a large popliteal cyst was entered which contained a considerable amount of clear viscous fluid and multiple irregular cartilagi-

Accepted for publication July 26, 1974.

Reprint requests: James D. Schlenker, Major, MC, USA, 2936A Summerall Circle, Fort Eustis, Va. 23604.

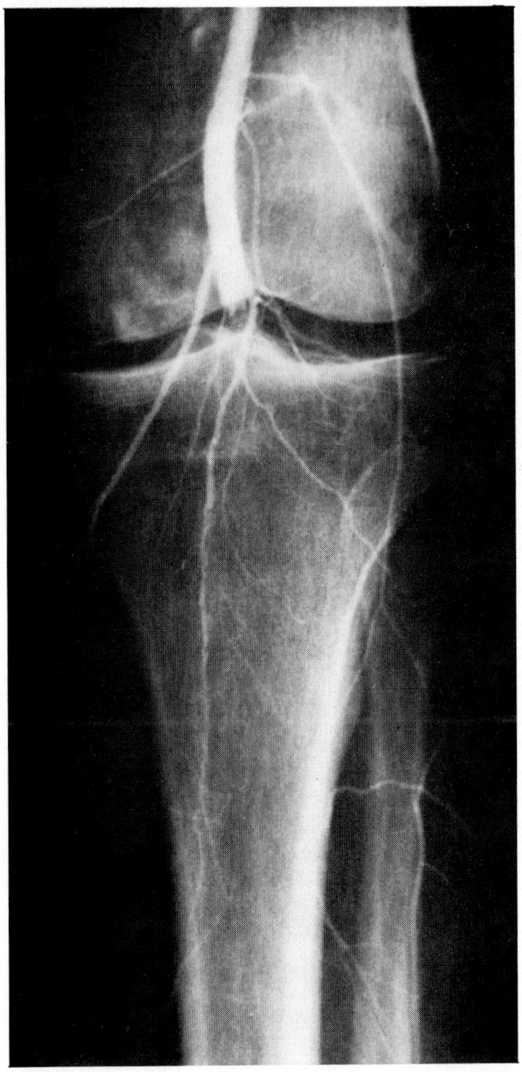

Fig. 1. The arteriogram shows occlusion of the popliteal artery at the level of the knee joint with poor runoff.

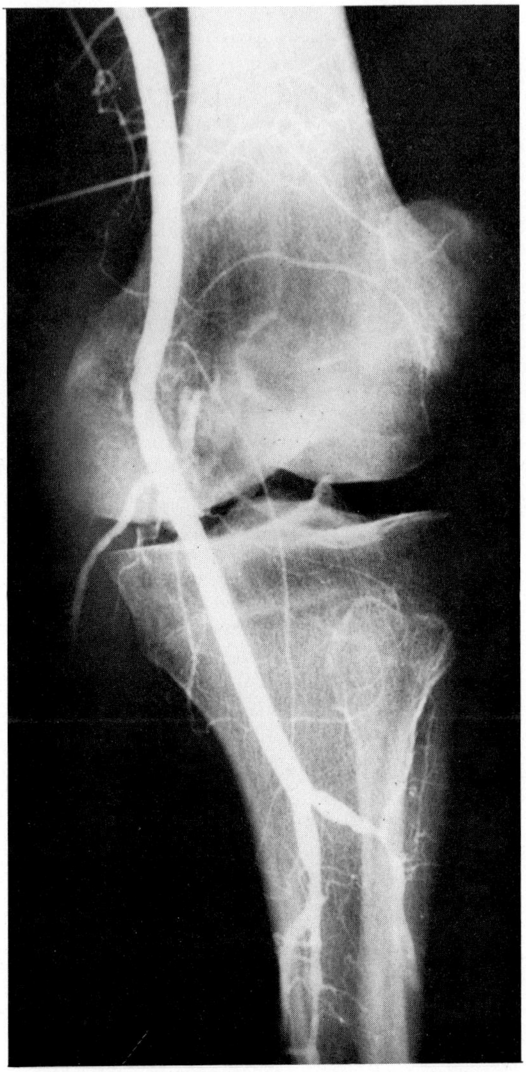

Fig. 2. Intraoperative arteriogram after excision of popliteal cysts and thrombectomy reveals re-establishment of flow through posterior tibial and peroneal arteries.

nous loose bodies. These were evacuated and the cyst was excised. It occupied the medial aspect of the popliteal space and tapered to a narrow neck, which was attached to the joint capsule between the medial head of the gastrocnemius muscle and the semimembranosus muscle. Lateral to this cyst, the popliteal vessels and nerve were identified. They were stretched and bowed medially by a laterally located mass. The thin fascia holding and compressing these structures against the mass was incised. The popliteal artery was freed and a pulse was restored. The mass was identified as another large popliteal cyst which contained viscous fluid and many cartilaginous bodies. This was dissected from the popliteal vessels and excised. The neck of the cyst appeared to communicate with the knee joint near the lateral head of the gastrocnemius muscle.

The patient was systemically anticoagulated with heparin and the popliteal artery was opened. The artery was pliable and the lumen was free of atheromatous material. By passing Fogarty catheters distally, recent and old thrombotic material was removed. Backflow was re-established. Subcutaneous fasciotomies of the posterior and anterior compartments of the leg were performed. An intraoperative arteriogram showed restoration of flow through the posterior tibial and peroneal arteries (Fig. 2).

Postoperatively the leg became warm and edematous. A posterior tibial but no dorsalis pedis pulse was present. The patient recovered his preoperative ability to ambulate. Pathologic examination confirmed the diagnosis of a synovial cyst containing loose osteochondromas. Prior to discharge, x-rays of the knee showed changes consistent with osteoarthritis. A pneumarthrogram of the left knee was normal.

DISCUSSION

The differential diagnosis on the basis of clinical presentation of this patient would include embolus, thrombosis of a segment of artery already narrowed by atheromatous plaques, popliteal aneurysm, and popliteal artery entrapment syndrome.[4, 6, 9] Popliteal aneurysm was considered initially in this patient because of the widened popliteal pulse. The inability to pass the Fogarty catheter distal to the knee led to exploration of the popliteal artery. This case indicates the importance of exploring the popliteal artery directly when thrombectomy through the femoral artery is not successful. The finding of cysts around the popliteal artery raised the possibility of cystic adventitial disease.[3, 8, 10, 11] Adventitial cysts are located between the adventitia and media of the artery, whereas the popliteal cysts in this patient were located outside the adventitia of the artery and vein. Histologically they are similar to popliteal cysts, but in only two cases has a connection with the joint space been demonstrated.[11] None has been reported to contain osteochondromas.

The cause-and-effect relationship between the popliteal cysts and occlusion of the popliteal artery was unmistakable at the time of the operation. Intrinsic disease of the arteries may have contributed to the thrombotic episode. Although the popliteal artery was grossly free of atherosclerosis, the arteriogram after thrombectomy showed that the arteries distal to the trifurcation of the popliteal were stenotic (Fig. 2). It cannot be stated with certainty whether the stenotic lesions seen on the arteriogram represented residual old thrombus or atherosclerotic plaques. It is interesting that a femoral arteriogram performed on the opposite leg after the operation was entirely normal. Polycythemia secondary to chronic obstructive pulmonary disease also predisposed this patient to thrombotic complications.

Popliteal cysts are thought either to arise from popliteal bursae or to be acquired herniations of synovium in the posterior part of the knee.[1, 12, 14] In our patient the two cysts originated in areas normally occupied by the gastrocnemio-semimembranosus bursa medially and the lateral gastrocnemius bursa laterally.[1, 14] The gastrocnemio-semimembranosus bursa has been thought to communicate with the knee joint in 50 percent of normal patients.[14] Wolfe and Colloff[15] found with pneumarthrograms that almost all clinically evident popliteal cysts communicated with the joint space. When popliteal cysts become acutely symptomatic, there is often an associated effusion of the knee joint.[5] In this patient the absence of symptoms related to the knee and the absence of knee joint effusion indicated that these cysts had not enlarged acutely.

Popliteal cysts in adults are often related to intra-articular disturbances of the knee such as damage to the menisci, osteoarthritis, and rheumatoid arthritis.[1, 2, 14] Since the pneumarthrograms showed no evidence of meniscal tears and the latex fixation test for rheumatoid factor was negative, the development of popliteal cysts in this patient was probably related to osteoarthritis and synovial osteochondromatosis.[7, 13] The osteochondromas may have formed by osteocartilaginous metaplasia of the synovium and may have been displaced out of the joint space into the popliteal bursae.[7, 13] Removal of the loose bodies, necessary to restore blood flow to the lower leg in this patient, is the recommended treatment for synovial osteochondromatosis.[7]

REFERENCES

1. Burleson, R. J., Bickel, W. H., and Dahlin, D. C.: Popliteal cyst, J. Bone Joint Surg. [Am.] **38:** 1265, 1956.
2. Childress, H. M.: Popliteal cysts associated with undiagnosed posterior lesions of the medial meniscus. The significance of age in diagnosis and treatment, J. Bone Joint Surg. [Am.] **52:** 1487, 1970.
3. Haid, S. P., Conn, J., Jr., and Bergan, J. J.:

Cystic adventitial disease of the popliteal artery, Arch. Surg. **101:** 765, 1970.
4. Harris, J. D., Jepson, R. P.: Entrapment of the popliteal artery, SURGERY **69:** 246, 1971.
5. Harvey, J. P., Jr., and Corcos, J.: Large cysts in lower leg originating in the knee occurring in patients with rheumatoid arthritis, Arthritis Rheum. **3:** 218, 1960.
6. Insua, J. A., Young, J. R., and Humphries, A. W.: Popliteal artery entrapment syndrome, Arch. Surg. **101:** 771, 1970.
7. Jeffreys, T. E.: Synovial chondromatosis, J. Bone Joint Surg. [Br.] **49:** 530, 1967.
8. Little, J. M., and Goodman, A. H.: Cystic adventitial disease of the popliteal artery, Br. J. Surg. **57:** 708, 1970.
9. Rich, N. M., and Hughes, C. W.: Popliteal artery and vein entrapment, Am. J. Surg. **113:** 696, 1967.
10. Robb, D.: Obstruction of popliteal artery by synovial cyst, Br. J. Surg. **48:** 221, 1960.
11. Shute, K., and Rothnie, N. G.: The etiology of cystic arterial disease, Br. J. Surg. **60:** 397, 1973.
12. Smillie, I. S.: Injuries of the knee joint, Baltimore, 1970, The Williams & Wilkins Company.
13. Spjut, H. J., Dorfman, H. D., Fechner, R. E., and Ackerman, L. V.: Tumors of bone and cartilage, Washington, D. C., 1972, Armed Forces Institute of Pathology.
14. Wilson, P. D., Eyre-Brook, A. L., and Francis, J. D.: A clinical and anatomical study of the semimembranosus bursa in relation to popliteal cyst, J. Bone Joint Surg. **20:** 963, 1938.
15. Wolfe, R. D., and Colloff, B.: Popliteal cysts, J. Bone Joint Surg. [Am.] **54:** 1057, 1972.

Successful balloon membranotomy for obstruction of the hepatic portion of the inferior vena cava

Shoji Eguchi, M.D., Yoshimi Takeuchi, M.D., *and* **Ken-ichi Asano, M.D.,** *Niigata, Japan*

A case of successful balloon membranotomy for obstruction of the hepatic portion of the inferior vena cava is presented. This method should be tried before proceeding to the operative treatment because of its simplicity and safety. Operative experience on six patients with this disease is reported.

From the Department of Thoracic and Cardiovascular Surgery, Faculty of Medicine, University of Niigata, Niigata, Japan.

In 1962 Kimura and his associates[4] reported the first successful corrective operation upon membranous obstruction of the hepatic portion of the inferior vena cava (IVC). Since then, an increasing number of obstructive lesions of that portion have been reported in which various surgical treatments were used. However, there are considerable operative mortality and morbidity rates. The purpose of this paper is to present a case which showed marked palliation by nonoperative intervention with the use of a balloon catheter.

CASE REPORT

A 39-year-old man was admitted to the University of Niigata Hospital on July 11, 1972, for evaluation of hematemesis. He had two episodes of hematemesis in January and February of that year and had been admitted to a local hospital for treatment. He had epigastric discomfort, a sensation of fullness, and loss of appetite.

On physical examination the patient appeared well nourished and was slightly jaundiced. No spider angioma was present. The back, flank, and abdominal walls showed dilated superficial veins draining cephalad. A small amount of ascites was present. The liver was palpable 2 cm. below the right costal margin in the midclavicular line. A few varicose veins were present in both legs which were slightly edematous.

Laboratory studies showed a red cell count of 4.0 million; hemoglobin, 12 Gm. per 100 ml.; hematocrit, 40 percent; white cell count, 3,200 per

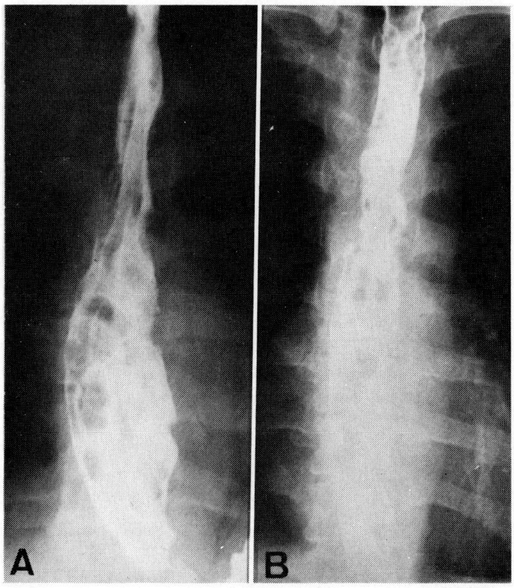

Fig. 1. Esophagogram. *A,* Before balloon membranotomy; *B,* after balloon membranotomy.

Accepted for publication July 26, 1974.

Reprint requests: Shoji Eguchi, M.D., Department of Thoracic and Cardiovascular Surgery, University of Niigata, Faculty of Medicine, Niigata, Japan.

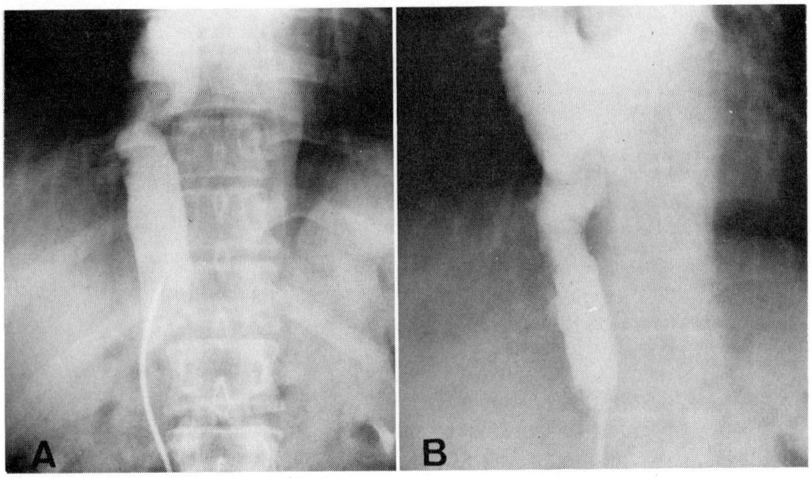

Fig. 2. Cavogram injecting dye in the inferior vena cava. *A,* Before membranotomy; *B,* after membranotomy.

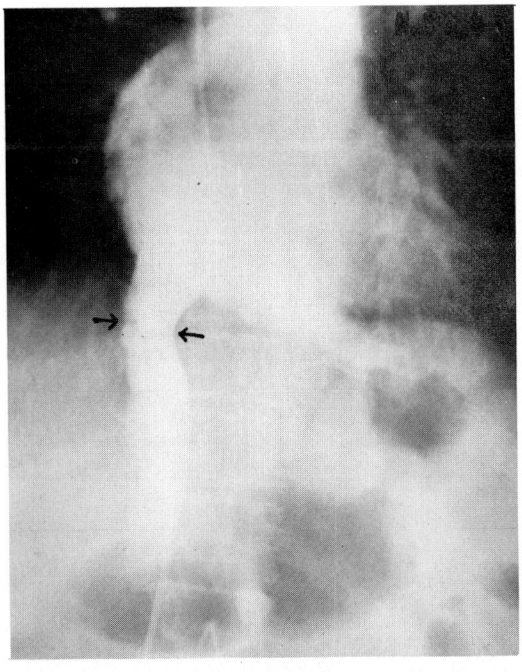

Fig. 3. Simultaneous visualization of the thoracic vena cava and abdominal vena cava with two catheters placed above and below the obstruction. Arrow indicates a membranous obstruction.

cubic millimeter, with a normal differential; platelet count, 84,000 per cubic millimeter; serum protein, 7.6 Gm. per 100 ml.; A/G ratio, 1.2; total serum bilirubin, 1.4 mg. per 100 ml.; serum alkaline phosphatase, 20.8 U. (King-Armstrong method); SGOT (serum glutamic oxalacetic transaminase) 37 U.; SGPT (serum glutamic pyruvic transaminase) 25 U.; and a negative Wassermann reaction. Upper gastrointestinal series revealed a marked degree of esophageal varices (Fig. 1, *A*). Peritoneoscopy showed a nodular liver, characterized by fine granular nodules and lymphectasia of the liver surface. Dilated veins were found in the hepatic round ligament.

Caval venography showed incomplete obstruction of the inferior vena cava at the level of the diaphragm (Fig. 2, *A*). The catheter could be passed into the right atrium and easily into the right hepatic vein. Pressures determined by catheter pull-back revealed a significant gradient across the obstruction. In order to determine the type of obstruction, simultaneous visualizations of the thoracic vena cava and abdominal vena cava were made with two catheters placed above and below the obstruction (Fig. 3). It revealed a membranous obstruction and no thrombus formation.

On Oct. 21, 1972, fracture of the membranous obstruction was performed with a Fogarty venous thrombectomy catheter inserted through a saphenous vein. Before fracture, the size of the opening of the membranous obstruction was measured by balloon inflation (Fig. 4, *A*). The calculated size was 5 mm. in diameter after correction for magnification. The fracture was carried out in a gradual fashion, until the inflated balloon (18 mm. in diameter) could pass up and down with only slight resistance (Fig. 4, *B*). The pressure gradient across the obstruction was reduced from 19 to 5 mm. Hg (Fig. 5). The cavogram after the procedure showed marked improvement of caval blood flow, but some residual ridge of the membrane was noted (Fig. 2, *B*). No pulmonary embolism occurred.

Following the procedure, abdominal complaints disappeared. The dilatation of the superficial veins

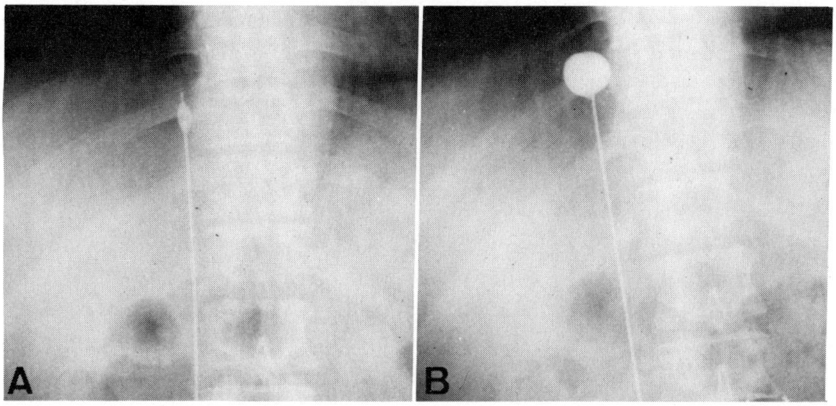

Fig. 4. *A,* The size of the opening of the membranous obstruction was measured by balloon inflation. *B,* After the fracture, the inflated balloon (18 mm. in diameter) could pass up and down with only slight resistance.

over the back, flank, and abdominal walls regressed markedly. The patient was re-examined 9 months after the procedure. No venous distension was noted over the abdomen, flank, or back. Although a few varicose veins were present in both legs, no edema was noted. The liver was palpable 2 cm. below the costal margin.

Laboratory studies showed improvement: red cell count, 4.4 million; hemoglobin, 16 Gm. per 100 ml.; hematocrit, 44 percent; white cell count, 4,800 per cubic millimeter; serum protein, 6.4 Gm. per 100 ml.; A/G ratio, 1.53; total serum bilirubin, 0.6 mg. per 100 ml.; serum alkaline phosphatase, 10.2 U.; SGOT, 29 U.; SGPT, 21 U. Esophagogram demonstrated some regression of esophageal varices (Fig. 1, *B*). Catheterization studies revealed a pressure gradient of 5 mm. Hg across the obstruction and essentially identical angiographic findings as those obtained just after the fracture. The patient is doing well 18 months after the procedure.

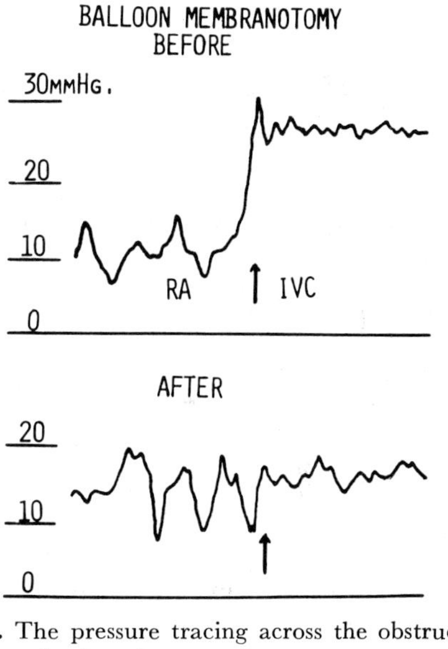

Fig. 5. The pressure tracing across the obstruction before and after the procedure.

DISCUSSION

Seven patients have been surgically treated by various procedures for obstruction of the hepatic portion of the inferior vena cava from 1964 through 1973 at the University of Niigata Hospital. According to our experience, the operative treatment of this disease should vary depending upon the type of obstruction, that is, membranous obstruction or diffuse obstruction[2].

In general, membranous obstruction has been treated by the established method—transcardiac membranotomy by means of a finger fracture technique, as Kimura and his associates reported previously. A Tubb's dilator may also be employed if digital dilation is unsatisfactory. As demonstrated by the present case, a balloon membranotomy may be beneficial when the membranous obstruction is thin and pliable and has an opening which can admit a catheter. Even in the case of complete obstruction, this method might be applicable with the similar technique of trans-septal left atrial puncture. It is conceivable that a balloon membranotomy might have been a better treatment for Case 2 reported by Lam, Green, and Gale.[7]

In an analysis of 89 cases of obstruction of

the hepatic veins and/or the corresponding portion of the inferior vena cava, 30 cases had caval obstruction caused by either a "membranous" or "valvelike" formation, less than 5 mm. in thickness.[5] In another 16, the membranous lesion was complicated by stricture or thrombosis. In 30, the hepatic portion of the vena cava was involved for a distance greater than 9 mm. In 12, the obliterative process was limited to the hepatic veins.

Six of our seven patients showed diffuse obstruction for which transcardiac fracture was impossible to perform and various surgical procedures were carried out. In one patient, a bypass operation was carried out with a crimped knitted Teflon graft between the thoracic and abdominal inferior vena cava through a tunnel fashioned by blunt finger dissection behind the liver and lateral to the course of inferior vena cava.[1] The patency of the graft was confirmed by venography 2 years after operation. In four patients, the digital-instrumental bidirectional dilatation was carried out. This procedure consisted of dilatation and/or thrombectomy of the obstructed portion with a Bakes dilator and/or a stone curette. These instruments were inserted through the inferior vena cava above the renal veins and manipulated, using an index finger as a guide through the right atrium. In two patients, dilatation of the obstructed portion was done only with a dilator, because stone curettes could not reach the lesion. These two patients showed early recurrence of the obstruction. In another two patients, thrombus at the lesion was curretted and removed through the inferior vena cava. The clinical condition improved and the cavogram at the time of discharge showed satisfactory patency. In one patient, a pericardial patch graft reconstruction was carried out for diffuse inflammatory narrowing of the inferior vena cava at the hepatic portion with the use of extracorporeal circulation under moderate hypothermia.

Although there was no operative death in our series, the immediate postoperative course was not always smooth because of relatively extensive operative intervention and malnutrition in several cases. Wound healing was retarded and wound dehiscence occurred in two cases. In the survey of 74 operations performed for occlusive lesions of the hepatic inferior vena cava, the operative mortality rate of transcardiac finger fracture was 20.7 percent, bypass grafting 40 percent, and excision of obstruction by inferior cavotomy 40 percent, respectively.[3] In a series of eight cases treated by transcardiac membranotomy, three operative deaths occurred, one due to bleeding and two due to anuria.[6] Accordingly, the balloon membranotomy should be tried on indicated cases before proceeding to operative treatment because of its simplicity and safety.

The ultimate prognosis after successful operation seems to depend upon pre-existent liver cirrhosis, the possibility of hepatoma from cirrhosis, and esophageal varices. Accordingly, early detection and early surgical treatment of this disease should be emphasized.

REFERENCES

1. Eguchi, S., Endo, S., Yamaguchi, A., and Asano, K.: Inferior caval occlusion associated with the Budd-Chiari's syndrome: Treatment with bypass operation, J. Cardiovasc. Surg. **7:** 490, 1966.
2. Eguchi, S., Takeuchi, Y., and Asano, K.: Surgical treatment of the inferior caval obstruction at the hepatic portion associated with the Budd-Chiari's syndrome, J. Cardiovasc. Surg. In press.
3. Hirooka, M., and Kimura, C.: Membranous obstruction of the hepatic portion of the inferior vena cava. Surgical correction and etiological study, Arch. Surg. **100:** 656, 1970.
4. Kimura, C., Shirotani, H., Kuma, T., et al.: Transcardiac membranotomy for obliteration of the inferior vena cava in the hepatic portion, J. Cardiovasc. Surg. **3:** 393, 1962.
5. Kimura, C., Shirotani, H., Hirooka, M., et al.: Membranous obliteration of the inferior vena cava in the hepatic portion, J. Cardiovasc. Surg. **4:** 87, 1963.
6. Kimura, C., Matsuda, S., Koie, H., and Hirooka, M.: Membranous obstruction of the hepatic portion of the inferior vena cava: Clinical study of nine cases, SURGERY **72:** 551, 1972.
7. Lam, C. R., Green, E., and Gale, H.: Transcardiac membranotomy for obstruction of the hepatic portion of the inferior vena cava, Circulation **32** (Suppl. I): 188, 1965.

Femorofemoral bypass

L. M. Gazzola, M.D., S. A. Hirsch, M.D., *and* G. I. Kaufer, M.D., *Pittsburgh, Penn.*

Femorofemoral bypass is an accepted procedure in vascular surgery. In the past it has been used primarily in those patients who had stenosis of one iliac vessel and an open iliac on the unaffected side. Patients chosen for this procedure generally were in the poor-risk category. We have added two new indications for this procedure. First is its use in the patient who has one limb of an aortofemoral bypass graft which occludes and cannot be opened by thrombectomy. We feel that using femorofemoral bypass in this instance is the procedure of choice. Second, it seems acceptable as an inflow tract for femoropopliteal bypass with a saphenous vein. Six patients in whom arterial reconstruction was performed in this fashion are presented. All of these patients had a satisfactory result.

From the Departments of Surgery, the University of Pittsburgh and Montefiore Hospital of Pittsburgh, Pittsburgh, Penn.

Femorofemoral bypass is now an accepted procedure in vascular surgery. First reported by McCaughan and Kahn[7] in 1960, it has been since supported by others as a procedure to be used in the poor-risk patient whose limb is in jeopardy. It is applicable when there is stenosis of one iliac system and an open iliac system on the unaffected side. This operation can be done under local or light general anesthesia. Aortofemoral bypass is still considered the procedure of choice in the usual patient with iliac disease, and femorofemoral bypass has been reserved as a desperation measure. Our reexamination of the procedure has led us to the belief that there are two circumstances in which it may be the procedure of choice. These are when one limb of a previously placed aortobilateral femoral bypass graft becomes occluded and cannot be reopened by simple thrombectomy through a groin approach, or to act as an inflow tract for a femoropopliteal bypass when there is iliac stenosis on the side for which the bypass is being considered.

The operation has previously been recommended[1-3] in elderly patients, patients who have abdominal sepsis, have had abdominal irradiation, or who are poor cardiac or respiratory risks, and in patients in whom the ischemia is caused by unilateral iliofemoral occlusive disease. We add the above two indications to this list and report six instances of femorofemoral bypass which demonstrate the usefulness of this approach.

Accepted for publication August 12, 1974.
Reprint requests: S. A. Hirsch, M.D., 22 S. Trenton Ave., Pittsburgh, Penn. 15221.

TECHNIQUE

Incisions are made in both groins and the common, superficial, and deep femoral vessels identified and dissected free. When a previously placed aortofemoral bypass graft is present, the dissection may be more difficult and the limb of the graft must also be

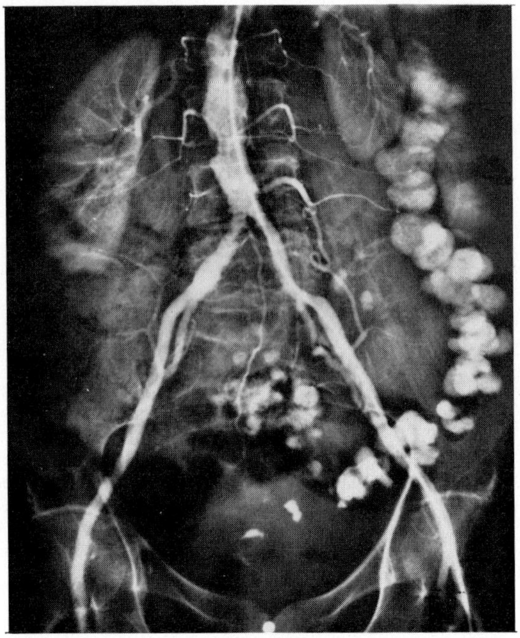

Fig. 1A. Arteriogram showing stenosis of right common iliac.

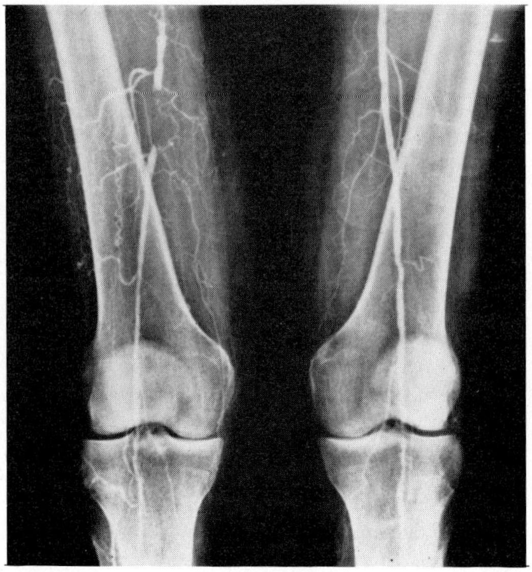

Fig. 1B. Arteriogram showing occlusion of right superficial femoral.

dissected free. A subcutaneous tunnel is created bluntly in the suprapubic area or deeper in the space of Retzius. An 8 or 10 mm. Dacron prosthesis is employed. The anastomoses are placed on the anteromedial aspect of the common femoral arteries or on the anteromedial aspect of the limb of the aortofemoral bypass graft. A long oblique anastomosis is created in order to decrease the angle between the artery and the graft. When a femoropopliteal bypass is to be done in addition, a saphenous vein is ordinarily utilized. The proximal anastomosis is done directly to the Dacron prosthesis of the femorofemoral bypass.

CASE REPORTS

There were six patients, three men and three women. Four had previously had bilateral aortofemoral bypass, and one had only a previous lumbar sympathectomy. The ages of the patients ranged from 68 to 79 years. The follow-up after femorofemoral bypass varied from 10½ to 18½ months. The patients were selected for operations because of impending gangrene, frank gangrene of an area of the foot or toe, or incapacitating rest pain. All the patients were unsuitable for aortofemoral bypass because of age, cardiopulmonary disease, or because an aortofemoral bypass had previously been performed and the patient presented with one limb of the graft occluded. Five patients had diabetes. The site of inflow obstruction was the common iliac artery in two cases and the limb of the aortofemoral bypass graft in the remaining four cases. All six underwent femorofemoral bypass. In four, an associated femoropopliteal bypass was carried out. In one, a deep femoral angioplasty was performed. In the patients with occluded limbs of their aortofemoral bypass, it was felt that this occlusion had occurred because of decrease in runoff due to progressive arteriosclerosis of the deep femoral artery.

There were no early or late graft failures in our six patients. One patient had a superficial wound infection of the left groin. All six patients are alive and well with functioning grafts 10½ to 18½ months following operation. Four had light general anesthesia; two had local anesthesia. In one case, a postoperative arteriogram 7 months after operation demonstrates the appearance of a femorofemoral bypass graft acting as the inflow to a femoropopliteal bypass graft (Fig. 1).

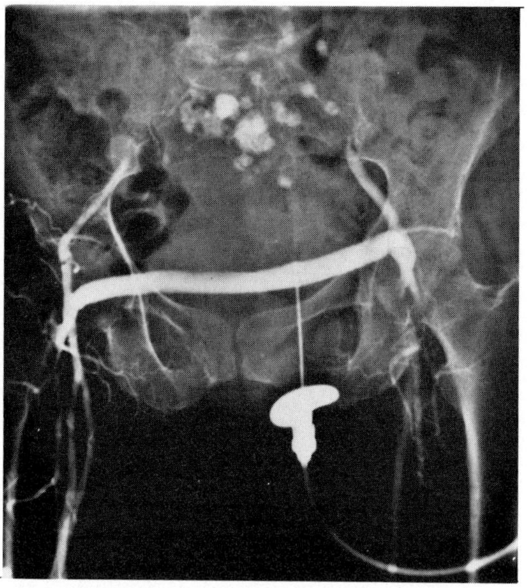

Fig. 1C. Postoperative arteriogram showing femorofemoral bypass.

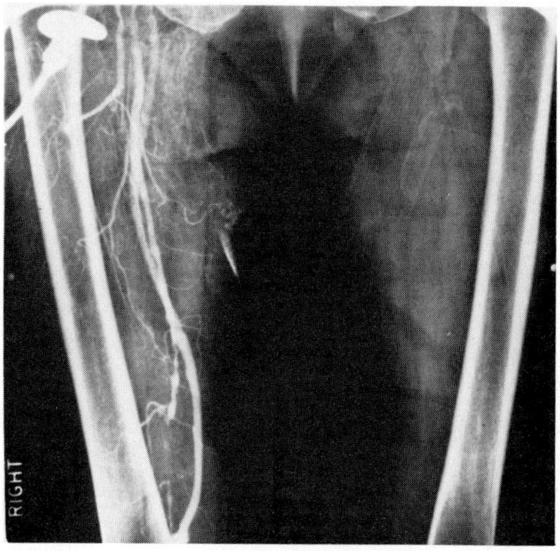

Fig. 1D. Postoperative arteriogram showing femoropopliteal bypass with saphenous vein whose inflow tract is the femorofemoral bypass.

All the rest of the patients have been followed by careful palpation of pulses. All six patients have palpable femoral and popliteal pulses and complete relief of pain.

DISCUSSION

At the present time femorofemoral grafts have not been used in preference to aortofemoral grafts in good risk patients.[1, 7, 10, 11] We generally agree with this, except in two instances. We feel that when a limb of an aortofemoral graft has occluded due to a decrease in the outflow tract, and when it is felt that a femoropopliteal bypass should be added to the procedure to improve the outflow tract, and when, further, one limb of the graft is open and has no stenotic area, a femorofemoral bypass graft is the procedure of choice. In our hands this has worked quite well, and we see no reason to subject these patients to another abdominal procedure. If a patient is seen soon after a limb of an aortofemoral bypass graft occludes, one can frequently restore the blood flow simply by using a Fogarty catheter. In all of the patients reported, thrombectomy was attempted but was unsuccessful due to organization of the thrombus. These poor-risk patients tolerated the procedure well. Four underwent mild general anesthesia, two local anesthesia, none spinal anesthesia. The procedures required 30 minutes for the femorofemoral bypass and an additional 65 minutes to perform the femoropopliteal bypass.

It has been suggested that the recipient artery will steal blood from the donor limb.[6] Studies have shown that this does not occur as long as the donor artery is not stenotic and there is a reasonably low peripheral vascular resistance.[9, 12] Ehrenfeld, Harris, and Wylie[4] demonstrated that flow through the donor artery can increase as much as 10 times. In experimental femorofemoral grafts in dogs, the flow of the donor artery doubled, and in the distal artery of the donor limb, the flow remained unchanged after the graft had been opened. In patients, flow studies have been done with opened and clamped femorofemoral grafts. When the graft was open there was a transient drop in pressure in the donor artery, but this rapidly returned to normal and was followed by an increase in inflow.[11]

Despite the fact that the angle between the donor artery and the femorofemoral bypass graft is close to 90°, this has not caused graft failure.

An angle of about 75° seems to provide the best flow pattern and the least transition from laminar to turbulent flow.[8, 12]

Our follow-up is, as yet, short, but the immediate results have been gratifying. Others have observed from 2 to 10 years patency of the graft and the donor vessels.[11]

CONCLUSIONS

1. In poor-risk patients femorofemoral bypass should be considered before amputation when the configuration of the arterial disease lends itself to this operation.

2. Femorofemoral bypass graft (four patients) is the procedure of choice in patients who have had occlusion of one limb of an aortofemoral bypass graft which cannot be opened by simple thrombectomy.

3. Femorofemoral bypass provides an adequate inflow tract for femoropopliteal bypass graft (four patients).

4. The procedure is subject to low morbidity and mortality rates. There were no immediate or late graft failures in our six patients. There was one superficial wound infection. No patients have exhibited a steal syndrome. All six patients are still alive.

REFERENCES

1. Blaisdell, F. W., DeMattei, G. A., and Gander, P. J.: Extraperitoneal thoracic aorta to femoral bypass graft as replacement for an infected aortic bifurcation prosthesis, Am. J. Surg. **102:** 583, 1961.
2. Blaisdell, F. W., Hall, A. D., Lim, R. C., et al.: Aorto-iliac arterial substitution utilizing subcutaneous grafts, Ann. Surg. **172:** 775, 1970.
3. DeAvila, R., Doyle, J., and Heaney, J. P.: Axillary-femoral bypass, Arch. Surg. **92:** 118, 1966.
4. Ehrenfeld, W. R., Harris, J. P., and Wylie, E. J.: Vascular "steal" phenomenon, an experimental study, Am. J. Surg. **116:** 192, 1968.
5. Mannick, J. A., and Mabseth, D. C.: Axillofemoral bypass graft. A safe alternative to aorto-iliac reconstruction, N. Engl. J. Med. **278:** 461, 1968.
6. May, A. G., DeWeese, J. A., and Rob, C. G.: Effect of sympathectomy on blood flow in arterial stenosis, Ann. Surg. **158:** 182, 1963.
7. McCaughan, J. J., and Kahn, S. F.: Crossover graft for unilateral occlusive disease of the iliofemoral arteries, Ann. Surg. **151:** 26, 1960.
8. Sauvage, L. R., and Wood, S. J.: Unilateral axillary bilateral femoral bifurcation graft: A procedure for the poor-risk patients with aortoiliac disease, SURGERY **60:** 573, 1966.
9. Trimble, I. R., Shonesifer, G. L., Shaw-Wilgis, E. F., et al.: Criteria for femoro-femoral bypass from clinical and hemodynamic studies, Ann. Surg. **175:** 985, 1972.
10. Vetto, R. M.: The treatment of unilateral iliac artery obstruction with a transabdominal subcutaneous femorofemoral graft, SURGERY **52:** 324, 1962.
11. Vetto, R. M.: The femoro-femoral shunt: An appraisal, Am. J. Surg. **112:** 162, 1966.
12. Warren, W. D., and Forman, J. J.: Rerouting arterial flow to relieve ischemia: Femorofemoral, axillary femoral and carotid-carotid artery bypasses, Ann. Surg. **163:** 131, 1966.
13. Wesolowski, S. A., Sauvage, L. R., Pinc, R. S., et al: Dynamics of blood flow in graft disproportion and in normal blood vessels, Surg. Forum **6:** 227, 1955.

ERRATUM

In a discussion by James A. O'Neill, Jr., M.D., Mark M. Ravitch, M.D., and Bruce A. Barton, M.S., entitled, "A model for evaluation of surgical manpower needs—Pediatric Surgery," in the July, 1974, issue of SURGERY, page 186, an incorrect figure was given for the ratio of pediatric surgeons to population in Great Britain. The authors wish the ratio to be corrected to read, "1:1,250,000."

Coronary artery aneurysms in a 9-year-old child

John E. Liddicoat, M.D., Szabolcs M. Bekassy, M.D., Manus J. O'Donnell, M.D., *and* Michael E. De Bakey, M.D., *Houston, Texas*

A 5-year-old girl suffered an acute episode of periarteritis nodosa and one year later developed signs of coronary artery insufficiency with strenuous exertion. Selective coronary arteriography revealed severe aneurysmal disease of the right and left coronary arteries. Because of the magnitude of the abnormalities in this relatively asymptomatic child, no surgical intervention was recommended. At present she is 9 years of age and, except for her inability to participate in strenuous activities, she continues to do well.

From the Cora and Webb Mading Department of Surgery, and the Department of Medicine, Baylor College of Medicine, Houston, Texas

PERIARTERITIS NODOSA is a rare disease of childhood and is usually associated with a high mortality rate with the leading cause of death secondary to coronary artery aneurysm.[1, 2] Since the majority of the cases have been diagnosed post mortem, an awareness of the signs and symptoms of this disease may make earlier diagnosis and treatment possible. The purpose of this report is to present the clinical findings and management of a 9-year-old female child with coronary artery aneurysms secondary to periarteritis nodosa.

CASE REPORT

This 9-year-old female child was the product of a normal pregnancy and delivery. She had a normal developmental history and was attending school when, in 1970 at 5 years of age, she had an episode of severe malaise, conjunctivitis with photophobia, and fever. Subsequently, she developed a macular rash over her face and body with painful inflammatory swelling of her joints. She was hospitalized and treated with prednisone and aspirin. During the ensuing 11 months she did well without any limitations. However, while climbing in the mountains with her family she suddenly complained of severe chest pains which

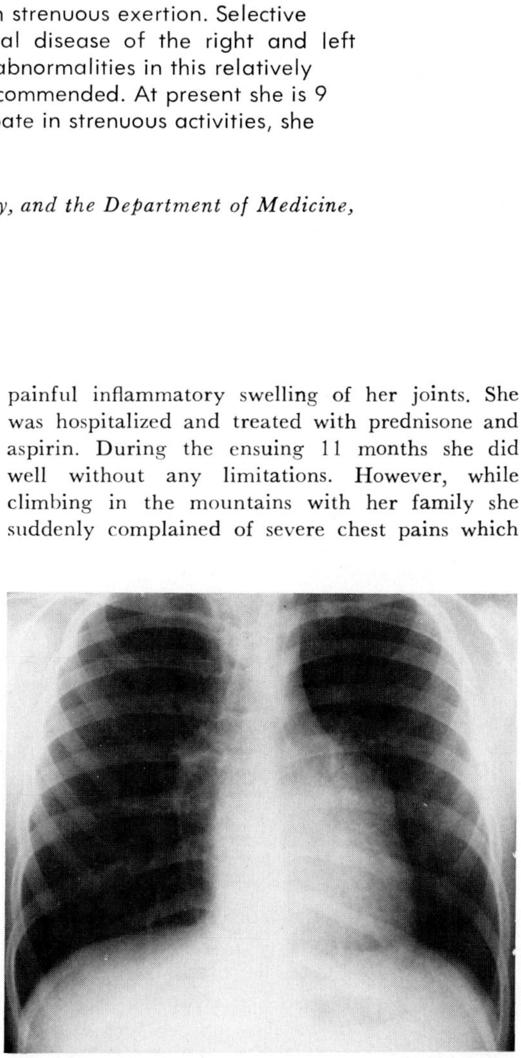

Fig. 1. Chest roentgenogram shows mediastinal mass on the left, at the level of the left auricular appendage, merging with the cardiac image, and containing eggshell-like calcification.

Accepted for publication on August 12, 1974.

Reprint requests: John E. Liddicoat, M.D., Cora and Webb Mading Department of Surgery, Baylor College of Medicine, Texas Medical Center, Houston, Texas 77025.

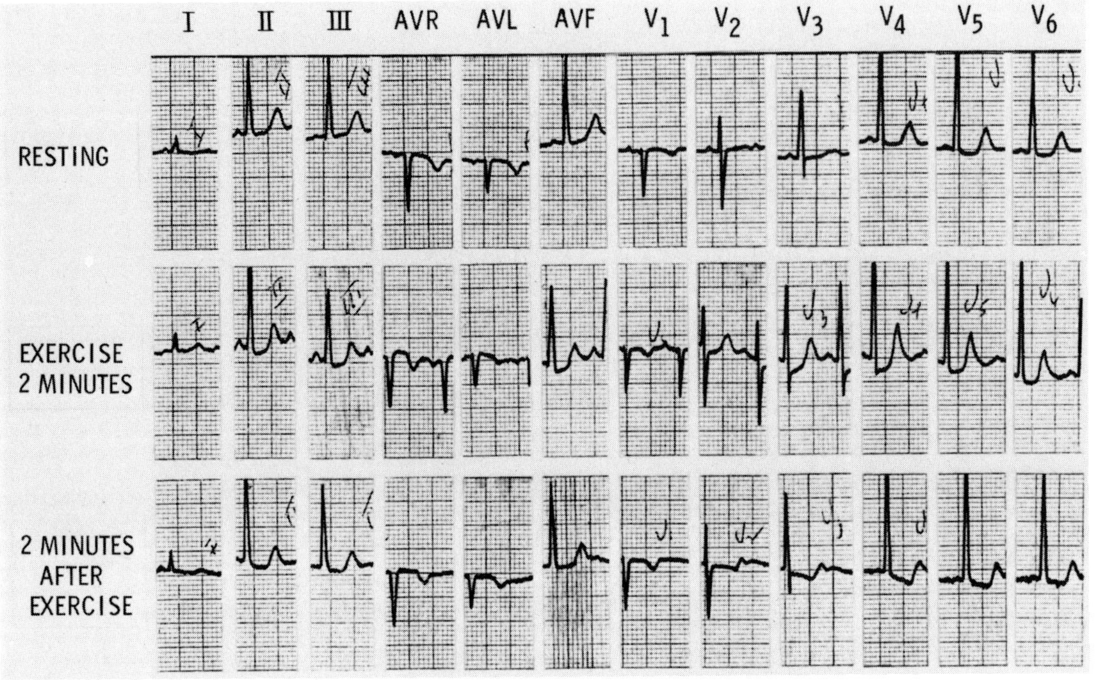

Fig. 2. Treadmill exercise test. S-T segment depression in Leads II, III, aV_F, V_3, and V_5 after 2 minutes of exercise.

were relieved by rest. An electrocardiogram (ECG) was performed at that time and was reportedly normal. Because of persistent exertional chest pains she was hospitalized and underwent complete evaluation.

The child was well developed and in no distress. The physical examination was entirely within normal limits with a blood pressure of 110/70 mm. Hg bilaterally. The laboratory studies were all within normal limits. The chest x-ray (Fig. 1) revealed a mediastinal mass on the left at the level of the left auricular appendage, merging with the cardiac image, and containing eggshell-like calcification. The resting ECG showed only minor ST-T segment changes. The treadmill exercise test demonstrated significant ischemic ECG changes (Fig. 2) after 2 minutes. Cardiac catheterization revealed normal left and right heart pressures except for the left ventricular end-diastolic pressure, which was elevated to 18 mm. Hg. Left ventricular angiography demonstrated good contractility, however. Selective coronary arteriography (Fig. 3) revealed severe aneurysmal disease of the proximal and middle portions of the right coronary artery. The left main coronary had a large aneurysm proximal to the origin of its bifurcation with very slow opacification of the left anterior descending and circumflex coronary arteries.

Because of the magnitude of the abnormalities in this child, who was symptomatic only with strenuous exercise, operative intervention was not recommended. Subsequently, she was discharged from the hospital to continue to have close follow-up and to return if her clinical condition were to change.

DISCUSSION

The true incidence of periarteritis nodosa is not known and, unfortunately, it still remains primarily a postmortem diagnosis.[2, 3, 4] It has been found to be a generalized process more frequently in the adult population, whereas in the younger patients there is a selective affinity for involvement of the coronary and renal arteries.[1] The aneurysmal dilatation of the coronary vessels is a progressive process and in most reported cases has resulted in death within a few months after the diagnosis has been established.[2] These patients primarily die from rupture of the aneurysm into the pericardial sac with pericardial tamponade.[4] Occasionally, death is attributed to massive myocardial infarction from embolization of the aneurysmal contents or thrombosis of the entire aneurysm.[2]

Adequate treatment of the disorder has not

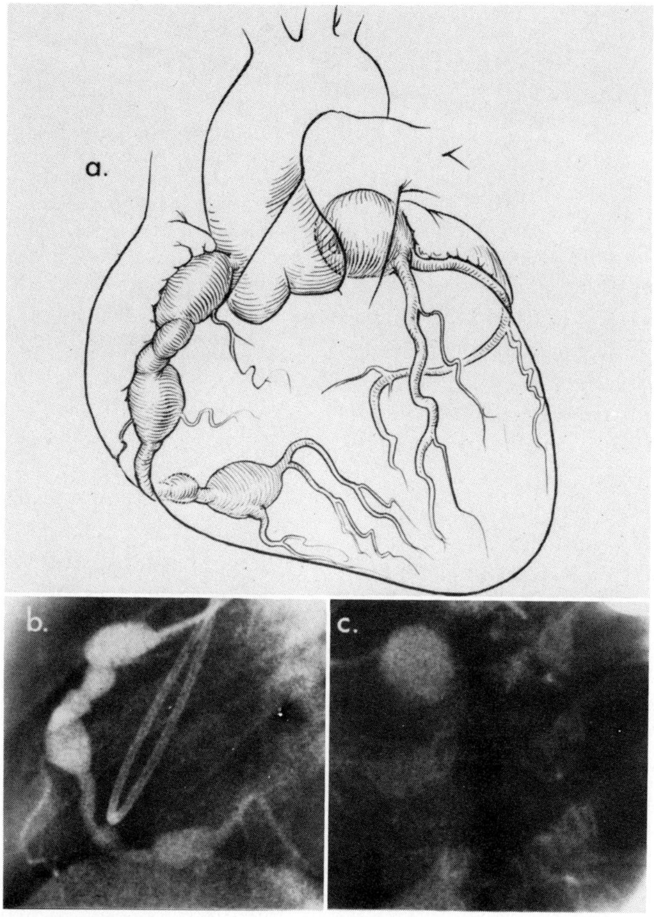

Fig. 3. *A,* Drawing illustrates severe aneurysmal disease of the right coronary artery and a large aneurysm of the left main coronary artery. *B,* Right coronary arteriogram in left anterior oblique position showing aneurysmal disease of the proximal and middle right coronary artery. *C,* Left coronary arteriogram in left anterior oblique position showing a large aneurysm of the left main coronary artery with calcification.

been accomplished; however, recently there seems to be some benefit from the prolonged use of steroids for the patients with systemic periarteritis nodosa.[1, 3]

With the availability of cardiac catheterization and coronary arteriography, earlier diagnosis may be possible and, when associated with the treadmill stress test, perhaps the magnitude of the problem can better be determined. Under these circumstances such patients may be candidates for coronary artery bypass to divert the coronary flow beyond the aneurysmal process.

Currently we are closely following this 9-year-old child who is now 4 years beyond the onset of the disease and off steroid therapy. At the time of this publication, she is leading a normal life except for her inability to participate in strenuous activities.

REFERENCES

1. Chamberlain, J. L., III, and Perry, L. W.: Infantile periarteritis nodosa with coronary and brachial aneurysms: A case diagnosed during life, J. Pediatr. **78:** 1039, 1971.
2. Crouch, J. A., and Diehl, A. M.: Periarteritis nodosa in infancy, J. Kan. Med. Soc. **74:** 78, 1973.
3. Frohnert, P. P., and Sheps, S. G.: Long-term follow-up study of periarteritis nodosa, Am. J. Med. **43:** 8, 1967.
4. Sinclair, W., Jr., and Nitsch, E.: Polyarteritis nodosa of the coronary arteries, Am. Heart J. **38:** 898, 1949.

Letters to the editors

Buerger's disease—the need for diagnostic criteria

To the Editors:

The report by Shionoya and associates[2] on the controversial Buerger's disease does not fulfill the promise of its title. It includes no definition of the criteria used to establish the diagnosis of Buerger's disease in 100 patients described and to differentiate them from other patients with peripheral vascular insufficiency seen by the authors.

Age, sex, and smoking habits are not definitive criteria for a given case. The typical anatomopathological lesion—as stated by the authors—is often not demonstrable. Arteriographic evidence of occlusion of vessels below the knee is suggestive but certainly not pathognomonic, as similar changes may be seen in some cases of atherosclerosis. The reduction in muscle blood flow is also not specific and merely reflects the severity of the ischemic process. In the absence of a known etiology or a specific laboratory test, the diagnosis of Buerger's disease remains a clinical one.

Mozes and associates[1] suggested well-defined clinical criteria for the diagnosis of Buerger's disease. These include lower extremity ischemia together with at least two of the following three symptoms or signs: migrating thrombophlebitis, upper extremity involvement, and Raynaud's phenomena. While these criteria may be open to criticism, and better criteria may well be suggested by others, the need for some definite criteria cannot be questioned. In the absence of a clear-cut definition of the diagnostic criteria even the most sophisticated blood-flow studies remain meaningless, the results of therapy cannot be evaluated, and the controversy regarding Buerger's disease will continue to rage.

Raphael Adar, M.D., F.A.C.S.
Department of General and Vascular Surgery
The Chaim Sheba Medical Center and
Tel Aviv University Medical School
Tel Aviv, Israel

REFERENCES

1. Mozes, M., Cahansky, G., Deutsch, V., and Adar, R.: The association of atherosclerosis and Buerger's disease: A clinical and radiological study, J. Cardiovasc. Surg. **11:** 52, 1970.
2. Shionoya, S., Ban, I., Nakata, Y., et al.: Diagnosis, pathology, and treatment of Buerger's disease, SURGERY **75:** 695, 1974.

Reply

To the Editors:

Three symptoms recognized by Mozes and associates are reliable in the diagnosis of Buerger's disease, although typical Raynaud's phenomenon does not occur commonly and is usually irregular and asymmetrical.

And it is frequently not easy to ascertain the occurrence of migratory phlebitis and the involvement of the arteries of the upper limbs.

^{133}Xe clearance method can reveal a peripheral arterial insufficiency that could not be recognized by arteriography. However, it goes without saying that the technique does not differentiate between Buerger's disease and other peripheral arterial disorders.

The ultimate criterion for the diagnosis of Buerger's disease is the finding of the typical histologic picture in the arteries of the extremities. The characteristic giant cells and remarkable infiltration of inflammatory cells in the thrombus are frequently seen if the specimen is in a series cut at different levels.

In our 100 patients diagnosed as having Buerger's disease, one or more of the systemic manifestations were present in addition to ischemic changes in the legs.

The details of their clinical features were not described in our article, for it was not the purpose of our paper.

"Diagnosis of Buerger's disease" in our title means a functional diagnosis of peripheral arterial insufficiency in Buerger's disease.

Shigehiko Shionoya, M.D.
Department of Surgery
Nagoya University Branch Hospital
2-1 Higashimonzen-cho, Higashi-ku
Nagoya, Japan

Volume 76 *Number* 6 SURGERY
DECEMBER, 1974

Society for Vascular Surgery

The beginnings of Vascular Surgery

W. Andrew Dale, M.D., *Nashville, Tenn.*

From the Department of Surgery, Vanderbilt University School of Medicine, St. Thomas Hospital and Baptist Hospital, Nashville, Tenn.

"To understand a science it is necessary to know its history."

—Auguste Comte (1798-1857)

The history of peripheral vascular disease dates to antiquity. While the brief average life span in early times no doubt precluded a high general instance of arteriosclerosis, evidence of the disease has been found in Egyptian mummies, and the Greeks recognized senile gangrene although its cause was unknown. The violence of the times made the results of traumatic vascular insufficiency quite evident, although the physiologic details were not understood.

THE ANCIENTS

A report by Susratas on the use of a ligature for the umbilical cord in 1500 B.C. is believed to begin the recorded history of vascular surgery. The ancients did use the ligature to control hemorrhage and even devised methods of ligation for peripheral aneurysms, but there was general loss of the main body of this knowledge during the Dark Ages. In 1552 Ambroise Paré revived control of bleeding by ligature (although this mass ligation of all tissues in the vicinity of the bleeding vessel was considerably more gross than the modern technique implied by the term). Thereafter, there was constant competition between ligature, cautery, compression, and other methods of hemorrhage control until the end of the eighteenth century when ligation became generally recognized as the best method for hemostasis. During this period of intellectual awakening, circulation of the blood was demonstrated by William Harvey in 1628 and many pathologic conditions were clearly described, including arteriosclerosis, by Leonardo da Vinci and the Italian anatomist, Gabriel Fallopius.

ARTERIAL REPAIR

In 1759 the first vascular repair was recorded. The land which would become the

President's address to the Twenty-eighth Annual Meeting of the Society for Vascular Surgery, Chicago, Ill., June 20 and 21, 1974.

Reprint requests: W. Andrew Dale, M.D., Mid State Medical Center, 2010 Church St., Nashville, Tenn. 37203.

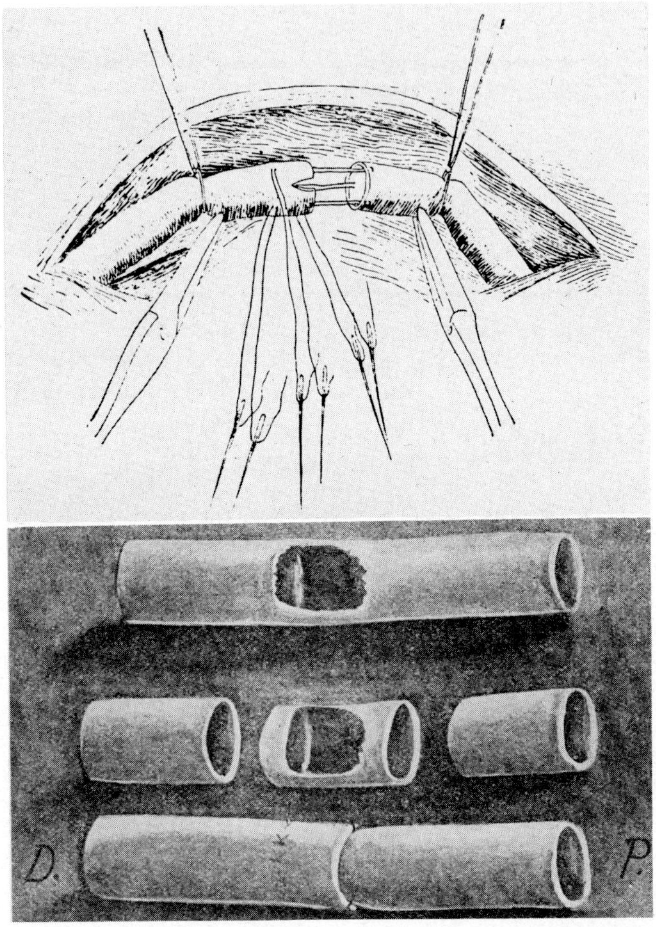

Fig. 1. The first end-to-end suture of a human artery by John B. Murphy of Chicago in 1897. The damaged segment of femoral artery was excised and the proximal end invaginated into the distal end and held in place by sutures.[70]

United States was still ruled by England. The political map of Europe, following the conclusion of the War of the Spanish Succession by the Treaty of Utrecht in 1715, featured the Hapsburg dominions in central Europe where Frederick the Great was attempting to form Germany during the Seven Years War. In England George II and his prime minister, William Pitt, continued the recurrent bloody struggle with France, where an aging Madame Pompadour comforted Louis XIV at Versailles, while he passed amiably from bed to bed. The average life span in France was 22 years. Surgeons had been officially separated from barbers for only 14 years.

In these surroundings brachial arteries were frequently injured during crude attempts at antecubital venesection for phlebotomy. On June 15, 1759, Hallowell in Yorkshire closed such an injury by running a pin through the edges of the arterial laceration and drawing a figure-eight ligature firmly about the protruding ends.[31] This ingenious method was like a lightning flash at midnight. It did not progress further and Asman effectively buried it several years later when he reported failure of the method in dogs,[85] no doubt due to the usual infection which produced either thrombosis or hemorrhage. This supported the generally accepted opinion that arterial injury always led to thrombosis and no further progress occurred until the

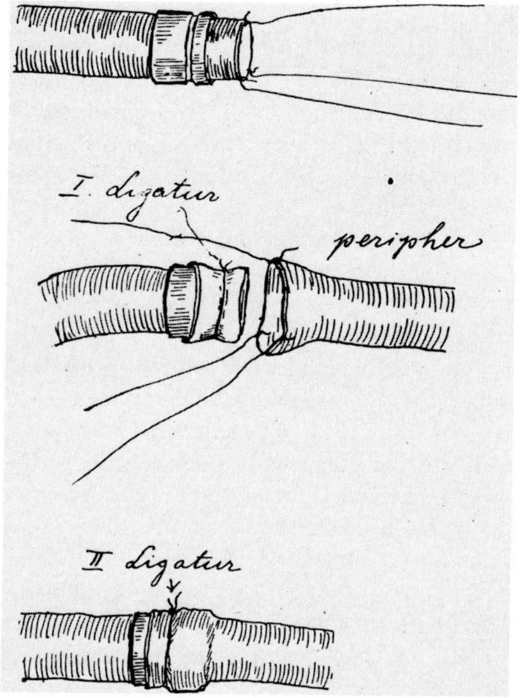

Fig. 2. Payr tubes, 1900. In 1900 Erwin Payr anastomosed arteries by pulling the distal end over the proximal end which was cuffed back on a metal tube.[77]

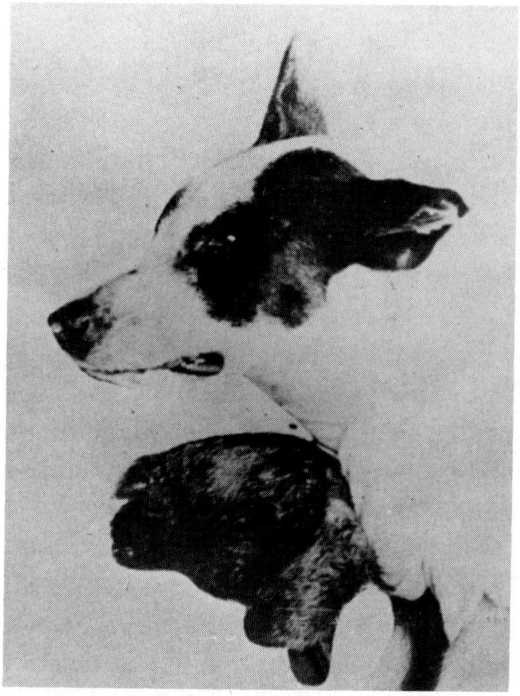

Fig. 3. In the early 1900's Alexis Carrel anastomosed arteries and veins both within and without species and here predated by 50 years the Russian claim for priority in transplanting a dog's head to the neck of a recipient animal.

cause of infection was discovered and Lister's ideas became known a century later. By then a time for progress had clearly arrived.

VASCULAR ANASTOMOSIS

In 1877 the United States was a century old. Ulysses S. Grant was being followed by Rutherford B. Hayes as president and baseball was 38 years old. Queen Victoria's England was placid.

In that year of 1877 a young Russian surgeon, Nikolai Eck, created the portacaval shunt which bears his name by suturing the two veins with continuous silk, and, thereafter, opening them blindly using special scissors. Six of his eight dogs lived from 2 to 7 days and one for 2½ months. Eck's fistula was really aimed toward a study of the effect of shunting blood away from the liver and his successful vascular technique was only a means to that end. His contribution was not recognized until much later and progress was terminated when he "had to postpone further experiments because I was called to join the active army."[17]

Soon there began attempts to rejoin vessels end to end. In 1889 Alexander Jassinowsky of Odessa reported that 22 of 26 carotid arteries of dogs, horses, and calves had remained patent after repair by interrupted suture. He stressed the importance of asepsis and recommended interrupted sutures of fine silk placed through the adventitia and media but avoidance of the intima in the anastomosis.[52] In 1896 the French surgeon, Mathieu Jaboulay, and his pupil, Briau,[50] failed to achieve patency among ten canine anastomoses but were successful using the larger artery of the donkey. Jaboulay confined his writing to the local journal, *Lyon Medical,* and after his early death in a train wreck,

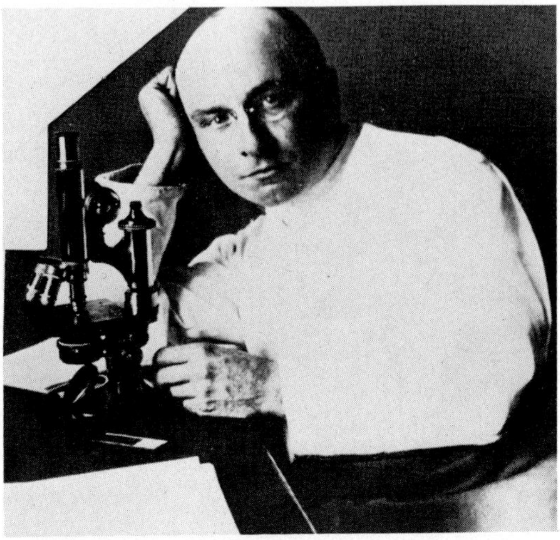

Fig. 4. Alexis Carrel at the Rockefeller Institute in New York received the Nobel Prize in 1912 for his continued experimental work in vascular surgery. (Courtesy of M.D., **17:** 129, April, 1973.) (Photograph by Culver Pictures.)

his work became known chiefly through his students.[34]

Silberg, Napalkow, and Heidenhain each independently described all-layer intima-to-intima anastomosis just at the end of the nineteenth century,[83] and at this distant time it is difficult to assign priority. Guthrie,[41] who was contemporary and knowledgeable, credited Julius Dorfler,[26] who recognized that a foreign body suture within the lumen did not cause thrombosis and indeed was well tolerated.

Other methods of junction were also studied. In 1897, John B. Murphy[70] of Chicago first rejoined a human artery by invaginating the proximal end into the distal femoral artery and holding it there by sutures (Fig. 1). Reunion of the vessel over an indwelling glass tube was reported by Robert Abbe[1] of New York in 1894. Later modifications of this principle included Nitze's ivory tubes in 1897,[90] the absorbable magnesium tubes of Payr[77] in 1900 (Fig. 2), and, as late as 1942, the vitallium tubes of Blakemore, Lord, and Stefko.[9] None of these proved worthwhile and this path led into a blind *cul de sac.*

If "fame is the spur" then "J. B." Murphy was a real horse! Lacking a background of security, he obtained a superior education by persistent hard work and determination from the start to rise above his fellows. Considerable egotism and hardness made him controversial but he did first perform and then popularize appendectomy, widened the field of intestinal surgery with the Murphy button for anastomoses, and maintained a dog laboratory in his barn for his surgical studies.[22] His entry into the vascular field was spectacular, if limited. Perhaps he did not go further because other areas appeared more likely to produce a jackpot!

The century ended. The few who had looked for the end of the millennium turned to other activities. Edward VII of England stamped royal approval upon conduct which Victoria had barely tolerated beneath the surface. The United States began recovery from the severe depression of 1897 with McKinley at the helm.

In 1890 in Lyon, France, there entered the medical school a young man destined to become a surgical giant, who would outstrip his contemporaries by decades and, as is commonplace, would become controversial in the process.

Alexis Carrel, while yet a student, became interested in the possibility of vascular repair. His interest was triggered by the fatal portal vein injury of the president of the French Republic, Sadi Carnot, the victim of assassination by the Italian anarchist, Santo Caseiro, in 1894. The student Carrel openly questioned the inability of his teachers to repair the vessel and at once set out to learn how to do this.[32]

He was soon rebuffed in France and, deeply hurt by his undeserved failure, moved to Canada and thence to Chicago in 1904. There he continued his vascular experiments and formed a fruitful association with Charles C. Guthrie.[41] In August, 1906, Guthrie moved to Washington University in St. Louis, and Carrel soon shifted his base to the Rockefeller Institute in New York, but the two continued correspondence about their mutual interests.

Carrel and Guthrie soon adopted an all-layer technique of vascular anastomosis and introduced their three-stay suture technique to stabilize the ends of the vessels and permit

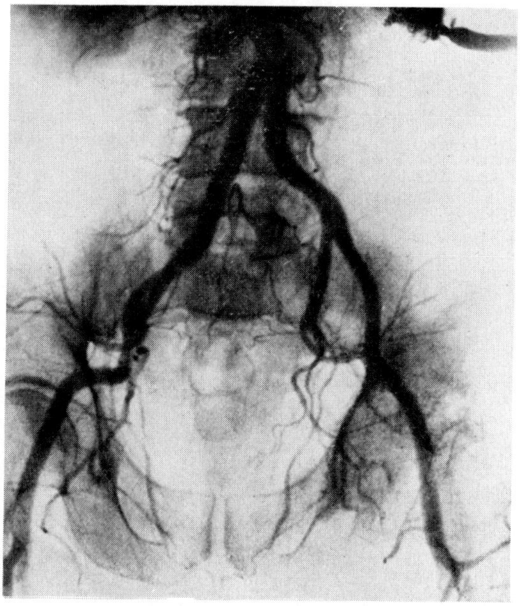

Fig. 5. Reynaldo dos Santos pioneered aortography in Portugal.[28]

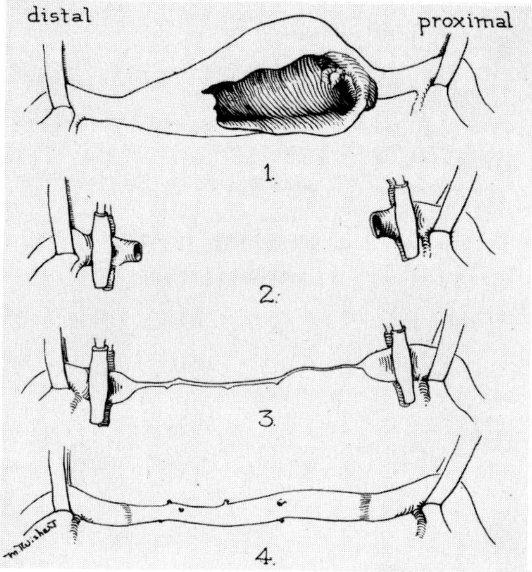

Fig. 6. Gordon Murray of Toronto resected a popliteal aneurysm and successfully replaced it with a vein graft in 1940, stressing the importance of intraoperative as well as postoperative anticoagulation by heparin.[71]

small anastomoses.[15] At the same time they stressed the importance of technical skill, atraumatic technique, the use of fine suture material, and the avoidance of drying of the vessels. Carrel's advice on vascular technique is still valid: "The vessels were handled very gently and endothelium was protected from drying by isotonic sodium chloride solution or by sterilized Vaseline. No dangerous metallic forceps were used. Great care was exercised to obtain accurate and smooth approximation of the endothelium of the vessels . . . stenosis or occlusion only occurs as a result of faulty technique." All forms of arterial and venous reconstructions were carried out, including free arterial and venous grafts both within the same animal and within and without the same species (Fig. 3).[14, 16] In 1912 Alexis Carrel was awarded the Nobel Prize in medicine "in recognition of his works on vascular suture and the transplantation of blood vessels and organs" (Fig. 4).[82] He remained a controversial figure throughout his life. Statements such as, "I am the creator of techniques; it is for others to use them," certainly did not win friends.[32]

While these laboratory studies progressed there were occasional successes in human patients by bold and knowledgeable surgeons, so that by 1908 Matas could collect 24 successful end-to-end arterial anastomoses and 120 lateral sutures.[59]

An occasional successful graft operation followed, such as Goyanes' vein graft for popliteal aneurysm in Madrid in 1906,[37] Erich Lexer's vein replacement of axillary aneurysm in Konigsberg in 1907,[56] and J. Hogarth Pringle's[79] two vein grafts for popliteal aneurysm in Glasgow in 1913. Pringle particularly understated his achievement and it lay unnoticed in *Lancet* and failed to spur efforts at repetition.

The brilliant promise of the early years of the twentieth century failed to materialize because surgical technique had far outstripped ancillary methods of diagnosis and support, and a long period of waiting followed.

The slaughter of World War I neither used nor stimulated progress in vascular surgery. Tuffier's paraffin-lined silver tubes were occasionally placed as temporary arterial splints,[86] but the very real fear of infection prohibited reparative vascular surgery along

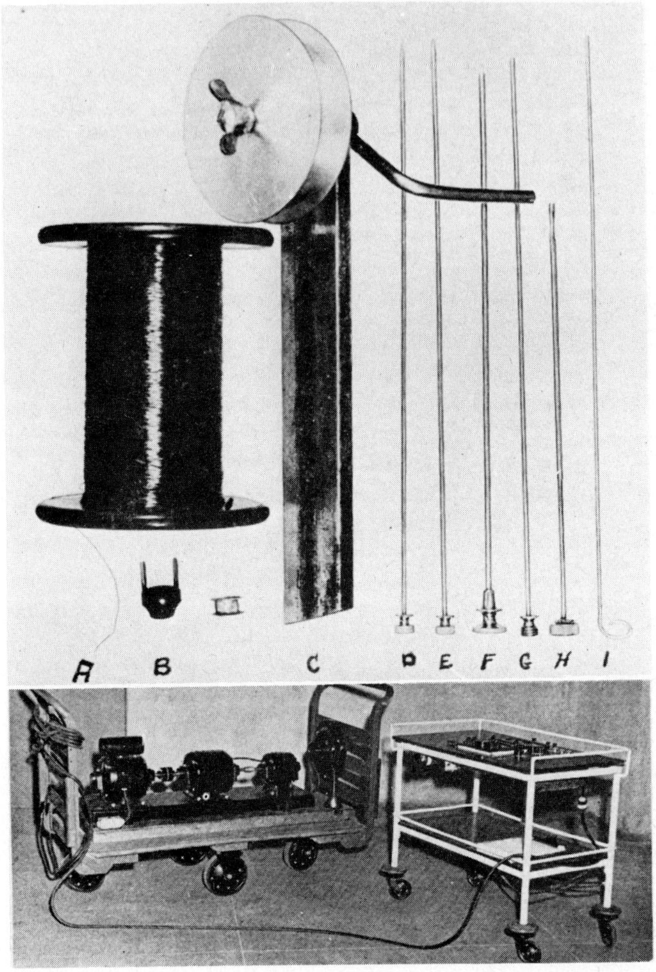

Fig. 7. Intra-aneurysmal wiring with electrocoagulation was the best method of treatment of abdominal and thoracic aneurysms as late as 1947. Arthur Blakemore of New York used this equipment and a few years later participated in the development of the first cloth prosthetic tube (Fig. 17). (From Blakemore, A. H.: Trans. South. Surg. Assoc. **59:** 27, 1947.)

with a general lack of knowledge of its possibilities.[6, 58] Weglowski's 1925 report of 51 vein grafts among German casualties of World War I escaped general attention[91] Wound treatment was chiefly in terms of a primitive (by present standards) debridement and amputation to save life. Incidentally, Alexis Carrel went to a front-line hospital in France where he developed the Carrel-Dakin sodium hypochlorite irrigation method of wound management.[32]

While there was little direct progress in vascular surgery between 1910 and the 1940's, there were important and necessary developments in anesthesia, blood replacement, angiography, surgical sympathectomy, and anticoagulants.

BLOOD TRANSFUSION

Blood transfusion had been sporadically attempted for centuries, but it required Landsteiner's discovery of blood groups in 1900 in Vienna to allow it to be done safely. Its practical use in the United States progressed at once and even surpassed that in Europe. Alton Ochsner recalled how, in 1923, transfusion was in disrepute in Zurich because of a 60 percent mortality rate. Their "biologische probe" test consisted of giving 25 c.c. of whole blood, and if the patient survived he would receive the main transfusion. Dr. Ochsner was allowed to treat an exsanguinated criminal, shot through the femoral artery, because "if he died it would be all right as they were anxious to get rid of him anyway!" He survived and the young surgeon was then allowed to type and transfuse a leading banker who also did well.[72] These cases altered their practice of blood transfusion.

ANGIOGRAPHY

The development of angiography began approximately 3 months after Roentgen's discovery of the x-ray, when Haschek and Lindenthal[44] injected a mixture of radiopaque material into the arteries of an amputated arm and demonstrated its radiopacity on an exposed film. Sicard and Forestier first reported injection into a live person in France when they injected poppy-seed oil (Lipiodol) into the antecubital vein and observed its passage toward the lungs fluoroscopically.[84] In the following year, 1924, Barney Brooks[11] initiated clinical angiography by injecting sodium iodide to study the femoropopliteal arterial system. Further developments largely occurred outside the United States, such as cerebral angiography by Egas Moniz in 1927 (who later in 1949 won the Nobel Prize for prefrontal lobotomy),[67] and aortography by Reynaldo dos Santos and associates[28] in 1929 in Portugal (Fig. 5) (reviewed by Dr. John Foster in his address to the International Cardiovascular Society).[36]

HEPARIN

In 1916 W. H. Howell[48] reported the discovery of the anticoagulant heparin, but, because of impurities, it was at first too toxic for use in patients.

In 1940 Gordon Murray[71] of Toronto administered a purified form[81] of heparin intravenously during and after embolectomy and also used it in the prevention and treatment of venous thromboembolism. He used intraoperative heparin during replacement of a popliteal aneurysm by vein graft (Fig. 6). Heparin—slowly at first and later rapidly—became widely accepted during the next 15 years.

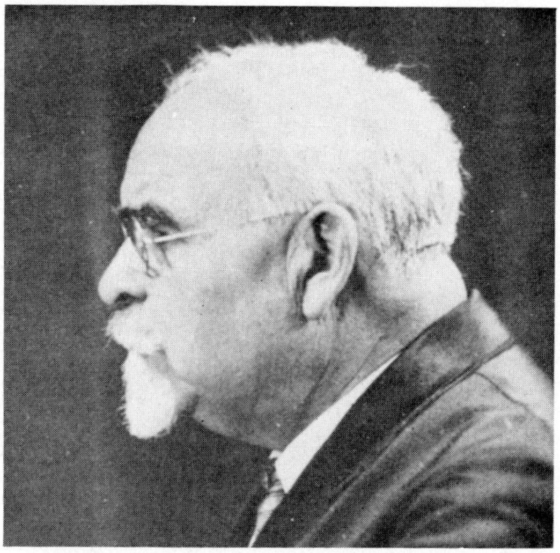

Fig. 8. Rudolph Matas of New Orleans.

ANEURYSMS

One of the major goals of vascular surgery had always been the cure of arterial aneurysms. Their early history is chiefly related to traumatic aneurysms of the peripheral arteries. Operation was quite dangerous in the preaseptic era, but it had long been recognized that intrasaccular thrombosis would alleviate the symptoms and prevent rupture of an aneurysm, although peripheral ischemia and even gangrene might occur. Over the centuries a variety of oral medications were advised and injections such as gelatin were given to encourage thrombosis. For example, Matas[62] described the injection of 12 oz. of sterile gelatin under the skin of the back of a patient and remarked upon the considerable pain and fever due to this. "The patient begged me not to repeat the injection!" No improvement followed.

Various forms of external compression, aimed at production of thrombosis and aneurysm were attempted, usually for those located in the limbs, but occasionally for aortic aneurysms. One method involved a series of assistants exerting proximal pressure for periods of 4 or more hours. A few successes were reported and poor results were generally overlooked.

The first recorded surgical treatment of an aneurysm is attributed to the Greek, Antyllus, who was a contemporary of Tiberius Caesar

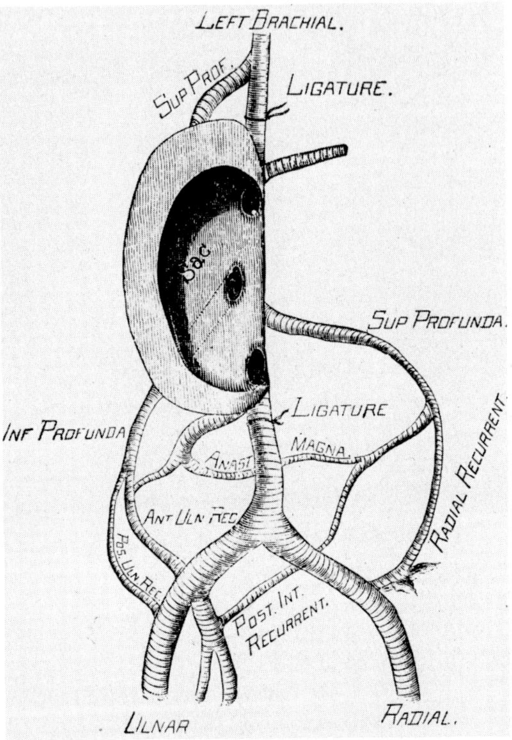

Fig. 9. Rudolph Matas' drawing of his initial endoaneurysmorrhaphy in 1888.[59] At the end of his lengthy career in 1940, he had operated on 620 aneurysms and treated 101 of these by endoaneurysmorrhaphy.[65]

in the first century. He performed proximal and distal ligation, followed by incision of the central portion and evacuation of the thrombus from the sac. Removal of all of the intervening aneurysm was avoided for fear of loss of the proximal ligature with uncontrollable hemorrhage.

This bipolar ligation remained the only treatment until a more simple proximal ligation was advocated in 1710 by the French surgeon Anel.[57]

Seventy-five years later John Hunter performed ligation of the proximal femoral artery in the adductor canal which bears his name, because more distal ligation at the neck of the popliteal aneurysmal sac often resulted in cutting through with uncontrollable bleeding. His first operation on Dec. 12, 1785, was performed on a coachman at St. George's Hospital in London. When the patient died 15 months later there was a solid thrombus within the sac.[47] His procedure was based on personally performed experiments. However, all methods of ligation usually failed because of collaterals bypassing the occlusion or the production of gangrene and only 5 percent had a good result.[65]

John Hunter found surgery little more than a trade but left it a science. He collapsed and died at the height of an argument with another surgeon. His relatives petitioned Parliament for funds to purchase his collection of pathologic specimens for the nation, but Prime Minister William Pitt was aghast and exclaimed, "What! Buy preparations! Why, I have not enough money to purchase gun-powder!"[38]

Aneurysms within the body cavities were not treated surgically at all. In 1831 the French surgeon, Velpeau,[87] did attempt to produce thrombosis by placing three pairs of sewing needles into an aneurysmal sac, and, in 1864, the British surgeon, Moore,[68] pushed 26 yards of fine iron wire into an aneurysm of the ascending aorta of a 27-year-old man in an attempt to form thrombus. When the patient died there actually was clot surrounding the wire. In 1879 Corradi of Pavia placed 42 cm. of iron wire into an aneurysm of the right upper chest and passed an electric current through this for 45 minutes, following which the aneurysm appeared to cease its pulsation. Such wiring and electrolysis thereafter were known as the Moore-Corradi treatment.[62] It did represent some progress and, in 1900, Hunner[49] collected 23 reported cases of wiring with electrocoagulation and stated that 17 percent had been "cured" in the sense that progression of the aneurysm ceased and the pain was relieved temporarily. However, this usually recurred with time so that the good result was temporary.

In 1947 Arthur Blakemore[8] of New York reported 63 cases treated by silver wiring and electrocoagulation (Fig. 7). Most were syphilitic thoracic aneurysms for which a death rate of under 10 percent was stated.[8] The development of arterial grafts ended this approach, but Eastcott's 1969 text described the continued occasional use of intrasaccular wiring for poor-risk patients in England.[31]

At the turn of the last century, when Alexis Carrel was still in medical school, a clinical

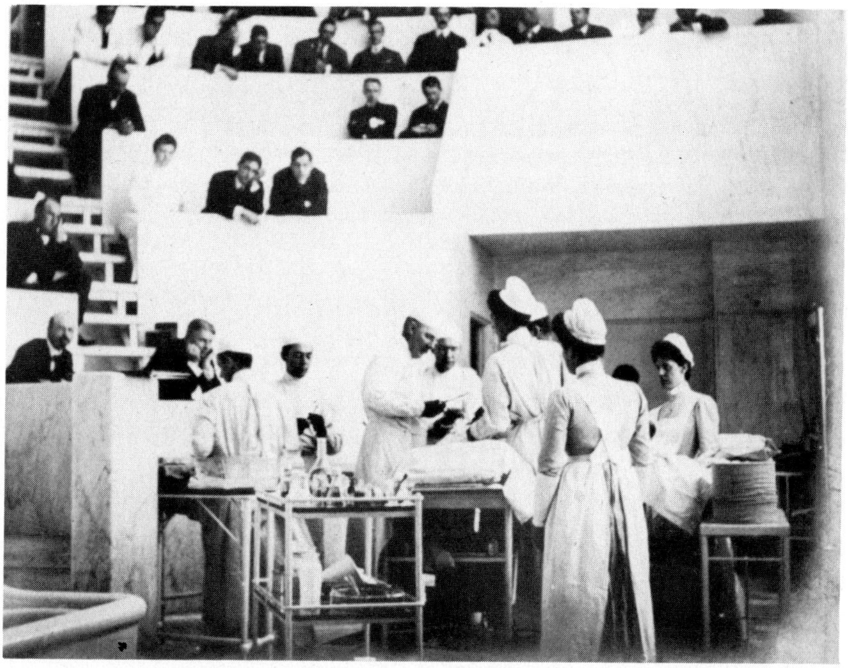

Fig. 10. William S. Halsted operating in the amphitheater at Johns Hopkins Hospital. (Photograph courtesy of Dr. George Zuidema.)

giant and legend in his own time developed in Dr. Rudolph Matas[73] of New Orleans (Fig. 8). On May 6, 1888, he performed his famous initial endoaneurysmorrhaphy for a large traumatic aneurysm of the brachial artery (Fig. 9). The new operation was inspired by the difficulties of the procedure when the aneurysm continued to pulsate following primary proximal and secondary distal ligation. A long incision was made into the aneurysm and laminated clot was removed. The large arterial orifices were closed by direct suture.[59] Dr. Matas[65] later stated that, although several opportunities for repetition of the procedure had occurred, it was not until 12 years later in 1900 that "I . . . mustered enough courage to battle with tradition," when a second case was similarly successful.

In 1900 Dr. Matas[62] also attempted treatment of abdominal aortic aneurysm by laparotomy with peritoneal exclusion of the sac followed later by wiring within the aneurysm and electrolysis. This procedure proved unsatisfactory but his experience increased yearly, and, in 1923, he ligated the aorta proximal to an aneurysm with survival of the patient. In his final extensive report to the American Surgical Association in 1940, he reported a total of 620 operations for aneurysms of which 101 had been treated by various methods of endoaneurysmorrhaphy. Among these latter the mortality rate was 4.9 percent.[64]

This remarkable individual also pioneered the use of intravenous saline infusions,[60] advocated nasogastric intubation as early as 1924,[64] and, in 1899, anesthetized a patient with spinal anesthesia.[61] He was a tireless worker throughout his 95 years of life, pioneered advances in many surgical fields, and was one of the 12 founders of the American Surgical Association.

An attempt to control an aneurysm of the aorta by ligation was first done by Sir Astley Cooper in 1817 but death occurred 3 days later.[7] Proximal ligation was generally unsuccessful, although in 1929 Vaughn's patient lived 2 years with continued expansion of the mass. Rudolph Matas[65] obtained the first success by this method in 1923, and Barney Brooks[12] of Nashville the second in 1925.

Imagine the scene in the operating room at Vanderbilt University Hospital in 1925. Dr. Brooks had just arrived from St. Louis as the first full-time chairman of the depart-

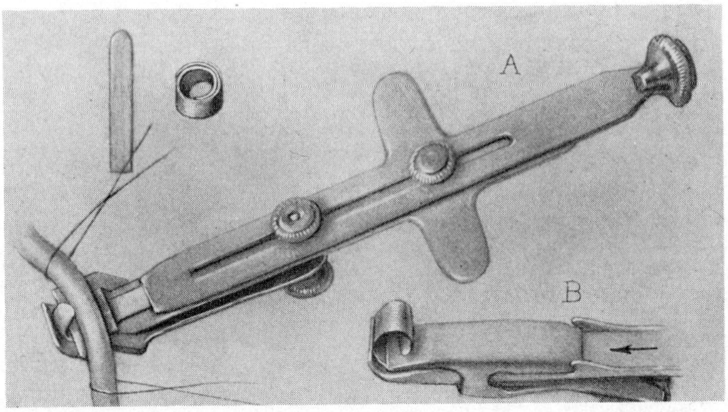

Fig. 11. Halsted's apparatus for banding an artery to produce gradual occlusion.

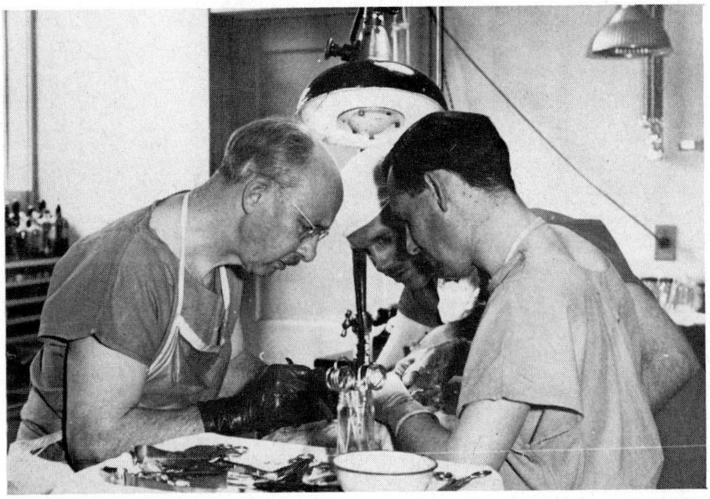

Fig. 12. Emile Holman (left) **studying arteriovenous fistula in the laboratory with Gerard Taylor of London** (opposite) **and Chester Herrod** (in background).

ment of surgery, and on this particular morning he found himself in a predicament while exploring a large aneurysm of the distal aorta and iliac arteries. Suddenly he found that his thumb was inside the sace and that he could feel the base of the vertebral bodies. There were no vascular instruments as we know them, little or no blood, and, worse, no previous experience. He improvised, cut a strip of fascia lata, and used it for proximal ligation of the aorta. He then removed his thumb and sutured the aneurysmal sac. The patient survived and returned to work as a truck driver but died of acute intestinal obstruction 3½ months later, at which time the aneurysm was found to be thrombosed. Dr. Brooks realized that good fortune had accompanied his effort and stated, "It is my belief that the ultimate satisfactory treatment of abdominal aneurysm . . . will be the development of methods to make it possible to excise completely the aneurysmal sac."

He immediately took the problem of ligation of the aorta to the laboratory and reported his experiences there to the Southern Surgical Association in 1926, as a young man following a masterful presentation by Dr. Rudolph Matas on surgery of the subclavian arteries. In discussion Dr. Matas regretted his inability to accept Brooks' conclusions since they contradicted previous concepts of the role of the heart and the prognosis of aortic ligation. Needless to say, Barney Brooks[13] defended his work vigorously and, in typical fashion, took exception to a point which Matas had just proposed in his paper!

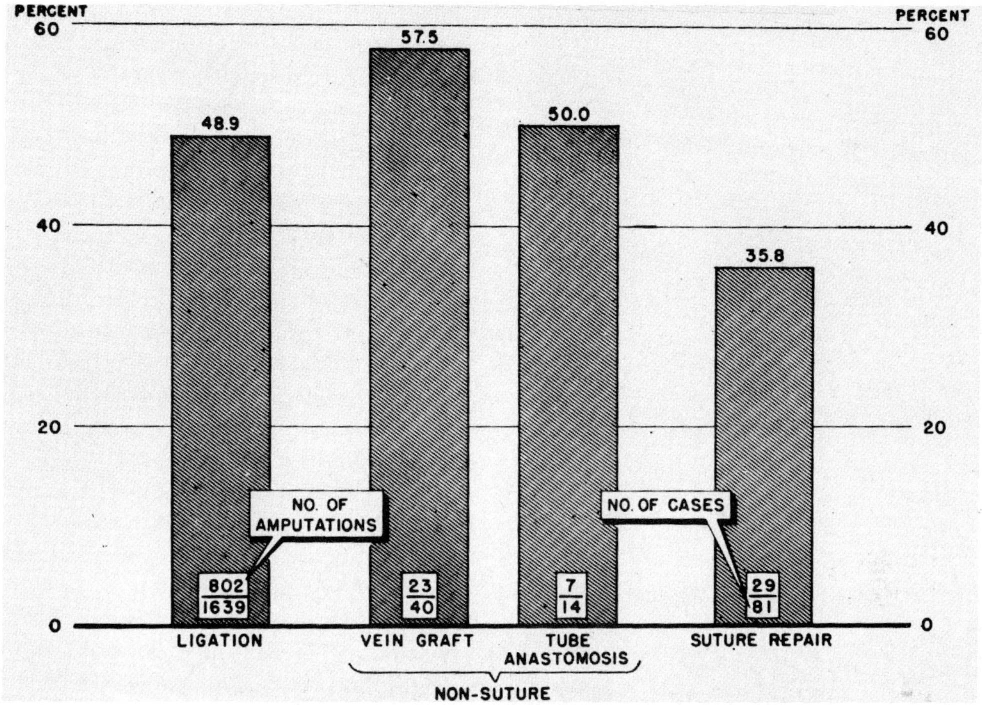

Fig. 13. Arterial reconstruction was uncommon during World War II and the series collected by De Bakey and Simeone showed more limb loss after vein graft than with simple ligation or direct suture repair.[25]

Barney Brooks never personally extirpated an aneurysm, yet his interest continued. He was well known to all of us as an absolutely strict teacher, who, despite his idiosyncrasies, impressed his students to the extent that the majority of my own medical class at Vanderbilt wished to become surgeons. Dr. Brooks' ability to state a clinical point so that it would be remembered is illustrated by his closing remarks after demonstrating a large femoral aneurysm at his teaching clinic, when he stated, "Never become so interested in an aneurysm that you forget the extremity, nor so much concerned with the extremity that you forget the patient."

The study of these surgical pioneers of arterial occlusion for aneurysm presents to us today an adventurous epic tinged with a heroic flavor where losses were minimized in relation to occasional successes.

William S. Halsted[43] of Baltimore had long maintained an interest in the problems of the arterial system and studied these both in the laboratory and clinically throughout his career (Fig. 10). The problems of the vascular system, especially of aneurysm, had a great fascination for Dr. Halsted and he particularly studied various methods of metallic banding and of ligation (Fig. 11). He stated, after one such preaneurysmal ligation, "The moment of tying the ligature is indeed a dramatic one. The monstrous booming tumor is stilled by a tiny thread, the tempest silenced by the magic wand." His and other methods of arterial banding and/or gradual occlusion failed because of infection or hemorrhage and, in 1940, Herman Pearse[78] concluded that no such method was really useful.

Many of Halsted's pupils continued to progress in the vascular field and Dr. Emile Holman,[46] in his 1937 monograph, delineated the physiologic pathology of arteriovenous fistula so that rational treatment could be done, at first by quadruple ligation and excision and more recently by repair (Fig. 12). The groundwork was thus laid for improvement in treatment of these communications during and after World War II.

Arterial repair during World War II was almost as rare as from 1914 to 1918. Indeed

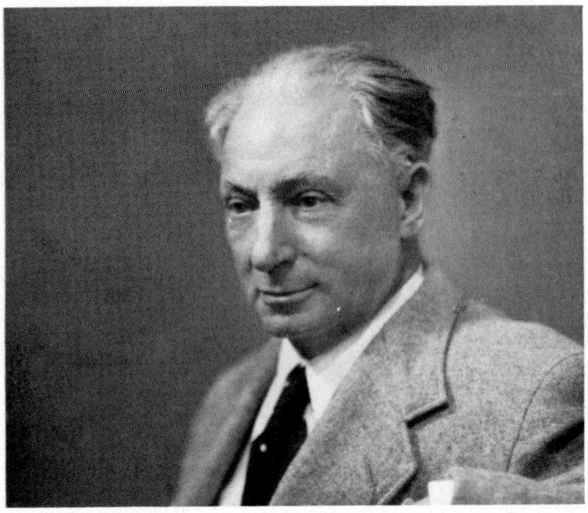

Fig. 14*A*. Reynaldo dos Santos, who pioneered aortography.

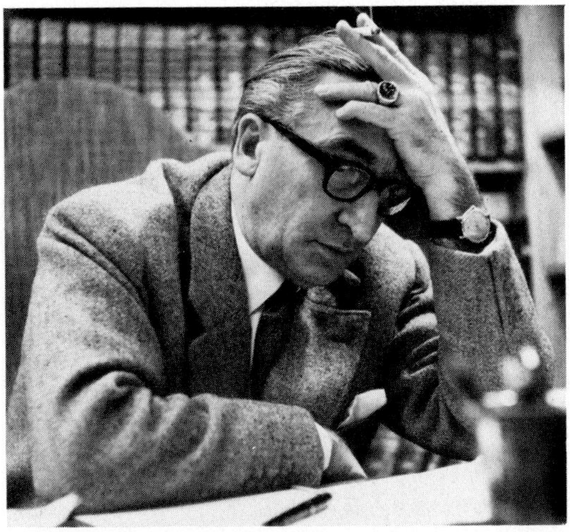

Fig. 14*B*. J. Cid dos Santos, the son of Reynaldo dos Santos, introduced thromboendarterectomy. The dos Santos were the only father and son to make important original contributions to vascular surgery independently.

the American series collected by De Bakey and Simeone[25] showed a slightly greater amputation rate among 54 cases repaired by vein graft (56 percent loss) than after arterial ligation (49 percent loss). Suture repair was associated with 36 percent limb loss among 81 cases (Fig. 13).

After World War II, accumulated knowledge exploded in a renaissance for vascular surgery, as imaginative and bold young men seized new knowledge in the animal laboratories and translated it into patient care in the wards and operating rooms. The rapid expansion of vascular surgery in one decade is staggering in relation to its slow progress for all of previous history.

Solution of a surgical problem by animal research is typified by Robert Gross' [39] report of the successful ligation of patent ductus arteriosus in 1938, based upon his work with dogs and human cadavers. In 1945 he resected and anastomosed two aortic coarctations in children, the first on June 28, 1945.[40] Crafoord and Nylin[21] of Stockholm had predated this with two successful coarctation cases in October, 1944.

In 1945 Blalock and Taussig[10] announced successful anastomosis of a systemic artery to the pulmonary artery in three patients for the relief of pulmonary stenosis or atresia.

The great Portuguese surgeon, J. Cid dos Santos, son of Reynaldo dos Santos[28] of angiographic fame, had studied in Strasbourg with René Leriche in the late 30's (Figs. 14*A* and 14*B*). At once he interested himself in vascular problems and repeated many of Carrel's early experiments. After wartime service in the Azores, he returned to Lisbon where, in June, 1946, he removed an acute femoral thrombosis from a patient dying of uremia. The specimen showed that he had unintentionally removed intima and a portion of media from the artery. Nevertheless this muscle-lined vessel remained patent. He concluded that the necessity of undamaged intima to allow patency was incorrect and that with heparin protection a "disobliterated" artery could remain patent. A longer-term success followed 6 months later when he performed subclavian-axillary thromboendarterectomy through two arteriotomies with continuing patency for over 28 years![27] Dos Santos thus destroyed the myth of intimal integrity as a necessity for luminal patency and provided a firm stance for the French surgeons who soon demonstrated that a variety of arterial grafts were feasible.

The long line of vascular developments by French surgeons dating back to Jaboulay continued. His pupil, Carrel, left France but retained citizenship there. René Leriche of Lyon then came to the fore in leading the

Travail du Service de M. le Pr R. LERICHE
(Hôpital Américain de Paris et Collège de France)

Le traitement de l'ischémie artéritique par la greffe veineuse longue

par J. KUNLIN
(Paris)

avec la collaboration
des Drs C. BITRY-BOÉLY, VOLNIÉ et BEAUDRY (1)

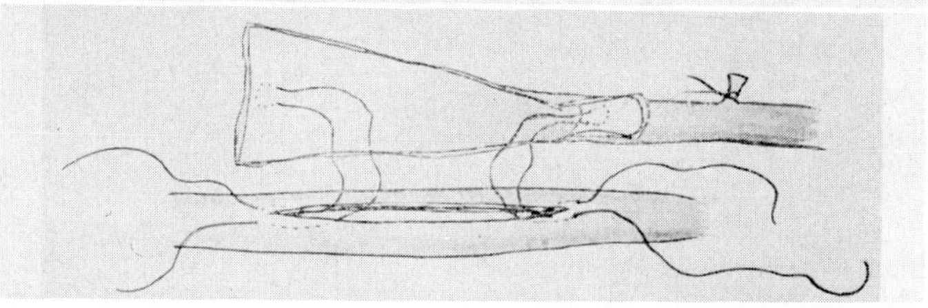

Fig. 15. Jean Kunlin's original description of long end-to-side anastomosis for a femoropopliteal venous bypass graft was published in 1949.[54]

vascular school of Strasbourg after 1924. He studied arterial disease and especially promoted sympathectomy along with his younger associate, René Fontaine,[34, 35] who later, in the mid 1940's, began to substitute vein grafts for obliterated peripheral arteries.

René Leriche, in collaboration with Carrel, attempted to graft two thrombosed arteries but they could not locate suitable sites for anastomosis since angiography was not available to them. Leriche thereafter mistrusted grafts and much preferred sympathectomy (and sometimes resection of the artery to interrupt other nerve fibers).

The bypass shunt graft, technically simple and functionally preserving collateral circulation, had been proposed by the German surgeon Ernest Jeger[51] in a long-forgotten book in 1913. The later history of Jeger and his idea is a mystery; perhaps he died in World War I.[55]

Jean Kunlin's[53] first bypass graft on a patient on Leriche's service occurred on June 3, 1948, as a 16 cm. femoral arterial replacement in a 54-year-old man (Fig. 15). By 1951 he had done 17 such cases with continued patency in seven.[54]

In 1923 Leriche had predicted that the "ideal treatment of thrombosis of the terminal abdominal aorta should consist of a resection of the occluded segment and reestablishment of arterial continuity by a graft."[55] In 1950—27 years later—this was first successfully performed by Jacques Oudot in France. He approached the aorta through a left extraperitoneal incision, and, after removing the distal aorta and common iliac arteries, placed a 24-hour-old homologous aortic graft. There was difficulty in performing the right anastomosis because of the exposure and because that side thrombosed. Six months later a secondary arterial graft was placed from the left external iliac artery to the right external iliac artery as a crossover graft, thus completing the two-stage revascularization of both lower extremities.

Jacques Oudot[76] was a man of parts. In that same year, 1950, he was a member of the great French mountain-climbing team which first ascended an 8,000 M. mountain—Annapurna in Nepal—23,493 ft. high. Maurice Herzog's[45] account of his intra-arterial anesthetic injections and digital amputations for frostbite while at high altitude are harrowing.

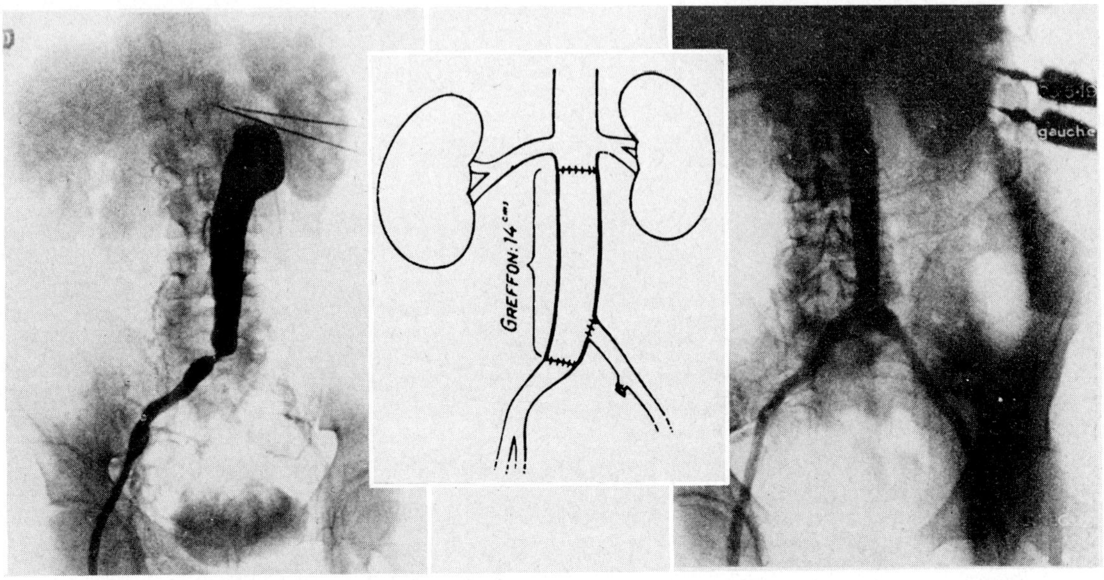

Fig. 16. Charles Dubost first placed an homologous arterial graft for aortic aneurysm in 1951. Because no bifurcation was available, the left iliac artery was anastomosed to the side of the graft.[29]

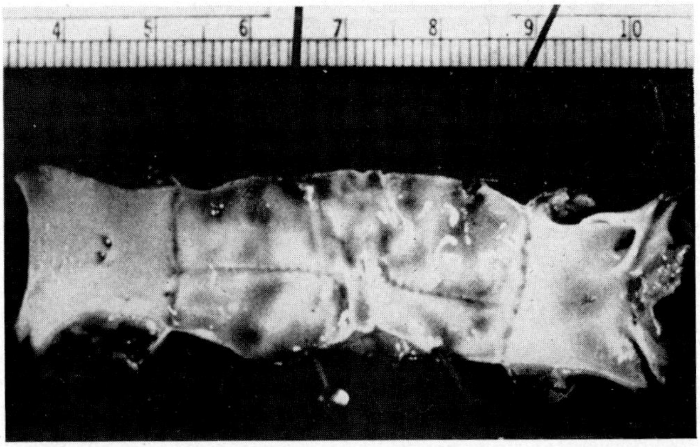

Fig. 17. In 1952 Voorhees, Jaretski, and Blakemore demonstrated that a porous fabric prosthesis would not only remain patent but would also develop a neointima. (From Voorhees, A. B., Jaretski, A., and Blakemore, A. H.: Ann. Surg. **135:** 332, 1952.)

His untimely death in 1953 occurred at age 48.

The French surgeons continued to prefer the extraperitoneal approach,[75] and the first resection of an abdominal aortic aneurysm was performed by Dubost, Allary, and Oeconomos[29] in Paris on March 29, 1951, via a left thoracoabdominal incision with resection of the eleventh rib. A large, atherosclerotic aneurysm was removed and a 3-week-old homologous thoracic aortic graft was anastomosed with No. 5-0 silk to the proximal aortic stump just below the renal arteries. Since a bifurcation graft was not available, the other end was anastomosed to the end of the right common iliac artery while the left reconstruction was carried out by joining that iliac artery to the side of the graft after removing some obstruction from within the left common iliac artery (Fig. 16).

Partial resection of a saccular aneurysm of the thoracic aorta was performed in 1944 by Alexander and Byron,[2] and the first complete excision with graft replacement by Michael

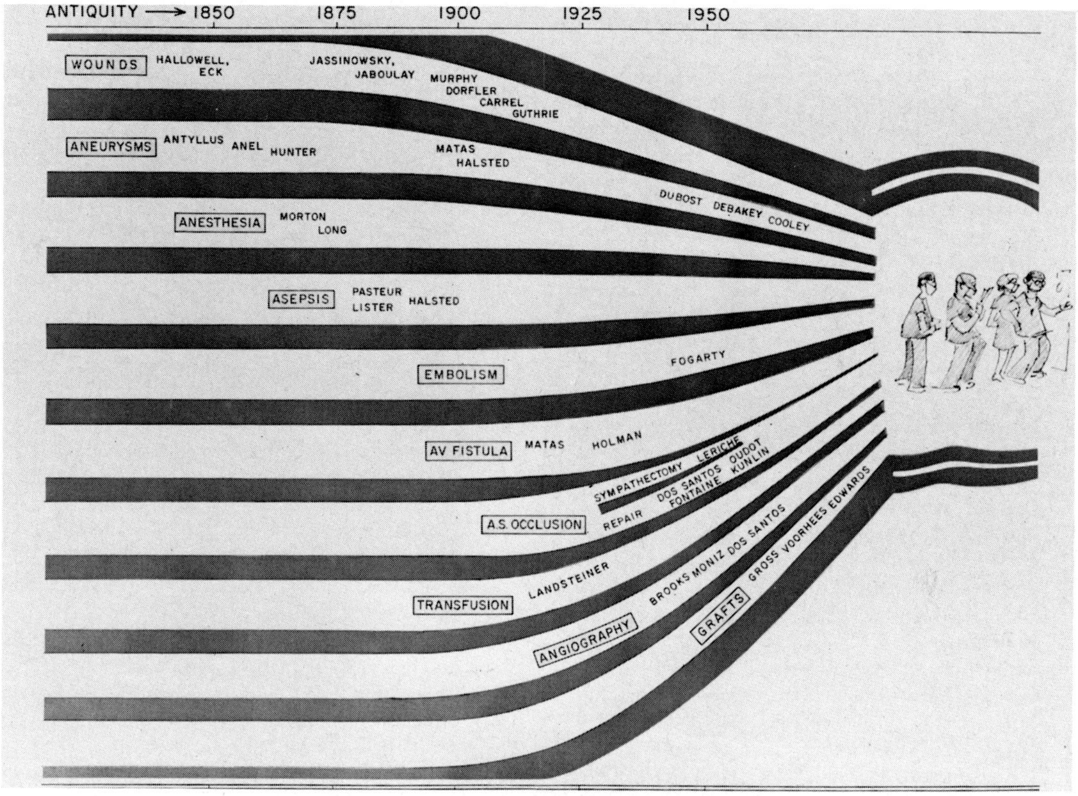

Fig. 18. The many origins of vascular surgery.

De Bakey and Denton Cooley[24] in 1953. They also successfully fenestrated the descending aorta for dissecting aneurysm in 1954,[23] totally excising the arch of the aorta in 1955[20] and the ascending aorta in 1956.[19] The Houston group soon developed the surgery of aneurysms into a routine, practiced successfully on thousands of patients.

The final explosive spread of vascular surgery throughout the world was triggered by what Charles Rob[80] termed one of the two great postwar innovations, namely, synthetic prosthetic grafts (the other being the Fogarty catheter). The then astonishing report in 1952 of Arthur Voorhees, Jaretski, and Blakemore[88] of New York that a vinyon-N cloth tube would remain open in a dog's aorta (Fig. 17) was soon confirmed and the further development of nylon, orlon, Teflon, and the presently famed Dacron prostheses requires no further comment.

As Will Durant[30] has advised, now we shall leave our history well behind the present, 20 years ago in the early 1950's, allowing each of you to assess it individually since then and to search for himself the continuing way along the broad highway that is vascular surgery in 1974 (Fig. 18).

The twisting paths from the past, beginning as unmarked trails in a jungle of ignorance, leading past many false sidetracks, built with imagination and courage but also with toil and tears, emerge upon the plateau of today, a broad and illuminated avenue teeming with surgical travelers.

REFERENCES

1. Abbe, R.: The surgery of the hand, N. Y. Med. J. Jan. 13, 1894.
2. Alexander, J., and Byron, F. X.: Aortectomy for thoracic aneurysm, J. A. M. A. **126:** 1139, 1944.
3. Allen, E. V., Barker, N. W., and Hines, E. A.: Peripheral vascular diseases, Philadelphia, 1955, W. B. Saunders Company.
4. Bazy, L., Huguier, J., Reboul, H., and Laubry, P.: Technique des "endarteriectomies" pour arterites obliterantes chroniques des

membres inferieurs, J. Chir. (Paris) **65:** 196, 1949.
5. Bernheim, B. M.: Surgery of the vascular system, Philadelphia, 1913, J. B. Lippincott Co.
6. Bernheim, B. M.: Blood-vessel surgery in the war, Surg. Gynecol. Obstet. **30:** 564, 1920.
7. Bigger, A.: The surgical treatment of aneurysm of the abdominal aorta, Ann. Surg. **112:** 879, 1940.
8. Blakemore, A. H.: Surgical aspects of aneurysm of the aorta, Trans. South. Surg. Assoc. **59:** 27, 1947.
9. Blakemore, A. H., Lord, J. W., and Stefko, P. L.: The severed primary artery in the war wounded, SURGERY **12:** 488, 1942.
10. Blalock, A., and Taussig, H. R.: Surgical treatment of malformations of the heart in which there is pulmonary stenosis or atresia, J. A. M. A. **128:** 189, 1945.
11. Brooks, B.: Injection of sodium iodide, J. A. M. A. **82:** 1016, 1924.
12. Brooks, B.: Ligation of the aorta: A clinical and experimental study, J. A. M. A. **87:** 722, 1926.
13. Brooks, B.: Ligation of the aorta: An experimental study, Trans. South Surg. Assoc. **39:** 228, 1926.
14. Carrel, A.: The surgery of blood vessels, Bull. Johns Hopkins Hosp. **18:** 18, 1907.
15. Carrel, A., and Guthrie, C. C.: Results of biterminal transplantation of veins, Am. J. Med. Sci. **132:** 415, 1906.
16. Carrel, A., and Guthrie, C. C.: Uniterminal and biterminal venous transplantation, Surg. Gynecol. Obstet. **2:** 266, 1906.
17. Child, C. G.: Eck's fistula, Surg. Gynecol. Obstet. **96:** 375, 1953.
18. Cooley, D. A., and De Bakey, M. E.: Surgical considerations of intrathoracic aneurysms of the aorta and great vessels, Ann. Surg. **135:** 660, 1952.
19. Cooley, D. A., and De Bakey, M. E.: Resection of entire ascending aorta in fusiform aneurysm using cardiac bypass, J. A. M. A. **162:** 1155, 1956.
20. Cooley, D. A., Mahaffey, D. E., and De Bakey, M. E.: Total excision of the aortic arch for aneurysm, Surg. Gynecol. Obstet. **101:** 667, 1955.
21. Crafoord, C., and Nylin, G.: Congenital coarctation of the aorta and its surgical treatment, J. Thorac. Surg. **14:** 347, 1945.
22. Davis, L.: J. B. Murphy: Stormy petrel of surgery, New York, 1938, G. P. Putnam's Sons.
23. De Bakey, M. E., Cooley, D. A., and Creech, O.: Surgical consideration of dissecting aneurysm of the aorta, Ann. Surg. **142:** 586, 1955.
24. De Bakey, M. E., and Cooley, D. A.: Successful resection of aneurysm of thoracic aorta and replacement by graft, J. A. M. A. **152:** 673, 1953.
25. De Bakey, M. E., and Simeone, F. A.: Battle injuries of the arteries in World War II, Ann. Surg. **123:** 534, 1946.
26. Dorfler, J.: Uber Arteriennaht, Beitr. Klin. Chir. **25:** 781, 1899.
27. dos Santos, J. C.: From embolectomy to thromboendarterectomy or the face of a myth, Address to Society for Clinical Vascular Surgery, Palm Springs, Calif. April, 1974.
28. dos Santos, R., Lanas, A., and Pereirgi, C. J.: L'arteriographie des membres de l'aorte et ses branches abdominales, Bull. Soc. Nat. Chir. **55:** 587, 1929.
29. Dubost, C., Allary, M., and Oeconomos, N. A.: Propos de traitement des aneurysmes de l'aorte ablauon de l'aneurysme. Retablissement de la continuité, Mem. Acad. Chir. (Paris) **77:** 381, 1951.
30. Durant, W., and Durant, A.: Rousseau and revolution, New York, 1967, Simon and Schuster.
31. Eastcott, H. H. G.: Arterial surgery, Philadelphia, 1969, J. B. Lippincott Co., p. 235.
32. Edwards, W. S., and Edwards, P. D.: Alexis Carrel: Visionary surgeon, Springfield, Ill., 1974, Charles C Thomas, Publisher.
33. Edwards, W. S., and Tapp, J. S.: Peripheral artery replacement with chemically treated nylon tubes, Surg. Gynecol. Obstet. **102:** 443, 1956.
34. Fontaine, R.: Letter, March, 1974.
35. Fontaine, R.: Early and late reoperation following reconstructive surgery for peripheral artery obliteration of atherosclerotic origin. An analytic synthesis of their causes, Ann. Chir. **27:** 897, 1973.
36. Foster, J. H.: Arteriography, the cornerstone of vascular surgery, Arch. Surg. In press.
37. Goyanes, J.: Neuvos trabajos de chirurgia vascular: Substiucion plastica de las arterias por las venas, o arterioplastia venosa, aplicado, como neuvo metodo, al traitamiento de los aneurismas, El Sigo. Med. **53:** 561, 1906.
38. Graham, H.: Surgeons all, New York, 1957, New York Philosophical Library.
39. Gross, R. E.: A surgical approach for ligation of a patent ductus arteriosus, N. Engl. J. Med. **220:** 510, 1939.
40. Gross, R. E.: Surgical correction for coarctation of the aorta, SURGERY **18:** 673, 1945.
41. Guthrie, C. C.: Blood vessel surgery and its application, New York, 1912, Longmans, Green Company.
42. Haimovici, H.: History of arterial grafting, J. Cardiovasc. Surg. **4:** 152, 1963.
43. Halsted, W. S.: Ligations of the left subclavian artery in its first portion, Johns Hopkins Hosp. Reports **21:** 5, 1924.

44. Haschek, E., and Lindenthal, O. T.: Ein Beitrag zur praktischen Verwerthung der Photographie nach Röntgen, Wien. Klin. Wochenschr. **9:** 63, 1896.
45. Herzog, M.: Annapurna; first conquest of an 8,000 meter peak, New York, 1953, E. P. Dutton Company.
46. Holman, E.: Arterio-venous aneurysm, New York, 1937, MacMillan Co.
47. Home, E.: An account of Mr. Hunter's method of performing the operation for popliteal aneurysm communicated in a letter to Dr. Simmons by Mr. E. Home. London Med. J. **7:** 391, 1786. (Reprinted in Med. Classics **4:** 449, 1939-40.)
48. Howell, W. H.: Two new factors in blood coagulation—heparin and proantithrombin, Am. J. Physiol. **47:** 328, 1918.
49. Hunner, G. L.: Aneurysm of the aorta treated by the insertion of a permanent wire and galvanism (Moore-Corradi method), Bull. Johns Hopkins Hosp. **11:** 263, 1900.
50. Jaboulay, M., and Briau, E.: Recherches expérimentales sur la suture et la greffe arterielle, Lyon Med. **81:** 97, 1896.
51. Jeger, E.: Die Chirurgie der Blut gefasse und des Herzens, Berlin, 1913, A. Hirschwald.
52. Jassinowsky, A.: Die Arteriennhat: Eine experimentelle Studie, Inaug. Diss. Dorpat., 1889.
53. Kunlin, J.: Le traitement de l'arterite obliterante par la greffe veineuse, Arch. Mal Coeur **42:** 371, 1949.
54. Kunlin, J.: Treatment of arterial ischemia by long vein grafts, Rev. Chir. **70:** 206, 1951.
55. Kunlin, J.: Personal letter, May 1974.
56. Lexer, E.: Die ideale Operation des arteriellen und des arteriellvenosen Aneurysma, Arch. Klin. Chir. **83:** 458, 1907.
57. Mahorner, H.: Historic and modern methods of treating aneurysms, Int. Abs. Surg. **105:** 105, 1957.
58. Makins, G. H.: Gunshot injuries to the blood vessels, New York, 1919, William Wood Company.
59. Matas, R.: Traumatic aneurysm of the left brachial artery. Failure of direct and indirect pressure; ligation of the artery immediately above tumor, return of pulsation on the tenth day; ligation immediately below tumor; failure to arrest pulsation: incision and partial excision of sac; recovery, Med. News New York **53:** 462, 1888.
60. Matas, R.: A clinical report on intravenous saline infusion in the wards of the New Orleans Charity Hospital from June, 1888, to June, 1891, New Orleans Med. Surg. J. **19:** 1, 1891.
61. Matas, R.: The growing importance and value of local and regional anesthesia in minor and major surgery, Trans. La. Med. Soc. 329 (April), 1900.
62. Matas, R.: The treatment of abdominal aortic aneurysm by a preliminary exploratory coeliotomy and peritoneal exclusion of the sac, followed at a later sitting by wiring and electrolysis with a report of two hitherto unpublished cases, Trans. South. Surg. Gynecol. **13:** 272, 1900.
63. Matas, R.: *In* Keen, W. W., and Da Costa, J. C., editors: Surgery: Its principles and practice, Philadelphia, 1914, W. B. Saunders.
64. Matas, R.: The continued intravenous drip: With remarks on the value of continued gastric drainage and irrigation by nasal intubation with a gastroduodenal tube (Jutte) in surgical practice, Ann. Surg. **79:** 643, 1924.
65. Matas, R.: Personal experiences in vascular surgery, Ann. Surg. **112:** 802, 1940.
66. Matas, R.: *In* Keys, T. E., editor: The history of surgical anesthesia, New York, 1945, Schuman, pp. 42, 43.
67. Moniz, E.: L'encephalographique arterielle; son importance dans la localization des tumeurs cérébrales, Rev. Neurol. **2:** 172, 1927.
68. Moore, C. H., and Murchison, C.: On a new method of procuring the consolidation of fibrin in certain incurable aneurysms, Med. Chir. Tr. **47:** 129, 1864.
69. Moore, H. D.: The replacement of blood vessels by polythene tubes, Surg. Gynecol. Obstet. **91:** 593, 1950.
70. Murphy, J. B.: Resection of arteries and veins injured in continuing end-to-end suture experimental and clinical research, Med. Rec. **51:** 73, 1897.
71. Murray, G.: Heparin in surgical treatment of blood vessels, Arch. Surg. **40:** 307, 1940.
72. Ochsner, A.: Personal letter, 1974.
73. Ochsner, A., and Batas, R.: Arch. Surg. **72:** 1, 1956.
74. Oudot, J.: La greffe vasculaire dans les thromboses du carrefour aortique, Presse Med. **59:** 234, 1951.
75. Oudot, J., and Beaconsfield, P.: Thrombosis of aortic bifurcation treated by resection and homograft replacement: Report of five cases, Arch. Surg. **66:** 365, 1953.
76. Oudot, J.: Necrology, Presse Med. **61:** 1181, 1953.
77. Payr, E.: Beitrage zur Technik der Blutgefasse und nervennaht nebst Mittheilungen über die vervendung eines resorbirbaren metalles in der Chirurgie, Arch. Klin. Chir. **62:** 67, 1900.
78. Pearse, H. E.: Experimental studies on the gradual occlusion of large arteries, Ann. Surg. **112:** 923, 1940.
79. Pringle, J. H.: Two cases of vein grafting for the maintenance of direct arterial circulation, Lancet **1:** 1795, 1913.

80. Rob, C. G.: A history of arterial surgery, Arch. Surg. **105:** 821, 1972.
81. Scott, D. A., and Charles, A. F.: Studies in heparin: The purification of heparin, J. Biol. Chem. **102:** 425, 1933.
82. Schuck, H., et al.: Nobel, the man and his prizes, Norman, Okla., 1951, University of Oklahoma Press, p. 256.
83. Shumacker, H. B., and Muhm, Y. Y.: Arterial sutures techniques and grafts: Past, present, and future, SURGERY **66:** 419, 1969.
84. Sicard, J. A., and Forestier, G.: Injections intra-vasculaires d'huile iodée sous controle radiologigue, C. R. Soc. Biol. (Paris), **88:** 1200, 1923.
85. Smith, S.: Studies in experimental vascular surgery, SURGERY **18:** 627, 1945.
86. Tuffier, T.: Intervention chirurgicale directe pour un aneurysme de la crosse de l'aorte, ligature du sac, Bull. Soc. Chir. (Paris) **28:** 326, 1902.
87. Velpeau, A. A. L. M.: Mémoire sur la figure de l'acupuncture des artères dans le traitement des aneurismes, Gaz. Med. (Paris) **2:** 1, 1831.
88. Voorhees, A. B., Jaretski, A., and Blakemore, A. H.: The use of tubes constructed from vinyon N cloth in bridging arterial defects, Ann. Surg. **135:** 332, 1952.
89. Warren, J. L.: The healing of arteries after ligature in man and animals, New York, 1886, William Wood Company.
90. Watts, S. H.: The suture of blood vessels. Implantation and transplantation of vessels and organs. An historical and experimental study, Bull. Johns Hopkins Hosp. **18:** 153, 1907.
91. Weglowski, R.: Uber die Gefass Transplantation, Zentralbl. Chir. **52:** 22441, 1925.

Long-term evaluation of the celiac band syndrome

William E. Evans, M.D., *Columbus, Ohio*

Follow-up of 59 patients with the celiac compression syndrome was carried out. Early surgical results (after one to 6 months) were excellent; long-term surgical results (after 3 to 12 years) showed only 41 percent of patients to be free of symptoms. Relief of symptoms occurred in 75 percent of nonoperated patients. A skeptical and cautious approach to these patients is suggested.

From the Department of Surgery, The Ohio State University Hospitals, Columbus, Ohio

THE EXISTENCE of the celiac compression syndrome, consisting of abdominal pain, epigastric bruit, and angiographic demonstration of compression of the artery, has been challenged by several authors.[2, 11] A clear demonstration of pathophysiologic significance of celiac compression has yet to be formulated. Although early results of operation on these patients appear encouraging, few long-term follow-up studies have been reported.[1-11] Fifty-nine patients, 47 of whom were operated on, have been re-evaluated 3 to 11 years after their initial diagnoses were made.

MATERIALS

From 1963 through 1971, 71 patients with celiac compression syndrome were studied. Of these, 59 could be traced for follow-up. Fifty returned for personal re-evaluation by the author. Six were re-evaluated by their personal physicians with full knowledge of the syndrome, and three were interviewed by the author by telephone. Ages ranged from 13 to 68 years. Only 10 were men. Forty-six (78 percent) were less than 50 years of age. Operation was done on 47, while 12 were treated nonsurgically. Operation consisted of division of the median arcuate ligament and clearing of all tissue overlying the celiac axis.

Fig. 1 shows the patients observed and operated on by year. The majority were seen in the 1963 to 1968 period. Table I shows the incidence of weight loss, diarrhea, and pain pattern. Weight loss occurred in only one third, diarrhea was rarely present, and postprandial pain occurred in fewer than half, the rest presenting with vague abdominal pain with no relation to meals. Over 70 percent had had a previous abdominal operation, and all had had a long history of abdominal complaints.

Operation was done on 47 patients; 44 had only celiac band release while three had cholecystectomy simultaneously. Thirteen underwent additional subsequent abdominal procedures.

RESULTS

Surgical group. Table II summarizes the initial surgical result from one to 6 months

Presented at the Twenty-eighth Annual Meeting of the Society for Vascular Surgery, Chicago, Ill., June 20 and 21, 1974.

Reprint requests: William E. Evans, M.D., Department of Surgery, The Ohio State University Hospitals, Columbus, Ohio 43210.

Table I. *Celiac band syndrome**

	Total		*Surgery*		*No surgery*	
	No.	*%*	*No.*	*%*	*No.*	*%*
Weight loss	21/59	36	17/47	36	5/12	41
Diarrhea	9/59	15	7/47	15	2/12	16
Postprandial pain	25/59	42	20/47	42	5/12	41
Previous operation	42/59	71	36/47	76	6/12	50

*Note the low incidence of diarrhea and weight loss. Pain related to meals in infrequent.

Table II. *Celiac band—initial results*

	No.	*%*
Asymptomatic	39	83
Improved	—	—
No change	8	17
Total	47	

Table III. *Celiac band—follow-up results**

	No.	*%*
Asymptomatic	18	41
Improved	4	9
No change	22	50
Total	44	

*Gallbladder initially: two asymptomatic, one improved.

following operation. Thirty-nine of 47 (83 percent) were asymptomatic, while eight (17 percent) were not improved. Results at the conclusion of the study, from 3 to 11 years after operation, are given in Table III. The three patients having simultaneous cholecystectomy were excluded, leaving 44 with only compression release. Of these, 41 percent were asymptomatic, less than half the number initially benefited by operation. Nine percent felt they were improved, although symptoms similar to the preoperative complaint persisted. Twenty-two (50 percent) were unchanged by operation and symptoms persisted.

Of the three patients with simultaneous cholecystectomy, two were relieved of symptoms while one claimed to be markedly improved. Contribution of the compression release is difficult to assess.

Of the 22 patients treated surgically without benefit, 13 had subsequent operations. Eight are now asymptomatic or improved, having had cholecystectomy (three), pyloroplasty (two), hysterectomy (two), and rerelease of a band (one). Five patients with subsequent surgery continued to be symptomatic. One had a gastrectomy 3 years later for carcinoma and died from the disease; one had a kidney stone removed; one had lysis of adhesions; one had rerelease of a band; and one had an unknown abdominal procedure.

In no patient was an abdominal bruit heard at the follow-up examination.

There was no correlation between presenting symptoms and results. Of the patients who were asymptomatic (18) or improved (four) by band release alone, 10 had weight loss and 12 had none. Diarrhea occurred in only three while postprandial pain was present in 10 of the 22. Twenty-two patients with no benefit from surgery had similar histories. Nine had weight loss while 13 did not; only three had diarrhea. Postprandial pain occurred in 12. Therefore no correlation could be found between symptoms and results of surgery.

Nonsurgical group. Twelve patients were treated nonoperatively, the majority having refused operation. Nine are free of abdominal pain, one is improved, and only two continue to have symptoms. Of the pain-free group, four responded to psychiatric treatment, two having had shock therapy. Three patients became symptom free when taken off milk products; symptoms recur whenever they are re-exposed to milk or milk products. Two, treated symptomatically, are now well and without complaint. There was no correlation between results and presenting symptoms.

DISCUSSION

Patients in this entire series appear to be similar to those previously reported.[1-11] As opposed to patients with true intestinal ischemia, few had diarrhea (15 percent), and weight loss occurred only in about one third (36 percent). The pain pattern was usually vague and in only 42 percent was it related to food intake. The majority had a long history of abdominal pain with extensive evaluations in the past. Over 70 percent had had a previous abdominal exploration without relief.

When evaluated soon after surgery, the majority were symptom free (83 percent), which is in agreement with most reports. Szilagyi and associates,[11] in 1972, summarizing collected reports, noted that 82 percent were asymptomatic with a mean follow-up of 20 months (range, one to 48 months).[11] However, when longer follow-up is evaluated, the results are less encouraging. In our surgically treated patients, only 41 percent were symptom free. Nine percent felt they were improved but, on close questioning, had symptoms quite similar to those recorded preoperatively. Twenty-two (50 percent) were not benefited at all. Eight of these underwent additional operations and are now symptom free.

Of great interest are the 12 patients who were not operated on. Nine (75 percent) are now asymptomatic, one is improved, and only two continue to be symptomatic. Their symptoms continue to be vague without specific pattern, suggesting organic disease.

In reviewing the data it was hoped that a pattern would emerge which might identify those patients likely to benefit from operation. None could be found. The presence of weight loss, diarrhea, and postprandial abdominal pain was no more frequent in those who did well than in those without benefit, nor did those factors vary in the nonsurgical group. Age, duration of symptoms, and presence or absence of previous operation also showed no correlation with results.

Although some patients appear to have benefited from operation, the predictability of response has been less than satisfactory. Because of the lack of a well-established pathophysiologic mechanism, and in light of these long-term results from release of celiac

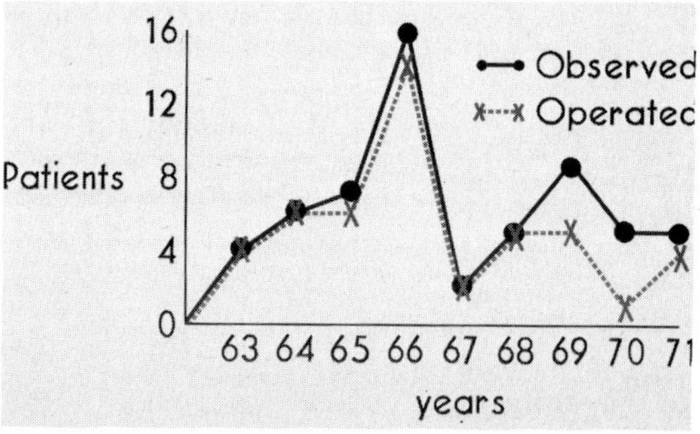

Fig. 1. Patients with the celiac band syndrome observed and operated on are summarized by year.

compression, it appears that a skeptical and cautious approach to these patients is justified. Unless a more definite formulation of etiology or a more favorable long-term result is forthcoming, it seems unlikely that compression of the celiac artery can be implicated as an identifiable syndrome causing abdominal pain.

REFERENCES

1. Carey, J. P., Stemmer, E. A., and Connolly, J. E.: Median arcuate ligament syndrome, Arch. Surg. **99:** 441, 1969.
2. Drapanas, T., and Bron, K. M.: Stenosis of the celiac artery, Ann. Surg. **164:** 1085, 1966.
3. Dunbar, J. D., Molnar, W., Beman, F. F., and Marable, S. A.: Compression of the celiac trunk and abdominal angina: Preliminary report of 15 cases, Am. J. Roentgenol. Radium Ther. Nucl. Med. **95:** 731, 1965.
4. Harjola, P. T., and Lahtiharju, A.: Celiac axis syndrome: Abdominal angina caused by external compression of the celiac artery, Am. J. Surg. **115:** 864, 1968.
5. Lord, R. S., Stoney, R. J., and Wylie, E. J.: Coeliac-axis compression, Lancet **2:** 795, 1968.
6. Marable, S. A., Kaplan, M. F., Beman, F. M., and Molnar, W.: Celiac compression syndrome, Am. J. Surg. **115:** 97, 1968.
7. Rob, C. G., and Owen, K.: Ligation of both the coeliac axis and superior mesenteric artery with survival of the patient, Br. J. Surg. **44:** 247, 1956-1957.
8. Snyder, M. A., Mahoney, E. B., and Rob, C. G.: Symptomatic celiac artery stenosis due to constriction by the neurofibrous tissue of the celiac ganglion, Surgery **61:** 372, 1967.
9. Stanley, J. C., and Fry, W. J.: Median arcuate ligament syndrome, Arch. Surg. **103:** 252, 1971.

10. Stoney, R. J., and Wylie, E. J.: Recognition and surgical management of visceral ischemic syndromes, Ann. Surg. **164:** 714, 1966.
11. Szilagyi, D. E., Rian, R. L., Elliott, J. P., and Smith, R. F.: The celiac artery compression syndrome: Does it exist? SURGERY **72:** 849, 1972.

DISCUSSION

Dr. D. Emerick Szilagyi (Detroit, Mich.). All those interested in the intriguing problem of the so-called celiac artery compression syndrome will readily recognize that Dr. Evans' study is a valuable one and one that has been greatly needed. His study gained particular importance from the fact that the patients on whom he reports form the group in which this syndrome was first described by Dunbar and his associates.

When my associates and I reported our analysis of this subject before this Society 2 years ago, we pointed out that all the anatomical, pathophysiological, and statistical evidence negated the existence of this syndrome, and that, indeed, the only proof consistently cited by its components was the nearly uniform symptomatic relief of the patients after the surgical correction of the celiac arterial narrowing. Dr. Evans' follow-up observations clearly show that, in at least half of the cases, even the symptomatic improvement was transient and, thus, these observations cast serious doubt on the assumption that the relief was due to the correction of an organic abnormality. This impression would have been further strengthened if Dr. Evans had shown by angiography that, in the cases with transient relief, the anatomical correction of the so-called celiac narrowing persisted. However, this proof is not essential since, in practically all instances reported in the literature, the results were expressed purely in terms of symptomatic relief and were not based on angiographic observations.

Thus I share completely the view that this so-called syndrome must be approached with great diagnostic skepticism. I would further like to repeat the plea that when a corrective operation is performed in a case diagnosed as celiac artery compression syndrome, all the pertinent objective tests and measurements should be carried out that are necessary to establish or disprove an etiological relationship between the angiographic deformity of the celiac artery and the clinical symptoms for which surgical treatment has been undertaken.

Dr. Ronald J. Stoney (San Francisco, Calif.). The first point I am concerned about deals with causes of failure. Immediate failures in our experience were usually due to persistent stenosis of the celiac axis at the area when the arcuate ligament compression existed. We found that, in more than half of our patients, release of the ligament was inadequate to restore to normal patency. These patients required an arterial reconstruction. I wonder if this cause of failure was discovered by anteriograms in Dr. Evans' patients.

The second point relates to the appearance of other intra-abdominal disease in this group of patients operated on. We, too, have observed this in a few instances. Careful preoperative screening for other diseases and, at operation, exploration of other possible visceral lesions should minimize the frequency of this problem.

Our own experience with this lesion included a similar size group of patients followed for 10 years. Thirty-five of the 43 patients remain cured or improved. Late arteriograms in selected patients document continuing patency of the celiac artery.

Dr. Gilbert S. Campbell (Little Rock, Ark.). This will be a short and ambivalent discussion. It is ambivalent in the sense that I am not sure what it will add, but it would subtract from my friendship with Dr. Raymond Read if I did not give it since he asked me to give this brief discussion for him.

A 50-year-old nurse had increasingly severe episodes of abdominal pain and syncope. Physical examination demonstrated an epigastic bruit. An x-ray showed the typical radiologic appearance of the arcuate ligament syndrome. At operation the abdominal aorta was covered for 2 or 3 inches below the diaphram by diaphragmatic musculature. It appeared that a hypertrophied left slip of the right crus had fused with the left crus, compressing the celiac artery for an inch or more on to the aorta and constricting it by the arcuate ligament. This containment was relieved by bisecting the abnormal crural musculature along the anterior surface of the aorta and dividing the arcuate ligament. The constriction in the celiac artery relieved itself. Pressure measurements showed no gradient before release.

Certainly in this patient hypertrophy of the diaphragmatic attachment to the spine distorted the celiac artery. We believe her symptomatology was related to intermittent complete obstruction of the celiac artery, whose flow was otherwise normal preventing collateralization from the superior mesenteric. As one would expect, the xylose absorption study was normal.

Dr. Edwin J. Wylie (San Francisco, Calif.). I am impressed by the large number of patients who had no postprandial pain, which I believe represented more than half of Dr. Evans' series.

In our own series virtually everybody had

significant postprandial pain; this was the reason for their operation. They would not eat because of the pain, and most had lost weight. In the series that Dr. Evans presented, very few have lost weight and a large percentage of them had no pain. Some of them had other diseases, as evidenced by cure from another subsequent operation. The whole problem is muddled in that a large number of people, particularly women, have this ligament compressing the celiac axis with no symptoms at all.

The problem would have been clarified better had Dr. Evans limited his patients to those who had genuine postprandial pain and who were losing weight.

Dr. William J. Fry (Ann Arbor, Mich.). I would like to emphasize a couple of things. I believe the group of patients that Dr. Evans reported, as Dr. Wylie remarked, were a "mixed bag" and were very difficult to interpret as to exactly what their primary symptomatology was.

In our series, our late good results are about 50 percent. As we look over these patients, we find that our initial enthusiasm is accounting for many of our failures with patients who really did not have marked weight loss, even though they had a distortion of their celiac axis.

More recently, with the advent of the provocative *d*-xylose test, we have at least found one thing we can use on these patients that will revert to normalcy, after operation, if there is a marked celiac stenosis.

I believe that as in all visceral ischemic diseases one must be very careful to make sure they do have postprandial pain and weight loss, indicating real visceral ischemia.

Vague abdominal pain is not enough.

The other thing I would like to ask Dr. Evans is, did he obtain arteriograms on the patients who were failures to see if there was a significant restenosis, or to see if he had really done as good a job as he thought at the time of the release of the arcuate ligament?

Dr. William E. Evans (Closing). In answer to Drs. Szilagyi, Stoney, and Fry, we do not have many postoperative arteriograms on these patients. The one piece of information we do have that relates to this is that, as we followed these patients and re-examined them, bruits were absent in all, so that at least this is evidence from physical examination that the stenosis was improved.

I was interested in Dr. Stoney's data as I looked at the slide quickly. It appears that 12 of his 16 patients treated only by decompression were improved, which is considerably better than we were able to do and not markedly different, I do not think, from those on whom bypass was done.

Dr. Fry, we did not do *d*-xylose testing in these patients.

In answer to Dr. Wylie's question as to the indications for the operation, we looked very closely at weight loss, diarrhea, and the presence of postprandial pain to see if we could identify patients who should do well from this group and those who might fail.

The presence or absence of postprandial pain in this particular series made absolutely no difference in terms of the results, nor did the diarrhea.

Deceptive patterns of renal artery stenosis

Richard H. Dean, M.D., Henry Burko, M.D., James P. Wilson, M.D., Joseph H. Mulherin, M.D., *and* **John H. Foster, M.D.,** *Nashville, Tenn.*

During the past 13 years, angiographic study of the renal arteries in over 1,700 hypertensive patients and intraoperative observations in 250 patients have shown many variations in the anatomy and morphology of the renal arteries. A number of deceptive patterns of renal artery stenosis have been recognized, many of which can be detected only by oblique and selective arteriograms. These patterns include (1) a main renal artery originating from the anterior or posterior aortic wall; (2) a main renal artery coursing from the aorta in an almost anterior-posterior plane; (3) two arteries to one kidney which are superimposed in the anterior-posterior plane, masking a stenosis in one; (4) complete occlusion of a segmental renal artery to a midrenal, anterior, or posterior segment of the kidney; and (5) masking of renal artery stenosis by other intra-abdominal arteries. Probably the most important lesion is the ventral right accessory lower pole renal artery. This artery originates from the anterior midline of the aorta, 1 to 2 cm. above the inferior mesenteric artery, and courses anterior to the vena cava to the lower pole of the right kidney. Demonstration of an orificial stenosis of this artery requires special oblique arteriograms. This artery also has special implications in patients who are undergoing operative treatment of abdominal aortic aneurysmal or occlusive disease. The primary purpose of this report is to show that oblique and selective arteriograms are required to demonstrate the anatomy and morphology of the renal arteries in patients with renovascular hypertension and in abdominal aortic disease as well.

From the Departments of Surgery and Radiology and the Specialized Center of Research in Hypertension, Vanderbilt University School of Medicine, Nashville, Tenn.

To RECOGNIZE the potentially deceptive patterns of renal artery stenosis and secondary renovascular hypertension (RVH), one must first have some concept of the normal variations which the renal artery exhibits in number, location, pathway to, and arborization within the kidneys. Most frequently the kidneys are supplied by single renal arteries originating from the lateral aspect of the aorta at the level of the lower border of the first lumbar vertebra. The artery then divides into five branches which supply the five segments of the kidney. There are, however, many variations from this anatomic pattern. In an autopsy review of 11,000 patients, Merklin and Michels[5] found multiple renal arteries in 28 percent of the patients. Boijsen[1] found a similar incidence (24 percent) of multiple renal arteries in 638 patients studied angiographically. These "aberrant" or "accessory" renal arteries have been

Supported in part by National Institutes of Health Grant No. 5 P17 HL 14192, Specialized Center of Research in Hypertension, and National Institutes of Health Grant No. MO1 RR00095, Clinical Research Center.

Presented at the Twenty-eighth Annual Meeting of the Society for Vascular Surgery, Chicago, Ill., June 20 and 21, 1974.

Reprint requests: John H. Foster, M.D., Department of Surgery, Vanderbilt University School of Medicine, Nashville, Tenn. 37203.

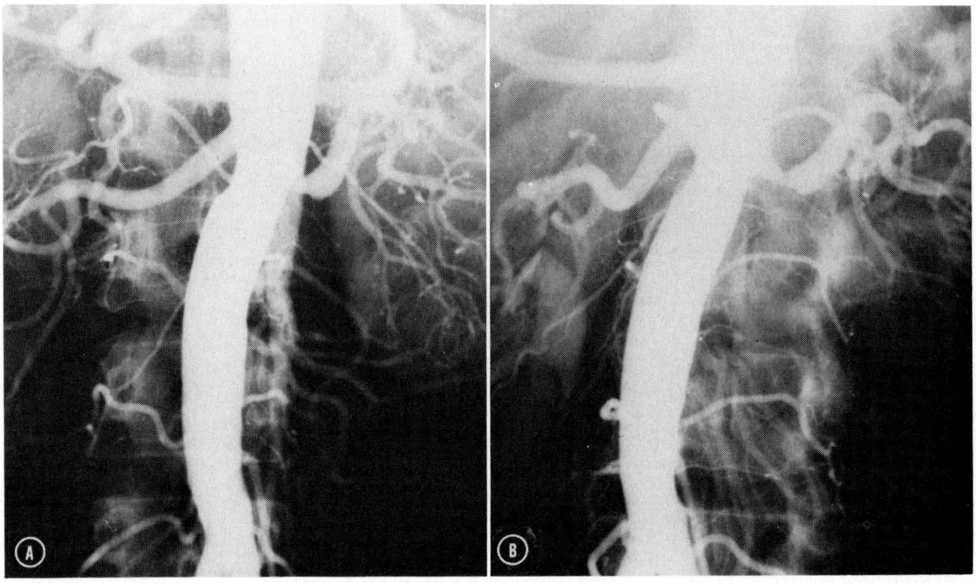

Fig. 1. *A,* A-P aortogram of N. N. showing only mild stenosis of left renal artery near orifice. *B,* Right posterior oblique projection of aortogram in N. N. revealing severe stenosis of left renal artery originating from posterolateral wall of aorta.

found to arise from the aorta as high as the eleventh thoracic vertebra to as low as the external iliac artery. Coupled with this presence of multiple arteries is a similar incidence of dorsal or ventral origin of a renal artery from the aorta. When atherosclerosis or fibromuscular dysplasia is associated with these "normal" variations, innumerable patterns of renal artery stenosis can be produced. In many instances, a simple anterior-posterior (A-P) midstream, flush aortogram will not provide adequate demonstration of all segments of the renal arteries.

During the past 13 years 1,750 hypertensive patients have had renal arteriography at Vanderbilt University Hospital; 250 of these patients proved to have RVH and have undergone operative treatment. This arteriographic experience combined with operative observations have led us to recognize a number of potentially deceptive patterns of renal artery stenosis, many of which undoubtedly went undetected when only a simple, A-P flush aortogram was done. We have previously described our criteria for the diagnosis of RBH.[4] The purpose of this report is to present illustrative cases of each of the deceptive patterns of renal artery stenosis. They are listed in Table I.

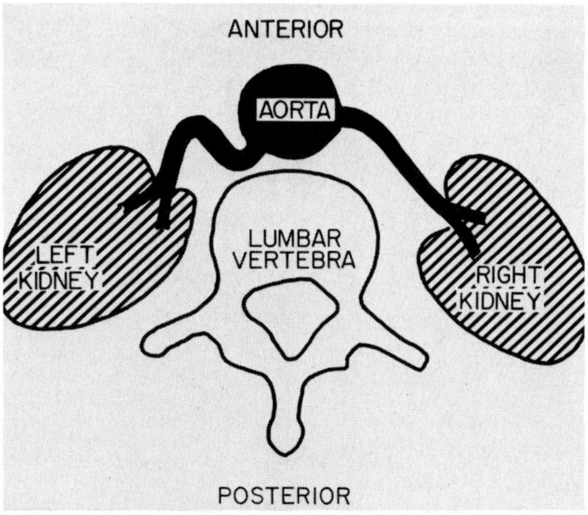

Fig. 2. The usual site of origin and course of renal arteries. (See text for comment.)

TYPES OF HIDDEN RENAL ARTERY STENOSIS

Main renal artery originating from anterior or posterior aortic wall. N. N., a 48-year-old white woman, had a 26 year history of hypertension. The diastolic blood pressure had recently increased (110 to 120 mm. Hg) on medications. She had a

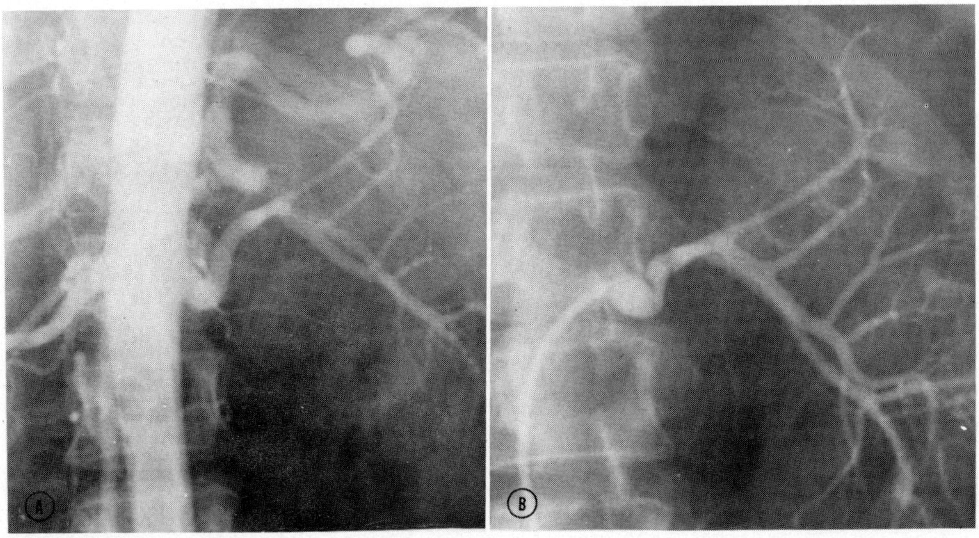

Fig. 3. *A,* Aortogram in A-P projection of J. H. showing apparent normal left renal artery. *B,* Selective oblique left renal arteriogram demonstrating severe stenosis of midportion of the left renal artery coursing in A-P direction.

Table I. *Common deceptive patterns of renal artery stenosis*

1.	Stenosis of main renal artery originating from anterior or posterior aortic wall
2.	Stenosis of a renal artery coursing in the anterior-posterior plane
3.	Superimposition of two renal arteries to the kidney with stenosis in one
4.	Masking of renal artery stenosis by other intra-abdominal arteries
5.	Total occlusion of a segmental or accessory renal artery
6.	Ventral right accessory lower pole renal artery

normal rapid sequence intravenous urogram. The A-P aortogram is shown in Fig. 1, *A*. A right posterior oblique aortogram is shown in Fig. 1, *B* and demonstrates a severe orificial stenosis. The renal venous renin assays (RVRA) showed a 4.01 ratio to the left and the split renal function studies (SRFS) lateralized to the left. Following saphenous vein aortorenal bypass she has remained normotensive and asymptomatic on low doses of antihypertensive medications for the past 3 years.

The left renal artery usually arises from the posterior-lateral side of the aorta (Fig. 2). Lesions situated in the orifice of the renal artery can be hidden in the A-P plane. Orificial lesions which are not seen or, as in this case, appear minor in the A-P plane are brought into profile when the patient is placed in the right posterior oblique position and the aortogram repeated. Frequently poststenotic dilatation of the renal artery will provide a clue to an orificial stenosis.

Stenosis of a renal artery coursing in an anterioposterior plane. J. H., a 39-year-old white woman, had a 2 year history of hypertension (210/110 mm. Hg). Intravenous pyelography (IVP) showed displacement of upper pole calyceal structure. On the A-P aortogram, the left renal artery appears to be normal (Fig. 3, *A*); however, the right posterior oblique aortogram shows a severe stenosis of the left renal artery in its midportion (Fig. 3, *B*). RVRA and SRFS showed that the stenosis was functionally significant; however, at laparotomy she was found to have a large leiomyosarcoma involving the left kidney, renal artery, adrenal gland, and encircling the celiac and superior mesenteric arteries.

As was shown in Fig. 3, the proximal third of the left renal artery usually courses anteriorly, the mid third transversely, and the distal third posteriorly, whereas the right renal artery pursues a more consistent posterior course. Lesions in the renal artery which are coursing anteriorly or posteriorly are frequently not seen or may appear insignificant in an A-P aortogram. Oblique aortography or oblique selective renal arteriography will project these portions of the vessels into profile and identify the stenosis. Fig. 4 shows how the delicate septal lesions of fibromuscular dysplasia may be unrecognizable or appear insignificant in the A-P projection, whereas in the oblique projection the true severity is demonstrated.

Superimposition of two renal arteries to one kidney. W. F. was a 31-year-old white man with hypertension of 2 years' duration (blood pressure, 170/105 mm. Hg). The rapid sequence IVP was interpreted as normal. The renal arteriograms were at first interpreted to be normal (Fig. 5). However, the RVRA and SRFS lateralized strongly to the left. Further study of the arteriograms revealed two superimposed left renal arteries with a severe stenosis in one of them. He underwent saphenous vein aortorenal bypass and became normotensive.

Superimposition of two renal arteries masking a stenosis of one in the A-P aortogram can easily be identified by several techniques. Oblique aortography will often separate these vessels and demonstrate the stenosis. Selective arteriography of each vessel will also show the lesion. Another variant of this condition is the superimposition of two branches of a single renal artery which masks a stenosis (Fig. 6). Selective oblique renal arteriograms may be necessary to elucidate the anatomy of such lesions.

Masking of renal artery stenosis by extrarenal arteries. M. D. was a 7-year-old white boy with a 4 year history of hypertension. Blood pressures were consistently measured at 150/100 to 105 mm. Hg, despite antihypertensive medication. Rapid sequence IVP was interpreted as normal. The A-P aortogram gave a suggestion of possible widening of the right renal artery. Selective right renal arteriography, however, clearly showed a severe stenosis with poststenotic aneurysmal dilatation of the right renal artery (Fig. 7). RVRA showed a 3:1 ratio to the right. The patient underwent an uneventful right Dacron aortorenal bypass and has subsequently been normotensive.

The superior mesenteric artery usually overlies the proximal third of the right renal artery in the A-P projection; occasionally it courses over the proximal left renal artery. Selective and oblique arteriography may be required to demonstrate lesions in these segments.

Occlusion of a segmental branch renal artery. J. B., a 56-year-old white man, was found to be

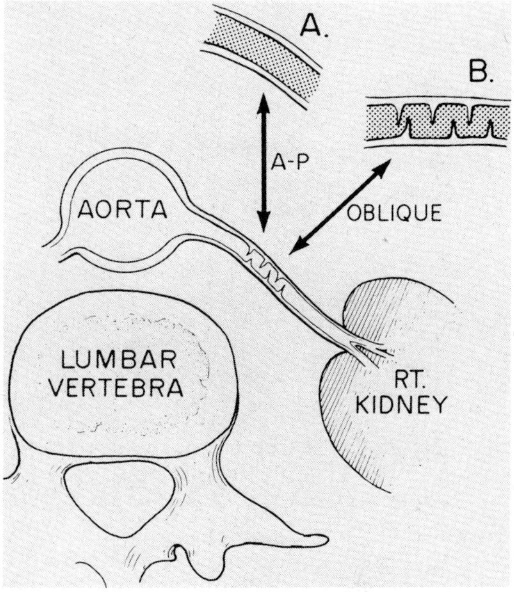

Fig. 4. Graphic illustration of how the septa of fibromuscular dysplasia can be missed. *A,* When the vessel is viewed with an A-P arteriogram, the septa are masked by the overlying dye column. *B,* They are demonstrated by oblique projections placing the direction of the vessel in a perpendicular direction and the septa parallel to the direction of the X-ray.

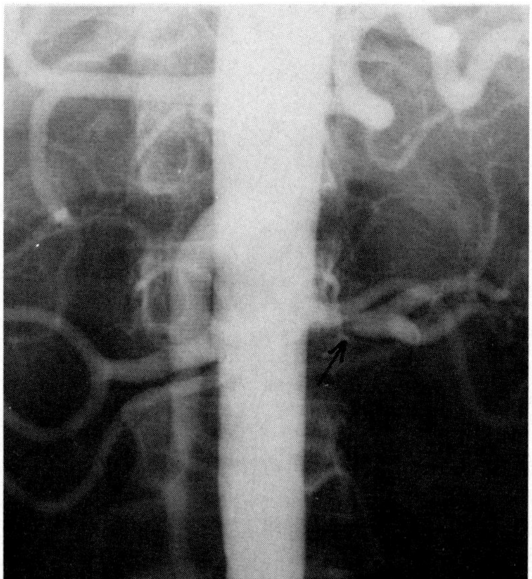

Fig. 5. Aortogram of W. F. showing poor definition of the stenosis in one of two superimposed renal arteries.

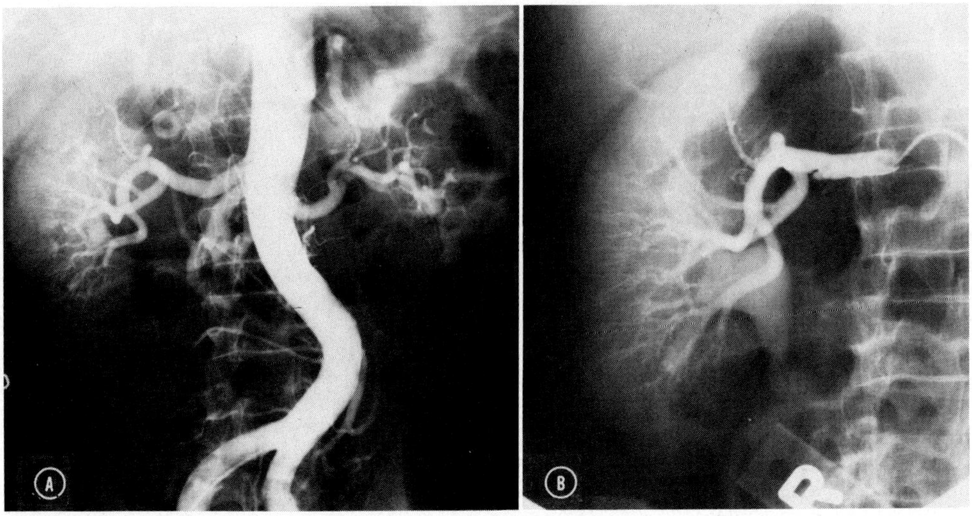

Fig. 6. Renal arteriograms of patient with fibromuscular dysplasia of the right renal artery. *A,* The A-P arteriogram on the right fails to visualize the obstruction because of superimposition of another segmental branch. *B,* By oblique projection the stenosis is graphically demonstrated.

hypertensive following blunt abdominal trauma. His blood pressure was 170/125 mm. Hg. The IVP showed only a delayed nephrogram and poor concentration of the contrast media bilaterally. The early films of the aortogram revealed apparently normal renal arteries bilaterally. However, the late films showed collateral filling of a segmental, accessory renal artery with occlusion at its origin from the aorta (Fig. 8). It is not possible to say whether this occlusion was due to trauma or to arteriosclerosis.

Occlusion of a segmental branch renal artery may be the most difficult type of hidden renal artery lesion to recognize. Ventral and dorsal segments of the kidney are often superimposed in the A-P projection. The artery to one of these segments can be occluded, and yet on the A-P aortogram the kidney may appear to have a normal arborization of the artery, and nephrogram may show a kidney of normal size and shape. Fig. 9 is a schematic drawing illustrating how a dorsal segmental branch artery can be occluded and will not usually be detected on an A-P aortogram. Inasmuch as a true lateral renal arteriogram is not feasible, some lesion such as this may be impossible to recognize.

Ventral right lower pole renal artery. Perhaps the most interesting type of hidden renal artery stenosis is an orificial stenosis of a ventral right lower pole renal artery (Fig. 10). This vessel originates from the midline of the aorta 1 to 2 cm. above the inferior mesenteric artery and courses anterior to the vena cava to supply the lower pole of the right kidney (Fig. 11). The usual right renal artery courses behind the vena cava to the kidney. To date, we have identified six patients with a very short, atherosclerotic, orificial stenosis of this artery which was responsible for the patient's hypertension. Five patients became normotensive following thromboendarterectomy and a vein patch graft. In the sixth patient, the artery thrombosed. Operative exposure of this artery is relatively simple, as is operative correction (Fig. 12). When the abstract for this report was submitted, we had been unable to find a previous report of this anatomic variation. It is not uncommon for an accessory right renal artery, which originates from the iliac artery, to pursue an antecaval course. However, we were unaware of a right renal artery which originated from the aorta and coursed anterior to the inferior vena cava. Since that time we have found a case report of a 10-month-old child who died of malignant hypertension.[2] The autopsy report described a right lower accessory renal artery which originated from the abdominal aorta above the inferior mesenteric artery and coursed anterior to the vena cava to the right kidney.

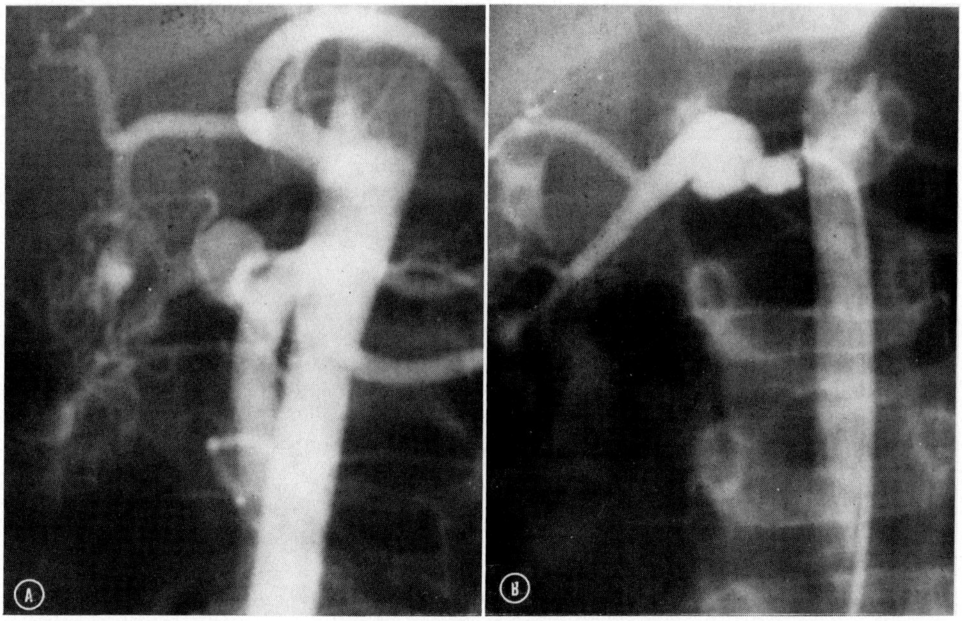

Fig. 7. *A,* Arteriograms of M. D. showing that superimposition of the opacified superior mesenteric artery by flush A-P aortography can mask severe right renal artery stenosis. *B,* Selective catheterization demonstrates the severe stenosis and poststenotic dilatation in this case.

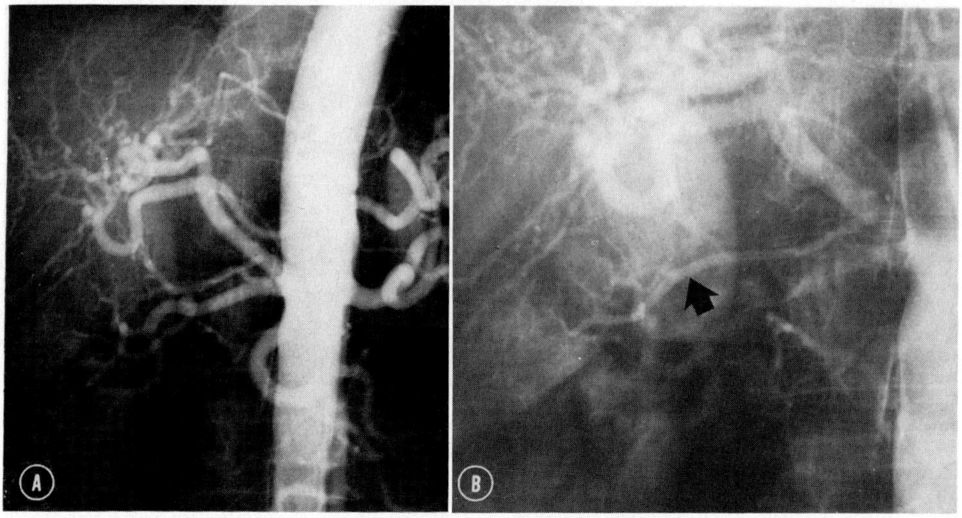

Fig. 8. *A,* Aortogram of J. B. showing apparent normal renal vasculature. *B,* Later films, however, show distal filling of a totally occluded accessory dorsal segmental artery.

This artery is frequently very difficult to recognize. Our first case was a 52-year-old white man with severe hypertension. The IVP and aortogram showed a relatively small left kidney, a normal size right kidney, but no discernable renal artery stenosis. Because of the small left kidney, RVRA were obtained. There was a 10:1 renin activity difference between the two kidneys, but the elevated renin activity came from the normal size right kidney. Close re-examination of the renal arteriograms revealed a very faintly opacificed right lower pole accessory renal artery with a severe orificial stenosis. At laparotomy, this artery was found to originate from the midline of the aorta 1 cm.

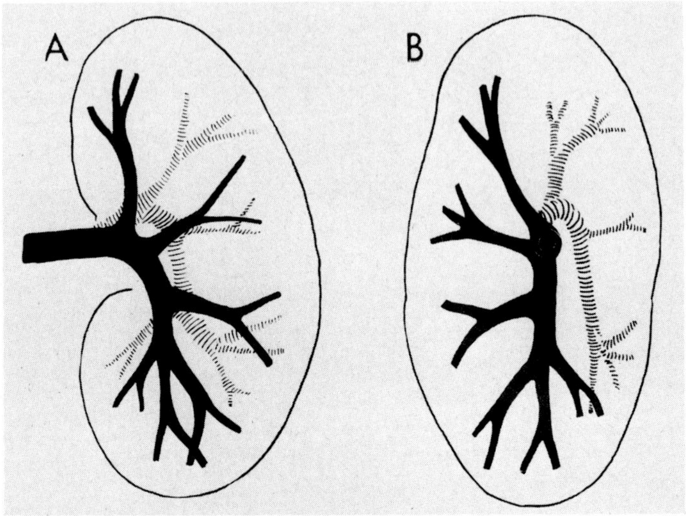

Fig. 9. Graphic illustration of how the posterior division branch can be totally thrombosed and on the A-P projection. *A,* The kidney would appear to have a normal outline of vessels. *B,* Lateral projections would show lack of perfusion to the posterior division. (From Renal Angiography by Kincaid, O. W., copyright 1966 by Year Book Medical Publishers, Inc., Chicago. Used by permission.)

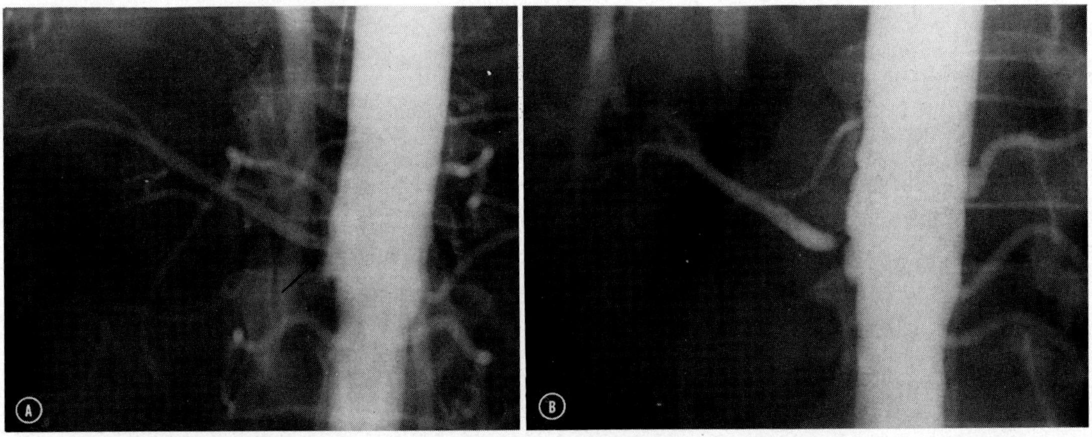

Fig. 10. *A,* Arteriograms of patients with ventral right accessory renal artery. A-P projection shows no obstruction while lateral aortogram, *B,* demonstrates severe orificial stenosis.

above the inferior mesenteric artery and was easily corrected by thromboendarterectomy and a vein patch graft. Patients with accessory renal arteries are now subjected to extensive oblique and selective renal arteriographic studies. It may require a true lateral aortogram to demonstrate an orificial stenosis of an accessory artery.

DISCUSSION

The illustrative cases presented demonstrate the need for multiple aortographic and selective renal arteriographic views in any study of patients with hypertension. Unless all areas of the renal artery are investigated, including the orifice and the intrarenal branches, one can easily miss significant renal artery lesions. This view is further supported by our experience with patients who have fibromuscular dysplasia of the renal arteries. In 1969, when we first reported our experience with fibromuscular dysplasia, we stated 60 percent of our patients had unilateral lesions and 40 percent had bilateral lesions.[3]

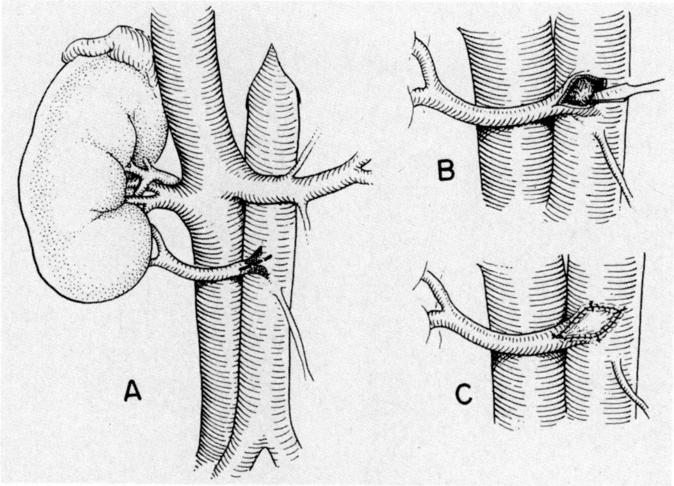

Fig. 11. Sketch showing usual relationships of ventral right accessory renal artery to inferior mesenteric artery and vena cava.

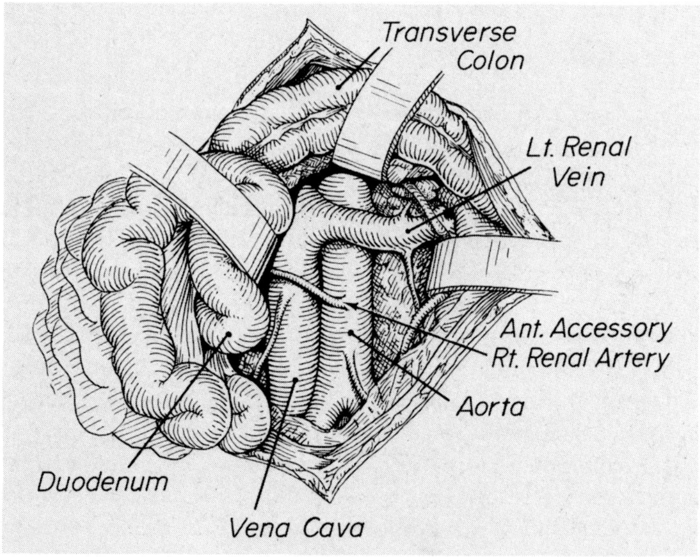

Fig. 12. Drawing depicting the operative approach to thromboendarterectomy and vein patch of a ventral right accessory renal artery.

Since we have been doing selective and oblique arteriograms, we have learned that the lesions are bilateral in over 80 percent of our patients. In our early experience most of the lesions presented in this report undoubtedly went undetected. It also may explain why some of our patients with well-documented hypertension and with what was thought to be severe unilateral stenosis had nonlateralizing functional studies (RVRA and SRFS). Many of these patients probably had bilateral renal artery stenosis, both of which were functionally significant.

As far as we can tell, the stenosis of the ventral right accessory lower pole renal artery as a cause of hypertension has not been previously reported. All of our cases were in adults and arteriosclerosis was the cause of the stenosis. The infant, who had such an artery discovered at autopsy, had intimal hyperplasia involving the distal portion of four renal arteries.

It is important to recognize this artery for two reasons. First, it may be causing hyper-

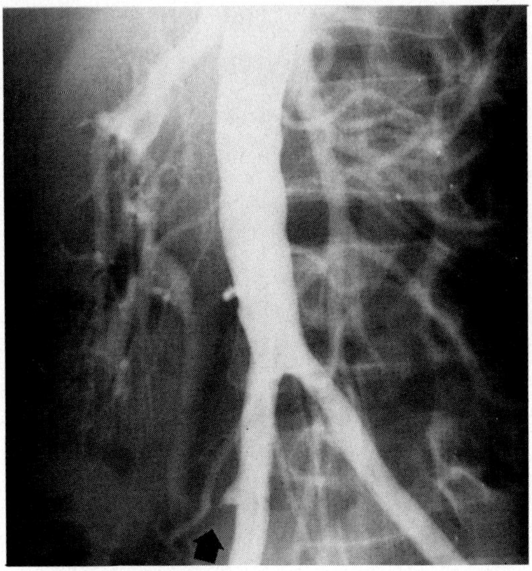

Fig. 13. Arteriogram demonstrating stump (arrow) of ligated accessory lower pole right renal artery arising from the right iliac artery.

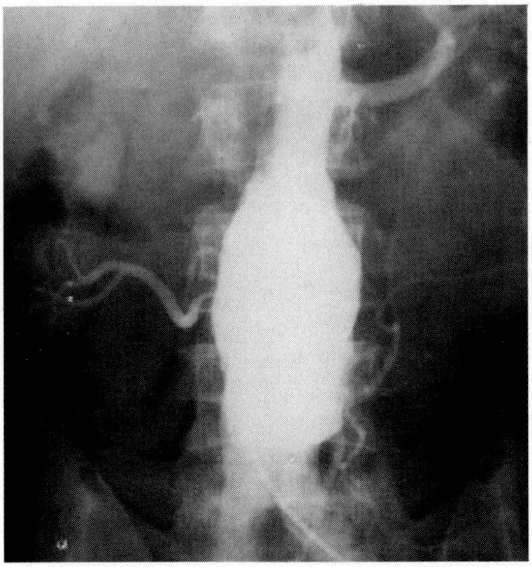

Fig. 14. Aortogram showing not only the abdominal aortic aneurysm but also a severely stenosed ventral accessory right renal artery arising from the wall of the aneurysm.

tension and is easily correctible. Second, in patients undergoing operative treatment of abdominal aorta aneurysm or aortoiliac occlusive disease, if the surgeon is unaware of the presence of this artery, it may be ligated and divided without his knowing what he has done. Of course this is true of any accessory renal artery, as is demonstrated in Fig. 13. This patient had undergone laparotomy for a pelvic mass. During the initial stages of the operation an "aberrant" artery arising from the right common iliac artery was ligated and divided. Later the mass was found to be a pelvic kidney. Postoperatively the patient developed severe hypertension and was referred to us. Aortography showed the stump of the ligated accessory renal artery and loss of perfusion of the lower pole of the kidney. Fig. 14 shows an example of a ventral right accessory lower pole renal artery arising from an abdominal aortic aneurysm. There is a severe orificial stenosis which was functionally significant. It was possible to implant this artery into the graft used to replace the aneurysm.

Typically, radiologists like to grade the severity of arterial stenoses. They report the severity in terms such as severe, insignificant, greater than 50 percent, less than 50 percent, etc. This is often extremely difficult to do with any degree of certainty. The reason for this difficulty is that an artery is a three-dimensional structure and on any one x-ray film only two dimensions can be appreciated. The severity of fibromuscular dysplasia is especially difficult to grade because the lesions are usually multiple. This is why the functional tests have become so important in patients with RVH. Even so, there are still serious problems with the patient who has bilateral renal artery stenosis and may have bilateral RVH.

Finally, there are two technical points that are important in the arteriographic evaluation of the renal arteries. If an orificial atherosclerotic stenosis is demonstrated on the A-P and oblique aortograms, then selective catheterization of such an artery may carry some risks. The catheter may injure the intima and create an intimal flap which leads to thrombosis, or it may dislodge material from the atherosclerotic plaque which embolizes into the branch renal arteries. For these reasons, if an orificial lesion is identified on the A-P and oblique aortograms, then selective catheterization is not done, and, by the same token, selective studies are not done until the A-P and oblique aortograms have been reviewed. The second technical point is that the placement of a catheter into a renal artery and injection of a contrast medium may cause a localized area of vasospasm. If this area has not been previously evaluated by aortography, one may incorrectly interpret the spasm to be a stenotic lesion of the renal artery.

REFERENCES

1. Boijsen, E.: Angiographic studies of the anatomy of single and multiple renal arteries, Acta Radiol. [Diagn.] [Suppl.] (Stockh.) **183:** 1, 1959.
2. Dawson, I. M. P., and Nabano, S.: A case of intimal hyperplasia of arteries with hypertension in a male infant, J. Pathol. **66:** 493, 1953.
3. Foster, J. H., Oates, J. A., Rhamy, R. K., et al.: Hypertension and fibromuscular dysplasia of the renal arteries, Surgery **65:** 157, 1969.
4. Foster, J. H., Dean, R. H., Pinkerton, J. A., et al.: Ten years experience with the surgical management of renovascular hypertension, Ann. Surg. **177:** 755, 1973.
5. Merklin, R. J., and Michels, N. A.: The variant renal and suprarenal blood supply with data on the inferior phrenic, ureteral and gonadal arteries: A statistical analysis based on 185 dissections and review of the literature, J. Int. Coll. Surgeons **29:** 41, 1958.

DISCUSSION

Dr. Calvin B. Ernst (Lexington, Ky.). It is universally agreed that the *single* most important study for diagnosis of renovascular hypertension is arteriography. Therefore, any improvements in recognition of renal arterial lesions, such as we have heard today, augment our ability to manage this most prevalent form of surgically remediable hypertension. Continuing emphasis on meticulous and precise arteriographic studies will significantly increase the yield of individuals who have surgically remediable renal artery lesions.

A subtle but helpful radiologic sign indicating a renal artery lesion requiring further study by oblique or selective views is identification of collateral vessels on the flush aortogram. This is the aortogram of a young woman with severe hypertension. Indication that "masked" renal artery stenosis was present, obscured by overlapping vessels, is presence of collateral channels in the renal hilum. Identification of such vessels should signal the angiographer to employ special techniques to detect a lesion.

In this instance, a selective renal arteriogram was performed. A webbed stenosis of the distal renal artery was documented and the patient underwent renal revascularization with an excellent result.

Perhaps this study underscores what Drs. Dean and Foster have said about oblique filming. This patient developed severe hypertension with deteriorating renal function 4½ years following renal transplantation. The renal artery appeared normal on the anterior-posterior projection of the aortogram.

With oblique filming, a pronounced stenosis was identified. Parenthetically, no collaterals were identified, indicating the possibility that transplanted kidneys cannot form collaterals. Resection and reanastomosis were performed with an excellent result.

I have two questions for Drs. Dean and Foster: First, with the use of sophisticated arteriographic techniques, how many patients do you estimate are found with surgically remediable renal artery lesions which might not have been discovered with standard aortography? Second, have you found identification of collateral channels to be helpful in this regard?

Dr. Richard H. Dean (Closing). Thank you, Dr. Ernst. We certainly agree that collaterals are extremely important in diagnosing renovascular hypertension. We also use this to a great advantage in patients who have nonlateralizing functional data and bilateral severe renal artery stenosis. Especially, we use it to get some index of which side to attack first by the degree of collateralization to that kidney on the arteriogram.

To hazard a guess as to how many patients whom we now pick up whom we previously had not found would be very difficult. Obviously, we do not have the data because we did not pick them up when we were only doing anterior-posterior aortography. However, I suspect it is probably in the range of 3 to 5 percent.

One other problem that is very difficult to resolve in patients with renovascular hypertension is the patient who has recurrent hypertension following a unilateral reconstruction.

On this arteriogram, one would think that there is left renal artery stenosis which would be the cause of the patient's recurrent renovascular hypertension. This patient did not have lateralizing functional data, however, and on the oblique projections one can appreciate the bilateral nature of the disease in the patient who had previously undergone reconstruction. He has a severe stenosis in the reconstructed right renal artery at the distal suture line and also a proximal lesion in the left renal artery.

Carotid cavernous fistula: Direct repair with preservation of carotid

Dwight Parkinson, M.D., Allan R. Downs, M.D., Lawrence L. Whytehead, M.D., *and* **Walter B. Syslak, M.D.,** *Winnipeg, Manitoba, Canada*

The standard treatment of carotid cavernous fistulas has been trapping or a combination of trapping and embolization. In either case the carotid is sacrificed and a certain percentage of fistulas persist in spite of complete trapping and embolization. Several years ago we began to devise a method of repairing the fistula and preserving the carotid. The first step involved finding the normal collateral vessels serving these persistent fistulas of the carotid, which is classically drawn in the anatomy texts as a nonbranching artery traversing a trabeculated venous cavern. The second problem involved finding an anatomically safe approach past the cranial nerves to the cavernous carotid and its branches. The third problem involved provision of periods of complete circulatory arrest in order that such an approach might be used and a repair effected. The significant arterial, venous, and neural anatomical findings are illustrated. The techniques are described as used in 11 fistula repairs with preservation of the carotid utilizing hyopthermia and circulatory arrest in increments up to 55 minutes. The operating microscope has greatly enhanced the technical feasibility.

From the Departments of Neurosurgery, Cardiovascular Surgery, and Anesthesia, Faculty of Medicine, University of Manitoba, Winnipeg, Manitoba, Canada

In 1942 a young soldier developed a pulsating exophthalmos secondary to a traumatic carotid cavernous fistula on the right. In 1947 he underwent ligation of his right common carotid, right internal and external carotids, and all available branches in the neck followed later by supraclinoid ligation of the right carotid, thus completing the trapping of the fistulous segment. As his lesion continued to progress, he later underwent ligation of the left external carotid and all available branches in the neck. Thereafter his impoverished face blanched considerably in the winter while his fistula prospered progressively, and, in 1953, he developed an exsanguinating epistaxis. Angiography at that time revealed a brisk fistula fed by numerous collaterals that were identifiable at their origin but not at their terminal confluence into the isolated segment of internal carotid.*

Research begins by asking Nature a question, and we asked, "What normally present arterial branches serve to receive the collateral supply to perpetuate a fistula in a

Presented at the Twenty-eighth Annual Meeting of the Society for Vascular Surgery, Chicago, Ill., June 20 and 21, 1974.

Reprint requests: Dwight Parkinson, M.D., Departments of Neurosurgery, Cardiovascular Surgery, and Anesthesia, Faculty of Medicine, University of Manitoba, Winnipeg, Manitoba, Canada.

*This first patient did not have his ophthalmic artery obliterated at its origin but the second patient did. It has long been recognized by neurosurgeons that fistulas may persist with the carotid trapped, even with the ophthalmic artery excluded from the system.[1, 4-7 17, 26] The presence of these connecting branches has long been suspected but the origin and destination were unknown, at least to us, and this included the carotico-tympanic artery.

trapped segment of internal carotid in cases such as this?" Such branches which become "recipient arteries" must be present normally because a fistula does not initiate arterial growth into or out of the lumen of a major artery such as the carotid, even though the fistula may cause existing channels to enlarge. A simple autopsy cadaver experiment verified the normal existence of these connecting arteries. With the external carotid ligated in the neck and the internal carotid and ophthalmic arteries ligated above the clinoid, water injected into the common carotid artery appears instantly at the cut ends of the external system (Fig. 1).

Finding these branches was not so easy. After the first month we nearly gave up in despair, but once we had learned how and where to look, these thin-walled arteries were found consistently. We dissected over 200 cavernous carotids and recognized three standard branches. These are, first, the meningohypophyseal artery and its three branches—the tentorial, the inferior hypophyseal, and the dorsal meningeal; second, the artery to the inferior cavernous sinus; and, third, McConnell's capsular artery. These have been previously described and photographed,[12, 15, 21] and a composite drawing was made by Nancy Joy, medical artist (Fig. 2). Each of these serves as a small-caliber, but short and hence effective, anastomosis between the two internal carotids and the internal and external systems proximal to the circle of Willis.[13-17, 31]

Having found these arterial connections, the next question was, "Is there a safe anatomic approach?" The anatomy books picture varying relationships of the third, fourth, fifth, and sixth cranial nerves in the parasellar region. We returned to the autopsy cadavers and found there is constantly present a triangular space with the third and fourth nerves above, and the sixth and first division of the fifth below.[13] A 2 cm. incision, carefully placed within this triangular space, avoids section of the cranial nerves and, on retraction, affords an exposure of the cavernous carotid and its branches (Figs. 3 to 6).

Previous work would indicate that the

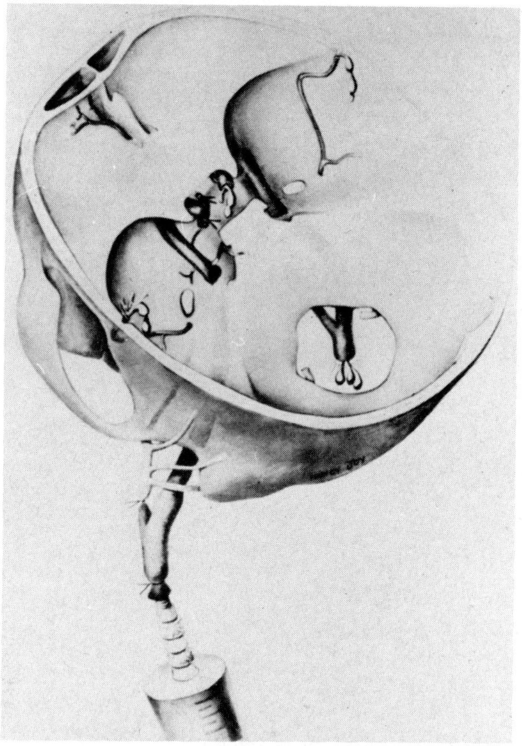

Fig. 1. Diagram of injection preparation. Left common carotid cannulated. Left external ligated. Left internal and ophthalmic ligated intracranially. Drawing depicts return through both ends of opposite carotid system and both middle meningeals. (From Parkinson, D., Can. J. Surg. **7:** 251, 1964, published by The Canadian Medical Association.)

brain would tolerate increments of total circulatory arrest up to 40 to 50 minutes under profound hypothermia.[18, 22, 30] We operated on this patient through this approach using open-chest bypass and total circulatory arrest of approximately 45 minutes. We merely clamped the structures at the lower end and the upper end of the space after separating the vascular elements from the cranial nerves.[13] He died 2 days after operation of a variety of complications, including intracranial and pericardial bleeding. We obliterated the fistula in the same manner in the next patient on whom we operated, but we used femoral bypass.[14, 16] He survived without any additional neurologic deficits. It became necessary to put him on total arrest two separate times with an interval of circulation of 20 minutes between.

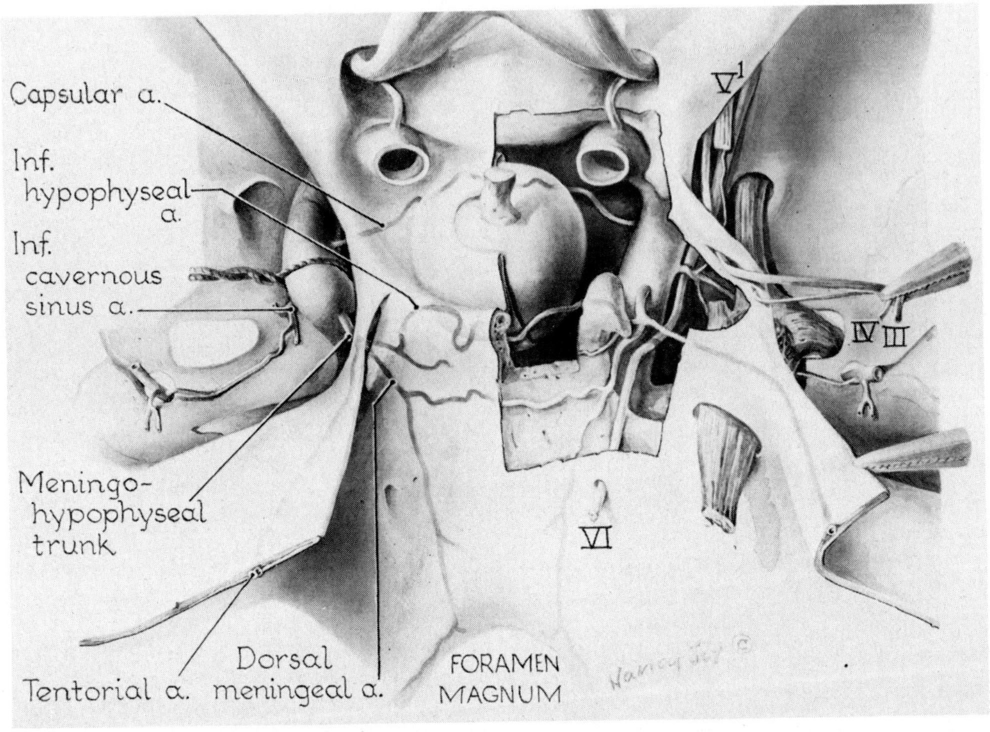

Fig. 2. Schematic drawing based on numerous photographs of two separate specimens in varying stages of dissection. Structures overlying an artery are drawn as though transparent. On the right the dura has been removed from half of the hypophyseal fossa and from a portion of the dorsum sellae as well as from the cavernous sinus and the entire middle fossa. A portion of the dorsum sellae itself has also been removed leaving only the posterior clinoid and the supporting bone. A portion of the first division of the fifth nerve has been resected to show the first portions of the artery to the inferior cavernous sinus, running over the sixth nerve on the right. The first portion of the inferior hypophyseal artery is viewed through the posterior clinoid. The minute branch of the inferior hypophyseal artery that wraps around the posterior clinoid is shown up to the region where the dorsum sellae has been cut away. The strip of dura enclosing the entrance of the third and fourth nerves has been preserved by the artist while the third and fourth nerves are pulled laterally. The point of departure of the tentorial artery from the space of the cavernous sinus to its course between the two dural layers is immediately beneath the entrance of the fourth nerve to its dural cleft. The trifurcation of the meningohypophyseal trunk is uncovered just adjacent to the lateral margin of the posterior clinoid. On the left, the trifurcation of the meningohypophyseal trunk is seen through the strip of dura left over the roof of the cavernous sinus. On this side the nerves are all removed as well as the dura of the middle fossa in order to demonstrate the entire length of the anastomosing portion of the artery of the inferior cavernous sinus. The carotid is pulled outwards to show the origin of the capsular artery. The first portion of the inferior hypophyseal artery on the right is viewed through the posterior clinoid. The minute branch of the inferior hypophyseal that wraps around the posterior clinoid is shown up to the region where the dorsum sellae has been cut away to better visualize the intrasellar portion of the inferior hypophyseal artery. The anastomosis between the two dorsal meningeal arteries is shown across the roof of the dorsum just beneath the cut away in the bone. Note that the tentorial artery is much closer to the undersurface than the superior surface owing to the difference in thickness of the two dural layers of the tentorium. On the right, the strip of dura enclosing the entrance of the third and fourth nerves has been preserved by the artist while the third and fourth nerves are drawn laterally. The actual departure of the tentorial artery from the space of the cavernous sinus to its course between the two dural layers is at a point immediately beneath the entrance of the fourth nerve to its dural cleft. (Reproduced courtesy of the Canadian Journal of Surgery **7:** 251, 1964.)

We found very early in the first case that it required more than total circulatory arrest because even then the venous blood tended to continually pool into the area, obliterating all landmarks. We solved this problem by having the head slightly elevated and by actually aspirating the venous blood from the body after the pump was stopped.

To our considerable astonishment, in neither case did we find an artery with a

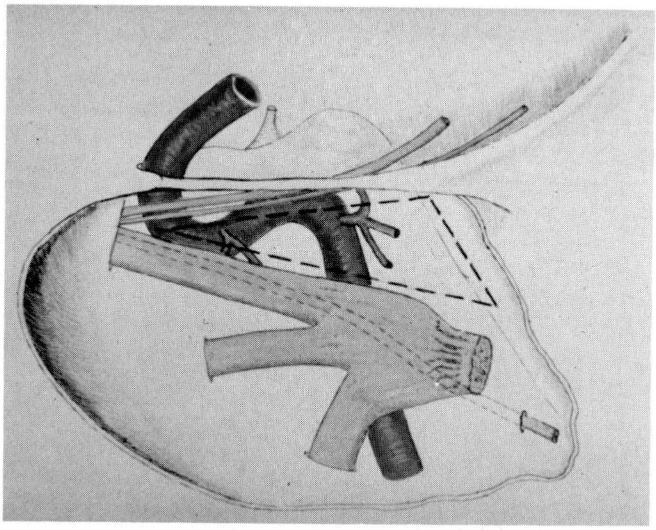

Fig. 3. Diagram of the left triangular space with the third and fourth nerves above, and the first division of the fifth and sixth below, showing how an incision placed within this triangular space affords access to the parasellar portion of the carotid artery and its branches, while avoiding incision of the cranial nerves. (From Parkinson, D., J. Neurosurg. **38:** 99, 1973.)

hole in it traversing a trabeculated venous cavern (Fig. 7), but instead a tangential fistulous connection (Fig. 8) similar in all respects to traumatic arteriovenous (A-V) fistulas elsewhere in the body,[8, 10, 29] with the adjacent, dilated, tortuous, adherent veins tightly compacted in this small dural space, indistinguishable in some segments both as to texture and size from the carotid itself (Figs. 5 and 6).

We returned to the autopsy cadavers and made venous corrosion specimens. We found, as we had suspected, that the parasellar venous pathways do not consist of bilateral trabeculated caverns but, instead, of irregular plexuses of varying sizes, shapes, and in variously located veins (Fig. 9).[27, 28]

By then we believed it should be possible, using the operating microscope, to repair a fistula and preserve the carotid, should a patient present without previous sacrifice of the carotid by a trapping procedure. Such a patient did present and his preoperative angiogram revealed a large caliber fistula.[17] He also required two increments of total circulatory arrest of 50 minutes each. His fistula was isolated with considerable difficulty and clipped, but the clip tore across and it was necessary to suture the opening in the artery. After operation his angiogram revealed complete obliteration of the fistula, but there was a small blister deformity at the site of our suturing. This disappeared within 2 weeks, leaving a normal contour of the carotid siphon. The next patient had an even larger caliber fistula and required two episodes of 50 minutes on total arrest and an additional episode of 25 minutes. His angiogram after operation revealed complete obliteration of his fistula. Again the artery was preserved (Figs. 10 and 11).

We operated on a total of 11 patients using this approach. The last nine had no prior sacrifice of their carotids by a trapping procedure and we were able to preserve the artery in each case. There has been one additional death and two patients remain partially aphasic. We have had a wide variety of very educational complications. All the other patients are now back at their usual occupations.

The difficulties encountered in these patients to date have been primarily associated with finding the carotid itself in the plexus of dilated veins, which, in some segments, resemble the carotid. With some of the very small fistulas this has not been a problem. By the time the fistula has been identified it

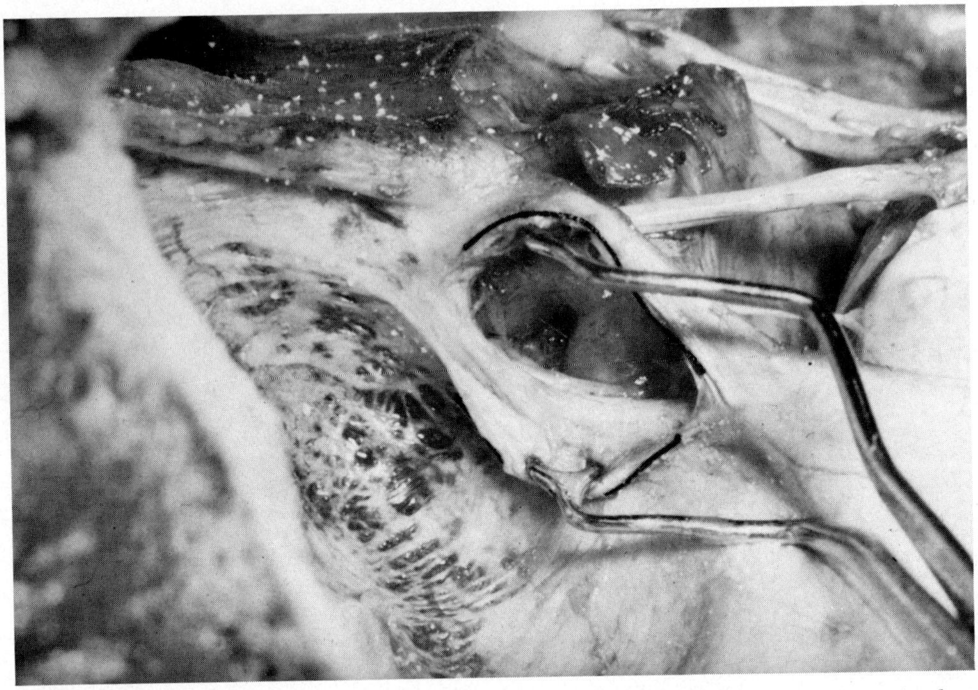

Fig. 4. Cadaver preparation showing incision in the left triangular space with retractor in place exposing the parasellar portion of the carotid artery. The third nerve is visible disappearing into the dura just lateral to the posterior clinoid. (From Parkinson, D., J. Neurosurg. **38:** 99, 1973.)

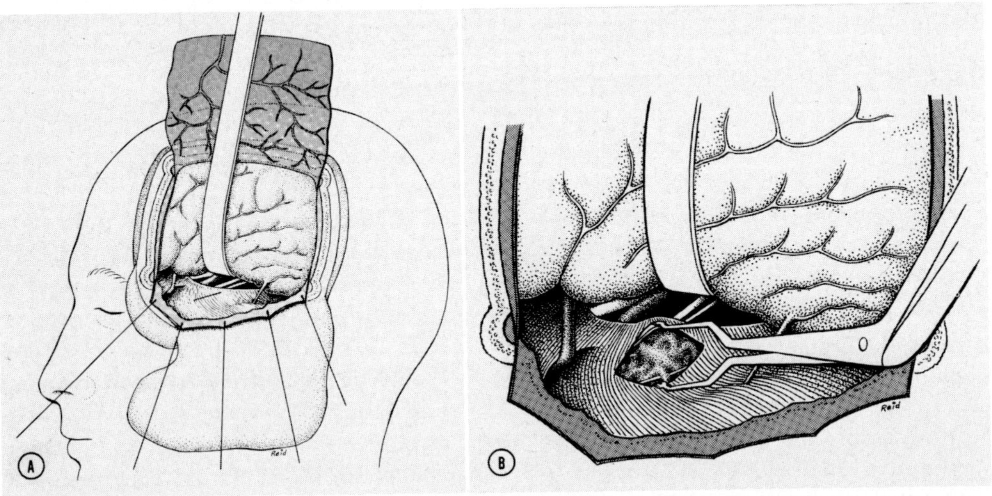

Fig. 5. *A,* Artist's sketch of operative exposure. On the left, descending vertically, is the greatly engorged Sylvian vein running down beneath the medial third of the sphenoid ridge. The next structure to the right is the optic nerve and immediately behind that is the supraclinoid portion of the carotid and next the third and fourth cranial nerves. The line of the incision is indicated in the triangular space of the lateral wall of the cavernous sinus. At the right hand side of the exposure is a vein bridging from the undersurface of the temporal lobe to the tentorium. *B,* A realistic diagram of the tangled appearance of the adherent, dilated, thickened, vascular channel as it first appears on retraction of the incision in the triangular space. The third and fourth nerves are indicated as just visible beneath the upper margin and the sixth nerve crosses the field inferiorly. (From Parkinson, D., J. Neurosurg. **38:** 99, 1973.)

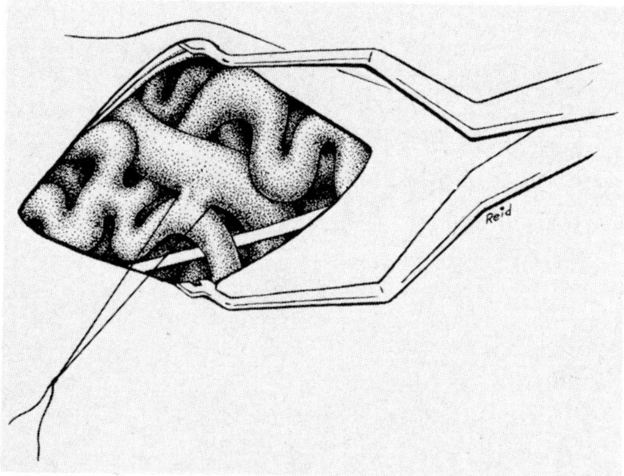

Fig. 6. A greater magnification indicating the appearance after the vessels have been teased apart. The veins which would normally overlay the carotid and obliterate it from view are not shown. The carotid itself is shown following its normal curvature upward and anteriorly to the left, whereas the venous channels are indicated as a tangle of multiple curved branches. The thread is looping around the fistula. (From Parkinson, D., J. Neurosurg. **38:** 99, 1973.)

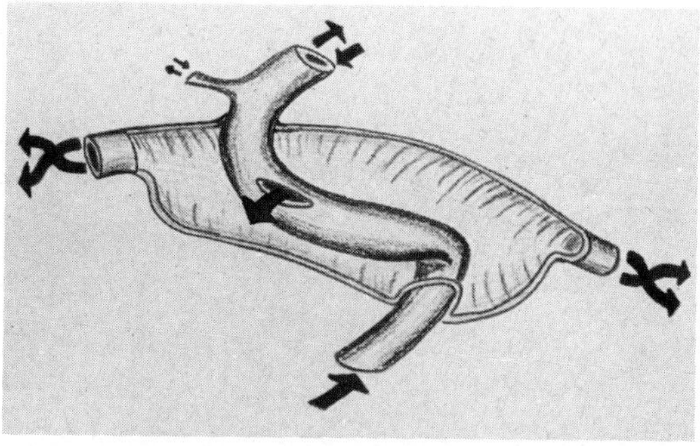

Fig. 7. Diagram of the original concept of the carotid cavernous fistula. The entire space within the dural walls of the "cavernous sinus" was considered to be a venous cavern surrounding the carotid. Hence, any rupture of the carotid spilled directly into this surrounding venous cavern. (From Parkinson, D., J. Neurosurg. **38:** 99, 1973.)

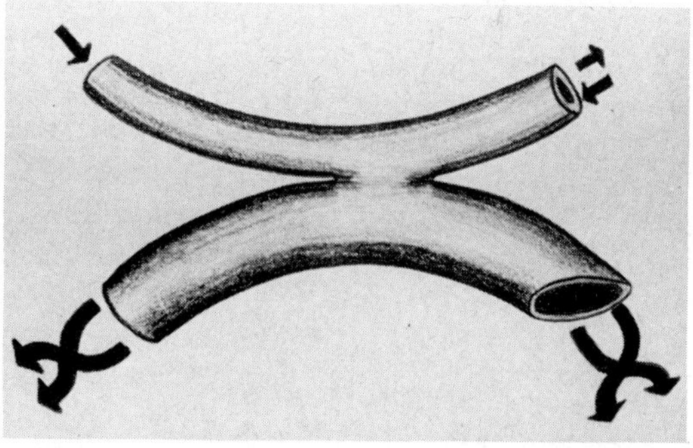

Fig. 8. Diagram of the actual mechanism of the fistulous connection between the carotid artery and any one of the many adjacent venous channels, all of which are enclosed within the dural coverings of the "cavernous sinus." The artery is depicted above as a smaller vessel and the arrows indicate the potential flow in either direction at the cranial end. The pathological vascular architecture thus differs in no way from that of a traumatic arteriovenous fistula elsewhere in the body. (From Parkinson, D., J. Neurosurg. **38:** 99, 1973.)

has usually been impossible to place a clip across its connection with the vein and it has been necessary to suture the opening or suture it and pack it from the outside. We have had to operate on two patients twice and one of these developed meningitis and later a communicating hydrocephalus requiring shunting of the cerebrospinal fluid in another center.

Three of the patients awakened in a matter of an hour or less and remained normal from that moment, with the exception of cranial nerve palsies from which it has taken up to 6 months to recover. Two others had very prolonged recovery periods, much longer and slower than one would anticipate continuing recovery to progress. Both of these also returned to their preoperative state.

Although our experience is limited, to date we believe that it is safer to put a patient on two or three increments of total circulatory arrest, each of no more than 50 minutes, rather than to try to prolong any one increment beyond 50 minutes.

We have learned four things: first, the normal anatomy of the arterial branches of the parasellar segment of the carotid artery; second, there is access through a triangular space to this region previously considered a surgical no-man's land; third, the normal venous anatomy is not that of a trabeculated cavern but a plexus; and, fourth, it is possible to go into this area and repair a fistula and preserve the carotid.

We do not contend that this is the ultimate in the treatment of these lesions. We are working on improvements and modifications such as preoperative placement of a catheter to aid in the localization and control of the

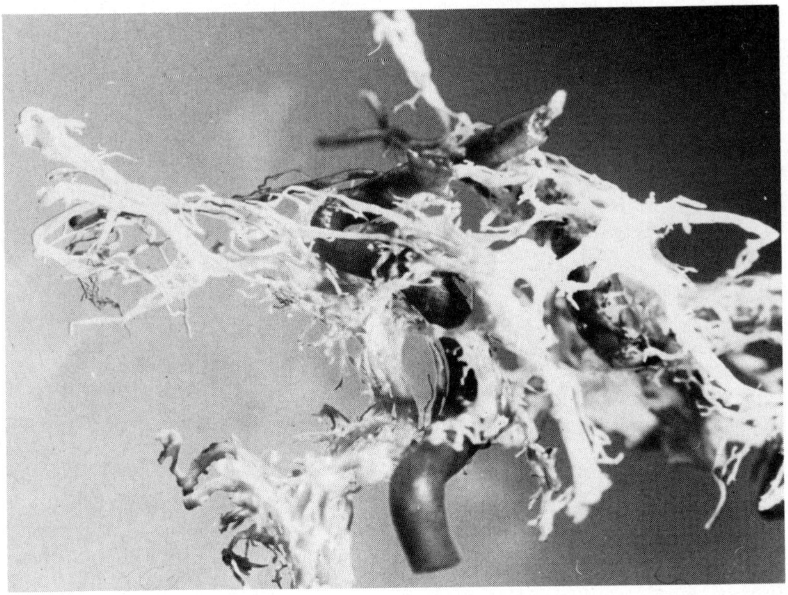

Fig. 9. Venous cast viewed obliquely from the side with the two carotid arteries in dark. The ophthalmic artery and orbital veins can be seen running forward to the left. The venous channels are white and show an irregular plexus incompletely surrounding the carotid siphon. (From Parkinson, D., J. Neurosurg. **38:** 99, 1973.)

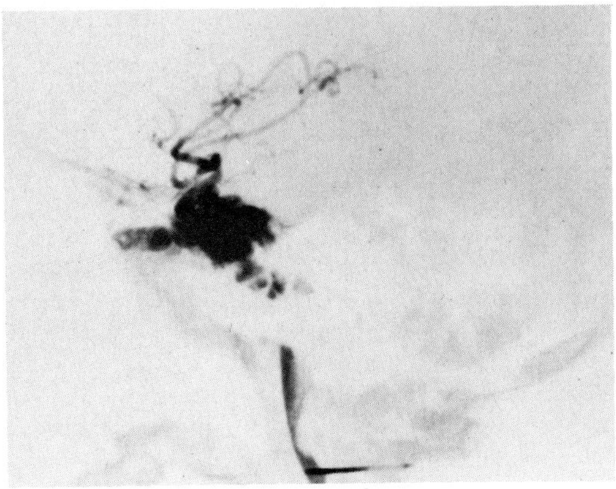

Fig. 10. Angiogram before operation, subtraction view film, showing the large-caliber fistula. (From Parkinson, D., J. Neurosurg. **38:** 99, 1973.)

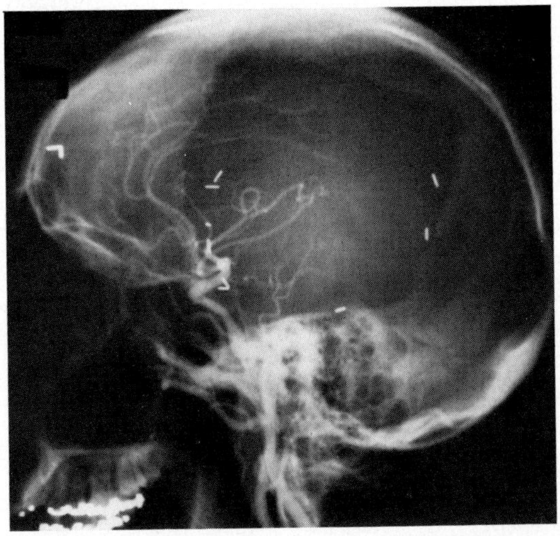

Fig. 11. Angiogram after operation showing the fistula obliterated and the carotid preserved. Note better filling of the cerebral circulation once it is removed from the shunting effect of the fistula.

opening.[2, 23-25] We anticipate that others with greater skills will reduce the operating time and hence the morbidity. We recognize the approaches being tried in other centers, such as the use of tethered emboli[3, 20] or wire electrocautery of the venous components.[9, 11, 19]

We are convinced, however, that it is no longer justifiable to sacrifice the carotid as the initial step in the treatment of one of these lesions.

REFERENCES

1. Adson, A. W.: Surgical treatment of vascular diseases altering function of eyes, Am. J. Ophthalmol. **25:** 824, 1942.

2. Arutiunov, A. I., Serbinenko, F. A., and Shlykov, A. A.: Surgical treatment of carotid cavernous fistulas, Prog. Brain Res. **30:** 441, 1969.
3. Black, P., Uematsu, S., Perovic, M., and Walker, A. E.: Carotid-cavernous fistula: A controlled embolus technique for occlusion of fistula with preservation of carotid blood flow, J. Neurosurg. **38:** 113, 1973.
4. Dandy, W. E.: Treatment of carotid cavernous arteriovenous aneurysms, Ann. Surg. **102:** 916, 1935.
5. Hamby, W. B.: Carotid cavernous fistulae, Springfield, Ill., 1966, Charles C Thomas, Publisher.
6. Hamby, W. B., and Dohn, D. F.: Carotid-cavernous fistulas: Report of 36 cases and discussion of their management, Clin. Neurosurg. **11:** 150, 1964.
7. Hayes, G. J.: Carotid cavernous fistulas; diagnosis and surgical management, Am. Surg. **24:** 839, 1958.
8. Holman, E.: The physiology of an arteriovenous fistula, Arch. Surg. **7:** 64, 1923.
9. Hosobuchi, Y.: Electrothrombosis of carotid cavernous fistula, presented at meeting of Am. Assoc. Neurolog. Surg., Boston Mass., April, 1972.
10. Hunter, W.: Quoted by Hamby.[5]
11. Mullan, S. F.: Results of innovations in the conservative and surgical treatment of intracranial aneurysms, presented at meeting of Am. Assoc. Neurolog. Surg., Houston, Texas, April, 1971.
12. Parkinson, D.: Collateral circulation of cavernous carotid artery: Anatomy, Can. J. Surg. **7:** 251, 1964.
13. Parkinson, D.: A surgical approach to the cavernous portion of the carotid artery: Anatomical studies and case report, J. Neurosurg. **23:** 474, 1965.
14. Parkinson, D.: Transcavernous repair of carotid cavernous fistula: Case report, J. Neurosurg. **26:** 420, 1967.
15. Parkinson, D.: Anatomy of the "cavernous sinus," *in* Smith, J. L., editor: Neuroophthalmology, vol. 6, St. Louis, 1972, The C. V. Mosby Company, pp. 73-101.
16. Parkinson, D.: Carotid cavernous fistula, *in* Vinken, P. J., and Bruyn, G. W., editors: Handbook of clinical neurology, vol. 12, Amsterdam, 1972, North-Holland Publishing Company.
17. Parkinson, D.: Carotid cavernous fistula: Direct repair with preservation of the carotid artery, J. Neurosurg. **38:** 99, 1973.
18. Patterson, R. H., and Ray, B. S.: Profound hypothermia for intracranial surgery using a disposable bubble oxygenator, J. Neurosurg. **23:** 184, 1965.
19. Peterson, E. W.: Personal communication, 1970.
20. Prolo, D. J., and Hanvery, J. W.: Intraluminal occlusion of a carotid-cavernous sinus fistula using a disposable bubble oxygenator, J. Neurosurg. **35:** 237, 1971.
21. Schnurer, L. B., and Stattin, S.: Vascular supply of intracranial dura from internal carotid artery with special reference to its angiographic significance, Acta Radiol. [Diagn.] (Stockh.) **1:** 441, 1963.
22. Sealey, W. C., Brown, I. W., Jr., and Young, W. G., Jr.: A report on the use of both extracorporeal circulation and hypothermia for open heart surgery, Ann. Surg. **147:** 603, 1958.
23. Serbinenko, F. A.: Balloon occlusion of a cavernous portion of the carotid artery as a method of treating carotid-cavitary anastomoses, Probl. Neurosurg. (Rus.) **6:** 3, 1971.
24. Serbinenko, F. A.: Catheterization and occlusion of major cerebral vessels and prospects for the development of vascular neurosurgery, Probl. Neurosurg. (Rus.) **5:** 17, 1971.
25. Serbinenko, F. A.: Personal communication, Sept. 1971.
26. Speakman, T. J.: Internal occlusion of a carotid-cavernous fistula, J. Neurosurg. **21:** 303, 1964.
27. Taptas, J. N.: Etiology et pathogénie des exophthalmies d'origine vasculaire dites exophthalmies pulsatiles, Arch. Ophthalmol. (Paris) **10:** 22, 1950.
28. Taptas, J. N.: La loge du sinus caverneux: Sa constitution et les rapports des éléments vasculaires et nerveux qui la traversant, Arch. Ophthalmol. (Paris) **14:** 404, 1956.
29. Treiman, R. L., Cohen, J. L., Gaspard, D. J., et al.: Early surgical repair of acute posttraumatic arteriovenous fistulas, Arch. Surg. **102:** 559, 1971.
30. Uihlein, A., Terry, N. R., Jr., Payne, W. S., et al.: Operations on intracranial aneurysms with induced hypothermia below 15° C. and total circulatory arrest, J. Neurosurg. **19:** 237, 1962.
31. Wallace, S., Goldberg, H. I., Leeds, N. E., et al.: The cavernous branches of the internal carotid artery, Am. J. Roentgenol. Radium Ther. Nucl. Med. **101:** 34, 1967.

Juxtarenal aortic occlusion

Richard W. Starrett, M.D., *and* **Ronald J. Stoney, M.D.,** *San Francisco, Calif.*

This report describes 55 patients treated at the University of California Medical Center, San Francisco, for atherosclerotic occlusion of the abdominal aorta to the level of the renal arteries. Only 13 patients presented with advanced ischemia and all of these patients had associated occlusive disease distal to the inguinal ligament. Suprarenal translumbar aortography provided adequate visualization of the distal arterial tree in 62 percent of the patients, even when the distal circulation was patent. An arterial reconstruction was performed in 40 patients, with the use of endarterectomy in 17 and prosthetic grafts in 21. In most of these patients, the occlusive atherosclerotic process centered at or below the level of the inferior mesenteric artery with proximal propagation of thrombus to the level of the renal arteries. Postoperative renal dysfunction occurred in only one patient operated on early in the series. Techniques to avoid this complication are described. There have been no late viscerorenal complications and patency at 10 years is 85 percent. Thirteen patients did not have an aortic reconstruction. Six of these patients developed thrombosis of the renal arteries, with associated superior mesenteric artery occlusion in two patients. Direct extension of the aortic thrombus was proved to have caused visceral arterial occlusion in five patients.

From the Department of Surgery, University of California Medical Center, San Francisco, Calif.

ATHEROSCLEROTIC occlusion of the abdominal aorta, which has progressed proximally to the level of the renal arteries, presents a continuing challenge in diagnosis and surgical management. Since abdominal aortic occlusion is rare (0.15 percent of 33,226 autopsies),[11] it is not surprising that no one has a reported large experience with this lesion. The following report describes the surgical experience with juxtarenal aortic occlusion and the outcome in a group of patients who were followed without operation at the University of California Medical Center, San Francisco, from 1951 to 1973.

Supported in part by the Keith Proud Memorial Fund.

Presented at the Twenty-eighth Annual Meeting of the Society for Vascular Surgery, Chicago, Ill., June 20 and 21, 1974.

Reprint requests: Ronald J. Stoney, M.D., Department of Surgery, University of California Medical Center, San Francisco, Calif. 94143.

Of 106 patients with chronic aortic occlusions documented arteriographically, there were 55 patients in whom the proximal level of occlusion was at or just distal to the renal arteries, or "juxtarenal" (Table I). The 40 men and 15 women ranged in age from 35 to 72 years with a mean age of 55 years. Symptoms were limited to claudication in 84 percent; only 16 percent presented with more advanced ischemia. In 80 percent of the patients, symptoms had been present longer than a year.

AORTOGRAPHY

All patients were studied by translumbar suprarenal aortography under epidural anesthesia. Fig. 1 shows some of the variations found in the proximal portion of the aortic thrombus. Ten patients had some degree of stenosis of the orifice of the renal artery.

Table I. *Abdominal aorta occlusion U.C.S.F. 1952 to 1973*

Aortic level	*No.*	*Male/female*	*Age*	*Claudication*	*Advanced ischemia*
Juxtarenal	55	40/15	55	42	13
Bifurcation	51	26/25	56	41	10

Since most of the radiological studies were confined to the anteroposterior projection, the extent of atherosclerotic involvement of the superior mesenteric and celiac arteries is unknown (Fig. 2). Two patients had symptoms suggestive of visceral ischemia. Supplementary lateral aortography via a transaxillary catheter disclosed stenosis of the superior mesenteric artery in one patient (Fig. 3).

Aortography clearly visualized the distal arterial tree bilaterally in only 62 percent of the patients with suprarenal occlusion. The distal arteries were visualized in 84 percent of the patients with distal aortic occlusion (Table I). Of the 21 patients with juxtarenal occlusion in whom one or both femoral arteries failed to visualize, 17 patients were explored surgically and only two of these patients had occlusion of the common femoral artery.

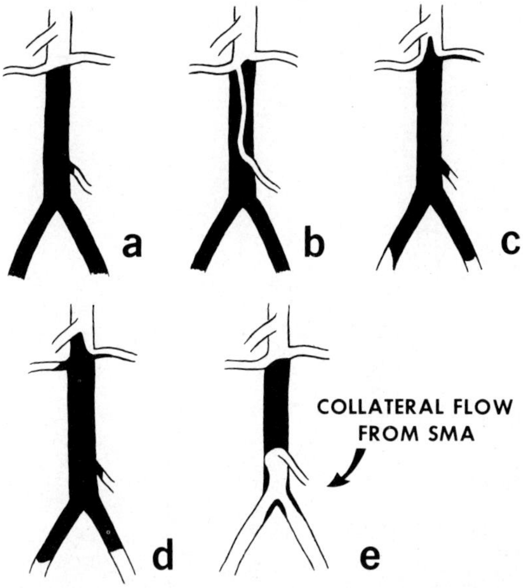

Fig. 1. Proximal configuration of aortic thrombus.

NONOPERATIVE GROUP

Revascularization of the lower extermities was not attempted in 15 patients. Most were seen early in our surgical experience, and except for two patients with inoperable outflow disease, the factors which then prompted us to decide against surgery could now be overcome. Only one of these patients had a demonstrated renal artery stenosis.

Two untreated patients were lost to follow-up study and two are currently living with functioning lower extremities, 64 and 105 months after their original diagnosis. Eleven patients have died (Fig. 4). At autopsy, six had occlusion of one or both renal arteries, the mechanism in at least five being a direct extension of the aortic thrombus. Two of the patients additionally had ascending thrombus which had occluded the superior mesenteric artery. All six of the patients died in partial or complete renal failure. An autopsy was not obtained in another patient who died after the relatively sudden onset of uremia. The interval between aortography and death in these patients varied from 15 days to 214 months. Three of the other four deaths in this group resulted from coronary or cerebrovascular atherosclerosis.

OPERATIVE GROUP

Forty patients with juxtarenal atherosclerotic occlusion underwent a revascularization procedure (Table II). The preoperative ischemic manifestations were claudication in 31 patients and rest pain or ulceration in nine. Five patients also underwent renal artery thromboendarterectomy.

Temporary suprarenal aortic control was utilized in all cases. The duration of renal ischemia averaged 14 minutes, and the longest period was 24 minutes in one of the five patients in whom transaortic renal endarterectomy was added to the primary operation.

An endarterectomy was performed in 17 patients. The distal level of endarterectomy

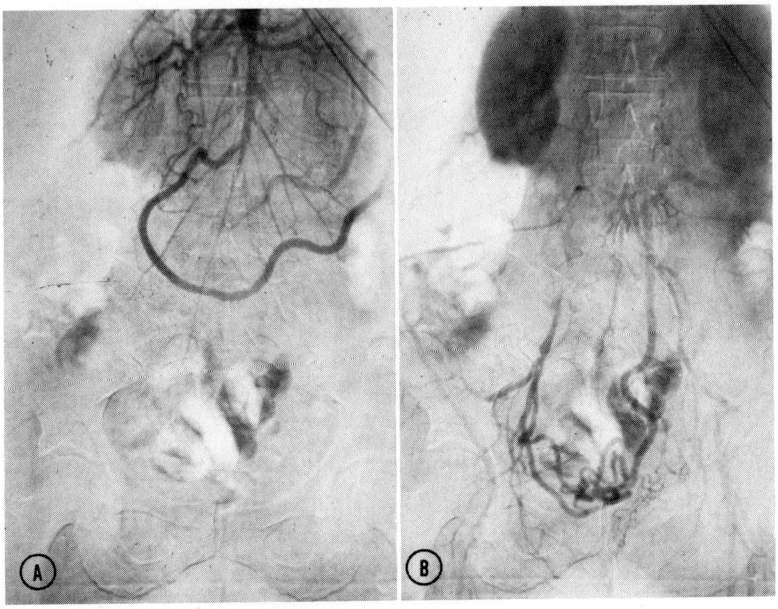

Fig. 2. Anterior-posterior aortogram demonstrating juxtarenal aortic occlusion.

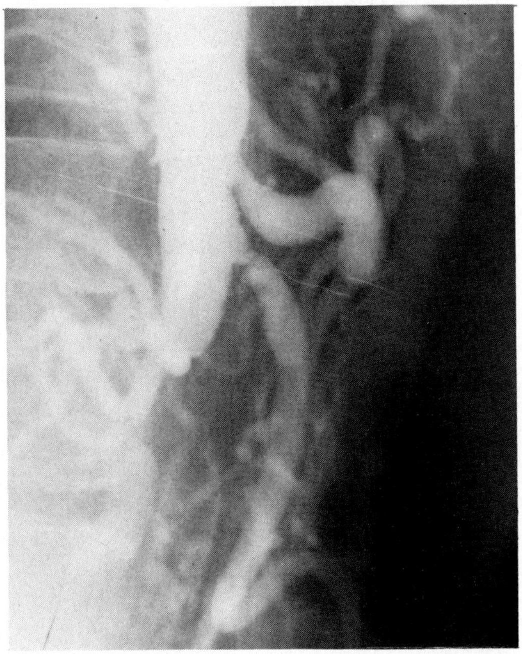

Fig. 3. Lateral aortogram showing superior mesenteric artery stenosis.

was the terminal common iliac artery in nine patients and the external iliac or common femoral in eight. The technique has undergone several modifications (Fig. 5). We currently approach first the upper segment using a full-length longitudinal aortotomy

Table II. *Reconstructive operation for juxtarenal aortic occlusion (40 patients)*

Type	*Aorto-iliac*	*Aorto-external iliac*	*Aorto-femoral*
Endarterectomy	9	6*	2*
Graft	1	4*	10*
Graft & distal endarterectomy	2	3	3

*Patient requiring bilateral renal endarterectomy.

after cross-clamping the proximal aorta and both renal arteries. The thrombus from the first few centimeters of the infrarenal aorta is removed under direct vision before the endarterectomy is begun. When the renal orifices are involved by atherosclerosis, the upper level of endarterectomy is proximal to the renal arteries. The removal of a sleeve of aortic intima at this level carries with it the renal lesions. When the renal arteries are not involved, the upper level of this endarterectomy is immediately distal to the renal artery orifices.

Following completion of the endarterectomy in the proximal half of the infrarenal aorta, the renal artery clamps are first removed and then the aortic clamp is repositioned at the subrenal level. The remainder of the procedure is then carried out in the

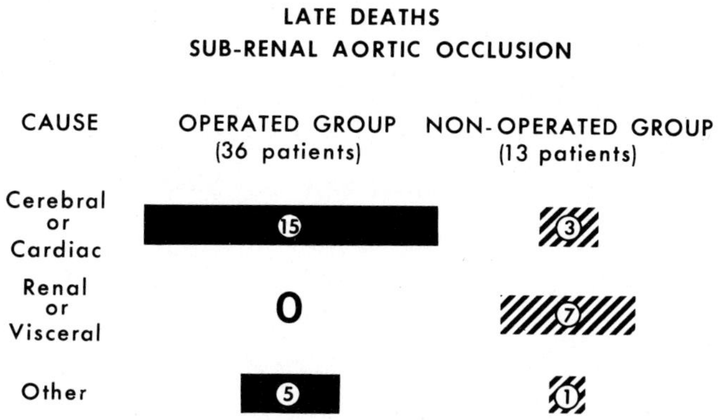

Fig. 4. Late deaths, subrenal aortic occlusion.

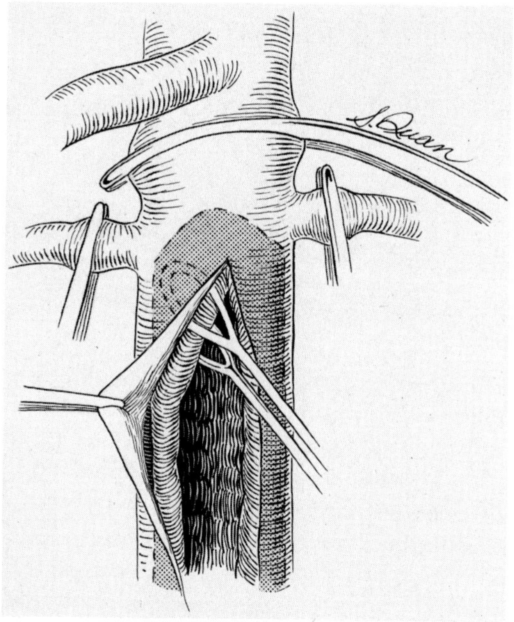

Fig. 5. Technique of thrombectomy in juxtarenal aortic occlusion.

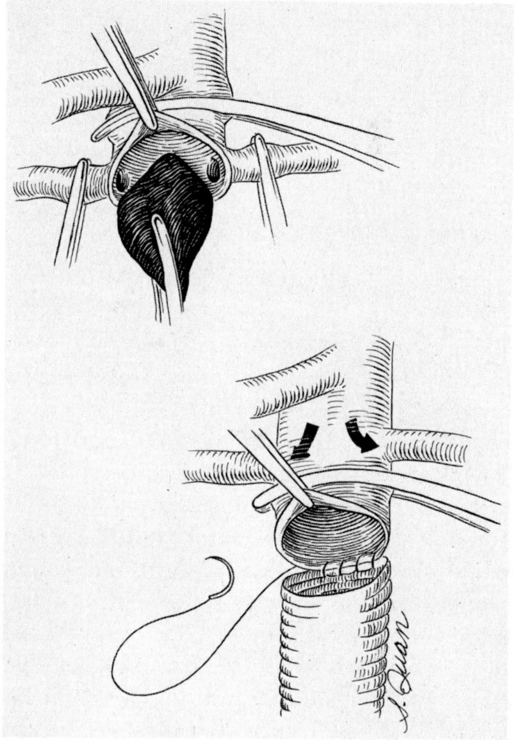

Fig. 6. Use of prosthetic grafts in juxtarenal aortic occlusion.

customary manner, using transverse terminal common iliac arteriotomies and interval arterial strippers.

Inspection of the endarterectomy specimens showed that the primary occlusive atherosclerotic lesion was in the segment of the aorta distal to the origin of the inferior mesenteric artery or in the orifices of the common iliac arteries. Occlusion proximal to these levels was by intraluminal thrombus, often in the absence of significant thickening of the aortic intima.

There were two postoperative deaths in the endarterectomy series early in our experience (1952), one from suture line disruption and hemorrhage and the other from renal infarction caused by atheromatous embolization. One patient required reoperation for postoperative iliac artery thrombosis.

In 23 patients a graft was used for reconstruction. Following renal artery and suprarenal aortic clamping, the aorta is transected 3 cm. distal to the renal level (Fig. 6). The thrombus in the proximal aorta is then ex-

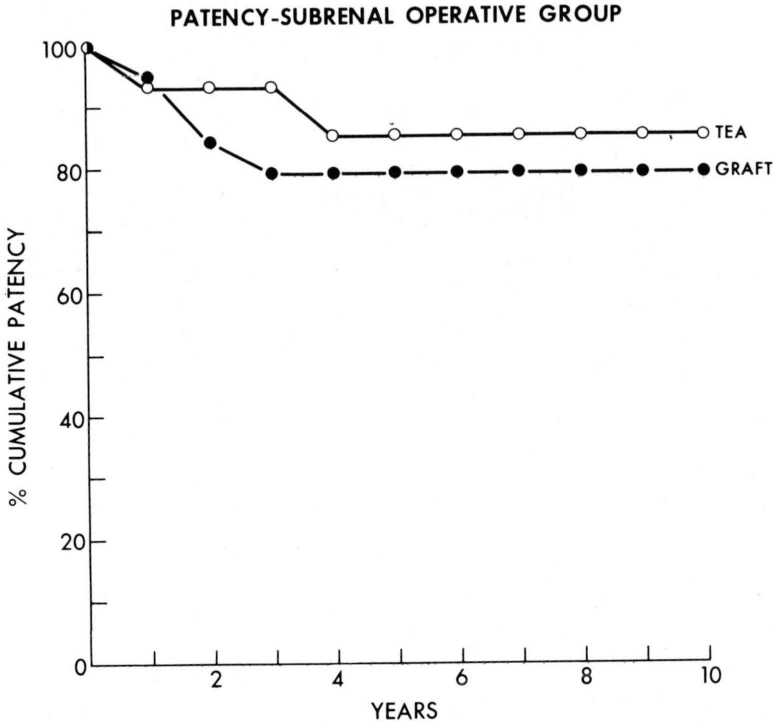

Fig. 7. Patency in operative group.

tracted. Following an end-to-end anastomosis of the graft to the aorta, the renal and suprarenal aortic clamps are removed and renal flow is re-established with the aortic clamp in a subrenal position.

Six of these grafts were aortic homografts, while 17 were knitted bifurcation Dacron prostheses. Four patients required renal endarterectomy in addition. The distal graft limbs were brought to the external iliac arteries in 10 patients and to the common femoral arteries in 13, utililzing end-to-side anastomoses. There were two postoperative deaths, both resulting from myocardial infarction; early graft thrombosis required a second operation in one patient.

Pedal pulses were restored after operation in 31 patients. Distal atherosclerotic occlusive lesions were present in those patients who failed to regain pedal pulses, but sufficient symptomatic relief resulted from the proximal operation to make further surgery unnecessary.

All 36 patients who survived have been followed with a mean follow-up period of 7.4 years. The survival and patency data computed according to the life table method are shown in Figs. 7 and 8.

Twenty patients have died. Two of these patients were operated on prior to 1960 when silk was still used for anastomosis and these patients died from rupture of false aneurysms. One death, 10 years after a successful endarterectomy, resulted from reocclusion of the aorta with subsequent superior mesenteric artery occlusion and visceral infarction. Three patients have required leg amputation following progression of distal atherosclerotic disease.

DISCUSSION

The frequent failure to obtain adequate radiographic definition of the distal arterial circulation presented less of a problem than one might expect. The presenting complaint in most patients was claudication, not advanced ischemia. When palpation of the groin failed to reveal the rigid tube of a thrombosed common femoral artery in a patient without advanced ischemia, exploration uniformly revealed an adequate lumen in the common femoral artery as well as in the

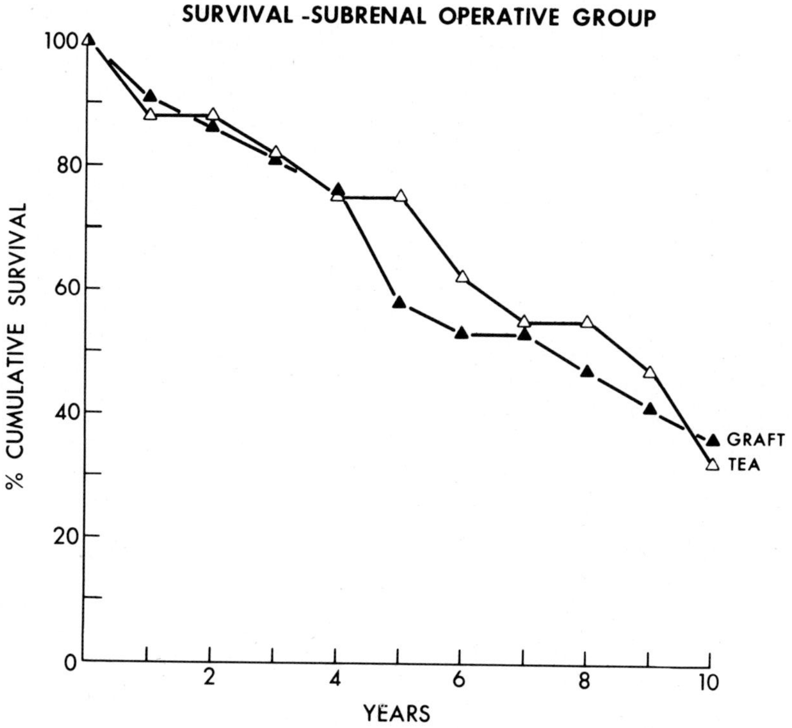

Fig. 8. Survival in operative group.

profunda femoris artery. Advanced disease at the profunda femoris level was a frequent finding, however, in patients with more severe ischemia. When the femoral artery can be felt as a hard, cylindrical, pulseless mass, it has been our custom to explore the groins prior to opening the abdomen. A local endarterectomy of the common femoral artery combined with profundaplasty may create an adequate outflow tract. This could not be accomplished in two patients, and operation was abandoned at that point.

Protection of the kidneys from atheromatous emboli by individually cross-clamping each renal artery is an essential aspect of aortic surgery in the presence of juxtarenal occlusion.[2] In 1952, prior to our recognition of this fact, one of our patients died from postoperative renal failure due to multiple renal arterial emboli.

Various authors have recorded cases of proximal propagation of thrombus in the aorta to obliterate the renal, and more rarely, the upper visceral arteries.[1, 3, 4, 8, 9, 11, 12] The frequency of this complication (six confirmed and one suspected) among the 13 patients in the series who were followed without surgery suggests that the threat of visceral arterial occlusion provides a strong indication for surgery, even in patients who experience only mild claudication.

Several remote bypass procedures for high aorta iliac occlusion have been recently described.[5-7, 10] Since these techniques do not remove the intraluminal aortic thrombus, they expose the patient to the risk of proximal extension of the thrombus. Furthermore, results obtained in this series indicate that a reconstructive operation can be safely performed at the subrenal level without resorting to the more extensive and complicated procedures.

SUMMARY

Fifty-five patients with juxtarenal atherosclerotic occlusion of the abdominal aorta have been studied in a 23 year period at the University of California, San Francisco. Of 13 patients followed without operation, six (46 percent) have died from proximal propagation of aortic thrombus with renal artery occlusion; a similar fate was suspected, but not confirmed, in a seventh patient who died of acute renal failure. Revascularization operations were performed on 40 patients. There were four postoperative deaths early in the series. Satisfactory results were obtained in 36 patients followed for a mean of 7.4 years.

REFERENCES

1. Beckwith, R., Huffman, E. R., Eiseman, B., and Blount, S. G.: Chronic aortoiliac thrombosis, N. Engl. J. Med. **258:** 721, 1958.
2. Bergan, J. J., and Trippel, O. H.: Management of juxtarenal aortic occlusions, Arch. Surg. **87:** 60, 1963.
3. Bron, K. M.: Thrombotic occlusion of the abdominal aorta, Am. J. Roentgenol. Radium Ther. Nucl. Med. **96:** 887, 1966.
4. Burt, C. C., Learmonth, J., and Richards, R. L.: On occlusion of the abdominal aorta, Edinburgh Med. J. **59:** 65, 1952.
5. De Bakey, M. E.: Basic concepts of therapy in arterial disease, Bull. N. Y. Acad. Med. **39:** 707, 1963.
6. Frantz, S. L., Kaplitt, J. J., Beil, A. R., and Stein, H. L.: Ascending aorta-bilateral femoral artery bypass for the totally occluded infrarenal abdominal aorta, Surgery **75:** 471, 1974.
7. Froysaker, T., Skagseth, E., Dundas, P., and Hall, K. V.: Bypass procedures in the treatment of obstructions of the abdominal aorta, J. Cardiovasc. Surg. **14:** 317, 1973.
8. Gomes, M. M. R., and Bernatz, P. E.: Aortoiliac occlusive disease. Extension cephalad to origin of renal arteries with surgical considerations and results, Arch. Surg. **101:** 161, 1970.
9. Johnson, J. K.: Ascending thrombosis of abdominal aorta as fatal complication of Leriche's syndrome, Arch. Surg. **69:** 663, 1954.
10. Nunn, D. B., and Kamal, M. A.: Bypass grafting from the thoracic aorta to femoral arteries for high aortoiliac occlusive disease, Surgery **72:** 749, 1972.
11. Starer, F., and Sutton, D.: Aortic thrombosis, Br. Med. J. **1:** 1255, 1958.
12. Wyatt, G. M., and Felson, B.: Aortic thrombosis as a cause of hypertension: An arteriographic study, Radiology **69:** 676, 1957.

DISCUSSION

Dr. James A. De Weese (Rochester, N. Y.). We have also observed five patients with thrombotic occlusion of the terminal aorta, who have gone on to develop and to propagate thrombus and, finally, to occlude their renal arteries.

In only one of these patients was this recognized prior to death, and, in that one, we were able to perform a delayed thrombectomy with survival.

I think it is important to realize this because it does add an additional reason for early operation on these patients. And this means that we would operate on anyone with a total occlusion of the terminal aorta, unless there was a serious medical contraindication.

Dr. Daniel B. Nunn (Jacksonville, Fla.). The surgical treatment of subrenal aortic occlusion is, indeed, a difficult and challenging problem. I wish to mention my own experience with an alternate surgical procedure—namely, bypass grafting from the descending thoracic aorta to the common femoral arteries. This procedure is performed through a left thoracoabdominal incision and bilateral groin incisions. Thus far, I have used this procedure in 10 patients, and the follow-up extends to a period of approximately 4 years. All patients have had an excellent result with respect to blood flow to the lower extremities and there have been no complications related to the renal arteries. At this time all of the grafts are patent.

With regard to the procedure described by Drs. Starrett and Stoney, I have been concerned about the advisability of performing an endarterectomy on the proximal infrarenal aorta when severe arteriosclerotic change is present and involves the media of the vessel. Certainly, when an endarterectomy is done under these circumstances, there is always the danger of recurrent disease and subsequent thrombosis with possible occlusion of one or both renal arteries. On the other hand, the use of a descending thoracic aortofemoral artery Dacron bypass graft would seem to minimize the possibility of this serious complication.

Finally, I wish to point out that bypass grafting from the descending thoracic aorta to the femoral arteries is particularly useful in the treatment of patients with high aortoiliac occlusive disease, who have had previous aortic operations resulting in considerable scar tissue formation in and around the aorta.

Dr. Anthony M. Imparato (New York, N. Y.). There are one or two facts about the surgical management of this particular group of patients which are extremely useful.

Having done almost exclusively endarterectomy on every one of our patients with this particular syndrome, it has been striking for me to observe that many of them have relatively little atherosclerosis but a maximum of thrombosis. I think this group of patients was recognized by Leriche as having these distinctive features.

The importance of the observation lies in the fact that the immediate infrarenal segment very often has very little atherosclerosis, and one can clear that segment by simply doing a thrombectomy without getting involved with doing endarterectomy of the renal segment.

The second point of interest to us has been that, in spite of the fact that a certain number of these patients have associated complete occlusions of the superficial femoral arteries, in our experience it has never been necessary to surgically correct these at the time of aortic operation in order to relieve the ischemia.

Dr. Alistair Karmody (Albany, N. Y.). We agree that operation is indicated because of the potential problem of extension of the thrombus proximally.

The point I want to make is very minor, and it involves the use of translumbar angiography in delineation of the lesions. I think a lot of collateral circulation to the lower limbs often derives from the intercostal vessels, and these are best visualized by thoracic aortic injection, possibly by axillary catheterization of the thoracic aorta.

Doing this, one sees in a number of such people that the external iliac arteries are in fact patent and it is possible, in most of these instances, to do an aorto-to-external iliac anastomosis and avoid femoral anastomoses.

Dr. Ronald J. Stoney (Closing). Dr. Dale, I believe extremity gangrene is not inevitable as two of our nonoperated patients have developed no advanced limb ischemia. I do think our results show that gangrene of the kidney and viscera is a more frequent sequela of untreated aortic occlusion than was previously suggested.

I have found no difference in the incidence of impotence in men with aortic occlusion and other forms of aortoiliac occlusion disease.

Dr. De Weese, we agree with your observation regarding progression of aortic thrombosis in untreated patients. This makes us concerned about the fate of patients subjected to remote bypass operations. As you know, this technique avoids removal of the intraluminal aortic thrombus and would not, therefore, alter the progressive thrombosis which is likely to ocur.

Dr. Nunn, we are aware of your technique for treating this lesion, but I am concerned that remote bypass procedures ignore the critical component of aortic occlusion, namely the juxtarenal aortic thrombosis.

Dr. Imparato, we agree that proximal aortic thrombectomy is often easily performed and does not require aortic endarterectomy in all instances. Also, the presence of residual occlusive lesions in the superficial femoral arteries did not require repair once the aortic occlusion was relieved.

Dr. Karmody, we have not been concerned if aortography failed to opacify distal vasculature, since in only 21 percent of the entire series were these vessels actually obliterated and nonreconstructable. We would agree, however, that there are several radiographic techniques which improve the chance to visualize vessels distal to the aortic occlusion.

In conclusion, we recognize that these objectives are not original. Well-documented case reports of ascending fatal aortic thrombosis have appeared. It does seem that this potential complication has been overlooked in treating this lesion in recent years. Hopefully, this report will focus attention on this overlooked but important aspect of juxtarenal aortic occlusion.

Pathogenesis and clinical significance of splenic artery aneurysms

James C. Stanley, M.D., *and* **William J. Fry, M.D.,** *Ann Arbor, Mich.*

Sixty patients (48 women and 12 men), 15 to 86 years of age, with splenic artery aneurysms were studied. Arteriosclerosis, a common histologic finding, was considered a secondary event rather than the initiating cause of most aneurysms. Factors relevant to the pathogenesis of these lesions included: arterial fibrodysplasia affecting eight patients, portal hypertension and splenomegaly in six patients, and inflammatory processes involving the vessel wall in three patients. Among the remaining 43 patients were 35 women, including 14 (40 percent) who had completed six or more pregnancies. Gestational alterations in the arterial wall due to hormonal and local hemodynamic events may have a causal relation to medial defects and aneurysmal formation. Pathogenic factors were less readily identified in eight men who completed the series, although arteriosclerosis was most suspect. Excluding three ruptured aneurysms associated with inflammatory disorders, aneurysmal rupture occurred in only three (5.3 percent) of the other 57 patients. All six patients with ruptured aneurysms survived operation, as did 33 patients with intact aneurysms. Specific risk factors producing aneurysmal expansion and rupture among older, asymptomatic patients are poorly understood. Symptomatic aneurysms and those in women of child-bearing age provide clear indications for operative intervention.

From the Department of Surgery, Section of General Surgery, University of Michigan Medical Center, Ann Arbor.

THE PATHOGENESIS of splenic artery aneurysms is unique in comparison to aneurysmal disease affecting other peripheral arteries. Etiologic mechanisms responsible for splenic artery aneurysms must account for their common occurrence in women—particularly grand-multiparous women—and the apparent predilection for splenic artery involvement in comparison with other splanchnic vessels. Considerable evidence exists to implicate hormonal and local hemodynamic events in the evolution of most of these aneurysms.

The clinical significance of splenic artery aneurysms resides in establishing their true incidence, the morbidity attributable to intact aneurysms, the risk of aneurysmal rupture, and the potential for death with rupture. Misconceptions concerning splenic artery aneurysms continue to be perpetuated in the literature. Reviews and reports of sporadic cases, frequently spectacular in nature, do not provide the basis for an accurate assessment of this disease entity. Among descriptions of more than 800 patients with splenic artery aneurysms, only two *clinical* series of more than 20 patients from a single institution have been reported.[15, 21] A reappraisal of the biologic character of splenic

Supported by the University of Michigan Peripheral Vascular Research Fund.

Presented at the Twenty-eighth Annual Meeting of the Society for Vascular Surgery, Chicago, Ill., June 20 and 21, 1974.

Reprint requests: James C. Stanley, M.D., Department of Surgery, Section of General Surgery, University of Michigan Medical Center, Ann Arbor, Mich. 48104.

artery aneurysms is in order. This paper reports on 60 patients with aneurysms of the splenic artery from the University of Michigan Medical Center.

CLINICAL MATERIAL

Over a 15 year period, 48 female and 12 male patients with splenic artery aneurysms were encountered. These patients ranged from 15 to 86 years of age. Factors relevant to suspected etiologic mechanisms were identified and provided for an arbitrary but useful categorization of patients. This classification includes aneurysms associated with (Group I) arterial dysplasia, (Group II) portal hypertension with splenomegaly, (Group III) focal arterial inflammatory processes, and (Group IV) hormonal and hemodynamic events in parous females. An additional group (V) was composed of aneurysms in men that were unassociated with clearly recognizable pathogenic factors, although arteriosclerosis was suspect in most instances. Examination of these groups individually revealed the uniqueness of certain splenic artery aneurysms.

Group I—arterial dysplasia. Eight female patients with dysplastic lesions of nonsplenic vessels were found to have asymptomatic splenic artery aneurysms (Table I). Seven patients had concomitant renal artery fibrodysplastic stenoses, including three with renal artery aneurysms. These seven patients represent 4.0 percent of the known cases of renal artery fibrodysplasia having arteriographic studies at this medical center. Dysplastic lesions and aneurysms affected multiple splanchnic arteries in the eighth patient. In no case were arteriograms of the splenic artery suggestive of arterial dysplastic stenotic disease. All but one patient had sustained arterial hypertension.

Group II—portal hypertension with splenomegaly. Splenic artery aneurysms were documented in five women and one man undergoing arteriographic assessment of portal hypertension (Table I). These six represent 7.1 percent of cirrhotic patients with portal hypertension recently subjected to arteriographic study at this medical center. Aneurysms in this group were asymptomatic, extrasplenic, and indistinguishable in shape or size from those occurring in nonportal hypertensive patients. Advanced cirrhosis with portal hypertension, varices, splenomegaly, and hypersplenism affected all six patients. Portal decompression was undertaken in each case, but aneurysms were removed only twice when splenorenal shunts were performed.

Group III—focal arterial inflammatory processes. Three men, unafflicted with arterial hypertension or arteriosclerosis, developed splenic artery aneurysms on the basis of focal inflammation of the vessel wall (Table I). Endarteritis, due to presumed septic emboli from a prosthetic aortic valve in a known drug user, led to rupture and intraperitoneal hemorrhage in one instance. An uneventful recovery followed emergent splenectomy. Two patients with pancreatitis had splenic artery aneurysms which ruptured into pancreatic pseudocysts. Bleeding—intraperitoneal in one case and intragastric in the other—resulted in both patients undergoing successful distal pancreatectomy and splenectomy. These three patients reflect primary disease processes unrelated directly to the splenic artery.

Excluding 17 patients described in Groups I, II and III, there remained 43 patients with splenic artery aneurysms unrelated to more obvious vascular or circulatory disorders. Women predominated, 35 to 8. When segregated (Group IV), they proved dissimilar in certain respects to other female patients in the series as well as to women in the general population.

Group IV—female patients: Ill-defined pathogenesis. An unusually high frequency of conception and completed pregnancies was observed among these 35 female patients (Table II). Thirty-four were Caucasian and one was Negro. Most had passed beyond the child-bearing portion of their lives at the time their aneurysms were discovered. Fourteen patients (40 percent) had completed six or more pregnancies. Arterial hypertension or arteriosclerotic cardiovascular disease affected a little more than half of this group.

Table I. *Splenic artery aneurysms: Pathogenesis associated with recognizable vascular disease*

Patient	*Age**	*Sex*	*Dysplastic lesion*	*Hepatic disease*
Arterial dysplasia (Group I):				
1	26	F	R renal FMD§	—
2	38	F	Pancreaticoduodenal, gastroduodenal, pancreatic magna FMD with aneurysms	—
3	42	F	L renal FMD	—
4	42	F	R renal FMD with aneurysm	—
5	48	F	R renal FMD	—
6	50	F	R renal FMD with aneurysm	—
7	53	F	R renal FMD with aneurysms	—
8	63	F	R renal FMD	—
Portal hypertension (Group II):				
9	50	F	—	Postnecrotic cirrhosis
10	55	F	—	Laennec's cirrhosis
11	61	F	—	Postnecrotic cirrhosis
12	64	F	—	Laennec's cirrhosis
13	69	F	—	Postnecrotic cirrhosis
14	56	M	—	Laennec's cirrhosis
Focal arterial inflammatory processes (Group III):				
15	25	M	—	—
16	28	M	—	—
17	62	M	—	—

*Age at time of diagnosis.
†Arteriosclerotic cardiovascular disease (excluding arteriosclerosis of splenic artery aneurysms).
‡S—splenectomy with aneurysmectomy; A—aneurysmectomy; P—distal pancreatectomy.
§Fibromuscular dysplasia.

Renal artery aneurysms, unassociated with fibrodysplastic lesions or hypertension, were discovered in two of these patients. Symptoms specifically attributable to splenic artery aneurysms occurred in 10 of the 35 patients. Left flank and left upper quadrant abdominal discomfort, often referred to the left subscapular area, were the most common complaints. Aneurysms ruptured into an adjacent splenic vein in one patient and into a parietal systemic vein in another. Both underwent uneventful splenectomy. Urgent splenectomy was successfully performed in one patient with a large, expanding aneurysm. Elective operations were undertaken in an additional 21 patients. None of these 24 patients died. Histologic examination of aneurysms often revealed arteriosclerotic changes with obscuration of the normal vessel architecture. Medial abnormalities without arteriosclerosis were evident in most of the specimens from younger patients and within the splenic artery adjacent to calcific aneurysms in many of the most elderly patients. Extensive arteriosclerotic involvement of the nonaneurysmal portion of the splenic artery was uncommon.

Group V—male patients: Ill-defined pathogenesis. Eight men completed the series of 60 patients with splenic artery aneurysms (Table II). Etiologic mechanisms were not obvious in six of the patients, although all had arteriosclerotic vascular disease and three were hypertensive. There was speculation that medionecrosis in the fifth patient and increased splenic blood flow due to hepatosplenomegaly in the sixth may have contributed to aneurysmal formation. Only one patient with a ruptured aneurysm was symp-

Cause of inflammation	*Pregnancy*	*Hypertension*	*ASCVD†*	*Operation‡*	*Comment*
—	G3P3	+	0	S	—
—	G4P2	+	0	A	Celiac artery occlusion, cause undetermined
—	G4P4	+	0	0	—
—	G4P4	+	0	S	—
—	G2P1	+	0	S	—
—	G2P2	+	0	0	Common hepatic artery stenosis, cause undetermined
—	G1P1	+	+	S	—
—	G7P7	0	+	S	—
—	G5P4	0	0	0	R hepatic artery–portal vein fistula, cause undetermined Splenomegaly
—	G3P3	0	0	0	Splenomegaly
—	G2P1	0	0	0	Splenomegaly
—	Nullip-arous	0	+	S	Splenomegaly
—	G1P1	0	0	0	Splenomegaly
—	—	+	0	S	Splenomegaly
bable mycotic embolism (aortic alve prosthesis–heroin user)	—	0	0	S	Aneurysmal rupture (intraperitoneal)
ute pancreatitis, pancreatic seudocyst	—	0	0	S, P	Aneurysmal rupture (pancreatic pseudocyst and intraperitoneal)
ronic pancreatitis, pancreatic seudocyst	—	0	0	S, P	Aneurysmal rupture (pancreatic pseudocyst and intragastric)

tomatic. This patient and three others underwent splenectomy without incident.

DISCUSSION

Pathogenesis. Splenic artery aneurysms associated with arterial fibrodysplasia of other vessels were encountered in 13 percent of our series (Group I). This has been an infrequently reported finding.[21, 25] Medial fibrodysplasia may account for the development of aneurysms in these patients. It is the most common form of arterial dysplasia to affect the renal and internal carotid arteries.[8, 22] The lesion is usually associated with alternate areas of medial thinning and fibrotic stenoses, resulting in small mural outpouchings. Larger aneurysms might be anticipated should bifurcations of muscular arteries like the splenic artery be involved. Supporting tissues including smooth muscle cells and elastic fibers are sparse at such branchings. Supporting this concept have been findings suggestive of medial fibrodysplasia in splenic arteries adjacent to aneurysms. Histologic findings include internal elastic lamina fragmentation, diminutions in elastic fibers, subendothelial and medial fibroplasia, and medial accumulations of sulfated acid mucopolysaccharides (Fig. 1, *A* and *B*). Hormonal factors peculiar to women and hypertension may influence the evolution of these aneurysms, although the exact mechanisms are not known.

Aneurysms of the splenic artery have been alleged to affect a significant percentage of patients having portal hypertension.[4, 14] Our more recent experience with arteriographic assessments of portal hypertensive

Table II. *Splenic artery aneurysms: Ill-defined pathogenesis*

Patient	*Age**	*Pregnancy*	*Hyper-tension*	*ASCVD†*	*Opera-tion‡*	*Comment*
Females (Group IV):						
1	29	G3P3	0	0	S	—
2	41	G2P2	0	0	S	—
3	42	G7P5	0	0	S	—
4	44	G5P4	0	0	0	—
5	44	G4P2	0	0	S	—
6	44	G8P8	0	0	S	—
7	48	G2P2	+	0	S	Splenomegaly
8	52	G5P2	0	0	0	—
9	52	G2P2	0	0	S	—
10	52	G3P3	0	+	S	—
11	53	G2P1	+	+	0	—
12	53	G10P10	+	+	A	Uterine artery–vein fistula
13	53	Nullip-arous	0	0	S	Splenomegaly, aneurysmal rupture (systemic vein)
14	54	G2P2	+	0	0	—
15	55	Nullip-arous	0	+	S	—
16	55	G10P9	0	0	S	R renal artery aneurysm
17	55	G6P5	0	0	S	
18	56	G10P6	0	+	S	Splenomegaly
19	57	G10P10	+	+	S	—
20	57	G13P10	0	0	0	L renal artery aneurysm
21	57	G4P4	+	0	S	—
22	57	G12P11	0	0	S	Splenomegaly, aneurysmal rupture (splenic vein)
23	60	G7P7	+	0	S	—
24	60	G4P3	0	0	S	—
25	61	G9P7	+	+	S	—
26	62	G3P3	0	+	0	—
27	62	G2P2	0	+	0	—
28	65	G7P6	0	0	S	
29	67	G3P3	+	+	S	—
30	68	G8P7	0	0	S	Acute aneurysmal expansion
31	69	G10P9	0	0	0	—
32	70	G3P3	+	0	0	—
33	73	G7P7	+	+	S	—
34	78	Nullip-arous	+	+	0	—
35	83	G9P9	+	+	0	—
Males (Group V):						
36	15	—	0	0	0	VonRecklinghausen's disease; stigmata of Marfan's syndrome
37	38	—	+	+	S	—
38	66	—	0	0	S	Hepatosplenomegaly (hereditary spherocytosis), inferior pancreatico-duodenal artery aneurysm, celiac artery occlusion—cause undetermined
39	69	—	+	+	0	—
40	74	—	+	+	0	Necropsy finding; splenomegaly
41	77	—	0	+	S	Aneurysmal rupture (intraperitoneal)
42	78	—	0	+	S	—
43	86	—	0	+	0	—

*Age at time of diagnosis.

†Arteriosclerotic cardiovascular disease (excluding arteriosclerosis of splenic artery aneurysm).

‡S—splenectomy with aneurysmectomy; A—aneurysmectomy.

patients lends credence to these observations (Group II). Increases in splenic artery diameter[3, 14] and increased volume flows through this vessel[3, 24] have been documented in cirrhosis and portal hypertension. Splenic arteriovenous shunting does not appear to exist in these cases, with blood flow per equal weight of splenic tissue usually being less than normal. Splenomegaly, affecting most severe portal hypertensive and many nonportal hypertensive patients with these aneurysms, probably accounts for the increased splenic artery flow that is observed. It is plausible that aneurysms may develop if the same process producing increases in splenic artery diameter affect its bifurcations, where reductions in supporting elements are known to exist. Dilations and aneurysmal changes are believed to be a sequela of the excessive blood volume and velocity flow rates. Medial alterations, as affected one of our patients, occurring secondarily to hormonal derangements seen in advanced cirrhosis is an intriguing but unfounded consideration. The absence of aneurysms affecting other muscular arteries lessens the likelihood that a generalized hormonal vasculopathy is the sole cause of these lesions. Intrasplenic aneurysms were not noted in our patients but have been reported to be associated with portal hypertension and splenomegaly in the cirrhotic patient.[18]

Occasional splenic artery aneurysms evolve as a consequence of an injury or disease process initially not associated with the vessel itself (Group III). Pancreatitis, especially with pseudocysts, penetrating gastric ulcers, septic emboli, and trauma are among the more common causes of the periarteritis or endarteritis in these patients that eventuate in mural injury and arterial dilatation. The often life-threatening complications of these splenic artery aneurysms overshadow their cause, which is usually easily recognized.

The pathogenesis of many splenic artery aneurysms is ill defined. Arteriosclerosis has been referred to as the most common cause, despite evidence that this is unlikely. Arteriosclerotic aneurysms in general affect men 4 to 5 times more frequently than they do women. Similarly, there was only one woman among 37 patients with peripheral arteriosclerotic aneurysms (excluding aortoiliac, renal, and splanchnic lesions) in a study of multiple arteriosclerotic aneurysms from this medical center.[6] Among patients without obvious causes of their splenic artery aneurysms (Groups IV and V), women, not men, predominated.

Most striking in the profiles of these female patients (Group IV) was an unusually high rate of parity. The *National Health Survey* offers rather reliable information concerning gravity and parity in respect to age and race.[1] Although sampling noninstitutionalized subjects, this study is representative of the United States population and provides a reasonable basis for comparison with our female patients having splenic artery aneurysms of undetermined etiology.

Mean gravity and parity among 34 selected women in Group IV (age adjusted to 1961 and excluding the series' one Negro) were 5.38 ± 0.62 (S.E.M.) and 4.71 ± 0.57 (S.E.M.). Gravity and parity in the 25 to 74 year age group of the *National Health Survey* were 3.02 ± 0.05 (S.E.M.) and 2.62 ± 0.04 (S.E.M.). The increased incidence of pregnancy associated with splenic artery aneurysms, considering age groups 35 to 44, 45 to 54, and 55 to 74 years, proved statistically significant ($p < 0.001$), as did the greater parity rates ($p < 0.001$). The uniqueness of these women continued to be apparent in comparison limited to the 45- to 64-year-old population. Six or more completed pregnancies were documented among 55 percent of patients so selected from Group IV, in contrast to only 11 percent of a similarly aged sample from the *National Health Survey*. This difference likewise proved highly significant ($p < 0.001$). Reproductive histories from other women in our series (Groups I and II) did not deviate from that expected of the general population. Although the association of pregnancy and aneurysmal rupture is recognized, the possible relation of pregnancy to the etiology of splenic artery aneurysms has received little attention in the past.

Gestational alterations in connective tissue, including that within the vascular wall, have been described in man and experimental animals.[5, 12, 13, 23] Internal elastic lamina disruption and duplication, elastic fiber fragmentation, and fibroplasia with accumulation of sulfated acid mucopolysaccharides in the media—all have been noted in splenic arteries adjacent to aneurysms (Figs. 2, *A* and *B*). Aneurysmal walls in many patients exhibited medial fibroplasia (Fig. 3), and those considered of long-standing duration often manifest extensive fibrosis with calcific atherosclerosis (Fig. 4). A number of patients with multiple aneurysms were found to have arteriosclerotic changes in some but not all of their aneurysms. This lends credence to the hypothesis that arteriosclerosis is a secondary event in the evolution of these aneurysms. Lesser alterations, particularly of elastic tissue and medial ground substance, probably occur regularly during pregnancy. In most individuals reparative processes are believed to follow parturition. Repeated pregnancies, perhaps, produce irreversible injury to vessels such as the splenic artery and cause aneurysms in certain individuals. To this end, 45 percent of female patients with splenic artery aneurysms described in the English literature from 1960 to 1970, in whom parity was stated, were grand-multiparous.[21] The findings of unusual parity rates in the present study reconfirm the importance of pregnancy in the genesis of these aneurysms.

Of all splanchnic artery aneurysms, 58 percent involve the splenic artery.[21] This apparent predilection for the splenic artery to become aneurysmal may possibly reflect excessive splenic arteriovenous shunting (anatomic or functional) during pregnancy, or it may represent pre-existing weaknesses of splenic artery bifurcations inherent to this particular vessel itself. Elevation of blood pressure may be an exceedingly important variable contributing to aneurysmal formation. However, it should be noted that women in the general population of similar age and parity to our patients (Group IV) appeared to have a higher incidence of hypertension. This may reflect differences in blood pressure determinations and definitions of hypertension.

Certain splenic artery aneurysms are seemingly the sequela of arteriosclerotic weakening of the vessel wall. Arteriosclerosis may be the basis for aneurysms in six male patients without other local vascular or circulatory disturbances (Group V). These aneurysms invariably involved branchings and perhaps are not related to calcific atherosclerosis which so often affects concave borders of tortuous splenic arteries. Congenital aneurysms and those associated with unusual arteritides such as periarteritis nodosa are very uncommon when compared with other types of splenic artery aneurysms.

Clinical significance. There is no unanimity in the literature as to the precise incidence of splenic artery aneurysms.[10] Cumulative findings from nearly 195,000 necropsies revealed aneurysms in 0.098 percent.[16] Over a 100-fold increase in this figure was reported from a careful necropsy study of elderly subjects.[2] Twenty-eight of our patients had true *incidental* recognition of splenic artery aneurysms during the course of an estimated 3,600 abdominal arteriographic studies where the splenic vessels were well visualized. This represents an incidence of 0.78 percent, which, despite the selected group of patients studied, probably comes closer to the actual frequency of splenic artery aneurysms in the general population than do the previously mentioned figures. An additional 29 patients had arteriographic documentation of aneurysms, but their lesions were suspected prior to arteriography and inclusion in the above calculations would inappropriately bias the result. One fact deserving mention is that at least 11 of the 51 patients in Groups I, IV, and V had multiple aneurysms.

Manifestations and methods of diagnosing splenic artery aneurysms have been thoroughly discussed in a number of earlier publications.[7, 9-11, 16, 17, 19-21] Most splenic artery aneurysms are asymptomatic. It is noteworthy that approximately 20 percent of our patients

1 A

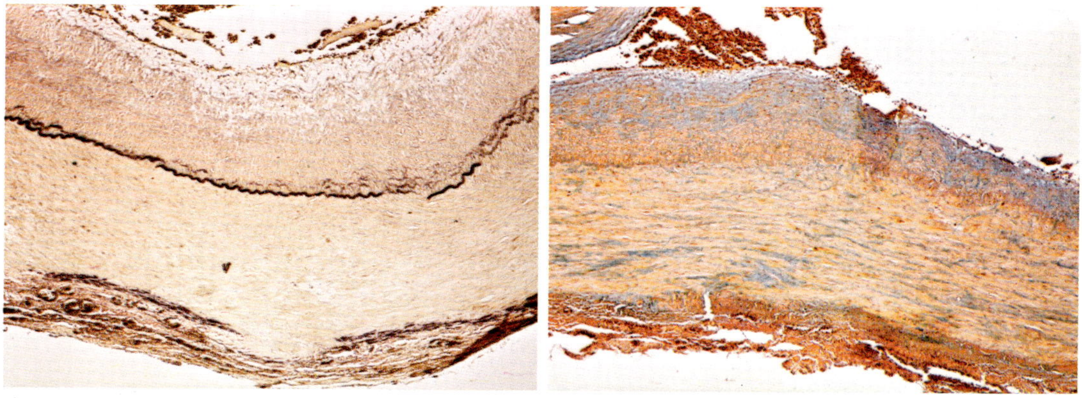

1 B

Fig. 1. Splenic artery cross section in a patient with arterial fibrodysplasia. *A,* Fragmentation of internal elastic lamina; subendothelial and medial fibroplasia are apparent. (Verhoeff's stain; original magnification ×32.) *B,* Accumulation of acid mucopolysaccharides (pale blue areas) can be noted throughout the vessel wall. (Abul Haj stain; original magnification ×32.)

2 A

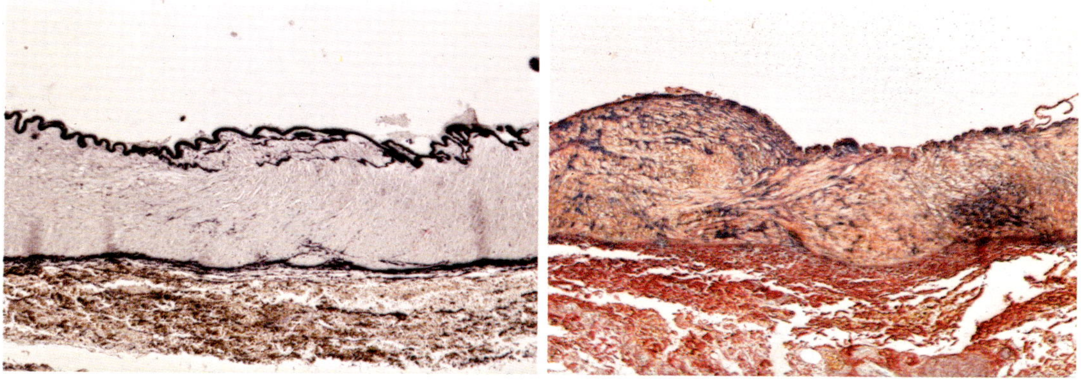

2 B

Fig. 2. Splenic artery cross section in a patient without demonstrable cause of aneurysmal disease. *A,* Fragmentation with duplication of internal elastic lamina and paucity of medial elastic tissue. (Verhoeff's stain; original magnification ×32.) *B,* Excessive acid mucopolysaccharides (dark blue areas) exist in the media. (Alcian Green stain; original magnification ×32.)

3

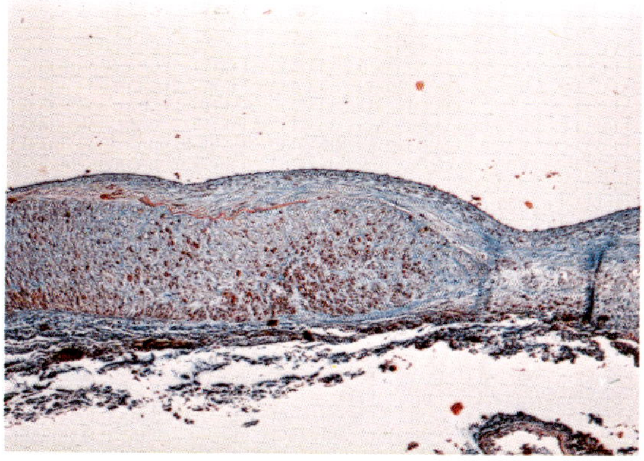

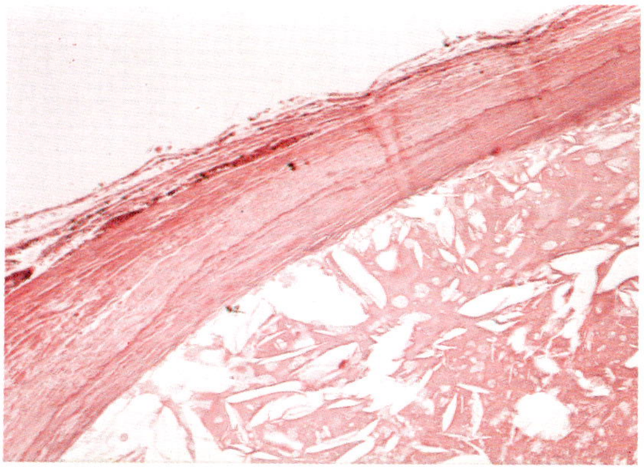

4

Fig. 3. Splenic artery aneurysm cross section revealing subendothelial fibroplasia and apparent medial hyperplasia adjacent to an area of fibroplasia. (Masson stain; original magnification ×32.)

Fig. 4. Splenic artery aneurysm cross section exhibiting marked fibrosis with cholesterol clefts and calcific atherosclerosis obscuring normal vessel wall architecture. (Hematoxylin and eosin stain—decalcified; original magnification ×32.)

had symptoms directly referable to their aneurysms. Suffice it to say that morbidity attributable to intact splenic artery aneurysms is minimal.

Risk of unexpected splenic artery aneurysm rupture is much less than earlier reports claimed. Data from a large group of patients at another institution revealed an incidence of rupture equaling 9.2 percent.[19, 20] Aneurysmal rupture affected 5.3 percent of our patients (excluding three patients with rupture associated with inflammatory processes which would have doubled this rate). Risk of life-threatening rupture is less among bland aneurysms. Two of three ruptures in our series were covert, involving adjacent venous structures for which nonemergent splenectomy was performed. Manifestations of splenic artery aneurysm rupture (double rupture, intestinal hemorrhage, etc.) and surgical therapy for ruptured as well as intact aneurysms have been thoroughly described in earlier reports.[7, 9, 11, 16, 17, 20, 21] It is important to recognize the fact that aneurysmal calcification, normotension, and age greater than 60 years *do not* preclude rupture of aneurysms. Death from ruptured aneurysms in nonpregnant patients from 1960 to 1970 was 25 percent,[21] and appears slightly less today. Symptomatic aneurysms warrant operation provided operative risks do not appear excessive. Elective surgical treatment of bland splenic artery aneurysms, to be justified, cannot engender an operative mortality rate much greater than 1 percent.

Hazards of splenic artery aneurysm rupture during pregnancy have been formidable.[11] Since our last review of the subject,[21] a 68 percent mortality rate ascribed to aneurysms occurring during pregnancy has not changed. All but one of the 77 cases in pregnancy have been associated with rupture. Operative intervention is strongly recommended in women of child-bearing age who may subsequently conceive and is mandatory in the patient already pregnant.

The authors wish to gratefully acknowledge contributions to this work by Millicent W. Higgins, M.D., D.P.H., and George W. Williams, Ph.D. (University of Michigan School of Public Health); and Gerald D. Abrams, M.D., Joseph J. Bookstein, M.D., and Vikrom Sottiurai, M.D., Ph.D. (University of Michigan Medical School).

REFERENCES

1. Baird, J. T., Jr., and Quinlivan, L. G.: National Center for Health Statistics: Parity and hypertension, *in* Vital and health statistics, Series II, No. 38, Washington, 1972, United States Public Health Service.
2. Bedford, P. D., and Lodge, B.: Aneurysm of the splenic artery, Gut **1:** 312, 1960.
3. Blendis, L., Kreel, L., and Williams, R.: The coeliac axis and its branches in splenomegaly and liver disease, Gut **10:** 85, 1969.
4. Boijsen, E., and Efsing, H.-O.: Aneurysm of the splenic artery, Acta Radiol. [Diagn.] (Stockh.) **8:** 29, 1969.
5. Danforth, D. N., and Buckingham, J. C.: Connective tissue mechanisms and their relation to pregnancy, Obstet. Gynecol. Surv. **19:** 715, 1964.
6. Dent, T. L., Lindenauer, S. M., Ernst, C. B., and Fry, W. J.: Multiple arteriosclerotic arterial aneurysms, Arch. Surg. **105:** 338, 1972.
7. Deterling, R. A.: Aneurysm of the visceral arteries, J. Cardiovasc. Surg. **12:** 309, 1971.
8. Harrison, E. G., Jr., and McCormack, L. J.: Pathologic classification of renal arterial disease in renovascular hypertension, Mayo Clin. Proc. **46:** 161, 1971.
9. Jones, E. L., and Finney, G. G.: Splenic artery aneurysms. A reappraisal, Arch. Surg. **97:** 640, 1968.
10. Kreel, L.: The recognition and incidence of splenic artery aneurysms. A historical review, Aust. Radiol. **16:** 126, 1972.
11. MacFarlane, J. R., and Thorbjarnarson, B.: Rupture of splenic artery aneurysm during pregnancy, Am. J. Obstet. Gynecol. **95:** 1025, 1966.
12. Manalo-Estrella, P., and Barker, A. E.: Histopathologic findings in human aortic media associated with pregnancy. A study of 16 cases, Arch. Pathol. **83:** 336, 1967.
13. Manalo-Estrella, P., Danforth, D. N., and Buckingham, J. C.: Regression rate of vascular effects induced by pregnancy and by norethynodrel-mestranol, Fertil. Steril. **16:** 81, 1965.
14. Manenti, F., and Williams, R.: Injection studies of the splenic vasculature in portal hypertension, Gut **7:** 175, 1966.
15. Moore, S. W., and Lewis, R. J.: Splenic artery aneurysm, Ann. Surg. **153:** 1033, 1961.
16. Moore, S. W., Guida, P. M., and Schumacher, H. W.: Splenic artery aneurysm, Bull. Soc. Int. Chir: **29:** 210, 1970.
17. Owens, J. C., and Coffey, R. J.: Aneurysm

of the splenic artery including a report of six additional cases, Int. Abst. Surg. **97:** 313, 1953.
18. Reuter, S. R., and Redman, H. C.: Intrasplenic arterial aneurysms, J. Can. Assoc. Radiol. **19:** 200, 1968.
19. Spittel, J. A., Fairbairn, J. F., Kincaid, O. W., and ReMine, W. H.: Aneurysm of the splenic artery, J. A. M. A. **175:** 452, 1961.
20. Spittel, J. A., Fairbairn, J. F., Sheps, S. O., Kincaid, O. W., and ReMine, W. H.: Splenic artery aneurysm, Surg. Clin. North Am. **41:** 1121, 1961.
21. Stanley, J. C., Thompson, N. W., and Fry, W. J.: Splanchnic artery aneurysms, Arch. Surg. **101:** 689, 1970.
22. Stanley, J. C., Fry, W. J., Seeger, J. F., Hoffman, G. L., and Grabrielsen, T. O.: Extracranial internal carotid and vertebral artery fibrodysplasia, Arch. Surg. **109:** 215, 1974.
23. Wexler, B. C.: Vascular degenerative changes in the uterine arteries and veins of multiparous rats, Am. J. Obstet. Gynecol. **107:** 6, 1970.
24. Williams, R., Condon, R. E., Williams, H. S., Blendis, L. M., and Kreel, L.: Splenic blood flow in cirrhosis and portal hypertension, Clin. Sci. **34:** 441, 1968.
25. Wylie, E. J., Binkley, F. M., and Palubinskas, A. J.: Extrarenal fibromuscular hyperplasia, Am. J. Surg. **112:** 149, 1966.

DISCUSSION

Dr. Ralph A. Deterling, Jr. (Boston, Mass.). Drs. Stanley and Fry's break with the traditional view that many splenic aneurysms are arteriosclerotic is indeed supported by their histologic studies and repeated demonstrations of medial fibrodysplasia in the splenic artery. Even when arteriosclerosis is present, it is convincing that another organic factor is in effect.

With regard to the sex incidence, we have found a 3:1 ratio of women to men in a group of 13. Two of seven multiparous patients had over six pregnancies. We, too, observed other patients with associated portal hypertension or arterial hypertension as described by the authors.

I suspect that a mechanical stress factor may also be significant in a tortuous long splenic artery. I call attention to perhaps similar hemodynamics as seen in the right carotid artery of hypertensive females where kinking and buckling develop. Some of us also can remember the high incidence of aneurysms in the long femoropopliteal homograft bypasses of the 1950's.

Hence, the stress factor associated with repeated pregnancies and elevated portal pressures or flow in arterial hypertension may have a selective effect on the splenic artery. The great majority of these lesions are single lesions at the bifurcation near the hilus.

A further study really should be made to determine the exact incidence of splenic aneurysm. The usual figures we see range from 1:1,000 to 1:100 autopsies. However, in 1960 Bedford and Lodge in England demonstrated a 10 percent incidence in 250 elderly patients with very careful autopsies. Many of these, however, were very minute lesions with no surgical implications.

We are greatly indebted to Drs. Stanley and Fry for helping us to determine more precise indications for surgical intervention and we agree that the female patient in childbearing age is at much greater risk for rupture and the attendant mortality rate is high.

Dr. Makis J. Tsapogas (Albany, N. Y.). As is apparent in certain instances of splenic artery aneurysm, vascular reconstruction following resection is not technically feasible nor indeed necessary. The splenic artery is also occasionally used for revascularization of neighboring viscera. In both instances this artery can be only ligated without necessarily removing the spleen. In one of our recent experimental studies in Albany, a segment of the splenic artery in dogs was ligated and resected, followed by splenectomy 16 weeks later. No significant changes were exhibited after ligation in the hematological picture, the scanning, and the histology of the spleen. However, in the splenectomized animals, the results of the hematological tests were markedly altered after operation.

In a second series of experiments, complete dearterialization of the spleen was performed. In about half of these animals, there were profound changes in the above parameters.

These experimental data have reinforced our clinical approach and that of others not to remove the healthy spleen when reconstruction of the artery is not feasible, when the artery is to be used for revascularization of other viscera, or if splenectomy is technically difficult. Care is taken during the dissection not to unduly disturb the short gastric vessels and other attachments to the spleen.

May I ask the authors what surgical procedures they employed in their series and if they observed any variation in the laboratory or other findings which could be correlated with the type of operation performed?

Dr. Donald R. Kahn (Madison, Wis.). I would like to change the subject to renal artery aneurysms just to make one point.

There has been speculation about the cause of hypertention in patients with renal artery aneurysms. We measured blood flows in the artery past the aneurysm before and after the aneurysm was resected. This renal artery aneurysm occurred just at the bifurcation of the renal artery. Flow in the uninvolved artery was 140 c.c. per minute and the artery of the same size past the aneurysm had a flow of only 60 c.c. per minute. After resection of the aneurysm and reanastomosis of this branch of the renal artery to the main renal artery, the flows became equal in the two branches.

This patient unquestionably had decreased blood flow to the lower pole of her kidney which was corrected by removing the aneurysm. She presented clinically with hypertension which was very difficult to control medically and now her hypertension is markedly improved. This observation suggests that, through some mechanism, there is a decrease in perfusion to the area of the kidney supplied by the artery involved in the aneurysm and that the patient's hypertension is on this basis.

Dr. Angelo Riberi (Youngstown, Ohio). In our cardiovascular service in Youngstown we have had about 13 cases of splenic artery aneurysms, 12 in women.

The standard operation has been through a subcostal incision by doing a splenectomy in continuity with the resection of the aneurysm as suggested by Dr. Tsapogas.

However, two patients showed very proximal aneurysms which lent themselves beautifully to simple resection and preservation of the spleen.

The only male patient showed portal hypertension by compression of the splenic vein from the aneurysm. Resection of the aneurysm and splenectomy resulted in a cure.

Dr. James C. Stanley (Closing). The importance of mechanical factors referred to by Dr. Deterling in the development of splenic artery aneurysms has been the subject of much speculation. Arteriosclerosis frequently appears to be more extensive in the main splenic artery than in other similar-size vessels. This may be a reflection of the relatively untethered splenic artery becoming tortuous, with accelerated arteriosclerosis occurring subsequently at sites of unusual physical stresses. Increased velocity and volume blood flow rates associated with pregnancy or portal hypertension would be expected to potentiate these events. Splenic artery arteriosclerosis can be attributed to such factors, but aneurysms are not believed to evolve as part of this pathologic process. Nonatherosclerotic medial derangements at bifurcations are considered to be the basis of most splenic artery aneurysms.

The actual incidence of these aneurysms is crucial to understanding their clinical significance. Reports of these lesions in nearly 10 percent of the population have not been borne out by recent arteriographic surveys. In discussing splenic artery aneurysms recognized by conventional diagnostic means, an incidence similar to the 0.78 percent presently reported seems realistic.

Arteriolosclerosis and stromal fibrosis were frequent histologic findings in spleens removed from patients with these aneurysms. As such, these changes were not unlike those in spleens from patients of similar age undergoing splenectomy for other reasons. Examination of spleens to determine effects of proximal splenic artery interruption in two patients of our series has not occurred, in that both retained their intact spleens without incident.

Distal splenic artery bifurcations, often within the splenic hilus, are the most common loci of aneurysms. Splenectomy in such instances is the preferred and most logical form of operative treatment. Proximal aneurysms, in contrast, can be excised locally with avoidance of hazardous dissection of the splenic artery in its entirety from retropancreatic tissues. Careful surgical technique and appropriate precautions, should postsplenectomy thrombocytosis occur, lessen the likelihood of significant operative morbidity attending treatment of these patients.

Renal artery aneurysms are intriguing and, interestingly, were encountered in five of our patients with similar splenic artery aneurysms. In collating data from the recent experience with more than 70 patients having renal artery aneurysms at the University of Michigan Medical Center, certain facts emerge. A cause-effect relation of these lesions to hypertension is very difficult to establish, and, not infrequently, the opposite appears equally plausible. Among many of these patients with renal artery aneurysms, intimal cushions or fibrodysplastic stenoses can be demonstrated as the cause of renovascular hypertension.

The intent of this work is to provide a better understanding of splenic artery aneurysms. Continued follow-up of patients harboring aneurysms *not* subjected to operative intervention should allow identification of still undefined risk factors leading to aneurysmal rupture. A more rational basis for operative treatment of bland splenic artery aneurysms will then be forthcoming.

Surgical therapy for venous stasis

Ralph G. De Palma, M.D., *Cleveland, Ohio*

Dermatitis, induration, and stasis ulcerations are common and distressing complications of venous insufficiency of the lower extremities. Since these skin changes are related to venous hypertension in superficial and communicating veins from the deep venous system, ideal therapy consists of elimination of the offending veins and skin grafting of ulcers or areas of advanced stasis. However, the traditional operative approaches are regarded as hazardous, owing to the need for creation of extensive longitudinal flaps which are prone to necrosis. Conservative therapy is often chosen; it is notoriously demanding of the time of both physician and patient. A modified operative approach to this problem was begun in 1966. Its long-term results have been gratifying in 38 operations. In this procedure, rather than an elevation of long longitudinal flaps, a series of "safe" parallel bipedicled skin flaps were created in the natural skin lines of the extremity. A ratio of flap surface to blood supply of at least 1:2 was used in planning flaps along with the location of ulcers and incompetent perforating veins. With this technique, perforating veins from the crest of the tibia to the Achilles tendon posteriorly could be ligated along with skin grafting of ulcers at the same operation. Postoperatively, the extremities were immobilized in a splint and elevated for 10 days, dependency with pressure support hose was begun on the twelfth to the fourteenth day, and ambulation begun by the fourteenth to the sixteenth day. The average hospital stay for 31 patients was 19 days. Necrosis of the flaps was absent; incisions healed with fine, inconspicuous scars. All patients were re-examined at least annually. Continued use of pressure support hose and triamcinolone cream to areas of pigmentation appeared to result in regression of induration and pigmentation. One minor recurrence was noted in a patient not using support; some of the patients spontaneously adopted lighter and more cosmetically attractive hose without ill effect. The safety and long-term sucess of this procedure have encouraged more liberal and prompt use of surgical treatment for advanced venous stasis of the lower extremities.

From the Department of Surgery, University Hospitals of Cleveland and Case Western Reserve University, Cleveland, Ohio.

DERMATITIS, induration, and stasis ulceration are common and distressing complications of chronic venous insufficiency of the lower extremities. These changes in the skin and subcutaneous tissue are caused by venous hypertension in superficial and communicating veins from the deep venous system. Ideal therapy consists of elimination of the offending veins and skin grafting of ulcers and areas of advanced stasis dermatitis. In 1938 Linton[2] described the anatomy of the communicating veins of the lower leg and techniques for their ligation. He recognized that it was imperative to interrupt

Presented at the Twenty-eighth Annual Meeting of the Society for Vascular Surgery, Chicago, Ill., June 20 and 21, 1974.

Reprint requests: Ralph G. DePalma, M.D., Department of Surgery, University Hospitals of Cleveland and Case Western University, 2065 Adelbert Rd., Cleveland, Ohio 44106.

incompetent communicating or perforating veins to control the effects of venous insufficiency. Subsequently, operations were described for both subfascial[3] and extrafascial[1, 5] ligation of communicating veins with grafting of ulcers and stripping of incompetent long and short saphenous veins.

Currently, with better understanding of the disordered anatomy and physiology leading to stasis changes and revised operative approaches, the results of operation for chronic venous insufficiency of the lower extremities have improved. In most descriptions of operation for chronic venous stasis, there has been a preference for longitudinal flaps. In spite of stress on meticulous handling of traditional extensive longitudinal flaps, these incisions have been regarded as hazardous because of the risks of necrosis and retarded primary healing.[3] Thus conservative therapy is often chosen for chronic venous insufficiency; however, it is notoriously demanding of time of both physician and patient. Because of dissatisfaction with time, expense, and difficulties of both conservative and traditional operative therapies, a modified operative approach to this problem was begun in 1966. The time used in preoperative and postoperative treatment was greatly shortened and long-term results were sufficiently gratifying to warrant this report.

TECHNIQUE

Postoperative care. The patient is admitted to the hospital for an interval of strict bed rest with the extremity elevated above the level of the right atrium. The ulcer is cultured and wet-to-dry one percent neomycin compresses are used every 6 hours. Tetracycline, 250 mg. four times a day, is begun; if betahemolytic streptococcus is isolated, or if cellulitis is present, penicillin is also given. Patients with pruritic dermatitis are treated with triamcinolone cream, 0.025 percent, applied to the areas of skin excoriation and discoloration. Soaks to areas of dermatitis are avoided since water almost always exacerbates the severity of stasis dermatitis. When systemic reaction or eczema is present, oral triamcinolone, 2 mg. three times a day, is also prescribed. After this preparation, usually lasting 3 to 5 days, operation is performed. No attempt is made to attain preliminary healing of the ulcer nor are preliminary debridements of skin grafts performed prior to operation. The usual methods of clinical examination[4] are used to localize superficial veins and communicators which are marked preoperatively with a ballpoint pen.

Operative technique. Ideally, the operation aims at complete interruption of communicating veins, complete removal of incompetent superficial veins, and skin grafting of ulcers. In this modified procedure, however, rather than creation of longitudinal flaps for ligation of communicating veins, a series of "safe" parallel bipedicled skin flaps are created in the natural skin lines of the extremity. With this technique, perforating veins from the crest of the tibia to the Achilles tendon posteriorly can be ligated along with skin grafting of ulcers and stripping of incompetent long or short saphenous veins at the same operation.

With the patient in a supine position for the usual medial dissection, the entire extremity is prepared with 5 percent Amphyl solution.* The ulcer is carefully isolated from the clean operative field and separately draped (Figs. 1*A* and 1*B*) Fig. 2 shows the usual anatomy of the incompetent long saphenous vein and incompetent medial communicating veins. For coverage of ulceration or replacement of severely involved skin, a 14 to 16 one thousandth inch skin graft is first taken from the lateral aspect of the thigh with a Brown dermatome; for more extensive skin replacement, a Reese dermatome is occasionally necessary.

The greater saphenous vein is then stripped from ankle to groin with incisions placed in the natural skin creases. This step is completed before entering the contaminated field of the ulcer. The transverse ankle incision for access to the long saphenous vein can be isolated from the ulcer since the

*Lehn and Fink Products Corp., 4934 Lewis Ave., Toledo, Ohio.

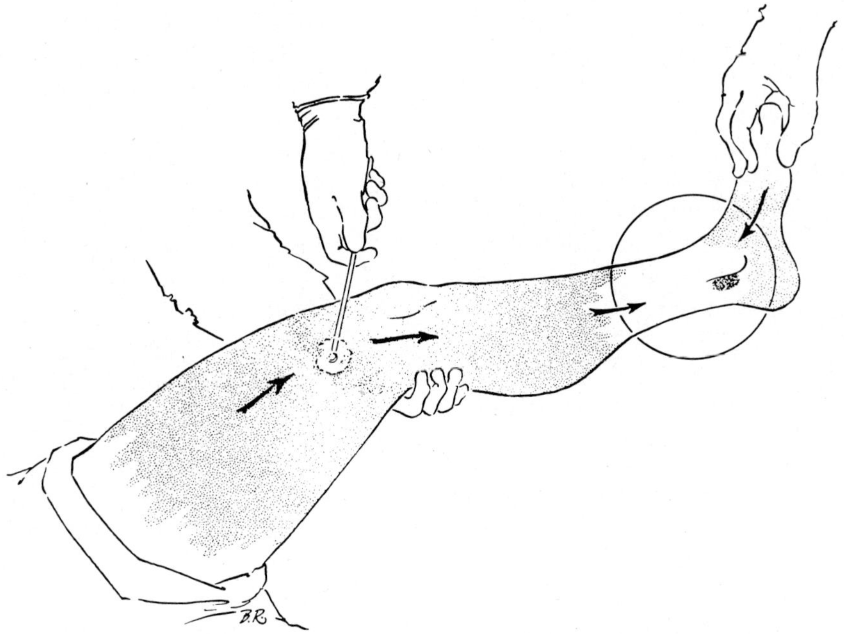

Fig. 1A. Preparation of skin of lower extremity to avoid contaminated field. Ulcer prepared last.

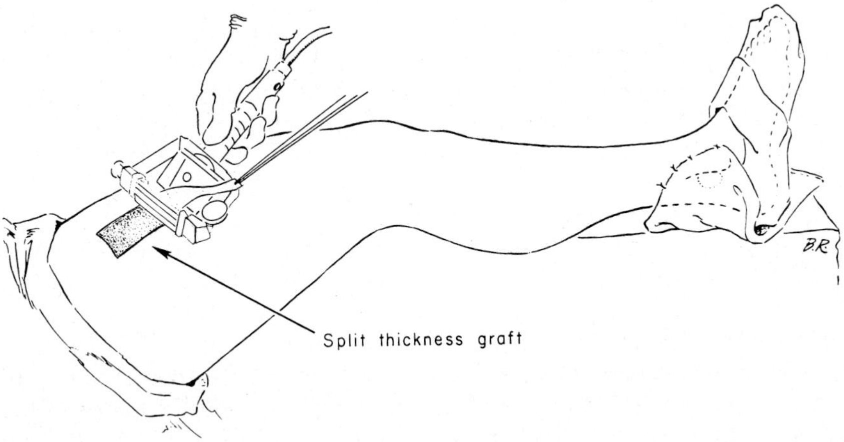

Fig. 1B. Draping to isolate ulcer from the clean operative field prior to long saphenous vein stripping. Split thickness graft taken prior to beginning dissection.

course of the main vein is almost always anterior to the ulcer. After stripping of the long saphenous vein, the ankle and groin incisions are then closed with fine Dermalon sutures.

A series of parallel flaps is designed according to the location of perforators and that of the ulcer (Fig. 2). The direction of the incisions is determined by the natural skin creases (Fig. 3). It has been found that these flaps on the lower leg will succeed if the dimensions of the flaps are maintained in a ratio of blood supply to length of at least 1:2. The excised border of the ulcer serves as the edge of a flap; access to the important lowest communicator is achieved through elevation of the edge of the ulcer as far as the Achilles tendon. In cases in which the subcutaneous tissue is not seriously effaced, the skin and subcutaneous tissue can be dissected from the deep fascia (Fig. 4). The extrafascial dissection must extend

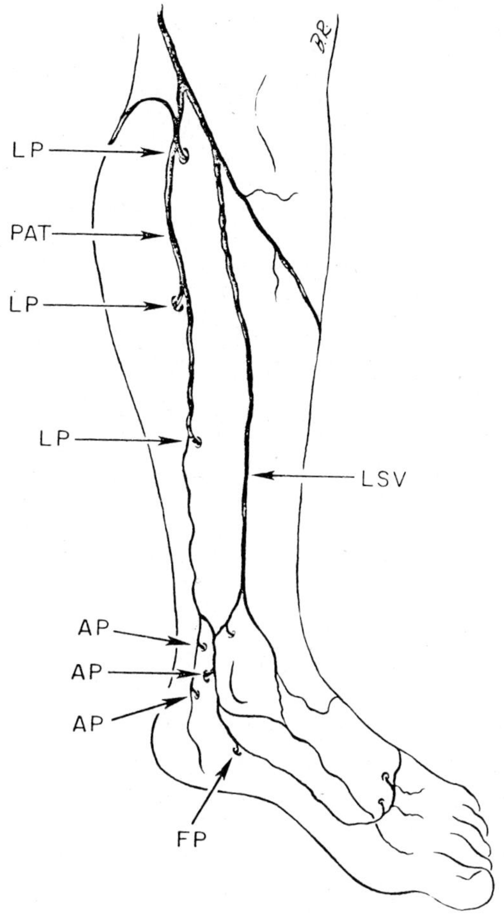

Fig. 2. Long saphenous vein (LSV) and representative arrangements of frequently observed communicating veins. PAT = posterior arch tributary connecting; LP = leg perforators; AP = ankle perforators; FP = foot perforators—may also be important. Adapted from Linton,[2] and Dodd and Cockett.[1]

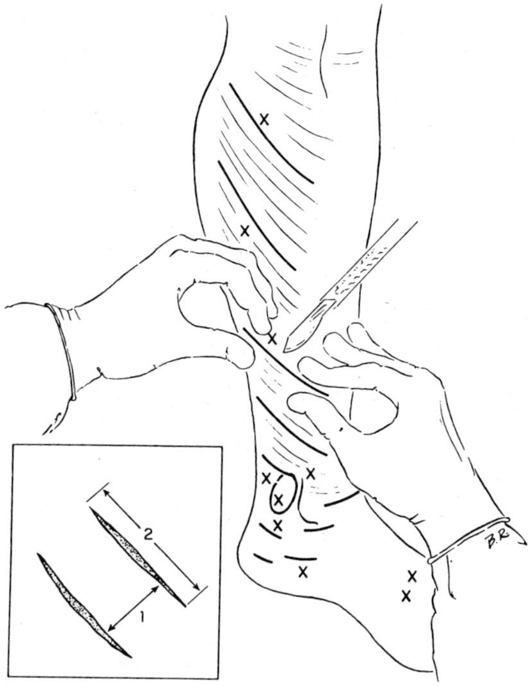

Fig. 3. Typical incisions for flaps in relation to skin lines and frequently encountered communicating veins. Insert: relative dimensions of safe parallel flaps.

from the crest of the tibia anteriorly to the Achilles tendon and to the soleus muscle posteriorly. Elevation of skin flaps will usually extend from a point 3 cm. below the medial malleolus to the upper third of the leg. By gently elevating and retracting the flaps with fine skin hooks, all communicating veins in undermined areas can be visualized and accurately ligated with No. 3-0 chromic catgut. Whether the dissection is to be subfascial or extrafascial is determined by the degree of subcutaneous fibrosis in the lower one third of the leg.

In cases in which the subcutaneous tissue in the lower leg has been effaced due to advanced stasis changes (bottle leg), the deep fascia can be entered through the excised ulcer bed as well as through parallel deep incisions under the flaps (Fig. 5). In this dissection, the posterior tibial artery and vein are visualized; perforating veins arising from the posterior tibial vein are ligated individually. Small branches of the posterior tibial artery often pass from the deep compartment with the communicating veins. These small arteries are ligated along with the veins, but care must be excercised to avoid damage to the posterior tibial artery. The dissection may be difficult due to inflammatory changes. Occasional fine silk arterial suture ligatures must be applied to the posterior tibial artery for control of short, friable, small arteries which accompany the perforating veins.

Upon completion of stripping of superficial veins, ligation of communicators under all flaps, and excision of the ulcer along with adjacent areas of severe stasis dermatitis, the skin graft is sutured into the ulcer defect with fine silk. This graft is dressed with

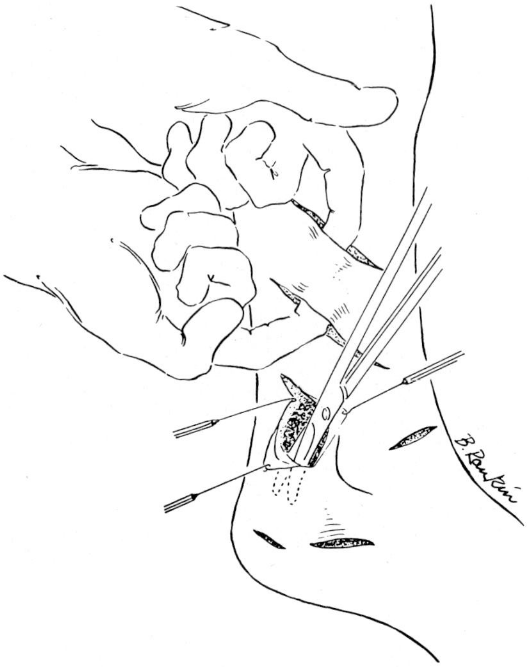

Fig. 4. Dissection of flaps and edge of ulcer for extrafascial ligation of perforators. The dissection extends from crest of tibia anteriorly to Achilles tendon posteriorly.

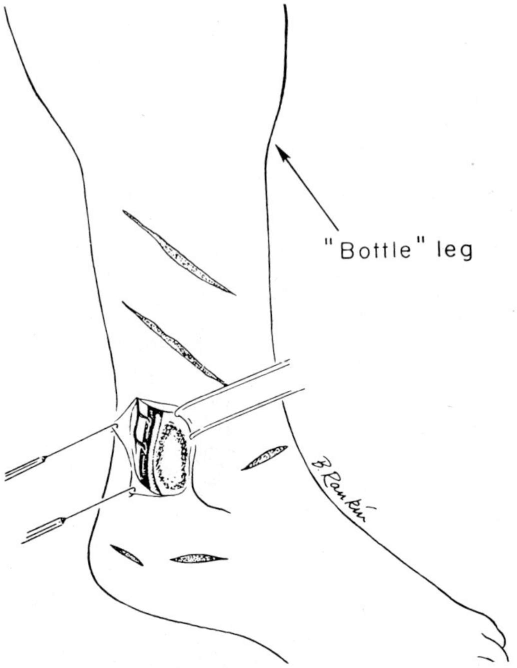

Fig. 5. Subfascial dissection and ligation of perforators from posterior tibial vein.

Xeroform gauze and a stent of a bolus of cotton (Fig. 6).

All incisions used for flaps are then closed with No. 4-0 Dermalon. No subcutaneous sutures are used, as these frequently extrude even when fine chromic catgut is used. The deep fascia is not sutured unless muscle obviously herniates through the incision. Parallel flaps can be extended easily to include anterior communicating veins when needed. The procedure for lateral involvement and for lateral ulcers is planned and accomplished in a similar fashion. The short sapheneous vein is usually stripped from the ankle to the popliteal fossa in these instances with the patient in the prone position.

Postoperative care. The leg is immobilized from foot to knee in a bulkily padded posterior molded splint. Strict bed rest is maintained with the extremity elevated for a period of 10 to 14 days—this is absolutely essential to ensure success of the flaps and skin graft. Antibiotics are continued for 7 to 10 days. To assist in prevention of thromboembolism, the patient is instructed to exercise his toes for 10 minutes each hour while awake. Since, in the past 12 months, two instances of pulmonary embolism were observed, low-dose heparinization, 2,000 U. intravenously or subcutaneously every 6 hours, is initiated on the second day after operation.

Unless fever or pain occur, the splint is not removed until the eighth day after operation. At this time the graft is dressed and sutures from the skin graft are removed. It is important to assure firm gentle pressure on the skin graft for a prolonged period. Flap sutures are removed from 12 to 14 days after operation and dependency of the extremity with pressure support hose is begun progressively on the twelfth to fourteenth day. Ambulation is started on the tenth to fourteenth day, depending on the status of the wounds. Prior to discharge, the patient is measured for permanent support hose* and preferably begins their use while hospitalized. The patient is instructed in their application during the day when

*Jobst, 30 to 40 mm. Hg.

Table I. *Anatomic distribution of lesions and procedures: 38 extremities*

	Women	*Men*	*Total limbs*
1. Medial communicators and incompetent long saphenous vein	20	6	26
2. Medial communicators only. Prior saphenous stripping	6		6
3. Lateral communicators and incompetent short saphenous vein	3	1	4
4. Lateral communicators only	1		1
5. Anterior communicators, medial communicators, and long saphenous vein		1	1
Total	30	8	38

first arising. Support is not used after retiring. Triamcinolone cream, 0.025 percent, is applied nightly to areas of darkened skin and bathing or soaking the extremity in water is avoided for at least 4 weeks.

RESULTS

The patients ranged in age from 36 to 78 years, with 10 in the sixth and seventh decades of life. Most of the older patients had suffered the pain, inconvience, and expense of "conservative" treatment for these stasis ulcers for over a decade. The older patients healed well in spite of extensive dissection required for ablation of venous insufficiency.

Thirty-eight procedures were performed from 1966 through 1973 on 31 patients with advanced stasis changes in the skin and subcutaneous tissues of the lower extremity due to the postphlebitic syndrome (Table I). In the majority of patients, the medial group of lower leg perforators described by Linton [2, 3] were involved.

The average hospital stay for all patients was 19 days. No major wound infections or sepsis were noted. In the last 15 patients (1969 through 1973), the preoperative preparation period ranged from 2 to 5 days, as it was found that it was possible to shorten this interval without risk of sepsis. Necrosis of flaps was absent; the skin line incisions favored primary healing of flaps since less tension occurs at the suture line.

Although sepsis was not a problem, pulmonary embolism occurred in two patients, one woman, 61 years of age, and one man, 37 years of age. In the former patient the clinical diagnosis was clear; in the latter, clinical manifestations were quite minor. Both diagnoses were confirmed by pulmonary scan using microspheres of human serum albumin tagged with technetium-99^m. Both patients recovered uneventfully with appropriate anticoagulation.

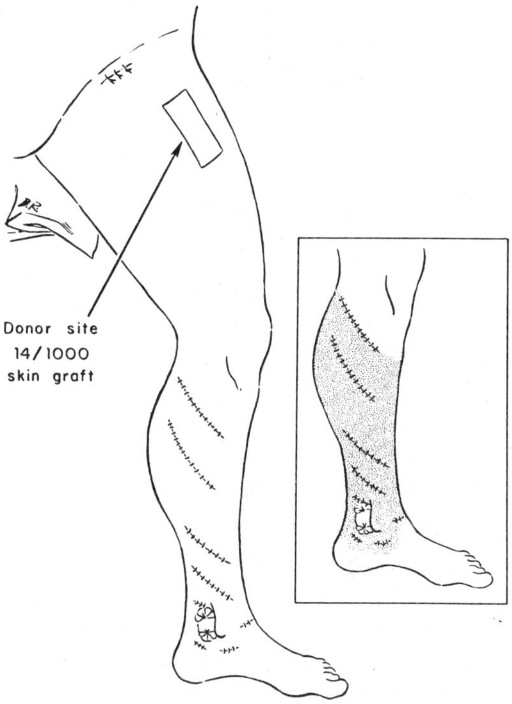

Fig. 6. Completed procedure for medial involvement. Incisions for flaps closed with fine nylon sutures. Insert: area dissected to ensure complete ligation of incompetent perforators.

DISCUSSION

The distressing amount of time, expense, and social disability associated with venous stasis of the lower extremities has been pointed out by Linton.[3] As yet, many physicians treat this problem with a variety of conservative, sometimes ineffective, and usually time-consuming methods. For many patients, a chronic venous leg ulcer becomes a way of life. In this experience, the safety and long-term success of surgical therapy encouraged more liberal operative intervention. Many patients can be relieved of invalidism, provided they understand the need for continued postoperative elastic support, learn to care for the affected skin properly, and report regularly for follow-up examinations.

The risks of operation appear to be minimal; with careful observation and use of prophylactic heparin therapy, the complications of pulmonary embolism can probably be averted. This risk is present in any circumstance requiring bed rest and is probably not peculiar to this particular operation. Thus for younger patients, the severe long-term economic and social disabilities of chronic venous stasis make clear the indication for surgical therapy. The present procedure avoids long periods of hospitalization and usually improves the appearance of the extremity.

Aged patients who are acceptable as anesthetic and operative risks should be more aggressively considered for surgical therapy than they have been in the past, since safety of primary healing and absence of sepsis can be achieved. A special problem of the aged patient is the occasional coexistence of arterial insufficiency with long-standing venous insufficiency. Since physical findings alone may not be reliable in these patients, femoral arteriography is required to plan treatment of chronic ulceration. Fortunately, combined arterial and venous ulcers are not the rule; when this combination occurs, quite obviously arterial reconstruction takes precedence over treatment of venous insufficiency.

REFERENCES

1. Dodd, H., and Cockett, F. B.: The pathology and surgery of the veins of the lower limb, Edinburgh and London, 1956, E. & S. Livingstone, Ltd., pp. 424-447.
2. Linton, R. R.: The communicating veins of the lower leg and the operative technique for their ligation, Ann. Surg. **107:** 582, 1938.
3. Linton, R. R.: The postthrombotic ulceration of the lower extremity: Its etiology and surgical treatment, Ann. Surg. **138:** 415, 1953.
4. Lofgren, K. A.: *In* Fairbairn, T. F., II, Juergens, J. L., and Spittell, J. A., editors: Peripneral vascular disease, Philadelphia, 1972, W. B. Saunders Company, pp. 607-609.
5. Lofgren, K. A.: *In* Fairbairn, T. F., II, Juergens, J. L., and Spittell, J. A., editors: Peripheral vascular disease, Philadelphia, 1972, W. B. Saunders Company, pp. 630-634.

DISCUSSION

Dr. Robert C. Lim (San Francisco, Calif.). We also have been interested in the postphlebitic syndrome for a long time and would like to share with you an alternative approach to handling this problem. We use a single posterior midline seam incision. The skin flaps are mobilized anteriorly around the subfascial plane. The communicating veins are identified, ligated, and divided.

Placement of the incision over the posterior midline area avoids making incisions over the areas of greater skin change, i.e., over pigmented, firm, brawny skin, which often led to wound complications. In the last 10 years we have used this posterior approach on more than 40 patients and have experienced only rare skin flap complications.

Dr. John J. Cranley (Cincinnati, Ohio). When we last presented our experience with the Linton procedure in 1960, one of the discussants, whose remarks were not recorded, chided us severely for discussing the subject with only a 7 year follow-up. So we have been quiet for 14 years!

The failure rate of 5.5 percent (of 174 operations) after excisional therapy could, I believe, be easily explained by error in diagnosis. In general, we consider these ulcers to be curable, by which we mean that the patient, following operation, leads a normal life without the use of elastic support.

The discussant in 1960 advised us correctly: we certainly have had recurrences, even after 10 years.

Our data present the results of the Linton procedure in the worst possible light for at least four reasons: (1) many of the recurrences were due to patient neglect; (2) some are due to recurrent disease or to recurrent trauma; (3) most of the recurrences are minor and are easily controlled by a pressure bandage; (4) but, primarily, the recurrence rate is skewed because this is a highly selective series, representing only 22 percent of patients seen with postphlebitic ulceration. The remaining 78 percent were treated conservatively. Only the worst cases, those difficult or impossible to manage by conservative measures, have been treated surgically.

Now I would like to review four cases showing extremities of patients photographed at 16, 17, two at 19, and two at 21 years postoperatively. One patient walked into our office this year with an ulcer on her right ankle, as shown in this photo, and said, "Well, doctor, it isn't nearly as bad as it was on my *left* side! Remember, you operated on me years ago, in 1955?" I think you can see the faint scar from that Linton procedure on the medial aspect of her *left* leg.

In another case we had a 21 year follow-up of an extremity that has remained healed throughout all that time.

Another case consists of a patient who had undergone two previous operations for her veins plus injection therapy. The induration was so tough that I broke two scalpels trying to penetrate it and finally had to cut it with scissors. The whole area sloughed, requiring a skin graft that was applied a short time after operation. This patient has now remained healed for 21 years, and the leg appears to be in excellent condition.

In concluding, I do believe that the principles and the technique recommended by Dr. Linton are still valid and are the most successful for the management of those patients who cannot be managed conservatively.

Dr. W. Andrew Dale (Nashville, Tenn.). How many of these people can be removed from elastic support or, conversely, from how many legs can the stockings be removed?

Dr. Ralph G. De Palma (Closing). Dr. Lim, I have not personally used the posterior approach though I am familiar with it. I have feared slough or skin loss over the Achilles tendon.

I agree that cutting into these areas of diseased skin frightens one at first. If one adheres to the skin lines and especially prepares this area with steroid cream, the operative approach is much more satisfactory.

Dr. Cranley, I, too, try to be quiet about the results of this kind of surgery, recognizing that here we have only an 8 year follow-up. All of these cases presented today were not simple saphenous incompetence, but post-thrombotic extremities. Patient neglect, I agree, Dr. Cranley, is the major cause for recurrence.

To answer Dr. Dale's question, the patients who are able to discard the gradient support stockings are not encouraged to do so. We fit them for pressure support stockings in the hospital, insisting that they leave the hospital with their stockings in hand and properly fitted.

However, the ladies will occasionally revert to lighter and cosmetically more attractive support hose. I permit this, provided there is absolutely no occurrence of edema in the late afternoon or evening.

The moment edema begins—one can anticipate recurrence—I recommend that these patients continue to wear carefully fitted support hose, though an occasional exception can be made for evening wear.

Finally, in reference to the hardness of the skin and the pigmentation that Dr. Cranley showed in his slides and also to his beautiful results with the conventional Linton procedure, if you continue to use 0.025 percent triamcinolone cream on the areas of pigmentation, after operation, the skin softens and the pigmentation fades over the years.

Sinusoidal shunt fraction by radioextraction ratio

E. L. Bradley, III, M.D., D. L. Quinton, B.S., L. G. Martin, M.D., Evangelos Kourias, M.D., *and* James Larose, M.D., *Atlanta, Ga.*

A new technique for the measurement of hepatic sinusoidal perfusion and shunt fraction based upon the degree of extraction of particulate material by the hepatic reticuloendothelial system (RES) is presented. Repeated control determinations were highly reproducible ($p > 0.40$). Using each animal as its own control, significant increases ($p < 0.001$) in nonsinusoidal perfusion were noted after either side-to-side or end-to-side portacaval shunting. While further development is necessary, the principles underlying this study appear promising.

From the Department of Surgery and Radiology, Emory University School of Medicine and Affiliated Hospitals, Atlanta, Ga.

While the hemodynamic consequences of portasystemic shunting procedures in man have long been recognized,[4] the possibility that such hemodynamic alterations might have prognostic significance was first suggested by Warren and his coworkers.[17] This hemodynamic hypothesis has received widespread clinical acceptance and, in essence, states that patients with good hepatic blood flow poorly tolerate portasystemic shunting due to the acute reduction in portal flow accompanying these procedures. Conversely, patients with restricted portal flow to the liver have already adjusted to decreased portal perfusion and will not suffer the same degree of hepatic deterioration following portal diversion. This hypothesis has seemed so "logical" that various operative procedures have been specifically designed to decompress esophageal varices without significantly reducing portal perfusion.[1, 7, 12]

However, the hemodynamic premise that hepatic tolerance to portasystemic shunting is based upon the existing state of portal perfusion has not been adequately tested. This apparent lack of objectivity has, for the most part, been caused by the conspicuous absence of a reliable technique for measuring hepatic perfusion suitable for widespread use in man. There would appear to be a pressing need for an objective technique capable of (1) estimating the preoperative degree of *cellular* perfusion, and (2) comparing the relative hemodynamic consequences of various shunting procedures. The description of such a technique, which bears considerable promise in its present state of development, is the subject of the present report.

MATERIALS AND METHODS

General procedure. Mongrel dogs weighing 20 to 30 kilograms were anesthetized with intravenous phenobarbital (20 mg. per

Supported by United States Public Health Service Grant 8AM15736.

Presented at the Twenty-eighth Annual Meeting of the Society for Vascular Surgery, Chicago, Ill., June 20 and 21, 1974.

Reprint requests: E. L. Bradley, III, M.D., Department of Surgery, 69 Butler St., S.E., Atlanta, Ga. 30303.

kilogram) and placed on positive-pressure respiration after endotracheal intubation. The superior mesenteric artery was then catheterized via the brachial artery by the Seldinger technique. A scintillation counter, with strip chart recorder and tape activity counter (Picker Multiprober, Model 1390), was placed over the region of the femoral artery and calibrated to minimize background activity.

Isotopes for injection through the catheter were prepared immediately prior to each study. A volume of ^{99m}Tc pertechnetate ($^{99m}TcO_4$) in normal saline was added to a constant mass of sulfur colloid supplied in kit form (Tesuloid, E. R. Squibb, Princeton, N. J.). The resultant particle size* permitted free passage through all capillary and sinusoidal systems in the absence of active extraction. After thorough mixing, a volume of the ^{99m}Tc sulfur colloid ($^{99m}TcSC$) calculated to contain 0.12 mg. of colloid was withdrawn and diluted to a total volume of 5 c.c. by the addition of normal saline. Activity was then determined in a well counter and the exact time recorded. Preparation of the $^{99m}TcO_4$ solution involved removing a sufficient quantity from the generator to yield an activity of approximately 500 μCi per cubic centimeter of solution. This amount was injected into a 30 c.c. bottle of sterile saline. After withdrawing 5 c.c. of the resultant mixture, the total syringe activity was measured in a well counter and the time recorded.

Initially, the $^{99m}TcSC$ mixture was injected through the arterial catheter and the catheter was flushed with heparinized saline. The exact time of sulfur colloid injection was marked on the digital recorder. Detected sulfur colloid activity was continuously monitored at one second intervals over the femoral artery in a graphic plot of activity and time. After a 4 to 5 minute delay, the previously prepared $^{99m}TcO_4$ solution was then injected through the catheter, the exact time noted, and the catheter flushed with heparinized saline solution. Counting at the femoral artery continued for 3 minutes following the second injection. All isotope injections were made by hand and an attempt was made to evenly space the 5 c.c. injections over a 3 second period of injection. All dogs received 1.2 million U. of Bicillin* and one gram of streptomycin intramuscularly.

This procedure was carried out in each of 43 animals and served as the control value. Similar procedures were subsequently repeated in 10 dogs for determination of control reproducibility and in 26 dogs after portacaval shunting. While intervals between studies ranged from 3 days to 4 weeks, the majority of the studies were repeated at one week intervals.

Both side-to-side and end-to-side shunts were performed with a continuous suture of No. 5-0 synthetic suture. All end-to-side anastomoses were performed above the entrance of the gastrosplenic vein into the portal vein. The orifice of the gastrosplenic vein was easily visible during all side-to-side shunts. The stoma of the side-to-side shunt was constructed to be at least 2 cm. long. Although the stoma of the portal vein was beveled, the primary limiting factor in the size of the end-to-side orifices was the diameter of the portal vein. Shunt patency was determined when the animal was put to death.

Methods of calculation. Absolute activities of the injected material were calculated with the standard decay equation† by knowing the initial total syringe activity at a specific time—the time of injection—and then subtracting the residual measured activity remaining in the syringe after injection at another known time. The actually injected activities were then expressed as a ratio of $^{99m}TcSC$ to $^{99m}TcO_4$ (injected activity ratio = IAR).

Appearance of the specific isotope at the femoral artery was heralded by a rapid rise in digital one second counts over the baseline. The initial injection of $^{99m}TcSC$ presented little difficulty in detection, as its ac-

*Colloidal particle size 100 to 500 mμ.

*Wyeth Laboratories, Philadelphia, Pa.

†$A_t = A_0 e^{-\lambda t}$

Where: A_t = activity at time t; A_0 = original activity; and λ = decay constant.

Table I. *Control reproducibility**

IAR_1	DAR_1	$CDAR_1$	IAR_2	DAR_2	$CDAR_2$
0.72	0.26	0.18	0.39	0.09	0.12
0.28	0.09	0.16	0.77	0.21	0.16
0.60	0.12	0.10	0.43	0.12	0.14
0.31	0.13	0.21	0.41	0.16	0.20
0.79	0.21	0.13	0.80	0.16	0.11
0.35	0.15	0.22	0.48	0.21	0.22
0.36	0.17	0.23	0.45	0.15	0.17
0.40	0.12	0.15	0.38	0.15	0.20
0.39	0.14	0.18	0.47	0.14	0.15
0.94	0.16	0.08	0.72	0.17	0.12
	Mean	0.16			0.16
	S.D.	0.05			0.04

*IAR = injected activity ratio; DAR = detected activity ratio; CDAR = corrected detected activity ratio.

tivity was greatly increased over the baseline. Arbitrarily we chose to sum the first 60 counts and to divide by 60, giving an average detected activity per second. The subsequent injection of $^{99m}TcO_4$ presented another problem in detection. The detected activity representing the $^{99m}TcO_4$ injection was superimposed upon residual ^{99m}TcSC activity, resulting in a combined activity. A computer program was developed to predict the area under the combined curve occupied by residual ^{99m}TcSC. This activity was subtracted from combined activity, resulting in detected $^{99m}TcO_4$ activity alone. The detected activity was then expressed as a ratio of ^{99m}TcSC to $^{99m}TcO_4$ (detected activity ratio = DAR).

Although it was possible to keep the colloid mass and the injection volumes constant, actual injected activities of ^{99m}TcSC and $^{99m}TcO_4$ varied due to potency of the technetium generator with time. Since the detected activity ratio is dependent upon the actual activities, it was necessary to normalize all injected activity ratios to a single arbitrary value in order to compare repeated studies within each animal and individual results with all animals. Accordingly, all raw DAR calculations were corrected by a normalized IAR value:

$$\frac{0.5}{\text{IAR}} \times \text{DAR} = \text{Corrected DAR (CDAR)}.$$

Since there was no known reason to expect that the data generated by this experiment would form a normal distribution, a two-tailed value of the nonparametric Wilcoxon Rank Sum for paired results was used as the test of significance.

RESULTS

General. Random samples of the labeled sulfur colloid were subjected to gel diffusion to detect separation of the label from the colloid. Such separation could not be demonstrated on repeated analyses. Therefore, any activity appearing at the femoral vessel represented colloid not being extracted by the hepatic reticuloendothelial system (RES).

Control studies. In two animals activity appeared at the femoral artery probe almost simultaneously with the beginning of injection into the superior mesenteric artery. Since these observations could only be explained by leakage of ^{99m}TcSC from the superior mesenteric artery back into the aorta, a falsely high DAR was expected and obtained. In another animal, the labeled colloid was injected into a lumbar artery. Results from these three animals have been excluded from calculations. In the remaining 40 animals, the mean CDAR was 0.17 and the standard deviation 0.07.

In 10 dogs the baseline control study was repeated after a minimum delay of 15 half-lives to determine control reproducibility (Table I). No significant difference existed between the paired initial $CDAR_1$ and the subsequent $CDAR_2$ ($p > 0.40$).

Postoperative studies. Of the 26 animals undergoing portasystemic shunting, 22 were found at postmortem to have a venous stoma larger than one cm. and are included in the calculation of results. We were impressed by the seeming tendency of the portasystemic stoma to decrease in size with the passage of time. Two animals among the group, which were kept as late survivors, had stomal orifices of 3 and 4 mm. at death. Since we could not be certain that these animals had stomas one cm. at the time of repeat isotope study, these data have been excluded from calculation.

A highly significant difference was found between the control study ($CDAR_1$) and the

Table II. *Increase in peripherally detected activity ratio as a result of side-to-side portacaval shunting**

Control			After shunt		
IAR_1	DAR_1	$CDAR_1$	IAR_2	DAR_2	$CDAR_2$
0.28	0.09	0.16	0.27	0.62	1.17
0.38	0.09	0.12	0.53	0.96	0.90
0.60	0.12	0.10	0.61	0.77	0.63
0.31	0.13	0.21	0.45	0.59	0.64
0.36	0.14	0.20	0.51	0.67	0.67
0.72	0.13	0.09	0.60	0.95	0.80
0.62	0.14	0.11	0.33	0.54	0.80
0.86	0.13	0.08	0.29	0.65	1.14
0.42	0.08	0.09	0.38	0.62	0.81
0.51	0.11	0.11	0.35	0.48	0.68
0.37	0.09	0.12	0.44	1.40	1.58
	Mean	0.13			0.89
	S.D.	0.04			0.29

*IAR = injected activity ratio; DAR = detected activity ratio; CDAR = corrected detected activity ratio.

Table III. *Increase in peripherally detected activity as a result of end-to-side portacaval shunting**

Control			After shunt		
IAR_1	DAR_1	$CDAR_1$	IAR_2	DAR_2	$CDAR_2$
0.33	0.15	0.23	0.78	1.17	0.75
0.43	0.19	0.22	0.52	0.64	0.62
0.27	0.14	0.26	0.21	0.31	0.75
0.79	0.25	0.16	0.28	0.58	1.03
0.61	0.18	0.15	0.39	0.44	0.56
0.44	0.15	0.17	0.44	0.56	0.63
0.40	0.12	0.15	0.49	0.61	0.61
0.35	0.13	0.20	0.41	0.46	0.57
0.40	0.12	0.15	0.40	0.42	0.52
0.39	0.13	0.17	0.46	0.71	0.77
0.38	0.14	0.18	0.40	0.82	1.04
	Mean	0.18			0.71
	S.D.	0.04			0.17

*IAR = injected activity ratio; DAR = detected activity ratio; CDAR = corrected detected activity ratio.

Table IV. *Demonstration of shunt thrombosis**

Control			After shunt		
IAR_1	DAR_1	$CDAR_1$	IAR_2	DAR_2	$CDAR_2$
0.36	0.16	0.22	0.80	0.43	0.27
0.31	0.13	0.21	0.38	0.14	0.19

*IAR = injected activity ratio; DAR = detected activity ratio; CDAR = corrected detected activity ratio.

post-shunt study ($CDAR_2$) for both side-to-side (Table II) and end-to-side shunted animals (Table III). $CDAR_2$ was found to be significantly greater than $CDAR_1$ ($p < 0.001$) for each of the shunted groups.

On two other occasions the corrected postshunt DAR ($CDAR_2$) was similar to the control DAR ($CDAR_1$), suggesting no change in shunting fraction following operation. Death confirmed the clinical impression and isotope demonstration of thrombosed shunts (Table IV).

Although no concerted attempt was made to evaluate the reproducibility of the postshunt values, on two occasions postshunt DAR's were repeated. In each animal the range of variation did not exceed 10 percent of the initial postshunt value.

DISCUSSION

Many *indirect* methods of estimating hepatic perfusion have been proposed: measurement of wedged hepatic vein pressure and hepatic venous oxygen saturation,[15] splenoportography with measurement of splenic pulp pressure and estimate of portal flow velocity,[8] wedged hepatic vein venography in conjunction with indirect portography by superior mesenteric arteriography,[18] and umbilical vein catheterization with pressure measurements and portography.[2] In a type of subjective discriminate analysis, Warren and his co-workers[16] have constructed hemodynamic "classes" based upon data derived from such tests and have reported a correlation between these subjective flow patterns in the cirrhotic and the clinical responses to portacaval shunting. However, the validity in nonrandomized series of these subjective criteria as determinants of hepatic blood flow has been challenged. Smith[14] and Burchell and his associates[5] were unable to find any correlation between such subjective tests and actual flows measured at operation, suggesting that little reliance should be placed upon such values. This same lack of correlation may account for the wide discrepancies between the results of surgical series using similar subjective methods of classification. Using similar indirect criteria in an unselected group of patients requiring emergency portacaval shunting, Orloff and his associates[10] reached the contrary conclusion that patients with the largest postoperative portal flow achieved the highest postoperative survival rate. Classification systems permitting such opposing conclusions are in need of revision. Recently McDermott[9] has discussed the great need for a more objective evaluation of hepatic perfusion and has re-emphasized the regrettable lack of data to support the indirect tests currently in use.

While seemingly most appropriate for determining the validity of the relationship between portal flow and the clinical response to portasystemic shunting, methods for the *direct* determination of hepatic blood flow have been infrequently used for this purpose. Reliability of these methods has been an important consideration. Major difficulties involved in the volumetric measurement of total hepatic blood flow have recently been summarized.[3] Of primary importance is the realization that indicator-dilution methods determine *total* volumetric flow only and can supply no information about the *nutritive* or effective cellular fraction of total flow. The fraction of total hepatic blood flow actually nourishing cells would be affected by the number and volume of shunts bypassing the sinusoidal areas. Since the existence of both intrahepatic[11] and extrahepatic shunts in cirrhosis is well established, under these conditions it is clear that the fraction of non-nutritive shunted blood may bear no necessary relation to absolute values of total hepatic flow. If postoperative hepatic function depends upon the maintenance of portal perfusion, then the fate of the hepatocyte will reflect only that fraction of total hepatic flow which can be regarded as nutritive. It is, therefore, of critical importance that nutritive flow be measured. Unfortunately no proved, reliable method for the objective estimation of hepatic cellular perfusion exists at present. Until such a method is found, the hemodynamic premise underlying the surgical care and treatment of portal hypertension will remain unproved and validation of operative procedures based upon this assumption will remain indirect or anecdotal.

Since the Kupffer cells of the RES line the hepatic sinusoids in close anatomic proximity to the hepatocytes, a method for determining sinusoidal perfusion based upon their location and function should provide information closely comparable to the actual nutritive hepatic flow. Rather than measuring the amount of a material extracted by these cells, it seemed more important to measure the amount *not* extracted. This latter value would represent the amount of material *not* presented to the Kupffer cells and, therefore, related to the degree of *both* extrahepatic and intrahepatic shunting. This would be true as long as total hepatic RES extraction was either independent of the number of injected particles or complete at the dosages involved. With the small amount of colloid used in this study, hepatic extraction is known to be virtually complete on the first pass through the liver.[6]

Because this study dealt with absolute levels of activity, it was necessary to provide a reference framework for the amount of colloid-bearing activity bypassing the Kupffer cells. Since $^{99m}TcO_4$ is for all practical purposes a freely circulating substance during the counting period involved in this study, a ratio of the peripherally detected activity of $^{99m}TcSC$ to $^{99m}TcO_4$ was established to eliminate the uncontrolled variables of blood volume, cardiac output, and variations in detector probe position when attempting to compare results at different points in time.

While it is our opinion that the principle of selective RES extraction of one agent referenced to a blood pool agent has merit for the determination of the sinusoidal shunt fraction, the practical application of this principle requires further investigation. Future refinements in methodology, particularly with regard to volumetric quantitation of the shunt fraction, appear both possible and desirable. The product of shunt fraction and total volumetric hepatic perfusion as determined by indicator-dilution methodology should result in volumetric estimations of both shunted blood and sinusoidal flow.

Other areas of future investigation should include the influence of particle size on sinusoidal and shunt passage, and the continued effectiveness of hepatic RES phagocytosis in hepatic disease. Without such continued function, this technique would become less reliable for volumetric cellular flow quantitation and more valuable as a hepatic RES function test. Some information exists to suggest that the hepatic RES does continue to function in extensive hepatic disease,[13] but further substantiation is necessary.

Although this technique as presently reported results in a dimensionless fraction, this fraction appears to be related to the amount of shunting around the hepatic sinusoids. Should this prove to be the case, elaboration of such a technique would permit the establishment of hemodynamic classes based upon the degree of *nutritive* perfusion. Since this method makes no distinction with regard to the anatomic shunting sites (intrahepatic or extrahepatic), it should be suitable not only for establishing the degree of preoperative perfusion but also capable of comparing the hemodynamic consequences of various types of shunting procedures. Clearly, this would permit adequate testing of the hemodynamic premise claimed to be the basis of the surgical physiology of portal hypertension.

REFERENCES

1. Adamsons, R. J., Kinkhabwala, M., Moskowitz, H., et al.: Portacaval shunt with arterialization of the hepatic portion of the portal vein, Surg. Gynecol. Obstet. **135:** 529, 1972.
2. Bayly, J. H., and Golzales, C.: The umbilical vein in the adult: Diagnosis, treatment, and research, Am. J. Surg. **30:** 56, 1964.
3. Bradley, E. L., III.: Measurement of hepatic blood flow in man, Surgery **75:** 783, 1974.
4. Bradley, S. E., MacPherson, A. I., Gammeltoft, A., et al.: Effects of portacaval anastomosis on hepatic oxygen extraction and estimated hepatic blood flow in patients with cirrhosis, J. Clin. Invest. **30:** 630, 1951.
5. Burchell, A. R., Moreno, A. H., Panke, W. F., et al.: Hemodynamic variables and prognosis following portacaval shunts, Surg. Gynecol. Obstet. **138:** 359, 1974.
6. Dobson, E. L., and Jones, H. B.: The behavior of intravenously injected particulate matter. Its rate of disappearance from the blood stream as a measure of liver blood flow, Acta Med. Scand. **144** (Suppl.): 273, 1952.
7. Johnson, G., Womack, N. A., Gabrielle, O. F., et al.: Control of the hyperdynamic circulation in patients with bleeding esophageal varices, Ann. Surg. **169:** 661, 1969.
8. Leger, L. H.: Splenoportography: Diagnostic phlebography of the portal venous system, Springfield, Ill., 1966, Charles C Thomas, Publisher.
9. McDermott, W. V., Jr.: Evaluation of the hemodynamics of portal hypertension in the selection of patients for shunt surgery, Ann. Surg. **176:** 449, 1972.
10. Orloff, M. J., Chandler, J. G., Charters, A. C., et al.: Emergency portacaval shunt treatment for bleeding esophageal varices. Prospective study in unselected patients with alcoholic cirrhosis, Arch. Surg. **108:** 293, 1974.
11. Popper, H., Elias, H., and Petty, D. E.: Vascular pattern of the cirrhotic liver, Am. J. Clin. Pathol. **22:** 717, 1952.
12. Salam, A. A., Warren, W. D., LePage, J. R., et al.: Hemodynamic contrasts between selective and total portal-systemic decompression, Ann. Surg. **173:** 827, 1971.
13. Shaldon, S., Chinundussi, L., Guevara, L., et al.: The estimation of hepatic blood flow and intrahepatic shunted blood flow by colloidal heat-denatured human serum albumin labeled with ^{131}I, J. Clin. Invest. **40:** 1346, 1961.
14. Smith, G. W.: An assessment of the validity of preoperative hemodynamic studies in portal hypertension, Surgery **74:** 130, 1973.
15. Taylor, W. J., and Myers, J. D.: Occlusive hepatic venous catheterization in the study of normal liver, cirrhosis of the liver and noncirrhotic portal hypertension, Circulation **13:** 368, 1956.
16. Warren, W. D., Fomon, J. J., and Zeppa, R.: Further evaluation of selective decompression of varices by distal splenorenal shunt, Ann. Surg. **169:** 652, 1969.
17. Warren, W. D., Restrepo, J. E., Respess, J. C., et al.: The importance of hemodynamic studies in management of portal hypertension, Ann. Surg. **158:** 387, 1963.
18. Warren, W. D., Fomon, J. J., Viamonte, M., et al.: Preoperative assessment of portal hypertension, Ann. Surg. **165:** 999, 1967.

DISCUSSION

Dr. Worthington G. Schenk, Jr. (Buffalo, N. Y.). This is indeed an exciting new approach by Dr. Bradley and his associates to this old but unsolved problem. I have been privileged to see the manuscript and can attest that the data separating the shunt animals from the normal animals are striking in their difference.

The authors arc careful to point out that this technique is not yet ready for clinical trial. While it has most probably occurred to them, it would seem of considerable value to repeat similar studies in animals subjected to dimethylnitrosamine cirrhosis.

Our studies have confirmed those of Madden and his associates concerning the histologic similarity of the canine cirrhosis so produced to that of the disease in man. In addition, our studies have confirmed the hemodynamic similarities to human cirrhosis, particularly the hyperdynamic state and a spontaneous portosystemic shunting approaching 40 percent of the splanchnic inflow.

Using this model, Dr. Bradley could tell us whether their noninvasive technique, which could be used in man, is capable of detecting similar degrees of shunting which can be independently measured by electromagnetic techniques, but only in animals.

It would also be most valuable for him to obtain hepatic vein samples while applying their measurements to the cirrhotic animal in order to confirm or refute that the particles are nearly 100 percent cleared by one pass through a cirrhotic liver as they are through a normal liver.

If Dr. Bradley and his co-workers can answer these two questions, this measurement described for us today may well be the way in which we select our shunt candidates in the future.

I would like to thank Dr. Bradley for bringing us that rare phenomenon, a new idea.

Dr. E. L. Bradley, III (Closing). We feel that Dr. Schenk's comments are quite pertinent. Our next primary goal is quantitation of this shunt fraction. We feel that this will be entirely possible by simply determining hepatic blood flow in the old style by indicator dilution techniques and by multiplying that value by the value derived from our shunt fraction. We should then end up with total hepatic blood flow, nutritive hepatic blood flow, and quantitation of the shunt fraction. Dr. Schenk is absolutely correct: this will require hepatic vein catheterization and we plan to do this in human subjects.

Of particular interest at the present time is the size of the injected particles. We feel that there will be an optimum size of the injected particles which will need to be standardized before we are ready to tell you that this technique will be helpful in man.

We are quite impressed now, but like so many developments which look good early, we are going to have to wait a while to find out whether this principle will prove to be of value in human physiology.

Objective assessment of late results of aortocoronary bypass operation

Hooshang Bolooki,* M.D., F.R.C.S.(C), Richard J. Thurer, M.D., Ali Ghahramani, M.D., Abelardo Vargas, M.D., Willis Williams, M.D., *and* **Gerard Kaiser, M.D.,** *Miami, Fla.*

Between May, 1969, and May, 1973, the procedure of aortocoronary bypass (ACB) was performed in 242 patients. A total of 42 patients (17 percent) had preinfarction angina or early acute myocardial infarction and others exhibited severe unremitting angina pectoris. There were 30 women (12.5 percent). The over-all operative mortality rate was 5.7 percent and the intraoperative infarction rate was 7 percent. On follow-up of the entire group of patients, 89 percent have remained angina free and at restudy 85 percent have patent grafts. Comparison of pre- and postoperative cardiac function and hemodynamics showed that 50 percent of patients, over all, had some improvement. This change in cardiac function was unrelated to the extent of intraoperative graft flow or number of grafts. In the preinfarction group there was no operative death but 20 percent developed intraoperative infarction. In the course of one to 4 years follow-up, 41 of these patients have remained angina free and have not had late myocardial infarction. Twenty-four of these patients have been restudied at 4 to 48 months after the operation and all but one (95 percent) have patent grafts. Female patients had an operative mortality rate of 10 percent, an intraoperative infarction rate of 18 percent, and only 65 percent have remained angina free at follow-up. Of 14 female patients studied postoperatively, only 64 percent have patent grafts. Three females (11 percent) developed myocardial infarction 10 days to 3 months after the operation and one has died. As these results indicate, the procedure of ACB produces a satisfactory long-term result in patients with preinfarction and chronic intractable angina. In women, however, the procedure has less satisfactory early and long-term results.

From the Division of Thoracic and Cardiovascular Surgery and Cardiovascular Laboratories, University of Miami School of Medicine, Jackson Memorial Hospital, Veterans Administration Hospital, Miami, Fla.

THE PURPOSE of this study was to evaluate our late results in patients who had received myocardial revascularization with a saphenous vein graft in the course of the past 4 years (1969 to 1973). Our aim was to assess objectively the long-term efficacy of this operation in various groups of patients and to evaluate the relation between graft flow and eventual change in cardiac function.

Supported in part by Grants from the National Heart and Lung Institute, Grants No. 13978-03, and the Greater Miami Heart Association.

Presented at the Twenty-eighth Annual Meeting of the Society for Vascular Surgery, Chicago, Ill., June 20 and 21, 1974.

Reprint requests: Dr. Hooshang Bolooki, P.O. Box 520875, Biscayne Annex, Miami, Fla. 33152.

*Research Career Development Awardee, National Heart and Lung Institute, Grant No. HL 70670-02.

PATIENT MATERIAL

Between May, 1969, and May, 1973, 242 patients who were suffering from coronary artery disease and its complications underwent direct myocardial revascularization with an aortocoronary vein bypass graft. Their ages ranged from 32 to 77 years (average, 54 years). All patients had extensive multivessel coronary artery disease and angina pectoris for months or years prior to admission to the hospital. More than half of them received potent coronary vasodilator agents (e.g., isosorbide dinitrate sublingual) and approximately 30 percent were also on beta-blocking agents (propranolol). The patients were cared for at the Jackson Memorial Hospital or at the Veterans Administration Hospital of Miami and were operated on conjointly by the authors.

METHODS

All patients were initially admitted to the hospital and were treated for 3 to 30 days with coronary vasodilators, with specific therapy for hypertension and anxiety, and with diuretics, as indicated. Preoperatively they received complete hemodynamic studies and cardiac catheterization with selective coronary angiograms under mild sedation. The hemodynamic studies included measurement of intracardiac pressures, left ventricular volumes, cardiac output, calculation of left ventricular diastolic compliance, and ejection fraction.[2]

Rigid criteria were used in selecting the patients for the operation. As a result, only those patients who were unresponsive to vigorous medical management were considered for cardiac catheterization. Among these, the patients who angiographically exhibited coronary artery lesions larger than 75 percent of the coronary artery diameter with acceptable distal vessel (more than one mm.) and runoff were selected for direct myocardial revascularization.

The operative procedure was done within a few days to one month after hemodynamic studies, except for patients with preinfarction. In this group the operation was done within a few hours after cardiac cathetherization studies. Aortocoronary bypass operation was performed under total cardiopulmonary bypass with mild hypothermia (28 to 32° C.). As far as possible, cardiac ischemia was not induced. The left ventricle was drained with a sump catheter through the left superior pulmonary vein. In most cases the proximal ends of the aortocoronary vein grafts were constructed initially without the use of cardiopulmonary bypass by using fine propylene suture material. The distal graft was always done with the heart supported on bypass. Continuous running sutures were used for the purpose of arterial anastomosis. Duration of cardiopulmonary bypass varied from 45 to 120 minutes.

The coronary graft blood flow was measured intraoperatively in 120 patients by an electromagnetic flow probe (Statham), which was positioned around the graft. Intraoperative monitoring of the left ventricular pressure was done in 52 of these patients by placing a left ventricular pressure transducer catheter (Millar, Houston) within the left ventricular cavity through the right superior pulmonary vein.[3] The pressure monitoring was continued postoperatively and was supplemented by 12 lead electrocardiograms for 3 consecutive days after the operation, simultaneous with serum enzyme analysis, in order to detect development of myocardial infarction.[6]

The patients discharged from the hospital were followed in an outpatient clinic, and upon development of any complications were readmitted to the hospital for the purposes of observation. Follow-up cardiac catheterization was done in 61 patients within 4 weeks to one year after the operation. Eleven patients were restudied at an interval of 2 to 4 years after the initial postoperative cardiac catheterization.

Excluded from this study were 36 patients who had an aortocoronary bypass procedure in association with other procedures, such as heart valve replacement, left ventricular resection, or closure of ventricular septal defect. Five of these patients were in cardiogenic shock preoperatively.

RESULTS

The over-all operative mortality rate for the entire group of patients was 5.7 per cent. In Table I detailed analysis of operative results for the entire group of patients is given and in Table II the annual frequency of this procedure as well as the operative mor-

Table I. *Early and late follow-up results of the entire group of patients undergoing direct myocardial revascularization*

	Patients		Mortality				Infarction			
			Operative		Late*		Perioperative		Late*	
	No.	%	No.	%	No.	%	No.	%	No.	%
Men	170	80.5	11	6.4	4	2.4	4	2.5	4	2.5
Women	30	12.5	3	10	1		5	18	3	11
Preinfarct	42	17	0	0	0	—	8	20	0	—
Total	242	100	14	5.7	5	2.1	17	7	7	3

*Late results were obtained in the course of average 2.5 years follow-up.

Table II

	1969		1970		1971		1972		1973		All years	
	No.	%	No.	%	No.	%	No.	%	No.	%	No.	%
No. patients	8		36		40		93		63		242	
Mortality rate	1	12	2	5	3	7	6	6	2	3	14	5.7
Single graft	2		5		4		8		6		20	8
Double graft	6		20		24		55		37		145	60
Triple graft	0		11		12		27		18		72	30
Quadruple graft	0		0		0		3		2		5	2

Table III. *Early postoperative complications in patients undergoing direct myocardial revascularization*

	Infarction		Dysrhythmia		Hypertension	
No. of patients	No.	%	No.	%	No.	%
242	17	7	17	7	50	20

Table IV. *Angiographic follow-up results in patients after direct myocardial revascularization*

Group	No. of patients	Interval (mo.)	No. of grafts	Grafts open		Patients with all or most grafts open	
				No.	%	No.	%
Men	23	1 to 12	52	43	84	20	86
Women	14	1 to 12	32	20	60	9	64
Preinfarct	24	1 to 12	42	39	93	23	95
Total	61	1 to 12	126	102	79	52	85
Late follow-up	11	24 to 28	15	14	93	9	81

tality rate in our hospital are indicated. Since 1970 the frequency of this procedure has increased but the mortality rate has remained the same. A single coronary graft was done in 8 percent, double grafts in 60 percent, triple in 30 percent, and quadruple in 2 percent (Table II). The operative mortality rate was highest for patients receiving triple grafts (10 percent) and lowest for patients with a single graft or quadruple graft (zero percent).

Graft flow. Graft flow was measured in 120 patients. It ranged from 30 to 280 ml., averaging 80 ml. per graft. Graft flow per patient, however, averaged 100 c.c. There was a direct relation between graft flow and graft patency. Among grafts with 60 ml. flow or greater, 96 percent were patent as

Table V. *Changes in cardiac function in patients undergoing direct myocardial revascularization**

Patients	No.	C.I. 1	C.I. 2	EDP 1	EDP 2
Patent grafts	32	2.9 ± 0.8	3.3 ± 1.0	14 ± 6	12 ± 4
Operative infarct	12	3.2 ± 0.2	2.5 ± 0.1†	9 ± 1	16 ± 1†
Males	17	2.6 ± 0.1	2.7 ± 0.1	23 ± 2	13 ± 1†
Females	14	3.1 ± 0.1	2.7 ± 0.1	8 ± 1	14 ± 1†
Preinfarct	24	3.4 ± 0.7	4.0 ± 1.2†	16 ± 7	13 ± 5

*C.I. = cardiac index in L./min./m;[2] EDP = end-diastolic pressure of left ventricle in mm. Hg; EF = ejection fraction. Diast and was obtained from the left ventricular pressure curves during the isometric contraction.[2] Preoperative data (1) and postopera

†p value < 0.05 indicates a significant difference between pre- and postoperative study.

Table VI. *Comparison of changes in cardiac function before and after successful direct myocard*

Group	No.	C.I. 1	C.I. 2	Vmax 1	Vmax 2
A†	8	2.8 ± 0.2	2.6 ± 0.2	1.8 ± 0.3	2.1 ± 0.3
B‡	7	2.8 ± 0.1	2.6 ± 0.2	1.7 ± 0.2	2.3 ± 0.2§

*C.I. = cardiac index in L./min./m;[2] EDP = end-diastolic pressure of left ventricle in mm. Hg; EDV = end-diastolic left ventric is an index of myocardial contractility in circ. per second and was obtained from the left ventricular pressure curves during

†Group A, mean graft flow 88 ml. per minute, 1.2 grafts per patient.

‡Group B, mean graft flow 227 ml. per minute, 2.6 grafts per patient.

§p value < 0.05.

compared with 50 percent when graft flow was less than 60 ml. A detailed analysis of the relation between graft flow and postoperative changes in cardiac function in 15 patients is given below.

Postoperative complications. Immediate postoperative cardiac complications occurred in 86 patients (35 percent). These included hypertension in 50 patients (20 percent) and dysrhythmia in 17 patients (7 percent), (Table III). By far the most important postoperative complication was that of development of acute myocardial infarction soon after operation in 17 patients (7 percent).[4]

Graft patency rate. On follow-up, 61 patients had postoperative angiographic studies within one to 12 months after operation. These 61 patients had received 126 grafts, of which 102 grafts (79 percent) were patent (Table IV). In 52 patients (85 percent) all or most grafts were open. Eleven of these patients had a second follow-up coronary angiography. They had received 17 grafts of which 15 (88 percent) were visualized at the initial studies. On restudy 2 to 4 years later, 14 (93 percent) of the grafts were patent (Table IV). As compared with early postoperative studies, there was a marked reduction in the size of the vein graft in most patients. Progression of the intrinsic coronary lesions were seen in approximately 20 percent of the patients. In the presence of a patent graft, more than half of the patients showed occlusion of the preoperative proximal stenotic coronary lesions.

Effects on cardiac function. Complete hemodynamic studies were done in 55 patients preoperatively and postoperatively. Among these patients 12 had developed intraoperative myocardial infarction and in this group there was a marked decrease in most parameters of cardiac function ($p < 0.05$) (Table V). Over all, 50 percent of patients without intraoperative infarction and patent grafts showed improvement in all parameters of cardiac function (Table V), with other patients showing no change (20 percent) or a decrease in cardiac function 30 percent).[2] There were no further significant changes in cardiac function in the 11 patients who were studied late (2 to 4 years) after operation.

Relation of graft flow to changes in cardiac function. In 15 patients who had intraoperative coronary blood flow studies, patent grafts postoperatively, and complete hemodynamic

EF%		Δ p/Δ v		Vmax	
1	2	1	2	1	2
70 ± 17	70 ± 16	0.24 ± 0.1	24 ± 0	2.5 ± 1	2.8 ± 0.9
70 ± 14	52 ± 13†	0.14 ± 0	0.32 ± 0†	2.9 ± 0.3	2.1 ± 0.1†
62 ± 5	65 ± 4	0.33 ± 0	0.38 ± 0	1.9 ± 0.1	2.3 ± 0.2
69 ± 4	64 ± 6	0.2 ± 0	0.3 ± 0	2.3 ± 0.2	2.1 ± 0.1
68 ± 15	80 ± 16†	0.16 ± 0	0.17 ± 0	2.6 ± 0.9	3.0 ± 0.9

ventricular stiffness is expressed by Δp/Δv in mm. Hg/per milliliter. Vmax is an index of myocardial contractility in circ. per second
ıes (2) are compared for those patients who had complete studies.

*ascularization in two groups of patients with low and high coronary graft flow**

EDP		Δ p/Δ v		EDV		EF (%)	
1	2	1	2	1	2	1	2
8 ± 4	12 ± 2§	0.22	0.33	353 ± 68	382 ± 68	61 ± 5	76 ± 3§
9 ± 4	14 ± 2	0.18	0.35	298 ± 84	335 ± 76	66 ± 7	62 ± 4

me in milliliters; EF = ejection fraction. Diastolic left ventricular stiffness is express by Δp/Δv in mm. Hg. per milliliter. Vmax
etric contraction.[2] Preoperative data (1) and postoperative values (2) are compared for those patients who had complete studies.

evaluation, the relation between the intraoperative coronary graft flow with changes in cardiac function were analyzed (Table VI). As shown in Table VI, these patients were divided into two groups depending on the extent of blood flow through the graft. In Group A (eight patients) the mean graft flow averaged 88 ml. per minute and there were 1.2 grafts per patient. In Group B, (seven patients) there were 2.6 grafts per patient and the mean coronary blood flow averaged 227 ml. per minute. Comparing the hemodynamic results from the preoperative and postoperative cardiac catheterization, there was no appreciable relation between the extent of coronary blood flow and the eventual improvement in resting cardiac function. In fact, as the data in Table VI indicate, the ejection fraction increased markedly ($p < 0.01$) and end-diastolic pressure decreased by 33 percent in patients in Group A, while myocardial contractility index (Vmax) increased (34 percent) in Group B ($p < 0.05$) who had higher coronary blood flow and a larger number of grafts per patient.

Follow-up results. All patients were followed for one to 5 years (average, 2.5 years). Late death due to acute myocardial infarction or congestive heart failure occurred in five patients (2 percent). Seven additional patients (3 percent) developed late postoperative myocardial infarction. Thus a total of 12 patients (5 percent) in an average of 2.5 years of follow-up had myocardial infarction late after coronary bypass (Table VII). On follow-up, 89 percent of the patients (205 of 228) were angina free and the remainder had either milder angina than before the operation (5 percent) or angina with the same severity as before the operation (6 percent). Interestingly, 40 percent of patients who developed intraoperative infarction are symptomatic.[4]

Results in females. Among 30 women (12.5 percent), the over-all operative mortality rate was 10 percent (three patients) and intraoperative infarction occurred in six (18 percent) (Table I). On follow-up 19 patients (65 percent) are angina free (Table VII). Three women (10 percent) developed myocardial infarction on follow-up (Table I) within 10 days to 3 months after the operation and one of them died despite a patent coronary graft.[5] Fourteen female patients had postoperative cardiac catheterization studies, and, of the 32 coronary bypass

Table VII. *Late postoperative results after direct myocardial revascularization*

Surviving patients	*No.*	*Without angina*		*Mild or severe angina*		*Late infarction and death*	
		No.	*%*	*No.*	*%*	*No.*	*%*
Men	159	145	91	14	9	8	5
Women	27	19	65	8	35	4	14
Preinfarction	42	41	97	1	3	0	—
Total	228	205	89	11	5	12	6

grafts, only 20 (60 percent) were patent (Table IV). None of the females have had long-term postoperative cardiac catheterization studies. The changes in cardiac function in the female patients were less striking than in males, with an over-all 40 percent of patients showing improvement in all parameters of cardiac function considering 10 percent change from preoperative value (Table V).

Results in preinfarction group. A total of 42 patients (17 percent) had preinfarction angina or early myocardial infarction which did not respond to 4 to 14 days of medical management in a coronary care unit. There was no operative death in this group but 20 percent of these patients developed intraoperative myocardial infarction (Table II). In an average follow-up period of 2.5 years, 41 of these patients have remained angina free and none has developed late myocardial infarction. Of these patients, 24 have had postoperative cardiac catheterization studies and 23 of them (96 percent) have patent coronary grafts (Table IV). Of 42 coronary bypass grafts in this group of patients, 39 (93 percent) are patent. Five patients have had second follow-up angiographic studies 2 to 4 years postoperatively. They had received six grafts which have remained patent to date. An analysis of the effects of aortocoronary bypass grafts in patients with preinfarction angina showed, over all, 60 percent of the patients to have an improvement in their cardiac function considering 10 percent change postoperatively as compared with preoperative values. The most striking improvement in cardiac function parameters, however, was in that group of patients who had low preoperative indexes of function, such as ejection fraction, cardiac index, myocardial contractility, and left ventricular end-diastolic pressure.[7]

DISCUSSION

Direct myocardial revascularization with the use of a reversed segment of a saphenous vein was initially applied clinically by Sabiston,[26] Cooley and associates,[12] and Kahn.[21] In all these patients the indication for operation was congenital anomaly of the left coronary artery. This procedure was used in adult patients with coronary artery disease in 1967 by Favaloro[14] and Johnson and associates,[20] and due to minimal operative risk and morbidity, it soon established its place as a routine cardiac procedure in the armamentarium of the cardiovascular surgeon. In the past 4 years this procedure has been applied with an increasing frequency for a variety of clinical manifestations instigated by coronary artery disease and it may remain, for some time to come, the most frequently performed operation in major cardiac surgery centers.

The initial reports on the results of this operation included a survey of its effect on angina pectoris and the operative mortality rate.[13, 25] Later a detailed analysis of results showed development of intraoperative and immediate postoperative complications as well as an appreciable (15 to 20 percent) incidence of graft closure on follow-up.[18, 27] Meanwhile a number of investigators questioned the long-term efficacy of this procedure on prevention of acute myocardial infarction and longevity.[15, 28] Their objection was based on the absence of double-blind clinical studies prior to the general acceptance of this operation, especially since the early results served as the basis for performing this operation more frequently.[29] Similar to the other clinical reports on myocardial revascularization, the present study lacks a control group with comparable extent of coronary artery disease. It is our opinion, however, that a survey such as this would improve our understanding of the effects of this procedure on late patient survival, graft patency, and cardiac function.

The early postoperative results in these patients, seen in the course of 4 years, indicate that the most favorable group are patients with preinfarction angina and men with chronic coronary artery disease. The overall perioperative myocardial infarction rate of 7 percent is somewhat a median figure as compared with other institutions.[23 24] Female patients, however, had a high incidence of perioperative infarction, which compared with patients undergoing myocardial revascularization for preinfarction angina. An analysis of earlier results also indicated development of a considerable number of other postoperative complications directly related to this operation, such as dysrhythmia in 7 percent and hypertension in 20 percent of the patients. Interestingly, however, these complications responded to conservative management, although recently we have had to use rapid-acting antihypertensive drugs (nitroprusside) in order to decrease the blood pressure to normal levels postoperatively. With this therapy the incidence of postoperative bleeding has also decreased considerably.

The results of coronary bypass graft in women were found to be inferior to those in men receiving the same operation. Our female patients had a smaller number of patent grafts per patient and had less improvement in cardiac function than did men postoperatively. Surprisingly, however, preoperative cardiac function in these patients was better than in men (Table V). Late results of this operation in females showed that only 65 percent of women were angina free as compared with 92 percent of men. A number of reasons were postulated as causes for these poor results; the presence of small-vessel coronary artery disease or microemboli was suggested by Glancy and associates.[17] Also, our female patients have had small and thin-walled coronary vessels and, over all, the operation was technically more difficult in this group than in men. The finding of a large left ventricular end-diastolic volume postoperatively and a smaller number of patent grafts could have served as other physiological factors contributing to over-all inferior results of this operation in females.[8]

The group of patients benefitting most from direct myocardial revascularization were those with preinfarction angina or intermediate coronary syndrome. We found that on long-term follow-up 97 percent of these patients were angina free and none had developed late myocardial infarction.[7] The incidence of intraoperative infarction based on serum enzyme analysis and electrocardiographic studies was directly related to a large number of patients operated on during an evolving infarction. In spite of this, the benefits gained from this operation were significant. In our hands there was no operative death among these patients, and this, we believe, was directly related to early operative intervention after cardiac catheterization studies. Other reports on similar types of patients indicate an operative mortality rate ranging from 5 to 22.5 percent,[10, 11] which we believe in most instances was due to a delay in operative intervention.

An important finding in this study, which confirms the previous reports,[19,27] was that of continued patency of the vein grafts after the initial studies. In our series in only one patient was a graft found closed 3 years later. In this case, during the initial studies, the graft to the right coronary artery was visualized but it did not fill the distal part of the coronary artery. This graft was not expected to remain patent for a long time. Our late (2 to 4 year) postoperative studies showed the size of most vein grafts, which were initially larger than the coronary artery, decreased considerably. This was perhaps due to the process of accommodation.

While blood flow through the graft had a direct relation to graft patency in our series, there was no relation between the number of coronary bypass grafts and the eventual change in cardiac function (Table VI). As shown in this table in group B patients there was an increase only in myocardial contractility index (Vmax). On the other hand, in patients in Group A, with an average mean graft flow of 88 ml. per minute and 1.2 grafts per patient, there was a significant improvement in ejection fraction and end-diastolic pressure. This finding does not deny the necessity and significance of multiple bypass grafts but confirms that complete myocardial revascularization was done in these patients. Thus patients in Group A were in need of a smaller number of grafts and patients in Group B had more vessels suitable for bypass grafting.

We have previously reported on the effects of aortocoronary bypass operation on early postoperative cardiac function.[2] Of the 11 patients who were studied for a second time after this operation, we found no further change in cardiac performance as compared with earlier study. This finding shows that the failure of successful coronary bypass operation to improve the cardiac function is not due to early postoperative studies and the effect of surgical stress.

Previous reports on patients with extensive coronary artery disease involving two and three vessels have indicated a 3 to 5 year mortality rate of 15 to 40 percent.[16, 22] While the extent of disease in our patients may not match that of patients reported by other investigators, a late infarction rate of 3 percent and late mortality rate of 2 percent favorably compare with those of patients treated by conservative management. Our results indicate the possibility of an improvement in statistics in patients with extensive coronary artery disease. Undoubtedly the final answer to the question of efficacy of myocardial revascularization for preventing myocardial infarction or longevity would come from that group of studies which uses randomized patient selection for medical and surgical therapy.[1]

REFERENCES

1. Aronow, W. S., and Stemmer, E. A.: Bypass graft surgery versus medical therapy of angina pectoris, Am. J. Cardiol. **33:** 415, 1974.
2. Bolooki, H., Mallon, S., Ghahramani, A., et al.: Objective assessment of the effects of aortocoronary bypass operation on cardiac function, J. Thorac. Cardiovasc. Surg. **66:** 916, 1973.
3. Bolooki, H.: Prolonged left ventricular pressure monitoring by a catheter transducer, SURGERY **73:** 97, 1973.
4. Bolooki, H., Sommer, L., Ghahramani, A., et al.: Complications of coronary bypass surgery, Circulation (Suppl. III) **47-48:** 120, 1973.
5. Bolooki, H., Ghahramani, A., Green, R., et al.: Results of coronary surgery in women. (In preparation.)
6. Bolooki, H., Sommer, L., Faraldo, A., et al.: The significance of serum enzyme studies in patients undergoing coronary bypass surgery, J. Thorac. Cardiovasc. Surg. **65:** 863, 1973.
7. Bolooki, H., Ghahramani, A., Vargas, A., et al.: Long-term follow-up of patients operated by emergency myocardial revascularization for intermediate coronary syndrome, J. Thorac. Cardiovasc. Surg. **68:** 90, 1974.
8. Braunwald, E.: The determinants of myocardial oxygen consumption, Physiologist **12:** 65, 1969.
9. Bruschke, A. V., Proudfit, W. L., and Sonesjr, F. M.: Progress study of 590 consecutive nonsurgical cases of coronary disease followed 5 to 9 years. I. Arteriographic correlations, Circulation **47:** 1147, 1973.
10. Cheanvechai, C., Effler, D. B., Loop, F. D., et al.: Emergency myocardial revascularization, Am. J. Cardiol. **32:** 901, 1973.
11. Conti, C. R., Brawley, R. K., Griffith, L. S., et al.: Unstable angina pectoris: Morbidity and mortality in 57 consecutive patients evaluated angiographically, Am. J. Cardio. **32:** 745, 1973.
12. Cooley, D. A., Hallman, G. L., and Bloodwell, R. D.: Definitive surgical treatment of anomalous origin of left coronary artery from pulmonary artery: Indications and results, J. Thorac. Cardiovasc. Surg. **52:** 798, 1966.
13. Effler, D. B., Favaloro, R. G., Groves, L. K., et al.: The simple approach to direct coronary artery surgery: Cleveland clinic experience, J. Thorac. Cardiovasc. Surg. **62:** 503, 1971.
14. Favaloro, R. G.: Saphenous vein graft in the surgical treatment of coronary artery disease, J. Thorac. Cardiovasc. Surg. **58:** 178, 1969.
15. Friedberg, C. K.: Caution and coronary surgery: Timeo chirurgos et dona ferentes, Circulation, **45:** 757, 1972.
16. Friesinger, G. C., Page, E. E., and Ross, R. S.: Prognostic significance of coronary arteriography, Trans. Assoc. Am. Physicians **83:** 78, 1970.

17. Glancy, D. L., Marcus, M. L., and Epstein, S. E.: Myocardial infarction in young women with normal coronary arteriograms, Circulation 44: 495, 1971.
18. Grondin, C. M., Castonguay, Y. R., Lesperance, J., et al.: Attrition rate of aorto-to-coronary artery saphenous vein grafts after one year: A study in consecutive series of 96 patients, Ann. Thor. Surg. 14: 223, 1972.
19. Grondin, C. M., Lesperance, J., Bourassa, M. G., et al.: Serial angiographic evaluation in 60 consecutive patients with aorto-coronary artery vein grafts 2 weeks, 1 year, and 3 years after operation, J. Thorac. Cardiovasc. Surg. 67: 1, 1974.
20. Johnson, W. D., Flemma, R. J., Lepley, D. W., Jr., et al.: Extended treatment of severe coronary artery disease: A total surgical approach, Ann. Surg. 170: 460, 1969.
21. Kahn, D.: Discussion of Effler et al.[13]
22. Kannel, W. B., and Feinleili, M.: Natural history of angina pectoris in the Framingham study—prognosis and survival, Am. J. Cardiol. 29: 154, 1972.
23. Karnegis, J. N.: Experience with the coronary artery bypass in a community hospital, Am. Heart J. 86: 51, 1973.
24. Morris, G. C., Reul, G. J., Howell, J. F., et al.: Late results following direct coronary artery surgery, Am. J. Cardiol. 29: 180, 1972.
25. Reul, G. J., Morris, G. C., Jr., Howell, J. F., et al.: Current concepts in coronary artery surgery: A critical analysis of 1,287 patients, Ann. Thorac. Surg. 14: 243, 1972.
26. Sabiston, B. C.: The role of the surgeon in the management of the patient with coronary atherosclerosis. Postgraduate course, cardiovascular surgery, Clinical Congress of American College of Surgeons: 41, 1973.
27. Sheldon, W. C., Rincon, G., Effler, D. D., et al.: Vein graft surgery for coronary artery disease: Survival and angiographic results in 1,000 patients, Circulation (Suppl. III) 47-48: 184, 1973.
28. Spodick, D. H.: Aortocoronary bypass, Chest 63: 80, 1973.
29. Spodick, D. H.: Revascularization of the heart: Numerators in search of denominators, Am. Heart J. 81: 149, 1971.

DISCUSSION

Dr. John Lockwood Ochsner (New Orleans, La.). The encouraging aspects of this paper were that there were no late or early deaths in the preinfarction group and the report also gives further support to the concept that, if a graft is open in one year, it will more than likely remain open.

It was worrisome to us, as to others, that there still remains greater than 20 percent graft closure of these veins.

We had had 24 percent occlude and 5 percent developed narrowing in the grafted veins. Consequently, we believe today that the procedure of choice, i.e., the primary operation, should be that of an internal mammary bypass because the results are far superior.

The other worrisome aspect of the paper was that there is still a significant intraoperative infarction rate, but there has been no correlation, at least in the paper, between the ischemic time at operation and graft patency.

There are two interesting points. First, there is an apparent difference in the benefits provided by operation in men and women, and, second, the authors have introduced a new concept of mean graft flow for assessing these grafts, which we do not think is correct, and which I think probably accounts for their great variation in the functions after operation—at least in the parameters that were measured.

We think that one must take into consideration not only the mean graft flow but also the morphology and the anatomy of the existing coronary circulation to make this have any real value.

Dr. Hooshang Bolooki (Closing). I believe, as Dr. Ochsner does, that mammary graft probably is better than saphenous vein. As you very well know, many surgeons are reluctant to do this operation, possibly because of lesser blood flow through the mammary artery as compared to the saphenous vein, but that probably is not a correct objection to this operation.

As to his question concerning the patients who had intraoperative myocardial infarction, in our experience infarction has happened in spite of patent grafts.

We published our experience in *Circulation,* supplement issue, July, 1973. There were 22 coronary bypass grafts in 10 patients who infarcted intraoperatively. Of the 22 grafts, 12 grafts were open, yet these patients had myocardial infarction based on angiographic studies. Based on hemodynamic studies, their cardiac function was totally deteriorated as compared with before operation.

The effects of graft flow and patency on cardiac function are points that I did not elaborate in the presentation mainly because of the time involved. This was a subject that we looked at a little bit carefully, as explained in the manuscript.

The idea was initiated because we noted the patient's cardiac function was not improving after the coronary bypass graft. We thought, perhaps, that the concept of so-called complete revascularization was an important thing to examine. We evaluated our patients and found one group of seven patients who had mean graft flow of 80 ml. per minute and another group who had mean graft flow of 200 ml. Then we looked at their cardiac function after the operation to see if the high graft flow group had a better function that the low graft flow group. It was not so at all.

Therefore, we have concluded that the number of grafts you do or the amount of blood flow in excess of 80 ml. per minute perhaps does not or is not going to affect the eventual change in cardiac function.

Again, this is something that is discussed in the manuscript but was not brought out in the presentation.

Total cardiopulmonary bypass with a new microporous Teflon membrane oxygenator

K. E. Karlson, M.D., Ph.D., W. R. Murphy, M.D., M. Kakvan, M.D., P. Anthony, B.A., G. N. Cooper, Jr., M.D., P. D. Richardson, Ph.D., *and* **P. M. Galletti, M.D., Ph.D.,** *Providence, R. I.*

A membrane oxygenator constructed from a microporous membrane with 3 to 5 μ pore size has been shown to have an O_2 transfer rate of 200 ml. per minute and and CO_2 transfer of up to 300 ml. per minute at 6 L. per minute blood flow. The nominal membrane area is 2.25 M.^{2} and the priming volume of the oxygenator is less than 400 ml. In vitro tests showed that CO_2 transfer decreases with increasing length of perfusion, but ventilating the oxygenator with dry O_2 and adjusting the "shim" pressure to equal input blood pressure minimizes this decay. Six sheep survived and were normal after 24 hours' partial perfusion at 2.5 L. per minute blood flow. Gas exchange and structural integrity have been found to be satisfactory in 40 clinical perfusions for cardiac surgery lasting up to 7 hours in patients up to 2.1 M.^{2} of body surface area.

From the Division of Biological and Medical Sciences, Brown University, and the Division of Cardiovascular and Thoracic Surgery, Department of Surgery, Rhode Island Hospital, Providence, R. I.

MEMBRANE OXYGENATORS have been shown to be physiologically superior to bubble oxygenators, particularly for long perfusions.[3, 10, 11, 13, 14] They have not gained widespread acceptance for cardiac surgery because they are not as efficient as bubblers in terms of gas transfer, and several units in parallel are often required for adequate support, resulting in an exceedingly large priming volume in the extracorporeal circuit. It has been shown recently that the incorporation of small pores in the membrane effectively eliminates the resistance of the membrane to gas transfer while retaining separation of blood and gas, thus making the microporous membrane oxygenator efficient and practical.[8, 9] This report relates our laboratory and initial clinical experience with such an oxygenator.*

The evaluation involved in vitro tests of pressure, volume, and gas transfer characteristics, followed by acute sheep perfusions to test gas transfer capacity in vivo. Long-term oxygenator performance was investigated in 24 hour partial perfusions in conscious sheep. Three hour open-chest total cardiopulmonary bypass was then performed in animals before the oxygenator was used clinically.

METHODS AND MATERIALS

The basic configuration of the oxygenator is an accordion-pleated design reported previously[1, 2, 4, 16] (Fig. 1). This results in a flat,

Presented at the Twenty-eighth Annual Meeting of the Society for Vascular Surgery, Chicago, Ill., June 20 and 21, 1974.

Reprint requests: Dr. Karl E. Karlson, Rhode Island Hospital, Providence, R. I. 02902.

*Model STX-434, Travenol Laboratories, Morton Grove, Ill.

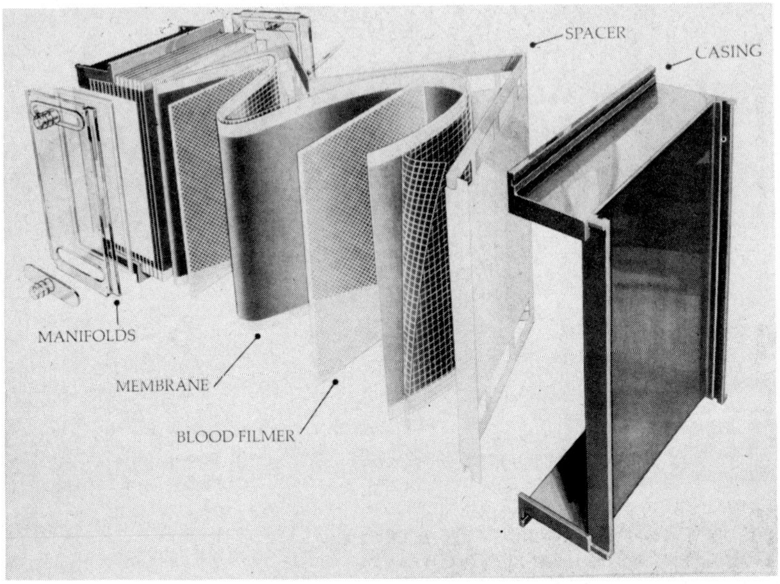

Fig. 1. Schematic view of the construction of the oxygenator. The manifolds distribute the blood to the blood envelopes (manifolds on the opposite side distribute gas to the gas envelopes). The blood filmer is a fine nylon screen separating the membranes in the blood phase. The spacer is a thin, stiff paperboard sheet which separates the membranes in the gas phase. The rigid casing completes the unit. Reproduced by permission of Travenol Laboratories, Inc.

rectangular oxygenator with 30 blood phase envelopes alternating with 30 gas envelopes. The membrane material is a sheet of expanded fibrillated tetrafluoroethylene, reinforced with a mesh of polyvinyl chloride-coated fiberglass. The effective pore size as measured by the ethanol bubble-point test is 3 to 5 μ. A fine nylon screen separates the membrane surfaces in the blood phase, and a thin, stiff paperboard sheet separates the folds in the gas phase. The nominal membrane surface is 2.25 $M.^2$, but the actual exchange area is less, in view of the masking effect of the various screens used in the blood and gas phases. A flat, rectangular polyvinyl chloride "shim" bag is inserted in the middle of the stack of envelopes. It serves to compress the blood layers and may be inflated to any desired pressure through a tube connecting it to an outside pressure source. The stack of membranes is enclosed in a rigid rectangular box 27.5 by 15 by 7.15 cm. The long, narrow side (27.5 by 7.15 cm.) facing the blood spaces contains blood inlet and outlet ports. The opposite side facing the gas phase contains gas inlet and outlet ports and egress for the "shim" access tube. The oxygenator fits into a steel frame on its pump console. Gas phase pressure is automatically limited by means of a vent through a water column. The oxygenator should be operated with about 10 percent blood recirculation to eliminate the possibility that gas pressure ever exceeds blood pressure. In the console furnished by the manufacturer, the arterial pump and the recirculation pump are "slaved" so that adjustment of the net perfusion rate automatically maintains the fraction of recirculation. During operation the "shim" pressure is manually adjusted; setting it equal to input blood pressure gives optimal oxygenator performance. Oxygen flow is variable up to 20 L. per minute and can be regulated manually to achieve the desired P_{CO_2} in the output blood.

The perfusion apparatus provided by the manufacturer includes four roller pumps (two of which are mechanically interlocked to rotate in constant speed relationship to each other), controls for O_2 flow and pressure and shim pressure, and appropriate tubing and reservoirs for total perfusion (Fig.

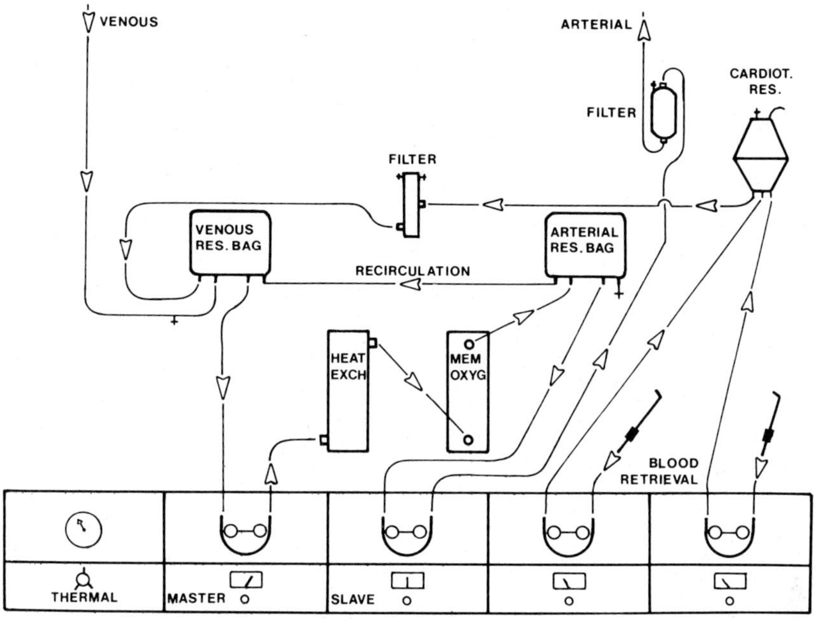

Fig. 2. Circuit configuration of clinical pump-oxygenator system.

2). In our evaluation, the apparatus was filled with heparinized whole blood for the normothermic sheep perfusions. For hemodilution perfusions the prime was Plasma-Lyte-148* (25 ml. per kilogram of body weight), 12 Gm. of dextrose (as 50 percent), blood and/or Plasmanate† added if necessary to yield an hematocrit of 25 percent during perfusion. The oxygenator requires 400 ml. prime with the shim deflated and 260 ml. prime with the shim inflated to 200 mm. Hg. The remainder of the circuit (with filters), as used clinically, requires a total of 2,200 ml. The O_2 used to ventilate the oxygenator in the clinical cases was not humidified, contrary to the initial suggestion of the manufacturer.

Nine sheep weighing 61 to 104 kilograms underwent total perfusion for 3 hours at flow rates up to 10.6 L. per minute. Hematocrit was maintained at 30 to 40 percent and the body temperature at 37° C. In all experiments oxygen transfer rates were calculated from the O_2 content of the input and output blood of the oxygenator and the blood flow rate. CO_2 transfer was calculated from the CO_2 concentration of output gas and the gas flow rate.

Six long-term partial perfusions were performed in conscious sheep weighing up to 104 kilograms at flow rates of 2.5 L. per minute and "shim" pressure of 200 mm. Hg. Venous drainage to the oxygenator occurred via a vena cava cannula inserted through the internal jugular vein. Arterial return was into a T tube in the common carotid artery. The sheep were allowed to stand and move within a restraining harness. Gas transfer rates, oxygenator input blood pressure, input gas pressure, plasma hemoglobin, fibrinogen, and platelet count were monitored. Hematocrit was 30 to 40 percent and body temperature was maintained at 37° C.

Eight further perfusions were performed in sheep weighing up to 101 kilograms to simulate the clinical conditions of open-chest total bypass, including coronary suction. These perfusions were of 3 hours' duration with hypothermia to 30° C. and hemodilution to 25 percent hematocrit.

To test the changes of CO_2 transfer over time, water at a fixed PO_2 and Pco_2 and 37° C. was run from a reservoir through the oxygenator at 4 L. per minute for 6 hours.

*Travenol Laboratories, Morton Grove, Ill.
†Cutter Laboratories, Inc., Berkeley, Calif.

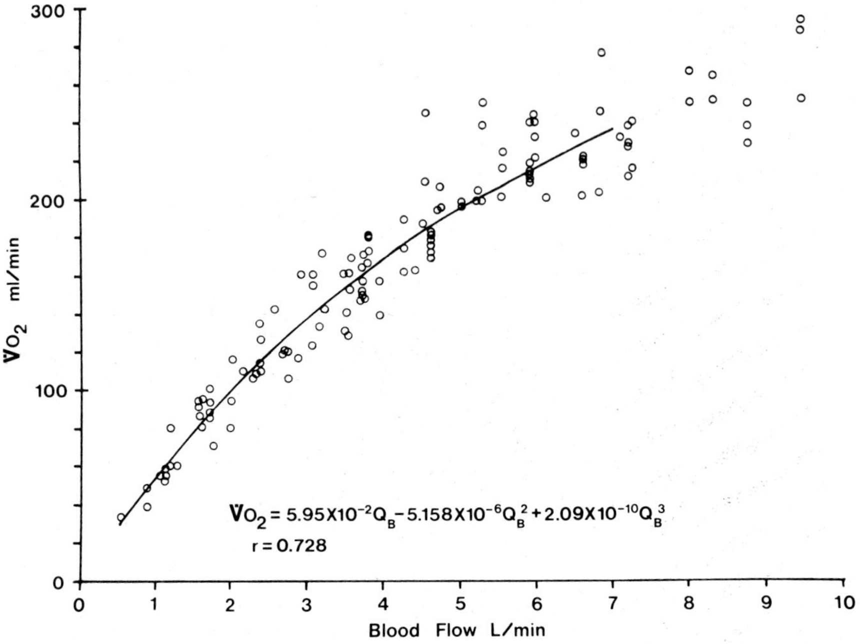

Fig. 3. O_2 transfer plotted against blood flow rate in acute sheep perfusions. $\dot{V}O_2$ oxygen transfer (milliliter per minute). Q_B = blood flow rate (milliliter per minute). Venous O_2 saturation was 60 to 70 percent, hematocrit 25 to 47 percent, temperature 36 to 38° C., O_2 flow rate 10 to 24 L. per minute, and shim pressure 130 to 300 mm. Hg. The regression curve is expressed by the equation.

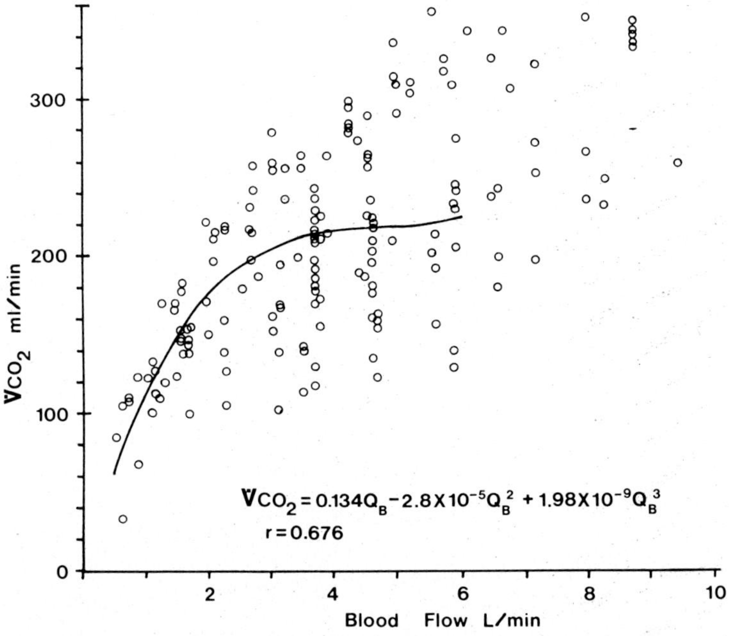

Fig. 4. CO_2 transfer plotted against blood flow rate in acute sheep perfusions. $\dot{V}CO_2$ = CO_2 transfer (milliliter per minute). Q_B = blood flow rate (milliliter per minute). Temperature 36 to 38° C., blood input P_{CO_2} 36 to 65 mm. Hg, O_2 flow rate 10 to 15 L. per minute, and shim pressure 150 to 300 mm. Hg.

The oxygenator was ventilated with oxygen at 10 L. per minute flow. The Pco_2 of the water in the reservoir was controlled at 100 mm. Hg using another microporous gas exchanger. The "shim" pressure was set either equal to input water pressure (entering the blood phase) or at 200 mm. Hg to compare the effect of this control mechanism on the gas transfer performance of the unit. Three oxygenators were tested at each shim pressure.

The pump-oxygenator system designed by the manufacturer was used for cardiac surgery in 40 patients (Table I). Blood O_2 saturation, Pco_2, and pH were determined at intervals during perfusion. Hypothermia to 30° C. and hemodilution (hematocrit 25 percent) were employed. All blood gas data were determined at 37° C. and corrected for temperature.

RESULTS

Oxygen transfer increased with blood flow rate as shown in Fig. 3. Carbon dioxide transfer also increased with blood flow rate and at any given flow was maximally larger than O_2 transfer (Fig. 4).

All six animals perfused for 24 hours (Table II) survived and were observed to be clinically normal for at least one week. During each of three perfusions, the oxygenators were replaced once following development of leaks or shunts. Mean oxygen transfer decreased 8 percent and mean CO_2 transfer decreased 1.5 percent over 24 hours in those three units which were mechanically reliable and did not leak or develop shunts. These changes were not statistically significant.

In open-chest procedures in sheep, gas transfer was satisfactory and the pump oxygenator system was mechanically effective (Table III). All animals recovered from anesthesia without apparent neurological sequelae.

To report the determinants of performance decay, the CO_2 transfer coefficient (a number that characterizes CO_2 transfer),[5, 6] was plotted against time (Fig. 5). Units with the "shim" pressure set at input blood pressure showed a 17 percent decrease in performance

Table I. *Cardiac patients*

	Mean	*Range*
No. of patients	40	
Age (yr.)	39.9	4 to 62
Procedures		
A-C bypass	24	
Valve replacement	5	
Congenital	11	
Size (body surface area) of patients ($M.^2$)	1.6	0.7 to 2.1
Weight of patients (Kg.)	61.4	16 to 94

Table II. *Partial perfusions in six sheep (24 hour)*

	Mean	*Range*
Weight (Kg.)	50	41 to 65
Perfusion flow (L./min.)	2.5	2.5
O_2 transfer (ml./min.)*		
Start	111	109 to 125
After 24 hr.	102	88 to 120
CO_2 transfer (ml./min.)*		
Start	219	210 to 228
After 24 hr.	216	170 to 265
Plasma hemoglobin (mg./100 ml.)		
Start	3	2.4 to 6.8
After 24 hr.	27	3.6 to 72
Plasma fibrinogen (mg./100 ml.)		
Start	450	300 to 670
After 24 hr.	200	42 to 293
Platelet count (per $mm.^3 \times 10^3$)		
Start	300	184 to 360
After 24 hr.	141	85 to 197

*These values are for the three oxygenators which were run 24 hours.

Table III. *Open-chest total bypass in eight sheep*

	Mean ± S.D.	*Range*	*N**
Weight (Kg.)	71 ± 15	53 to 101	8
Duration of perfusion (hr.)	3		
Flow rate (L./min.)	4.6 ± 0.7	2.6 to 5.8	43
Oxygen saturation (%)			
Venous	85 ± 8	66 to 96	43
Arterial	99 ± 1	95 to 100	43
Pv_{CO_2} (mm. Hg)	42 ± 10	29 to 69	43
Pa_{CO_2} (mm. Hg)	37 ± 8	25 to 62	43
Arterial pH	7.45 ± 0.07	7.28 to 7.57	43

*N = number of observations during the course of these eight perfusions.

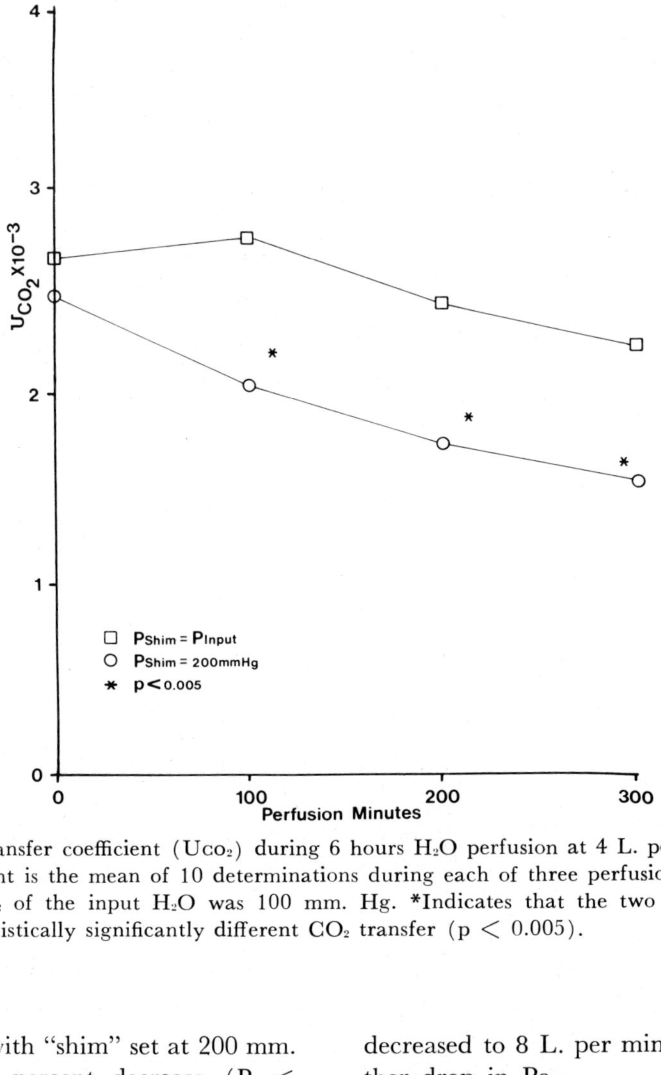

Fig. 5. CO_2 transfer coefficient (U_{CO_2}) during 6 hours H_2O perfusion at 4 L. per minute flow. Each data point is the mean of 10 determinations during each of three perfusions (total of 30 samples). P_{CO_2} of the input H_2O was 100 mm. Hg. *Indicates that the two shim pressures resulted in statistically significantly different CO_2 transfer ($p < 0.005$).

at 6 hours. Units with "shim" set at 200 mm. Hg showed a 40 percent decrease ($P < 0.005$) after the same interval.

In the first 40 consecutive clinical perfusions with this pump-oxygenator system, arterial oxygen saturation was 95 percent or more at each sampling during all perfusions (Table IV). Arterial P_{CO_2} was acceptable (48 mm. Hg or lower) in all cases except one (Fig. 6). In this patient the Pa_{CO_2} rose to 60 mm. Hg in spite of a high oxygen flow and a venous-arterial P_{CO_2} difference of 19 mm. Hg. Blood staining was noted at the gas outlet port at the end of this perfusion, which was the fourth in the clinical series. In contrast, the final Pa_{CO_2} during the longest perfusion (7 hours) was 34 mm. Hg, and the gas flow through the oxygenator had to be decreased to 8 L. per minute to prevent further drop in Pa_{CO_2}.

DISCUSSION

The rated blood flow*[7] of this oxygenator is about 4 L. per minute with an oxygenator priming volume of less than 400 ml.[12] At 6 L. per minute blood flow and venous O_2 saturation of 65 percent, O_2 transfer is approximately 200 ml. per minute and CO_2 transfer up to 300 ml. per minute. Long-term experimental perfusions indicated a small, but gradual loss in gas transfer (particularly for CO_2) with time, but this phenomenon was

*Rated blood flow: amount of blood which an artificial lung can arterialize at 37° C. to 95 percent saturation when the input (venous) blood has an oxygen saturation of 65 percent and a hematocrit of 40 percent.

not discernible up to 7 hours in human perfusions. The decrease in CO_2 transfer observed is probably related to details of oxygenator design, specifically the condensation of water vapor in certain areas of the gas phase.

Inflating the pneumatic "shim" bag reduces the thickness of the blood film but also affects the resistance to oxygen flow through the gas envelopes. A fraction of gas is probably shunted around the edges of the "shim" bag, resulting in an imbalance of perfusion and ventilation of the oxygenator with the current design. Carbon dioxide transfer appears to be lessened if the pressure in the "shim" exceeds the blood pressure at the input port of the oxygenator. We therefore operate the oxygenator with "shim" pressure equal to input blood pressure. Oxygen transfer is increased only to a minor extent by raising the "shim" pressure much above the input blood pressure. The "shim" pressure was increased to raise the Pa_{O_2} in occasional clinical cases.

CO_2 transfer increases greatly with the increases in the rate of ventilation of the oxygenator. Most of the clinical perfusions were carried out with an oxygen flow below that recommended by the manufacturer in an attempt to prevent hypocapnia.

In vitro tests demonstrated an accumulation of water in the gas phase with passage of time, particularly while ventilating the apparatus with humidified oxygen. Decreasing CO_2 transfer was associated with this water accumulation and its affect on the support structures in the gas phase. H_2O accumulation was less noticeable when heated, dry oxygen was used. Therefore the ventilating O_2 was not humidified in our clinical experience. Because the CO_2 transfer tended to decrease with time, the oxygenator was not primed until immediately before the start of bypass. (Priming can proceed very rapidly since air trapped in the unit can be forced through the pores of the membrane into the gas phase by the priming fluid.) We modified the apparatus to measure input blood pressure during perfusion to enable us to operate the "shim" at the lowest effective

Table IV. *Clinical total bypass*

	Mean ± S.D.	*Range*	*N**
Bypass duration (min.)	143 ± 86	17 to 425†	40
Blood flow rate (L./min.)	3.53 ± 0.81	1.25 to 5.80	136
O_2 flow (L./min.)	14.5 ± 4.6	5 to 22	127
Oxygen transfer (ml./min.)	115 ± 35.7	55 to 227	123
Oxygen saturation (%)			
Venous	72.3 ± 9.2	38 to 90	136
Arterial	99 ± 0.9	95 to 100	136
P_{CO_2} (mm. Hg)			
Venous	34 ± 9.8	18 to 79	136
Arterial	27 ± 7.7	14 to 60	136
Arterial pH	7.50 ± 0.11	7.16 to 7.78	
Platelet count (per mm.^{3} × 10^3)			
Start of perfusion	86.9 ± 29.1	34 to 132	18
End of perfusion	92.0 ± 50.3	34 to 190	18
Plasma fibrinogen (mg./100 ml.)			
Start of perfusion	203 ± 108	65 to 410	15
End of perfusion	190 ± 88	50 to 380	15

*N = number of observations during the course of these 40 perfusions.

†The longest perfusion was terminated with the death of the patient due to uncontrollable hemorrhage associated with a technical problem.

pressure since laboratory experience suggested least deterioration of CO_2 transfer under these conditions.

With an oxygenator characterized by minute pores in the membrane, it is essential to prevent blood seepage into the gas phase as well as the release of gas bubbles through the membrane into the blood phase. Limited blood staining of the gas phase occurred only once during an early clinical perfusion. Gas microemboli were not detected as long as the gas input pressure was kept below the blood phase output pressure. The pump-oxygenator assembly is designed to maintain these conditions throughout the range of operation of the unit, but these can be overridden if the circuit arrangement is different from that recommended. Typically recirculation keeps the output blood pressure sufficiently high and the O_2 blowoff keeps the gas phase pressure low.

The oxygenator has been shown to be atraumatic to erythrocytes in in vitro tests of hemolysis. Recirculation of 2,000 ml. of

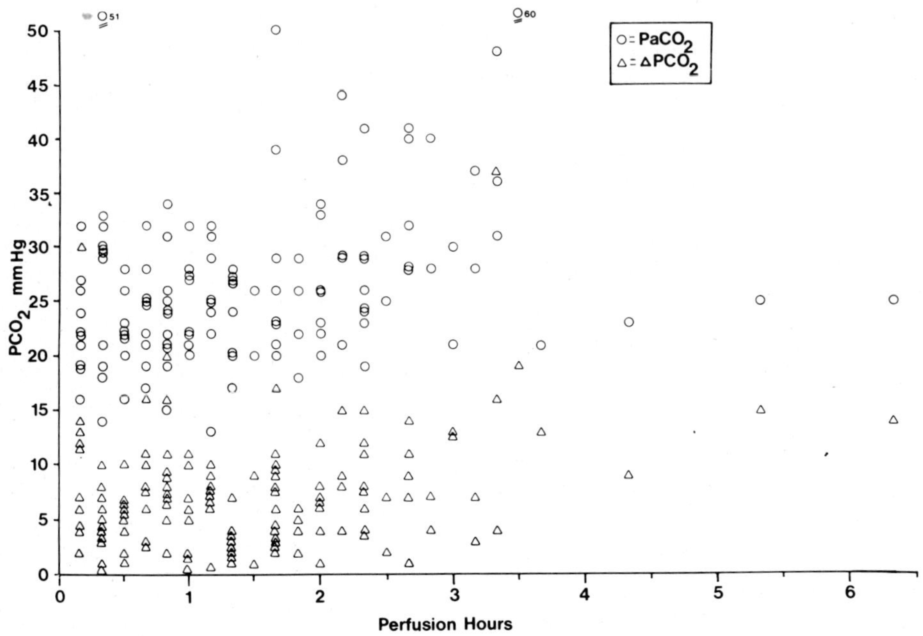

Fig. 6. Arterial P_{CO_2} and venous-arterial P_{CO_2} difference (ΔP_{CO_2}) plotted against length of perfusion in 40 clinical cases. The two values above 48 mm. Hg were from a case in which blood staining of the gas phase occurred.

dog blood through the oxygenator with a roller pump at 6 L. per minute for 150 minutes resulted in a mean increase of plasma hemoglobin of 57 mg. per 100 ml. Similar experiments with recirculation of the same amount of blood from the same mixed pool through a similar circuit but without the oxygenator resulted in a mean increase of plasma hemoglobin of 43 mg. per 100 ml. This results in an hemolysis index for the oxygenator, after subtracting the hemolysis from the pump alone, of 0.00034 Gm. per liter pumped.[15]

The oxygenator has proven to be safe and reliable for clinical use in total bypass up to 7 hours. Oxygenation has been satisfactory in all instances. Carbon dioxide transfer decreases with time, but the unit has an inherently large excess of CO_2 transfer capacity and CO_2 transfer has been adequate in all units except that which developed "hemoptysis." The use of a microporous membrane has improved gas transfer in this configuration of membrane oxygenator significantly. The oxygenator is structurally reliable and has a comfortable margin of safety during operation.

To achieve optimal results, the oxygenator should be primed immediately before bypass starts. Dry, heated oxygen should be used to ventilate the oxygenator, and the "shim" pressure should equal input blood pressure. During most clinical perfusions of 7 hours or less, the flow of O_2 through the oxygenator has been adjusted downward to prevent hypocapnia.

The authors wish to thank Dr. Harold Harrower and Mrs. G. F. Lewis for the fibrinogen determinations in the clinical cases and Wilbur Murray, John Martin, and Ronald Massimino for their technical collaboration.

REFERENCES

1. Birnbaum, D., and Eiseman, B.: Laboratory evaluation of a new silicone membrane oxygenator, J. Thorac. Cardiovasc. Surg. **64:** 441, 1972.
2. Boyd, J. C., Moran, J. F., and Clark, R. E.: An analysis of the operating characteristics of the 0.25 M.[2] Travenol infant membrane oxygenator, SURGERY **71:** 262, 1972.

3. Carlson, R. G., Landé, A. J., Ivey, L. W., et al.: Total cardiopulmonary support with disposable membrane oxygenator during aortocoronary artery-vein graft operations, Chest **62:** 424, 1972.
4. Douglas, M., Birnbaum, D., and Eiseman, B.: Biological evaluation of a disposable membrane oxygenator, Arch. Surg. **103:** 89, 1971.
5. Friedman, L. I., Richardson, P. D., and Galletti, P. M.: Blood oxygenator testing and evaluation, part II. Procedures and results, Annual report, Contract No. NIH-NHLI **69:** 2047, Medical Devices Applications Program, 1973.
6. Galletti, P. M., Richardson, P. D., and Snider, M. T.: Blood oxygenator testing and evaluation, part I. Evaluation techniques, Annual report, Contract No. NIH-NHLI **69:** 2047, Medical Devices Application Program, 1971.
7. Galletti, P. M., Richardson, P. D., Snider, M. T., and Friedman, L. I.: A standardized method for defining the overall gas transfer performance of artificial lungs, Trans. Am. Soc. Artif. Intern. Organs **18:** 359, 1972.
8. Gille, J. P., Trudell, L., Snider, M. T., et al.: Capabilities of microporous membrane-lined capillary oxygenator in hypercapnic dogs, Trans. Am. Soc. Artif. Intern. Organs **16:** 365, 1970.
9. Hill, J. D., Iatridis, A., O'Keefe, R., and Kitrilakis, S.: Technique for achieving high gas exchange rates in membrane oxygenation, Trans. Am. Soc. Artif. Intern. Organs **20,** 1974. In press.
10. Hill, J. D., deLeval, M. R., Fallat, R. J., et al.: Acute respiratory insufficiency. Treatment with prolonged extracorporeal oxygenation, J. Thorac. Cardiovasc. Surg. **64:** 551, 1972.
11. Kolobow, T., Zapol, W. M., Sigman, R. L., and Peirce, J.: Partial cardiopulmonary bypass lasting up to seven days in alert lambs with membrane lung blood oxygenation, J. Thorac. Cardiovasc. Surg. **60:** 781, 1970.
12. Murphy, W., Trudell, L. A., Friedman, L. I., et al.: Laboratory and clinical experience with a microporous membrane oxygenator, Trans. Am. Soc. Artif. Intern. Organs **20:** 1974. In press.
13. Peirce, E. C.: Is the blood-gas interface of clinical importance? Ann. Thorac. Surg. **17:** 526, 1974.
14. Peirce, E. C., Thebaut, A. L., Kent, B. B., et al.: Techniques of extended perfusion using a membrane lung, Ann. Thorac. Surg. **12:** 451, 1971.
15. Sassetti, R., Kloppal, R., and Yameshita, S.: Personal communication.
16. Trudell, L. A., Friedman, L. I., Kakvan, M., et al.: Evaluation of a disposable membrane oxygenator, Trans. Am. Soc. Artif. Intern. Organ **18:** 538, 1972.

DISCUSSION

Dr. Robert G. Carlson (New York, N. Y.). I congratulate Karl Karlson in pioneering the first clinical use of this microporous membrane oxygenator. I would like to ask two questions and make one comment. This microporous oxygenator has demonstrated an excellent ability to transfer oxygen and carbon dioxide gas. It probably is about twice as effective as the silicone membrane for gas transfer.

1. Is it possible to transfer too much gas in the form of gas emboli across the membrane? The first slide shows our experience comparing the Landé membrane oxygenator with the Bentley bubble oxygenator (presented at this meeting 2 years ago). With an ultrasonic counter, we counted 18,000 to 35,000 microemboli, 50 μ or larger, per minute with a bubble oxygenator and almost no microemboli counts with the silicone membrane. In our clinical studies, the Bender-Gestalt visual motor test scores taken before and after heart operation with either the Landé membrane or the Bentley bubble oxygenator correlated with emboli counts.

In 47 patients, the postoperative scores were worse in 63 percent of the patients after use with bubble oxygenator but worse in only 36 percent of the patients after using the Landé membrane. Adding a 40 μ barrier screen filter in the arterial line reduced the percentage of worse scores to 43 percent of the bubble and only 13 percent of membrane patients with a filter. It would be interesting to perform these tests on your patients receiving the microporous membrane.

2. Is this truly a membrane oxygenator? Does this apparatus reduce the denaturation of protein as described by Dr. Lee or does the excellent gas transfer result in more denaturation of the protein similar to the bubble oxygenator?

Dr. Arthur C. Beall, Jr. (Houston, Texas). We have likewise used the Teflon membrane oxygenator on sheep and would only say that our results confirm the results that Dr. Karlson presented. There are excellent transfer characteristics to this membrane oxygenator. We have now used the oxygenator in roughly 150 clinical cases and have been quite impressed with it. One major advantage we have seen is that one has independent control of carbon dioxide elimination and oxygenation.

As Dr. Karlson pointed out, one controls oxygenation by the shim pressure, which varies the thickness of the blood film, and controls CO_2 elimination by the oxygen flow rate through the oxygenator. In comparison to the bubbler, where these two are interrelated, one has the ability to control them separately.

The other advantage we have seen is better establishment of hemostasis following neutralization of heparin. We cannot say exactly why this occurs, but there is no question that there is quite a difference.

We believe it relates, not to the number of platelets, but to platelet function. In our laboratory Dr. Salise now is studying this and, hopefully, within the next few months we will have some answers. It would appear that the function of the platelets is better maintained when using the membrane oxygenator.

My other reason for rising is to give a warning that use of this membrane can be tricky until one learns some of the problems. I would encourage anyone planning to use this membrane to gain some experience with it in the laboratory and, perhaps even further, to have the pump technicians visit one of the centers where it is being used for a few days, prior to using it clinically.

Dr. E. Converse Peirce, II (New York, N. Y.). Early membrane lungs used membranes of low gas permeability. Drs. George Clowes and William Neville were so intrepid that they did some human studies using polyethylene, which has a maximum oxygen transfer of only 8 ml. per square meter of membrane. Later, of course, we all used Teflon, which is five or six times more permeable to oxygen. Silicone and related membranes have since made it possible to build full-capacity lungs but these require 4 square meters or more of membrane and are consequently expensive.

Microporous Teflon has virtually no resistance to gas flow. It cannot be given a meaningful value for oxygen or carbon dioxide transfer because it has an essentially infinite permeability even for membranes up to 2 mm. thick. This makes possible construction of much smaller and less expensive devices.

Membrane lungs are clearly less traumatic to blood than nonmembrane devices, and they have been used for successful clinical pulmonary support for periods up to 21 days.

This new device raises some questions: First, is it really a membrane lung? It does not start out as one but, as soon as blood enters it, a protein film forms over the micropores and converts it to one.

Second, it has a very high blood flow relative to the membrane area and it uses screens between the membranes to provide blood mixing. My earlier data from comparative 6 hour in vitro tests, where dog blood passed through a membrane device more than 300 times, showed that screens between the membranes caused more hemolysis even than a disk oxygenator. Low hemolysis was the rule when screens were not used. If I understand correctly, the microporous lung is intended to function up to 6 L. of blood flow per minute, although most of your perfusions were at a good bit lower flow. I would like to ask how much hemolysis occurs in the lung if it is used at its maximum recommended flow?

And, third, I note that, although the rated flow is about 4 L. per minute, lower flows were employed clinically for most of the cases and that hypothermia was used. Oxygen exchange averaged only 116 ml. per minute, which is perhaps half the expected basal uptake. Is this new lung suitable for full flow at normal body temperature?

This is an excellent paper and an important contribution. I congratulate Dr. Karlson and the other authors on an unusually comprehensive description of this new microporous Teflon lung which should help greatly to revolutionize the field.

Dr. Glenn Kelly (Denver, Colo.). In Dr. Eiseman's laboratory, in Denver, we have been working with the Travenol Laboratories in designing a membrane oxygenator for 5 years. In 1971 we published the design and efficiency of this unit subsequently used by us and described by Dr. Karlson today.

At that time it appeared that the silicone membrane adequate for oxygen transfer was of little use in carbon dioxide transfer.

After a number of experimental studies in 1972, we first published our results in the use of expanded Teflon or Gore-Tex membrane in a membrane oxygenator. Since that time Dr. Esato, in our laboratory, has evaluated both the 0.75 $M.^2$ silicone membrane unit and a 2.25 $M.^2$ oxygenator, using a Gore-Tex membrane. The latter is exactly the same as the one we have just heard described today.

In 15 animals perfused for 3 hours by Dr. Esato, we have arrived at many results similar to those just described by Dr. Karlson. CO transfer was up to 500 ml. per minute. This is, of course, in excess of conceivable physiologic demand in contrast to very limited carbon dioxide permeability through other membranes. Dr. Esato has also found up to 400 ml. of oxygen transfer per minute using the Gore-Tex unit.

When we used the silicone membrane at the mile-high altitude of Denver, we found it necessary to recirculate the blood through the oxygenator. In contrast, when we used the more permeable Gore-Tex membrane, no such recirculation was required.

These membrane oxygenators seem kinder to the blood elements than are those containing a gas-blood interface.

Our prime interest has been in developing a membrane oxygenator for prolonged use in supporting patients with respiratory insufficiency who cannot be supported with mechanical respirators. Our experience shows that the Travenol Gore-Tex 2.25 M^2 unit is ideal for such purposes.

The paper we have just heard adds important supporting evidence as to the efficiency of this unit and, for the first time, documents the clinical use of this promising device.

Dr. Karl E. Karlson (Closing). I thank Dr. Peirce for answering Dr. Carlson's question regarding whether this was really a membrane oxygenator.

As you saw from our data, the oxygen transfer levels off at about 200 ml. per minute. If we consider that the average anesthetized patient will consume about 120 ml. of oxygen per square meter, this oxygenator, in its present configuration, is just barely suitable for full-flow perfusion in a patient of 2 square meter size.

In our clinical experience, we almost never see these types of oxygen consumption at full flow at normothermia. In our practice we use hypothermia according to the clinical indications of the cardiac operation.

I did not present any hemolysis data, but there are hemolysis data available which would indicate that the hemolysis with this oxygenator would be somewhere in the low part of Dr. Peirce's curve.

I believe that all of the authors have emphasized that this modification of membrane oxygenators appears to have increased the gas-transfer properties of membrane oxygenators significantly. We believe that the unit, as we are using it at the present time, is safe and reliable for clinical perfusion, although there no doubt will be improvements and modifications coming along rapidly.

Complications following the contoured Dacron baffle in correction of transposition of the great arteries

George J. Reul, Jr., M.D., Denton A. Cooley, M.D., Frank M. Sandiford, M.D., *and* **Grady L. Hallman, M.D.,** *Houston, Texas*

Over a 15 month period, a contoured Dacron patch was utilized as the primary material for the intra-atrial baffle in repair of both complex and simple transposition of the great arteries (TGA) in 32 patients. The mortality rate for the entire group was six of 32, with two late deaths. A high incidence of postoperative pulmonary venous obstruction (PVO) occurred. Seven of the 24 survivors required reoperation because of PVO. Five of the seven patients had superior vena caval obstruction. In six more patients mild obstruction of the vena cava and/or pulmonary veins was found during the postoperative evaluation The obstruction occurred late (mean, one year). It was the result of fibrosis, contracture, and formation of a thick neointima on the Dacron material. The diagnosis was made by cardiac catheterization and pulmonary scanning. Early operative repair was done from 6 to 17 months following the first operation. In five patients a pulmonary venous atrioplasty was done by enlargement of the pulmonary venous atrium with a patch graft. One patient had pulmonary atrioplasty with reinsertion of a pericardial intra-atrial baffle and the last patient had left pneumonectomy because of severe obstruction of the left pulmonary veins. In a similar series of 112 patients operated with the same technique except for use of pericardium rather than Dacron for the intra-atrial baffle, no patients required reoperation because of PVO. We, therefore, favor the use of pericardium as the primary material for an intra-atrial baffle in correction of TGA. If Dacron must be utilized, a pulmonary venous atrioplasty by enlargement of the pulmonary venous atrium may prevent PVO caused by late stricture of the Dacron baffle.

From the Division of Surgery of the Texas Heart Institute of St. Luke's Episcopal and Texas Children's Hospital, Houston, Texas

TEN YEARS have passed since modifications of the technique of Albert[3] were advanced by Mustard and associates[22, 23] for correction of transposition of the great arteries (TGA). More recent modifications of of the intra-atrial baffle operation have been helpful in reducing the mortality rate. The high incidence of conduction disturbances has been decreased by avoiding the sinoatrial node in cannulation, the intra-atrial conduction fibers in septectomy, and the atrioventricular bundle in patch placement.[1, 2, 7] Early correction in infancy has been urged because of an acceptable mortality rate when compared to early palliation and late operation.[1, 5, 6, 14, 15, 26]

Although operative death has been substantially reduced, the early and late complication of venous obstruction, tricuspid insufficiency, and arrhythmia have made the procedure far from curative.[4, 12, 19] Obstruction of venous return to the new atrial chambers has been the most challenging compli-

Presented at the Twenty-eighth Annual Meeting of the Society for Vascular Surgery, Chicago, Ill., June 20 and 21, 1974.

Reprint requests: Denton A. Cooley, M. D., P. O. Box 20345, Houston, Texas 77025.

cation.[9, 13, 17, 18, 25] Shape, size, placement, and material of the intra-atrial baffle have been the determining factors of venous return. Because of laboratory[21] and clinical evidence of late pericardial contracture, use of Dacron as the primary material for the intra-atrial baffle has been proposed.[1, 8, 9, 13, 18, 20] Although our results with pericardium as the primary patch material had been good, we proposed a contoured knitted Dacron baffle for the repair.[8] This report is an analysis of the late complications of this technique.

CLINICAL MATERIAL

At the Texas Heart Institute from April, 1972, through July, 1973, a contoured Dacron baffle fashioned from a 16 mm. weave-knit graft was utilized as the primary intra-atrial patch material in the repair of TGA in 32 children. This represented our entire series of patients repaired with the contoured Dacron baffle according to the techniques previously described.[8] The patients ranged in age from 7 weeks to 8 years, with a mean age of 2.8 years. There were 23 boys and 9 girls (Fig. 1). There were five children under the age of one year and 12 from one to 2 years of age. Thus 17 patients were under the age of 2. The weight distribution was from 8 to 68 pounds, with a mean weight of 27.9 pounds. Most patients weighed from 21 to 30 pounds (Fig. 2).

All patients had balloon atrial septostomy prior to surgical intervention. In addition, there were 13 palliative operative procedures prior to the intra-atrial baffle operation (Table I). Ten patients had previous atrial septectomies (Blalock-Hanlon procedure). Two patients with left ventricular outflow tract obstruction (LVOTO) had intrapericardial aorta to right pulmonary artery shunts. One patient had closure of a ductus arteriosus along with a Blalock-Hanlon procedure. Simple TGA alone was present in 14 patients. Ten patients had TGA plus LVOTO. Five patients had associated TGA with LVOTO and ventricular septal defect (VSD). Three patients had TGA with VSD.

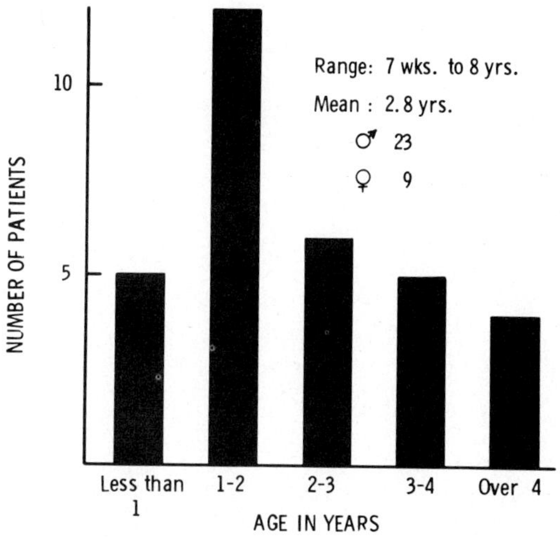

Fig. 1. The age distribution of the 32 patients who underwent Dacron intra-atrial baffle correction of transposition of the great vessels.

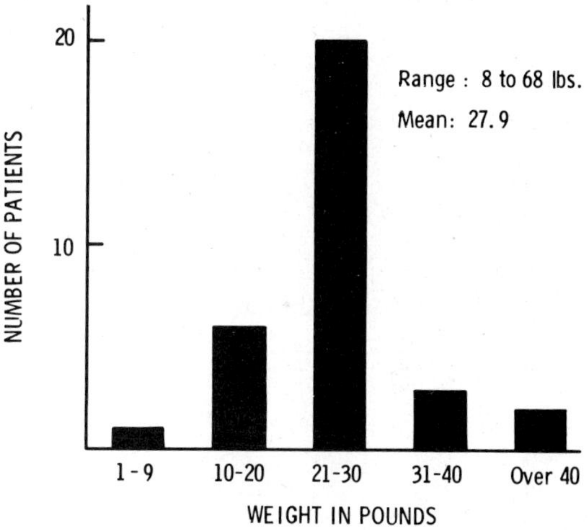

Fig. 2. The weight distribution of the patients who underwent Dacron intra-atrial baffle repair.

RESULTS

Of the 32 patients undergoing intra-atrial baffle procedure for correction of TGA, six died in the 30 day postoperative period. Five of the six patients died early because of low cardiac output following repair of their lesions (Table II). The other died because of disseminated intravascular coagulation. Only one patient with simple TGA died following operation. The remaining five patients had complex TGA. There were two late deaths. In one patient, superior vena caval obstruction may have played a role.

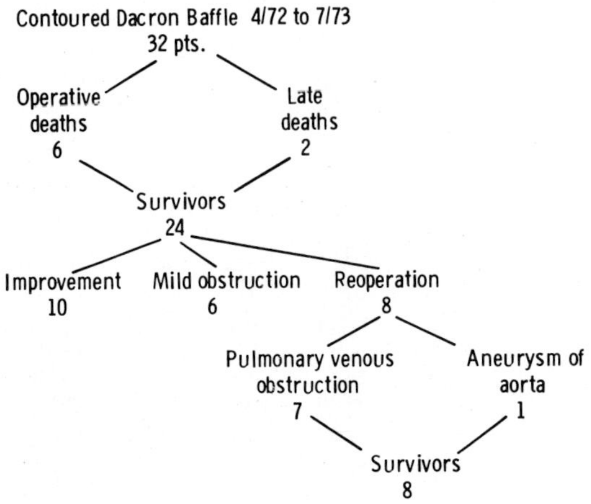

Fig. 3. The results in the 32 patients following Dacron intra-atrial baffle repair of TGA. Of the 24 survivors, seven required reoperation because of pulmonary venous obstruction from the Dacron baffle. All of the reoperated patients survived.

Of the 24 survivors, 10 had improvement following the operation, six had mild obstruction of the superior or inferior vena cava, and eight patients required reoperation (Fig. 3). One of these patients had an aneurysm of the ascending aorta at the cannulation site, preceded by a bout of bacterial endocarditis. The remaining seven patients were operated on for severe pulmonary venous obstruction (PVO). All eight patients survived following the second surgical procedure.

The late occurrence of PVO was quite dramatic in the seven patients. The age range was from one to 4 years, with a mean of 2.4 years. (Table III). The weight range was from 20 to 31 pounds, with a mean weight of 25.3 pounds. Of major importance was the late occurrence of obstruction in these patients. Symptoms first occurred from 4 to 12 months following operation. The reoperation was done from 6 to 17 months following the original operation and the mean reoperation time was one year postoperatively. After the first operation, there was little evidence of early obstruction of the pulmonary veins in the postoperative course.

All patients who had suspicion of PVO or inferior or superior vena caval obstruction (SVCO) following operation had cardiac

Table I. *Preoperative pathology*

		*Previous surgery**		
		Atrial septectomy	*Shunt*	*Ductus closure*
TGA† (simple)	14	2		
TGA† + LVOTO‡	10	3		
TGA† + LVOTO‡ + VSD§	5	3	2	
TGA† + VSD§	3	2	—	1
Total	32	10	2	1

*All patients had previous balloon atrial septostomy.
†TGA—transposition of great arteries.
‡LVOTO—left ventricular outflow tract obstruction.
§VSD—ventricular septal defect.

Table II. *Results**

	All patients	*Mortality*		*Reoperation*
		30 days	*Late*	
TGA† (simple)	14	1	1	4
TGA† + LOVOTO‡	10	1	1	2
TGA† + LVOTO‡ + VSD§	5	3		
TGA + VSD§	3	1	—	1
Total	32	6	2	7

*All survived.
†TGA—transposition of great arteries.
‡LVOTO—left ventricular outflow tract obstruction.
§VSD—ventricular septal defect.

catheterization. The hemodynamics in the seven patients consisted of elevated pulmonary artery pressure, elevated pulmonary artery mean wedge pressure, and, in most instances, elevation of the superior vena caval mean pressure (Table IV). Three of seven patients had minimal SVCO with good azygous vein drainage in addition to the PVO. Two others had severe SVCO with azygous drainage. The systemic arterial saturation was satisfactory following the intra-atrial baffle repair. One patient had moderate tricuspid insufficiency and poor systemic ventricular contraction in addition to the PVO.

In some instances at cardiac catheterization the pulmonary veins could be directly injected and the flow of blood was shown to

Table III. *Characteristics in 7 patients reoperated on after intra-atrial baffle repair of TGA because of pulmonary venous obstruction*

Case	Type	Age (yr.)	Weight (lbs.)	Time after surgery (mo.)	Pathology	Operation	Result
1	TGA*	4	27	16	PVO§ SVCO‖	Atrioplasty revision	Good
2	TGA*	1 10/12	20	10	PVO§ SVCO‖	Atrioplasty intra-atrial baffle redo	Fair
3	TGA*	3	28	6	PVO§ SVCO‖	Atrioplasty	Good
4	TGA*	1 8/12	26	17	PVO§	Atrioplasty	Good
5	TGA* + LOVOTO†	1	21	10	PVO§ SVCO‖	Atrioplasty	Fair
6	TGA* + LVOTO†	1 4/12	24	17	PVO§	Atrioplasty	Good
7	TGA* + VSD‡ (PHBP)	4	31	9	Left PVO§ SVCO‖	Left pneumonectomy	Poor

*TGA—transposition of great arteries.
†LVOTO—left ventricular outflow tract obstruction.
‡VSD—ventricular septal defect.
§PVO—pulmonary venous obstruction.
‖SVCO—superior vena cava obstruction.

be markedly decreased in the obstructed veins (Fig. 4). Other evidence of obstruction by angiogram was obtained by recirculation through the left atrium (Fig. 5). All patients had dye injection of the superior and/or inferior vena cava to demonstrate the systemic venous return. Kinking of the Dacron graft appeared to be responsible for obstruction in most of the cases of SVCO (Fig. 6).

Operation for pulmonary venous obstruction. Once severe PVO was demonstrated by angiographic and hemodynamic studies, reoperation was indicated. One patient (Case 7, Table III) had severe left PVO with very little pulmonary arterial flow and evidence of pulmonary damage by lung scan. This patient underwent left thoracotomy and the left lung was found to be severely diseased. A pneumonectomy was done. Marked bronchial venous varices were present, indicating the high degree of obstruction which caused significant destruction of the lung. Reoperation in the remaining six patients consisted of enlargement of the new pulmonary venous atrium by Dacron patch graft (Fig. 7). The patients were placed on cardiopulmonary bypass by direct cannulation of both venae cavae. The pulmonary venous atrium was opened and the patch examined for evidence of kinking. In

Table IV. *Hemodynamics in 7 patients with Dacron baffle obstruction*

	Range	Mean
Pulmonary artery pressure	42/20 to 130/80	75/40
P.A. mean wedge pressure	10 to 32	24.4
Superior vena cava mean pressure*	7 to 20	11.8
Systemic arterial saturation (room air) (%)	80 to 95	90

*Five of seven had SVC obstruction.

most instances fibrosis, thickened neointima, and kinking with buildup of fibrotic tissue were demonstrated at the orifices adjacent to the venous return. Reconstruction of the pulmonary venous atrium was done by placement of a woven Dacron patch enlarging the pulmonary venous atrium to enlarge both inferiorly between the pulmonary veins and superiorly on the surface of the pulmonary venous atrium. This allowed for a larger drainage chamber bordered by the kinked thickened baffle. No evidence of persistent PVO was present following this type of repair. One patient (Case 1, Table III) had a pulmonary atrioplasty at the first operation and this was enlarged with an additional patch. In Case 2 (Table III) there was kinking of the baffle at the superior vena

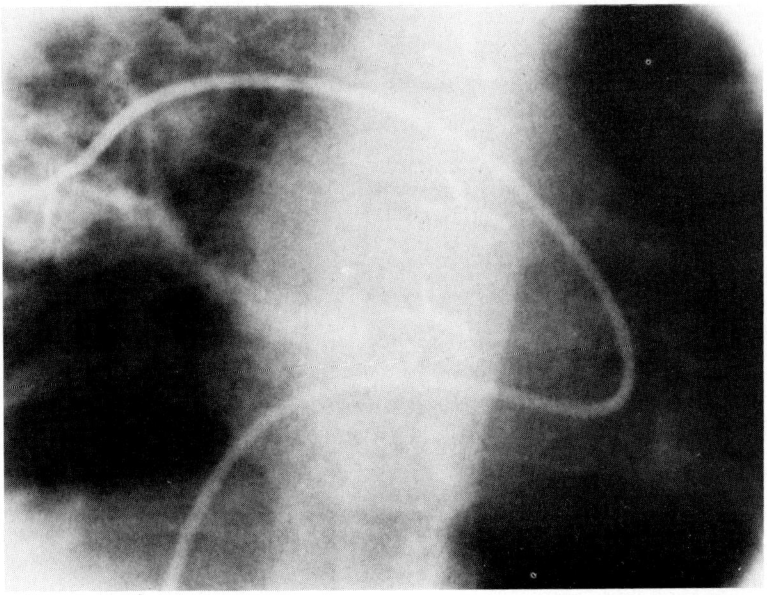

Fig. 4. The angiogram shows the slow drainage of the pulmonary veins of a 1-year-old girl, 16 months following intra-atrial Dacron baffle repair (Case 1, Table III). There is severe obstruction of the superior right pulmonary vein as it empties into the new pulmonary venous atrium.

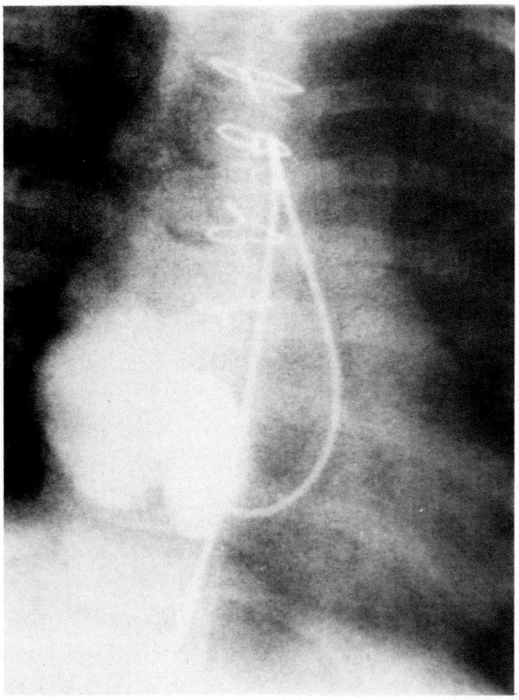

Fig. 5. This is the new pulmonary venous atrium of a 1-year-old boy, 9 months following correction by an intra-atrial baffle of Dacron (Case 5, Table III). Note the ridge on the inferior surface caused by kinking of the Dacron baffle. The boy had pulmonary venous obstruction and underwent atrioplasty 14 months following the original operation.

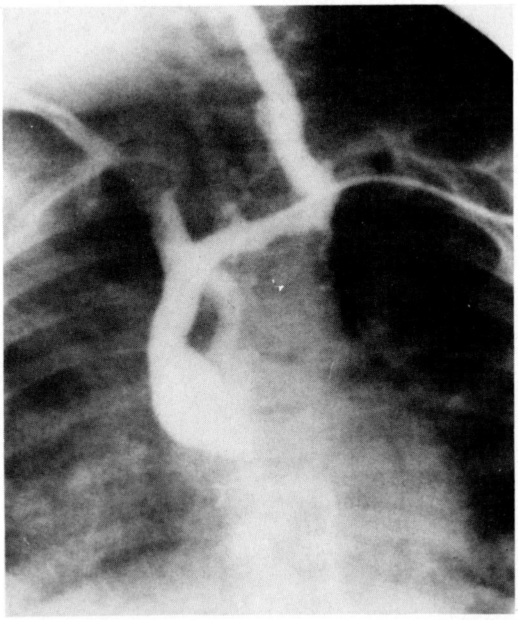

Fig. 6. This is a contrast injection into the superior vena cava of a 22-month-old boy, 10 months following previous Dacron intra-atrial baffle repair for transposition of the great arteries (Case 2, Table III). There is obstruction to the drainage of the superior vena cava in the area of the septectomy and baffle. This was caused by a kink in the Dacron. Note the large azygous vein. The child underwent pulmonary atrioplasty with reconstruction of the baffle with a good result.

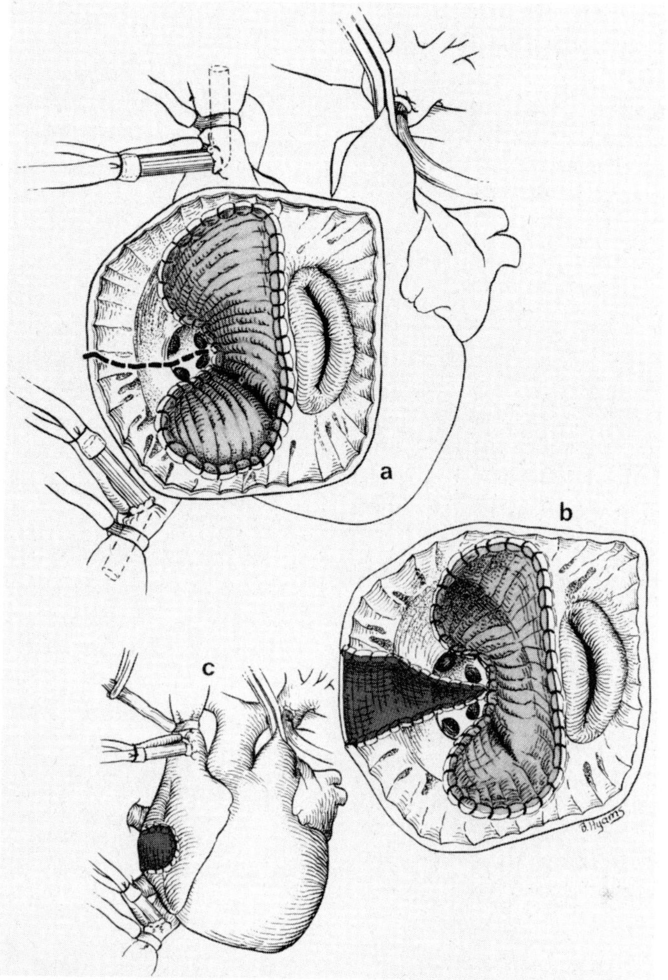

Fig. 7. This is a diagrammatic representation of the technique for pulmonary venous atrioplasty utilized to correct pulmonary venous obstruction caused by the Dacron baffle. The view is into the pulmonary venous atrium. The pulmonary vein orifices show posteriorly below the tricuspid valve. The old Dacron baffle is seen with a kink in its inferior portion. Cannulation for drainage has been done through both venae cavae. A Dacron patch has been used to enlarge the pulmonary venous atrium. The patch extends between the pulmonary veins into the new pulmonary venous atrium. This technique was used for most reconstructions of the pulmonary venous atrium.

cava inlet. The Dacron baffle was removed and a baffle of pericardium replaced. All patients survived the operative procedure and in follow-up have shown improvement.

DISCUSSION

The incidence of the serious complication of PVO was high in the patients in whom a contoured Dacron baffle was used for correction of TGA. Rather than decreasing the incidence of late fibrosis, as had been hoped, by substituting Dacron for pericardium, PVO was markedly increased. In fact, of the 112 patients who had pericardium as the intra-atrial baffle in repair of TGA, no patients required reoperation for early or late pulmonary venous obstruction. Only three patients with pericardial baffles were reoperated on, all for complications other than those related to late patch fibrosis. Thus the theoretical problems of pericardial stricture have not occurred in our series of pericardial baffles. On the other hand, severe PVO was common following the use of the Dacron baffle.

The characteristics of PVO were easily

Table V. *Comparison of Dacron to pericardium for the intra-atrial baffle in correlation of TGA*

Dacron	*Pericardium*
Stiff	Pliable
Thick neointima	Thin neointima
Kinking common	Conforms to atrial pressure
Difficult to tailor	Easily shaped to contour
High incidence of late obstruction	Rare late obstruction

recognized in the postoperative evaluation of the patient. The late occurrence of this complication was the result of progressive fibrosis and kinking of the Dacron baffle. Others have reported this same phenomenon.[10, 12, 25] In fact, our incidence of obstruction closely parallels that reported by Stark and associates[25] following use of a Dacron baffle.

The minor factor altered in our Dacron baffle series when compared to the series of patients who had a pericardial baffle was the material itself. The shape and patch placement were similar in both groups. Actual kinking, fibrosis, and thickening of the Dacron patch were observed at reoperation. Thus in this series the patch material itself has been shown to be responsible for late PVO. Dacron is stiff when compared to pericardium and, despite the predetermined contour or loose weave of the Dacron, it is difficult to tailor it to the numerous bends and curves of the intra-atrial baffle. In fact, immediately after inserting a Dacron baffle, the appearance is deceiving. Later contraction of the atrial septectomy site, changes in intra-atrial pressure, ventricular volume, and/or growth contractility may cause kinking of the Dacron graft. Pericardium, on the other hand, is quite pliable and does not kink easily (Table V). In addition, a thickened neointima was found on the Dacron baffle. This fibrous material filled some of the spaces in the kinked areas.

The operative mortality rate following surgical repair of TGA is quite acceptable at most centers, but late complications remain a difficult problem. We have continued to reserve early operative repair for the critically ill infant. Death from atrial septectomy for palliation of TGA has been quite low. Death due to medical problems such as cerebral vascular accidents while awaiting operation has not been as high as described by others.[1, 3] More reports of long-term follow-up after intra-atrial baffle repair in infants are urged. Due to this unexpected high incidence of PVO and/or SVCO following placement of a Dacron baffle, we have abandoned its use as a primary patch material since July, 1973. In the few patients in whom a pericardial patch is not possible for various reasons, a knitted Dacron patch is used with an awareness of the possibility of increased postoperative complications. In the case of the small or questionably small new pulmonary venous atrium, we prefer to do a primary pulmonary atrioplasty. For those in whom PVO does develop, early correction by pulmonary atrioplasty is suggested before permanent lung destruction occurs.

REFERENCES

1. Aberdeen, E.: Correction of uncomplicated cases of transposition of the great arteries, Br. Heart J. **33** (Suppl.): 66, 1971.
2. Aberdeen, E., Waterston, D. J., Carr, I., et al.: Successful "correction" of transposed great arteries by Mustard's operation, Lancet **1:** 1233, 1965.
3. Albert, H. M.: Surgical correction of transposition of the great vessels, Surg. Forum **5:** 74, 1954.
4. Balderman, S. C., Athanasuleas, C. L., and Anagnostopoulos, C. E.: The atrial baffle operation for transposition of the great arteries: A review of 591 reported cases. Ann. Thorac. Surg. **17:** 114, 1974.
5. Barratt-Boyes, B. G., Simpson, M., and Neutze, J. M.: Intracardiac surgery in neonates and infants using deep hypothermia with surface cooling and limited cardiopulmonary bypass, Circulation **43:** 44, 1971.
6. Bonchek, L. L., and Starr, A.: Total correction of transposition of the great arteries in infancy as initial surgical management, Ann. Thorac. Surg. **14:** 376, 1972.
7. Breckenridge, I. M., Oelert, H., Stark, J., et al.: Mustard's operation for transposition of the great arteries, Lancet **1:** 1140, 1972.
8. Cooley, D. A., Wukasch, D. C., and Sandiford, F. M.: Contoured knitted Dacron baffle for repair of transposition of the great vessels, Ann. Thorac. Surg. **15:** 640, 1973.

9. Danielson, G. K., Mair, D. D., Ongley, P. A., et al.: Repair of transposition of the great arteries by transposition of the venous return: Surgical considerations and results of operation, J. Thorac. Cardiovasc. Surg. **61:** 96, 1971.
10. Doty, D. B., and Ehrenhaft, J. L.: Editorial on Mustard procedure, Ann. Thorac. Surg. **17:** 210, 1974.
11. El-Said, G., Rosenberg, H. S., Mullins, C. E., et al.: Dysrhythmias after Mustard's operation for transposition of the great arteries, Am. J. Cardiol. **30:** 526, 1972.
12. Grehl, T. M., and Shumway, N. E.: Transposition of the great arteries: Reoperation for dysfunctional intra-atrial baffle, J. Thorac. Cardiovasc. Surg. **67:** 863, 1974.
13. Indeglia, R. A., Moller, J. H., Lucas, R. V., Jr., and Castaneda, A. R.: Treatment of transposition of the great vessels with an intra-atrial baffle (Mustard procedure), Arch. Surg. **101:** 797, 1970.
14. Kilman, J. W., Williams, T. E., Jr., Kakos, G. S., et al.: Surgical correction of the transposition complex in infancy, J. Thorac. Cardiovasc. Surg. **66:** 387, 1973.
15. Kirklin, J. W.: Surgery for transposition of the great arteries and other types of malpositions of the great arteries, *in* Barratt-Boyes, B. G., Neutze, J. M., and Harris, P. D., editors: Heart disease in infancy: Diagnosis and surgical treatment, Edinburgh, 1973, Churchill Livingstone, p. 253.
16. Lindesmith, G. G., Meyer, B. W., Stanton, R. E., et al.: Surgical treatment of transposition of the great vessels, Ann. Thorac. Surg. **8:** 12, 1969.
17. Massei, E. A., and Mulder, D. G.: Superior vena cava syndrome following complete correction (Mustard repair) of transposition of the great vessels, Ann. Thorac. Surg. **11:** 243, 1971.
18. McGoon, D. C.: Technics of open-heart surgery for congenital heart disease, Curr. Probl. Surg. **3:** 42, 1968.
19. McGoon, D. C.: Surgery for transposition of the great arteries, Circulation **45:** 1147, 1972.
20. Merendino, K. A., Jesseph, J. E., Herron, P. W., et al.: Interatrial venous transposition: A one-stage intracardiac operation for the conversion of complete transposition of the aorta and pulmonary artery to corrected transposition, Surgery **42:** 898, 1957.
21. Mohri, H., Barnes, R. W., Rittenhouse, E. A., et al.: Fate of autologous pericardium and Dacron fabric used as substitutes for total atrial septum in growing animals, J. Thorac. Cardiovasc. Surg. **59:** 501, 1970.
22. Mustard, W. T.: Recent experiences with surgical management of transposition of the great arteries, J. Cardiovasc. Surg. (Torino) **9:** 532, 1966.
23. Mustard, W. T., Keith, J. D., Trusler, G. A., et al.: The surgical management of transposition of the great vessels, J. Thorac. Cardiovasc. Surg. **48:** 953, 1964.
24. Stark, J., de Leval, M. R., Waterston, D. J., et al.: Corrective surgery of transposition of the great arteries in the first year of life: Results in 63 infants, J. Thorac. Cardiovasc. Surg. **67:** 673, 1974.
25. Stark, J., Tynana, M. J., Ashcraft, K. W., et al.: Obstruction of pulmonary veins and superior vena cava after the Mustard operation for transposition of the great arteries, Circulation **45-46** (Suppl.): 1, 1972.
26. Waldhausen, J. A., Pierce, W. S., Park, C. D., et al.: Physiologic correction of transposition of the great arteries: Indications for and results of operation in 32 patients, Circulation **43:** 738, 1971.

DISCUSSION

Dr. Harris Shumacker, Jr. (Indianapolis, Ind.). I should like to call attention to the use of another structure for creation of the intra-atrial tube. In November, 1961, I operated on a 12-month-old infant with transposition and an inconsequential ventricular septal defect. An intra-atrial baffle was created utilizing the patient's right atrial wall. The anterior atrium was reconstructed with pericardium. This case was reported in Surgery in 1961, approximately 3 years before Mustard published the method of utilizing pericardium for the same purpose.

The child did well and was restudied several times, the last time in June, 1968, at 8 years of age. He was quite healthy and the catheterization and angiographic observations indicated that the repair was complete, that no stenosis existed, and that the tiny ventricular septal defect persisted in a harmless fashion. These follow-up observations were reported in the *Journal of Thoracic and Cardiovascular Surgery* in 1969.

One of my former residents, Dr. Kenneth Tyson, Director of the Division of Pediatric Surgery at Galveston, has recently adopted the use of the right atrial wall for creating the intra-atrial baffle, employing a modification of the atrial incision I originally used in a way which seemingly makes the procedure easier to perform. He tells me that he has had excellent success and looks forward to further experiences with it.

The precise method of making the atrial wall incision can be conceivably altered in a variety of ways in an effort to facilitate ease of creation of the tunnel and avoidance of stenosis and other troubles.

I point out, for what it is worth, therefore, the alternative utilization of the right atrial wall for making the tunnel and reconstruction of the anterior atrium with pericardium.

Dr. Robert G. Carlson (New York, N. Y.). As a boy, I was taught that two wrongs do not make a right. If transposition results in the great vessels being wrongly placed, and then if we do an operation to convert the two atria the "wrong way," as in the "Mustard" operation, that does not make a "right." This is demonstrated by the worldwide high incidence of postoperative arrhythmias and venous obstruction, etc., after the "Mustard" operation.

At Cornell Medical Center, we have the same postoperative problems. I would like to mention a new method of *correcting* transposition of the great arteries (TGA). As a medical student 20 years ago, I observed Dr. Varco and associates trying to retranspose the aorta and the pulmonary artery in transposition hearts. They had trouble because of the coronary arteries.

With the advent of coronary artery bypass surgery, things have changed a bit. Two years ago, Dr. Renate Dische and I began working in the necropsy room trying to analyze transposition of the great vessel in view of the possibility of adding coronary artery surgery. We transposed "two thirds" of the aorta with "two thirds" of the pulmonary artery by leaving a wedge of one third attached laterally. We found that in all but two of 12 autopsy specimens, we could satisfactorily transpose the great vessels along with the coronary arteries.

In two of the necropsy specimens with TGA that we operated on, simple insertion of a subclavian artery graft would compensate for the shortness of the coronary artery. This idea has recently been published in the *Journal of Thoracic and Cardiovascular Surgery* by another group in Syracuse, N. Y.

I think that the medical giants in this room who are performing a lot of transposition surgery perhaps could consider this primary method of correcting the "wrong," rather than making an additional "wrong."

Dr. George J. Reul (Closing). In response to Dr. Shumacker, we have not used the right atrial tube in place of the Mustard operation. He is certainly to be congratulated for this long-term result. Using his technique, it would seem difficult to obtain good atrial tissue for the critical tailoring of the intra-atrial baffle.

In reponse to Dr. Carlson, we have attempted to surgically transpose the great vessels instead of the atria in transposition of the great arteries. These attempts have not been successful. Needless to say, we, as well as others, are constantly in search of a more physiologic technique for surgical repair and, perhaps, some time in the near future, a better operation will be developed.

Management of carotid artery injuries

Erwin R. Thal, M.D., William H. Snyder, III, M.D., *Dallas, Texas,* **Robert J. Hays, M.D.,** *Amarillo, Texas, and* **M. O. Perry, M.D.,** *Dallas, Texas*

Sixty patients with common or internal carotid artery injuries were reviewed. Indications for surgery included hemorrhage, hematoma, presence of a bruit, pulse discrepancy, proximity of wound, and positive arteriography. The patients were divided into three groups according to their neurologic status prior to surgery. Six of 41 patients with no preoperative neurologic symptoms developed a postoperative deficit. Five of six patients with mild deficits prior to operation had complete recovery. Four of 13 patients with severe deficits prior to operation died. The over-all mortality rate was 8.3 per cent. It is suggested from this series that vascular repair may be undertaken with reduced risk to the patient presenting with a mild neurologic deficit in the absence of a frank stroke. When the injury is accompanied by a severe neurologic deficit, it is important to assess the carotid flow. Operative arteriography is very helpful in these patients. Restoration of flow in a patient with a severe neurologic deficit may be hazardous and an anemic infarct may become hemorrhagic. If the arterial injury is accompanied by a cerebral infarct, it is probably advisable to ligate rather than repair the artery.

From the Department of Surgery, University of Texas, Southwestern Medical School, Dallas, Texas

THE QUESTION of whether and when to perform an exploratory operation on patients with penetrating and blunt trauma to the neck has not been resolved. An increasing number of these injuries are being seen and, as experience is gained, principles and methods of management evolve. During the early days of vascular surgery, vigorous attempts were made to restore arterial flow to the cerebral circulation. These concepts are now slowly changing because of information acquired from patients undergoing vascular reconstruction for cerebral vascular insufficiency syndromes.

Presented at the Twenty-eighth Annual Meeting of the Society for Vascular Surgery, Chicago, Ill., June 20 and 21, 1974.

Reprint requests: Erwin R. Thal, M.D., 5323 Harry Hines Blvd., Dallas, Texas 75235.

Improvement in diagnostic studies, in particular angiography, has permitted more accurate preoperative evaluation of patients sustaining potential vascular injuries in the neck. Whereas some authors are advocating conservative management of patients with penetrating neck trauma, the real dilemma centers around the individual with a neurologic deficit prior to the time of surgical intervention.

CASE MATERIAL

The charts of 60 patients with common carotid or internal carotid artery injuries who were operated on at Parkland Memorial Hospital in Dallas, Texas, between 1956 and February, 1974, were reviewed. The etiology of these injuries included penetrating as well as blunt trauma.

Table I. *Neurologic status prior to operation*

Group	*Patients*	*Percent*
I	41	68.3
II	6	10.0
III	13	21.7

Table II. *Frequency of indications*

Indication	*Percent*
Hematoma alone or in conjunction with another indication	67.0
Hemorrhage	25.0
Arteriography	8.0
Proximity	6.7
A-V fistula	5.0

Table III

Hypotension	*%*
At time of admission	43.3
Group I	41.5
Group II	50
Group III	46

During this study an aggressive approach was used in handling neck injuries. Following rapid resuscitation and stabilization, patients were operated on for the following indications: (1) major hemorrhage, (2) expanding or significant hematoma, (3) the presence of a bruit at or distal to the wound, (4) a diminished or absent pulse, or (5) anatomical proximity of the wound to the carotid artery. Arteriography was not routinely used during the period of this study but was frequently employed in patients developing neurologic deficits after admission or in those instances where solid indications for exploration were not present. Isolated neurologic deficits without other indication or evidence of injury by arteriography did not constitute absolute indications for surgical exploration.

The patients were divided into three groups: Group I had no neurologic deficit prior to operation, Group II had mild neurologic deficits prior to operation, and Group III had severe neurologic deficits prior to operation. Mild deficits were defined as weakness of either the upper or lower extremity in the absence of other neurologic injuries, such as closed head injuries or spinal cord trauma. Severe deficits were defined as aphasia, spastic or flaccid hemiplegia, or neurologic injuries accompanied by an altered state of consciousness.

All patients with external carotid and venous injuries of the neck were eliminated from the study.

RESULTS

Neurologic status prior to surgery. Of the 60 patients included in the study, evaluation of the neurologic status was made prior to operation in every case. The majority of patients had no neurologic deficit, as shown in Table I.

Indications. The presence of a hematoma was the most common indication for operation; 11.7 percent of the patients had only a single indication. The frequency of other indications is shown in Table II.

Distribution of injuries. A total of 65 percent of the injuries occurred on the left side, with 80 percent involving the common carotid artery and 20 percent the internal carotid; 6.7 percent of the injuries were located at the bifurcation.

Ninety-three percent of the injuries were sustained as a result of penetrating trauma; 73.3 percent were due to gunshot wounds, 20 percent due to stab wounds, and 6.7 percent due to blunt trauma.

Type of injury. Arterial lacerations were the most common injury found at operation and were seen in 70 percent of the patients. Complete vessel transection was seen in 18.3 percent, contusion in 10 percent, and spasm in 1.7 percent. The distribution of these injuries was seen with equal frequency in all three groups.

Associated injuries. Sixty percent of the patients had other injuries besides the carotid artery. In Group 3, 10 of 13 patients (77 percent) had an additional injury. Venous injuries, usually the internal jugular vein, were found in over half of the cases with additional injuries.

Shock. Upon arrival in the emergency room, 43.3 percent of the patients had a

Table IV. *Blood flow assessment*

	Recovered completely	*Deficit improved*	*No improvement*	*Death*
Group I, postoperative neurologic deficit (6):				
Flow present—vessel repaired (5)	2	2	1	
Flow absent—vessel repaired (1)	1			
Group II, mild deficit (6):				
Flow present—vessel repaired (5)	4			1
Flow absent—vessel repaired (1)	1			
Group III, severe deficit (13):				
Flow present—vessel repaired (9)	2	3	2	2
Flow present—vessel not repaired (1)				1
Flow absent—vessel not repaired (3)	1		1	1

systolic blood pressure below 100 mm. Hg (Table III). Three of the patients in Group I developed a postoperative neurologic deficit.

Three patients in Group II arrived at the hospital in shock. Two recovered completely without neurologic deficit and one died. The patient who died was involved in a motor vehicle accident and had several associated injuries, including liver, lung, and multiple long-bone fractures.

Six patients in Group III were hypotensive upon arrival. Two recovered completely without neurologic defect, two had postoperative neurologic deficits which did not improve, and two patients died.

Assessment of flow. The presence or absence of blood flow to the brain at the time of exploration is shown in Table IV.

Five of the six patients in Group I who developed a postoperative deficit did not have a significant reduction of flow. The one patient with no flow was repaired because of the absence of a preoperative deficit and subsequently recovered completely.

Flow was present in five of the six patients in Group II. The one patient in Group II with no flow was repaired because the preoperative deficit was mild.

Flow was absent in three (23 percent) of the 13 patients in Group III. Of the patients with adequate flow who were repaired, 77.8 percent either recovered completely, improved, or remained the same, but they did not deteriorate postoperatively.

Method of repair. Small lacerations were debrided and closed with a lateral suture technique so as not to narrow the lumen. More serious injuries were resected and reanastomosed. Interposition grafts were used in patients with extensive injuries (Table V).

Two patients in Group I had ligation of the injured vessel without neurologic sequelae. Three patients in Group III had ligation. One patient died, one patient had a residual deficit which improved postoperatively, and one patient was unchanged following ligation.

Cerebral support. Heparin and/or inlying shunts were used to protect the cerebral circulation in selected patients. The decision to use a shunt was based on the type of injury, presence or absence of flow, presence or absence of hypotension, and evaluation of backflow from the distal carotid.

Both heparin and a shunt were used in only six patients (10 percent). Heparin was used without a shunt in 14 (23.3 percent) and a shunt alone in 21 patients (35 percent).

In Group I a shunt was used in eight patients (19.5 percent) and both heparin and a shunt in four (9.8 percent). There were no postoperative neurologic deficits in the patients in this group.

In Group II four of the six patients had a shunt inserted and all recovered without evidence of neurologic deficit. One patient had both heparin and a shunt and did well postoperatively.

In Group III a shunt was used in three patients (23.1 percent). One had both heparin and a shunt with no change in the

Table V

Method of repair	%
Resection & anastomosis	40
Lateral	33.3
Interposition graft	15
Ligation	8.3
Anastomosis	1.7
No repair	1.7

Table VI

Complications	*No. of patients*
Neurologic deficit	3
Embolization with deficit	2
Occlusion with deficit	1
Wound infection	1
Pulmonary infection	1
Bleeding	1
Mycotic aneurysm	1
Total	10

neurologic status postoperatively. Two patients showed improvement of their preoperative neurologic deficits and one demonstrated no change.

In Group I heparin was used alone in five patients (12.2 percent), in Group II in no patients, and in Group III in three patients (23.1 percent). One patient in Group I developed a neurologic deficit for unexplained reasons. In none of the patients in Group III did the neurologic status change postoperatively.

RESULTS

In Group I six of 41 patients (14.6 percent) developed a postoperative neurologic deficit. In five of the six patients the deficit was noted immediately after operation. One developed a deficit 60 hours after operation. Two of these patients had emboli demonstrated by arteriography. The patient that developed the delayed deficit was found to have a completely occluded carotid artery by arteriography. One patient developed two cardiac arrests, one preoperatively and one during operation, so that the deficit may not have been the result of the carotid injury. The etiology of the deficit was uncertain in the remaining three patients. Of these six patients, two cleared their deficit completely, three improved but were left with a residual deficit, and one showed improvement.

In Group II six patients had mild deficits prior to operation. Five (83.3 percent) had complete recovery following operation and one died.

Nine of the 13 patients in Group III had primary repair of the injured vessel. Two (22.2 percent) recovered completely, three (33.3 percent) improved but were left with a residual deficit, two (22.2 percent) showed no improvement, and two (22.2 percent) died. Three patients in Group III had ligation of the artery; one improved but did not recover completely, one showed no improvement, and one died. One patient with spasm had no repair and subsequently died.

Complications. Ten patients (16.7 percent) sustained a complication directly related to the surgical procedure (Table VI). Three patients in Group I developed a neurologic deficit for undetermined reasons. One repair occluded and two patients had embolization to the cerebral circulation.

Mortality rate. Five patients in the series died—a mortality rate of 8.3 percent. The one death in Group II was apparently caused by cerebral edema and fat embolism following multiple injuries sustained in a motor vehicle accident. The other four deaths occurred in Group III and represented 31 percent of the patients who were seen in that group. Three patients had severe deficits before operation and died of cerebral damage. The fourth patient developed left hemiplegia after admission, and arteriography showed occlusion of the right internal carotid artery. At operation the patient had intense spasm of the artery which did not respond to therapy.

DISCUSSION

An aggressive approach to penetrating neck trauma often leads to the discovery of unsuspected injuries of other than vascular origin, as described by Jones, Terrell, and Salyer.[6] Better methods of preoperative evaluation have reduced the number of negative explorations. Bleeding and the presence of a hematoma continue to be the most reliable indicators of significant injury. The presence of a bruit is reliable but did not occur frequently in this series. Proximity as the sole indication was rarely seen. Arteriography, while not extensively used, proved helpful in those cases of suspected injury without other solid indications. Its usefulness is especially noted in potential injuries at the base of the skull that may be relatively inaccessible. Arteriography has also been helpful in those cases where neurologic manifestations occur some time after the initial injury. Arteriograms are frequently used to evaluate the distal circulation following operative repair.

Hypotension does not appear to have a predictable deleterious effect on the eventual neurologic status of the patient. This is especially true if the condition is rapidly reversed prior to operation. Of those patients with no neurologic deficit before or after operation, 37.1 percent were admitted in shock. It cannot be concluded from this study that shock by itself adversely influences the neurologic status of the patient. This may, in part, be due to cerebral vascular autoregulation in the absence of profound or sustained hypotension.

Most carotid injuries are not accompanied by neurologic deficits and repair can be safely accomplished. Bradley[1] has demonstrated the similarity between acute arterial obstruction due to trauma and that due to atherosclerosis. There are now convincing data to support the concept that a danger exists when revascularization is accomplished in patients with acute cerebral vascular insufficiency. The question then arises how best to manage the trauma patient with a preoperative neurologic deficit that is caused by the interruption of blood flow to the brain.

It is suggested from this series that vascular repair may be undertaken with reduced risk to the patient presenting with a mild neurologic deficit in the absence of a frank stroke. By contrast, those patients with severe neurologic deficits prior to operation present a poor risk and are analogus to the patient with an acute severe stroke. It is often difficult to separate those patients with primary cerebral injuries, such as closed head injuries and contusions, from those with brain damage due to diminished arterial flow. Often other indications exist that warrant operative intervention in spite of the neurologic status. The risk of converting an anemic infarct to a hemorrhagic infarct with progressive neurologic deterioration or even death is a real hazard in this group of patients.

The following approach to the management of the carotid injury associated with a neurologic deficit is suggested. If the deficit is mild and the carotid circulation can be freed of all obstruction, such as thrombi and emboli, restoration of flow appears to be safe. Likewise, if an embolus is present in the distal cerebral circulation, it is probably safe to restore flow. If, however, the carotid is occluded or clots cannot be removed from the distal carotid, it may be safer to ligate the vessel rather than attempt repair. If collateral circulation is adequate, these patients can be expected to recover.

If the patient presents with a severe neurologic deficit, it is important to assess the carotid flow before deciding upon further management. Operative arteriography is helpful in these patients. If flow is uninterrupted, it is probably safe to repair the vessel. If, however, distal patency does not exist, repair with restoration of flow appears to offer too great a risk to the patient. It may be hazardous to attempt removal of clots from the distal carotid. It is difficult to completely evacuate all clots and leaving some behind predisposes to embolization or thrombosis. The risk of perforation exists as well.

The effect of cerebral support was inconclusive from the data gathered in this review. It is believed that heparin in modest amounts either systemically or regionally is helpful if not otherwise contraindicated.

Many authors, such as Thompson, Austin, and Patman[12] and Gaspar,[4] recommend the routine use of shunts with elective carotid surgery. Shunts may be useful in the trauma patient and are considered if backflow is not adequate. Measurement of stump pressures, as described by Hays, Levinson, and Wylie,[5] and Moore and Hall,[8] serves as an excellent guide to the usefulness of a shunt.

It appears that trauma patients with carotid injuries are best managed by following the principles learned from a vast experience of elective carotid artery surgery.

REFERENCES

1. Bradley, E. L., III: Management of penetrating carotid injuries: An alternative approach, J. Trauma **13:** 248, 1973.
2. Cohen, A., Brief, D., and Mathewson, C., Jr.: Carotid artery injuries. An analysis of eighty-five cases, Am. J. Surg. **120:** 210, 1970.
3. Crissey, M. M., and Bernstein, E. F.: Delayed presentation of carotid intimal tear following blunt craniocervical trauma, SURGERY **75:** 543, 1974.
4. Gaspar, M.: Personal communication.
5. Hays, R. J., Levinson, S. A., and Wylie, E. J.: Intraoperative measurement of carotid back pressure as a guide to operative management for carotid endarterectomy, SURGERY **72:** 953, 1972.
6. Jones, R. F., Terrell, J. C., and Salyer, K. E.: Penetrating wounds of the neck: An analysis of 274 cases, J. Trauma **7:** 228, 1967.
7. Meyer, J. S., and Marx, P.: Cerebral autoregulation and "dysautoregulation" and their relation to cerebral vascular symptoms, Cur. Concepts Cerebrovasc. Dis. Stroke **6:** 1, 1971.
8. Moore, W. S., and Hall, A. D.: Carotid artery back pressure: A test of cerebral tolerances to temporary carotid occlusion, Arch. Surg. **99:** 702, 1969.
9. Moore, W. S., Yee, J. M., and Hall, A. D.: Collateral cerebral blood pressure, Arch. Surg. **106:** 520, 1973.
10. Perry, M. O., Thal, E. R., and Shires, G. T.: Management of arterial injuries, Ann. Surg. **173:** 403, 1971.
11. Rich, N. M., and Hughes, C. W.: Vietnam vascular registry: A preliminary report, SURGERY **65:** 218, 1969.
12. Thompson, J. E., Austin, D. J., and Patman, R. D.: Carotid endarterectomy for cerebrovascular insufficiency: Long-term results in 592 patients followed up to thirteen years, Ann. Surg. **172:** 663, 1970.
13. Towne, J. B., Neis, D. D., and Smith, J. W.: Thrombosis of the internal carotid artery following blunt cervical trauma, Arch. Surg. **104:** 565, 1972.
14. Williams, J. W., and Sherman, R. T.: Penetrating wounds of the neck: Surgical management, J. Trauma **13:** 435, 1973.

DISCUSSION

Dr. Max R. Gaspar, (Long Beach, Calif.). From our experiences at the Los Angeles County–University of Southern California Medical Center with a considerable number of vascular injuries, we would have to agree with almost everything that the authors have said.

I think it is interesting that they classified the patients into three different groups. I would agree completely with their management for the first and third groups. We know it is dangerous to restore flow if the patient has had a complete stroke. Probably the most important aspect of their paper was the proposal that, if there is a mild neurological deficit, the restoration of flow appears to be safe. From their data it seems to be so, although I think this is dangerous and that restoration of flow may cause a hemorrhagic infarct in some cases. The management of Groups I and III is clear-cut, but the management of Group II is still a gray area and clinical judgment is important.

The authors did not employ preoperative arteriography in all cases. We do this almost routinely in all but the most obvious vascular injuries. Very often minute defects in the arteriogram lead us to operate when physical examination indicates a minor wound. Also, the site of an arteriovenous fistula can be located and often is far removed from the site indicated by the wound and physical examination.

Intraoperative arteriography after repair of an artery is even more important. In routine carotid endarterectomy, we find defects in 8 percent of cases. Intimal flaps, stenotic suture lines, and distal thrombi are found alarmingly often after repair of traumatized arteries, and they must be corrected or the repair will be unsuccessful. We admonish our residents to use arteriography after repair on a routine basis.

Dr. Norman M. Rich, (Washington, D. C.). The authors have not only brought us their generally good results, but they have emphasized that we do not have all of the answers to this very complex problem.

Our military experience in Southeast Asia ended approximately 18 months ago. A number of you helped participate in the care of many patients in our ongoing registry project. Our statistics are not complete, but I believe that our results, in general, and our approach to this problem are similar to those outlined by the authors.

One important aspect that I would emphasize, which the authors alluded to, is the presence of concomitant head trauma. I would ask the authors about several of their patients in Group I, where they mentioned a neurological deficit from undetermined etiology. I wonder if some of these patients might not have had intracranial trauma. Several patients in our series were found at autopsy to have subdural hematomas, which actually created the problems, and not restoration of flow into ischemic brain.

I was a little concerned by the six of 41 patients (or 14.6 percent) in the authors' Group I who did have post-repair neurological deficits. We still have to answer the problems in that group.

My last comment concerns long-term follow-up. We have operated on seven patients at Walter Reed for late failures of treatments of these vascular injuries. It is important to follow patients because we might correct repair failures.

Dr. Kenneth Mattox, (Houston, Texas). I would like to re-emphasize several points. The vascular trauma registry of the Ben Taub General Hospital in Houston now has 81 carotid injuries and 72 patients who have been analyzed.

In recent years, gunshot wounds, as in Dallas, have prevailed as the predominant type of injury, with 83 percent causing the injuries in this location. Comparing our statistics to those in Dallas, the mortality rate is higher in our series—most of the deaths being in patients who were moribund at the time of arrival or died from associated injuries. The methods of repair were quite similar, ligation being reserved for those people with irreversible brain damage.

The incidences of neurologic deficits, as well as I can correlate from our series and the abstract of the Dallas series, are quite similar. Interluminal shunts were used in only five patients in our series and heparinization was not utilized.

I would like to emphasize that, in analyzing our cases, it seems that the period of hypotension does play some role in the development of neurologic deficits.

I would like to conclude with three points. First, neck exploration is performed usually to look for vascular injuries and those persons performing neck exploration must be prepared to fix a vascular injury. Second, with prehospital care now being available to many of us through trained emergency medical technicians, the period of hypotension can, perhaps, be lessened by prehospital administration of Ringer's lactate or normal saline solution. Finally, in our institution repair is carried out in all instances possible, in an attempt to perhaps reverse some neurologic injuries. In none of the cases with mild-to-moderate neurologic deficit was progression of a neurologic condition seen.

We would ask, has there been evidence in the Dallas series to support the premise that revascularization of an injured carotid in a patient with marked neurologic deficit results in a worsening of the patient's condition?

Dr. E. L. Bradley, III, (Atlanta, Ga.). Early in 1973 we reported on a group of patients in a retrospective study of penetrating carotid injuries with conclusions similar to those drawn by Dr. Thal. It was our contention that cerebral infarction was rendered hemorrhagic by reconstitution of carotid flow in patients with severe preoperative neurologic deficits. In an effort to avoid this excessive mortality rate we are prospectively looking at two groups of patients, much as Dr. Thal described to you this morning. Patients who have mild or no pre-existing neurologic deficit are all repaired. All patients with severe deficits, as manifested by coma or quadraplegia, are not being repaired; they are being ligated.

We do not have enough patients to give you any reliable prospective information this morning. Should any of you working in major trauma centers like to join the study, we would be most happy to have you.

I have one other comment to make and that is in regard to the classification of the patients for whom you might consider ligation. I think it is very important that the patient not be hypotensive when you perform the neurologic examination. We have had three patients whom we would have classified as very severe neurologic deficits. Once their hypotension was corrected, the rapid improvement in neurologic status permitted primary carotid repair.

Dr. Stuart A. Levinson, (Richmond, Va.). We have also seen an increased incidence of penetrating carotid artery injuries in the last several years. Dr. Halloran reviewed our 3½ year experience and found that we had treated 12 patients with carotid artery injuries secondary to stab wounds or gunshots.

Our policy regarding the management of this type of injury is determined by the condition of the artery and the condition of the patient. By this I mean, if flow is still present in the carotid artery at the time of exploration, or as demonstrated by preoperative angiography, then the artery needs to be repaired regardless of the neurologic findings in the patient. Conversely, if the artery is totally occluded at exploration, or if arteriography does not demonstrate prograde flow, then, in a patient with a neurologic deficit, the artery is ligated. If the patient does not have a neurologic deficit at the time of exploration and the artery is occluded, then the burden is entirely on the surgeon to revascularize this vessel without subjecting the patient to any neurologic insult. Obviously, this type of patient is one who has selected himself as being able to withstand carotid artery interruption without sustaining a neurologic injury, and carotid artery ligation, therefore, seems justifiable in this situation.

Utilizing this philosophy, we have ligated the carotid artery in three patients without extending their preoperative neurologic deficits. In addition, one patient who was neurologically sound but had a carotid transection also tolerated arterial ligation.

Dr. Malcolm O. Perry (Closing). It is obvious that the critical question is, when does the patient depart the ischemic and enter the infarct stage of his illness? At present we have imperfect means of determining this.

Several years ago I embarked upon a study of the elaboration of spinal fluid enzymes and amino acids. Their appearance in the spinal fluid is, perhaps, a method of detecting when this change occurs.

Unfortunately, the study was not completely satisfactory because the standard deviation was too large. This is the important dilemma, as Dr. Thal mentioned.

The patient's outcome appears to be determined by the severity of the deficit prior to repair, unless technical misadventures occur.

As Dr. Rich noted, of Group I patients (those with no neurologic deficit at the time of operation) six subsequently had what appeared to be an operatively related deficit.

In four of those patients, there appeared to be a reason. One had multiple cardiac arrests. One had a postoperative technical failure which resulted in occlusion of the carotid artery. Two had emboli in the distal circulation.

One of these patients with embolus was a 16-year-old boy who had an immediate craniotomy and removal of the middle cerebral embolus with complete recovery.

The other two patients, perhaps, had, as Dr. Rich mentioned, some cerebral injury other than we identified as resulting from interrupted blood flow. They were, however, the victims of penetrating rather than blunt trauma and we deemed this unlikely.

The deficit may have been due, however, to interruption of blood flow because a shunt was not used. That was not answered by our study.

We know that arteriography is very important, as Dr. Gaspar pointed out. We did not use it often preoperatively and, perhaps, not even often enough operatively. I would like to re-emphasize the point he made about the importance of immediate operative angiography.

Like others, we found that obtaining arteriograms at the termination of vascular procedures tends to make honest surgeons of us. One often found that an "impeccable and pristine" repair was not quite as good as one thought. I think this is an important concept, particularly in cerebral vascular surgery.

Dr. Rich also mentioned a problem about a late follow-up. Unfortunately, as Dr. Mattox noted, in Dallas and in Houston war is endemic and follow-up is not too good. Many casualties fail to return to the place of initial care.

We also, as Dr. Gaspar mentioned, have had an arteriovenous fistula at the base of the skull that was identified preoperatively by arteriograms, and this was very helpful. Otherwise, it can get quite colorful if one just goes in there unsuspectingly.

Dr. Beall said he believed that we might not, from our data, be able to support our conclusion about not operating on the people with severe neurologic deficits. I would agree with him. However, we attempted not to operate on those people with severe deficits and complete carotid occlusion in whom it was necessary to try to remove the clots.

We believe that in many instances one cannot get all the clots out and the risk of perforation into the cavernous sinus is significant. When flow is interrupted and severe neurologic deficits are present, we have elected not to repair the vessel. We repaired the artery when there was uninterrupted flow.

We would make a plea for repair of injuries in these people and, as Dr. Bradley mentioned, for initiation of a prospective study. Ours was retrospective and, as a result, the use of shunts, heparin, and many of the methods employed in this series were at the discretion of the individual staff surgeon, so there was considerable variation.

The modified bovine arterial graft: A clinical study

Bruce S. Cutler, M.D., Jesse E. Thompson, M.D., R. Don Patman, M.D., Alfred V. Persson, M.D., *and* **Philip D. Manfredi, M.D.,** *Dallas, Texas*

During a 44 month period, 43 bovine grafts were implanted in 39 patients. Elective operations were performed on 43.7 percent, limb salvage procedures on 56.3 percent. Distal runoff was judged good in 31.2 percent, while in 68.8 percent runoff was fair or poor. Eleven grafts were used in miscellaneous locations. All aortic, iliac, and femorofemoral grafts are patent. Only one of four axillofemoral grafts has achieved long-term patency. All 32 femoropopliteal grafts terminated above the knee. A striking correlation between the severity of ischemic symptoms and the quality of distal runoff was observed. In elective situations with good runoff, patency was 100 percent, while in salvage operations with poor runoff, patency dropped to 35.7 percent. The cumulative patency rate for bovine femoropopliteal grafts calculated by the life-table method was 59.4 percent (± 8.7 percent) at 36 months. This compares favorably with other reported series of similar grafts in the same location. The cumulative patency rate of bovine femoropopliteal bypass after one year parallels that of autologous veins. The late failure rate is approximately 3 percent per year. Major amputations were required in 11 of 14 graft failures (79 percent). These preliminary studies indicate that bovine grafts are acceptable arterial substitutes when cloth or autologous grafts are unavailable or undesirable.

From the Department of General Surgery, Baylor University Medical Center, Dallas, Texas

ALTHOUGH the ideal arterial substitute has not been found, the knitted Dacron prosthesis in most instances serves as the best large vessel replacement, while the autologous saphenous vein is most satisfactory for medium and small vessel reconstruction, especially in the lower extremity.[4, 8, 14] The vascular surgeon not infrequently encounters situations in which the saphenous vein is unsatisfactory or has been removed and a Dacron graft is undesirable; under these circumstances the bovine graft may be a suitable alternative.

Presented at the Twenty-eighth Annual Meeting of the Society for Vascular Surgery, Chicago, Ill., June 20 and 21, 1974.

Reprint requests: Jesse E. Thompson, M.D., 3434 Swiss Ave., Dallas, Texas 75204.

Arterial grafts of bovine origin were first used by Rosenberg and associates[18, 20] in experimental animals in 1956 and in man in 1962. Carotid arteries from freshly slaughtered cattle are modified by ficin enzymatic digestion to remove elastic tissue, leaving a collagen tube which is then tanned with dialdehyde starch. Grafts prepared in this manner are nonantigenic, biocompatible, and have been used successfully in dogs for up to 7 years and in man for 6¾ years.[6, 15, 19, 20]

The early clinical success of bovine arterial grafts reported by Rosenberg, Glass, and Rosenberg,[17] Keshishian and associates,[13] and Dale and Lewis[3] encouraged us to undertake a cautious clinical trial in September, 1970.

Table I. *Anatomic location and patency rates for bovine grafts*

Location	No. of patients	No. of extremities	Grafts occluded (total)	Early patency (%)	Late patency (%)
Aortofemoral	1	2	0	100	100
Axillofemoral	3	4	3	75	25
Femorofemoral	2	2	0	100	100
Iliac	3	3	0	100	100
Femoropopliteal	31	32	14	93.8	56.3
Total	40*	43	17	93	60.5

*One patient had both axillofemoral and femoropopliteal grafts.

Table II. *Comparison of indications and runoff status—femoropopliteal bypass operations*

	Bovine grafts, present series (%)	Vein grafts, DeWeese et al.[8] (%)	Vein grafts, Darling et al.[4] (%)	Dacron grafts, Kouchoukos et al.[14] (%)
Salvage operations	56.3	41.1	43.2	60.5
Fair-poor runoff	68.8	33.9	37.4	37.5

MATERIALS AND METHODS

During a 44 month period, 43 bovine grafts were implanted in 39 private patients. Thirty patients were men and 9 were women. The average age was 67 years (range, 47 to 83). Ten patients had diabetes and 16 had hypertension. More than half gave a history of cardiac or cerebrovascular disease. Only four denied the use of tobacco. Commercially available bovine grafts (Artegraft, Johnson & Johnson, New Brunswick, N. J.), 7.5 to 11 mm. in outer diameter, were used.

Bovine grafts were considered for femoropopliteal bypass if the saphenous vein was absent or was inadequate in length or caliber or for failure of a previous autologous vein graft. In addition, they were used in patients with iliac occlusive disease whose cardiopulmonary, cerebral, or renal status posed such an operative hazard that an expeditious, extra-abdominal procedure with minimal blood loss was preferable to the standard intra-abdominal procedure.

All patients had preoperative arteriograms and the runoff status was estimated. Operative arteriograms were frequently carried out, especially with femoropopliteal grafts. In an attempt to ascertain causes of graft failure, histologic studies of thrombosed grafts were performed whenever possible.

At the time of operation, all traces of preservative (alcohol and propylene oxide) were removed from the graft by triple washing in normal saline. Local and systemic heparinization were employed during arterial clamping. Standard vascular operative techniques were employed. Parenteral and topical antibiotics were routinely used. The usual size of femoropopliteal grafts was 7.5 to 8.0 mm., outside diameter.

The anatomic location of the 43 grafts is shown in Table I. Seven procedures were secondary operations following failure of previous autologous vein grafts. It should be emphasized that all femoropopliteal grafts terminated proximal to the knee joint.

RESULTS

The patency of each arterial reconstruction was determined by the presence or absence of distal pulses and was confirmed by oscillometry, Doppler pressure measurements, or arteriography. End points for follow-up were death of the patient, occlusion of the graft, or May, 1974. No patient was lost to follow-up.

There were no deaths associated with operation. Seven patients died during the follow-up period, five of whom were operated on for limb salvage. There were no wound

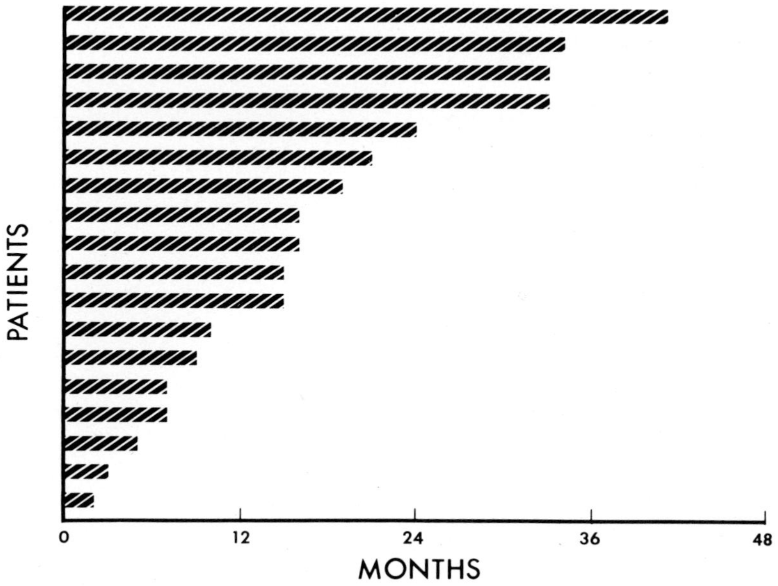

Fig. 1. Bar graphs of all patients with patent femoropopliteal bovine grafts, showing length of follow-up for each case.

infections and no anastomotic aneurysms. One patient with diabetes developed a false aneurysm in the midportion of a femoropopliteal graft 3 months following implantation and eventually required amputation.

Early and late patency of all grafts is shown in Table I. Among seven grafts in the aortic, iliac, and crossover femoral locations, all have remained patent. One axillofemoral graft occluded in the early postoperative period, while two occluded at 3 and 15 months, leaving only one graft to achieve long-term patency.

In analyzing the results of femoropopliteal grafts, we agree with those who have suggested that immediate and long-term patency is largely determined by the severity of ischemic symptoms and the quality of distal runoff.[8, 14, 21, 22] Therefore we have divided our indications for femoropopliteal surgery into two categories on the basis of presenting complaints. Operations for claudication were termed *elective* procedures, while those for rest pain, gangrene, or ulceration were designated *salvage* procedures. Elective operations for incapacitating claudication were performed on 43.7 percent of extremities; limb salvage procedures for rest pain were performed on 56.3 percent.

Quality of runoff was estimated from the arteriograms. Runoff was said to be good if two or three vessels distal to an open popliteal segment were patent. Runoff was judged fair to poor if the distal popliteal was narrowed or occluded and/or fewer than two distal vessels were patent. Only 31.2 percent of our patients were considered to have good runoff, while 68.8 percent were judged to have fair or poor runoff (Table II).

Among 32 femoropopliteal grafts were two immediate occlusions which could not be reopened, yielding an early patency rate of 93.8 percent. The complete postoperative course for each femoropopliteal bypass is shown graphically in Figs. 1 and 2.

Table III lists the patency rates for femoropopliteal grafts classified as to elective or salvage procedures and good or fair-to-poor runoff. In elective operations with good runoff, patency was 100 percent, while in salvage situations with poor runoff, patency dropped to 35.7 percent, with an overall patency rate of 56.3 percent.

The life-table method is the best way to report long-term graft patency.[4, 20, 23] The long-term patency of the present series of bovine femoropopliteal bypass grafts has been

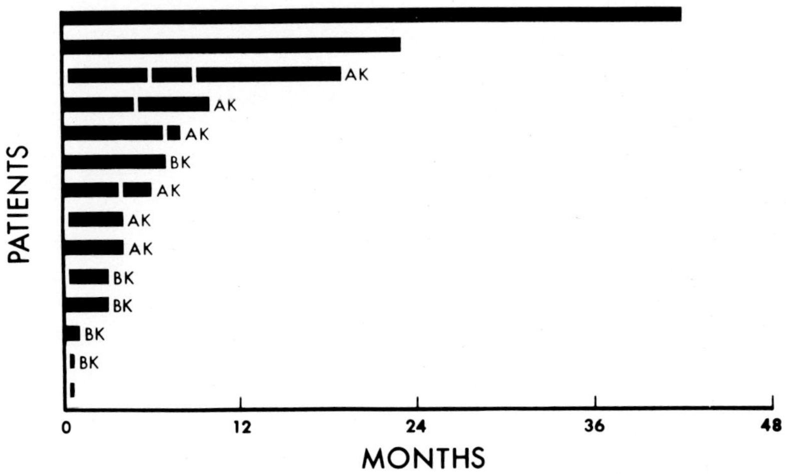

Fig. 2. Bar graphs of all patients with occluded femoropopliteal bovine grafts, showing the time at which each graft became occluded during the follow-up period. Amputations required are shown as AK or BK. Interruptions on the bars indicate the times of secondary operations.

Table III. *Patency rates for bovine grafts in femoropopliteal location*

Clinical situation	*No. of extremities*	*Grafts occluded (total)*	*Patency (%)*
Elective			
Good runoff	6	0	100
Fair-poor runoff	8	3	62.5
Salvage			
Good runoff	4	2	50
Fair-poor runoff	14	9	35.7
Total	32	14	56.3

calculated by the life-table method and is shown for comparison with several other widely quoted series taken from the literature (Figs. 3 and 4). The cumulative patency rate for our femoropopliteal grafts at 36 months is 59.4 percent (± 8.7 percent).

Fourteen re-explorations were performed on 11 patients, seven for immediate graft occlusion, and seven for late thrombosis. Three of five femoropopliteal and one of two axillofemoral re-explorations for immediate occlusion resulted in restoration of flow. However, these procedures provided an average of only 6.5 months of additional patency before reocclusion of the graft. Similarly, although five of seven reoperations for late thrombosis were initially successful, they resulted in an average of 4.3 months of additional patency before thrombosis recurred.

All patients with patent femoropopliteal grafts have had satisfactory relief of symptoms and healing of ischemic lesions. However, a distressingly large number of graft failures have been followed by amputation. Of failures in the elective group, two have required amputation, both in the same 47-year-old black male patient with rapidly progressive and widespread atherosclerotic disease. In the salvage group, nine of 11 graft failures have required amputation. Among the miscellaneous procedures, one amputation followed occlusion of an axillofemoral graft in a patient with a severely occluded profunda femoris system.

DISCUSSION

Patency rates approaching 100 percent can be expected when bovine grafts are used for large vessel reconstructions. In this series all aortic, iliac, and crossed femoral grafts have remained open, with follow-up to 44 months. This experience parallels that of others.[13, 17] Rosenberg and associates[20] have reported a bovine iliac graft functioning for nearly 7 years with no evidence of deterioration or aneurysm formation.[20] Bovine grafts have the advantage over Dacron in these situations in that they do not require preclotting; the time and blood saved may thus make the bovine preferable in certain high-risk patients.

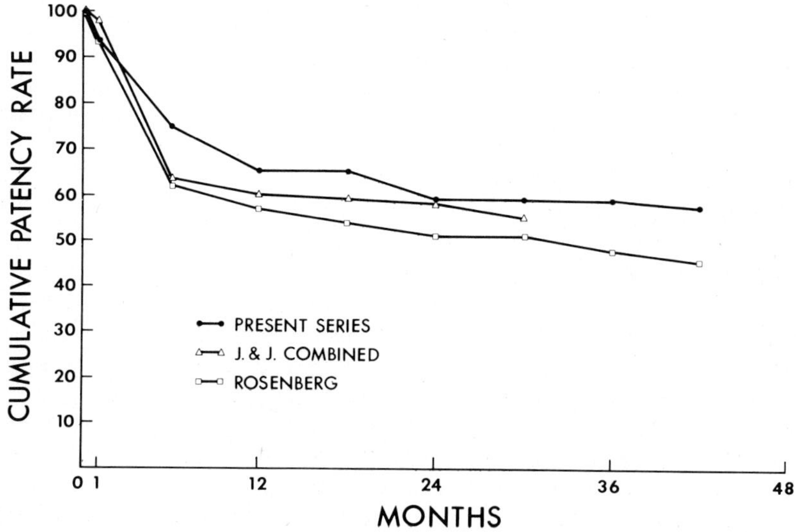

Fig. 3. Curves showing cumulative patency of two representative series[12, 17] of femoropopliteal bovine grafts together with the present series, calculated according to the life-table method. All cases, both elective and salvage, are included.

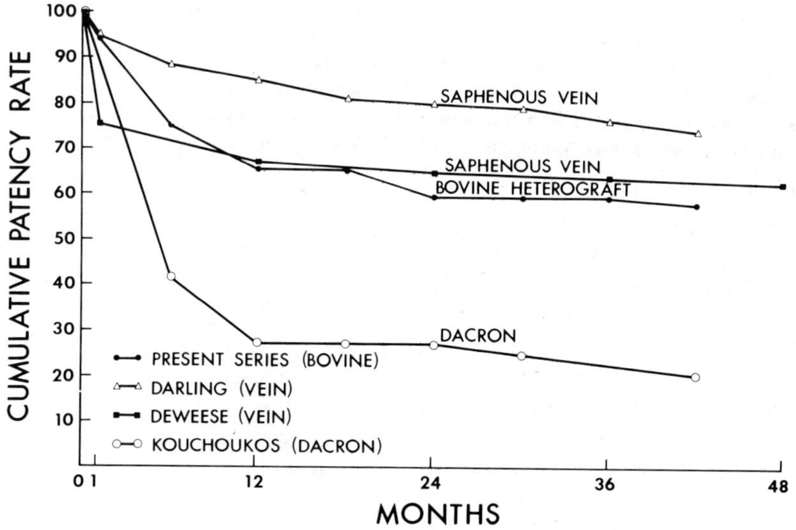

Fig. 4. Curves showing cumulative patency of several series of femoropopliteal reconstructions using autologous veins[4, 7] and Dacron prostheses,[14] and the present series using bovine grafts, calculated according to the life-table method. All cases, both elective and salvage, are included regardless of runoff status.

Bovine grafts for small and medium vessel reconstructions were initially employed by us only for limb salvage, but with experience, indications were liberalized to include selected patients with claudication and good runoff. Our long-term results with the bovine graft in the femoropopliteal position compare favorably with a group of 50 grafts reported by Rosenberg, Glass, and Rosenberg[17] and with a series of 255 grafts collected by the manufacturer[12] (Fig. 3).

Any comparison of femoropopliteal results using different graft materials should take into account the proportion of operations for claudication versus limb salvage and the quality of distal runoff. Table II shows these

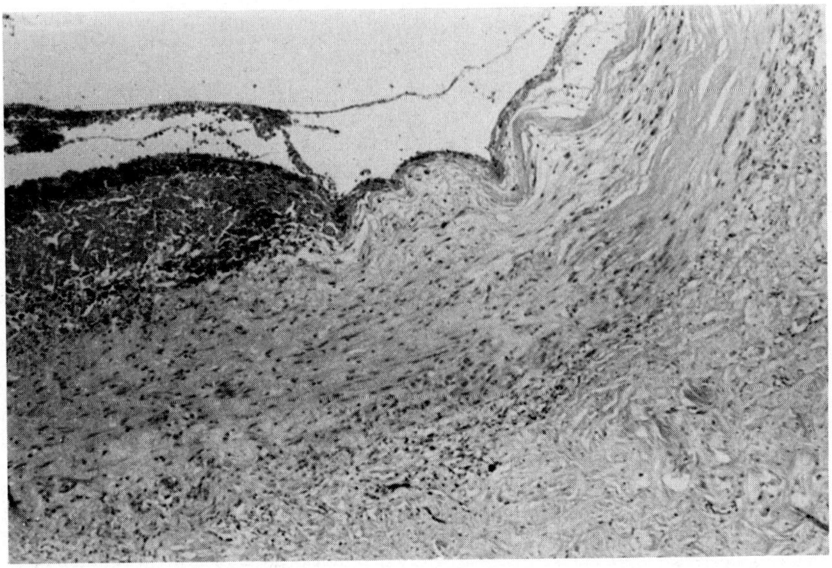

Fig. 5. Photomicrograph of bovine graft removed following occlusion 7 months postoperatively, showing the development of an atherosclerotic plaque in the graft wall, with superimposed thrombus formation. (Original magnification ×10; reduced by one third.)

indices for the curves of bovine grafts, autologous veins, and Dacron prostheses compared in Fig. 4. Although the cumulative patency rate for bovine grafts appears inferior to that of autologous veins, a higher percentage of our patients had salvage procedures and poor distal runoff. The bovine results appear better than the Dacron figures at 3 years.

The arteriogram does not give an infallible estimate of the quality of distal runoff[16]; nonetheless, in the present series those patients with claudication and good runoff have enjoyed 100 percent patency. Of those operated on for limb salvage with fair or poor runoff, only 35.7 percent have remained patent.

It has been shown that over a period of several months the host surrounds the implanted bovine graft with a dense layer of collagen.[9, 18] This encasement may be responsible for the kinking seen on flexed-knee arteriograms of grafts to the distal popliteal artery. For this reason we have not used the bovine graft below the level of the knee joint.

Immediate graft failure is usually attributed to technical factors. Although five of seven early occlusions were successfully reopened, all have subsequently gone to rethrombosis. This suggests that the quality of runoff may have been overestimated initially, or that other factors inherent in the graft may have contributed to early failure.[11]

Late graft failure in femoropopliteal grafts occurs when progressive atherosclerotic narrowing of the distal outflow tract reduces the flow rate in the graft below a critical level and thrombosis occurs. Szilagyi[23] has stated that 3 percent of vein grafts fail each year due to progressive occlusion of runoff vessels. After the first year the rate of occlusion of the bovine grafts parallels that of autologous vein grafts and approximates 3 percent per year (Fig. 4).

Late failure in bovine grafts can also be due to the development of atherosclerotic plaques in the graft itself. Dillon and associates[9] have demonstrated that blood can dissect into the media of bovine grafts and, after a period of organization, may develop into typical atherosclerotic plaques. At least three grafts in our series exhibited atheromas within the graft wall (Fig. 5).

We have been concerned by the high rate of amputation following occlusion of femoropopliteal bovine grafts. In this series, among 14 graft failures, 11 major amputations were required (79 percent). Nine of 11 amputations occurred in patients operated on for limb salvage and nine of the 11 also had only fair-to-poor runoff. Rosenberg, Glass, and Rosenberg[17] reported amputations on 30 percent and Keshishian and associates[13] on 36 percent of failed bovine grafts.

Are there factors other than poor runoff and progression of distal disease which may increase this incidence of amputation following failure of a bovine graft? Several studies have shown that when graft diameter exceeds that of the outflow vessel, layering of thrombotic material occurs, which tapers the lumen to the size of the distal artery.[3, 9] We have observed this phenomenon on postoperative arteriograms (Fig. 6). Dillon and associates[9] have shown that no ingrowth of fibroblasts occurs in the bovine graft, and, consequently, there is no firm attachment of luminal thrombus to the vessel wall. The loose adherence of concentric thrombus is corroborated by the clinical observation that recent and late thromboses in bovine grafts can frequently be removed intact with the Fogarty catheter.

It may well be that repeated embolic episodes caused by dislodgement of luminal thrombi progressively occlude both collateral and runoff vessels, especially in situations where there is marked disproportion between the size of the graft and that of the host artery. When final graft occlusion occurs, the limb is considerably more ischemic than before the graft was implanted. The reduced runoff capacity limits the success of further reconstructive efforts and may lead to an increased amputation rate.

Bovine grafts may be successfully employed in a variety of anatomic areas. The best results are seen in large vessel replacements in high flow situations. In femoropopliteal reconstructions, they appear inferior to autologous veins but superior to Dacron. It should be emphasized, however, that grafts of appropriate size (8 mm. or smaller) should be used in the femoropopliteal position, since an oversize graft may lead to thrombosis and and increased rate of amputation. Ease of handling, minimal blood loss, and shortened operating time favor their use in selected cases. Bovine grafts are acceptable arterial substitutes when veins are unavailable and cloth is undesirable.

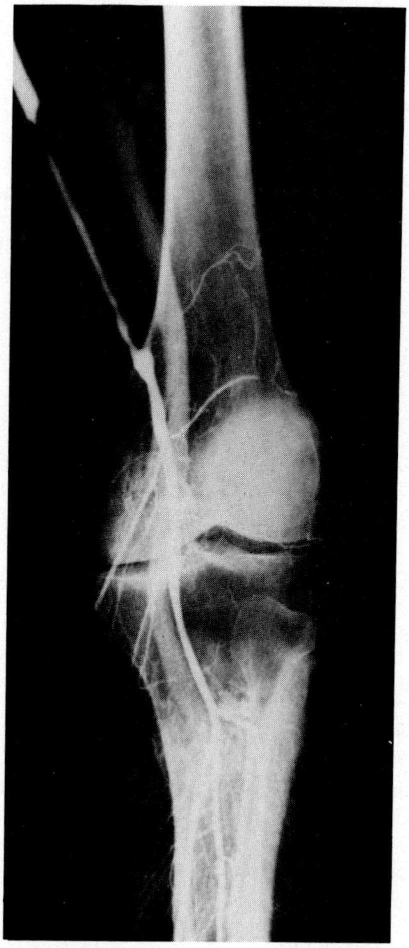

Fig. 6. Arteriogram of femoropopliteal bovine graft 6 months postoperatively, showing concentric thrombus formation at distal end of graft. Thrombectomy restored flow.

We are grateful to Johnson & Johnson, Inc., New Brunswick, N. J., who kindly furnished some of the Artegrafts used in this study.

REFERENCES

1. Austin, D. J., Thompson, J. E., Wheeler, C. G., and Patman, R. D.: Arteriosclerotic occlusive disease of superficial femoral and popliteal arteries, Am. J. Surg. **108:** 636, 1964.
2. Baier, R. E., and DePalma, V. A.: The relation of the internal surface of grafts to thrombosis. Management of arterial occlusive disease, Chicago, 1971, Year Book Medical Publishers, Inc., pp. 147-163.
3. Dale, W. A., and Lewis, M. R.: Modified

bovine heterografts for arterial replacement, Ann. Surg. **169:** 927, 1969.
4. Darling, R. C., and Linton, R. R.: Durability of femoropopliteal reconstructions, Am. J. Surg. **123:** 472, 1972.
5. DeBakey, M. E., Crawford, E. S., Morris, G. C., et al.: Late results of vascular surgery in the treatment of atherosclerosis, J. Cardiovasc. Surg. **5:** 473, 1964.
6. DeFalco, R. J.: Immunologic studies of untreated and chemically modified bovine carotid arteries, J. Surg. Res. **10:** 95, 1970.
7. DeWeese, J. A.: Results of thromboendarterectomy vs. venous bypass grafts. Management of arterial occlusive disease, Chicago, 1971, Year Book Medical Publishers, Inc., pp. 119-145.
8. DeWeese, J. A., and Rob, C. G.: Autogenous venous bypass grafts five years later, Ann. Surg. **174:** 346, 1971.
9. Dillon, M. L., Scott, S. M., Vasquez, M. D., et al.: Tissue response to an arterial substitute of bovine origin, Arch. Surg. **105:** 577, 1972.
10. Edwards, W. S.: Late occlusion of femoral and popliteal fabric arterial grafts, Surg. Gynecol. Obstet. **110:** 714, 1960.
11. Imparato, A. M., Bracco, A., Kim, G. E., and Zeff, R.: Intimal and neointimal fibrous proliferation causing failure of arterial reconstructions, SURGERY **72:** 1007, 1972.
12. Johnson & Johnson, Inc., Collected data: Bovine heterograft, New Brunswick, N. J., 1973. Unpublished.
13. Keshishian, J. M., Smyth, N. P. D., Adkins, P. C., et al.: Clinical experience with the modified bovine arterial heterograft, J. Cardiovasc. Surg. **12:** 433, 1971.
14. Kouchoukos, N. T., Levy, J. F., Balfour, J. F., and Butcher, H. R.: Operative therapy for femoral-popliteal arterial occlusive disease. A comparison of therapeutic methods, Circulation **1:** (Suppl. 35) 174, 1967.
15. Matilla, S. P., and Fogarty, T. J.: Antigenicity of vascular heterografts, J. Surg. Res. **15:** 81, 1973.
16. Mundth, E. D., Darling, R. C., Moran, J. M., et al.: Quantitative correlation of distal arterial outflow and patency of femoro-popliteal reversed saphenous vein grafts with intraoperative flow and pressure measurements, SURGERY **65:** 197, 1969.
17. Rosenberg, D. M. L., Glass, B. A., and Rosenberg, N.: Experiences with modified bovine carotid arteries in arterial surgery, SURGERY **68:** 1064, 1970.
18. Rosenberg, N., Gaughran, E. R. L., Henderson, J., et al.: The use of segmental arterial implants prepared by enzymatic modification of heterologous blood vessels, Surg. Forum **6:** 242, 1956.
19. Rosenberg, N., Lord, G. H., Henderson, J., et al.: Collagen arterial craft of bovine origin: Seven year observations in the dog, SURGERY **67:** 951, 1970.
20. Rosenberg, N.: The modified bovine arterial graft, Arch. Surg. **105:** 547, 1972.
21. Stoney, R. J., James, D. R., and Wylie, E. J.: Surgery for femoropopliteal atherosclerosis, Arch. Surg. **103:** 548, 1971.
22. Szilagyi, D. E.: Ten years' experience with aorto-iliac and femoro-popliteal arterial reconstruction, J. Cardiovasc. Surg. **5:** 502, 1964.
23. Szilagyi, D. E.: Discussion of Rosenberg et al.[17]
24. Szilagyi, D. E., Elliott, J. P., Hageman, J. H., et al.: Biologic fate of autogenous vein implants as arterial substitutes: Clinical, angiographic and histopathologic observations in femoro-popliteal operations for atherosclerosis, Ann. Surg. **178:** 232, 1973.

DISCUSSION

Dr. John A. Mannick (Boston, Mass.). I would like to congratulate Drs. Cutler and Thompson for attempting to put the bovine heterograft in clinical perspective. However, I am still a little confused as to the indications for its use and I have some questions for Dr. Cutler.

I would gather that the bovine graft in your series, Dr. Cutler, functioned quite well in the femoropopliteal position when the distal anastomosis was placed above the knee joint and the runoff was good.

Now, it is our experience that the knitted Dacron graft functions reasonably satisfactorily under those circumstances as well. It does not function well when the distal anastomosis is placed below the knee joint or when the runoff is poor. I gather from your data that the bovine graft functions better than the Dacron one under these circumstances. Is this correct?

With regard to the use of bovine heterografts for axillofemoral and femorofemoral grafts, I must say that I am not really convinced. In our series of approximately 70 femorofemoral grafts and 75 axillofemoral grafts using knitted Dacron, we find well over a 90 percent patency rate at a 3 year interval in the former group and a 75 percent patency rate in the latter group. Since knitted Dacron is less expensive, in Boston anyway, than the bovine heterograft, and since it is not that much more difficult to suture and can be preclotted successfully with 30 ml. of blood, I do not think we are ready to abandon the Dacron graft just yet.

Dr. W. Andrew Dale (Nashville, Tenn.). My experience totals 75 bovine grafts placed for one of three reasons. First, the saphenous vein was not suitable or had been used previously. Second, a crossover femorofemoral graft was needed. Third, a very rapid operation was required, such as for a critically ill patient whose leg was in immediate danger.

There have been two grafts which have formed wall aneurysms and required removal. Another graft became infected, blew out, and required removal. The rest have remained in situ with approximately a 60 percent patency rate at varied time intervals up to 8 years.

We are presently engaged in follow-up studies.

There is a real need to answer certain questions. First, are bovine grafts better, equal to, or worse than synthetic Dacron grafts in various positions? Second, is there any difference between the subcutaneous placement of a bovine graft and placement beneath the fascia? Third, why do occasional bovine grafts suddenly clot but remain open for long periods after immediate thrombectomy? The easy explanation that preliminary washing was incomplete is not good enough since blood flow must at once wash the interior of the graft far better than any amount of saline irrigation. The fourth question is whether there is any decrease in the long-term results if length requires that two segments of bovine graft be sutured together end to end.

Meanwhile, we still prefer autogenous vein as first choice for peripheral grafts but find that the bovine graft is often a useful backup material.

Dr. William Tompkins (Long Beach, Calif.). At the University of California at Irvine's affiliated hospitals, we have employed bovine heterografts over the past 4 years in preference to cloth grafts when the saphenous vein is not available. They have been used in the iliofemoral, femorofemoral, and femoropopliteal areas as well as for arteriovenous shunts for hemodialysis.

We have noted one characteristic of the bovine heterograft which Dr. Dale has just mentioned which is worthy of report. We have had two bovine heterografts in the femoropopliteal position which have become infected postoperatively. An attempt was made for about 3 to 4 weeks in each case to allow the wound to granulate over the graft. Although healthy granulation tissue did develop around the grafts with wet-to-dry dressings, the granulation failed to cover the graft and the graft eventually ruptured in each case, necessitating removal. So the graft apparently acts as a foreign body in an infected field. Saphenous vein grafts usually withstand infection and heal.

Our experience to date makes us cautiously optimistic about the ultimate place of bovine heterografts in vascular surgery, but we would strongly recommend early removal of the heterograft if infection occurs.

Dr. Julius H. Jacobson, II (New York, N. Y.). I rise not to present another series but to simply state that in the past month we have sent in the page proofs to the *Annals of Surgery* on the similar size series of bovine heterografts, which proved to be entirely satisfactory in all areas but the femoropopliteal position. They were particularly good for dialysis grafts, but, in the former area, they were a disaster!

The problems included aneurysm formation, infection, false aneurysm formation, the need for frequent thrombectomy immediately following the operation, and poor long-term patency.

This is in marked contrast to the present study. We started somewhat earlier than this study. Many of our grafts were in the 11 and 12 ml. diameter range, which is definitely bad. Below the knee placement was common and most cases were patients who failed with other procedures.

I do not want to damn the bovine heterograft but simply say that our experience was so poor that we have switched from the type of situation where we need autogenous vein and do not have it to the autogenous mandril type of graft which, so far in our hands over a period of 18 months, has held up far better than did the bovine heterograft over the same period.

Dr. Jere W. Lord (New York, N. Y.). Our experience, too, with bovine grafts is a small one and it mirrors the data presented today. However, I would like to speak about the use of the bovine graft below the knee. We had four patients with a graft placed to the distal popliteal artery and three of them thrombosed within one year. Because of this experience, we were forced in July, 1973, to improvise a technique wherein a vein graft, which is of good size from the groin to near the knee, became a small one below the knee. In this patient the graft was joined to the distal popliteal and to the proximal superficial femoral artery. The graft thrombosed under vision before we closed the wound. We then realized that a portion of the vein was too small.

Fortunately, or unfortunately, we missed the meeting last year and did not hear Dr. Linton's excellent paper on the composite Dacron vein graft. Our previous experience with end-to-end fluted technique had not been satisfactory, similar to Dr. Dale's experience reported in 1961.

What we did was tie the vein graft down to the adductor fascia at its proximal end where it was still of good size. A knitted Dacron prosthesis 6 ml. in diameter was joined to the side of the vein graft with a 25 ml. opening. The vein graft immediately proximal to this anastomosis was tied and then the Dacron prosthesis was sutured to the side of the common femoral artery.

This seemed to work well and since that time we have now employed this composite graft from the common femoral to an artery below the knee in 21 patients. There have been four closures over a period of 11 months. Four of the bypasses extended to the peroneal and posterior tibial arteries distally.

I would like to show you angiograms of one patient. This 66-year-old man was admitted to the hospital in early March, 1974, with rest pain and an open ulcer of the metatarsophalangeal joint, which would not heal over a period of many months. He had diabetes, was a heavy smoker, and had suffered a myocardial infarction.

His aorta appeared normal from angiographic study, except for a little sclerosis, without serious narrowing. The proximal common iliac artery on the right was stenotic with poststenotic dilatation. There was narrowing of the external iliac artery, a block of the superficial femoral artery, and stenosis of the profunda femoral artery. The distal popliteal artery was completely occluded and the peroneal artery showed patency beyond a zone of obstruction. The anterior tibial was blocked from its origin. The composite graft was inserted and an angiogram was made 2 weeks later when the foot was doing well. There was anastomosis between the prosthesis and the vein graft. At this point the popliteal artery was still patent. The only runoff was from one collateral artery and the graft was still functioning without closure.

Following that a vein graft was then joined from the popliteal vein graft to the peroneal artery in mid leg. A good anterior tibial pulse appeared and is functioning well 3 months later.

Dr. Norman Rosenberg (Highland Park, N. J.). Placing a graft in the iliac position is a pure test of its ability to function as a long-term conduit, since the runoff and the run-in can be expected to remain adequate for years and the only stress is that of pulsatile arterial pressure. Dr. Cutler's group has had no failures in that location nor have we. Quite a few years ago we placed eight grafts in the iliac area, which have functioned in place from 4 to almost 7 years.

On the other hand, the more distally placed femoropopliteal implant is additionally subject to a diminished flow syndrome, secondary to progression of distal arterial disease. As the total cross-sectional diameter of the outflow decreases, *all* grafts find themselves functionally oversized and only those with a living intima, such as autogenous veins, can avoid the deposition of some mural thrombus on their inner aspects.

Our own indications for and observations on this graft material essentially parallel those of the authors.

We have always preferred autogenous veins in femoropopliteal situations, reserving the bovine graft for indications described by them.

We have used composite grafts of bovine artery and autogenous vein when we have been forced to go below the knee to either the distal popliteal or tibial vessels and sufficient vein is not available.

On polling those investigators with the largest series of bovine grafts, there is approximately a 3 percent incidence of aneurysms over the long-term, which dissuaded us from its use for the indications described.

Some 10,000 of these grafts have been distributed to date. The paucity of complaints received by the manufacturer probably bespeaks the high degree of sophistication of those who use them.

Dr. Victor M. Bernhard (Milwaukee, Wis.). We, too, have been working in this area and have come up with conclusions quite similar to those of the authors.

We have employed bovine grafts since March, 1971, and have rigidly restricted our indications to those patients without a suitable vein who require revascularization for limb salvage. All of our patients would fall into their worst group.

We have implanted 22 heterografts and all but one were immediately patent. The large arteries with high volume runoff permit excellent long-term results. However, in all of our femoropopliteal and femorotibial bypasses, runoff was poor and this is reflected in the high rate of graft attrition. These findings are similar to those noted by Dr. Cutler.

Grafts which were initially successful became failures at about 2 to 3 months in most instances.

One failure was related to infection following attempted thrombectomy and a second infection occurred in the vein segment of a composite graft. Severe heart failure precipitated occlusion in two, and in eight no reason for thrombosis was apparent other than poor runoff.

Stenosis at the anastomosis from progressing atheroma development resulted in thrombosis in one tibial graft, and this was successfully repaired with a long-term good result.

In five instances, thrombectomy was performed to restore flow, one rethrombosed at 3 months; two failures, as noted before, were due to infection, and two have remained open but one is too recent for anything more than casual comment.

In each instance the material removed consisted of a gelantinous sheet of white thrombus conforming to the inner diameter of the heterograft and was filled with a currant jelly–like fresh thrombus. This specimen is an example of the material which we have removed and which the authors have described.

This finding and the authors' contention that thrombotic lining material may be prone to embolize would lead one to speculate on potential value of long-term anticoagulant therapy in these patients. In this regard we now agree with Dr. Rosenberg, and all of our recent graft patients have been placed on long-term anticoagulants.

Recent reports of the use of heterografts for hemodialysis support the notion that these may be less prone to infection. I would like the author's comment.

Dr. John M. Keshishian (Washington, D. C.). Let me bring you up to date rather quickly on some interesting figures. We are now following about 100 patients at this time. At the femoropopliteal position we presently enjoy a 70 percent success rate. My colleague, Dr. Slovin, has followed a small number of patients—14 patients from zero to 39 months with extension of the graft below the knee. His patency rate at this time is 62 percent.

We should like to urge you to use 6 to 7 mm. grafts and abandon anything larger than that simply because you obtain higher velocity flow with this smaller sized graft.

We are following 24 patients who have had patch grafts in the carotid artery following endarterectomy and who have had no complications.

We have had three aneurysms, two true aneurysms of the graft at 3 years. These were replaced; one limb was lost. We had one infection following the unrecognized resection of a mycotic aneurysm. The leg was salvaged.

Dr. Bruce S. Cutler (Closing). In answer to the questions asked by Drs. Mannick and Lord regarding the use of bovine grafts below the level of the knee joint, we have been guided by the observations of Drs. Dillon and Rosenberg. They have shown that the host surrounds the graft with an inflexible layer of collagen, which may be responsible for the kinking seen on flexed knee arteriograms of grafts placed to the distal popliteal artery. We have not used bovine grafts below the level of the knee joint. A composite graft using a proximal segment of bovine and distal segment of saphenous vein may be the best solution to this particular problem.

We would agree with the remarks of Drs. Tompkins and Keshishian with regard to the behavior of the bovine graft in the septic wound. None of our patients operated on for occlusive disease has developed a wound infection. We have had experience with a single interposition graft, not included in this series, which was used to replace a segment of the superficial femoral artery because of a gunshot wound of the thigh. The patient developed a staphlococcal wound infection and the graft literally dissolved 6 weeks following implantation. From our limited experience, we cannot advocate the use of the bovine graft in a contaminated wound.

In response to Dr. Dale's question, all of our grafts have been placed subfascially. The manufacturer, in a collective review of 255 bovine femoropopliteal grafts, has reported a 20 percent incidence of aneurysm formation among 30 grafts placed subcutaneously. The incidence of true aneurysm formation among subfascial grafts was 2.2 percent.

All of us who have used the bovine graft owe Dr. Rosenberg a debt of gratitude for his pioneer work in this field.

In closing this discussion about the pro's and con's of bovine grafts, I am reminded of the nursery rhyme that goes something like this: "There was a little girl who had a little curl right in the middle of her forehead; when she was good, she was very, very good, but when she was bad, she was horrid."

Experience with open mitral commissurotomy in 100 consecutive patients

Michael J. Mullin, M.D., Richard M. Engelman, M.D., O. Wayne Isom, M.D., Arthur D. Boyd, M.D., Ephraim Glassman, M.D., *and* **Frank C. Spencer, M.D.,** *New York, N. Y.*

A total of 100 open mitral commissurotomies (OMC) were performed at New York University Hospital between January, 1966, and July, 1973: 71 patients had OMC alone and 29 had additional cardiac procedures. There were eight male (36 to 63 years of age) and 92 female (15 to 69 years of age) patients. The technique employed included extracorporeal circulation with a Temptrol oxygenator, ventricular fibrillation, and ischemic arrest for 10 to 15 minutes at 30° C. Fused commissures were carefully incised in each of the 100 patients. Leaflet mobility was improved by separation of fused chordae, incision into papillary muscle, and debridement of calcium and fibrous tissue from thickened leaflets (30 percent). The valve was opened as widely as possible, striving not only to abolish the gradient but also to minimize turbulent blood flow, the latter being a suspected factor in the phenomenon of late "restenosis." Mitral regurgitation was assessed prior to closing the left atrium by manipulating a catheter across the aortic valve to create controlled aortic insufficiency, which filled the left ventricle and closed the mitral valve, allowing identification of focal areas of insufficiency. The left atrial appendage was routinely excluded to prevent postoperative embolization. In 94 patients who had OMC alone or in combination with aortic or tricuspid operation, there were no operative deaths. One patient died following reoperation and tricuspid valve replacement 5 months later. Two patients were reoperated on for mitral regurgitation and had mitral valve replacement with subsequent recovery. Three of six patients who had OMC and coronary revascularization died in the postoperative period. Ninety-six patients are alive and well. It seems probable that late analysis of these patients will demonstrate substantially better long-term results than can be obtained with closed commissurotomy.

From the Department of Surgery, New York University School of Medicine, New York, N. Y.

As EXTRACORPOREAL circulation has become simpler and safer in recent years, especially with nonblood primes and disposable oxygenators, there has been a progressive increase in the use of an "open" approach with extracorporeal circulation for mitral stenosis, rather than the traditional closed digital commissurotomy. The term "open commissurotomy" has become established through common usage, though actually the term is somewhat misleading. With an open technique, as emphasized in this report, considerably more may be done than with simple commissurotomy, such as separation of fused chordae tendineae, splitting of papillary muscles, or debridement of calcium from stiffened leaflets. Both techniques, open or closed, have an operative mortality rate of less than 3 to 4

Presented at the Twenty-eighth Annual Meeting of the Society for Vascular Surgery, Chicago, Ill., June 20 and 21, 1974.

Reprint requests: Richard M. Engelman, M.D., Department of Surgery, New York University School of Medicine, 550 First Ave., New York, N. Y. 10016.

percent and little morbidity. A crucial question, analyzed in this report, is whether better long-term results can be obtained with the open approach. At New York University an open approach has been used for most patients undergoing mitral commissurotomy during the past 7 years. These experiences form the basis of this report.

METHODS AND MATERIALS

One hundred patients (92 women, 8 men), from 15 to 69 years of age, underwent open mitral commissurotomy between January, 1966, and July, 1973. Seventy-one patients had only commissurotomy, while 29 had additional procedures performed on either the aortic or tricuspid valve or the coronary arteries (Table I). Eighty-four percent of patients were operated on for symptoms of congestive failure, ranging in severity from moderate dyspnea with daily activities to frank cardiac decompensation with dyspnea at rest, azotemia, anasarca, and pulmonary hypertension (Table II). Sixteen percent were operated on because of peripheral embolization. Seventy-three percent of the patients were in New York Heart Association Class III or IV; 27 percent were in Class II. Seven percent had undergone previous closed commissurotomy.

Right and left heart catheterization was done on all patients beforehand, including a ventriculogram to assess the degree of mitral regurgitation and contractility of the left ventricle. Coronary angiography was routinely performed on patients over 30 years of age.

Prosthetic valve replacement, usually with a ball-valve prosthesis, was almost always done for patients with significant regurgitation combined with stenosis. Also massive calcification of valve leaflets was usually treated by replacement. Otherwise valvuloplasty was regularly attempted when it appeared that a satisfactory opening would result, usually a cross-sectional area of 3 cm.^{2} or greater, without producing significant insufficiency. An opening of this size, though not normal, equals that of a No. 3 Starr-Edwards mitral prosthesis. It is estimated that currently about 75 percent of patients with mitral stenosis are treated by valvuloplasty rather than prosthetic valve replacement, but significant comparable data are not available.

Table I. *Operative procedures performed on 100 patients undergoing open mitral commissurotomy*

Procedure	*No.*
OMC*	71
OMC and tricuspid annuloplasty	7
OMC and tricuspid valve replacement	2
OMC and aortic commissurotomy	3
OMC and aortic valve replacement	10
OMC and tricuspid and aortic valve replacement	1
OMC and coronary bypass	5
OMC and coronary bypass & AVR†	1
Total	100

*OMC—open mitral commissurotomy.
†AVR—aortic valve replacement.

Table II. *Clinical characteristics of 100 patients undergoing operation*

	No.
Operative indications:	
Symptoms of congestive failure	84
Peripheral embolization	16
New York Heart Association Classification:	
Class II	27
Class III	69
Class IV	4

OPERATIVE TECHNIQUE

The bypass technique was a uniform one with a Temptrol bubble oxygenator, De Bakey roller pumps, and a nonblood prime with a balanced electrolyte solution, similar in composition to plasma. Blood was often not necessary but was used if the hematocrit decreased below 20 percent. The perfusion rate was often near 3.0 L. per minute per square meter, carefully maintaining blood pressure near the preoperative mean pressure. A median sternotomy was customarily used and the tricuspid valve was regularly palpated for insufficiency or stenosis before bypass was started. Operation was performed with electrically induced fibrillation, blood temperature of 30° C., and intermittent clamping of the aorta for 10 to 15 minutes.

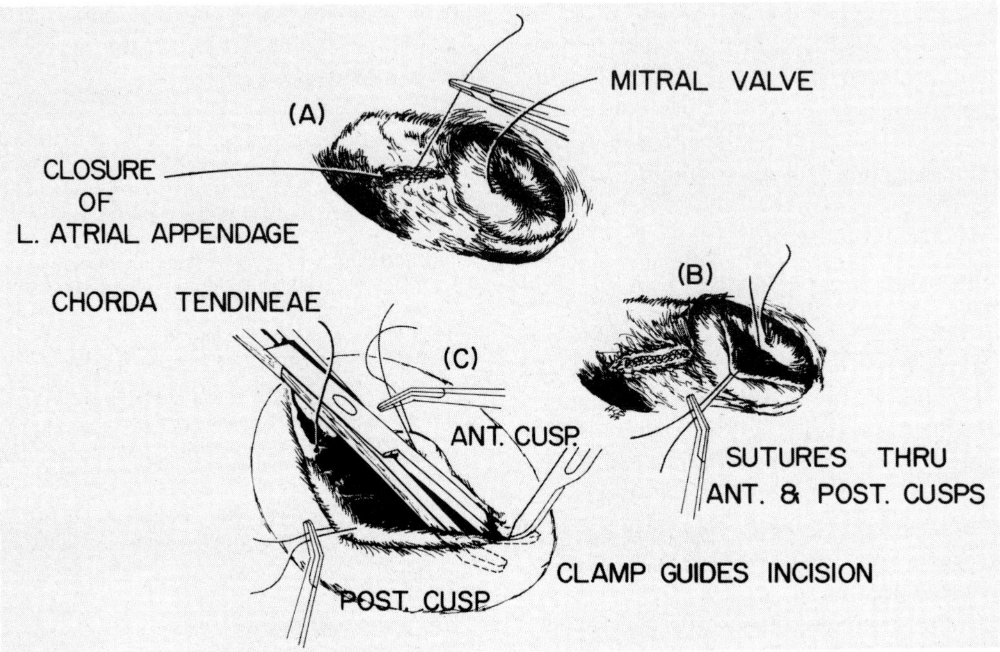

Fig. 1. *A,* closure of left atrial appendage; *B,* exposure of mitral valve with horizontal traction on sutures; *C,* third right-angle clamp guides incision.

Both the aorta and the left ventricle were vented to remove air.

The left atrium was opened with a long incision posterior to the interatrial groove, extending the atriotomy when necessary beneath and over to the left of both the superior and inferior venae cavae. By appropriate insertion of a malleable retractor, carefully adjusting the tip to produce maximum traction about 2 cm. superior to the mitral annulus, adequate exposure usually could be obtained. Initially the atrial cavity was carefully examined for thrombi, especially noting the interior of the atrial appendage. For the past 3 years, the atrial appendage has been carefully excluded from the left atrium because of the possibility of late embolization from chronic atrial fibrillation. This policy was developed after finding that each of four patients sustained a cerebral embolus 6 weeks, 1½, 2, and 5 years, respectively, following operation. The probable importance of this technique was vividly shown in one patient who suffered a devastating cerebral embolus 6 weeks following an uneventful commissurotomy, when the cardiac rhythm abruptly changed from atrial fibrillation to a sinus rhythm. It seems likely that the thrombus was lying in the fibrillating atrial appendage and was probably expelled when the atrium began to contract. This potential mechanism has been visualized in at least three patients, who, at the time of operation, were found to have 3 to 5 mm. fragments of thrombus lying *free* in the atrial appendage. Why the thrombi were not fused to the endocardium, as is customarily seen, was not certain, but the alarming probability that such thrombi would be readily expelled from the appendage if sinus rhythm returned seemed clear.

Several methods of exclusion of the left atrial appendage were evaluated, including external clamping and amputation, but closure of the orifice with a continuous suture from within the atrium seemed preferable. Care was taken to avoid insertion of sutures to a depth that might injure the underlying circumflex coronary artery in the atrioventricular groove. This method has been used satisfactorily in 75 patients undergoing mitral commissurotomy or valve replacement during the past 18 months without complications.

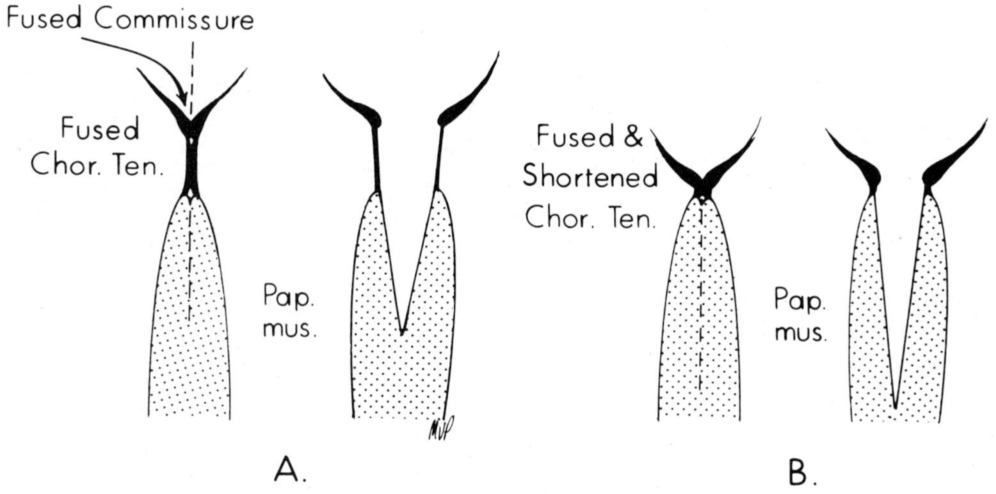

Fig. 2. *A,* separation of fused chordae tendineae with incision into papillary muscle; *B,* deeper incision into papillary muscle when valve leaflets are fused to underlying papillary muscle.

Exposure of the mitral valve was best obtained by insertion of a heavy suture, such as Dacron, in each leaflet, which in turn was grasped with a right-angle clamp to apply traction to the leaflet in a *horizontal* direction, as opposed to simple vertical traction by pulling up on the valve. Application of horizontal traction stretched the leaflets and considerably facilitated identification of the precise site of commissural fusion. Usually the fused commissure could be readily identified as a wrinkled furrow, considerably thicker on palpation than adjacent valve leaflets. A third right-angle clamp was introduced beneath the fused commissure, between the chordae, and the blade was slightly opened (Fig. 1).

Incision of a commissure was cautiously done, 2 to 3 mm. at a time, checking the separated margins to be certain that chordae tendineae inserted into the edge of each leaflet were separated. This precaution minimized the risk of incision in an incorrect area.

Occasionally landmarks were grossly distorted, especially when the leaflets were directly fused to an underlying papillary muscle because of shortening or obliteration of chordae tendineae. The correct area for incision was then uncertain. In such instances the initial incision was often begun through the fused commissure beyond the site of fusion to the papillary muscle, after which the incision was extended back to the free margin, splitting the underlying papillary muscle for 5 to 10 mm. (Fig. 2).

Both commissures were opened as widely as possible without producing insufficiency, stopping a few millimeters from the valve annulus. A more limited commissurotomy was done if fibrotic contraction and calcification suggested that insufficiency would result.

After the commissural incisions were completed, leaflet mobility was assessed. Restricted motion was sometimes improved by separation of fused chordae and further incision of papillary muscles beneath the shortened chordae. In a few patients cautious debridement of calcium and fibrous tissue from the leaflet itself, carefully avoiding perforation, improved mobility.

A particularly critical point in comparing open and closed methods was discovered when review of the operative techniques disclosed that at least 30 percent of patients had more than simple commissurotomy, with either separation of chordae tendineae and papillary muscles or removal of calcium from stiffened leaflets. It is the potential for utilizing these different valvuloplasty techniques that constitutes one of the great advantages of the open approach.

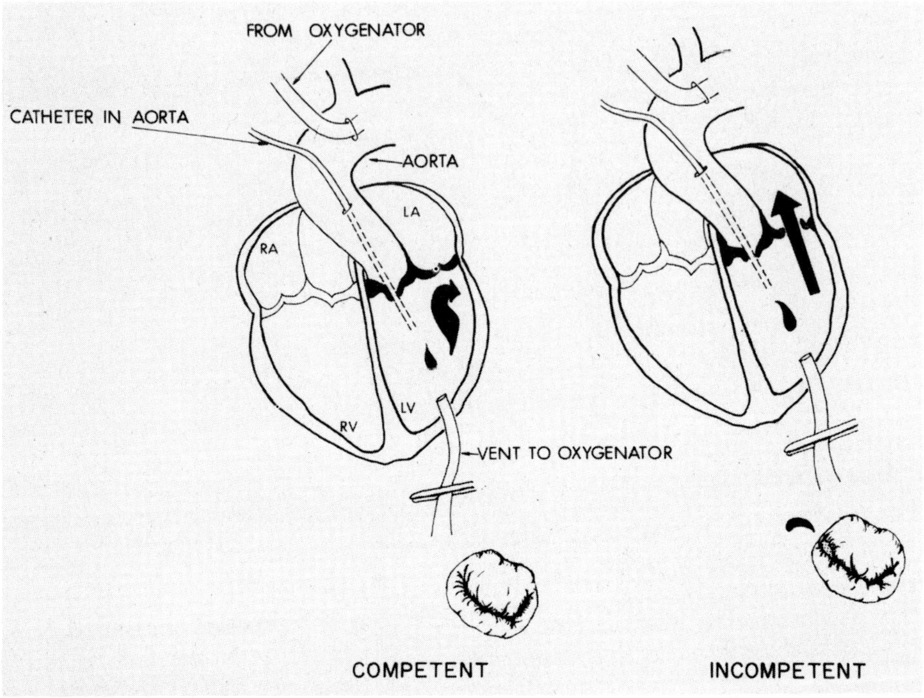

Fig. 3. Assessment of mitral regurgitation utilizing controlled aortic insufficiency to close mitral valve.

The troublesome question of production of mitral insufficiency from radical commissurotomy has been assessed in the past two years by selective induction of aortic insufficiency to fill the left ventricle, balloon the aortic leaflet upward, and seat the mitral valve. This technique has been considerably more effective than retrograde flushing of fluid through the left ventricular vent. The method is shown in Fig. 3. A small plastic cannula (No. 10 Fr.) with multiple side perforations over a distance of 6 to 7 cm. was introduced into the ascending aorta through a stab wound and manipulated across the aortic valve into the left ventricle, usually while the aorta was clamped to permit collapse of the aortic valve leaflets. In the final position of the catheter, some of the perforations were in the aorta while the remainder were in the outflow tract of the left ventricle. When the aortic clamp was released, carefully removing intra-aortic air, blood would reflux into the ventricle, ballooning the aortic leaflet of the mitral valve and seating it firmly against the mural leaflet. Focal areas of regurgitation could be readily identified and corrected, usually with one or two sutures between leaflets. In a few patients annuloplasty was performed across one or both commissures. This method of assessing regurgitation before closing the left atrium has been used in over 20 patients in the past 2 years. It has greatly simplified valvuloplasty and has permitted a bolder approach to commissurotomy than previously seemed feasible. The reliability of this method of assessing regurgitation has been routinely checked by digital palpation of the mitral valve subsequently, with the heart beating, the systolic pressure equal to or above preoperative level, and bypass either slowed or stopped. To date, the method appears to have been uniformly reliable, as measured by both the results found on digital palpation and the subsequent clinical course of the patient.

Following bypass, when normal cardiac contractility and blood pressure had been re-established, adequate correction of the mitral stenosis was confimed by measuring left

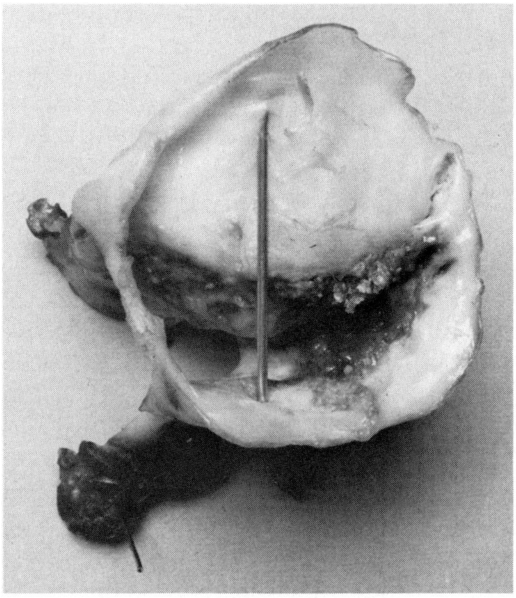

Fig. 4. Mitral valve removed from patient who underwent closed mitral commissurotomy 12 years previously.

Table III. *Operative and late results after open mitral commissurotomy alone or with aortic or tricuspid valve surgery (94 patients)**

	Early (30 days postoperatively)	*Late*
Death	0	1
Morbidity:		
Reoperation for bleeding	4	
Arrhythmia	12	
Hemothorax	2	
Mitral valve replacement		2
Systemic embolus		4
Hepatitis		1

*Three of six patients died following combined mitral commissurotomy and coronary bypass.

atrial and left ventricular diastolic pressure, demonstrating that no significant gradient between left atrium and ventricle remained.

RESULTS

There were no deaths following commissurotomy alone (71 patients) (Table III). Three deaths occurred in the group of six patients who had both mitral commissurotomy and coronary bypass. All died in the early postoperative period from a low cardiac output. Four of the 100 patients required reoperation for postoperative bleeding in the immediate postoperative period.

In 17 patients a thrombus was found in the left atrium, although 12 of the 17 had no prior history of embolization. No patient sustained an embolus in the early postoperative course. As mentioned earlier, four patients operated on early in the series, who did not have the left atrial appendage closed at operation, had a peripheral embolus 6 weeks to 5 years later.

Late evaluation of the 100 patients was made either by periodic visits to the postoperative cardiovascular clinic, where most patients are seen at regular intervals, or by direct contact with the patient's physician for the few patients no longer living in the area. No patient was lost to follow-up examination. Of the original 100 patients, 96 are alive and well, though one third of the group have a slight apical systolic murmur of uncertain significance. Sixty-four patients are now between one and 7 years since commissurotomy, while 32 are less than one year. Three patients have been re-operated on. Two patients early in the series, who required annuloplasty in addition to commissurotomy, subsequently required valve replacement for progressive mitral insufficiency. One patient was re-operated on 5 months following mitral commissurotomy and tricuspid annuloplasty, at which time tricuspid valve replacement was done with subsequent death. One patient currently has symptoms of congestive heart failure that will require evaluation by cardiac catheterization.

DISCUSSION

The choice between open and closed mitral commissurotomy is based on operative death and morbidity and the quality of the long-term result. Although previously open-heart operations were associated with greater mortality and morbidity rates than closed digital commissurotomy, ample data now show that open commissurotomy approaches in simplicity that of closed commissurotomy and may have less morbidity.[4, 5, 11] There were no operative deaths in this series among the 71 patients who required commissurotomy alone. Similarly, Gerami and associates[5] reported a series of 100 patients with no deaths, Nichols and associates[11] a series of 100 with two deaths, and Finnegan and associates[4] a group of 139 with one death.

Morbidity from bleeding associated with extracorporeal circulation has become infrequent with the use of nonblood primes. Only 4 percent of this group of 100 patients required reoperation for bleeding, all recovering uneventfully. The complete absence of any clinical evidence of neurologic injury was significant, indicating both the safety of extracorporeal circulation and the protection from intraoperative embolization. A significant number of patients (10 to 20 percent) have a thrombus within the left atrium, often with no clinical symptoms. Ullal and associates[15] reported that 50 percent of patients with left atrial thrombus had no prior history of embolization. An occasional patient had the frightening combination of no history of embolization, a grossly normal left atrial appendage, and a large, free-floating thrombus which could readily embolize with even slight digital manipulation.

Separate from operative mortality and morbidity rates is the important question of whether a better valvuloplasty can be performed by an open rather than a closed technique. There are at least three considerations in this regard. As mentioned earlier, at least 30 percent of the patients in this series had procedures in addition to simple commissurotomy. These included separation of fused chordae tendineae, incision of papillary muscles, debridement of valve leaflets, and correction of focal areas of insufficiency. None of these is feasible with the closed technique. In addition, the ability to evaluate mitral insufficiency during the procedure by manipulating a catheter across the aortic valve made bolder techniques of reconstruction feasible without the fear of finding significant insufficiency at the conclusion of the procedure.

Second, there is a 15 to 20 percent frequency of significant mitral regurgitation after closed commissurotomy, suggesting that many valves are injured. This may be due to opening stenotic valves that would have been replaced with an open technique or to injury to valves that could have been avoided with an open approach.

Finally, a third consideration concerns the advantage of precisely incising a fused commissure under direct vision rather than separating it blindly with a mechanical dilator. A concept often quoted is that a mitral valve can be opened more effectively and physiologically with a mechanical dilator in the beating heart rather than under direct vision by sharp incision in a nonbeating heart. The origin of this concept is difficult to determine. Probably it is simply a myth, originally quoted as a hypothesis, then requoted over a period of time by others until it unwittingly became considered an established fact. Although the good results obtained for years in many patients with mechanical dilators are recognized by everyone, we would sharply disagree with this concept and strongly prefer precise identification of anatomical structures before incising a fused commissure.[6] We have not used the mechanical dilator on the mitral valve during an open operation for several years.

LONG-TERM CONSIDERATIONS

Of even greater significance, though, than immediate operative mortality and morbidity rates is the quality of long-term results. A significant question for future studies is whether the frequency of subsequent restenosis or insufficiency is less with the open than with the closed approach. A separate question, which cannot be analyzed here, is when a densely scarred, partly calcified valve is encountered, is there a greater tendency for valve replacement with open approach than with the closed commissurotomy? This question has been analyzed in the report by Olinger, Rio, and Maloney.[12]

Although the follow-up period is short, no patient in this series has been recognized to have significant mitral stenosis, and only two, both operated on early in the series, have required valve replacement for mitral regurgitation. These results are comparable to those reported by Roe and associates[13] and Finnegan and associates.[4] It seems probable that long-term analysis of these patients will demonstrate a substantially lower frequency of restenosis and regurgitation than the 17 to 40 percent frequency reported for closed commissurotomy.[3, 9, 10, 12]

Two objectives can be considered with mitral commissurotomy. The immediate consideration is to abolish the gradient without creating regurgitation. A second, somewhat theoretical objective is to open the mitral valve as widely as possible to minimize turbulent flow of blood, which may be the most significant factor in the phenomenon of late "restenosis." A normal mitral valve has an opening of 3 to 4 cm.,[2] but significant symptoms may not develop until the opening is reduced below 1.5 cm.[2] A limited commissurotomy enlarging the opening to 1.5 or 2.0 cm.[2] can relieve symptoms temporarily, but continued turbulent flow of blood may promote restenosis. Selzer and Cohn[14] studied the natural history of mitral stenosis and emphasized the similarity to that of the congenitally bicuspid aortic valve. Both conditions commonly progress to a rigid, calcified valve, perhaps the result of chronic turbulent flow of blood across a stenotic orifice. Hence, the concept that restenosis is an inevitable consequence of the rheumatic process may be erroneous. Indeed, Harken and associates,[7] Higgs and associates[8] and others[1, 2] have shown that true restenosis of the mitral valve was uncommon if the commissures were completely opened at the first operation. If this concept of turbulent blood flow is correct, an early open commissurotomy may greatly lessen the likelihood of more extensive destruction of the valve with eventual prosthetic replacement.

The specimen shown in Fig. 4 is from a woman who had a closed commissurotomy 12 years earlier. At repeat operation, the anterolateral commissure was widely patent, with a perfectly normal subvalvular mechanism. However, the posteromedial commissure and adjacent leaflets had calcified to an extensive degree with fusion to the underlying papillary muscle, resulting in a rigid, stenotic, and insufficient valve. This selective involvement of one commissure strongly suggests that at the previous closed commissurotomy 12 years earlier only the anterolateral commissure was opened completely. Now, because of extensive destruction of the valve, prosthetic replacement was necessary.

In summary, a serious question is whether or not insufficiency or late restenosis must be expected in many patients after commissurotomy. Is this progressive valve destruction an inevitable consequence of rheumatic valvulitis or is it related to chronic turbulent blood flow? If the latter concept is correct, a valvuloplasty that widely opens the mitral orifice and minimizes turbulent blood flow may lead to much better long-term results than have been reported with closed techniques. For these reasons we strongly prefer an open approach upon virtually all patients undergoing operation for mitral stenosis.

REFERENCES

1. Aronstam, E. M., Geiger, J. P., and Gillespie, J. T.: Reoperation for mitral stenosis, J. Thorac. Cardiovasc. Surg. **55:** 784, 1968.
2. Belcher, J. R.: Restenosis of the mitral valve: An account of fifty second operations, Lancet **1:** 184, 1960.
3. Ellis, L. B., Singh, J. B., Morales, D. D., and Harken, D. E.: Fifteen to twenty-year study of one thousand patients undergoing closed mitral valvuloplasty, Circulation **48:** 357, 1973.
4. Finnegan, J. O., Gray, D. C., MacVaugh, H., et al.: The open approach to mitral commissurotomy, J. Thorac. Cardiovasc. Surg. **67:** 75, 1974.
5. Gerami, S., Messmer, B. J., Hallman, G. L., et al.: Open mitral commissurotomy, J. Thorac. Cardiovasc. Surg. **62:** 366, 1971.
6. Gott, V. L., Revilla, A., Donahoo, J. S., et al.: Closed mitral commissurotomy on cannulated pump stand-by through a sternal-split incision, J. Thorac. Cardiovasc. Surg. **67:** 66, 1974.
7. Harken, D. E., Black, H., Taylor, W. J., et al.: Reoperation for mitral stenosis, Circulation **23:** 7, 1961.
8. Higgs, L. M., Glancy, D. L., O'Brien, K. P., et al.: Mitral restenosis: An uncommon cause of recurrent symptoms following mitral commissurotomy, Am. J. Cardiol. **26:** 34, 1970.
9. Keith, T. A., and Noble, O. F.: Closed mitral

commissurotomy complications and their effect on survival, Chest **61:** 24, 1972.

10. Nathaniels, S. K., Moncure, A. C., and Scannell, J. G.: A fifteen year follow-up study of close mitral valvuloplasty, Ann. Thorac. Surg. **10:** 28, 1970.
11. Nichols, H. T., Blanco, G., Morse, D. P., et al.: Open mitral commissurotomy, J. A. M. A. **182:** 268, 1962.
12. Olinger, G. N., Rio, F. W., and Maloney, J. V., Jr.: Closed valvulotomy for calcific mitral stenosis, J. Thorac. Cardiovasc. Surg. **62:** 357, 1971.
13. Roe, B. B., Edmunds, H., Jr., Fishman, N. H., and Hutchinson, J. C.: Open mitral commissurotomy, Ann. Thorac. Surg. **12:** 483, 1971.
14. Selzer, A., and Cohn, K. E.: Natural history of mitral stenosis: A review, Circulation **45:** 878, 1972.
15. Ullal, S. R., Kluge, T. H., Hill, J. D., et al.: Left atrial thrombi in mitral valve disease. J. Thorac. Cardiovasc. Surg. **62:** 932, 1971.

DISCUSSION

Dr. Safuh Attar (Baltimore, Md.). At the University of Maryland we feel that a closed mitral commissurotomy can give an excellent result over a long-term follow-up.

However, I rise to discuss one point regarding the prevention of air embolism during open commissurotomy as well as during mitral valve replacement.

I think a beating heart provides a better opportunity for evaluation of the degree of mitral stenosis and insufficiency than does a fibrillating heart. And an approach to the mitral valve through a right thoracotomy is easier than median sternotomy.

However, the main objection to the right-sided approach for the mitral valve has been the high incidence of air embolism. I have found that if one uses the right-sided approach and cross-clamps the ascending aorta immediately prior to opening the left atrium, one will avoid the incidence of any air embolism.

The technique we use to protect the myocardium is moderate hypothermia to about 30° C. with ice slush around the heart, leaving the heart beating. The aorta is cross-clamped and a needle is inserted below it. On some occasions, when we opened the left atrium prior to clamping of the aorta, we found that air had already escaped, although there was only about a minute elapsing between the opening of the left atrium and occlusion of the aorta.

In subsequent cases we followed this technique of cross-clamping the aorta for 10 to 15 minutes at a time and no air embolism occurred. We feel that a commissurotomy through a right-sided approach is much easier and can afford probably a better evaluation of the mitral valve than can a midline sternal approach in a fibrillating heart.

Dr. Frank C. Spencer (Closing). The basic hypothesis proposed in this paper is that a much more effective commissurotomy can be performed with the open technique. The objective should be not only to abolish the gradient across the mitral valve but also to minimize or eliminate the turbulent flow of blood. Fortunately, both mortality and morbidity rates are small with either the open or closed approach, so a choice cannot be made on this basis alone.

A normal mitral valve has a cross-sectional area of 4 to 6 $cm.^2$. Symptoms are minimal unless the cross-sectional area is less than 2 $cm.^2$, and severe symptoms are often associated with an area of less than 1 $cm.^2$. Hence excellent palliation can be obtained by surgically opening the valve to 2 or 2.5 $cm.^2$, though turbulent flow of blood, with an audible murmur, remains. It seems plausible that this long-continued turbulent flow may eventually result in progressive fibrosis and calcification, termed "restenosis."

A particularly important point in support of the open technique is the frequency with which something additional can be done to open the stenosed valve besides separation of fused commissures. The additional techniques include separation of fused chordae, incision of papillary muscles, and debridement of calcium from leaflets. These additional manuevers were performed to some extent in 25 to 30 percent of the patients operated on in this series. Certainly these techniques cannot be performed to any degree with a closed approach.

Finally, one of the myths in cardiac surgery is that a better commissurotomy can be done with a finger or a mechanical instrument in a beating heart, as opposed to incising the fused commissures under direct vision in a still heart. Previously, the main virtue of the closed technique, aside from simplicity, was that insufficiency could be detected as a commissure was opened. This advantage disappears, however, with a reliable method for evaluating insufficiency with an open technique. As emphasized in this report, with confidence in the ability to recognize and correct the insufficiency during an open procedure, a progressively more radical valvuloplasty has been performed in recent years.

In summary, a long-term evaluation, probably 5 or 10 years, on the comparative frequency of late "restenosis" or insufficiency after commissurotomy will permit a final decision about the relative merits of the two techniques. Our decision from experiences over the past 4 years is that, for the vast majority of patients, the closed digital approach is an inferior operation.

Clinical and hemodynamic comparisons of Kay-Shiley, Starr-Edwards No. 6520, and Reis-Hancock porcine xenograft mitral valves

John W. Brown, M.D., P. David Myerowitz, M.D., Michael S. Cann, M.D., Stephen B. Colvin, M.D., Charles L. McIntosh, M.D., *and* Andrew G. Morrow, M.D., *Bethesda, Md.*

Mitral valve replacement (MVR) in a patient with a small or normal-size left ventricle necessitates the use of a low-profile prosthesis or a porcine xenograft. This retrospective study summarizes the clinical and hemodynamic findings in 88 patients in whom such valves were implanted. Isolated MVR was performed in 74 patients and MVR plus tricuspid valve replacement with the same type of prosthesis in 14 patients. Preoperative hemodynamic findings and the number of patients in each group were comparable. Early ($<$ 30 days) and 6 month mortality rates were Kay-Shiley (KS) 33 and 48 percent, Starr-Edwards No. 6520 (SE) 14 and 25 percent, porcine xenografts (P) 6 and 12 percent. The incidence of fatal postoperative arrhythmias was 11 percent with KS valves, 11 percent with SE valves, and 6 percent with P valves. Postoperative thromboembolic complications occurred in 33 percent of patients with KS valves, 28 percent with SE valves, but were not observed in any patient with a P valve. The hemodynamic performance of all three valve types was similar as measured at postoperative catheterization; the calculated orifice areas and diastolic gradients were not significantly different in the three groups. However, the significantly lower early mortality rate and the absence of thromboembolic complications make the porcine xenograft a superior choice for patients with normal or small-size left ventricles.

From the National Heart and Lung Institute, Clinic of Surgery, National Institutes of Health, Bethesda, Md.

NUMEROUS atrioventricular valve prostheses have been introduced since the first successful mitral valve replacement performed at the National Heart and Lung Institute in March, 1960.[1] The cardiac surgeon has at his disposal numerous prosthetic devices which claim improved hemodynamic performance, increased durability, low profile, and decreased hemolysis. The complication of thromboembolism remains the most significant cause of postoperative morbidity and death with all mechanical valves, in spite of the use of anticoagulation. Composite tissue valves (fresh or formaldehyde-fixed homologous or heterologous aortic valves, fascia lata, or pericardium) enjoy the combined advantages of good hemodynamic function and low thrombogenicity, but late postoperative tissue failure has caused a decrease in their popularity.[2, 4, 5, 11]

The problem of mitral valve replacement in the patient with a small or normal-size left ventricle requires the choice of a prosthesis small enough to be easily accomodated within the left ventricle. This report attempts to compare clinical and hemodynamic aspects of three prosthetic valves which have been used at the National Heart and Lung Insti-

Presented at the Twenty-eighth Annual Meeting of the Society for Vascular Surgery, Chicago, Ill., June 20 and 21, 1974.

Reprint requests: John W. Brown, M.D., National Heart and Lung Institute, Clinic of Surgery, National Institutes of Health, Bethesda, Md. 20014.

Table I. *Preoperative clinical findings in 88 patients who underwent mitral valve replacement**

	Kay-Shiley		Starr-Edwards No. 6520		Porcine	
	No.	%	No.	%	No.	%
Total patients	27	100	28	100	33	100
Operative dates	Jan. 1966 to Oct. 1970		Aug. 1971 to Dec. 1972		July 1970 to Sept. 1973	
Operation performed:						
MVR	19	70	17	61	15	45
MVR & TA	1	4	7	25	5	15
MVR & TVR	4	15	4	14	6	18
MVR & aortic valvotomy	1	4	0	0	6	18
MVR & other	2	7	0	0	1	3
Mitral lesion:						
Pure MS	9	33	3	11	4	12
Pure MR	4	15	4	14	6	18
Combined MS & MR	14	52	21	75	23	70
Associated cardiac lesions:						
TR	12	44	14	50	16	48
AS	4	15	0	0	7	21
AR	4	15	6	21	13	39
Other	1	4	0	0	0	0
Functional Class (NYHA):						
Class III	15	56	19	68	25	76
Class IV	8	30	9	32	7	21
Average age	43	—	47	—	49	—
Mitral valve cal.	19	70	13	46	16	48
Left atrial thrombus	6	22	5	18	4	12
Previous mitral Commissurotomy	7	26	9	32	9	27
Previous MVR	1	4	0	0	2	6

*Abbreviations: AR = aortic regurgitations; AS =aortic stenosis; cal. = calcification; LA = left atrial; MR = mitral regurgitation; MS = mitral stenosis; MVR = mitral valve replacement; NYHA = New York Heart Association; TA = tricuspid annuloplasty; TR = tricuspid regurgitation; TVR = tricuspid valve replacement.

tute for atrioventricular valve replacement in patients who were felt to have ventricular cavities too small for a caged-ball prosthesis. Eighty-eight patients underwent mitral valve replacement with one of these prostheses, and 14 of the 88 required tricuspid valve replacement with the same prosthetic type. Patients also requiring aortic valve replacement and patients who had two prostheses of different types were excluded from the study. Twenty-seven patients received Kay-Shiley (KS) valves between January, 1966, and October, 1970.[8] Twenty-eight patients received Starr-Edwards No. 6520 (SE) disc valves between August, 1971, and December, 1972. Porcine xenografts (P) (Hancock Laboratories, Anaheim, Calif.) were used in 33 patients between July, 1970, and September, 1973. Other reports on the clinical results with the P valves have been presented.[7, 10, 12]

PATIENTS AND METHODS

Table I summarizes the preoperative clinical data subdivided according to the type of prosthesis used. The average ages of patients in the three groups were 43, 47, and 49 years, respectively. Rheumatic valvular disease was the etiology in 81 of the 88 patients. Three patients who received KS valves, two patients who received SE valves, and one of the two patients who received a P valve had congenital mitral abnormalities. The other P valve recipient had papillary muscle dysfunction secondary to coronary artery disease with severe mitral regurgitation. Thirty-four of the 88 patients had associated aortic valvular disease that did not require aortic valve replacement (eight KS, six SE, and 20 P, respectively). Pure or predominant mitral stenosis was the primary valvular lesion in nine patients who received KS valves, three pa-

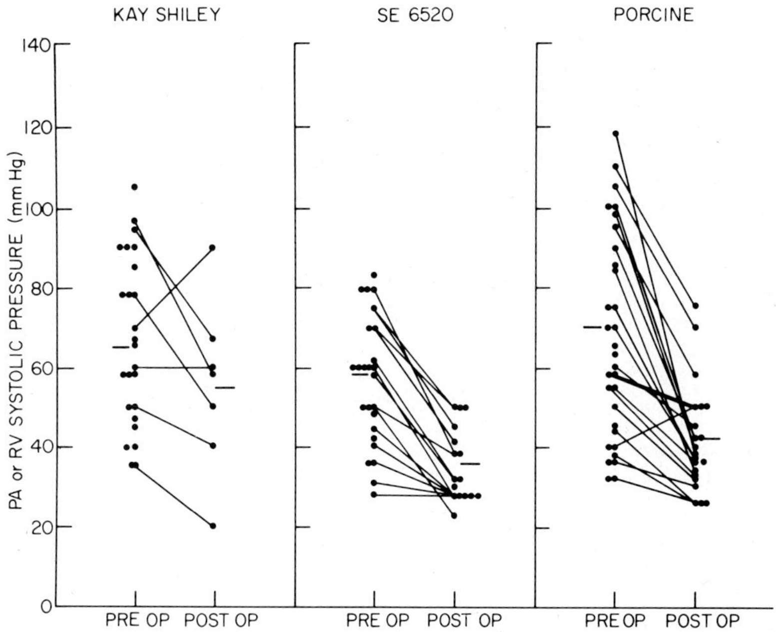

Fig. 1. Pre- and postoperative pulmonary artery (PA) or right ventricular (RV) systolic pressure in patients who underwent mitral valve replacement (MVR) with Kay-Shiley, Starr-Edwards No. 6520 (SE 6520), and porcine xenograft mitral valves. Connected circles indicate that values were obtained both preoperatively and postoperatively. Unconnected circles indicate that only the preoperative value was obtained. The mean values are represented by the horizontal line.

tients who received SE valves, and four patients who received P valves. Pure mitral regurgitation was the preoperative lesion in four KS, four SE, and six P patients. Fourteen KS, 21 SE, and 23 P patients had combined mitral stenosis and regurgitation. Associated tricuspid regurgitation prompted tricuspid annuloplasty in one KS, seven SE, and five P patients and tricuspid valve replacement with the same type valve in four patients who received KS, four who received SE, and six patients who received P valves.

Pre- and postoperative right heart catheterization was performed either through an antecubital cutdown or from a femoral vein using the Seldinger technique. Left atrial pressure was measured directly by trans-septal catheterization or indirectly by pulmonary artery wedge pressure. The left ventricle was entered by retrograde arterial catheterization preoperatively. In patients with tricuspid prostheses, right ventricular pressure was measured by percutaneous puncture. The mean pressure gradient between left atrium and left ventricle or between right atrium and right ventricle was obtained by planimetric integration of the area between the simultaneously recorded phasic pressure tracings during diastole. Cardiac output was determined by the indicator (indocyanine green) dilution technique. The effective orifice areas of the prostheses were calculated using the formula of Gorlin and Gorlin.[6]

The results of preoperative cardiac catheterization showed an average pulmonary artery systolic pressure of 65, 58, and 70 mm. Hg for the KS, SE No. 6520, and P valves, respectively (Fig. 1). The left atrial mean ($\overline{LA}$) or pulmonary artery wedge mean ($\overline{PAW}$) pressure for each group of patients was 24 mm. Hg (Fig. 2). Left ventricular end-diastolic pressure was 12.5, 14, and 12 mm. Hg for the respective groups preoperatively (Fig. 3). Cardiac index (Fig. 4) for KS patients was 2.0 L. per minute per square meter and was 2.3 L. per minute per square

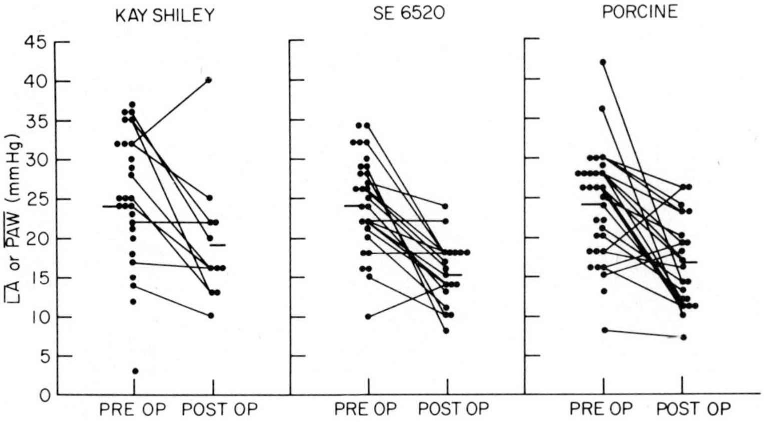

Fig. 2. Mean left atrial ($\overline{LA}$) or mean pulmonary artery wedge ($\overline{PAW}$) pressure pre- and postoperatively. (See Fig. 1 for explanation of symbols.)

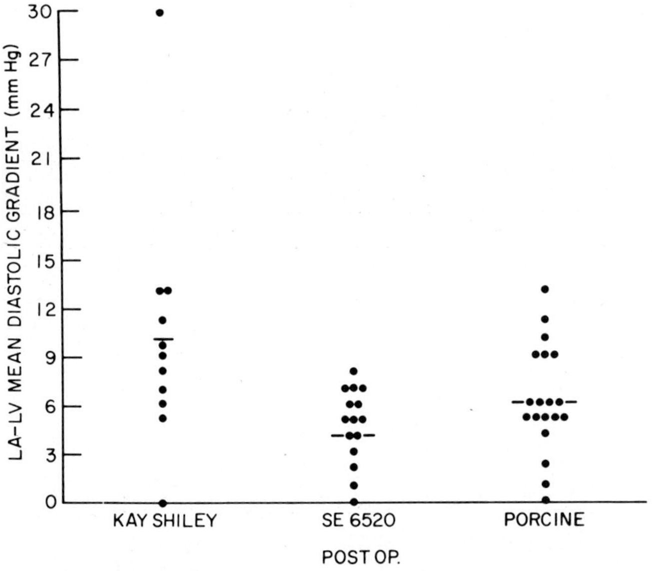

Fig. 3. Postoperative left atrial (LA)–left ventricular (LV) mean diastolic gradient. (See Fig. 1 for explanation of symbols.)

meter for SE and P patients. The preoperative average left atrial–left ventricular mean diastolic gradients were 13, 11, and 14 mm. Hg for the groups. Preoperative mitral valve area for KS patients was 0.75 cm.^{2} and 1.1 cm.^{2} for both SE and P valve patients.

OPERATIVE METHODS

Standard techniques for cardiopulmonary bypass utilizing the Kay-Cross disc oxygenator were employed. Aortic crossclamping was used only when necessary for visualizing the mitral annulus. All valves were placed in the supra-annular position. Left ventricular decompression was maintained with a wire whisk or Foley catheter through the prosthetic orifice until closure of the left atriotomy was accomplished. Residual air was removed via a stab wound in the apex of the left ventricle. The average size KS valve used in the mitral position was size 4, which had a mounting diameter of 27 mm. and an in vitro orifice area of 220 mm.^{2} The average SE valve size used was 3 M., which had a

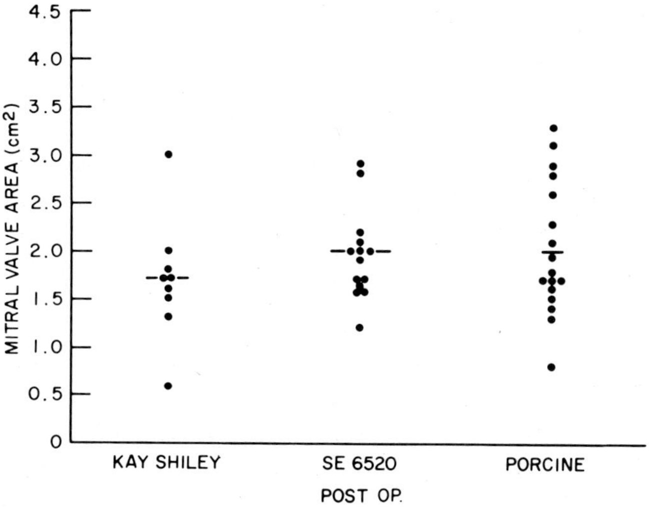

Fig. 4. Postoperative mitral valve area. (See Fig. 1 for explanation of symbols.)

Table II. *Early (< 30 days) and late (6 months) postoperative mortality rate in patients who underwent mitral valve replacement**

	Kay-Shiley				*Starr-Edwards No. 6520*				*Porcine*			
	Early		*Late*		*Early*		*Late*		*Early*		*Late*	
	No.	*%*	*No.*	*%*	*No.*	*%*	*No.*	*%*	*No.*	*%*	*No.*	*%*
Operation:												
MVR	4	15	3	11	0	0	1	4	2	6	1	3
MVR and TVR	2	7	0	0	1	4	1	4	0	0	0	0
MVR and miscellaneous	3	11	1	4	3	11	1	4	0	0	1	3
Total	9	33	4	15	4	15	3	12	2	6	2	6
Total months of postoperative follow-up			467				433				437	

*Abbreviations: MVR = mitral valve replacement; TVR = tricuspid valve replacement.

mounting diameter of 30 mm. and an orifice area of 285 mm.[2] The average size and mounting diameter of porcine xenograft valve was 29 mm. and it had an orifice area of 490 mm.[2]

Anticoagulation with warfarin in standard doses was started on the third postoperative day in patients who received KS and SE No. 6520 valves and continued indefinitely. Patients who received porcine xenograft valves received no anticoagulants postoperatively unless they had had a left atrial thrombus removed at the time of operation. In such patients warfarin was used in standard doses for 6 months postoperatively and then discontinued.

Postoperative evaluation, including cardiac catheterization, was carried out in most patients who survived postoperatively. Ninety-three percent of surviving patients who received KS valves, 81 percent of surviving patients who received SE valves, and 86 percent of surviving patients receiving P valves were catheterized at an average of 6 months postoperatively.

RESULTS

The early (< 30 days) mortality rate for patients who obtained KS valves was 33 percent (9 of 27 patients) (Table II). Two died at operation as a result of technical errors. One patient (4 years of age) with subaortic

Table III. *Cause of death in patients who underwent mitral valve replacement*

	Kay-Shiley		*Starr-Edwards No. 6520*		*Porcine*	
	No.	*%*	*No.*	*%*	*No.*	*%*
Thromboembolic	1	4	1	4	0	0
Arrhythmias	3	11	3	11	2	6
Low cardiac output	4	15	2	7	1	3
Technical at operation	3	11	0	0	1	3
Coronary artery disease	1	4	0	0	0	0
Infection	1	4	1	4	0	0
Total	13	49	7	26	4	12

stenosis and marked mitral regurgitation died early after operation as a result of poppet impingement by ventricular muscle. Another child (10 years of age) who underwent repair of an incomplete A-V canal and mitral valve replacement died as a result of third-degree heart block. One patient died of an acute myocardial infarction. Four patients died early after operation secondary to severely low cardiac output.

The early postoperative mortality rates for SE and P valve patients were 14 and 6 percent, respectively. Two of the four early postoperative deaths in patients who received SE valves were the result of severely low cardiac output. Another patient died of sepsis and the fourth of an arrhythmia. One of the two early deaths in patients with P valves occurred as a result of a technical problem at operation and the other followed a drug-resistant ventricular arryhthmia. There were four late deaths (> one month) in patients with KS valves, one of pneumonia, one of an embolus, and two of sudden and unexplained etiology. A cerebrovascular accident was the cause of late death in one of the two patients with the SE valves and the other death was sudden and unexplained. One of the two late deaths in patients with P valves was due to chronic congestive heart failure. The other was sudden and of unexplained etiology. To date no deaths have occurred beyond 6 months in any group.

Comparative pre- and postoperative hemodynamic data are shown in Figs. 1 to 4. The average postoperative pulmonary artery systolic (PA) pressure was 55 mm. Hg for patients who obtained KS valves, 36 mm. Hg for patients receiving SE valves, and 42 mm. Hg for patients who received P valves (Fig. 1). The average $\overline{LA}$ or $\overline{PAW}$ pressures for the groups were 19, 15, and 16.5 mm. Hg postoperatively (Fig. 2). The average cardiac index rose from 2.0 to 2.8 L. per minute per square meter in patients with KS valves, stayed the same at 2.3 L. per minute per square meter in patients with SE valves, and increased from 2.3 to 2.5 L. per minute per square meter in patients with P valves. The postoperative mean LA-LV diastolic gradient was 10 mm. Hg for patients with KS valves, 4 mm. Hg for patients with SE valves, and 6 mm. Hg for patients with P valves (Fig. 3). The mitral valve area was 1.7, 2.0, and 2.0 cm.^{2} postoperatively for the respective groups (Fig. 4).

There were nine postoperative thromboembolic complications (33 percent) in the patients with KS valves in 467 postoperative months. Three patients obstructed their prostheses with thrombi and underwent prosthetic replacement with P valves. Six patients had peripheral emboli, four of which were cerebral. Thromboembolic complications occurred in eight patients (28 percent) with SE valves in 433 postoperative patient-months. Six of the seven peripheral emboli were cerebral. The remaining patient underwent replacement of his mitral prosthesis, which was obstructed with thrombus. There have been no thromboembolic complications with the P valve in 437 postoperative patient months.

The postoperative average (New York Heart Association) functional classification was 1.4 for patients surviving with KS valves, 1.3 for patients surviving with SE valves, and 1.2 for patients surviving with P valves.

DISCUSSION

All three valves discussed in this report meet the criteria for use in the atrioventricular position in patients with small ventricular cavities. Preoperative hemodynamic and clinical characteristics of each group of patients are comparable, as are the postoperative hemodynamic findings in surviving patients. The significant difference in early mortality rates may, in part, reflect more recent improved surgical techniques and improved techniques of bypass and postoperative care in patients who received SE and P valves. Clearly, sepsis, coronary artery disease, and technical problems at operation cannot be attributed to the prosthesis (Table III). Postoperative low cardiac output syndrome is probably not the fault of the prosthesis in this series of patients since these prostheses do not produce obstruction of ventricular emptying as is postulated to occur with the caged-ball prosthesis.

Postoperative ventricular arrhythmias caused by impingement of an atrioventricular prosthesis on the interventricular septum would seem to be almost nonexistent in patients with the low profile KS or SE valves. The fact that 11 percent of patients with these prostheses died of ventricular arrhythmias probably means that the stimulus for these arrhythmias is other than interventricular septal impingement. Although the struts of the porcine prosthesis extend into the ventricular cavity and one strut lies parallel to and may contact the septum, our incidence of fatal ventricular arrhythmias was only 6 percent.

Thromboemboli are the major complications which directly relate to the prosthesis. The 33 percent incidence of thromboembolic complications with the KS valve and the 28 percent incidence with the SE valve (both groups of patients being maintained on therapeutic doses of warfarin) are in clear contrast to our experience with the Hancock porcine xenograft, with which no thromboembolic complications have appeared. All three groups have been followed for a comparable period.

Cooley, Bloodwell, and Hallman[3] reported an operative mortality rate of 11 percent and a one year mortality rate of 17 percent in a series of 130 patients who received KS valves. The thromboembolic rate was 14 percent in the first year. Shepherd and associates,[8] from this institution, reported a 29 percent early mortality rate and a 45 percent late mortality rate in 48 patients with KS valves in the atrioventricular position. Several of those patients, however, had an aortic valve replacement and others had mixed prosthetic types inserted. Starr[9] has observed a 14 percent incidence of thromboembolic complications in 21 patients with the SE valve.

Excellent early results have been reported with other tissue valves in the atrioventricular position. The unacceptably high rate of late tissue degeneration, however, has caused virtual abandonment of their use.[5-8] The Hancock porcine xenograft in the atrioventricular position has enjoyed nearly a 4 year follow-up with no reported cases of tissue degeneration.[7, 10, 12] Stinson, Griepp, and Shumway[10] and Zuhdi and associates[12] have recently discussed the increased long-term durability of this tissue prosthesis and have attributed it to the more biostable intermolecular bonds formed by the stabilized gluteraldehyde process used during its preparation and storage.

Good hemodynamic results and a low incidence of thromboembolic complications have recently been reported by other institutions using the Hancock prosthesis. Long and associates[7] reported a 3 percent early and 8.5 percent late mortality rate in 117 patients undergoing atrioventricular valve replacement. Their incidence of thromboemboli was 2 percent and all instances occurred in the first 3 months postoperatively. Stinson, Griepp, and Shumway[10] reported a 5 percent early and 8 percent 2 year mortality rate in 103 patients undergoing mitral valve replacement with the Hancock porcine xenograft with a 1.7 percent incidence of thromboemboli. Zuhdi and associates[12] have reported no thromboemboli in 48 patients followed up to 42 months postoperatively.

The results of the present study show that there was little significant difference in the hydraulic function of the three prostheses discussed in this report. The strikingly lower thromboembolic rate, without anticoagulation, with the Hancock porcine valve makes it a superior choice in patients with small ventricular cavities.

REFERENCES

1. Braunwald, N. S., Cooper, T., and Morrow, A. G.: Complete replacement of the mitral valve. Successful clinical application of a flexible polyurethane prosthesis, J. Thorac. Cardiovasc. Surg. **40:** 1, 1960.
2. Buch, W. S., Kosek, J. C., and Angell, W. W.: Deterioration of Formalin-treated aortic valve heterografts, J. Thorac. Cardiovasc. Surg. **60:** 673, 1970.
3. Cooley, D. A., Bloodwell, R. D., and Hallman, G. L.: Mitral valve replacement with a discoid prosthesis, Ann. Thorac. Surg. **3:** 487, 1967.
4. Edwards, W. S.: Late results with autogenous tissue heart valves, Ann. Thorac. Surg. **12:** 385, 1971.
5. Gerbode, F., editor: Proceedings of the First International Workshop on Tissue Valves, Ann. Surg. **172**(Suppl.): 1, 1970.
6. Gorlin, R., and Gorlin, S. G.: Hydraulic formula for calculation of the area of the stenotic mitral valve, other cardiac valves, and central circulatory shunts, Am. Heart J. **41:** 1, 1951.
7. Long, J. W., Reis, R. L., Bolton, M. R., et al.: Clinical and hemodynamic assessments of porcine heterograft prostheses mounted on flexible stents, Circulation (abst.) **8** and **9:** 75, 1973.
8. Shepherd, R. L., Glancy, L. D., Reis, R. L., et al.: Hemodynamic function of the Kay-Shiley prosthetic cardiac valve, Chest **63:** 323, 1973.
9. Starr, A.: Unpublished data.
10. Stinson, E. B., Griepp, R. B., and Shumway, N. E.: Clinical experience with a porcine aortic valve xenograft for mitral valve replacement, Presented at the Society of Thoracic Surgeons, Los Angeles, Calif., 1974.
11. Yarbrough, J. W., Roberts, W. C., and Reis, R. L.: Structural alterations in tissue cardiac valves implanted in patients and in calves, J. Thorac. Cardiovasc. Surg. **65:** 364, 1973.
12. Zuhdi, N., Hawley, W., Voehl, V., et al.: Porcine aortic valves as replacement for human heart valves, Ann. Thorac. Surg. **17:** 479, 1974.

DISCUSSION

Dr. Robert L. Reis (Kansas City, Kan.). I rise to make one point regarding hydraulic function. The measurement of cardiac output and transvalvular gradient permits calculation of valve orifice area. When a pressure gradient is not measured or is not present, it is not possible to calculate a valve orifice area. In a significant number of patients with heterografts, pressure gradients were not present. However, in none of the patients with a ball valve was there an absence of obstruction.

If we compare the 3 M Starr-Edwards ball valve to the 29 mm. porcine valve, the in vitro orifice areas are very similar. Similarly, the calculated orifice area in patients is quite similar.

The 31, 33, and 35 mm. porcine valves have larger in vitro than in vivo orifice areas; that is, the orifice area calculated in patients is also larger.

Therefore, I agree with Dr. Brown that when valves of varying design but of similar size are compared, the hydraulic function of the disk valve, the ball valve, and the tissue valve are the same. However, since in similar size patients, a larger tissue valve can be implanted, the tissue valve has hydraulic advantage.

Dr. Arthur C. Beall, Jr. (Houston, Texas). It was interesting to note that there were few significant differences in the three groups of valves compared except for thromboembolism. I was a little concerned that there were no embolic episodes with porcine valves in this paper, after having listened to the previous paper on mitral commissurotomy where there was a 4 percent incidence of thromboembolism, even though a prosthetic valve was not used. Also, Dr. Bruno Messmer and Ake Senning reported a series of mitral annuloplasties where there was a 5 percent incidence of emboli.

I think what this means is that any time we go in the left atrium and do anything to the mitral valve, there is going to be a certain percentage of emboli and that we can now do valve replacement with a similar incidence as with reparative techniques. I think we have achieved as low an incidence of thromboembolism as we can accomplish.

It has been demonstrated in numerous reports and with over 20,000 valves with the entire cloth-covered base and sewing ring that this can be achieved.

There has been a problem within the last couple of years of some broken struts that I think has been overemphasized. The grand total now is six out of some 3,500 or an incidence of less than two tenths of one percent.

What we have done about this is to thicken the struts slightly so that it is three times as hard to crack the struts.

This valve, the Model 106, has now been put in a package that has a seal to show that it has not been opened. This assures that the valve has not been damaged, as it cannot be damaged as long as it stays in the package. It can be either gas or steam autoclaved in the package without breaking the seal.

Once the package is opened, the valve can be lifted out with the valve holder.

With these cloth-covered prostheses, we have been able to demonstrate as low an incidence of thromboembolism without anticoagulants as with valve repair. I have not used anticoagulants with these patients since 1967.

I think we will find a similar incidence of thromboembolism with the porcine grafts as we do with reparative techniques once they are followed long enough.

Dr. Philip N. Sawyer (Brooklyn, N. Y.). When considering the type of prosthetic valves to use, it probably is important to make sure that we are all considering the same prostheses. They should be kept as clean and thromboresistant as when received from the manufacturer.

What we must know is the shelf life, the handling that the valve receives, the type of glove that one uses, and how many people touch the valve before it is implanted. All are essential parts of the subsequent history of the valve.

A spectrograph, which uses an x-ray beam of electrons, can identify the material on a starch-covered glove.

It tells us that there is zinc, magnesium, aluminum, silicone, sulfur, and calcium on the glove, as replicable and identifiable as a fingerprint.

If we wash the gloves very hard, we still have the same material on the gloves. Added to this is the foreign material which is used to sterilize the water. So now we have, in addition to the zinc, magnesium, aluminum, silicone, sulfur, and calcium, chloride potassium and some additional calcium.

If one looks at a strut on a prosthesis before one puts it in, one can see that the strut of the Starr-Edwards valve, as received from industry, is not particularly clean. It has a little bit of chlorine and calcium on the surface. Then it is autoclaved, and all the dirt, steam, iron oxide, rust, filth, and grease are added. Next, the scrub nurse takes it in her clean, sterile, dirty hand and gives it to the surgeon, who takes it in his clean, sterile, dirty hand, and then the valve is sewn in. What is very interesting to note is that if one has less than about two particles per 20 μ^2 of metallic surface the valve continues to remain relatively resistant to thrombosis. When one gets into the steam-sterilized valve, one is definitely in a rather thrombogenic area.

Dr. John W. Brown (Closing). In response to Dr. Beall, I would like to say that thromboemboli were not the only difference observed in these series of valves. The early mortality rate with the Kay-Shiley valve was significantly higher than for the other two groups. The incidences of low output syndrome and ventricular arrhythmias were also higher for the Kay-Shiley and Starr-Edwards valve patients.

I would like to thank Dr. Sawyer, for calling our attention to these important matters of valve handling and valve cleanliness. I think it would have been interesting to see what one of the Starr-Edwards valves would have looked like after it had been dipped in blood.

The deleterious effect of immediate postoperative prosthesis in below-knee amputation for ischemic disease

Steven I. Cohen, M.D., Leon D. Goldman, M.D., Edwin W. Salzman, M.D., *and* **Donald J. Glotzer, M.D.,** *Boston, Mass.*

The results of 97 consecutive amputations for lower extremity ischemia were analyzed, including 20 full metatarsal amputations, 39 below-knee (BK) amputations with conventional dressings and physiotherapy, 9 BK amputations with immediate postoperative prosthesis (IPOP) and 29 above-knee (AK) amputations. The ratio of successful BK to AK amputations was 2:1. Eighty-four percent of patients with transmetatarsal amputations (TMA) healed, and all were able to walk. The mortality rate for AK amputation was 22 percent, and all survivors healed; however, only 42 percent of these patients regained the ability to walk. In conventional BK amputation, there was a 97.3 percent healing rate and a rehabilitation rate of 80 percent. The one failure required a supracondylar amputation. In nine patients selected to have IPOP, only two amputations healed while still in plaster. Moreover, three of the seven failures of the plaster technique required supracondylar amputation (33 percent failure rate requiring higher amputation). In follow-up, five of six BK (IPOP) patients (83 percent) were able to walk. In our hands BK with IPOP had a complication rate requiring higher amputation 10 times that for conventional technique with no advantage in eventual rehabilitation rate.

From the Departments of Surgery, Harvard Medical School and Beth Israel Hospital, Boston, Mass.

THE LAST TWO DECADES have witnessed a remarkable transformation in the surgical approach to the treatment of ischemic disease of the lower extremity. Preservation of limbs by vascular reconstruction is now commonplace. A less dramatic, but nonetheless important advance in preservation of function has occurred in the last 10 years with the realization that the knee joint need not be sacrificed in the majority of patients with irreversible ischemia requiring amputation.[15, 16, 25, 28, 33] In some centers these efforts have resulted in a ratio of successful below-knee (BK) to above-knee (AK) amputations as high as 3:1,[24, 27] a reversal of the prior proportion.[29, 31]

During this same decade, the concept of immediate postoperative prosthesis (IPOP) was introduced by Berlemont[2] and by Weiss[41] and brought into this country by Burgess.[5] Improved primary healing and an increased rate and percentage of patient rehabilitation have been cited as advantages of this method.[5, 6, 10, 14, 19, 24, 25, 33, 36, 38] Moreover, this technique has the potential of mitigating the psychological trauma of amputation and of lessening the mortality and morbidity rates associated with prolonged bed rest in the elderly amputee, including venous throm-

Presented at the Twenty-eighth Annual Meeting of the Society for Vascular Surgery, Chicago, Ill., June 20 and 21, 1974.

Reprint requests: Donald J. Glotzer, M.D., Beth Israel Hospital, 330 Brookline Ave., Boston, Mass. 02215.

Table I. *Results of amputations for peripheral vascular disease*

Site*	No. of patients	No. of amputations	First-degree healing (%)	Eventual healing (%)	Failure (%)	Conversion to higher level (%)	Rehabilitation rate (%)	Mortality rate (%)	Mean age (yrs.)	Mean hospital stay (days)
TMA	20	20	73.6	84.2	15.8	15.8	100	5	70.4 ± 9.1‡	43.4 ± 25.2
BK (conventional)	38	39	89.5	97.3	2.7	2.7	79.8	2.7	73.7 ± 11.4	45.1 ± 21.6
BK (IPOP)	9	9	44.4	66.7	77.7†	33.3	83.3	0	68.8 ± 8.0	58.2 ± 7.6
AK	27	29	86.9	100	0	0	42.1	22	78.8 ± 9.1	39.3 ± 22.5

*TMA = transmetatarsal amputation; BK = below-knee amputation; IPOP = immediate postoperative prosthesis; AK = above-knee amputation.

†In IPOP failure defined as discontinuation of plaster.

‡± One standard deviation.

bosis, pulmonary embolism, decubitus ulceration, and pneumonia. Although most reports stress the benefits of IPOP, a few have expressed dissatisfaction with this method when applied to the treatment of peripheral vascular disease.[13, 22, 24, 34]

The purpose of this study is to review our recent experience with lower extremity amputation for peripheral vascular disease to assess the impact of these new concepts and methods on our results.

CASE MATERIAL

The records of all patients undergoing amputation for peripheral vascular disease during the period Jan. 1, 1968, to Sept. 31, 1973, were reviewed. Single-toe amputations and those for neoplasm and trauma were excluded from consideration. Full transmetatarsal amputations were included to gain a full perspective of lower extremity amputation for severe ischemia.

The influence of age, pulse status, diabetes mellitus, amputation level, and the use of IPOP on healing and rehabilitation were assessed. It was possible to determine the current status and the ability to walk of 100 percent of the patients from the charts, the patients, or their physicians.

During this period 97 amputations were performed in 94 patients, the sites of which are listed in Table I. The amputations were performed by attending surgeons and residents under their supervision, with various operative techniques. In general, however, drains were not used and myodesis was not employed. Simple (not mattress) sutures, usually of stainless steel or other monofilament material, were used to approximate skin edges. In BK amputations the fascia of the posterior muscles was approximated to that over the anterior compartment and tibia.

IPOP was used in nine of 47 patients undergoing BK amputation. Although patients having IPOP were not systematically selected, they were generally younger and were considered to be better operative risks and better candidates for primary healing on the basis of their circulatory status than those in whom conventional technique was used.

RESULTS

Transmetatarsal amputations. Twenty patients with a mean age of 70.4 years underwent full transmetatarsal amputation (TMA). The amputation was preceded by a vascular reconstruction in 14 patients as follows: aortoiliac seven, axillofemoral two, femoropopliteal four, and femorotibial one. Prior sympathectomy as an isolated procedure was used in one patient. Eventual healing occurred in 16 of 19 surviving patients, a healing rate of 84.2 percent, 14 by primary and two by secondary intention. One patient whose amputation was healing satisfactorily died of an acute myocardial infarction nine days following operation, giving an over-all mortality rate of 5 percent (Table I). Eighty percent of the patients had diabetes mellitus. The most distal palpable pulse in patients

Table II. *Comparative data on patients having amputations at various levels*

Site*	Age (yrs.)	Diabetes mellitus (%)	Most distal palpable pulse			
			Aortic	Femoral	Popliteal	Pedal
TMA	70.4	80	0	10	8	2
BK (conventional)	73.7	57.8	4	21	13	0
BK (IPOP)	68.8	77.7	0	5	4	0
AK	78.8	55.5	2	24	3	0

*TMA = transmetatarsal amputation; BK = below-knee amputation; IPOP = immediate postoperative prosthesis; AK = above-knee amputation.

with successful TMA's was pedal in two patients, popliteal in seven, and femoral in seven (Table II). Upon follow-up all patients in this group who survived and healed were ambulatory. None of the patients whose healing was by second intention had pulses distal to the femoral. In all three failures of TMA, the most distal palpable pulse was the femoral. Among three patients whose amputations failed, two underwent a successful BK amputation while the third refused a higher amputation and was discharged to a nursing home.

Below-knee amputations.

1. Conventional dressings and physiotherapy. Of the 38 patients who underwent 39 conventional BK amputations, 37 survived and one died—a mortality rate of 2.7 percent. In the 37 survivors, 37 of 38 amputations healed (97.3 percent), 34 (89.5 percent) by primary intent. In three patients developing wound complications (two infections and one hematoma), healing nevertheless occurred by secondary intention (Table I). Only one patient required reamputation at the AK level because of nonhealing, a failure which resulted from iliofemoral venous thrombosis and a wound infection. The one death occurred in a patient who developed a massive cerebrovascular accident in the postoperative period. The mean age of patients in this group was 73.7 years and diabetes mellitus was present in 57.8 percent. The most distal palpable pulse in successful amputations was popliteal in 13 limbs, femoral in 20, and aortic in four (Table II). In the one failure only the femoral pulse was palpable. In follow-up 79.8 percent of the conventional BK amputees have been fitted with a prosthesis and were able to walk.

2. Immediate postoperative prosthesis (IPOP). The surgical technique was essentially the same as that for conventional BK amputation, utilizing a long posterior flap. The plaster technique was identical to that of Burgess and Romano.[6] Patients were allowed to stand but not to bear significant weight for the first 7 postoperative days and, in those successfully completing the program, progressive weight bearing was allowed after this.

In this group, two of the nine patients healed primarily while still in plaster. Two additional patients had primary healing but were considered failures of the technique inasmuch as severe erythema of the wound led to discontinuance of the rigid cast after removal to investigate excessive pain. In four patients necrosis and/or inflammation at the suture line were noted upon removal of the cast. In two of these patients healing took place by second intention while the remaining two required reamputation at the AK level. In four of the seven patients in whom plaster was removed, blistering was noted upon removal of a primary or secondary plaster. In one instance this blistering led to full thickness skin loss proximal to an intact suture line, a complication which led to the third AK amputation in this group. Thus the failure rate leading to higher amputation was 33 percent and the over-all failure rate of the technique was 77.7 percent (Table I). The mean age of the nine patients in this group was 68.8 years, 5 years younger on the average than the group in whom conventional BK amputation was employed. Diabetes mellitus was present in 77.7 percent, a higher proportion than those treated by conventional technique (57.8 percent). Despite the higher incidence of diabetes, the most distal palpable pulse was popliteal in four patients and femoral in five, a distribution of palpable pulses presumably more favorable for healing than that in the conventional group (Table II). The most distal pulse in three patients requiring reamputation at the above-knee level was the femoral in two and popliteal in one. In follow-up five of six patients with eventually successful BK amputation in this group were able to walk, a rehabilitation rate of 83 percent in successful amputations. Two of the three patients in this group requiring conversion to an AK amputation were able to walk, giving an over-all rehabilitation rate in their group of 78 percent.

Above-knee amputations. Twenty-nine AK amputations were performed in 27 patients. The supracondylar level was primary in 25 instances but was required because of failure of a prior BK amputation in four limbs, three following IPOP and one following conventional BK amputation. Six of 27 patients died, a mortality rate of 22 percent. The high fatality rate can reasonably be attributed to the precarious status of some of these patients, since the policy during this period was to elect the BK level if the local skin nutrition appeared adequate for healing and if the general condition of the patient would permit this somewhat more time-consuming procedure. There were no deaths in the group of four patients having AK amputation following a failure of BK amputation. All amputations at this site in surviving patients healed, 20 by first intention and three secondarily (Table I). The most distal palpable pulse in the patients surviving amputation was popliteal in three of 29 limbs, femoral in 18 of 29, and aortic in two of 29. The average age of the patients in this group was 78.8 years. Fifty-five percent had diabetes mellitus (Table II). Of 19 patients surviving with a unilateral amputation, eight (42.1 percent) were able to walk on a prosthesis at the time of follow-up. Neither patient with bilateral amputation at the AK level was able to walk.

DISCUSSION

It has become evident not only that major amputation is followed by substantial mortality and morbidity rates but also that even after BK amputation surprisingly few patients are able to walk. Warren and Kihn[37] found an in-hospital mortality rate of 10 percent for BK amputation and 28 percent for AK amputation. Moreover, only 46 percent of patients with unilateral AK amputations and 76 percent of unilateral BK amputees were able to walk again. Warren and Record,[39] in a review of the literature, found that between 50 and 92 percent of healed BK amputees were able to walk with a prosthesis. Clearly there is much room for improvement.

Immediate postoperative application of a prosthesis was introduced into this country by Burgess, and its use has been reported in over 1,000 cases. This method appears generally to be regarded as a step forward in the rehabilitation of patients. It was in this context that the use of immediate postoperative prosthesis was cautiously introduced into our institution. Because of some adverse experience with IPOP, this review of our recent experience with all types of lower extremity amputation was undertaken.

Our high rate of success with the TMA popularized by McKittrick, McKittrick, and Risley[23] bears out the applicability of this procedure to patients with peripheral vascular disease and its obvious superiority in preserving function. Moreover, our roughly 2:1 successful BK-to-AK ratio confirms the opinion that BK can be done in the majority of patients requiring major amputation for peripheral vascular disease who can thus gain the benefits of the greater potential of BK amputation for ambulation. Our 97 percent success rate of healing of conventional BK amputation compares favorably with published reports,[37, 39] as does the rehabilitation rate of almost 80 percent.

Table III. *Results of below-knee amputation treated with immediate postoperative prosthesis*

Reference	*No. of below-knee amputations*	*Average age*	*Peripheral vascular disease (%)*	*Primary first degree healing (%)*	*Eventual healing (%)*	*Below knee to above knee (%)*	*Rehabilitation rate (%)*	*Mortality rate (%)*	*Hospital stay*
Moore[25]	20	57	100	90	90	10	90	0	Not given
Warren and Moseley[38]	10	62.2	90	80	90*	0	70	20	28§
Sarmiento et al.[33]	134	—	86†	—	90	7.4	73.2	5.2†	35
Condon and Jordan[10]	38	64	100	82	89	11	65	5	Not given
Kihn et al.[19]	116	—	100	—	83	13	78	1	Not given
Burgess, Traub, and Wilson[7]	103	—	47	87	93	6.8	—	0	Not given
Mooney et al.[24]	106	66.4	100	—	65/74‡	10/6‡	52/59‡	9/6‡	Not given
Burgess et al.[8]	157	—	100	80.3	93	7.6	93	3.8	Not given
Silverstein and Kadish[34]	62	—	—	—	74	—	—	10	Not given
Jones and Burniston[17]	21	—	100	66.7	71	29	63	0	Not given

*Forty percent of patients did not complete the program.
†Includes Syme amputations.
‡Plaster dressing/plaster and pylon.
§Figure given only for successfully rehabilitated patients.

Our hopes that IPOP would aid healing and improve rehabilitation have not been realized. Fully one third of a somewhat more favorable group of patients required a higher level of amputation and only two of nine patients successfully completed the program. In net terms neither the rehabilitation rate nor the length of hospitalization were improved.

It does not appear that surgical technique *per se* can be indicted as the cause of the failures in view of our success rate for conventional technique. Patient selection also does not seem to be responsible, since, on the average, patients chosen for IPOP were 5 years younger than the group treated conventionally and had comparable or superior peripheral circulation. It seems very likely that either the plaster technique itself or its application must be faulted. In the four patients in whom blisters developed, the lesion resembled second-degree burns. Measurement of temperatures at the inner surface of the stretchable plaster during setting revealed values up to 137° F. Thermal injury thus may have contributed to failures in some instances, although we have not seen previous reference to this possibility. Clearly our own relative inexperience with the plaster technique must also have played a significant role.

Regardless of the cause, the high failure rate for IPOP in our institution has caused us to question the wisdom of this technique. We have not found that the plaster favors healing as has been claimed,[24, 25] but, as observed in the setting of a 400 bed general hospital, it proved detrimental. In special centers with a larger volume of amputee patients, where a high degree of expertise with the plaster technique can be developed, one might argue that IPOP would be superior to conventional methods. Yet the recently completed Boston Interhospital Amputation Study[40] did not support the contention that the superimposition of a team of experts in IPOP in various hospitals would be beneficial in the rehabilitation of amputee patients. As a practical matter, our healing rate of 97 percent with conventional technique of BK amputation is higher than the best success rate reported in any experience with IPOP, which does not exceed 93 percent, even in series including patients without ischemic disease (Table III). In addition it can be seen from Table III that the reported rate of conversion of BK to AK in amputation with IPOP

Table IV. *Results of below-knee amputation treated with conventional technique**

Reference	*No. of below-knee amputations*	*Average age (yrs.)*	*Primary first degree healing (%)*	*Eventual healing (%)*	*Below knee to above knee (%)*	*Rehabilitation rate (%)*	*Mortality rate (%)*	*Hospital stay*
Warren and Kihn[39]	121	—	48.8	66.9	18.2	70.9	4.1	Not given
Bradham and Smoak[4]	84	—	—	85	15	—	—	Not given
Block and Whitehouse[3]	43	—	88	95	2.5	57.5	0	Not given
Baddeley and Fulford[1]	42	—	—	81	19	59.4	—	Not given
Lempke et al.[20]	81	—	—	72	—	—	—	Not given
Perry[29]	15	—	40	93	7	30	0	Not given
Robb, Jacobson, and Jordon[30]	15	—	80	100	0	73	0	Not given
Smith and Casingal[35]	41	—	—	100	0	94	0	Not given
Cranley et al.[11]	101	—	76	86	10	75	7	Not given
Lim et al.[21]	55	64	—	83	17	78	16	Not given
Ecker and Jacobs[12]	69	62.5	77	—	—	—	8.7	Not given
Chilvers et al.[9]	53	60	50.9	67.9	32.1	89	7	Not given

*All for peripheral vascular disease.

Table V. *Comparison of hospital days in below knee (conventional) and below knee (immediate postoperative prosthesis)*

	Patients with primary healing and/or completion of plaster technique if used	*Patients with failure of primary healing and/or plaster technique*	*All patients*
Below knee (conventional)	43.1 ± 17.8*	71.0 ± 25.1	45.1 ± 21.6
Below knee (immediate postoperative prosthesis)	28.5 ± 2.1	66.4 ± 31.8	58.2 ± 7.6

*± One standard deviation.

ranges from zero to 29 percent (average 10 percent), rehabilitation rates from 63 to 93 percent (average 80 percent), and mortality rates from zero to 20 percent (average 4 percent). These results, which are the figures cited to stress the advantages of IPOP, do not appear in fact to differ appreciably from those culled from a review of reports of conventional amputations, all for peripheral vascular disease (Table IV). In these studies failures ranged from zero to 32 percent (average 11 percent), rehabilitation rates from 30 to 94 percent (average 73 percent), and mortality rates from zero to 16 percent (average 6 percent). These figures support the conclusion from comparative studies that IPOP does not increase the ultimate percentage of patients rehabilitated[10, 24] and does not decrease the failure rate of BK amputations.[33] Our successful cases do confirm the claim that successful IPOP reduces rehabilitation time, but this was not true for the group as a whole (Table V).

It seems appropriate to question whether IPOP is superior to conventional technique in the treatment of ischemic disease even in specialized centers, since the potential benefits of IPOP seem to be achievable by traditional methods with fewer opportunities for complications.

REFERENCES

1. Baddeley, R. M., and Fulford, J. C.: A trial of conservative amputations for lesions of the

feet in diabetes mellitus, Br. J. Surg. **25:** 38, 1965.
2. Berlemont, M.: Notre expérience de l'appareillage précoce des amputés des membres inférieurs aux établissements Heliomarins de Berck, Ann. Med. Physique **4:** 213, 1961.
3. Block, M. A., and Whitehouse, F. W.: Below-knee amputations in patients with diabetes mellitus, Arch. Surg. **87:** 682, 1963.
4. Bradham, R. R., and Smoak, R. D.: Amputations of the lower extremity, Arch. Surg. **90:** 60, 1965.
5. Burgess, E. M.: Immediate post surgical prosthetic fitting, J. Bone Joint Surg. **48A:** 1022, 1966.
6. Burgess, E. M., and Romano, R. L.: The management of lower extremity amputees using immediate postsurgical prosthesis, Clin. Orthop. **57:** 137, 1968.
7. Burgess, E. M., Traub, J. E., and Wilson, A.B., Jr.: Immediate postsurgical prosthetics in the management of lower extremity amputees, Technical Report TR 10-5, Washington, D. C., 1967, Veterans Administration.
8. Burgess, E. M., Romano, R. L., Zettl, J. H., et al.: Amputations of the leg for peripheral vascular insufficiency, J. Bone Joint Surg. **53A:** 874, 1971.
9. Chilvers, A. S., Briggs, J., Brouse, N. L., et al.: Below- and through-knee amputations in ischemic disease, Br. J. Surg. **58:** 824, 1971.
10. Condon, R. E., and Jordan, P. H.: Immediate postoperative prosthesis in vascular amputations, Ann. Surg. **170:** 435, 1969.
11. Cranley, J. J., Krause, R. J., Strasser, E. S., et al.: Below-the-knee amputations for arteriosclerosis obliterans, Arch. Surg. **98:** 77, 1969.
12. Ecker, M. L., and Jacobs, B. S.: Lower extremity amputation in diabetic patients, Diabetes **19:** 189, 1970.
13. Friedman, L. W.: The prosthesis—immediate or delayed fitting, Angiology **23:** 518, 1972.
14. Golbranson, F. L., Asbelle, C., and Strand, D.: Immediate postsurgical fitting and early ambulation: A new concept in amputee rehabilitation, Clin. Orthop. **56:** 119, 1968.
15. Haimovici, H.: Criteria for and results of transmetatarsal amputation for ischemic gangrene, Arch. Surg. **70:** 45, 1955.
16. Hoar, C. S., and Torres, J.: Evaluation of below knee amputation in the treatment of diabetic gangrene, N. Engl. J. Med. **266:** 440, 1962.
17. Jones, R. F., and Burniston, G. G.: A conservative approach to lower limb amputations, Med. J. Aust. **2:** 711, 1970.
18. Kraeger, R. R.: Amputation with immediate fitting prostheses, Am. J. Surg. **120:** 634, 1970.
19. Kihn, R. B., Golbranson, F. L., Hutchinson, R. H., et al.: The immediate postoperative prosthesis in lower extremity amputations, Arch. Surg. **101:** 40, 1970.
20. Lempe, R. E., King, R. D., Kaiser, G. D., et al.: Amputation in arteriosclerosis, Arch. Surg. **86:** 406, 1963.
21. Lim, R. C., Jr., Blaisdell, F. W., Hall, A. D., et al.: Below knee amputations for ischemic gangrene, Surg. Gynecol. Obstet. **125:** 493, 1967.
22. Little, J. M.: Amputation of the leg—a dull topic revisited, Med. J. Aust. **2:** 442, 1973.
23. McKittrick, L. S., McKittrick, J. B., and Risley, T. S.: Transmetatarsal amputation for infection or gangrene in patients with diabetes mellitus, Ann. Surg. **130:** 826, 1949.
24. Mooney, V., Harvey, J. P., Jr., McBride, E., et al.: Comparison of postoperative stump management: Plaster vs. soft dressings, J. Bone Joint Surg. **53A:** 241, 1971.
25. Moore, W. S., Hall, A. D., and Wylie, E. J.: Below knee amputation for vascular insufficiency, Arch. Surg. **97:** 886, 1968.
26. Moore, W. S., Hall A. D., and Lim, R. C., Jr.: Below the knee amputation for ischemic gangrene, Am. J. Surg. **124:** 127, 1972.
27. Olejniczak, S.: Summary of leg amputations and prosthetic replacement at Wayne County General Hospital during the five year period 1961 through 1965, Mich. Med. **66:** 723, 1967.
28. Pederson, H. E., Lamont, R. L., and Ramsey, R. H.: Below knee amputation for gangrene, South. Med. J., **57:** 820, 1964.
29. Perry, T.: Below-knee amputation, Arch. Surg. **86:** 199, 1963.
30. Robb, H. J., Jacobson, L. F., and Jordan, P.: Midcalf amputation in the ischemic extremity, Arch. Surg. **91:** 506, 1965.
31. Romano, R. L., and Burgess, E. M.: Level selection in lower extremity amputations. Clin. Orthop. **74:** 174, 1971.
32. Sarmiento, A., and Warren, W. D.: A re-evaluation of lower extremity amputations. Surg. Gynecol. Obstet. **129:** 799, 1969.
33. Sarmiento, A., May, B. J., Sinclair, W. F., et al.: Lower extremity amputation—the impact of immediate postsurgical prosthetic fitting, Clin. Orthop. **68:** 22, 1970.
34. Silverstein, M. J., and Kadish, L.: A study of amputation of the lower extremity, Surg. Gynecol. Obstet. **137:** 579, 1973.
35. Smith, A. G., and Casingal, E. L.: Management of diabetic patients with foot lesions, Surg. Gynecol. Obstet. **128:** 85, 1969.
36. Warren, R.: Early rehabilitation of the elderly lower extremity amputee, Surg. Clin. North Am. **48:** 807, 1968.
37. Warren, R., and Kihn, R. B.: A survey of

lower extremity amputations for ischemia, SURGERY **63:** 107, 1968.
38. Warren, R., and Moseley, R. V.: Immediate postoperative prosthesis for below the knee amputations: A preliminary report, Am. J. Surg. **116:** 429, 1968.
39. Warren, R., and Record, E.: Lower extremity amputations for arterial insufficiency, ed. 1, Boston, 1969, Little, Brown & Company.
40. Warren, R., James, R. C., Banks, H. H., et al.: The Boston Interhospital amputation study, Arch. Surg. **107:** 861, 1973.
41. Weiss, M.: The prosthesis on the operating table from the neurophysiological point of view, Report of the Workshop Panel in Lower Extremity Prosthetics Fitting, Committee on Prosthetics Research and Development, National Academy of Science Meeting, February 6 to 9, 1966.

DISCUSSION

Dr. Wesley S. Moore (San Francisco, Calif.). Few topics in surgery have as many emotional overtones or carry such serious medical, social, and economic implications as does lower extremity amputation. In the past 15 years, there have been significant advances in amputation management, the most important of which has been recognition that the knee joint can be preserved in most patients. This assures the maximum opportunity for successful prosthetic rehabilitation of the geriatric dysvascular amputee. The technique of immediate postoperative application of a prosthesis with ambulation, as introduced by Weiss of Poland, later to be modified and popularized by Burgess in the United States, was an attempt to shorten the period of rehabilitation by utilizing the postoperative healing phase for prosthetic training. Improved healing has been a secondary benefit observed by many investigators, presumably due to edema prevention. There has also been a corresponding reduction in morbidity and mortality rates that has come about by avoiding the complications related to immobility in an elderly patient following amputation operation.

At issue here today is a report describing nine attempts at below-knee amputation with immediate postoperative prosthesis that resulted in poor healing. The authors complemented their presentation with a splendid series of transmetatarsal and conventional below-knee amputations, indicating that the failures with immediate postoperative prosthesis were not due to lack of surgical expertise. Their unhappy experience with immediate postoperative prosthesis, while not unique, does represent a minority experience when one reviews the experience of many amputation centers.

Our experience with below-knee amputation at the Veterans Administration Hospital, San Francisco, dates back to 1961, when, under the leadership of Bill Blaisdell, an aggressive program was begun to perform below-knee amputation in patients with advanced occlusive disease who would have previously been considered candidates for above-knee amputation. In this protocol, no patient underwent a primary above-knee amputation regardless of level of distal palpable pulse or angiographic findings. The only contraindication to below-knee amputation was extension of the gangrenous process to involve the skin at the level of below-knee incision. In 1966 it was my privilege to assume the responsibility for the amputation program and, following a visit with Ernie Burgess in Seattle, I started a trial of immediate postoperative prosthesis. Our indications for below-knee amputation remained the same, so that no primary above-knee amputations were performed. The time intervals between 1961 and 1966 and between 1967 and 1971 provided two distinct series with similar indications and operative technique but differing only in the postoperative management in regard to the use of immediate postoperative prosthesis. A retrospective comparative analysis provided information as to the effect of immediate fitting with ambulation on the results of amputation. Fifty-five amputations in the first series were compared with 53 amputations in the second series. The two groups of patients were carefully analyzed for age distribution, incidence of diabetes, level of distal palpable pulse, and angiographic patterns of disease. The two series were found to be suitably comparable with regard to these parameters.

The healing failure rate with the immediate fitting was only 11 percent as compared to 24 percent with conventional technique. There were no deaths in the immediate postoperative prosthesis (IPOP) group as compared to a 15 percent mortality rate with conventional amputation. These deaths were due to pulmonary and cardiac complications. All patients with immediate fitting became ambulatory on a prosthesis in an average of 32 days, as compared to an 81 percent rehabilitation rate requiring an average of 125 days with conventional amputation.

These data are not unique since several other groups have reported comparable results with appropriate use of IPOP. Why, then, did Dr. Cohen and his colleagues experience poor results with their trial of this technique? In order to gain some insight into the problem, it is important to emphasize that amputation with IPOP is a team effort which requires close cooperation and interaction between the surgeon, prosthetist, and the physical therapist. Any weakness among members of this team can lead to poor results. No amount of expertise on the part of the surgeon can make up for a poorly applied prosthesis and vice versa. The authors have demonstrated outstanding surgical competence in their conventional amputation series. Therefore, one has to question either the ability of the individuals applying the prosthesis or the supervision of the efforts of the physiatrist in order to explain these untoward results. Dr. Cohen also makes the point that conventional below-knee amputation in their series resulted in primary healing in 97.3 percent of the cases as an argument against using any additional modality, such as IPOP, to achieve successful results. However, his ratio of 47 below-knee amputations to 29 above-knee amputations is only 1.6/1. While this is certainly a step in the right direction, considering the days when the below-knee/above-knee (BK/AK) ratio used to be the reverse, it still indicates considerable clinical selection, which resulted in performance of 29 primary above-knee amputations. In neither of our own series was a primary above-knee amputation performed. The only above-knee amputations done were failures following attempted below-knee amputation. If you use these failed cases to calculate the BK/AK ratio, we find that in our first series the BK/AK ratio was 4/1 and this has been further improved with immediate postoperative prosthesis to a BK/AK ratio of 9/1.

Human nature among investigators usually dictates the reporting of only good results; for this reason I am grateful to the authors for their courage in bringing to our attention their problems with a new technique, for only in this manner can we suitably analyze the factors leading to failure so that other surgeons, about to embark on an immediate fitting program, can profit from this experience. The data presented here today should drive home the point that success with the technique cannot be obtained by the unilateral efforts of the surgeon, for each member of the team must have a corresponding level of competence in managing his or her respective contribution to this valuable technique.

Dr. Richard Warren (Boston, Mass.). In the first place, a 97 percent over-all healing rate for below-knee (BK) amputations for ischemia is, to me, unique. I do not know of any other group that reported higher than 85 percent.

We used to say that if one is getting that many successes, one is selecting one's patients too well, but certainly this is not true in the authors' presentation because they got a 2/1 below-knee/above-knee (BK/AK) ratio, which is very respectable.

I have watched the Beth Israel group over the years because, when I did a survey of the BK/AK ratios in the Boston area, of all the hospitals doing amputations there, Beth Israel had the best record, and I think at that time it was 4/1.

Similarly, their transmetatarsal record is better than any I know, 84 percent success. Very few people have gotten better than 75 percent in transmetatarsal amputation.

These records fall into the good and bad news categories. They have really broken the record in bad news as far as these nine patients with immediate postoperative prosthesis (IPOP) go—three of nine failures. I really do not know the reason for this.

I would like to ask them to make an objective comment on why they feel these results have been so much worse than those of other people. Because if they cannot do this, I do not think that we ought to use their record as a condemnation of the technique. Most people feel that the main contribution of the IPOP technique has been its spinoff. It has oriented people toward early walking after amputation. And, since this technique was introduced, people have used other techniques to get the patients out of the hospital within 3 to 4 weeks.

Another spinoff is that it can give you a method to test walking in a debilitated patient without buying an expensive prosthesis.

There are various methods of inducing early walking. If one is going to pick the plaster technique, one must put it on carefully. And I cannot close without making a plug for the courses that teach you how to do this. The New York University course is a 2 day course for general surgeons. It is very popular with those who have taken it and all have felt that they profited from it. This same course is also given at Northwestern University and UCLA.

Dr. Anthony M. Imparato (New York, N. Y.). I am almost in total agreement with the conclusions of the authors.

At New York University, I became disenchanted with immediate postoperative prosthesis (IPOP) for end-stage arterial disease amputees, either above-knee (AK) or below-knee (BK), following an approximately 3 year trial.

Disenchantment was due to the high incidence of local wound complications, even though the fittings were performed by a highly sophisticated group. I think there is very little question that, in those individuals in whom the immediate fitting was successful, the period between amputation and total rehabilitation was considerably shortened.

So I think I would agree with Dr. Warren and, perhaps, with Dr. Moore that the key to the whole business is how the immediate fitting is done.

Our present technique is a rather simple one and employs application of a stockinette to the limb as the first surgical dressing, with one pound of traction without compression dressing. This controls pain and prevents contractures.

Our results are similar to the authors'. The ratio of BK to AK is 2.2/1. The decision to do a BK amputation is made at the operating table when incising the pretibial skin. If arterial bleeding is recognized, the operation is continued, and if it is not, we simply go to the AK site. No anterior flap is made.

Immediate healing in our hands is lower than

in the authors'—it is in about the 85 percent range, but eventually about 90 to 93 percent of the patients heal.

Delayed healing has almost invariably been due to the breakdown of the skin anteriorly over the tibia where no skin flap is made.

Rehabilitation is quite a variable thing and is not entirely related to the surgical procedure. Interestingly enough, approximately two thirds of the BK and AK amputees manage to find their way to Rusk Institute, and whether they have a BK or an AK operation, 87 to 90 percent, respectively, of these patients are rehabilitated, a tribute to both the patients and the rehabilitation group.

The key questions I would ask the authors are how do they select their patients for transmetatarsal amputation? What guidelines would they offer for making a final decision to perform a BK amputation?

Dr. Steven I. Cohen (Closing). Dr. Moore has reported an important series, and there is no doubt that his reduction of healing failures from 24 to 11 percent is admirable. We believe that an 11 percent failure rate is still too high when one can do as well or even better with conventional techniques. Even the reduction from 24 percent failures may be due to other factors, since the comparison group was not concurrent.

As to the accusation of poorly fitting prostheses, we agree that, if the prosthesis does not fit, no amount of technical expertise in performing the operation will suffice. However, our prostheses were fitted by experienced orthopedic surgeons who had been trained under Burgess or his students, and we believe they were highly competent. Also, we believe that if the immediate plaster technique is that exacting, its general adoption in cases with marginal circulation is hazardous.

Dr. Warren, thank you for your comments, but you give us too much credit. Our failure rate with immediate postoperative prosthesis (IPOP) does not really appear to be a new record. If one reads the discussion after previous presentations of IPOP patients, it is clear that there have been many unsatisfactory experiences in patients with ischemia. It is not easy to report a series of failures, and we do not stand here today without some soul searching, but we hope that by calling attention to the problems with this procedure in patients with ischemia, we may have performed a service.

The reasons for the failures are probably several and include the very advanced age of our patients and our practice of electing the lowest possible level of amputation as a matter of policy. We have also been struck by one aspect of the use of IPOP not previously mentioned. In four of the patients we noted blistering when their casts were removed to investigate excessive pain. The blisters resembled second-degree burns. We subsequently measured the temperature at the inner surface of the setting, stretchable plaster and found temperatures as high as 137° F. We postulate that thermal injury in association with severe ischemia may have contributed to the failures in some cases.

Dr. Imparato, we have no absolute rules for selection of the level of amputation but tend to go as distal as possible. We are influenced primarily by skin nutrition at the site of incision, and we are influenced not at all by the most distal palpable pulse. If we have decided preoperatively that a patient will heal a below-knee amputation, and this prediction is based chiefly on the appearance and temperature of the skin, we generally proceed with the below-knee amputation regardless of any lack of skin or muscle bleeding at the time of incision, and I think our results support this rather optimistic position.

The acutely ischemic upper extremity: Selective management

Charles R. Sachatello, M.D., Calvin B. Ernst, M.D., *and* Ward O. Griffen, Jr., M.D., *Lexington, Ky.*

Etiology of the acutely ischemic upper extremity is variable and demands a specific diagnosis for optimum management. From a retrospective review of 12 years' experience encompassing 62 patients, treatment methods were standardized. Cardiac emboli are best treated by brachial embolectomy; emboli of arterial origin demand exclusion of the arterial focus and bypass grafting. Complications of invasive arterial studies require individualized management. Pre- and postcatheterization assessment of radial, ulnar, and interdigital pressure patterns employing the Doppler apparatus may permit more standardized treatment.

From the Department of Surgery, University of Kentucky Medical Center, Lexington, Ky.

THE PRESENTATION and natural history of vascular disease of the upper extremity differ from those of vascular disease in the lower extremity in that embolic incidents and arterial complications of invasive diagnostic techniques far exceed symptomatic arteriosclerotic occlusive disease.

This present study of upper extremity arterial ischemia was initiated to define more clearly its natural history and treatment results. The clinical, operative, and arteriographic data of 62 patients seen at the University of Kentucky Medical Center from 1962 to 1974 form the basis of this report.

CLINICAL MATERIAL

Thirty-eight patients had arterial emboli to the upper extremity. In 26 of these, the embolus originated in the heart, whereas in the other 12 there was a demonstrable arterial source for the embolus (Tables I and II). An additional 24 patients were operated on for complications of invasive arterial diagnostic studies (Table III).

Emboli of cardiac origin (Table I). Among the 26 patients whose emboli were of cardiac origin were 16 patients with atrial fibrillation, three with recent myocardial infarction, and one with ventricular aneurysm. Two other patients had decompensated heart disease with intractable heart failure. Four patients had no recognizable heart disease. In these four, emboli were presumed of cardiac origin either because of the anatomic distribution of other emboli or failure to document an arterial source by arteriographic study.

The majority were over 65 years of age and six were more than 80 years old. Males and females were affected with approximately equal frequency. There was no significant lateralization of the emboli to either arm.

Pain and numbness prompted admission

Presented at the Twenty-eighth Annual Meeting of the Society for Vascular Surgery, Chicago, Ill., June 20 and 21, 1974.

Reprint requests: Charles R. Sachatello, M.D., Department of Surgery, University of Kentucky Medical Center, Lexington, Ky. 40506.

Table I. *Upper extremity emboli of cardiac origin*

	No.	Operative Rx	Radial ulnar pulse restored	Comments
Atrial fibrillation	16	13	10	One patient died from superior mesenteric embolus 2 days following brachial embolectomy One patient developed embolus following cardioversion—unsuccessful embolectomy One patient, age 16, developed embolus following closed mitral commissurotomy One patient underwent amputation of 3 fingertips —good radial pulse
Myocardial infarction	3	2	1	Only brachial pulse restored in one patient; 3 months later only subclavian pulse detected; patient had an ischemic painful hand
Ventricular aneurysm	1	—	—	Patient treated with heparin with return of normal radial and ulnar pulse; serum lipids 2,000 mg. per 100 ml.
Undetermined	4	4	3	One patient with successful delayed embolectomy developed painless wasting of muscles of hand and forearm One patient with unsuccessful embolectomy had ischemic disabling hand 2 of 4 patients have history of other arterial emboli; 1 had prior pulmonary embolus
Severe heart failure	2	1	0	Both patients underwent amputation; both died 3 weeks later of intractable heart failure
Total	26	20	14	Postoperative deaths—3 patients Major amputations—2 patients Digit amputations—1 patient Symptomic ischemia—3 patients

for most patients. Duration of symptoms varied from a few hours to 6 weeks, with the majority presenting between 8 and 16 hours after onset of symptoms. Patients with prior strokes or cerebrovascular disease had especially late recognition of symptoms. Midbrachial or axillary artery pulses were palpable in the majority on admission. In two patients, the most distal palpable pulse was at the supraclavicular-subclavian artery. The only laboratory finding of significance was an elevated hematocrit; 10 patients had an initial hematocrit of 45 or greater.

Two patients noted transient blindness associated with their upper extremity emboli. Two others developed severe abdominal pain. Both individuals underwent exploratory celiotomy. Gangrenous small and large bowel resulted in death in one. In the other, abdominal exploration was normal.

Embolectomy was performed in 20 of 26 patients and primary amputation in one patient (Table I). The remaining five had either no treatment, stellate ganglion block, or heparin. Embolectomy initially restored wrist pulses in 17 of 20 patients, but three of these patients lost wrist pulses after operation and one required an amputation. One patient who had restoration of normal wrist pulses developed painless muscle wasting of his hand.

The two patients with intractable heart failure had a similar clinical course. Both required amputation and both died 3 weeks after operation. One patient was autopsied but no intracardiac thrombus was found.

Three patients who underwent embolectomy had persistent disabling ischemia. One had a palpable brachial pulse in the antecubital fossa while the other two had palpable supraclavicular-subclavian pulses only. Of the five patients treated nonoperatively, one had return of wrist pulses on heparin

Table II. *Upper extremity emboli of arterial origin*

Diagnosis	*No. of patients*	*Operative procedures*	*Pulses restored*
Poststenotic aneurysm (cervical rib)	1	Resection of cervical and first rib, clavicle, and aneurysm; embolectomy of axillary, brachial, radial	Yes—8 weeks only. Thrombosis of brachial artery
False subclavian aneurysm	1	Resection of clavicle and aneurysm with vein graft. Brachial embolectomy	Yes
Dissecting aortic aneurysm	1	Amputation	No
Thoracic outlet syndrome; no cervical rib or aneurysm	1	Dacron bypass or subclavian; occlusion 3 months	
		Carotid subclavian vein bypass	Yes
Arteriosclerotic plaque 1 cm. proximal to left subclavian	1	Brachial embolectomy × 3; amputation; succumbed to superior mesenteric embolus 4 months later	No
Clavicular fracture nonunion; callus	2	Claviculectomy	No
		Vein graft subclavian—brachial	No
Crutch thrombosis, axillary artery	2	Vein graft	No
Proximal arterial operation	3	Embolectomy (1); 2 patients had spontaneous return of pulses	No

Table III. *Upper extremity thromboemboli after catheterization*

	No.
Patients	24
Operative procedures	26
Pulses restored	23
Procedures:	
Embolectomy alone	14
Revision of arteriotomy	3
Vein patch graft	3
Resection and end-to-end anastomosis	4
Vein graft interposition	2
Procedures within 24 hours	24
Delayed procedures (vein grafts 12 cm.)	2
Major complications:	
Median nerve injury	2

therapy alone. The other four had detectable pallor but were asymptomatic.

Emboli of arterial origin (Table II). Among the 12 patients with emboli of arterial origin, two were considered to have complications of the thoracic outlet syndrome (Fig. 1). A third had a post-traumatic subclavian pseudoaneurysm (Figs. 2 and 3). A fourth patient presented with a pregangrenous hand and required amputation despite having embolectomy and vein graft. He died 4 months later of a superior mesenteric embolus. At autopsy examination he had a 2 cm. raised, ulcerated arteriosclerotic plaque just proximal to the origin of the left subclavian artery. The remaining aorta had minimal arteriosclerotic streaking but no other plaques.

Two patients with nonunited clavicular fractures associated with extensive callus presented with ischemic hands. In each, arteriograms documented intimal irregularity of the subclavian artery and evidence of extensive distal embolization. Two patients who had used crutches for more than 50 years presented with ischemic hands and absent wrist pulses. In three individuals, arm emboli followed proximal reconstructive arterial procedures. Although ten of twelve were operated on, only two had return of pulses after operation.

Postcatheterization brachial artery obstruction (Table III). Twenty-four patients underwent 26 operative procedures for arterial complications following invasive diagnostic studies. Indications for operation varied from asymptomatic loss of distal pulses to severe ischemia. Operation was performed within 12 hours of brachial catheterization in the majority of patients. Chronic ischemia prompted operative treatment 2

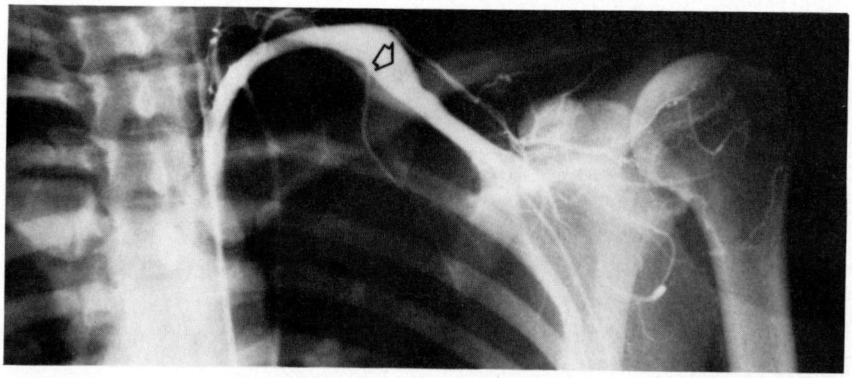

Fig. 1. A 27-year-old female patient with a severely ischemic left hand and arm secondary to a cervical rib. The arrow points to an intraluminal filling defect in the poststenotic subclavian aneurysm. Repetitive embolization led to complete brachial and axillary artery occusion.

months after catheterization in two individuals. Wrist pulses were restored in 23 of 24.

DISCUSSION

Baird and Lajos'[3] report details the natural history of emboli to the arm in 95 patients seen from 1932 to 1962. Their patients were elderly and had heart disease. Only 19 percent survived 5 years. Eighteen percent underwent embolectomy. Twenty-six patients had disabled or useless arms and seven required amputation. These authors did not recognize arterial emboli of arterial origin. Patients in the present study were equally elderly; and, similarly, atrial fibrillation was the most common heart abnormality. Twelve of 38 patients, 32 percent, had emboli of arterial origin. Seventy-four percent of the patients reported herein underwent operations. Three required amputation and three others had symptomatic ischemia.

Upper extremity embolectomy can be performed through a medial bicipital or antecubital approach.[11] Inconstant bifurcation of the brachial artery at the antecubital fossa precludes exclusive use of either approach. Failure to restore wrist pulses warrants catheterization or both radial and ulnar arteries using Nos. 2F and 3F Fogarty catheters. As catheters are passed distally and withdrawn, movement of the overlying skin

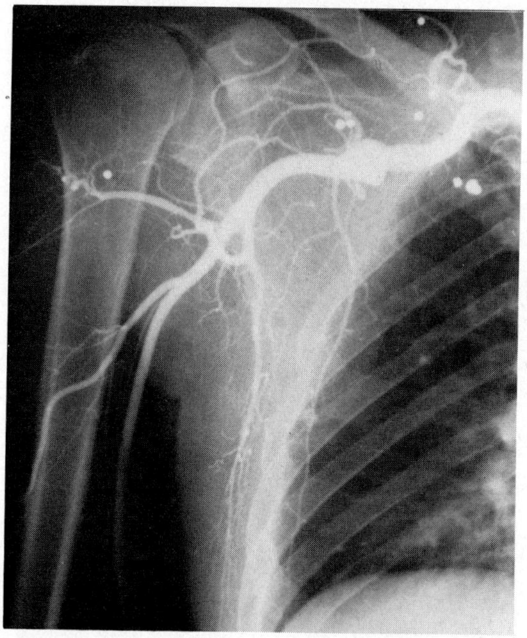

Fig. 2. The asymptomatic pseudoaneurysm resulted from a shotgun injury 15 years previously.

indicates either a radial or ulnar placement. Manipulation of the arm may permit alternate placement of the catheter into either the radial or ulnar arteries without exposing the bifurcation. In some patients the catheter will consistently pass down one or the other artery in spite of persistent attempts at selective passage. In such instances the brachial bifurcation must be exposed, but a second arteriotomy is unnecessary.[11]

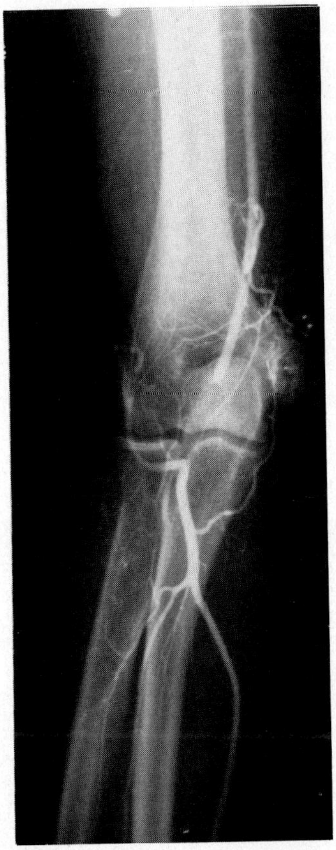

Fig. 3. Brachial embolus from pseudoaneurysm seen in Fig. 2. The origin of the radial was occluded from prior silent embolization.

The recent introduction of the No. 2F size Fogarty balloon catheter facilitates radial or ulnar embolectomy at the wrist. This catheter may be introduced 3 to 4 cm. into the hand from a transverse arteriotomy at the wrist. Embolectomy of the proximal palmar arch should be attempted when wrist pulses are present but the hand appears nonviable. The use of magnification aids in precise closure of the arteriotomy.

Forearm fasciotomy has a definite role following embolectomy. When fasciotomy is indicated, it should extend beyond the transverse carpal ligaments.

Postoperative administration of intravenous heparin (500 to 1,500 U. per hour) is advisable and may prevent distal thrombosis from residual thrombi or catheter-related intimal damage.[6]

Experience suggests that an aggressive operative approach to brachial emboli, use of intraoperative arteriograms, selective catheterization of both radial and ulnar arteries, palmar arch embolectomy, fasciotomy, and postoperative heparin therapy are important in treating the acutely ischemic hand.[13]

Arterial emboli of arterial origin presented difficult management problems. Repetitive silent embolization from a proximal arterial focus may occur for years. The progressive obliteration of distal vessels, not the arterial focus *per se,* produces ischemic symptoms. Extensive obliteration of the distal arterial tree all but precludes successful revascularization.

Abbott and Darling[1] recently reported seven patients with crutch trauma and axillary aneurysms, noting that the literature contained case reports of only 11 other such patients, two of whom had aneurysms. They advocated saphenous vein bypass of axillary aneurysms because of the high incidence of distal embolization. Neither patient reported herein had aneurysms. That repetitive arterial trauma can lead to extensive distal embolization was illustrated by each. Observations in these two patients would support axillary artery bypass, even prior to aneurysm formation, once distal embolization is recognized.

Vascular complications of the thoracic outlet syndrome further emphasize that *small* proximal aneurysms and fragmented or ulcerated intima of repetitively traumatized arteries frequently cause distal embolization.[7]

Comprehensive evaluation of patients with ischemic hand symptoms is mandatory to preserve both tissue and function.[5] Even when there is little hope of *complete* revascularization, optimal treatment dictates operative intervention to prevent progressive embolic obliteration of the distal arteries.

Although wrist pulses were restored in 23 of 24 individuals suffering arm ischemia following arterial invasive diagnostic studies, two incurred major complications involving the median nerve (Table III). Both had percutaneous mid brachial arterial puncture and both developed acutely ischemic extremities. Initially, the brachial artery was explored in the antecubital fossa and the puncture site was not visualized. Following passage of embolectomy catheters, brisk bleeding was noted from the upper part of the incision, necessitating hurried proximal extension of the incision to expose the bleeding puncture site. Wrist pulses were restored in both, but each was noted to have median nerve deficit in the postoperative period.

The two median nerve injuries emphasize the following points: (1) percutaneous mid brachial puncture may be associated with an increased frequency of vascular or neurologic complications; (2) nerve function should be assessed independently of arterial patency before and after operation; (3) surgical exposure should be designed to visualize directly and to control the puncture site; and (4) balloon catheter dilatation can lead to extensive bleeding from a previously sealed arterial puncture site.

Factors predisposing to brachial artery occlusion following invasive diagnostic studies may be classified as (1) a low flow, (2) catheter related, and (3) arterial wall complications.[2, 4, 8-10]

Low flow states accompany inadequate cardiac output, proximal subclavian stenosis, and use of oversized catheters. Absence of wrist pulses in these patients is usually on a thrombotic basis but may be due to ischemic, edematous muscle. Fasciotomy is mandatory for nonthrombotic arterial occlusion.[12]

Catheter-generated thrombi may embolize distally during the procedure or may be scraped off upon catheter withdrawal. Oversized catheters, multiple catheter changes, prolonged duration of study, and lack of heparin administration correlate directly with increased embolic incidents.

Arterial wall complications are related to the technique of puncture, manner of inserting and removing catheters, and the preciseness of suture placement. All relate to the experience and gentleness of the examiner.

The decision to operate on a patient with imperceptible wrist pulses following arterial catheterization can only be made on an individual basis. Intravenous heparin therapy should be initiated immediately following recognition of absent wrist pulses. Patients in whom symptomatic ischemia persists for an hour or two require arterial exploration. On the other hand, patients having asymptomatic loss of wrist pulses in whom cardiac disease precludes long-term survival may not require arterial exploration.

Criteria for operating on asymptomatic patients who lack wrist pulses following brachial catheterization must be developed utilizing the following guidelines:

1. Comparison of pre- and postcatheterization Doppler measurements of radial, ulnar, and interdigital pressure levels.[8] Specific precatheterization assessment of the collateral adequacy of both wrist and palmar arch vessels is mandatory for precise postcatheterization evaluation. Obliteration of one wrist pulse coincident with compression of its companion pulse indicates proximal obstruction. Loss of interdigital pulses during compression of either wrist artery characterizes the inadequacy of palmar arch collaterals.[8]

2. Re-examination 4 to 6 hours later to evaluate changing interdigital pressure patterns while on heparin therapy.

3. Careful follow-up studies of the Doppler pressure patterns of asymptomatic versus symptomatic patients.

Until such specific criteria are developed and confirmed, it would appear reasonable to be liberal in advising brachial artery exploration following loss of wrist pulses in patients with a favorable prognosis or dominant hand involvement.[2, 4, 10] Arterial exploration performed within 12 to 24 hours of cathterization will restore wrist pulses in over 90 percent of patients. Delayed exploration is technically more demanding and usually less successful.

REFERENCES

1. Abbott, W. M., and Darling, R. C.: Axillary artery aneurysms secondary to crutch trauma, Am. J. Surg. **125:** 515, 1973.
2. Armstrong, P. W., and Parker, J. O.: The complications of brachial arteriotomy, J. Thorac. Cardiovasc. Surg. **61:** 424, 1971.
3. Baird, R. J., and Lajos, T. Z.: Emboli to the arm, Ann. Surg. **160:** 905, 1964.
4. Brener, B. J., and Couch, N. P.: Peripheral arterial complications of left heart catheteri-

zation and their management, Am. J. Surg. **125:** 521, 1973.
5. Chase, R. A.: Surgery of the hand (Part II), N. Engl. J. Med. **287:** 1227, 1972.
6. Holm, J., and Schersten, T.: Anticoagulant treatment during and after embolectomy, Acta Chir. Scand. **138:** 683, 1972.
7. Judy, K. L., and Heymann, R. L.: Vascular complications of thoracic outlet syndrome, Am. J. Surg. **123:** 521, 1972.
8. Little, J. M., Zylstra, P. L., West, J., et al.: Circulatory patterns in the normal hand, Br. J. Surg. **60:** 652, 1973.
9. Nachnani, G. H., Lessin, L. S., Motomiya, T., et al.: Scanning electron microscopy of thrombogenesis on vascular catheter surfaces, N. Engl. J. Med. **286:** 139, 1972.
10. Page, C. P., Hagood, C. O., Jr., and Kemmerer, W. T.: Management of postcatheterization: Brachial artery thrombosis, SURGERY **72:** 619, 1972.
11. Sachatello, C. R.: Technique for subclavian, axillary, and brachial artery embolectomy, Arch. Surg. **97:** 836, 1968.
12. Sharzer, L. A., and Baker, W. H.: Nonthrombotic arterial occlusion, Arch. Surg. **106:** 344, 1973.
13. Thompson, J. E.: Acute peripheral arterial occlusions, N. Engl. J. Med. **290:** 950, 1974.

DISCUSSION

Dr. Thomas J. Whelan (Honolulu, Hawaii). I rise to emphasize one particular aspect of this paper and that is the difficulty in management of extremities which become ischemic in an insidious way, namely, those in which arterial thrombosis and embolism complicate the thoracic outlet syndrome.

In 1957 Schein, Haimovici, and Young found 29 cases in the literature showing arterial complications of the thoracic outlet syndrome. Two patients required major amputation and nine required minor amputations of digits.

For years the etiology of the pulseless, cold extremity, complicating a cervical rib or thoracic outlet syndrome, was argued, regarding a neurogenic origin vs. vascular origin. In 1933 Lewis and Pickering summed up the vascular etiology, "The hypothesis of sympathetic stimulation, however, is too difficult in its application to be acceptable. As an alternative we suggest the hypothesis of local thrombosis and resultant embolism." And they were quite correct.

The chronicity of these lesions, when diagnosed, leads to the difficulty in their surgical management because small distal emboli arising from a mural thrombus in the subclavian artery are not recognized early until major arteries are occluded. By that time many of the thrombosed arterial segments are already organized and thrombectomy is not possible.

The second point is that the arteriogram of the subclavian artery very often is negative for the mural thrombus. Usually in such cases of arterial complication of the thoracic outlet syndrome, there is a bony anomaly, either a complete cervical rim, an anomolous first rib, or an anomaly or callus of the clavicle.

An 18-year-old sailor, who presented to us with a 4 month history of episodic coldness, parasthenia, and pain in this extremity, had ischemic fingers of the left hand. Gradually the pain complex became more constant and nail-edge gangrene of the index and ring fingers supervened. Arteriogram of the subclavian artery was negative; however, he was explored because he had an anomalous first rib and evidence of distal emboli.

The arteriogram of the involved extremity revealed a normal brachial artery, completely occluded radial and ulnar arteries at mid forearm, and the radiolucent densities of arterial emboli within the nonoccluded lumen of the volar interosseous artery.

This patient had removal of the anomalous first rib, cervicodorsal sympathectomy, and resection of the artery bearing the mural thrombus.

I should like to conclude by asking a question. Was cervicodorsal sympathectomy utilized in any of the authors' patients in whom distal arteries could not be disobliterated? We have been impressed by the benefit of this additional procedure in these late cases.

Dr. David B. Pilcher (Burlington, Vt.). Cardiac catheterization with its many catheter changes is performed at many institutions by the technique of an open brachial arteriotomy, which is closed with an adventitial purse string suture. I have seen two patients at two separate institutions in whom this technique was used with resulting forearm amputation.

In the first patient, delay in recognition of the severity and the complications of ischemia and delay in consultation with the vascular service resulted in a late treatment of this problem. A vein graft was required to bypass an elevated plaque in the artery, which was proximal to the area of the arteriotomy. Despite revascularization, gangrene had set in and forearm amputation was necessary. This lady had her lawyer in the room before the amputation was performed.

In the second patient, a delay in recognition and consultation again played a serious role. It was 2½ days following cardiac catheterization before the vascular surgeons were called. Severe venous hypertension with low cardiac output led to limb loss in this patient, despite restoration of pulses in the hand.

Vascular surgical consultation and education

of medical services in the recognition and evaluation of ichemia, rather than reliance on presence or absence of pulses is vitally important. The vascular surgeon should share technical advances with other medical people to avoid such disasters.

Dr. William Abbott (Boston, Mass.). At the New England Surgical Society a couple of years ago, Dr. Clem Darling and I reported eight cases of aneurysms of the axillobrachial artery seen over a period of 7 years. The final common denominator in all of these patients was that they had been using crutches in an improper fashion.

Six of these eight patients presented with acute arterial occlusion of the upper extremity. The one thing that really impressed us, however, was that during the same time period of 7 years, there were 66 cases of acute arterial occlusion in the upper extremity in our institution. This means that these aneurysms represented about 10 percent of the total.

The message is that should you see a patient who is a chronic crutch user present with acute arterial occlusion, this diagnosis should be considered because the operative approach is going to be very different.

We would be very curious to hear the authors' experience with this entity.

Dr. Charles R. Sachatello (Closing). I believe Dr. Whalen and I are in substantial agreement. Sympathectomy was performed in two of the six patients but neither had significant beneficial effect.

Dr. Pilcher's unfortunate complications probably are much more common than any of us believe. Few will ever be published because of medicolegal implications. Precatheterization assessment of the adequacy of palmar arch collateral circulation may help identify patients prone to develop ischemic complications.

With respect to Dr. Abbott's comments, our patients did not have aneurysms. We suggest in our paper that vein graft bypass be performed once embolization is recognized even without a demonstrable aneurysm. It is quite clear that embolization results from intimal damage prior to the development of aneurysms in some patients.

Reoperation for residual defects after repair of tetralogy of Fallot

Aldo R. Castaneda, M.D., Robert M. Sade, M.D., John Lamberti, M.D., *Boston, Mass.,* *and* **Demetre M. Nicoloff, M.D.,** *Minneapolis, Minn.*

Forty patients required reoperation after corrective surgery for tetralogy of Fallot. Indications for reoperation included residual ventricular septal defect (VSD) with $Q_p/Q_s > 2:1$, right ventricular outflow gradient (ΔP) of 60 mm. Hg or more, and aneurysm of the right ventricular outflow tract. VSD alone was found in nine patients (22.5 percent) and ΔP alone in seven patients (17.5 percent). VSD and ΔP occurred together in an additional 19 patients (47.5 percent). In 19 of the 29 patients with VSD, disruption of the patch suture line was located at the posteroinferior quadrant. Five patients had a right ventricular aneurysm; all had ΔP and one also had a VSD. An outflow patch had been placed at the first operation in four of the five. Thirty-eight patients (95 percent) survived: complete heart block occurred in one patient; transection of an anomalous descending coronary artery led to myocardial infarction and chronic heart failure in another. Twenty patients have been recatheterized. Two have a residual VSD and three a residual gradient of 40, 50, and 70 mm. Hg, respectively. Reoperation for residual lesions after tetralogy repair can be associated with mortality and morbidity rates no greater than with the original operation.

From the Department of Cardiac Surgery, The Children's Hospital Medical Center and Harvard Medical School, Boston, Mass., and the University of Minnesota Health Sciences Center, Minneapolis, Minn.

"THE ONLY LOGICAL GOAL in any individual patient, and hence the one we all seek, is the complete correction of all the existing cardiac defects. After having thus restored the circulation to normal anatomically and physiologically, one can for the first time hope that life expectancy can be lengthened to its full span. In this regard it is pertinent to point out that virtually the entire mortality in corrective surgery is the initial one."[5]

Presented at the Twenty-eighth Annual Meeting of the Society for Vascular Surgery, Chicago, Ill., June 20 and 21, 1974.

Reprint requests: Aldo R. Castenada, M.D., Department of Cardiac Surgery, The Children's Hospital Medical Center and Harvard Medical School, Boston, Mass. 02115.

This imaginative and bold approach to the correction of tetralogy of Fallot was enunciated in 1954 by the University of Minnesota cardiac surgical team, headed by C. Walton Lillehei; its rationale has stood the test of time. Now, 20 years later, the pathological anatomy of tetralogy of Fallot is well enough understood, the surgical techniques for its correction are sufficiently standardized, and the principles of postoperative management clearly enough defined to produce a low hospital mortality rate and generally good long-term results.

Postoperative heart catheterization studies demonstrate residual hemodynamic abnormalities in some patients, however. This review details our experience with 40 patients who underwent an open operation for tetralogy of Fallot and postoperatively had significant residual hemodynamic abnormalities which were identified by cardiac catheterization. The original operations were carried out over an 18 year period by 12 different surgeons; some of these patients were referred from other centers.

CLINICAL MATERIAL

Forty patients, ranging in age from 11 months to 27 years, required a second operation after an initial attempt at correction of tetralogy of Fallot. The residual abnormalities included ventricular septal defects (VSD) with $Q_p/Q_s > 2$, right ventricular outflow gradients (VOG) greater than 60 mm. Hg, and right ventricular outflow tract aneurysm. They were found alone or in various combinations. The distribution of residual lesions is summarized in Table I; the time intervals between operations, in Table II.

Nine patients (22.5 percent) had an isolated VSD, and the time between the first and second operations ranged from one day to 120 months (mean, 28 months). Seven patients (17.5 percent) had isolated VOG; reoperation was carried out from 13 to 92 months after the original operation (mean, 30 months). Nineteen patients (47.5 percent) had both a VSD and VOG. Time between operations in this group varied from 12 days to 92 months (mean, 32 months). Aneurysms of the right ventricular outflow tract occurred in five patients (12 percent), all of whom also had VOG of 60 to 100 mm. Hg. One patient had an aneurysm with both VOG and VSD. The second operation in patients with aneurysms (Table III) took place between one and 80 months after the original operation (mean, 22 months). The three true aneurysms were diagnosed at 1, 6, and 24 months after the initial operation, and reoperation was carried out at 1, 12, and 80 months, respectively. The two false aneurysms were detected at 2 and 7 months after operation. One was reoperated on immediately when the diagnosis was made because of the large size of the aneurysm; the other expanded rapidly one month after detection and was then removed at operation.

Table I. *Types and distribution of residual defects (ventricular septal defect [VSD] and right ventricular outflow gradient [RVOG])*

Lesions	*No. of patients*
VSD (Q_p/Q_s 2:1)	9
RVOG ($\Delta P > 60$ mm. Hg)	7
VSD + RVOG	19
Aneurysm + RVOG	4
Aneurysm + RVOG + VSD	1
Total	40

Table II. *Time interval between operations (ventricular septal defect [VSD] and right ventricular outflow gradient [RVOG])*

Lesion	*No. of patients*	*Time between first and second operations*	
		Δ time	*$\bar{m}$ time (mo.)*
VSD	9	1 day to 120 mo.	28
RVOG	7	13 mo. to 92 mo.	30
VSD + RVOG	19	12 day to 91 mo.	32
Aneurysm	5	1 mo. to 80 mo.	22

Among the 29 patients with VSD, 17 (59 percent) had disruption of the patch suture line at the posteroinferior quadrant (Table IV). The recurrence included both the posteroinferior and posterosuperior quadrant in three patients (10.5 percent). The posteroinferior quadrant was, therefore, involved in approximately 70 percent of these patients.

In the group of 31 patients with VOG, the residual obstruction was due to inadequate resection of the infundibular outflow tract in 16 (51.6 percent), a hypoplastic pulmonary valve annulus in eight (25.8 percent), and residual stenosis of the pulmonary valve in seven (22.6 percent) (Table V).

METHODS

All reoperations were done on cardiopulmonary bypass using the Bentley bubble oxygenator with moderate hemodilution. During total bypass, flows of 100 to 125 ml. per square meter were maintained, and moderate

Table III. *Reoperation for right ventricular aneurysm*

	No. of patients	Time of diagnosis (mos.)	Time of operation (mos.)
Aneurysms:	5		
True aneurysm	3	1, 6, 24	1, 12, 80
False aneurysm	2	2, 7	2, 8
Residual ΔP (mm. Hg)	5 (60, 70, 70, 80, 100)		
Residual shunt	1		

Table IV. *Location of residual VSD at patch suture line*

	No.
PI*	17 } (70%)
PI + PS†	3 }
PS	2
PS + AS‡	3
AS	2
Circumferential	2

*Posteroinferior.
†Posterosuperior.
‡Anterosuperior.

Table V. *Reoperation for residual RVOG*

Residual obstruction	31
Infundibulum	16
Hypoplastic annulus	8
Pulmonary valve	7

First operation	No. of patients	Second operation	No. of patients
Infundibuloplasty	21	Outflow patch	17
		Valvotomy	4
Outflow patch	10	Extension of patch	7
		Valvotomy	3

hypothermia in the range of 28 to 30° C. was utilized, except as noted below.

All isolated VSDs were closed through a right atriotomy approach. The technique of closure was resuture of the original patch to the septal rim in 18 of the 29 patients (62.1 percent), insertion of a small additional piece of prosthetic material in seven patients (24.1 percent), and total replacement of a completely disrupted patch in two patients (6.9 percent).

Of the 31 patients with VOG, 21 had only infundibuloplasty at the first operation, 17 of the 21 required insertion of a right ventricular outflow patch at the second operation, and five needed a pulmonary valvotomy. Ten of the 31 patients with VOG had a right ventricular outflow patch placed at the first operation. Four of the 10 required distal extension of the patch to cross the annulus of the pulmonary valve, and two were found to need a proximal extension of the patch in order to relieve obstruction at the level of the parietal band. Pulmonary valvotomy alone was sufficient to relieve the outflow obstruction in three patients (Table V).

Special precautions were taken to reopen the original midline sternotomy incision in three patients. An 11-month-old boy, whose first operation was done under combined surface and core cooling with circulatory arrest, developed a large, rapidly expanding right ventricular outflow tract aneurysm within one month of operation. At the second operation, the child underwent surface cooling to a rectal temperature of 25° C.; the sternum was then reopened without incident and cooling was completed on cardiopulmonary bypass to a nasopharyngeal temperature of 20° C. At this point the circulation was arrested, a large true aneurysm involving the region of the transverse ventriculotomy incision was resected, and a right ventricular outflow patch was placed across the hypoplastic pulmonary annulus. The second patient was a 6-year-old boy with a large anteriorly projecting pseudoaneurysm. He was placed on peripheral cardiopulmonary bypass utilizing the femoral artery and vein, and, at 25° C., the sternum was cautiously opened without incident. An additional venous cannula was placed in the superior vena cava for total bypass and the pseudoaneurysm was successfully repaired. In the third patient, a 16-year-old-boy, a large patch of Ivalon had been used to widen the right ventricular outflow patch. During opening of the midline sternotomy it became apparent that the Ivalon was intimately adherent to the periostium of the sternum and, while a plane of dissection was being developed, the right ventricle was entered. Since bleeding could not be controlled, the patient was placed on peripheral cardiopulmonary bypass using the femoral artery and vein, and two cardiotomy suction tips were placed within the laceration of the right ventricle. Only then could the sternum be opened. After the patient was placed on total bypass, the Ivalon patch was removed, the residual VSD was closed, and a Dacron patch was used to widen the right ventricular outflow tract.

RESULTS

Two of the 40 reoperated patients (5 percent) died in the hospital. An 8-year-old girl, reoperated on for a large pseudoaneurysm originating from an outflow tract patch suture line, died of massive hemorrhage due to mediastinal sepsis 2 weeks after repair of the pseudoaneurysm. The other patient was a 12-year-old boy who remained in a low cardiac output state after closure of a large VSD and proximal extension of a right ventricular outflow patch. He died 3 days after operation. At postmortem examination the area of proximal extension of the outflow patch seemed to have compromised the sinus portion of the right ventricle.

Of the 38 surviving patients, 36 are asymptomatic. One 16-year-old boy suffered a large myocardial infarction after inadvertent transection of the anterior descending coronary artery which originated from the right coronary artery.[8] This patient has remained in chronic congestive heart failure. Another boy, 17 years old, still has a left-to-right shunt ($Q_p/Q_s = 2$) after a third attempt at closure. Although markedly improved, he is still mildly symptomatic.

An 8-year-old boy developed permanent complete heart block after replacement of his VSD patch. He now has a permanent implanted pacemaker. Another patient developed left anterior hemiblock in addition to a pre-existing right bundle branch block after placement of three sutures to close a defect along the posteroinferior margin of his VSD. He may eventually require an implanted pacemaker.

Twenty patients have had a heart catheterization after the second operation. A left-to-right shunt ($Q_p/Q_s > 2{:}1$) persisted in two patients. In both, the residual defects were localized to the posteroinferior quadrant and were closed by reattaching the original patch to the rim of the septum. Three patients have residual outflow gradients of 40, 50, and 70 mm. Hg, respectively.

DISCUSSION

Repair of tetralogy of Fallot can now be accomplished by those experienced in the treatment of this complex congenital heart defect with a risk of death less than 5 percent. Long-term function and results are excellent: many patients lead a symptom-free existence and pursue a physically and intellectually active life. A few, however, remain symptomatic or are found to have hemodynamically significant residual abnormalities at repeat heart catheterization. Routine cardiac catheterization studies one year after operation serve the important function of providing the surgeon with objective data concerning long-term results, thus permitting adjustments in technique where necessary.

The most common residual lesions in our patients were (1) a shunt at the VSD site and (2) a gradient across the right ventricular outflow tract. Aneurysms related to the ventriculotomy, pericardial outflow patch, or its suture line occur less often. Criteria concerning the functional significance of residual defects have not been clearly defined. Our indications for reoperation have been an outflow gradient greater than 60 mm. Hg, a residual shunt with $Q_p/Q_s > 2$, or an expanding aneurysm.

The most common location of residual obstruction was the right ventricular outflow tract. The parietal band was usually found to have been inadequately mobilized and the need for a patch across the right ventricular outflow tract, particularly across the pulmonary valve ring, had often been misjudged.

Intraoperative measurement of right ventricular–to–left ventricular peak pressure ratio, as suggested by Kirklin and Karp,[3] does provide a helpful guide in determining the need for an outflow gusset, particularly during the early stages of surgical experience with this lesion. We have been sensitized by the finding at recatherterization of a number of residual gradients across the infundibulum and have, therefore, become more agressive in the use of outflow patches. In our last 100 patients with tetralogy of Fallot, we have used outflow patches in 63 percent. Although the patch produced free insufficiency of the pulmonary valve, we have so far seen few long-term ill effects in our group of patients. Nevertheless, we are not yet complacent with these results. Pulmonary artery hypertension and other hemodynamic alterations have been found after long-standing pulmonary regurgitation.[1, 2, 7]

Unexpectedly, the pulmonary valve was the site of residual obstruction in a number of patients. In each of those cases, the pulmonary valve had been exposed and incised from below, through the ventriculotomy incision. We now prefer to approach the stenotic valve through a separate pulmonary arteriotomy.

Detachment of the VSD patch most frequently occurs along its posteroinferior margin, near the fibrous base of the tricuspid valve. This is probably related to several factors: the difficulty of exposing that corner of the VSD, the flimsiness of the tissue that is often available for suturing, and the surgeon's eagerness to avoid damaging the bundle of His. Despite the seemingly dangerous location of most residual VSD's, the risk of causing permanent heart block at reoperation is no greater than at the initial intracardiac procedure. This may be due to the scar tissue that develops along the margins of the disrupted suture line, allowing for more solid anchoring of stitches. In order to allow the scar tissue to mature, we try to delay reoperation for 6 months; however, early reoperation is sometimes precipitated by the effects of increased pulmonary artery pressure and flow.

The technique of closing the residual VSD is important. In the two patients who still had a residual interventricular shunt after reoperation, the original patch had been directly resutured to the margin of the defect; therefore, we now utilize an additional patch to obliterate every residual defect.

The transatrial approach to the repair of residual VSD's has proven most advantageous. Exposure of the posteroinferior quadrant is excellent. In addition, the hazard of injuring a coronary artery, often difficult to visualize because of dense epicardial adhesions, is eliminated. Transection of an anomalously orginating anterior descending coronary artery from the right coronary artery can be lethal or of great hemodynamic consequences—the one patient with this complication has remained in chronic congestive heart failure. If a ventriculotomy is necessary to relieve a residual gradient, we strongly recommend coronary angiography (aortic root injection) in all patients before reoperation. Selective coronary angiography should not be performed since anomalous vessels can be easily missed by that technique.

Outflow tract aneurysms are usually detected within the first 6 months after surgery. Pseudoaneurysms tend to increase rapidly in size and usually require operation soon after diagnosis.[6] True aneurysms, on the other hand, expand slowly and often stabilize; they can be followed with periodic chest x-rays.

The development of aneurysms has been attributed to high pressure (residual outflow obstruction) and to high flow (residual VSD). In our series all patients with ventricular aneurysm had significant residual obstruction to right ventricular outflow. We therefore believe that increase in pressure load plays an important role in the genesis and expansion of these aneurysms. For example, the true aneurysm that developed in our 11-month-old infant a month after operation probably resulted from a combination of two factors: transection of a large preventricular branch of the right coronary artery (enlarging the area of infarction that commonly occurs around the ventriculotomy site),[4] and the presence of a residual gradient of 80 mm. Hg across a hypoplastic pulmonary valve ring. High pressure exerted on the infarcted ventricular muscle produced a rapidly expanding aneurysm. Special techniques, such as deep hypothermic circulatory arrest or peripheral (femoral artery and femoral vein) cardiopulmonary bypass, sucreopening a sternotomy incision in the prescessfully obviated the potential hazards of ence of a large right ventricular aneurysm.

Complete right bundle branch block with left anterior hemiblock occurs in about 8 percent of patients after repair of tetralogy of Fallot; these patients are at risk of sudden death, as high as 12.5 percent within 12 years after operation in one series.[9] Although we have not as yet had an opportunity to treat such a patient, we presently would recommend a demand pacemaker at the slightest indication of a Stokes-Adams attack.

It is now 20 years since the first report of total correction of tetralogy of Fallot; it continues to be one of the most challenging congenital heart lesions for the surgeon. Because of improvements in techniques, the incidence of residual defects after repair has become progressively lower. The current incidence cannot be calculated from our series, since these patients had been operated on since 1955 by 12 different surgeons at different levels of training, and several of the patients were referred from other institutions. Even when residual defects are found, however, it is encouraging that reoperation is associated with mortality and morbidity rates no greater than with the original operation.

REFERENCES

1. Birks, W., Loogen, F., and Wilke, K. E.: Haemodynamic findings after surgical correction of tetralogy of Fallot, J. Cardiovasc. Surg. **11:** 15, 1970.
2. Gotsman, M. S.: Hemodynamic and cineangiographic findings after one-stage repair of Fallot's tetralogy, Br. Heart J. **28:** 448, 1966.
3. Kirklin, J. W., and Karp, R. B.: The tetralogy of Fallot from a surgical viewpoint, Philadelphia, 1970, W. B. Saunders Co., pp. 73-74.
4. Korus, M. E., Schwartz, C. J., Lillehei, C. W., et al.: Sequelae and complications of ventriculotomy: A pathological study, Circulation **40** (Suppl. III): 124, 1969 (abst.).
5. Lillehei, C. W., Cohen, M., Warden, H. E., et al.: Complete anatomical correction of the tetralogy of Fallot defects. Report of a successful surgical case, Arch. Surg. **73:** 526, 1956.
6. Rosenthal, A., Gross, R. E., and Pasternac, A.: Aneurysms of the right ventricular outflow patches, J. Thorac. Cardiovasc. Surg. **63:** 735, 1972.
7. Weldon, C. S., Rowe, R. D., and Gott, V. L.: Clinical experience with the use of aortic valve homografts for reconstruction of the pulmonary artery, pulmonary valve, and outflow portion of the right ventricle, Circulation **37** (Suppl. II): 51, 1968.
8. White, R. I., Fredi, R. S., Castaneda, A. R., et al.: The nature and significance of anomalous coronary arteries in tetralogy of Fallot, Am. J. Roentgenol. Radium Ther. Nucl. Med. **64:** 350, 1972.
9. Wolff, G. S., Rowland, T. W., and Ellison, C. R.: Surgically induced right bundle branch block with left anterior hemiblock, Circulation **46:** 587, 1972.

DISCUSSION

Dr. Gordon K. Danielson (Rochester, Minn.). Dr. Castaneda has mentioned a number of important factors which are related to the development of residual defects after repair of tetralogy of Fallot. In regard to right ventricular aneurysms, it should be emphasized that all of his patients had significant residual right ventricular outflow gradients. This is probably much more important in the development of outflow aneurysms than the presence or absence of an outflow patch or the type of patch used.

I would agree with the authors that an operation should be considered incomplete without measurement of the gradient between the right ventricle and the pulmonary artery at the conclusion of bypass and before decanulation.

At the present time, approximately 50 percent of our patients undergo outflow tract reconstruction, a figure comparable to that of the authors. We have not noted a problem with aneurysm formation from pericardial patches and continue to prefer that material when outflow tract reconstruction is required.

We still perform pulmonary valvotomy through the right ventriculotomy. The authors have mentioned that they prefer now to do that through the pulmonary artery. I do not believe the approach is as important, perhaps, as the fact that it is necessary to widely open and even partially detach the pulmonary valve, when indicated, to provide a maximum opening. Most of these valves are bicuspid and partial detachment or incision of the valve is required to provide a good result.

We have noted a disturbing finding of late in

some of these patients, namely that thickening and decreased mobility of the pulmonary valve resulting in a recurrence of pulmonary stenosis. Increasingly, we are totally excising the more abnormally formed pulmonary valves encountered at the time of primary repair.

As the authors' series was a collected one, the incidence of residual defects that require reoperation cannot be determined. To derive some data in this regard, a review was made of 1,091 patients who underwent repair of tetralogy of Fallot at the Mayo Clinic. Reoperation was required in 31 patients, an incidence of 3.1 percent. Proper attention to the technical details outlined by the authors in their manuscript should permit primary repair of tetralogy of Fallot with an incidence in this range or less.

I would like to ask the authors whether they ever consider a patient with a pulmonary-systemic flow ratio of less than 2 or a gradient across the outflow tract of less than 60 mm. Hg as sometimes needing reoperation.

Dr. Nicholas T. Kouchoukos (Birmingham, Ala.). Dr. Castaneda's excellent presentation has focused on three major complications requiring operation after definitive correction of the tetralogy of Fallot: residual ventricular septal defects, residual outflow tract obstruction, and development of ventricular true and false aneurysms.

At the University of Alabama we have also noted that the majority of residual septal defects after primary repair occur at the inferior margin of the defect, as Dr. Castaneda has emphasized. In an attempt to reduce the incidence of this complication, we have modified our technique for the primary repair. We presently prefer a continuous suture rather than an interrupted technique and, utilizing Proline suture, have placed a number of the stitches through this critical area and through the patch, leaving the patch *outside* the right ventricle to allow adequate exposure of the rim of the defect, before setting it in the proper position. We feel that this maneuver allows a more secure closure of the defect in this area.

The problem of residual outflow tract obstruction is an important one. We still rely heavily on the intraoperative measurement of right-sided and left-sided pressures in helping us to decide whether an outflow patch is required. Although these pressure measurements are not absolutely accurate in predicting pressure relationships late postoperatively, we feel they are fairly representative, and that they have provided us with a satisfactory set of guidelines for deciding whether or not a patch is necessary.

In our experience with previously unoperated children over 4 years of age and in adults, we have inserted outflow patches in 11 percent of the patients. In infants and children under 4 years of age, the percentage requiring patches has been higher, but it has not exceeded 25 percent to date. This is a slightly lower incidence than that reported by Dr. Castaneda. As he noted, the use of an outflow patch does not guarantee complete relief of outflow obstruction, since 10 of the 31 patients with residual gradients in his series had an outflow patch placed at the first operation.

Our preferred technique for inserting an outflow patch is to extend the incision to the bifurcation of the pulmonary artery. We have employed one half of the circumference of a tubular, woven Dacron graft, whose diameter is approximately that of the size of the outflow tract desired. Insertion of the patch in this manner has reduced the occurrence of residual outflow tract obstruction and should hopefully minimize the incidence of aneurysm formation.

The right and left ventricular pressure measurements were obtained at operation in eight consecutive patients requiring outflow patches in which this technique was used. The mean right ventricular–to–left ventricular pressure ratio at the completion of this procedure was 0.35/1.

Dr. Castaneda and his associates are to be commended for carrying out these secondary operations at such a low operative mortality rate and with such excellent long-term results. As he and Dr. Danielson pointed out, increasing experience and refinements in the operative procedure should further reduce the incidence of these complications.

Dr. Frank C. Spencer (New York, N. Y.). Dr. Castaneda's low operative mortality rate—only two deaths among 40 patients reoperated on—certainly supports his recommendation that the great majority of patients with a significant residual defect should be operated on again.

The question arises when a defect is found on a postoperative catheterization whether the defect is a residual one, not closed at the original operation, or a "recurrent" defect, representing dehiscence of the original repair. I doubt that this distinction can be made from the data Dr. Castaneda presented, for, as he indicated, his experiences were over a period of 15 years, with operations performed by several different surgeons.

Multiple defects are supposed to be rare with tetralogy of Fallot. In the large series just mentioned by Dr. Danielson from the Mayo Clinic, the frequency in over 1,000 cases was only 2.5 percent. About 3 years ago, multiple defects were the cause of death in a 16-year-old patient with tetralogy operated on at New York University, who died from congestive failure within 18 hours after operation because of a large additional undetected defect. Subsequently, for the past 3 years we have regularly used the technique of placing a small catheter in the apex of the left ventricle, then clamping the aorta just above the coronary arteries, and forcefully injecting saline retrograde through the catheter into the left ventricle with sufficient force to distend visibly the ventricular septum.

With the forceful injection, leaks in the suture line can be readily detected, as can multiple defects. To our surprise, the frequency of multiple defects with tetralogy, in a series of about 60 patients, has been nearly 6 percent. The additional defect has usually been a separate 3 to 4 mm. defect located within a centimeter of the large defect. I am certain that previously these have been detected at postoperative catheterization and simply reported as "residual shunt."

Since using this method routinely for detection of additional defects, no "residual" defects have been recognized. Separate from tetralogy, the method has been especially valuable when operating on an infant with known multiple defects, especially those with so-called "Swiss cheese" septum.

Separately, I would like to ask Dr. Castaneda if he employs any method of buttressing the posterior suture line in the vulnerable area of the posterior-inferior part of the septum, where sutures are inserted superficially to avoid the conduction bundle.

Dr. Aldo R. Castaneda (Closing). Dr. Danielson, the surprisingly low incidence of residual defects in the Mayo Clinic series is most impressive. However, it is important to know whether routine postoperative catheterization studies were done on these patients. If these figures are based solely on clinical examinations, rather than on postoperative catheterization studies, then the incidence of residual defects may well prove somewhat higher at recatheterization.

Concerning our policy for reoperation, we have arbitrarily selected a 60 mm. gradient and a 2/1 shunt as minimal indications for reoperation. We are following a number of patients with lesser gradients or smaller shunts. Eventually, we hope to have sufficient data to define the need for reoperation more accurately.

Dr. Kouchoukos, I am surprised at the low (11 percent) incidence of outflow patches used in Alabama. Our incidence is 63 percent. I should add that this radical approach has evolved from a careful review of our postoperative catheterization data. Residual gradients used to be quite common despite, what we considered, extensive infundibuloplasties.

Dr. Spencer, I must disagree with you about the 5 percent incidence of additional ventricular septal defects in tetralogy of Fallot. I doubt that the incidence exceeds a fraction of one percent. I have encountered only two additional defects. One was awkwardly located within the septal band and the other was a low-lying, small muscular defect. I am excluding from this discussion those patients who have both a tetralogy of Fallot and an endocardial cushion defect.

Concerning the technique of VSD closure, we do not buttress the sutures. Lately, we are more prone to use a running suture technique, as mentioned by Dr. Kouchoukos.

Since we rarely use a left ventricular vent, it is usually quite easy to detect persistent leaks along the suture line after removal of the aortic clamp.

To facilitate postoperative care, we now routinely leave a right atrial, a left atrial, and a pulmonary artery catheter in place. Blood samples from these locations permit calculations of cardiac output and of residual shunts. We also record a pullback tracing across the pulmonary valve and right ventricular outflow tract to measure gradients.

A 6 year clinical experience with arteriovenous fistulas and bypasses for hemodialysis

Victor R. Zerbino, M.D., David A. Tice, M.D., Lois A. Katz, M.D., *and* Bernard D. Nidus, M.D., *New York, N. Y.*

Subcutaneous arteriovenous fistulas or bypasses have eliminated the need for Scribner's shunts and are recommended for all patients undergoing hemodialysis and/or transplantation. Since long-term patency is important, certain technical aspects and alternative methods for construction of the fistula are considered essential in the management of these patients. A total of 163 patients underwent the following types of procedures: radial artery fistula (at different levels), ulnar artery fistula, brachial artery fistula, autogenous or allograft saphenous vein bypass fistula from the radial artery to the cephalic vein, saphenous vein loop to the femoral artery, translocation of the superficial femoral artery, superficialization of the basilic vein in the arm, and thrombectomy for acute occlusion in short- and long-standing fistulas. Our experience suggests that a single fistula, properly constructed, will be sufficient for 90 percent of the patients. The success rate for radial artery-cephalic vein fistulas is 91.2 percent. All deaths in this series (41) were due to diseases complicating prolonged renal failure. The complication rate was 9.8 percent (16 of 163 patients) and in no instance was it responsible for death.

From the Departments of Surgery and Medicine, New York University School of Medicine, and the New York Veterans Administration Hospital, New York, New York

INTERNAL ARTERIOVENOUS fistulas constitute a simple and safe route of repetitive access for successful hemodialysis. Although the fistula described by Brescia and Cimino[3] in 1966 is the preferred technique, there are many patients who require alternative procedures when the radial arteriovenous fistulas fail.

In addition, the calcified arteries and thrombosed superficial veins in old or diabetic patients may present serious problems in creating the usual fistula at the wrist.

Presented at the Twenty-eighth Annual Meeting of the Society for Vascular Surgery, Chicago, Ill., June 20 and 21, 1974.

Reprint requests: Victor R. Zerbino, M.D., Department of Surgery and Medicine, New York University School of Medicine, and the New York Veterans Administration Hospital, 550 First Ave., New York, N.Y. 10016.

The increasing availability of dialysis demands the establishment and maintenance of an adequate fistula so that survival and improved quality of living may result from chronic hemodialysis alone or in conjunction with kidney transplantation. The following is the experience with a variety of internal arteriovenous fistulas.

METHODS AND MATERIALS

Since 1968, 163 patients have had a total of 212 vascular procedures performed for hemodialysis. Of these patients 161 were men and 2 were women between 19 and 77 years of age. There were 21 diabetic patients. During this period 41 patients died from other diseases complicating the renal failure—congestive heart failure, myocardial infarction, malignant hypertension, stroke, and infection with sepsis. There were no deaths related to the surgical procedure. Of the 163 patients, 18 required more than one operation (two to seven procedures). Table I lists the procedures used. It is important to select the type of fistula that will remain patent and provide easy access to long segments of veins.

Preoperative evaluation includes careful examination of the arterial and superficial venous system by measuring blood flow with the Doppler flowmeter, determination of the flow through the radial and ulnar arteries, and the Allen test. Arteriography and venography can help to determine patency. Soft tissue x-rays of the extremities can show significant arterial calcifications especially in older or diabetic patients.

No external shunts were used in this series. Patients in end-stage renal failure were dialyzed initially with percutaneous femoral puncture before a permanent fistula was constructed.

As 158 patients underwent a side-to-side radial artery–cephalic vein fistula, important details of this technique are emphasized. The procedure was performed under local anesthesia. The radial artery and cephalic vein were dissected for an adequate distance and left in the anatomical position. The vein was never clamped and the vessels were never clamped together since this might have caused twisting which could result in turbulent flow or kinking with early thrombosis. Magnification loops (×4)[10, 13] were always used. Heparin-saline and papaverine solutions were used locally for irrigation to prevent thrombus formation and arterial spasm. Regional heparinization was used for brachial fistulas or bypasses. A No. 3 Fogarty catheter and/or coronary dilators (1.5 to 2.5 mm.) were very useful in determining venous patency and in dilating the vein when necessary. At the time of arteriotomy, a small ellipse was removed if the artery was firm or calcified. The radial fistulas were made with a diameter of 6 to 8 mm., while the diameter of the brachial fistulas was 4 to 5 mm. For the anastomosis, No. 7-0 tycron suture was used in running fashion. If a thrill was absent

Table I. *Procedures performed on 163 patients*

	No.
Radial artery–cephalic vein side to side	158
Cephalic vein–radial artery end to side	2
Radial artery–cephalic vein upper forearm	6
Ulnar artery–basilic vein side to side	2
Autogenous saphenous vein bypass in forearm	6
Preserved allograft vein bypass in forearm	3
Brachial artery–basilic vein side to side	17
Superficialization of basilic vein	5
Saphenous loop to femoral artery	2
Translocation of superficial femoral artery	2
Thrombectomy for acute and chronic fistulas	9
Total	212

at the completion of the anastomosis or there was doubt about the patency of the fistula, the distal limb of the vein was opened, a Fogarty catheter was used to remove any possible clot, and the anastomosis was dilated with the Fogarty balloon. If the bruit or thrill disappeared, the fistula was re-explored as soon as possible. A successful fistula may be used for dialysis within 24 hours, if necessary.

RESULTS

1. Radial artery–cephalic vein side-to-side fistula was performed in 158 patients with 14 failures and a success rate of 91.2 percent. The long-term patency of this fistula is shown in Fig. 1. After 5 to 6 years, 12 fistulas remain open.

2. Cephalic vein–radial artery end-to-side fistula was performed in two patients. Both are patent after 8 and 11 months.

3. Radial artery–cephalic vein fistula in the upper forearm was performed in six patients. Two of them occluded after 2 months; the other four remain patent up to 19 months.

4. Ulnar artery–basilic vein side-to-side fistula was used in two patients. One remains patent after 6 years; the other patient died 24 months after operation with a patent fistula.

5. Brachial artery–cephalic vein side-to-side fistula was performed in 17 patients and 11 have remained patent up to 56 months. The six closures occurred between 2 and 9

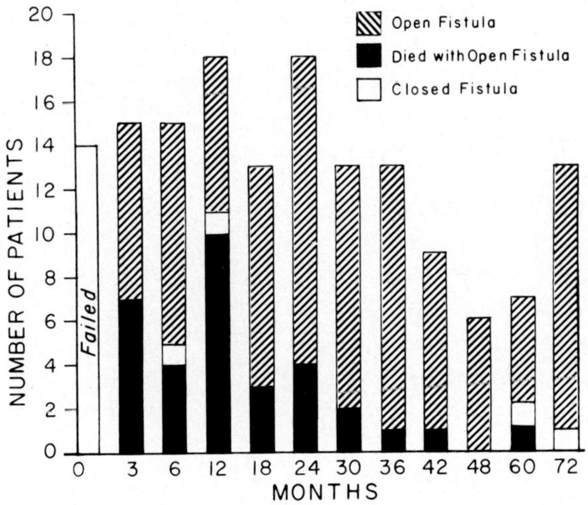

Fig. 1. Results in 158 patients with radial artery–cephalic vein side-to-side fistula.

months. With this type of fistula, the Fogarty catheter was used to dilate the distal veins in the forearm at the time of operation. These veins filled subsequently and were easier to use for dialysis. The size of the fistula was never over 5 mm. in diameter.

6. Autogenous saphenous vein bypass in the forearm was used in seven patients. Two fistulas closed after 3 and 5 months, respectively. The other five remain patent after 5 and 45 months. The lower saphenous vein (below the knee) was used initially in order to preserve the proximal segment, in case it was needed at a later date for another fistula.

7. Superficialization of the basilic vein was carried out as a second procedure in five patients with brachial fistulas to facilitate dialysis.[12]

8. Preserved frozen allograft vein bypass in the forearm was used in three patients.[9, 15, 16, 17] One patient died one year later with a patent graft which was used over 170 times for dialysis. The second patient (a former drug addict) has a patent graft in use for 18 months. The third patient's graft occluded after 3 months due to an outflow obstruction in the cephalic vein.

9. Saphenous vein loop to the common femoral artery was used in two patients and remained patent for 2 weeks and 2 months, respectively.

10. Translocation of the superficial femoral artery was used in two patients using the technique described by Brittinger.[4] One of the patients has been dialyzed by this technique for over 5 years without complications.[12] The second patient had this procedure 7 months ago, and it is still used successfully.

11. Thrombectomy for recent or longstanding fistulas was performed in six patients within 24 hours after occlusion. Flow was re-established in all and five remain patent. Thrombectomy was performed in three patients more than 24 hours after occlusion. One failed immediately; the other two remained open for 5 and 12 months, respectively.

COMPLICATIONS

The following complications occurred:

1. Infection of arteriovenous (A-V) fistula was seen in four patients within the first 8 weeks. Two of the patients had acute bleeding from the fistula area. All the patients underwent proximal and distal ligation and resection of the fistula with re-establishment of a fistula in the other extremity at a later date.

2. Cardiac failure due to A-V fistula was seen in four patients with fistula blood flows between 1.8 and 3 L. per minute. An attempt to reduce the size of the fistula in one patient was partially successful. In a second patient the brachial fistula was closed with complete

recovery from heart failure. A new fistula of smaller size was constructed at a later date. The other two patients are being treated medically.[2]

3. Lymphocele occurred in one patient 4 months following a brachial A-V fistula. After a preoperative arteriogram which was normal, the lymphocele was excised without difficulty.

4. Moderate steal syndrome occurred in four patients during the first few months but disappeared in all without any specific treatment.[5]

5. Aneurysmal dilatation at the level of the fistula area was present in five patients. None of these required operation. During dialysis, care was taken not to puncture in the aneurysmal area. One of these fistulas has been in use for over 5 years.

6. Edema of the hand and fingers was seen in some patients during the first few months, but no ischemic changes of the hand and fingers have occurred in this series.[11]

DISCUSSION

More than 20 techniques have been described due to the lack of available superficial veins or the short patency time of previous fistulas.[1, 4, 7-9] This outlines the importance of preserving and handling the veins in all patients with great care.

There are also great discrepancies among statistics, patency of fistulas, and complications. Failure rates can range from 12 to 25 percent in radial fistulas[6, 11] and up to 100 percent in brachial fistulas.[6, 14]

There is certainly a great difference in performing fistulas in children, women or men, young or old patients, diabetic patients, or those formerly addicted to drugs. The A-V fistulas in the upper extremity offer better chances of success and length of patency than those performed in the lower extremity.

Straight saphenous vein bypass fistulas seem to offer longer patency than the "loop-type" bypasses.[11] Bovine xenograft bypass fistulas are being used by several groups with variable success.[11] They have not been used in our series, and it is felt that they need further long-term evaluation. Frozen preserved homograft veins can be useful when patients' veins are not available.[17]

Fistulas constructed in the presence of hypotension, significant dehydration, obstructed venous outflow, or arterial spasm have little chance of success.

We performed 212 internal A-V fistulas in 163 patients in chronic renal failure requiring prolonged hemodialysis. Our experience suggests that a single fistula, properly constructed, will be sufficient for 90 percent of patients. The success rate for radial artery–cephalic vein fistulas is 91.2 percent. No external shunts have been used since 1968. All deaths (41) in this series were due to diseases complicating prolonged renal failure. The complication rate was 9.8 percent (16 of 163 patients), and in no instance was it responsible for death.

The authors acknowledge gratefully the technical assistance of Ms Judith Mable.

REFERENCES

1. Adar, R., Siegel, A., Bogokowsky, H., and Mozes, M.: The use of arterio-venous autograft and allograft fistulas for chronic hemodialysis, Surg. Gynecol. Obstet. **136:** 941, 1973.
2. Ahearn, D. J., and Maher, J. F.: Heart failure as a complication of hemodialysis arteriovenous fistula, Ann. Intern. Med. **77:** 201, 1972.
3. Brescia, M. J., Cimino, J. E., Appel, K., and Hurwitch, B. J.: Chronic hemodialysis using venipuncture and a surgically created arteriovenous fistula, N. Engl. J. Med. **275:** 1089, 1966.
4. Brittinger, W. D., von Henning, G. E., Huber, W., et al.: Shuntlose Hämodialyse durch punktion der subcutan fixierten Arteria femoralis superficialis, Klin. Wochenschr. **47:** 393, 1969.
5. Bussell, J. A., Abbott, J. A., and Lim, R. C.: A radial steal syndrome with arteriovenous fistula for hemodialysis, Ann. Intern. Med. **75:** 387, 1971.
6. Byrne, J. P., Stevens, L. E., Weaver, D. H., et al.: Advantages of surgical arteriovenous fistulas for hemodialysis, Arch. Surg. **102:** 359, 1971.
7. Cerilli, J., and Limbert, J. G.: Technique and results of the construction of arterio-venous fistulas for hemodialysis, Surg. Gynecol. Obstet. **137:** 922, 1973.
8. Cohn, H. E., and Solit, R. W.: Arteriovenous

fistulas for chronic hemodialysis, Surg. Clin. North Am. **53:** 673, 1973.

9. Ehrenfeld, W. K., Grausz, H., and Wylie, E. J.: Subcutaneous arterio-venous fistulas for hemodialysis, Am. J. Surg. **124:** 200, 1972.
10. Glenn, W. L.: Magnification and coronary surgery, Surgery **75:** 629, 1974.
11. Haimov, M., Burrows, L., Baez, A., et al.: Alternatives for vascular access for hemodialysis: Experience with autogenous saphenous vein autografts and bovine heterografts, Surgery **75:** 447, 1974.
12. Nidus, B. D., Tice, D. A., Matalon, R., and Eisinger, R. P.: Repositioning of the basilic vein and superficial femoral artery for chronic hemodialysis, Kidney Int. **1:** 124, 1972.
13. Spencer, F. C.: Binocular loupes (microtelescopes) for coronary artery surgery, J. Thorac. Cardiovasc. Surg. **62:** 163, 1971.
14. Thompson, B. W., Barbour, G., and Bissett, J.: Internal arterio-venous fistulas for hemodialysis, Am. J. Surg. **124:** 785, 1972.
15. Tice, D. A., and Santoni, E.: Use of saphenous vein homografts for arterial reconstruction. A preliminary report, Surgery **67:** 493, 1970.
16. Tice, D. A., and Zerbino, V. R.: Clinical experience with preserved human allografts for vascular reconstruction, Surgery **72:** 260, 1972.
17. Zerbino, V. R., and Tice, D. A.: Successful use of preserved allograft vein for chronic hemodialysis, Nephron **10:** 61, 1973.

DISCUSSION

Dr. Dennis Rosenberg (New Orleans, La.). I rise to suggest the use of the bovine graft in selected instances for creation of an arteriovenous (A-V) fistula.

Three years ago, when we presented our material on the bovine graft before this Society, I had no idea that it would ever be used for A-V fistulas. Now, with more than 200 bovine grafts in the femoropopliteal region, we have rather cautiously started to use the bovine graft for the creation of A-V fistulas.

In all our cases, we have used it where no satisfactory autogenous vessel has been available. I would suggest that, if the bovine graft is to be used, it be used from a large artery to a large vein. The bovine graft can be used from the brachial artery to any of the larger veins lower in the forearm or arm and also for poplitosaphenous or femorosaphenous fistulas.

Direct needling of the bovine artery is carried out, although we do not know what the long-term result of this repeated trauma will be. We have had no aneurysms in those cases where the bovine artery has been used in the arm, but we have seen aneurysms in other locations, such as the femoropopliteal bypass.

Dr. William K. Ehrenfeld (San Francisco, Calif.). Whereas we are in agreement with many of the things that were stated, we have some difference of opinion both in method and approach.

We have, by and large, favored the saphenous vein fistula in women. I noted in reading the manuscript that all but two of the patients in this series were men. In our series, we have a large number of women and have had some difficulty in creating a durable and satisfactory Brescia-Cimino fistula in many of them.

We have performed 197 operations on 164 patients. There were a total of 154 graft fistulas and 43 Brescia-Cimino type fistulas. We like graft fistulas because they are easy to puncture and can be used right away. When the saphenous vein autograft was not available, we originally went to the saphenous vein homograft, but our enthusiasm has been tempered quite a bit. All of our six homografts have occluded within 12 months due to accelerated intimal fibrosis. At the suggestion of Dr. John Hutton of Letterman General hospital, we switched to the bovine heterograft and now have over 40 patients using this graft for dialysis with good results. I do not think it is as good as the saphenous vein, but it is an acceptable substitute.

One of the interesting phenomena that we have observed has been diffuse aneurysmal dilatation of the vein. Our biggest problem, however, has been intimal fibrosis.

At three years, we have a 65 percent patency rate for the saphenous fistulas. Regarding the Brescia-Cimino fistulas, which we have been doing for 4 years, the long-term patency rate is in the range of 50 percent.

Dr. Paul De Camp (New Orleans, La.). I am not here today to peddle a technique. I am here to state that it is most significant that this matter is being discussed before this Society today. This problem has been around for over a decade, and because it was born in nephrology and was not very exciting, most of us have tried to keep it under the carpet—and at the very best turn it over to junior members of the staff.

It is apparent from the experience that all of us have had that you cannot treat this problem this way. I am delighted to find that somebody was paying attention to this at least 6 years ago, and I think the most significant feature of this paper is that, with the proper care, they have had these truly amazing results.

Now, of course, most of us are not in the Veterans Administration and we cannot have 99 percent men, so we will have to have some other techniques, but I want to congratulate these men on the fact that, with extreme care, they have developed a technique which is certainly one of the simplest and, as they can prove in a high percentage of cases, a highly successful one.

Dr. Jack A. Cannon (Phoenix, Ariz.). I would like to talk about the work of my associate, Dr. John M. Johnson. In this regard, I act as his assistant and kibitzer in terms of a technique which has already been mentioned but one which we have adopted totally as our method of preference for chronic hemodialysis, namely, the use of the heterograft.

We have a 2 year experience with 58 cases and our method of choice is a modified bovine heterograft interposed between the radial artery and cephalic vein.

The complications are mainly five instances of thrombosis occurring anywhere from 2 weeks to 8 months. The majority of thromboses have been from fibrous intimal proliferation at the venous anastomosis in the cephalic vein. All have been reopened and reconstituted. There has been one incidence of infection due to a puncture from a cat claw and two instances of hemorrhage when the bovine graft was punctured from front to back by the nurse, and the patient had to be returned to the operating room and the hemorrhage controlled. The seven deaths have been unrelated to the graft.

We have found that the patient acceptance has been so universal that most people who have fistulas of other types are asking to be converted to the bovine graft.

I had misgivings initially because of the philosophy of the situation and, yet, in terms of palliation, we find that these people by and large are very pleased with this method and are eager to go on living by this method.

Dr. Moshe Haimov. I want to make one comment regarding the retrograde venous arterialization. This may be followed by complications. Breaking the valves, as the authors suggested, will result in arterializing of the veins in a retrograde fashion. Some of these patients will develop chronic venous insufficiency in the hand, similar to the one we see in the lower extremity. You see swelling, hyperpigmentation, and even beginning ulceration associated with a considerable amount of pain and discomfort. Therefore, I do not consider retrograde arterialization of the veins to be advisable.

Regarding the use of bovine heterografts, we have used them to date in 82 patients, the longest one being used now for more than 2 years. The results have been very satisfactory.

I would not use it instead of the standard arteriovenous fistula, which is the simplest procedure, but, when peripheral veins are not available for the standard arteriovenous fistula, the bovine heterograft is a very satisfactory substitute.

Dr. Victor R. Zerbino (Closing). We seem to come again to the problem of the bovine heterografts. We have one in our locker just in case, which does not mean that we are against them. We are awaiting other results, similar to these, which appear rather convincing so far, such as Dr. Haimov just mentioned, a long-term patency of 2 years in some cases.

In reference to the homograft occlusion, our longest experience is 18 months with the homograft bypass fistula. We do not know if the early occlusion or the failures of Dr. William Ehrenfeld are related to the preservation method. We think that homografts can vary in their behavior, according to how they are treated, how they are preserved, and how long they are preserved.

Our series does not involve as many women. Probably saphenous vein bypass is a better procedure than bypass of fistulas in the upper extremities in this group.

We are also concerned with the bovine graft in reference to complications such as infections, hemorrhage, and thrombosis. We know there are cases in which it is difficult to stop the bleeding after dialysis.

But we also feel that very important for the success of these fistulas is the way in which the renal unit and the internists and their team handle the dialysis of these patients. I think that a lot of the closures and the failures are related to the management of the fistulas during the period of dialysis.

Caution regarding autotransfusion

S. Edwin Duncan, M.D., William H. Edwards, M.D., *and* **W. Andrew Dale, M.D.,**
Nashville, Tenn.

Intraoperative autotransfusion was utilized on 20 patients undergoing elective and emergency vascular surgical procedures. There were eight deaths. Six deaths were in patients with ruptured aortic aneurysms. Three deaths were thought to be related to the use of the autotransfusor unit and these patients suffered from abnormal coagulation studies prior to their deaths. Autotransfusion in the survivors was completely uneventful. It is concluded that autotransfusion is an effective means of reinfusing blood lost at operation, but, until the specific indications and proper anticoagulation regimen are determined, caution regarding the use of autotransfusion is urged.

From the Department of Surgery, Vanderbilt University School of Medicine, and St. Thomas Hospital, Nashville, Tenn.

INTRAOPERATIVE autotransfusion provides an effective means of returning blood lost at the operating site directly into the patient without the recognized complications and disadvantages of stored bank blood, but it is not without its own hazards.

Autotransfusion has been described as safe and efficient in both traumatic and elective surgery in providing immediate blood replacment. Reports by Duncan and associates,[6, 7] Reul,[11] Dowling,[5] and others[10] have described the usefulness of autotransfusion in making immediately available reusable blood replacement during operation for penetrating and blunt trauma. This was particularly evident in those reported patients who required less than 3,000 c.c. autotransfusion and whose morbidity and mortality rates were not increased by the use of intraoperative autotransfusion. This technique in elective surgical procedures has been advocated by Symbas and associates[12-14] and by Brener, Raines, and Darling,[3, 4] who suggested that autotransfusion may be applicable where large blood losses are anticipated. Last year we decided to evaluate autotransfusion in elective and emergency vascular surgery in the light of this favorable experience.

METHOD OF STUDY

Twenty patients admitted to the vascular surgery service at St. Thomas Hospital in Nashville, Tenn., from July to December, 1973, were chosen for intraoperative autotransfusion. The decision to use autotransfusion was strictly on an elective basis and no form of patient selection was carried out, except that large blood losses were anticipated. Trained operating room cardiopulmonary pump technicians operated the autotransfusor unit as their sole responsibility in

Presented at the Twenty-eighth Annual Meeting of the Society for Vascular Surgery, Chicago, Ill., June 20 and 21, 1974.

Reprint requests: W. Andrew Dale, M.D., Mid-State Medical Center, 2010 Church St. Nashville, Tenn. 37203.

Table I. *Twenty patients who underwent vascular operations*

Sex		*Age*					*Intraoperative autotransfusion*		*Deaths*	
Male	*Female*	*Under 50*	*51 to 60*	*61 to 70*	*71 to 80*	*80+*	*Diagnosis*	*No.*	*No.*	*%*
18	2		6	9	4	1	Aortic aneurysms			
							Elective	8	2	
							Ruptured	6	6	
							Aortoiliac graft	1	0	
							Aortofemoral graft	4	0	
							IVC ligation	1	0	
								20	8	40

accordance with the previous recommendations.[6, 7]

The ATS-100 Bentley Autotransfusion Unit* was primed with 200 c.c. of heparinized Ringer's lactate aspirated from a solution containing 1,000 c.c. of Ringer's lactate plus 5,000 U. of aqueous heparin. The priming solution removed air from the reservoir and the inflow lines. The unit was connected to the patient by two 14 gauge venous catheters and these lines and tubings were periodically flushed with priming solution following aspirations of blood. Besides the use of the heparin in the priming solution, the patients were given intravenous heparin in doses of 2,500 to 5,000 U. prior to aortic crossclamping. The patients were not otherwise systemically heparinized.

The 20 patients consisted of 14 having grafts for abdominal aortic aneurysm (six ruptured), one having aortoiliac bypass, four having aortofemoral bypasses, and one patient with a vena caval umbrella removal and vena caval ligation. There were 18 males and two females. The ages ranged from 51 to 85 years, with a mean age of 64 years (Table I). The patients exhibited the usual array of prior myocardial injury, pulmonary insufficiency, and renal abnormalities that are characteristic of the elderly patient suffering from peripheral vascular problems. Fourteen patients had undergone extensive preoperative evaluations consisting of sequential multiple analyzer (with 12 different vital determinations), complete blood count, electrolytes, platelet count, prothrombin time (PT), partial thromboplastin time (PTT), and specific arteriographic procedures prior to autotransfusion. Six patients with emergency admissions for ruptured aortic aneurysms did not undergo these studies.

*Autotransfusion Unit, Bentley Laboratories, Inc., Santa Ana, Calif.

RESULTS

There were eight deaths among the 20 patients who received autotransfusion (40 percent). All deaths followed operation for aortic aneurysms, six patients having ruptured aneurysms who had received large volumes of autotransfused blood but had also received total blood replacement (banked blood plus intraoperative autotransfusion) of greater than 7,000 c.c. This was true in all cases except one patient with a ruptured aortic aneurysm who was moribund on admission and received only 300 c.c. of autotransfusion. Among the eight deaths, there were three instances of marked hemolysis, prolongation of PT and PTT, and reduction of platelet counts, which were thought to be related to the use of the autotransfusion unit (Table II).

There were two intraoperative deaths occurring in patients with ruptured aortic aneurysms, with one patient receiving 10,000 c.c. autotransfusion and 12,000 c.c. banked blood before dying from hypotension when the Dacron graft prosthesis failed to clot at the conclusion of the procedure. His bleeding and clotting studies were grossly abnormal. The other intraoperative death occurred in the moribund patient with only 300 c.c. autotransfusion.

There were six immediate postoperative deaths. Four of these patients were operated

Table II. *Coagulation abnormalities in three patients who died*

Patient	*Volumes of auto-transfused blood (c.c.)*	*Bank blood (c.c.)*	*Serum*	*Prothrombin time (sec.)*	*Partial thromboplastin time (sec.)*	*Platelets*
1. C. D.	10,000	12,000	Hemolyzed	24/11	90	86,000
2. W. F.	500	10,500	Not hemolyzed	18/11	90	100,000
3. F. M.	1,000	7,000	Hemolyzed	19/11	90	46,000

on as emergency procedures for ruptured aortic aneurysms. They received an average of 1,000 c.c. autotransfusion but from 5,000 to 10,000 c.c. of banked blood during the course of the operation and in the postoperative course until their deaths. Three of these four deaths were from hypotension and one was from renal failure on the third day after operation. The other two postoperative deaths were in patients with elective aneurysm resections. One also had a recognized renal cell carcinoma and underwent nephrectomy at the time of resection. He received 1,150 c.c. autotransfusion as well as 21,500 c.c. of banked blood in the following 3 days for continuous bleeding from the nephrectomy and unresected tumor site; he died from continued bleeding. His bleeding and clotting studies following autotransfusion had been normal. The other death was in a patient with a resected aneurysm, whose graft thrombosed on the second day after operation. These two deaths were thought not to be related to the use of the autotransfusor.

The 100 percent mortality rate for these ruptured aneurysms is not the general experience of the vascular surgical service at St. Thomas Hospital where the average mortality rate for ruptured aneurysms is 40 to 50 percent.

The six survivors of elective aneurysmectomy received an average of 1,000 c.c. of autotransfusion and had normal coagulation studies. One patient received autotransfusion during an aortoiliac bypass graft. He received 700 c.c. autotransfusion. Four patients with aortofemoral bypass all survived with average ranges of 600 c.c. autotransfused. The one case of vena caval ligation received 300 c.c. of autotransfusion. All these patients had no difficulty from the use of the unit and suffered no consequences of blood coagulation abnormalities. Before their discharge from the hospital, the survivors received slightly more than one unit of blood on the average. This usually occurred on the second or third day after operation for the indication of a low hematocrit level in the range of 28 to 34 percent. Otherwise, all the survivors had normal bleeding and clotting studies and had no evidence of hemoglobinuria, hemolysis, or postoperative renal failure.

DISCUSSION

Intraoperative autotransfusion has been used effectively in elective as well as in trauma surgery. The report of the use of autotransfusion in elective vascular surgery by Brener, Raines, and Darling[3, 4] points out the usefulness of this unit in a controlled situation where large volumes of blood may be lost and where rapid replacement is needed without apparent side effects. In their report, full heparinization was used for the patients undergoing autotransfusion in a dose of 300 U. per kilogram to prevent any clot formation in the reservoir and suction lines. It was their conclusion that this full heparinization did not increase the need for blood transfusions but made hemostasis tedious. This was the same observation of Rakower and Worth[10] who also used full heparinization and arrived at the same conclusions. Likewise, Brener, Raines, and Darling reported that 50 percent of their patients did not receive any banked blood either intraoperatively or prior to discharge following autotransfusion. However, we did not hesitate to give additional banked blood in the postoperative period. This was done to replace

Table III. *Coagulation diagram*

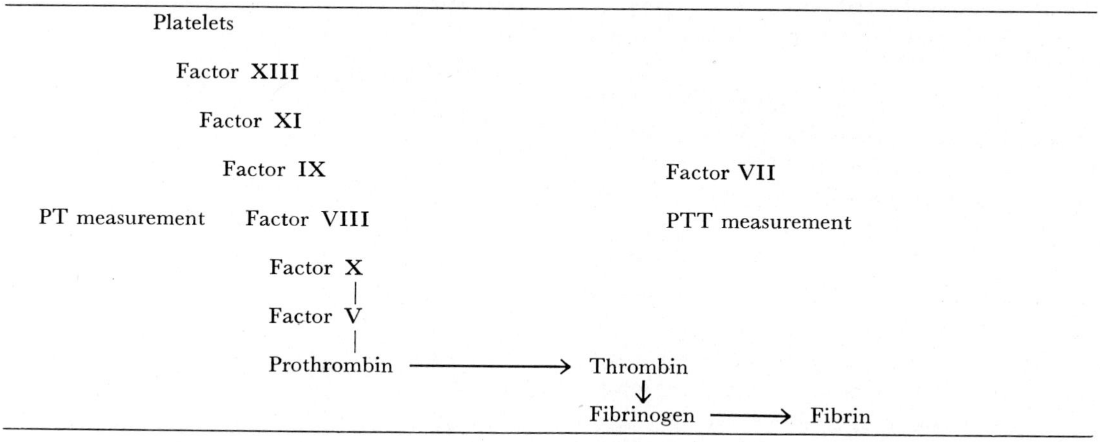

the red cell mass that had been diminished by the use of the autotransfusor. This postoperative anemia is not from hemodilution but from simple red cell destruction, as has been demonstrated by Cr-tagged red cells and evaluation of the diminished half-life.[2, 14] The cell destruction is due to the trauma of the suction apparatus, reservoir and filtering systems, and the pumping mechanism. This is clinically obvious by the appearance of serum hemolysis, hemoglobinuria, and elevated, plasma-free hemoglobin levels. However, there have been no reports of renal failure as a consequence of this hemolysis alone if the patients were well perfused, but recent reports question its benignity.[1]

The use of autotransfusion seemed to be a factor in the coagulation abnormalities that existed in three of our patients. All exhibited bleeding and clotting disorders, thrombocytopenia, gross serum hemolysis, and positive urine hemoglobinuria. It was apparent that patients who received large volumes of autotransfusion had the collecting reservoir filled with clotted blood. This would seem to indicate that trapping of the circulating platelets as well as labile clotting factors did occur and added to the bleeding problems. This phenomenon of platelet destruction has been described by Wright[16] and others,[1, 14, 15] who showed in their canine models that microaggregation of platelets did occur following contact of extravasated blood with the body tissues and that these were removed by reservoir filtration. The platelet counts following autotransfusion were diminished in our survivors but returned to normal within 24 hours, as has been the experience of previous investigators.[2-7 11-14]

It would appear, therefore, that the abnormal coagulation might have been decreased if more effective anticoagulation had been achieved. Such anticoagulation proposals have been offered by Klebanoff[9] and others,[4, 8] who suggest acid-citrate-dextrose (ACD) anticoagulation in the reservoir. They recommend the use of 40 c.c. of ACD solution added to each 500 c.c. of aspirated blood with manual mixing of the reservoir to prevent any clot formation. This alternate mode of anticoagulation is perhaps a better method for the patient with traumatic hemorrhage in whom the use of total body heparinization would not be acceptable.

The stage was set for a duplication of coagulation problems when the patient received large volumes of banked blood plus the autotransfused blood. This occurred because of the combination of lowered platelets and Factor V and Factor VIII deficiencies in stored banked blood and in autotransfused blood which had passed the reservoir filter more than once (Table III). Likewise, the same patients who required the additional banked blood plus autotransfusion were involved in severe surgical situations and suffered from the added insults of hemorrhagic shock, acidosis, hypothermia, and renal ischemia to complicate their hemostatic mechanisms.

Nonetheless, the autotransfusor was believed to contribute and possibly to be at the source of the coagulation difficulties in three of our patients. However, there is a need for autotransfusion in the over-all blood salvage program as a means of reducing the shortages facing blood banks in situations of massive transfusions often necessary for elective surgery as well as for trauma surgery. It is apparent that the theory of simply returning blood lost at the operating site directly back into the patient is feasible, and the practice of autotransfusion can be carried out in our modern surgical setting. This will be more practical when the proper anticoagulation for intraoperative autotransfusion is absolutely determined. It appears that reservoir heparinization is inadequate for large volume anticoagulation, as demonstrated in this report. Likewise, the use of total body heparinization is not practical for trauma surgery and may contribute to excessive blood loss and lengthy elective vascular surgical procedures. However, the favorable reports of ACD anticoagulation deserve further laboratory and clinical investigation as a means of possible solution to the anticoagulation difficulties.

UNANSWERED QUESTIONS

1. What are the indications for autotransfusion? Should it always be available for each operative procedure or should the technique be abandoned?

2. Should autotransfusion be used only in emergency traumatic surgery?

3. What are the indications in elective vascular procedures?

4. Beyond what autotransfusion volumes is the procedure unsafe in terms of continued cell destruction and alteration of platelets and coagulation factors?

5. What is the proper anticoagulation regimen for autotransfusion?

We conclude that autotransfusion is an effective means of reinfusing blood lost at operation but, until the specific indications and proper anticoagulation regimen are determined, caution regarding the use of autotransfusion is urged.

REFERENCES

1. Aaron, R. K., Beazley, R. M., and Riggle, G. D.: Hematologic integrity after intraoperative allotransfusion, Arch. Surg. **108:** 831, 1974.
2. Bennett, S. H., Geelhoed, G. W., Gralnick, H. R., et al.: Effects of autotransfusion on blood elements, Am. J. Surg. **125:** 273, 1973.
3. Brener, B. J., Raines, J. K., and Darling, R. D.: Intraoperative autotransfusion in abdominal aortic resections, Arch. Surg. **107:** 73, 1973.
4. Brener, B. J., Raines, J. D., and Darling, R. D.: Intraoperative autotransfusion in clinical surgery: A progress report, Proc. 2nd Ann. Bentley Autotrans. Sem. Oct. 1973, Chicago, Ill.
5. Dowling, J. B.: Clinical experience with intraoperative autotransfusion in the trauma patient, Proc. 2nd Ann. Bentley Autotrans. Sem., Oct. 1973, Chicago, Ill.
6. Duncan, S. E., Klebanoff, G., and Rogers, W.: Clinical experience with intraoperative autotransfusion, Ann. Surg. Accepted for publication.
7. Duncan, S. E., Klebanoff, G., and Rogers, W.: Patient experience with intraoperative autotransfusion, Rev. Surg. **31:** 121, 1974.
8. Kingsley, J. R., Valeri, C. R., Peters, H., et al.: The use of citrate anticoagulation and cell-washing for intraoperative autotransfusion in the baboon, Proc. 2nd Ann. Bentley Autotrans. Sem., Oct., 1973, Chicago, Ill.
9. Klebanoff, G.: Summary of Second Annual Bentley Autotransfusion Seminar, Proc. 2nd Ann. Bentley Autotrans. Sem., Oct. 1973, Chicago, Ill.
10. Rakower, S. R., and Worth, M. H., Jr.: Perspective and critical problems, J. Trauma, **13:** 573, 1973.
11. Reul, G. J., Jr.: A safe technique for autotransfusion in the surgical treatment of trauma, Proc. 2nd Ann. Bentley Autotrans. Sem., Oct. 1973, Chicago, Ill.
12. Symbas, P. N., Levin, J. M., Ferrier, F. L., et al.: A study on autotransfusion from hemothorax, South. Med. J. **62:** 671, 1969.
13. Symbas, P. N.: Autotransfusion from hemothorax: Experimental and clinical studies, J. Trauma **12:** 689, 1972.
14. Symbas, P. N., Levin, J. M., Ferrier, F. L., et al.: Autotransfusion and its effects upon the blood components of the recipient, Curr. Top. Surg. Res. **1:** 386, 1969.

15. Swank, R. L.: Alteration of blood on storage: Measurement of adhesiveness of "aging" platelets and leukocytes and their removal by filtration, N. Engl. J. Med. **265:** 728, 1961.
16. Wright, C. B.: Microaggregates in autotransfusion: The canine model, Proc. 1st Ann. Bentley Autotrans. Sem., Sept. 1972, San Francisco, Calif.

DISCUSSION

Dr. R. Clement Darling (Boston, Mass.). I agree entirely with Dr. Duncan's message regarding the use of caution with intraoperative autotransfusion. On an elective basis, we have studied over 52 patients at the Massachusetts General Hospital undergoing planned resection and grafting of large, extensive, or complicated aortic aneurysms where more than one liter of blood loss was expected. Dr. Raines, who directs the vascular laboratory, has modified the Bentley apparatus to include dual 4.5 inch Sarnes occlusive roller pumps, additional Swank filters, and a photoelectric air antiembolism device for greater safety. In our early experience we found, as did Dr. Duncan, that with low-dose heparin, clots formed in the filters. We quickly moved to using between 200 and 250 mg. (300 U. per kilogram) of beef-lung heparin and learned the following:

1. Patients did not bleed significantly more during operations with high-dose heparin than with the conventional low dosage.
2. Filters did not clog.
3. Beef-lung heparin, although hard to obtain, seemed superior to heparin obtained from other sources in its ability to be adequately neutralized with protamine.
4. Disseminated intravascular coagulation did not occur and was not noted in any of our 52 patients, all of whom have been studied hematologically.
5. Massive free hemoglobinemia occurred in all patients and gross hemoglobinuria in one half; plasma levels returned to normal within 24 hours in each instance, however.
6. No case of renal failure secondary to hemolysis has been noted in this group of patients. In our experience this should be anticipated as long as the patient's blood volume has been adequately maintained, acidosis was avoided, brisk urinary diuresis was induced using mannitol and furosemide, and if adequate filtration of any agglutinated red cell ghosts were carried out.
7. Hemolysis rates averaged between 30 and 50 percent in five patients undergoing an average of 3.5 L. of autotransfusion. Platelet counts were somewhat lowered in autotransfused blood, but as long as the autotransfusion was limited to 6 L. or under, no diminution in the patient's platelet count or platelet function was noted.

If you are fortunate enough these days to be able to operate on your own patients and can move along without complications and are willing to accept a mild postoperative anemia, most aortic aneurysm surgery can be carried out without the use of banked blood. Intraoperative autotransfusion, however, may be helpful if it is restricted to volumes between one and 6 L. This has been a safe procedure in our hands when used electively by a well-trained technician in selected patients. However, autotransfusion of more than one blood volume introduces the potential problem of dilutional coagulopathy, which may require urgent treatment with fresh blood, fresh frozen plasma, or fresh platelets.

Despite destruction of some red cells, it is apparent that autotransfused blood probably is more physiologic than banked blood in many ways. In a severely traumatized patient, however, total body heparinization is usually not feasible. Further investigation in the use of local anticoagulation either using heparin or acid-citrate-dextrose solution is under way at our institution.

Dr. George Noon (Houston, Texas). The contribution of the autotransfusion to the coagulation disorders and the hemolysis that the authors describe is hard to determine, because these same disorders could result from the large volumes of banked blood that the patients also received.

Clotting of blood in their collecting reservoir indicates that too little anticoagulation was used. When coagulation occurs in the autotransfuser, there will be an increased tendency to develop disseminated intravascular coagulation because of coagulation abnormalities resulting from the increased levels of fibrin split products or fibrinolysis.

Heparin in small doses can be easily reversed by the antiheparins released by platelet destruction. The potent thromboplastins resulting from hemolysis of red blood cells and destruction of leukocytes and platelets will also produce clotting despite heparin. This will not occur, however, if the calcium has been chelated, as with citrate.

I would like to show you a simple method of intraoperative autotransfusion I have developed in conjunction with the Sorenson Research Laboratories. This is an easy system to use and can be applied in any operating room, which can provide a suction apparatus with 30 mm. Hg of suction to a cannister with two collecting reservoirs. The suction tip has a mixing chamber to which a C.P.D. solution is added to mix with aspirated blood—even in the heparinized patient. The canister contains two collecting bags. The blood goes into the upper collecting bag through a filter, then drains by gravity into the lower collecting system. When the collected blood has reached a quantity that is sufficient for autotransfusion, the bags are removed from the canister. The two bags are then separated and the autotransfusion is administered through a Swank filter. All the air can be removed from this bag, thereby eliminating any problems of air embolism.

I have used this system of intraoperative autotransfusion in nearly 50 patients on whom I have performed vascular surgical procedures. Autotransfusion varied between 500 and 10,000 c.c. of blood. Most patients received 150 U. of heparin per kilogram, which was reversed with protamine sulfate at the end of the procedure.

Elevation of fibrin split products and fibrolynic activity was eliminated in these heparinized patients when C.P.D. was added at the sucker tip. I have had difficulty in preventing clot formation in the autotransfuser in patients who have not been heparinized.

We are now working on a special suction tip with a chamber for mixing of the aspirated blood and the C.P.D. before it enters the suction tubing and the autotransfuser. No clotting occurred in initial trials with this in the nonheparinized patients.

I have had no significant coagulation disorders or hemolysis occurring in any of the patients with the autotransfusion, and all air can be removed from the bag prior to reinfusion, eliminating the possibility of air embolism.

Dr. P. N. Symbas (Atlanta, Ga.). We, too, have been interested for the last several years in autotransfusion. Our initial interest was with extraoperative autotransfusion from traumatic hemothorax and, so far, we have autotransfused more than 500 patients with an average of 1,800 ml. with no side effects.

Subsequently, we become interested in the intraoperative autotransfusion and initially we studied three groups of dogs in which one third of the blood volume was allowed to bleed sequentially twice in the peritoneal cavity. In the first group it was left in for 45 minutes before it was suctioned; in the other two groups it was suctioned immediately. All three groups were autotransfused through the Bentley Autotransfusion System. In the first two groups only 10 mg. of heparin was added in the priming solution, whereas in the third group only 3 mg. per kilogram of body weight of heparin was given intravenously. The best preservation of the fibrinogen and platelets was observed in the fully heparinized group as well as the least elevation of the free plasma hemoglobin. These results concur with those observed by the authors that coagulation and other abnormalities do occur during autotransfusion and suggest that the abnormalities are greater in the animals not fully heparinized. However, it is well known that stored bank blood has an imperfect clotting package, i.e., lacking platelets and ionized calcium with low levels of factors V and VIII and that coagulopathy does occur following massive transfusion of homologous blood. Therefore, from a coagulability point of view, it appears that we gain little by giving old banked homologous blood instead of autotransfusing autologous blood.

Although there is work to be done for the perfection of the intraoperative autotransfusion technique, it is unfair to imply that the coagulopathy and high mortality rate observed by Dr. Duncan and his associates were due to autotransfusion, since the patients who succumbed intraoperatively or postoperatively were autotransfused with an average amount of 1,000 ml., but received, in addition, from 8,000 to 21,000 ml. of banked blood.

Before I close, I would like to stress two points: first, autotransfusion of less than half or two thirds of the patients' blood volume, in our experience, does not result in a clinically significant coagulopathy; and, second, whenever intraoperative autotransfusion is used, the patients' coagulation factors should be monitored and, when critically deranged, should be appropriately corrected.

Dr. S. Edwin Duncan (Closing). Dr. Symbas, we also recognize that the large volume autotransfusion beyond one blood volume is when we did get into trouble.

Dr. Noon, we now realize that our coagulation problems have been related to the low-dose heparin and we look forward to further reports about your new device and, particularly, the information about the bags that prevent any sort of air embolism.

Structural changes during preparation of autogenous venous grafts

William M. Abbott, M.D., Steven Wieland, B.S., *and* **W. Gerald Austen, M.D.,** *Boston, Mass.*

This study evaluated two preparative maneuvers for autogenous venous grafts in terms of their effects on structural properties. With the use of an in vitro analytic system, stress/strain curves of fresh canine jugular vein segments and those modified by hydrostatic dilatation or short-term immersion were compared. Hydrostatic dilatation was carried out to 300 and 1,000 mm. Hg. Short-term immersion experiments explored the variables of media composition, temperature, pH, immersion time, and the presence of homologous protein and enzymatic effects. The following conclusions were drawn. Hydrostatic dilatation was associated with stiffening of the vessel wall and should be avoided or minimized. Immersion in various crystalloid solutions exhibited increased distensibility of the venous wall, whereas a balanced salt solution was better. Changes were exaggerated by warm temperature; therefore, a chilled (4° C.) solution seems important. Optimum pH was 7.0 in view of stiffening associated with acidic solutions and distensibility related to alkaline solutions. According to these results, the best preinsertion medium seems to be a balanced salt solution with 10 percent serum at 4° C. with a pH adjusted to 7.0. The most likely cause for alterations in structural characteristics rests in changes in the functional ratio of elastin and collagen.

From the Department of Surgery and General Surgical Services, Massachusetts General Hospital, Boston, Mass.

Autogenous venous bypass grafts have become widely accepted as a technique for arterial reconstructive surgery in the modern era. The original application was as a conduit to circumvent atherosclerotic occlusive disease in the superficial femoral artery. More recently they have also been employed as conduits from the aorta to the distal coronary arteries for coronary artery insufficiency. Although originally thought to be associated with reasonably good long-term patency rates,[4] it has become increasingly apparent that venous bypass grafts sustain a significant and substantial loss of patency with time.[2, 14] In spite of little incisive data to explain this loss of patency, critical concern with vein grafting techniques has been growing. Recently veins grafted into the aorta-to-coronary artery position were found to undergo a poorly understood degenerative process manifested as a subintimal fibrous hyperplasia.[16] This process has also been described in autogenous vein grafts in the femoropopliteal position.[15] These findings have also raised the level of concern.

Of many probable factors involved in the etiology of the above-mentioned problems, one possibility is that changes are induced in the veins themselves by the methods used for preparation prior to insertion into the ar-

Presented at the Twenty-eighth Annual Meeting of the Society for Vascular Surgery, Chicago, Ill., June 20 and 21, 1974.

Reprint requests: William M. Abbott, M.D., Department of Surgery and General Surgical Services, Massachusetts General Hospital, Boston, Mass. 02114.

terial circulation. The purpose of this investigation was to evaluate the effects of two preparative maneuvers, short-term immersion and hydrostatic distension, on the structural properties of the venous wall in accordance with the theory that eliminating preinsertion changes may hopefully lower the incidence of degenerative and other patency-limiting processes in newly arterialized vein grafts.

METHODS

Venous wall structural properties were evaluated in canine jugular veins by a modified in vitro stress/strain analytic system developed in this laboratory. A specially designed hydraulic chamber was filled with saline after elimination of all air by CO_2 insufflation. A pressure transducer was mounted on a sideport and calibrated. A small segment of longitudinally opened vein was mounted onto the chamber between circular washers, which allowed a 1 cm. diameter section to protrude. Via another port, a measured constant volume infusion was begun and the resulting increments of pressure recorded on a standard multiple-channel recorder. The infusion was continued throughout a pressure range of 0 to 250 mm. Hg, and the original and final arc radius of the expanding vein segments was measured with a modified caliper. From the changes in arc radius and the pressure/volume curves, both wall tension or stress and resulting elongation or strain were geometrically computed, as previously described.[11]

The stress/strain characteristics of any material have been classically expressed as a modulus of elasticity or Young's modulus, which is the quotient of dividing stress by its resulting strain according to Hooke's law. However, in biologic systems which are nonlinear, a single modulus of elasticity is, of course, inaccurate. Therefore, an incremental modulus of elasticity has been used to denote varying elasticities throughout a wide pressure range,[9] as in previous experiments in this laboratory where the incremental moduli have been described for normal artery, vein, and heart valve cusps.[1, 11] Even normal tissue, however, varies considerably between individual animals. We have recently found that a more accurate expression of elasticity is gained from graphing tension or stress as a function of strain, that is, a stress/strain curve. Comparison of the stress/strain curves of fresh and modified specimens, not only from the same animal but also from the same vein, have provided meaningful data in small numbers of experiments. Paired t tests from equivalent data points were performed by stress/strain comparisons at arbitrary stress levels of 10, 40, 100, and 200 dynes per square centimeter $\times$ 10.[4]

Two preparative measures, hydrostatic dilatation and short-term immersion, were studied in such a system. Long lengths of excised canine jugular vein had a specially tipped needle inserted into one end and were gently cleared of blood with heparinized saline solution. One segment of the vein was immediately tested for its stress/strain characteristics as a fresh, undistended control. The remaining segment was ligated and then hydrostatically dilated with a syringe containing heparinized normal saline. The syringe was coupled to a pressure monitor, and hydrostatic pressure controlled under direct vision. In the first group of experiments hydrostatic dilatation was carried out to 300 mm. Hg with a single injection. In a second group hydrostatic dilatation was carried out to 1,000 mm. Hg.

Veins for immersion experiments were similarly prepared with one portion immediately tested as a fresh control. A series of variables was then studied. Immersion media composition was analyzed by comparing the effects of immersing the vein in chilled (4° C.) normal saline, Ringer's lactate, and Hanks Balanced Salt Solution with 10 percent homologous serum (HBSSP) for periods of 4 and 24 hours. The effect of temperature was evaluated by comparing 4 hour immersions in 4° and 37° C. HBSSP. The effect of media pH was studied by varying the pH of HBSSP with hydrochloric acid or sodium hydroxide titrations. Immersions in media of pH 4.7,

Table I. *The effect of 300 mm. Hg dilatation on venous elasticity*

	Tension (dynes/cm.²)			
	10^5	4×10^5	10^6	2×10^6
Control	1.33	1.55	1.63	1.67
300 mm. Hg	1.26	1.40	1.45	1.48
P	< 0.01	< 0.01	< 0.01	< 0.05

Table II. *The effect of 1,000 mm. Hg dilatation on venous elasticity*

	Tension (dynes/cm.²)			
	10^5	4×10^5	10^6	2×10^6
Control	1.29	1.41	1.45	1.45
1,000 mm. Hg	1.20	1.26	1.28	1.31
P	< 0.01	< 0.01	< 0.01	< 0.01

5.9, 7.0, 7.4, and 8.1 for 4 hours at 4° C. were evaluated. To better understand the changes observed, veins were exposed to 0.05 percent solutions of collagenase and elastase for 60 minutes at 37° C. and compared to untreated controls. Finally, the effects of the homologous serum added to the HBSS were tested by comparing 24 hour immersions in 4° C. balanced salt solution with and without added protein.

RESULTS

Hydrostatic dilatation. Hydrostatic dilatation of canine jugular vein to both 300 and 1,000 mm. Hg was associated with significant ($p < 0.01$) stiffening of the vein, as can be seen in Tables I and II, which was indicated by a lessened strain or elongation with each given increment of stress. The relationship between the two distending pressures is more clearly seen in Fig. 1, where stiffening appears as a shift to the left in the curve with a steeper, flatter slope. Although the alterations were considerable after 300 mm. Hg distension, they were even more pronounced after distension to 1,000 mm. Hg. However, even minimal distension of the vein to pressures slightly greater than arterial levels is potentially harmful.

Table III. *The effect of media composition on venous elasticity*

	Tension (dynes/cm.²)			
	10^5	4×10^5	10^6	2×10^6
Control	1.26	1.34	1.37	1.40
HBSS*	1.28	1.35	1.38	1.40
NS†	1.31	1.40	1.43	1.46
P (NS vs. HBSS)	NS	NS	< 0.05	< 0.05

*Immersed 4 hours at 4° C. in Hanks Balanced Salt solution (HBSS).

†Immersed 4 hours at 4° C. in normal Saline (NS).

Table IV. *The effect of media pH on venous elasticity*

	Tension (dynes/cm.²)			
	10^5	4×10^5	10^6	2×10^6
Acidic (pH 4.7)*	1.19	1.26	1.29†	1.32†
Control	1.24	1.32	1.35	1.37
Neutral (pH 7.0)*	1.28	1.35	1.38	1.40
Alkaline (pH 8.0)*	1.38	1.59†	1.66†	1.69†

*Immersed 4 hours at 4° C.

†Different from control P < 0.05.

Media composition. In contrast to hydrostatic dilatation, the effects on venous wall properties after immersion were manifested in the opposite direction, i.e., increased distensibility. Table III shows that even after 4 hours significant changes ($p < 0.05$) were detected. The changes after immersion in chilled Ringer's lactate solution were virtually identical (data not shown). Fig. 2 illustrates that the increases in distensibility or elasticity were cumulative with time, since they were exaggerated after the longer (24 hour) period. Table III also shows a better retention of normal stress/strain relationships after immersion in balanced salt solution (HBSS).

Media temperature. The previous experiments were conducted at 4° C. Fig. 3 compares the curve after immersion in HBSSP for 4 hours at 4° C. with that after similar immersion at 37° C. Warm temperature immersion produced greater increases in distensibility than did immersion in any chilled

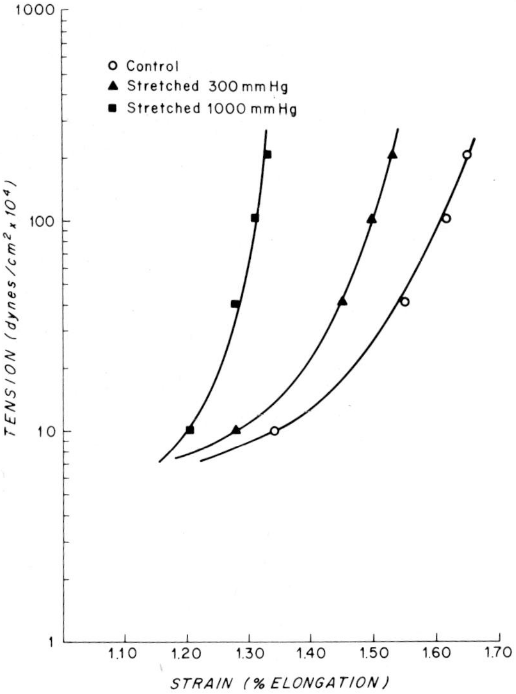

Fig. 1. The effect of dilatation on venous elasticity. Curves after hydrostatic dilatation show an increased stiffening in veins after 300 mm. Hg distension, which is even more marked after 1,000 mm. Hg distension.

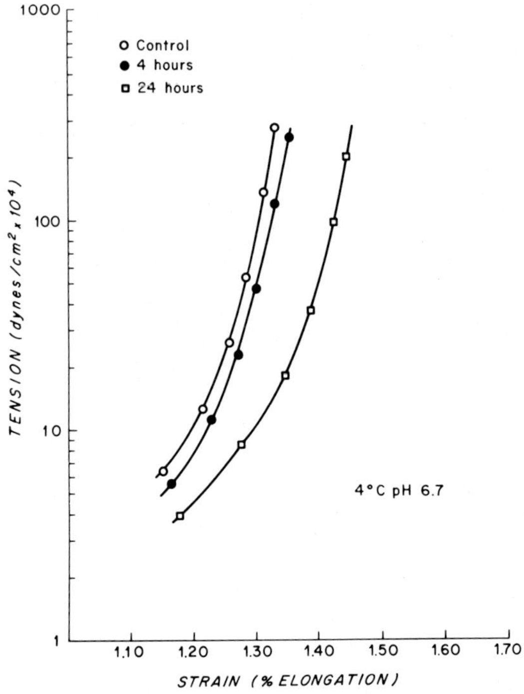

Fig. 2. The effect of normal saline storage on venous elasticity. Curves after immersion in 4° C. normal saline for 4 to 24 hours reveal an increased distensibility which is cumulative with time.

solution, in spite of what previous experiments have shown to be an excellent media composition.

Media pH. Studies in which the pH of the immersion media was varied provided interesting results, as illustrated in Table IV. Acidity was associated with increased stiffness, and alkalinity was associated with increased distensibility ($p < 0.05$). In experiments where balanced salt solution seemed superior to simple crystalloid solution, its pH was 7.4. Fig. 4, however, shows the optimum pH for immersion of venous structures was 7.0, where the curve after immersion most approximated that of the fresh control and was certainly superior to a pH of 7.4 in this regard.

Enzymatic effects. Fig. 5 depicts the effects after exposure to enzymatic solutions for short periods. Treatment with elastase was associated with marked stiffening of the vein, whereas collagenase induced as great a degree of increased distensibility as was observed in any experiment. Both of these effects illustrate the relative contributions of the two main structural components of the venous wall.

Media protein. In all previous experiments using balanced salt solution, such media contained 10 percent homologous protein. The final experiment compared immersion of veins in HBSS, pH 7.0, with and without 10 percent serum for 24 hours at 4° C. Fig. 6 illustrates that even prolonged immersion in either solution, longer than that ever employed clinically, was not associated with changes in stress/strain relationships. Since deletion of the protein was not associated with any significant difference, it might be concluded that its presence is not important.

DISCUSSION

Of the several explanations for the now well-documented failures of autogenous venous bypass grafting, two have received the

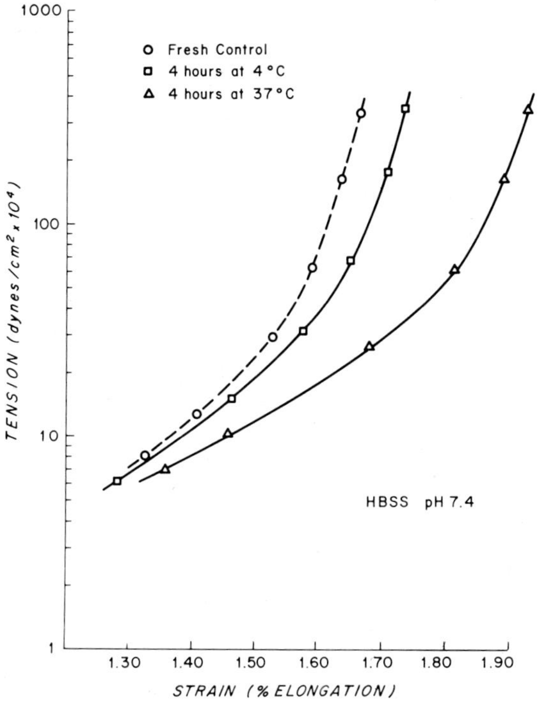

Fig. 3. The effect of temperature on venous elasticity. Curves comparing immersion in HBSSP for 4 hours at 4° and 37° C. reveal a marked exaggeration of changes in the warm media, as compared to the chilled.

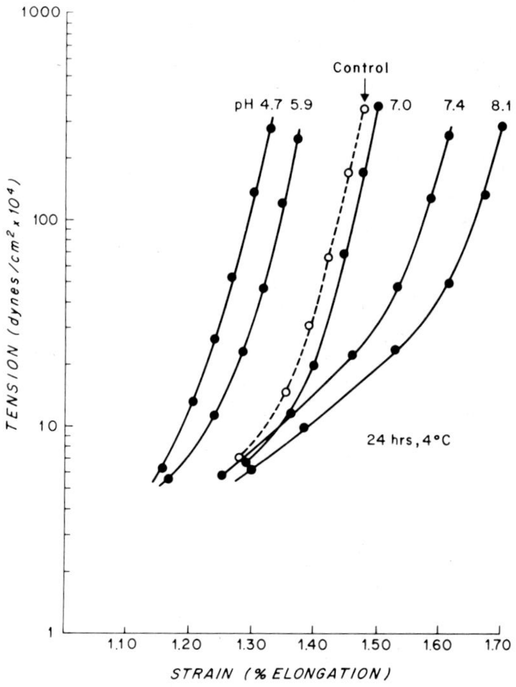

Fig. 4. The effect of media pH on venous elasticity. Curves after immersion in HBSSP of varying pH. Acidic media are associated with stiffening; alkaline media are associated with increased distensibility. The curve for pH 7.0 medium most nearly approximates that of the fresh control.

most attention: progression of the atherosclerotic disease process in proximal and distal arterial segments and degenerative changes in the vein grafts themselves. Of the two, disease progression has been supposed to be the more likely contributive factor, in view of the fact that the saphenous vein serves very satisfactorily for up to 10 years or longer in situations such as trauma, i.e., those not associated with atherosclerosis obliterans.[8] However, since vein grafts are now known to undergo degenerative processes in both the femoropopliteal[15] and the aortocoronary[16] positions in patients with occlusive disease, part of the problem may well lie within the vein grafts themselves after placement into a disease-prone arterial circulation. This possibility is supported by observations that femoropopliteal reconstruction in patients under 50 years of age has a much less satisfactory result than in those over 60.[2] In general, coronary artery reconstruction is carried out in a younger age group than is femoropopliteal bypass reconstruction. This may explain why the previously mentioned subintimal proliferative processes have been documented in the former anatomic location more frequently than in the latter.

The studies reported herein attempt to gain better understanding of the failures of venous bypass grafts. They are based upon an hypothesis that preinsertion preparative techniques may in some way be implicated in subsequent events. Indirect support for this hypothesis comes from the recent report by Grondin and associates,[7] who showed radiographically that changes in coronary artery vein grafts seemed to occur early and then stabilized at something less than one year.[7] Direct support for this hypothesis comes from the results reported here, which illustrate that two preparative maneuvers are acutely associated with changes in venous wall structural properties or elasticity, as

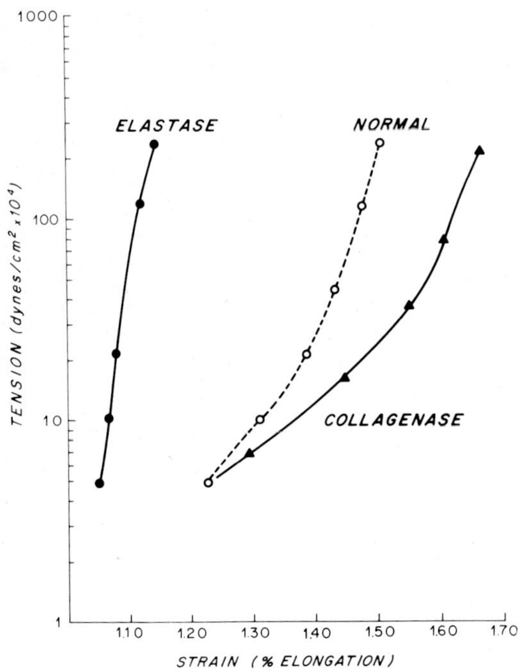

Fig. 5. Tension-strain. Curves after exposure to enzymes illustrate stiffening with elastase and increased distensibility with collagenase.

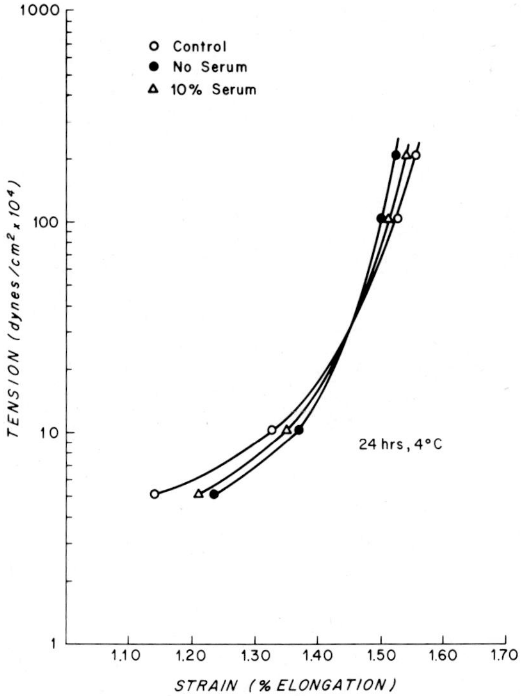

Fig. 6. The effect of serum on HBSS storage. Curves after 24 hour immersion in HBSS with and without 10 percent serum. No significant differences from fresh control are seen with either medium.

measured in an in vitro system. The experiments not only outline these changes but also illustrate simple means of minimizing or eliminating them.

Hydrostatic dilatation, which is commonly employed to allow ligation of side branches and enlargement to facilitate anastomoses, was associated with stiffening of the vein wall. In preliminary experiments we did not look directly at the pressure monitor but used a distending pressure similar to that which we had heretofore employed in the operating room. We found that pressures of 500 to 700 mm. Hg were generated with surprisingly little effort. Using scanning electron microscopy, Ramos and Sauvage[13] have described changes in the intimal surfaces of veins after hydrostatic dilatation. These observations, plus those described above, provide sufficient evidence to recommend avoiding distension or minimizing it by pressure monitoring to within the arterial pressure range—a technique easily applied in the clinical setting.

The results of the immersion experiments show effects opposite to those of hydrostatic dilatation. With less than ideal immersion media composition, the stress/strain curves showed an increased distensibility, which reflected a loss of the ability of the vein wall to resist stretch due to pressure. This was noted more in the higher pressure or tension levels, which is not surprising, since with greater stresses there is always a greater corresponding strain. Both of the simple crystalloid solutions (normal saline and Ringer's lactate) were associated with changes and these were directly related to the duration of the immersion. It is also important that temperature seemed a more critical factor than did media composition.

Experiments altering the pH provided further understanding of the above results. With increasing acidity the vein became stiffer, whereas the opposite occurred with increasing alkalinity. It is interesting that a pH of 7.0, demonstrating the least change in structural properties, is also that of canine venous blood. The pH experiments do not wholly explain the results, since immersion in normal saline, with a usual pH of 6.6 to 6.7 was associated with increased distensibility, a result which was seen not with acidic but with alkaline solution. Thus slight acidity is not responsible for the changes after normal saline immersion.

The explanation for the changes observed probably rests with alterations in the functional ratio of collagen to elastin, which is known to control the so-called elastic properties of the vessel.[3] The enzyme studies support this, since treatment with elastase was associated with stiffening similar to that after hydrostatic dilatation. Both of these, albeit by different means, probably disrupt the fine fibrillar elastin network, leaving collagen as the sole functioning supporting element. After collagenase treatment, the curves show marked increases in distensibility similar to that seen after immersion in the alkaline, crystalloid, and warm temperature media. A common mechanism of disruption or dissolution of the collagen supporting network may also exist here. Raising the pH is known to increase the solubility of collagen,[5] which solubility may not only elucidate the findings after immersion in alkaline media but also in crystalloid and warm media as well. The fact that the changes after immersion are cumulative with time fits well into this rationale. At the outset, the crystalloid media were slightly acidic, which, on the basis of pH evidence, should lead to stiffening. However, collagen solubility is much less sensitive to acidic than to alkaline change,[5] and evidently the effects of slight acidity in saline are not as potent as those of the loss of soluble collagen. The critical experiment to clarify this was not done, i.e., to compare the changes after immersion in saline at a pH of 7.4 to those at a pH of 6.6. The interpretation is thus incomplete, since it does not fully indicate what is involved in the loss of soluble collagen nor the reasons for the fact that balanced salt solution must, therefore, favorably effect collagen solubility. Nevertheless, on the basis of available data, collagen loss does seem to be the most likely explanation.

There was little change in stress/strain characteristics in the balanced salt solution experiments with or without 10 percent homologous serum. Both curves were virtually identical to those of fresh control experiments, even after immersion for 24 hours. This might lead to an interpretation that the addition of protein is unimportant. Serum was originally included for two reasons. (1) It has definite nutrient properties and, therefore, Hanks Balanced Salt Solution with protein should be an excellent nutrient medium for veins similar to that used for storage of other soft tissues.[12] (2) In addition, the presence of protein provides osmolar or oncotic properties which should be helpful in preventing tissue swelling and electrolyte transfer, as well as in promoting the stabilization of—especially—the endothelial cell layer. Other studies have supported this rationale.[6, 10] Although the addition of protein provided little benefit in terms of stress/strain characteristics, it probably warrants inclusion for the above reasons. Thus on the basis of available evidence, probably the best solution for preinsertion immersion of veins is a balanced salt solution with 10 percent serum at 4° C. with a pH adjusted to 7.0.

The ultimate goal of these studies has been directed toward the prevention of patency-limiting changes in vein grafts. Solid conclusions in this regard are not possible from these experiments, since they were done only acutely and the veins studied were not implanted. Therefore, the changes observed may well be temporary and reversible, reverting to normal after insertion. Experiments to determine this are in progress. Long-term studies are also needed to identify whether the acute changes are associated with recognizable degenerative changes after prolonged residence within the arterial circulation. Nevertheless, since the principles described above are simple to apply and seemingly may obviate potentially hazardous alterations in venous structural properties, it would seem logical to adopt them.

REFERENCES

1. Abbott, W. M., Mundth, E. D., and Austen, W. G.: Autogenous vein grafts: Effects of simple storage on structural properties, Surg. Forum **24:** 260, 1973.
2. Bouhoutsos, J., and Martin, P.: The influence of age on prognosis after arterial surgery for atherosclerosis of the lower limb, SURGERY **74:** 637, 1973.
3. Burton, A. C.: Physiology and biophysics of the circulation, ed. 2, Chicago, 1972, Year Book Medical Publishers, Inc., Chap. 7.
4. Darling, R. C., and Linton, R. R.: Durability of femoro-popliteal reconstructions: Endarterectomy versus vein bypass grafts, Am. J. Surg. **123:** 472, 1972.
5. Elden, H. R., and Boucek, R. J.: The successive extraction of collagen from hide powder, J. Colloid Sci. **15:** 97, 1960.
6. Enerson, D. M., and Merola, J.: Cellular swelling. III. Effects of hypothermia and addition of low molecular weight dextran on oxygen consumption and electrolyte composition of isolated tissues, Ann. Surg. **165:** 244, 1967.
7. Grondin, C. M., Lesperance, J., Bourassa, M. G., et al.: Serial angiographic evaluation in 60 consecutive patients with aorto-coronary artery vein grafts 2 weeks, 1 year, and 3 years after operation, J. Thorac. Cardiovasc. Surg. **67:** 1, 1974.
8. Hershey, F. B., and Spencer, A. D.: Autogenous vein grafts for repair of arterial injuries, Arch. Surg. **86:** 836, 1963.
9. Krafka, J.: Comparative studies of the histophysics of the aorta, Am. J. Physiol. **125:** 1, 1939.
10. Mansfield, P. B.: Personal communication.
11. Mundth, E. D., Wright, J. E. C., and Austen, W. G.: Development of a method for stress/strain analysis of cardiac valvular tissue, Curr. Top. Surg. Res. **3:** 67, 1971.
12. Perry, V. P.: A review of skin preservation, Cryobiology **3:** 109, 1966.
13. Ramos, J. R., and Sauvage, L. R.: Effects of pressure and distending medium upon venous autografts in femoral artery of dog, 1974. In press.
14. Stoney, R. J., James, D. R., and Wylie, E. J.: Surgery for femoro-popliteal atherosclerosis, Arch. Surg. **103:** 548, 1971.
15. Szilagyi, D. E., Elliott, J. P., Hageman, J. H., et al.: Biologic fate of autogenous vein implants as arterial substitutes: Clinical, angiographic, and histopathologic observations in femoro-popliteal operations for atherosclerosis, Ann. Surg. **178:** 232, 1973.
16. Vlodaver, Z., and Edwards, J. E.: Pathologic changes in aortic-coronary arterial saphenous vein grafts, Circulation **44:** 719, 1971.

DISCUSSION

Dr. John Vasko (Columbus, Ohio). We, too, have been interested in this problem and have conducted some experiments that may add support to what Dr. Abbott has presented.

In our laboratories, we have examined the influences of harvesting techniques, distending pressure, and hemodynamic variables on the chronic histologic and hemodynamic changes in arterialized veins in animal preparations.

In our experience, it appears that the insults that Dr. Abbott has presented do indeed induce greater subintimal proliferation and fibrosis in the chronic animal preparation. We have also looked at the influences of angulation and have not seen any significant difference, whether the grafts originate at 90° or greater angles to the parent vessel. In short, our studies tend to corroborate the information presented by Dr. Abbott indicating that destructive chronic changes can be produced by traumatic preparation of view grafts which may be important to all of us working with vein grafts, either in the heart or peripheral circulation.

Dr. James C. Stanley (Ann Arbor, Mich.). Dr. Abbott and his colleagues have presented a unique method to assess effects of preparation media upon the physical properties of vein grafts. The conditions of their experiment bring one obvious question to mind. At pressures of 300 to 1,000 mm. Hg, what anatomic component of the vein wall is altered such that one storage solution may be identified as causing less physical derangement in comparison to others? It is intriguing to speculate on what happens to adventitial collagen and sparse elastic tissue in veins subjected to such extreme stresses. Second, I wonder if they have correlated their results with conventional length-tension studies, or, perhaps, even with tests of smooth muscle reactivity? Third, were the authors able to demonstrate a relation between altered physical properties and histologic or morphologic changes within the veins?

In this latter regard, Drs. Fry and Sottiurai and I have just completed a light and electron microscopic study of 169 canine vein segments, following storage for periods of 30, 60, 90, and 120 minutes in a balanced salt solution at 5° C., buffered culture medium at 20° C., and whole blood at 20° C. Subtle increases in ground substance and reductions in adventitial compactness were most apparent by light microscopy after salt solution storage. More obvious differences were revealed with transmission electron microscopy. Disruption of smooth muscle cell membranes, mitochondrial swelling, increases in intracellular vesicles, accumulation of interstitial fluid and cellular debris, and frequent disintegration of vasa vasoral endothelial cells all developed early and were consistently more severe after salt solution storage. These changes were less severe following culture media storage and infrequent until after 90 minutes of storage in whole blood.

It is only reasonable to keep in mind that fewer histopathologic changes following whole blood storage, as has been our experience—like the lessening of physical changes with buffered balanced salt solution to which serum has been added as just reported—represent *acute* experimental findings. Extraplolation of such findings to late graft abnormalities would appear premature. Certainly, a critical reassessment of usual vein graft procurement and preparation techniques is in order.

Dr. John A. Mannick (Boston, Mass.). I would also like to congratulate Dr. Abbott and his co-workers on an interesting paper which certainly suggests that many of us have been dialating vein grafts at the wrong pressure with the wrong solution at the wrong temperature.

And with regard to that, I have one question. Since most autogenous vein grafts in ordinary clinical practice are sutured in place with blood flowing through the lumen within one hour of removal from the body, I would like to ask Dr. Abbott if he has any studies on the effects of variations in storage conditions, i.e., crystalloid composition, temperature, and pH if the in vitro time is less than 4 hours.

Dr. D. E. Szilagyi (Detroit, Mich.). There is hardly any need to emphasize the importance of Dr. Abbott's study. It is conservatively estimated that 20,000 to 30,000 coronary and about 5,000 femoropopliteal autogenous venous bypasses are inserted every year by American surgeons. And yet, very little solid information has been published regarding the practical details of harvesting, temporarily preserving, and handling saphenous graft material. These considerations make clear the significance of the study of Dr. Abbott and his associates.

I am not certain how reliable it is to transfer information expressing the physical behavior of venous grafts in terms of stress-strain analysis to the prediction of biological behavior after implantation. It would seem to me that correlation of these findings with the results of studies dealing with more nearly biologic parameters would be desirable.

For this reason among others, it might be of interest to summarize briefly our own observations on the effects of variations in the preserving medium and ambient temperature on the physiologic and anatomic properties of vein grafts in the dog.

Observations in a series of human femoropopliteal autogenous vein grafts, recently reported by us, suggest that the untoward intrinsic changes of these implants depend on histological alterations in the smooth muscle and in the intimal complex—the endothelium and subendothelial membranes. We studied the effect of ambient temperature and various preserving media on the smooth muscle—a histologic element of high metabolic activity—by measuring oxygen consumption of appropriately prepared venous segments, and those on the intima by light and electron microscopy. We concluded that the best method for short-term preservation of the vein grafts is immersion in heparinized whole blood at a temperature of about 4° C. This method of preservation has now become a part of our routine for harvesting the greater saphenous vein for grafting. Extreme carefulness in mechanical handling and leaving the vein in situ until its dissection is completed are also details of importance. It should be added that we do not hesitate to distend the venous trunk—which is always in a state of varying degrees of spasm—by forcing blood through under sufficient pressure to restore the normal diameter of the vein.

Dr. William Abbott (Closing). The whole thrust of our laboratory effort these days is toward a better understanding of the biologic fate of the autogenous vein graft. And, so, this work really is consistent with Dr. Szylagyi's remarks, although I would certainly agree that looking at physical parameters cannot be easily translated into the biologic system.

However, the work to do that translation is in progress. And I think that Dr. Vasko's work suggests that it is going to be translatable information, since he has observed subintimal proliferative changes in veins which have been abused.

In response to Dr. Mannick's question, the answer is yes, at least as far as temperature is concerned. After one hour at 37°, if the immersion medium is saline, there are changes which are clearly demonstrable. It is more difficult to definitively demonstrate them in that short period of time using a pH-adjusted balanced salt solution.

As far as Dr. Stanley's comments are concerned, he obviously is working along the same lines as we are. First, as far as tension-length studies are concerned, we evaluated this method some time ago but were not really able to make it succeed in giving meaningful data in venous preparations.

Regarding the hydrostatic pressures, I think he is absolutely right: 300 mm. Hg pressure is a very serious insult to a structure as delicate as the vein. However, I think that you would all be surprised if you would couple the distending syringe to a pressure transducer and distend the vein, as we sometimes do in the operating room, to find what the pressures generated are. In our hands, we found we were generating pressures of 500 mm. Hg with surprising ease.

Finally morphologic studies are in progress in our laboratory and we are also seeing some of the changes that Dr. Stanley described. But it is really too premature to make much more of a correlation than that.

Index to volume 76

AUTHOR INDEX*

A

ABBOTT, WILLIAM M., WIELAND, STEVEN, AND AUSTEN, W. GERALD. Structural changes during preparation of autogenous venous grafts, 1031

ACKERMAN, LAUREN V. (*See* Donaldson et al.), 771

ACKERMAN, NORMAN B. Duodenal duplication cysts: Diagnosis and operative management, 330

ADAR, R. Bifurcation of canine abdominal aorta, 358

ADAR, RAPHAEL. Buerger's disease—the need for diagnostic criteria (letter to editors), 848

ALEXANDER-WILLIAMS, J. (*See* Donovan et al.), 729

ALKSNE, JOHN F. Myonecrosis in chronic experimental vasospasm, 1

ANTHONY, P. (*See* Karlson et al.), 935.

ARIEL, IRVING M. The use of lymphangiography in melanoma, 654

ARIMA, EITOKU. (*See* Fonkalsrud et al.), 527

ARRINGTON, PAUL J., AND McNAMARA, J. JUDSON. Effect of aspirin on microaggregate formation in banked blood, 295

ASANO, KEN-ICHI. (*See* Eguchi, Takeuchi, and Asano), 837

ASCH, MORRIS J., COHEN, ARTHUR H., AND MOORE, THOMAS C. Hepatic and splenic lymphangiomatosis with skeletal involvement: Report of a case and review of the literature, 334

ASKANAZI, JEFFREY. (*See* Neville et al.), 65

AUSTEN, W. GERALD. (*See* Abbott, Wieland, and Austen), 1031

B

BACH, J. F. (*See* Lacombe et al.), 556

BALDERSON, GLENDA. (*See* Battersby et al.) 617

BALLINGER, WALTER F. (*See* Wise and Ballinger), 811

BARSAMIAN, ERNEST M. (*See* Harken et al.), 786

BARTON, BRUCE A. (*See* O'Neill et al.), 185

—. (*See* Ravitch and Barton), 754

BATTERSBY, C., EGERTON, W. S., BALDERSON, GLENDA, KERR, J. F., AND BURNETT, W. Another look at rejection in pig liver homografts, 617

BEACH, C. (*See* Groves et al.), 533

BEBIN, JOSE. (*See* Kondo et al.), 439

BECKER, HORST, D. (*See* Watson et al.), 419

BECKER, MATHIS L. (*See* Hewitt et al.), 715

BEKASSY, SZABOLCS M. (*See* Liddicoat et al.), 845

BENFIELD, JOHN R. (*See* Drews et al.), 80

BERGENTZ, SVEN-ERIK, ERICSSON, BJÖRN, HEDNER, ULLA, LEANDOER, LENNART, AND NILSSON, INGA MARIE. Thrombosis in the superior mesenteric and portal veins: Report of a case treated with thrombectomy, 286

*July, pp. 1-198; August, pp. 199-358; September, pp. 359-526; October, pp. 527-684; November, pp. 685-848; December, pp. 849-1062.

BERGLAND, RICHARD M. "We have met the enemy and he is us" (panel discussion), 183

BERNSTEIN, DOROTHY M. (*See* DeShazo et al.), 461

BIALOSTOZKY, LEON. Painless removal of sutures, 356

BLACKBURN, GEORGE L. Myocardial glycogen, 346

BLUMENBERG, ROBERT M. (See Gelfand and Blumenberg), 504

BOLINGER, ROBERT E. (*See* Friesen, Bolinger, and Kyner), 804

BOLOOKI, HOOSHANG, THURER, RICHARD J., GHAHRAMANI, ALI, VARGAS, ABELARDO, WILLIAMS, WILLIS, AND KAISER, GERARD. Objective assessment of late results of aortocoronary bypass operation, 925

BOYD, ARTHUR D. (*See* Mullin et al.), 974

BOYDEN, CARYL MAGNUS. (*See* Moore et al.), 376

BRADLEY, E. L., III, QUINTON, D. L., MARTIN, L. G., KOURIAS, EVANGELOS, AND LAROSE, JAMES. Sinusoidal shunt fraction by radioextraction ratio, 918

BRENNAN, MURRAY F. (*See* Harken et al.), 786

BRETTSCHNEIDER, LAWRENCE. (*See* Holper et al.), 423

BROWN, ANNE. (*See* Donovan et al.), 729

BROWN, JOHN W., MYEROWITZ, P. DAVID, CANN, MICHAEL S., COLVIN, STEPHEN B., MCINTOSH, CHARLES L., AND MORROW, ANDREW G. Clinical and hemodynamic comparisons of Kay-Shiley, Starr-Edwards No. 6520, and Reis-Hancock porcine xenograft mitral valves, 983

BURKHOLDER, P. M. (*See* Malek et al.), 272

BURKO, HENRY. (*See* Dean et al.), 872

BURNETT, W. (*See* Battersby et al.), 617

BUSCH, GEORGE J. (*See* Wren et al.), 112

BUTSCH, JOHN L., AND BUTSCH, WINFIELD L. Lower abdominal tenderness following traumatic rupture of the spleen, 524

BUTSCH, WINFIELD L. (*See* Butsch and Butsch), 524

BUTTERFIELD, W. C. (*See* Rasche and Butterfield), 764

C

CALDWELL, W. L. (*See* Malek et al.), 272

CALLENDER, CLIVE O. (*See* Toledo-Pereyra et al.), 121

—, SIMMONS, RICHARD L., YUNIS, EDMUND J., TOLEDO-PEREYRA, LUIS H., DESHAZO, MAUREEN T. M., AND NAJARIAN, JOHN S. Anti-HL-A antibodies: Failure to correlate with renal allograft rejection, 573

CANAAN, SAMUEL A., JR. (*See* Donaldson et al.), 771

CANN, MICHAEL S. (*See* Brown et al.), 983

CASTANEDA, ALDO R., SADE, ROBERT M., LAMBERTI, JOHN, AND NICOLOFF, DEMETRE M. Reoperation for residual defects after repair of tetralogy of Fallot, 1010

CHARNEY, J. (*See* Lo Gerfo et al.), 16

CHEUNG, LAURENCE Y., ENGLERT, EDWIN, JR., MOODY, FRANK G., AND WALES, ENGENE E. Dissolution of gallstones with bile salts, lecithin, and heparin, 500
CLARKE, R. J. (*See* Donovan et al.), 729
COALSON, JACQUELINE J. (*See* Greenfield et al.), 560
COCKRELL, JOHN V. (*See* Kondo et al.), 447
COHEN, ARTHUR H. (*See* Asch, Cohen, and Moore), 334
COHEN, STEVEN I., GOLDMAN, LEON D., SALZMAN, EDWIN W., AND GLOTZER, DONALD J. The deleterious effect of immediate postoperative prosthesis in below-knee amputation for ischemic disease, 992
COLVIN, STEPHEN B. (*See* Brown et al.), 983
COOLEY, DENTON A. (*See* Reul et al.), 946
COOPER, G. N., JR. (*See* Karlson et al.), 935
COOPERBAND, S. R. (*See* Glasgow et al.), 35
COX, JIMMY L. (*See* Oldham et al.), 160
CRONAU, L. H. (*See* Gillis et al.), 608
CROSIER, JAMES H. (*See* Hickman et al.), 601
CUTLER, BRUCE S., THOMPSON, JESSE E., PATMAN, R. DON, PERSSON, ALFRED V., AND MANFREDI, PHILIP D. The modified bovine arterial graft: A clinical study, 963

D

DALE, W. ANDREW. The beginnings of Vascular Surgery, 849
—. (*See* Duncan, Edwards, and Dale), 1024
DALY, BENEDICT D. T., HUGHES, DAVID A., AND NORMAN, JOHN C. Alveolar morphometrics: Effects of positive end-expiratory pressure, 624
DARDENNE, M. (*See* Lacombe et al.), 556
DARDIK, HERBERT, AND DARDIK, IRVING. Axillo-axillary bypass with cephalic vein for correction of subclavian steal syndrome, 413
DARDIK, IRVING. (*See* Dardik and Dardik), 413
DEAN, RICHARD H., BURKO, HENRY, WILSON, JAMES P., MULHERIN, JOSEPH H., AND FOSTER, JOHN H. Deceptive patterns of renal artery stenosis, 872
DE BAKEY, LOIS. Reply: Authorship in scholarly journals (letter to editors), 344
DE BAKEY, MICHAEL J. (*See* Liddicoat et al.), 845
DELANCY, HERMAN, AND HITCH, WILLIAM STROUD. Solitary rectal ulcer: A cause of life-threatening hemorrhage, 830
DEMETRIOU, ACHILLES A., SEIFTER, ELI, AND LEVENSON, STANLEY M. Effect of sera obtained from normal and partially hepatectomized rats and patients on the growth of cells in tissue culture, 779
DE PALMA, RALPH G. Surgical therapy for venous stasis, 910
DESHAZO, CLAUDE V., SIMMONS, RICHARD L., BERNSTEIN, DOROTHY M., DESHAZO, MAUREEN T. M., WILLMERT, JUSTINE, AND NAJARIAN, JOHN S. Results of renal transplantation in 100 children, 461
DESHAZO, MAUREEN T. M. (*See* DeShazo et al.), 461
—. (*See* Callender et al.), 573
DEGENSHEIN, GEORGE A. Choledochoduodenostomy: An 18 year study of 175 consecutive cases, 319.
DICKSON, L. G. (*See* Filo et al.), 88
DI LUZIO, NICHOLAS R., OLCAY, ISIK, AND DRAPANAS, THEODORE. Reply to letter to editors by Gans, 353
—. (*See* Holper et al.), 423
—. (*See* Olcay et al.), 643
DONALDSON, ROBERT C., CANAAN, SAMUEL A., JR., MCLEAN, ROBERT B., AND ACKERMAN, LAUREN V. Uveitis and vitiligo associated with BCG treatment for malignant melanoma, 771
DONG, E., JR. (*See* Morris et al.), 150
DONOVAN, I. A., GUNN, I. F., BROWN, ANNE, ALEXANDER-WILLIAMS, J., AND CLARKE, R. J. A comparison of gastric emptying before and after vagotomy with antrectomy and vagotomy with pyloroplasty, 729
DOWLING, JAMES B. (*See* Hewitt et al.), 715
DOWNS, ALLAN R. (*See* Parkinson et al.), 882
DRAPANAS, THEODORE. (*See* Hewitt and Drapanas), 346
—. (*See* Di Luzio, Olcay, and Drapanas), 353
—. (*See* Holper et al.), 423
—. (*See* Olcay et al.), 643
—. (*See* Hewitt et al.), 715
DREWS, JOHN A., TIERNEY, DONALD F., AND BENFIELD, JOHN R. Effect of immunosuppression and lung transplantation upon surfactant, 80
DUNCAN, S. EDWIN, EDWARDS, WILLIAM H., AND DALE, W. ANDREW. Caution regarding autotransfusion, 1024
DUTKA, MARY F. (*See* Elizinga et al.), 482

E

EBERT, PAUL A. (*See* Ellis et al.), 142
EDWARDS, BRUCE G. (*See* Gordon et al.), 405
EDWARDS, WILLIAM H. (*See* Duncan, Edwards, and Dale), 1024
EGERTON, W. S. (*See* Battersby et al.), 617
EGUCHI, SHOJI, TAKEUCHI, YOSHIMI, AND ASANO, KEN-ICHI. Successful balloon membranotomy for obstruction of the hepatic portion of the inferior vena cava, 837
EHRLICH, H. PAUL, TARVER, HAROLD, AND HUNT, THOMAS K. Proteolysis of preformed protein in wound nutrition, 263
EISEMAN, B. The academic surgical body count, 367
EKWUEME, O., AND FORREST, A. P. M. Lymphocyte output by the isolated perfused rabbit thymus, 794
ELIAS, E. G. (*See* Karakousis and Elias), 674
ELKINS, RONALD C., PEYTON, MARVIN D., AND GREENFIELD, LAZAR J. Pulmonary vascular impedance in chronic pulmonary hypertension, 57
—. (*See* Greenfield et al.), 560
ELLIS, ROBERT J., ZABRISKIE, JOHN B., AND EBERT, PAUL A. Tolerance to myocardial tissue allografts by pretreatment with cross-reactive streptococcal membrane antigen, 142
ELIZINGA, WILLIAM E., SKINNER, DAVID B., DUTKA, MARY F., AND GOTT, VINCENT L. Coronary blood flow and myocardial reactive hyperemia in the ischemic dog heart, 482
ENGELMAN, RICHARD M. (*See* Mullin et al.), 974
ENGLERT, EDWIN, JR. (*See* Cheung et al.), 500
ERICSSON, BJÖRN. (*See* Bergentz et al.), 286
ERNST, CALVIN B. (*See* Sachatello, Ernst, and Griffen), 1002
EVANS, WILLIAM E. Long-term evaluation of the celiac band syndrome, 867

F

FARACI, ROBERT P. In vitro demonstration of altered antigenicity of metastases from a primary methylcholanthrene-induced sarcoma, 469
FILO, R. S., DICKSON, L. G., SUBA, E. A., AND SELL, K. W. Immunologic injury induced by ex vivo perfusion of canine renal autografts, 88
FINK, RICHARD W. (*See* Schwartz et al.), 325
FITE, FULTON W. (*See* Hagood, Mozersky, and Fite), 671
FLAXMAN, B. A. (*See* Goldman et al.), 50
FONKALSRUD, ERIC W., HIGASHIJIMA, ISAO, SARWAT, ABDEL K., ARIMA, EITOKU, AND SANCHEZ, MANUEL. Evaluation of pulmonary function in the ischemic, nonventilated canine lung, 527
FORREST, A. P. M. (*See* Ekueme and Forrest), 794
FORTNER, JOSEPH G. (*See* Kim and Fortner), 357
FOSTER, JOHN H. (*See* Dean et al.), 872
FRIEDMAN, ELI A. (*See* Girardet, Friedman, and Karlson), 267
FRIEDMAN, EUGENE W. (*See* Schwartz et al.), 325
FRIESEN, STANLEY R., BOLINGER, ROBERT E., AND KYNER, JOSEPH L. The influence of glucose on gastrin and insulin release in the enteroinsular axis, 804
FRY, WILLIAM J. (*See* Stanley and Fry), 898

G

GAJL-PECZALSKA, KAZIMIERA Y. (*See* Miller et al.), 129
GALLETTI, P. M. (*See* Karlson et al.), 935
GANS, H. Phagocytosis, 352
GAZZOLA, L. M., HIRSCH, S. A., AND KAUFER, G. I. Femorofemoral bypass, 841
GELFAND, MICHAEL L., AND BLUMENBERG, ROBERT M. A technique for in situ repair of bipolar transvenous pacemaker electrode, 504
GHAHRAMANI, ALI. (*See* Bolooki et al.), 925
GILDER, HELENA, AND MCSHERRY, CHARLES K. Mechanisms of oxygen inhibition of pulmonary surfactant synthesis, 72
GILLIS, C. N., CRONAU, L. H., GREENE, N. M., AND HAMMOND, G. L. Removal of 5-hydroxytryptamine and norepinephrine from the pulmonary vascular space of man: Influence of cardiopulmonary bypass and pulmonary arterial pressure on these processes, 608
GIRARDET, ROLAND, FRIEDMAN, ELI A., AND KARLSON, KARL E. Rabbit anti–rat lymphocyte serum-induced lymphopenia in thoracic duct lymph and peripheral blood, 267
GLASGOW, A. H., MENZOIAN, J. O., NIMBERG, R. B., COOPERBAND, S. R., SCHMID, K., AND MANNICK, J. A. An immunosuppressive peptide fraction in the serum of cancer patients, 35
GLASSMAN, EPHRAIM. (*See* Mullin et al.), 974
GLOTZER, DONALD J. (*See* Cohen et al.), 992
GOETZ, FREDERICK C. (*See* Spanos et al.), 741
GOLDBERG, MARVIN E. (*See* Spanos et al.), 252
GOLDMAN, LEON D. (*See* Cohen et al.), 992
GOLDMAN, LEONARD I., FLAXMAN, B. A., WERNICK, G., AND ZABRISKIE, J. B. Immune surveillance and tumor dissemination: In vitro comparison of the B_{16} melanoma in primary and metastatic form, 50
GOODWIN, DAVID A. (*See* Vistnes et al.), 291
GORDON, MICHAEL J., SKILLMAN, JOHN J., EDWARDS, BRUCE G., AND SILEN, WILLIAM. Effect of ethanol, acetylsalicylic acid, acetaminophen, and ferrous sulfate on gastric mucosal permeability in man, 405
GOTT, VINCENT L. (*See* Elzinga et al.), 482
GRANGER, GALE A., AND MOORE, THOMAS C. Accumulation of lymphotoxin-secreting lymphoid cells in rat heart allografts, 542
GREENBERG, S. DONALD. (*See* Reul et al.), 546
GREENE, N. M. (*See* Gillis et al.), 608
GREENFIELD, LAZAR J. (*See* Elkins et al.), 57
—. JACKSON, RICHARD H., ELKINS, RONALD C., COALSON, JACQUELINE J., AND HINSHAW, LERNER B. Cardiopulmonary effects of volume loading of primates in endotoxin shock, 560
GRIFFEN, WARD O., JR. (*See* Sachatello, Ernst, and Griffen), 1002
GRIFFITH, CHARLES A. Anatomic approach to vagotomy, 350
GRIFFITHS, CERI M. (*See* Knight and Griffiths), 238
GROVES, A. C., WOOLF, L. I., O'REGAN, P. J., BEACH, C., HASINOFF, C., AND SUTHERLAND, W. H. Impaired gluconeogenesis in dogs with *E. coli* bacteremia, 533
GRUBER, RONALD P. (*See* Vistnes et al.), 291
GULLICKSON, MILES J. Value of intraoperative tests in vagotomy, 357
GUNN, I. F. (*See* Donovan et al.), 729

H

HAAGENSEN, C. D. The choice of treatment for operable carcinoma of the breast, 685
HAGOOD, CLYDE O., JR., MOZERSKY, DAVID J., AND FITE, FULTON W. Staged palliative resection of recurrent carcinoma of the neck using an extra anatomic carotid bypass, 671
HALLER, J. ALEX, JR. (*See* White, Oh, and Haller), 398
HALLMAN, GRADY L. (*See* Reul et al.), 946
HALMAGYI, DENIS F. J., KARIS, J. H., STENNING, F. G., AND VARGA, D. Pulmonary hypertension in acute hemorrhagic pancreatitis, 637
HAMMOND, G. L. (*See* Gillis et al.), 608
HANG-LONG, ZHENG. (*See* Satomura et al.), 581
HARA, KEIBUN. (*See* Satomura et al.), 581
HARDAWAY, ROBERT M., III. Disseminated intravascular coagulation (letter to editors), 682
HARDY, JAMES D. (*See* Kondo et al.), 439
—. (*See* Kondo et al.), 447
HARKEN, ALDEN H., BRENNAN, MURRAY F., SMITH, BEVERLY, AND BARSAMIAN, ERNEST M. The hemodynamic response to positive end-expiratory ventilation in hypovolemic patients, 786
HASINOFF, C. (*See* Groves et al.), 533
HATTLER, BRACK G., JR. (*See* Miller et al.), 129
HAYES, MICHAEL. (*See* Moore and Hayes), 587
HAYS, ROBERT J. (*See* Thal et al.), 955
HEDNER, ULLA. (*See* Bergentz et al.), 286
HEWITT, ROBERT L., AND DRAPANAS, THEODORE. Reply to letter to editors by Blackburn, 346
—, —, SMITH, ARNETT D., BECKER, MATHIS L., LINDSEY, EDWARD S., AND DOWLING, JAMES B. Penetrating vascular injuries of the thoracic outlet, 715

HICKMAN, ROSEMARY, CROSIER, JAMES H., SAUNDERS, STUART J., AND TERBLANCHE, JOHN. Transhepatic metabolism after end-to-side portacaval shunt in the young pig, 601
HIGASHIJIMA, ISAO. (*See* Fonkalsrud et al.), 527
HINSHAW, LERNER B. (*See* Greenfield et al.), 560
HIRSCH, S. A. (*See* Gazzola, Hirsch, and Kaufer), 841
HITCH, WILLIAM STROUD. (*See* Delancy and Hitch), 830
HOLCOMBE, R. GORDON, JR., A splendid statement on a taboo subject, 345
HOLPER, KLAUS, OLCAY, ISIK, KITAHAMA, AKIO, MILLER, ROBERT H., BRETTSCHNEIDER, LAWRENCE, DRAPANAS, THEODORE, TREJO, RAFAEL A., DI LUZIO, NICHOLAS R. Effect of ischemia on hepatic parenchymal and reticuloendothelial function in the baboon, 423
—. (*See* Olcay et al.), 643
HOWARD, R. J. (*See* Nowygrod et al.), 630
HUGHES, DAVID A. (*See* Daly, Hughes, and Norman), 624
HUGHES, EDWARD F. X. The demand for surgical residents: Some preliminary observations (panel discussion), 176
HUMPHREYS, J. W., JR. Changes and trends in graduate medical education nd credentialling, 243
HUNT, THOMAS K. (*See* Ehrlich, Tarver, and Hunt), 263

I

IKEDA, KEIICHI. (*See* Koga, Ikeda, and Inokuchi), 278
INOKUCHI, KIYOSHI. (*See* Koga, Ikeda, and Inokuchi), 278
ISOM, O. WAYNE. (*See* Mullin et al.), 974

J

JACKSON, RICHARD H. (*See* Greenfield et al.), 560
JESSEPH, JOHN E. (*See* Lowe, Winegarner, and Jesseph), 511
JOHNSTON, KENT. (*See* Schlenker, Johnston, and Wolkoff), 833

K

KAISER, GERARD. (*See* Bolooki et al.), 925
KAKVAN, M. (*See* Karlson et al.), 935
KALEMBA, JÓZEF, AND LAZARKIEWICZ, BOGDAN. New method of reconstruction of the alimentary canal after total gastrectomy, 748
KANE, PETER B. (*See* Neville et al.), 65
KARAKOUSIS, G. P., AND ELIAS, E. G. Spontaneous (pathologic) rupture of spleen in malignancies, 674
KARIS, J. H. (*See* Halmagyi et al.), 637
KARLSON, K. E., MURPHY, W. R., KAKVAN, M., ANTHONY, P., COOPER, G. N., JR., RICHARDSON, P. D., AND GALLETTI, P. M. Total cardiopulmonary bypass with a new microporous Teflon membrane oxygenator, 935
—. (*See* Girardet, Friedman, and Karlson), 267
KATSKE, GORDON E. (*See* Wren et al.), 112
KATZ, LOIS A. (*See* Zerbino et al.), 1018
KAUFER, G. I. (*See* Gazzola, Hirsch, and Kaufer), 841
KAWAI, YOSHIO. (*See* Matsumoto, Kawai, and Kimura), 827
KAWARADA, Y., SATINSKY, S., AND MATSUMOTO, T. Ischemic colitis following rectal prolapse, 340
KAWASHIMA, YASUNARU, YAMAMOTO, ZENGO, AND MANABE, HISAO. Safe limits of hemodilution in cardiopulmonary bypass, 391
KAY, JEROME HAROLD. (*See* Yamamoto et al.), 678
KELLY, KEITH A. British surgery today: Perspective of a James IV surgical traveler, 433
KERN, DAVID H. (*See* Pilch et al.), 23
KERR, J. F. (*See* Battersby et al.), 617
KERSTEIN, M. D. (*See* Sherck, Kerstein, and Stansel), 209
KIM, DONG K., AND FORTNER, JOSEPH G. Central venous catheter maintenance, 357
KIMURA, KEN. (*See* Matsumoto, Kawai, and Kimura), 827
KINOSHITA, KENICHI. (*See* Satomura et al.), 581
KISAKA, YOSHIHIKO. (*See* Satomura et al.), 581
KITAHAMA, AKIO. (*See* Holper et al.), 423
—. (*See* Olcay et al.), 643
KJELLSTRAND, CARL M. (*See* Spanos et al.), 741
KNIGHT, MICHAEL J., AND GRIFFITHS, CERI M. Attitudes of British graduates on surgical research fellowships in the United States, 238
KNUTSON, CARL O., AND WATSON, FRANCIS R. Preliminary results of a computer logic program for the operative management of colon cancer, 298
KOGA, YOSHIKO, IKEDA, KEIICHI, AND INOKUCHI, KIYOSHI. Effect of complete parenteral nutrition including fat emulsion on plasma lipid, 278
KOMAKI, KATSUHIKO. (*See* Satomura et al.), 581
KONDO, YOSHIO, TURNER, M. DON, BEBIN, JOSE, AND HARDY, JAMES D. Body responses and recovery after 2½ hour hypothermic circulatory arrest, 439
—, —, COCKRELL, JOHN V., AND HARDY, JAMES D. Ischemic tolerance of the canine autotransplanted lung, 447
KOPPENHEFFER, THOMAS L. (*See* Wren et al.), 112
KOURIAS, EVANGELOS. (*See* Bradley et al.), 918
KSANDER, GEORGE A. (*See* Vistnes et al.), 291
KUMADA, KAORU. (*See* Satomura et al.), 581
KYNER, JOSEPH L. (*See* Friesen, Bolinger, and Kyner), 804
KYRIAKIDES, GEORGE. (*See* Miller et al.), 129

L

LACOMBE, M., PERNER, F., DARDENNE, M., AND BACH, J. F. Thymectomy in the young pig: Effects on the level of circulating thymic hormone, 556
LAGRONE, LAVENIA. (*See* Watson et al.), 419
LAMBERTI, JOHN. (*See* Castaneda et al.), 1010
LAMPE, ERNEST. (*See* Spanos et al.), 741
LANDING, BENJAMIN H. (*See* Mahour et al.), 309
LAROSE, JAMES. (*See* Bradley et al.), 918
LAVIN, JOHN H. Is the author the writer? Who cares, 344
LAZARKIEWICZ, BOGDAN. (*See* Kalemba and Lazarkiewicz), 748
LEANDOER, LENNART. (*See* Bergentz et al.), 286
LEAPE, LUCIAN L. Physician supply, residency programs, and the foreign medical graduate, 372
LEDDICOTTE, GEORGE W. (*See* Schwartz et al.), 325
LEE, HYUNG M. (*See* Pierce and Lee), 101
LEMMI, CARLOS A. E. (*See* Moore et al.), 733
LEVEEN, HARRY H. Reply to letter to editors by Mozersky, 355
LEVENSON, STANLEY M. (*See* Demetriou, Seifter, and Levenson), 779

LIDDICOAT, JOHN E., BEKASSY, SZABOLCS M., O'DONNELL, MANUS J., AND DE BAKEY, MICHAEL E. Coronary artery aneurysms in a 9-year-old child, 845
LIFTON, JUDITH. (*See* Miller et al.), 129
LILLY, J. R. (*See* Weintraub, Lilly, and Randolph), 490
LINDSEY, EDWARD S. (*See* Hewitt et al.), 715
LOGERFO, FRANK W. An inverted Dacron patch graft, 525
—, AND MASON, G. ROBERT. Directional Doppler studies of supraorbital artery flow in internal carotid stenosis and occlusion, 723
LO GERFO, P., SILVERSTEIN, G., AND CHARNEY, J. Radioimmunoassay for mouse mammary tumor virus–associated antigen, 16
LOKICH, JACOB. (*See* Moore et al.), 376
LOWE, DANIEL K., WINEGARNER, FREDERICK G., AND JESSEPH, JOHN E. Cystic adventitial degeneration of the common femoral artery, 511

M

MADDEN, JOHN W., MORTON, DUNCAN, JR., AND PEACOCK, ERLE E., JR. Contraction of experimental wounds. I. Inhibiting wound contraction by using a topical smooth muscle antagonist, 8
MAGIDSON, OSCAR. (*See* Yamamoto et al.), 678
MAHOUR, G. HOSSEIN, WOOLLEY, MORTON M., TRIVEDI, SULOCHANA N., AND LANDING, BENJAMIN H. Teratomas in infancy and childhood: Experience with 81 cases, 309
MALEK, G. H., RICHARDS, M. J. S., BURKHOLDER, P. M., AND CALDWELL, W. L. Effect of single dose irradiation on isolated perfused canine kidney, 272
MANABE, HISAO. (*See* Kawashima, Yamamoto, and Manabe), 391
MANFREDI, PHILIP D. (*See* Cutler et al.), 963
MANNICK, J. A. (*See* Glasgow et al.), 35
MARTIN, L. G. (*See* Bradley et al.), 918
MARTINS, ANTONIO C. P. (*See* Wren et al.), 112
MATHES, STEPHEN J., AND SALAM, ATEF A. Subclavian artery aneurysm; sequela of thoracic outlet syndrome, 506
MATSUMOTO, T. (*See* Kawarada, Satinsky, and Matsumoto), 340
MATSUMOTO, YOICHI, KAWAI, YOSHIO, AND KIMURA, KEN. Aberrant pancreas causing pyloric obstruction, 827
MATTOX, KENNETH L. (*See* Reul et al.), 546
MASON, G. ROBERT. (*See* LoGerfo and Mason), 723
MCALPIN, COLUMBUS D. (*See* Moore et al.), 733
MCDONALD, JOHN C. (*See* Tajima and McDonald), 259
MCGOON, DWIGHT C. (*See* Satava and McGoon), 454
MCINTOSH, CHARLES L. (*See* Brown et al.), 983
MCLEAN, ROBERT B. (*See* Donaldson et al.), 771
MCNAMARA, J. JUDSON. (*See* Arrington and McNamara), 295
MCSHERRY, CHARLES K. (*See* Gilder and McSherry), 72
MENDEZ, A. MICHAEL. (*See* Yamamoto et al.), 678
MENZOIAN, J. O. (*See* Glasgow et. al.), 35
MILLER, JOSHUA, LIFTON, JUDITH, ROOD, FAYE, KYRIAKIDES, GEORGE, GAJL-PECZALSKA, KAZIMIERA Y., YUNIS, EDMOND J., AND HATTLER, BRACK G., JR., Functional characterization of blocking antibody after human renal transplantation, 129
MILLER, LEONARD D. The training of surgeons: How many, in what, and by whom? (panel discussion), 170
MILLER, ROBERT H. (*See* Holper et al.), 423
—. (*See* Olcay et al.), 643
MIYATA, MASAHIKO, SATANI, MINORU, UEDA, TAKASHI, AND OKAMOTO, EIZO. Long-term results of hepatic portoenterostomy for biliary atresia: Special reference to postoperative portal hypertension, 234
MOORE, FRANCIS D. Reduction in the surgical training program of the United States: Warnings for the unwary (panel discussion), 192
—, VANDEVANTER, SUSAN BLAND, BOYDEN, CARYL MAGNUS, LOKICH, JACOB, AND WILSON, RICHARD E. Adrenalectomy with chemotherapy in the treatment of advanced breast cancer: Objective and subjective response rates; duration and quality of life, 376
MOODY, FRANK G. (*See* Cheung et al.), 500
MOORE, THOMAS C. (*See* Asch, Cohen, and Moore), 334
—. (*See* Granger and Moore), 542
—, AND HAYES, MICHAEL. Combined use of ^{131}I hippurate blood clearance and bladder/kidney ratio data in the early detection, classification, and management of accelerated rejection of human renal transplants, 587
—, SINCLAIR, MICHAEL C., MCALPIN, COLUMBUS D., WEBER, GRIFFITH A., AND LEMMI, CARLOS A. E. Effect of aging, organ allografting, and surgical stress on rat thymus histidine decarboxylase activity, 733
MORRIS, R. E., SOUTHER, S. G., DONG, E., JR., VISTNES, L. M., AND SHUMWAY, N. E. Prolongation of rat cardiac allograft survival by a new immunosuppressant: Chicken anti–rat lymphoocyte globulin, 150
MORROW, ANDREW G. (*See* Brown et al.), 983
MORTON, DUNCAN, JR. (*See* Madden et al.), 8
MOZERSKY, DAVID J. Subclavian steal syndrome, 355
—. (*See* Hagood, Mozersky, and Fite), 671
MULHERIN, JOSEPH H. (*See* Dean et al.), 872
MULLIN, MICHAEL J., ENGELMAN, RICHARD M., ISOM, O. WAYNE, BOYD, ARTHUR D., GLASSMAN, EPHRAIM, AND SPENCER, FRANK C. Experience with open mitral commissurotomy in 100 consecutive patients, 974
MURPHY, W. R. (*See* Karlson et al.), 935
MYEROWITZ, P. DAVID. (*See* Brown et al.), 983

N

NAJARIAN, JOHN S. (*See* Toledo-Pereyra et al.), 121
—. (*See* Spanos et al.), 252
—. (*See* Toledo-Pereyra et al.), 474
—. (*See* DeShazo et al.), 461
—. (*See* Nowygrod et al.), 630
—. (*See* Callender et al.), 573
—. (*See* Spanos et al.), 741
NEVILLE, JOHN F., JR., ASKANAZI, JEFFREY, KANE, PETER B., AND WEBB, WATTS R. Airway resistance regulation of dynamic compliance, 65
NICOLOFF, DEMETRE M. (*See* Castaneda et al.), 1010
NIDUS, BERNARD D. (*See* Zerbino et al.), 1018
NILSSON, INGA MARIE. (*See* Bergentz et al.), 286

NIMBERG, R. B. (*See* Glasgow et al.), 35
NORMAN, JOHN C. (*See* Daly, Hughes, and Norman), 624
NOWYGROD, R., SUTHERLAND, D. E. R., HOWARD, R. J., AND NAJARIAN, J. S. Allograft tolerance in the absence of circulating antibodies, 630

O

O'DONNELL, MANUS J. (*See* Liddicoat et al.), 845
OKAMOTO, EIZO. (*See* Miyata et al.), 234
OH, KOOK SANG. (*See* White, Oh, and Haller), 398
OHNISHI, SATOSHI. (*See* Satomura et al.), 581
OLCAY, ISIK. (*See* Di Luzio, Olcay, and Drapanas), 353
—. (*See* Holper et al.), 423
—, HOLPER, KLAUS, KITAHAMA, AKIO, MILLER, ROBERT H., DRAPANAS, THEODORE, TREJO, RAFAEL A., DI LUZIO, NICHOLAS R. Reticuloendothelial function: Determinant for survival following hepatic ischemia in baboon, 643
OLDHAM, H. NEWLAND, JR., COX, JIMMY L., PASS, HARVEY I., WECHSLER, ANDREW S., AND SABISTON, DAVID C., JR. Effects of pulmonary embolism on regional myocardial blood flow, 160
O'NEILL, JAMES A., JR., RAVITCH, MARK M., AND BARTON, BRUCE, A. A model for evaluation of surgical manpower needs—Pediatric Surgery (panel discussion), 185
O'REGAN, P. J. (*See* Groves et al.), 533

P

PARKINSON, DWIGHT, DOWNS, ALLAN R., WHYTEHEAD, LAWRENCE L., AND SYSLAK, WALTER B. Carotid cavernous fistula: Direct repair with preservation of carotid, 882
PARKS, LEON C., SMITH, WILLIAM J., AND WILLIAMS, G. MELVILLE. Distinction of allogeneic immunity from tumor-specific immunity in man, 43
PATMAN, R. DON. (*See* Cutler et al.), 963
PASS, HARVEY I. (*See* Oldham et al.), 160
PATEY, DAVID. Debridement, 347
PEACOCK, ERLE E., JR., (*See* Madden et al.), 8
PERNER, F. (*See* Lacombe et al.), 556
PERRY, M. O. (*See* Thal et al.), 955
PERSSON, ALFRED V. (*See* Cutler et al.), 963
PEYTON, MARVIN D. (*See* Elkins et al.), 57
PIERCE, JAMES C., AND LEE, HYUNG M. The kidney cell crossmatch in retransplantation, 101
PILCH, YOSEF H., VELTMAN, LARRY L., AND KERN, DAVID H. Immune cytolysis of human tumor cells mediated by xenogeneic "immune" RNA: Implications for immunotherapy, 23
PLESSAS, S. N. (*See* Sechas, Plessas, and Skalkeas), 666
POSNER, CHRISTIAN. (*See* Yamamoto et al.), 678

Q

QUINTON, D. L. (*See* Bradley et al.), 918

R

RAIJ, LEOPOLDO, (*See* Toledo-Pereyra et al.), 474
RANDOLPH, J. G. (*See* Weintraub, Lilly, and Randolph), 490
RASCHE, R., AND BUTTERFIELD, W. C. The effect of sepsis on acute gastric ulcerations in the rat, 764
RATTAZZI, LUCA C. (*See* Spanos et al.), 252
—. (*See* Spanos et al.), 741
RAVITCH, MARK M. (*See* O'Neill et al.), 185
—. A computer logic program in the operating room, 202
—, AND BARTON, BRUCE A. The need for pediatric surgeons as determined by the volume of work and the mode of delivery of surgical care, 754
RAY, PRASANTA K. (*See* Toledo-Pereyra et al.), 121
REEDER, DAVID D. (*See* Watson et al.), 419
REUL, GEORGE J., JR., SOLIS, R. THOMAS, GREENBERG, S. DONALD, MATTOX, KENNETH L., AND WHISENNAND, HARTWELL H. Experience with autotransfusion in the surgical management of trauma, 546
—, COOLEY, DENTON A., SANDIFORD, FRANK M., AND HALLMAN, GRADY L. Complications following the contoured Dacron baffle in correction of transposition of the great arteries, 946
RICHARDS, M. J. S. (*See* Malek et al.), 272
RICHARDSON, P. D. (*See* Karlson et al.), 935
RITCHIE, W. P., JR. Ischemia and the gastric mucosal barrier: A note of caution, 363
ROOD, FAYE. (*See* Miller et al.), 129

S

SABISTON, DAVID C. (*See* Oldham et al.), 160
SACHATELLO, CHARLES R., ERNST, CALVIN B., AND GRIFFEN, WARD O., JR. The acutely ischemic upper extremity: Selective management, 1002
SADE, ROBERT M. (*See* Castaneda et al.), 1010
SALAM, ATEF A. (*See* Mathes and Salam), 506
SALZMAN, EDWIN W. (*See* Cohen et al.), 992
SANCHEZ, MANUEL. (*See* Fonkalsrud et al.), 527
SANDIFORD, FRANK M. (*See* Reul et al.), 946
SARWAT, ABDEL K. (*See* Fonkalsrud et al.), 527
SATANI, MINORU. (*See* Miyata et al.), 234
SATAVA, RICHARD M., JR., AND MGOON, DWIGHT C. A model for cardiogenic shock by coronary artery microembolization in calves, 454
SATINSKY, S. (*See* Kawarada, Satinsky, and Matsumoto), 340
SATOMURA, KISAKU, HANG-LONG, ZHENG, OHNISHI, SATOSHI, KUMADA, KAORU, KISAKA, YOSHIHIKO, YAMAZAKI, HIDEHIRO, KOMAKI, KATSUHIKO, TANIGAWA, NOBUHIKO, HARA, KEIBUN, TOMINAGA, SUMIO, KINOSHITA, KENICHI. Follow-up study of the endorectal pull-through operation for the treatment of Hirschsprung's disease, with special reference to intestinal anastomosis, 581
SAUNDERS, STUART J. (*See* Hickman et al.), 601
SAXBE, WILLIAM B., JR. The surgeon-in-training: A preview (panel discussion), 172
SCHLENKER, JAMES D., JOHNSTON, KENT, AND WOLKOFF, JERRY S. Occlusion of popliteal artery caused by popliteal cysts, 833
SCHMID, K. (*See* Glasgow et al.), 35
SCHWARTZ, ARTHUR E., LEDDICOTTE, GEORGE W., FINK, RICHARD W., AND FRIEDMAN, EUGENE W. Trace elements in normal and malignant human breast tissue, 325
SCHWARTZ, SEYMOUR I. Reply to letter to editors from Hardaway, 684
SECHAS, M. N., PLESSAS, S. N., AND SKALKEAS, G. D. Post-traumatic renovascular hypertension, 666
SEIFTER, ELI. (*See* Demetriou, Seifter, and Levenson), 779
SELL, K. W. (*See* Filo et al.), 88
SHAIPANICH, THONGDEE. (*See* Wren et al.), 112

Sherck, J. P., Kerstein, M. D., and Stansel, H. C., Jr. The current status of vena caval replacement, 209
Shionoya, Shigehiko. Reply to letter to editors from Adar, 848
Shumway, N. E. (*See* Morris et al.), 150
Silen, William. (*See* Gordon et al.), 405
Silverstein, G. (*See* Lo Gerfo et al.), 16
Simmons, Richard L. (*See* Toledo-Pereyra et al.), 121
—. (*See* Spanos et al.), 252
—. (*See* DeShazo et al.), 461
—. (*See* Toledo-Pereyra et al.), 474
—. (*See* Callender et al.), 573
—. (*See* Spanos et al.), 741
Sinclair, Michael C. (*See* Moore et al.), 733
Skalkeas, G. D. (*See* Sechas, Plessas, and Skalkeas), 666
Skandalakis, John E. Reply: The vagaries of the vagus, 352
Skillman, John J. (*See* Gordon et al.), 405
—. Pathogenesis of peptic ulcer: A selective review, 515
Skinner, David B. (*See* Elzinga et al.), 482
Smith, Arnett D. (*See* Hewitt et al.), 715
Smith, Beverly. (*See* Harken et al.), 786
Smith, William J. (*See* Parks et al.), 43
Snyder, William H., III. (*See* Thal et al.), 955
Solis, R. Thomas. (*See* Reul et al.), 546
Souther, S. G. (*See* Morris et al.), 150
Spanos, Panayiotis K., Simmons, Richard L., Rattazzi, Luca C., Goldberg, Marvin E., and Najarian, John S. The fate of kidney transplants from donors with minor renal abnormalities, 252
—, —, Lampe, Ernest, Rattazzi, Luca C., Kjellstrand, Carl M., Goetz, Frederick C., and Najarian, John S. Complications of related kidney donation, 741
Spencer, Frank Cole. Should the total number of surgical residency training programs be regulated? (panel discussion), 188
—. (*See* Mullin et al.), 974
Stanley, James C., and Fry, William J. Pathogenesis and clinical significance of splenic artery aneurysms, 898
Stansel, H. C., Jr. (*See* Sherck, Kerstein, and Stansel), 209
Starrett, Richard W., and Stoney, Ronald J. Juxtarenal aortic occlusion, 890
Stenning, F. G. (*See* Halmagyi et al.), 637
Stoney, Ronald J. (*See* Starrett and Stoney), 890
Suba, E. A. (*See* Filo et al.), 88
Sutherland, D. E. R. (*See* Nowygrod et al.), 630
Sutherland, W. H. (*See* Groves et al.), 533
Syslak, Walter B. (*See* Parkinson et al.), 882

T

Tajima, Tomoo, and McDonald, John C. Adjuncts to the abdonimal wall reconstruction following extensive cancer surgery, 259
Takeuchi, Yoshimi. (*See* Eguchi, Takeuchi, and Asano), 837
Tanigawa, Nobuhiko. (*See* Satomura et al.), 581
Tarver, Harold, (*See* Ehrlich, Tarver, and Hunt), 263
Tenery, John H. (*See* Vistnes et al.), 291
Terblanche, John. (*See* Hickman et al.), 601
Thal, Erwin R., Snyder, William H., III, Hays, Robert J., and Perry, M. O. Management of carotid artery injuries, 955
Thompson, James C. (*See* Watson et al.), 419
Thompson, Jesse E. (*See* Cutler et al.), 963
Thurer, Richard J. (*See* Bolooki et al.), 925
Tice, David A. (*See* Zerbino et al.), 1018
Tierney, Donald F. (*See* Drews et al.), 80
Tominaga, Sumio. (*See* Satomura et al.), 581
Trejo, Rafael A. (*See* Holper et al.), 423
—. (*See* Olcay et al.), 643
Trivedi, Sulochana N. (*See* Mahour et al.), 309
Toledo-Pereyra, Luis H., Ray, Prasanta K., Callender, Clive O., Najarian, John S., and Simmons, Richard L. Renal allograft prolongation using phytomitogens to mask graft antigens, 121
—, Raij, Leopoldo, Simmons, Richard L., and Najarian, John S. Role of endotoxin and bacteria in long-term survival of preserved small-bowel allografts, 474
—. (*See* Callender et al.), 573
Turner, M. Don. (*See* Kondo et al.), 439
—. (*See* Kondo et al.), 447

U

Ueda, Takashi. (*See* Miyata et al.), 234

V

VanDevanter, Susan Bland. (*See* Moore et al.), 376
Varga, D. (*See* Halmagyi et al.), 637
Vargas, Abelardo. (*See* Bolooki et al.), 925
Veltman, Larry L. (*See* Pilch et al.), 23
Vistnes, Lars M. (*See* Morris et al.), 150
—, Goodwin, David A., Tenery, John H., Ksander, George A., and Gruber, Ronald P. Control of capillary bleeding by topical application of microcrystalline collagen, 291
Von Haefen, Ulrich. (*See* Wren et al.), 112

W

Wales, Eugene E. (*See* Cheung et al.), 500
Walker, L. G., Jr. The Carrel-Guthrie letters revisited, 359
Walker, W. Allan. (*See* Warshaw and Walker), 495
Wangensteen, Owen H. Boris Petrov, great Russian surgeon, and the Sklifosovsky Institute of Emergency Surgery, 204
—. The role of debridement—Reply to Mr. Patey's Interrogatory, 347
Warshaw, Andrew L., and Walker, W. Allan. Intestinal absorption of intake antigenic protein, 495
Watson, Francis R. (*See* Knutson and Watson), 298
Watson, Larry C., Reeder, David D., Becker, Horst D., LaGrone, Lavenia, and Thompson, James C. Gastrin concentrations in upper gastrointestinal mucosa in dogs, 419
Webb, Watts R. (*See* Neville et al.), 65
Weber, Griffith A. (*See* Moore et al.), 733
Wechsler, Andrew S. (*See* Oldham et al.), 160
Weintraub, W. H., Lilly, J. R., and Randolph, J. G. A chickenpox epidemic in a pediatric burn unit, 490
Welch, Claude E. Too many surgeons, 199
Wernick, G. (*See* Goldman et al.), 50
Whissennand, Hartwell H. (*See* Reul et al.), 546
White, John J., Oh, Kook Sang, and Haller, J. Alex, Jr. Positive-contrast peritoneography for accurate delineation of diaphragmatic abnormalities, 398
Whytehead, Lawrence L. (*See* Parkinson et al.), 882
Wieland, Steven. (*See* Abbott, Wieland, and Austen), 1031

WILLIAMS, G. MELVILLE. (*See* Parks et al.), 43
WILLIAMS, WILLIS. (*See* Bolooki et al.), 925
WILLMERT, JUSTINE. (*See* DeShazo et al.), 461
WILSON, JAMES P. (*See* Dean et al.), 872
WILSON, RICHARD E. (*See* Wren et al.), 112
—. (*See* Moore et al.), 376
WINEGARNER, FREDERICK G. (*See* Lowe, Winegarner, and Jesseph), 511
WISE, LESLIE, AND BALLINGER, WALTER F. The elective surgical treatment of chronic duodenal ulcer: A critical review, 811
WOLKOFF, JERRY S. (*See* Schlenker, Johnston, and Wolkoff), 833
WOOLF, L. I. (*See* Groves et al.), 533
WOOLLEY, MORTON M. (*See* Mahour et al.), 309
WREN, SIMON F. G., MARTINS, ANTONIO C. P., VON HAEFEN, ULRICH, BUSCH, GEORGE J., KATSKE, GORDON E., KOPPENHEFFER, THOMAS L., SHAIPANICH, THONGDEE, AND WILSON, RICHARD E. Passive enhancement of Canine renal allografts with polyspecific $F(ab')_2$ fragments, 112

Y

YAMAMOTO, NORIAKI, MAGIDSON, OSCAR, POSNER, CHRISTIAN, MENDEZ, A., MICHAEL, ZUBIATE, PABLO, AND KAY, JEROME HAROLD. Salmonella endocarditis treated with prosthetic valve replacement: A case report, 678
YAMAMOTO, ZENGO. (*See* Kawashima, Yamamoto, and Manabe), 391
YAMAZAKI, HIDEHIRO. (*See* Satomura et al.), 581
YUNIS, E. J. (*See* Miller et al.), 129
—. (*See* Callender et al.), 573

Z

ZABRISKIE, JOHN B. (*See* Goldman et al.), 50
—. (*See* Ellis et al.), 142
ZERBINO, VICTOR R., TICE, DAVID A., KATZ, LOIS A., AND NIDUS, BERNARD D. A 6 year clinical experience with arteriovenous fistulas and bypasses for hemodialysis, 1018
ZUBIATE, PABLO. (*See* Yamamoto et al.), 678

SUBJECT INDEX*

A

Abdominal aorta, canine, bifurcation of (Adar) (letter to editors), 358
  tenderness, lower, following traumatic rupture of spleen (Butsch and Butsch) (letter to editors), 524
  wall reconstruction following extensive cancer surgery, adjuncts to (Tajima and McDonald), 259
Aberrant pancreas causing pyloric obstruction (Matsumoto, Kawai, and Kimura), 827
Abnormalities, minor renal, fate of kidney transplants from donors with (Spanos et al.), 252
Absorption, intestinal, of intake antigenic protein (Warshaw and Walker), 495
Academic surgical body count (Eiseman) (editorial), 367
Acetaminophen, ferrous sulfate, ethanol, and acetylsalcylic acid, effect of, on gastric mucosal permeability in man (Gordon et al.), 405
Acetylsalicylic acid, acetaminophen, ferrous sulfate, and ethanol, effect of, on gastric mucosal permeability in man (Gordon et al.), 405
Adjuncts to abdominal wall reconstruction following extensive cancer surgery (Tajima and McDonald), 259
Adrenalectomy with chemotherapy in treatment of advanced breast cancer: objective and subjective response rates; duration and quality of life (Moore et al.), 376
Adventitial degeneration, cystic, of common femoral artery (Lowe, Winegarner, and Jesseph), 511
Aging, organ allografting, and surgical stress, effect of, on rat thymus histidine decarboxylase activity (Moore et al.), 733
Airway resistance regulation of dynamic compliance (Askanazi et al.), 65
Alimentary canal, new method of reconstruction of, after total gastrectomy (Kalemba and Lazarkiewicz), 748
Allogeneic immunity, distinction of, from tumor-specific immunity in man (Parks et al.), 43
Allograft(s), canine renal, passive enhancement of, with polyspecific $F(ab')_2$ fragments (Wren et al.), 112
  myocardial tissue, tolerance to, by pretreatment with cross-reactive streptococcal membrane antigen (Ellis et al.), 142
  preserved small-bowel, role of endotoxin and bacteria in long-term survival of (Toledo-Pereyra), 474
  rat cardiac, prolongation of survival by new immunosuppressant: chicken anti–rat lymphocyte globulin (Morris et al.), 150
    heart, accumulation of lymphotoxin-secreting lymphoid cells in (Granger and Moore), 542
  rejection, renal, failure of anti–HL-A antibodies to correlate with (Callender et al.), 573

*July, pp. 1-198; August, pp. 199-358; September, pp. 359-526; October, pp. 527-684; November, pp. 685-848; December, pp. 849-1062.

Allograft(s)—Cont'd
  renal, prolongation using phytomitogens to mask graft antigens (Toledo-Pereyra et al.), 121
  tolerance in absence of circulating antibodies (Nowygrod et al.), 630
Alveolar morphometrics: effects of positive end-expiratory pressure (Daly, Hughes, and Norman), 624
Amputation, below-knee, for ischemic disease, deleterious effect of immediate postoperative prosthesis in (Cohen et al.), 992
Anastomosis, intestinal, special reference to, in follow-up study of endorectal pull-through operation for treatment of Hirschsprung's disease (Satomura et al.), 581
Anatomic approach to vagotomy (Griffith) (letter to editors), 350; reply (Skandalakis), 352
  extra-, carotid bypass, staged palliative resection of recurrent carcinoma of neck using (Hagood, Mozersky, and Fite), 671
Aneurysm(s), coronary artery, in 9-year-old child (Liddicoat et al.), 845
  splenic artery, pathogenesis and clinical significance of (Stanley and Fry), 898
  subclavian artery; sequela of thoracic outlet syndrome (Mathes and Salam), 506
Antibody(ies), anti–HL-A: failure to correlate with renal allograft rejection (Callender et al.), 573
  blocking, functional characterization of after human renal transplantation (Miller et al.), 129
  circulating, allograft tolerance in absence of (Nowygrod et al.), 630
Antigen(s), cross-reactive streptococcal membrane, tolerance to myocardial tissue allografts by pretreatment with (Ellis et al.), 142
  graft, using phytomitogens to mask in renal allograft prolongation (Toledo-Pereyra et al.), 121
  mouse mammary tumor virus–associated, radioimmunoassay for (Lo Gerfo et al.), 16
Antigenic protein, intake, intestinal absorption of (Warshaw and Walker), 495
Antigenicity, altered, of metastases from primary methylcholanthrene-induced sarcoma, in vitro demonstration of (Faraci), 469
Anti–HL-A antibodies: failure to correlate with renal allograft rejection (Callender et al.), 573
Anti–rat lymphocyte, rabbit, serum-induced lymphopenia in thoracic duct lymph and peripheral blood (Girardet, Friedman, and Karlson), 267
Antrectomy, vagotomy with, and vagotomy with pyloroplasty, comparison of gastric emptying before and after (Donovan et al.), 729
Aorta, canine abdominal, bifurcation of (Adar) (letter to editors), 358
Aortic occlusion, juxtarenal (Starrett and Stoney), 890
Aortocoronary bypass operation, objective assessment of late results of (Bolooki et al.), 925
Arterial graft, modified bovine: clinical study (Cutler et al.), 963

Arterial—Cont'd
pressure, pulmonary, and cardiopulmonary bypass, influence of, on these processes: removal of 5-hydroxytryptamine and norepinephrine from pulmonary vascular space of man (Gillis et al.), 608
Arteriovenous fistulas and bypasses for hemodialysis, 6 year clinical experience with (Zerbino et al.), 1018
Artery(ies), carotid, injuries, management of (Thal et al.), 955
common femoral, cystic adventitial degeneration of (Lowe, Winegarner, and Jesseph), 511
coronary, aneurysms in 9-year-old child (Liddicoat et al.), 845
microembolization in calves, model for cardiogenic shock by (Satava and McGoon), 454
great, transposition of, complications following contoured Dacron baffle in correction of (Reul et al.), 946
popliteal, occlusion of, caused by popliteal cysts (Schlenker, Johnston, and Wolkoff), 833
renal, stenosis, deceptive patterns of (Dean et al.), 872
splenic, aneurysms, pathogenesis and clinical significance of (Stanley and Fry), 898
subclavian, aneurysm; sequela of thoracic outlet syndrome (Mathes and Salam), 506
supraorbital, flow in internal carotid stenosis and occlusion, directional Doppler studies of (LoGerfo and Mason), 723
Aspirin, effect of, on microaggregate formation in banked blood (Arrington and McNamara), 295
Atresia, biliary, long-term results of hepatic portoenterostomy for: special reference to postoperative portal hypertension (Miyata et al.), 234
Author the writer, is the? Who cares? (Lavin) (letter to editors), 344; reply (De Bakey), 345
Authorship in scholarly journals: reply (De Bakey) (letter to editors), 344
Autogenous venous grafts, structural changes during preparation of (Abbott, Wieland, and Austen), 1031
Autografts, canine renal, immunologic injury induced by ex vivo perfusion of (Filo et al.), 88
Autotransfusion, caution regarding (Duncan, Edwards, and Dale), 1024
in surgical management of trauma, experience with (Reul et al.), 546
Autotransplanted lung, canine, ischemic tolerance of (Kondo et al.), 447
Axillo-axillary bypass with cephalic vein for correction of subclavian steal syndrome (Dardik and Dardik), 413
Axis, enteroinsular, influence of glucose on gastrin and insulin release in (Friesen, Bolinger, and Kyner), 804

B

B_{16} melanoma, in vitro comparison of, in primary and metastatic form: immune surveillance and tumor dissemination (Goldman et al.), 50
Baboon, effect of ischemia on hepatic parenchymal and reticuloendothelial function in (Holper et al.), 423
hepatic ischemia in: reticuloendothelial function as determinant for survival following (Olcay et al.), 643
Bacteremia, *E. coli,* impaired gluconeogenesis in dogs with (Groves et al.), 533
Bacteria and endotoxin, role of, in long-term survival of preserved small-bowel allografts (Toledo-Pereyra et al.), 474
Baffle, contoured Dacron, complications following, in correction of transposition of great arteries (Reul et al.), 946
Balloon membranotomy, successful, for obstruction of hepatic portion of inferior vena cava (Eguchi, Takeuchi, and Asano), 837
Band, celiac, syndrome, long-term evaluation of (Evans), 867
Banked blood, effect of aspirin on microaggregate formation in (Arrington and McNamara), 295
Barrier, gastric mucosal, and ischemia: note of caution (Ritchie) (editorial), 363
BCG treatment for malignant melanoma, vitiligo and uveitis associated with (Donaldson et al.), 771
Below-knee amputation for ischemic disease, deleterious effect of immediate postoperative prosthesis in (Cohen et al.), 992
Bifurcation of canine abdominal aorta (Adar) (letter to editors), 358
Bile salts, lecithin, and heparin, dissolution of gallstones with (Cheung et al.), 500
Biliary atresia, long-term results of hepatic portoenterostomy for: special reference to postoperative portal hypertension (Miyata et al.), 234
Bladder/kidney ratio data and ^{131}I hippurate blood clearance, combined use of, in early detection, classification, and management of accelerated rejection of human renal transplants (Moore and Hayes), 587
Bleeding, capillary, control of, by topical application of microcrystalline collagen (Vistnes et al.), 291
Blood, banked, effect of aspirin on microaggregate formation in (Arrington and McNamara), 295
clearance, ^{131}I hippurate, and bladder/kidney ratio data, combined use of, in early detection, classification, and management of accelerated rejection of human renal transplants (Moore and Hayes), 587
flow, coronary, and myocardial reactive hyperemia in ischemic dog heart (Elzinga et al.), 482
regional myocardial, effects of pulmonary embolism on (Oldham et al.), 160
peripheral, and thoracic duct lymph, rabbit anti–rat lymphocyte serum-induced lymphopenia in (Girardet, Friedman, and Karlson), 267
Body count, academic surgical (Eiseman) (editorial), 367
Boris Petrov, great Russian surgeon, and Sklifosovsky Institute of Emergency Surgery (Wangensteen), 204
Bovine arterial graft, modified: clinical study (Cutler et al.), 963
Bowel, preserved small-, allografts, role of endotoxin and bacteria in long-term survival of (Toledo-Pereyra), 474
Breast cancer, advanced, adrenalectomy with chemotherapy in treatment of: objective and subjective response rates; duration and quality of life (Moore et al.), 376
choice of treatment for operable carcinoma of (Haagensen), 685

Breast—Cont'd
tissue, normal and malignant human, trace elements in (Schwartz et al.), 325
British graduates, attitudes of, on surgical research fellowships in United States (Knight and Griffiths), 238
surgery today: perspective of James IV surgical traveler (Kelly), 433
Buerger's disease—need for diagnostic criteria (Adar) (letter to editors), 848; reply (Shionoya), 848
Burn unit, pediatric, chickenpox epidemic in (Weintraub, Lilly, and Randolph), 490
Bypass(es), aortocoronary, operation, objective assessment of late results of (Bolooki et al.), 925
axillo-axillary, with cephalic vein for correction of subclavian steal syndrome (Dardik and Dardik), 413
cardiopulmonary, and pulmonary arterial pressure, influence of, on these processes: removal of 5-hydroxytryptamine and norepinephrine from pulmonary space of man (Gillis et al.), 608
safe limits of hemodilution in (Kawashima, Yamamoto, and Manabe), 391
carotid, extra anatomic, staged palliative resection of recurrent carcinoma of neck using (Hagood, Mozersky, and Fite), 671
femorofemoral (Gazzola, Hirsch, and Kaufer), 841
and fistulas, arteriovenous, for hemodialysis, 6 year clinical experience with (Zerbino et al.), 1018
total cardiopulmonary, with new microporous Teflon membrane oxygenator (Karlson et al.), 935

C

Calves, model for cardiogenic shock by coronary artery microembolization in (Satava and McGoon), 454
Canal, alimentary, new method of reconstruction of, after total gastrectomy (Kalemba and Lazarkiewicz), 748
Cancer, advanced breast, adrenalectomy with chemotherapy in treatment of: objective and subjective response rates; duration and quality of life (Moore et al.), 376
colon, preliminary results of computer logic program for operative management of (Knutson and Watson), 298
patients, serum of, immunosuppressive peptide fraction in (Glasgow et al.), 35
surgery, extensive, adjuncts to abdominal wall reconstruction following (Tajima and McDonald), 259
Canine abdominal aorta, bifurcation of (Adar) (letter to editors), 358
autotransplanted lung, ischemic tolerance of (Kondo et al.), 447
kidney, perfused, effect of single-dose irradiation on (Malek et al.), 272
lung, ischemic, nonventilated, evaluation of pulmonary function in (Fonkalsrud et al.), 527
Capillary bleeding, control of, by topical application of microcrystalline collagen (Vistnes et al.), 291
Carcinoma, operable, of breast, choice of treatment for (Haagensen), 685
recurrent, of neck, staged palliative resection of, using extra anatomic carotid bypass (Hagood, Mozersky, and Fite), 671
Cardiac allograft, rat, prolongation of survival by new immunosuppressant: chicken anti–rat lymphocyte globulin (Morris et al.), 150
Cardiogenic shock by coronary artery microembolization in calves, model for (Satava and McGoon), 454
Cardiopulmonary bypass and pulmonary arterial pressure, influence of, on these processes: removal of 5-hydroxytryptamine and norepinephrine from pulmonary space of man (Gillis et al.), 608
safe limits of hemodilution in (Kawashima, Yamamoto, and Manabe), 391
total, with new microporous Teflon membrane oxygenator (Karlson et al.), 935
effects of volume loading of primates in endotoxin shock (Greenfield et al.), 560
Carotid artery injuries, management of (Thal et al.), 955
bypass, extra-anatomic, staged palliative resection of recurrent carcinoma of neck using (Hagood, Mozersky, and Fite), 671
cavernous fistula: direct repair with preservation of carotid (Parkinson et al.), 882
direct repair of carotid cavernous fistula with preservation of (Parkinson et al.), 882
internal, stenosis and occlusion, directional Doppler studies of supraorbital artery flow in (LoGerfo and Mason), 723
Carrel-Guthrie letters revisited (Walker) (editorial), 359
Catheter maintenance, central venous (Kim and Fortner) (letter to editors), 357
Cavernous fistula, carotid: direct repair with preservation of carotid (Parkinson et al.), 882
Celiac band syndrome, long-term evaluation of (Evans), 867
Cells, lymphoid, lymphotoxin-secreting, accumulation of, in rat heart allografts (Granger and Moore), 542
in tissue culture, growth of, effect of sera obtained from normal and partially hepatectomized rats and patients on (Demetriou, Seifter, and Levenson), 779
Central venous catheter maintenance (Kim and Fortner), 357
Cephalic vein, axillo-axillary bypass with, for correction of subclavian steal syndrome (Dardik and Dardik), 413
Changes and trends in graduate medical education and credentialling (Humphreys), 243
Chemotherapy with adrenalectomy in treatment of advanced breast cancer: objective and subjective response rates; duration and quality of life (Moore et al.), 376
Chickenpox epidemic in pediatric burn unit (Weintraub, Lilly, and Randolph), 490
Child, 9-year-old, coronary artery aneurysms in (Liddicoat et al.), 845
Childhood and infancy, teratomas in: experience with 81 cases (Mahour et al.), 309
Children, 100, results of renal transplantation in (DeShazo et al.), 461
Choledochoduodenostomy: 18 year study of 175 cases (Degenshein), 319
Chronic duodenal ulcer, elective surgical treatment of: critical review (Wise and Ballinger), 811
Circulatory arrest, 2½ hour hypothermic, body responses and recovery after (Kondo et al.), 439
Coagulation, disseminated intravascular (Hard-

Coagulation—Cont'd
away) (letter to editors), 682; reply (Schwartz), 684
Colitis, ischemic, following rectal prolapse (Kawarada, Satinsky, and Matsumoto), 340
Collagen, microcrystalline, control of capillary bleeding by topical application of (Vistnes et al.), 291
Colon cancer, preliminary results of computer logic program for operative management of (Knutson and Watson), 298
Commissurotomy, open mitral, experience with, in 100 consecutive patients (Mullin et al.), 974
Compliance, dynamic, airway resistance regulation of (Askanazi et al.), 65
Computer logic program in operating room (Ravitch) (editorial), 202
preliminary results of, for operative management of colon cancer (Knutson and Watson), 298
Contoured Dacron baffle, complications following, in correction of transposition of great arteries (Reul et al.), 946
Coronary artery aneurysms in 9-year-old child (Liddicoat et al.), 845
microembolization in calves, model for cardiogenic shock by (Satava and McGoon), 454
blood flow and myocardial reactive hyperemia in ischemic dog heart (Elzinga et al.), 482
Credentialling and graduate medical education, changes and trends in (Humphreys), 243
Crossmatch, kidney cell, in retransplantation (Pierce and Lee), 101
Culture, tissue, growth of cells in, effect of sera obtained from normal and partially hepatectomized rats and patients on (Demetriou, Seifter, and Levenson), 779
Cystic adventitial degeneration of common femoral artery (Lowe, Winegarner, and Jesseph), 511
Cysts, duodenal duplication: diagnosis and operative management (Ackerman), 330
popliteal, occlusion of popliteal artery caused by (Schlenker, Johnston, and Wolkoff), 833
Cytolysis, immune, of human tumor cells mediated by xenogeneic "immune" RNA: implications for immunotherapy (Pilch et al.), 23

D

Dacron baffle, contoured, complications following, in correction of transposition of great arteries (Reul et al.), 946
patch graft, inverted (Lo Gerfo), 525
Debridement (Patey) (letter to editors), 347; reply (Wangensteen), 347
role of—reply to Mr. Patey's Interrogatory (Wangensteen) (letter to editors), 347
Diagnosis and operative management of duodenal duplication cysts (Ackerman), 330
Diagnostic criteria, need for—Buerger's disease (Adar) (letter to editors), 848; reply (Shionoya), 848
Diaphragmatic abnormalities, positive-contrast peritoneography for accurate delineation of (White, Oh, and Haller), 398
Directional Doppler studies of supraorbital artery flow in internal carotid stenosis and occlusion (Lo Gerfo and Mason), 723
Disease, Buerger's—need for diagnostic criteria (Adar) (letter to editors), 848; reply (Shionoya), 848

Disease—Cont'd
Hirschsprung's, follow-up study of endorectal pull-through operation for treatment of, with special reference to intestinal anastomosis (Satomura et al.), 581
Disseminated intravascular coagulation (Hardaway) (letter to editors), 682; reply (Schwartz), 684
Dog(s), gastrin concentrations in upper gastrointestinal mucosa in (Watson et al.), 419
heart, ischemic, coronary blood flow and myocardial reactive hyperemia in (Elzinga et al.), 482
with *E. coli* bacteremia, impaired gluconeogenesis in (Groves et al.), 533
Donation, related kidney, complications of (Spanos et al.), 741
Donors with minor renal abnormalities, fate of kidney transplants from (Spanos et al.), 252
Doppler studies, directional, of supraorbital artery flow in internal carotid stenosis and occlusion (Lo Gerfo and Mason), 723
Duodenal duplication cysts: diagnosis and operative management (Ackerman), 330
ulcer, chronic, elective surgical treatment of: critical review (Wise and Ballinger), 811
Duplication cysts, duodenal: diagnosis and operative management (Ackerman), 330
Dynamic compliance, airway resistance regulation of (Askanazi et al.), 65

E

E. coli bacteremia, impaired gluconeogenesis in dogs with (Groves et al.), 533
Education, graduate medical, and credentialling, changes and trends in (Humphreys), 243
Elective surgical treatment of chronic duodenal ulcer: critical review (Wise and Ballinger), 811
Electrode, bipolar transvenous pacemaker, technique for in situ repair (Gelfand and Blumenberg), 504
Embolism, pulmonary, effects of, on regional myocardial blood flow (Oldham et al.), 160
Emergency Surgery, Sklifosovsky Institute of, and Boris Petrov, great Russian surgeon, (Wangensteen), 204
Emptying, gastric, before and after vagotomy with antrectomy and vagotomy with pyloroplasty, comparison of (Donovan et al.), 729
Emulsion, fat, effect of complete parenteral nutrition including, on plasma lipid (Koga, Ikeda, and Inokuchi), 278
End-expiratory pressure, positive, effects of, on alveolar morphometrics (Daly, Hughes, and Norman), 624
ventilation, positive, hemodynamic response to, in hypovolemic patients (Harken et al.), 786
Endocarditis, salmonella, probable, treated with prosthetic valve replacement: case report (Yamamoto et al.), 678
Endorectal pull-through operation, follow-up study of, for treatment of Hirschsprung's disease, with special reference to intestinal anastomosis (Satomura et al.), 581
Endotoxin and bacteria, role of, in long-term survival of preserved small-bowel allografts (Toledo-Pereyra et al.), 474
shock, cardiopulmonary effects of volume loading of primates in (Greenfield et al.), 560
End-to-side portacaval shunt in young pig, transhepatic metabolism after (Hickman et al.), 601

"Enemy, we have met, and he is us" (Bergland), 183
Enteroinsular axis, influence of glucose on gastrin and insulin release in (Friesen, Bolinger, and Kyner), 804
Epidemic, chickenpox, in pediatric burn unit (Weintraub, Lilly, and Randolph), 490
Ethanol, acetylsalicylic acid, acetaminophen, and ferrous sulfate, effect of, on gastric mucosal permeability in man (Gordon et al.), 405
Extra-anatomic carotid bypass, staged palliative resection of recurrent carcinoma of neck using (Hagood, Mozersky, and Fite), 671
Extremity, upper, acutely ischemic: selective management (Sachatello, Ernst, and Griffen), 1002

F

F(ab')$_2$ fragments, polyspecific, passive enhancement of canine renal allografts with (Wren et al.), 112
Fallot, tetralogy of, reoperation for residual defects after repair of (Castaneda et al.), 1010
Fat emulsion, effect of complete parenteral nutrition including, on plasma lipid (Koga, Ikeda, and Inokuchi), 278
Fellowships, surgical research, in United States, attitudes of British graduates on (Knight and Griffiths), 238
Femoral artery, common, cystic adventitial degeneration of (Lowe, Winegarner, and Jesseph), 511
Femorofemoral bypass (Gazzola, Hirsch, and Kaufer), 841
Fistula(s) and bypasses, arteriovenous, for hemodialysis, 6 year clinical experience with (Zerbino et al.), 1018
  carotid cavernous: direct repair with preservation of carotid (Parkinson et al.), 882
Flow, supraorbital artery, in internal carotid stenosis and occlusion, directional Doppler studies of (LoGerfo and Mason), 723
Foreign medical graduate, physician supply, and residency programs (Leape) (editorial), 372

G

Gallstones, dissolution of, with bile salts, lecithin, and heparin (Cheung et al.), 500
Gastrectomy, total, new method of reconstruction of alimentary canal after (Kalemba and Lazarkiewicz), 748
Gastric emptying before and after vagotomy with antrectomy and vagotomy with pyloroplasty, comparison of (Donovan et al.), 729
  mucosal barrier and ischemia: note of caution (Ritchie) (editorial), 363
    permeability in man, effect of ethanol, acetylsalicylic acid, acetaminophen, and ferrous sulfate on (Gordon et al.), 405
Gastrin and insulin release in enteroinsular axis, influence of glucose on (Friesen, Bolinger, and Kyner), 804
  concentrations in upper gastrointestinal mucosa in dogs (Watson et al.), 419
Gastrointestinal mucosa, upper, in dogs, gastrin concentrations in (Watson et al.), 419
Globulin, chicken anti-rat lymphocyte: prolongation of rat cardiac allograft survival by new immunosuppressant (Morris et al.), 150
Gluconeogenesis, impaired, in dogs with *E. coli* bacteremia (Groves et al.), 533
Glucose, influence of, on gastrin and insulin release in enteroinsular axis (Friesen, Bolinger, and Kyner), 804
Glycogen, myocardial (Blackburn) (letter to editors), 346; reply (Hewitt), 346
Graduate(s), British, attitudes of, on surgical research fellowships in United States (Knight and Griffiths), 238
  foreign medical, physician supply, and residency programs (Leape) (editorial), 372
  medical education and credentialling, changes and trends in (Humphreys), 243
Graft(s) antigens, using phytomitogens to mask in renal allograft prolongation (Toledo-Pereyra et al.), 121
  autogenous venous, structural changes during preparation of (Abbott, Wieland, and Austen), 1031
  inverted Dacron patch (LoGerfo), 525
  modified bovine arterial: clinical study (Cutler et al.), 963
Great arteries, transposition of, complications following contoured Dacron baffle in correction of (Reul et al.), 946
Guthrie-Carrel letters revisited (Walker) (editorial), 359

H

Heart, ischemic dog, coronary blood flow and myocardial reactive hyperemia in (Elzinga et al.), 482
  rat, allografts, accumulation of lymphotoxin-secreting lymphoid cells in (Granger and Moore), 542
Hemodialysis, arteriovenous fistulas and bypasses for, 6 year clinical experience with (Zerbino et al.), 1018
Hemodilution in cardiopulmonary bypass, safe limits of (Kawashima, Yamamoto, and Manabe), 391
Hemodynamic and clinical comparisons of Kay-Shiley, Starr-Edwards No. 6520, and Reis-Hancock porcine xenograft mitral valves (Brown et al.), 983
  response to positive end-expiratory ventilation in hypovolemic patients (Harken et al.), 786
Hemorrhage, life-threatening, cause of: solitary rectal ulcer (Delancy and Hitch), 830
Hemorrhagic pancreatitis, pulmonary hypertension in (Halmagyi et al.), 637
Heparin, bile salts, and lecithin, dissolution of gallstones with (Cheung et al.), 500
Hepatectomized, partially, and normal rats and patients, effect of sera obtained from, on growth of cells in tissue culture (Demetriou, Seifter, and Levenson), 779
Hepatic and splenic lymphangiomatosis with skeletal involvement: report of case and review of literature (Asch, Cohen, and Moore), 334
  ischemia in baboon: reticuloendothelial function as determinant for survival following (Olcay et al.), 643
  parenchymal and reticuloendothelial function in baboon, effect of ischemia on (Holper et al.), 423
  portion of inferior vena cava, obstruction of, successful balloon membranotomy for (Eguchi, Takeuchi, and Asano), 837
  portoenterostomy for biliary atresia, long-term results of: special reference to postoperative portal hypertension (Miyata et al.), 234
Hippurate, ^{131}I, blood clearance and bladder/kidney ratio data, combined use of, in

Hippurate—Cont'd
early detection, classification, and management of accelerated rejection of human renal transplants (Moore and Hayes), 587
Hirschsprung's disease, follow-up study of endorectal pull-through operation for treatment of, with special reference to intestinal anastomosis (Satomura et al.), 581
Histidine decarboxylase activity, rat thymus, effect of aging, organ allografting, and surgical stress on (Moore et al.), 733
HL-A antibodies, anti–: failure to correlate with renal allograft rejection (Callender et al.), 573
Homografts, pig liver, another look at rejection in (Battersby et al.), 617
Hormone, circulating thymic, effects of thymectomy in young pig on level of (Lacombe et al.), 556
Human breast tissue, normal and malignant, trace elements in (Schwartz et al.), 325
renal transplants, accelerated rejection of, combined use of ^{131}I hippurate blood clearance and bladder/kidney ratio data in early detection, classification, and management of (Moore and Hayes), 587
5-Hydroxytryptamine and norepinephrine, removal of, from pulmonary vascular space of man: influence of cardiopulmonary bypass and pulmonary arterial pressure on these processes (Gillis et al.), 608
Hyperemia, myocardial reactive, and coronary blood flow in ischemic dog heart (Elzinga et al.), 482
Hypertension, chronic pulmonary, pulmonary vascular impedance in (Elkins et al.), 57
postoperative portal, special reference to: long-term results of hepatic portoenterostomy for biliary atresia (Miyata et al.), 234
pulmonary, in acute hemorrhagic pancreatitis (Halmagyi et al.), 637
renovascular, post-traumatic (Sechas, Plessas, and Skalkeas), 666
Hypothermic circulatory arrest, 2½ hour, body responses and recovery after (Kondo et al.), 439
Hypovolemic patients, hemodynamic response to positive end-expiratory ventilation in (Harken et al.), 786

I

^{131}I hippurate blood clearance and bladder/kidney ratio data, combined use of, in early detection, classification, and management of accelerated rejection of human renal transplants (Moore and Hayes), 587
Immune cytolysis of human tumor cells mediated by xenogeneic "immune" RNA: implications for immunotherapy (Pilch et al.), 23
surveillance and tumor dissemination: in vitro comparison of B_{16} melanoma in primary and metastatic form (Goldman et al.), 50
Immunity, allogeneic, distinction of, from tumor-specific immunity in man (Parks et al.), 43
tumor-specific, distinction of allogeneic immunity from, in man (Parks et al.), 43
Immunologic injury induced by ex vivo perfusion of canine renal autografts (Filo et al.), 88
Immunosuppressant, new, prolongation of rat cardiac allograft survival by: chicken anti–rat lymphocyte globulin (Morris et al.), 150
Immunosuppression and lung transplantation effect of, upon surfactant (Drews et al.), 80
Immunotherapy, implications for, in immune cytolysis of human tumor cells mediated by xenogeneic "immune" RNA (Pilch et al.), 23
Impedance, pulmonary vascular, in chronic pulmonary hypertension (Elkins et al.), 57
Infancy and childhood, teratomas in: experience with 81 cases (Mahour et al.), 309
Inferior vena cava, successful balloon membranotomy for obstruction of hepatic portion of (Eguchi, Takeuchi, and Asano), 837
Influence of glucose on gastrin and insulin release in enteroinsular axis (Friesen, Bolinger, and Kyner), 804
Injury(ies), carotid artery, management of (Thal et al.), 955
immunologic, induced by ex vivo perfusion of canine renal autografts (Filo et al.), 88
penetrating vascular, of thoracic outlet (Hewitt et al.), 715
Institute of Emergency Surgery, Sklifosovsky, and Boris Petrov, great Russian surgeon (Wangensteen), 204
Insulin and gastrin release in enteroinsular axis, influence of glucose on (Friesen, Bolinger, and Kyner), 804
Internal carotid stenosis and occlusion, directional Doppler studies of supraorbital artery flow in (Lo Gerfo and Mason), 723
Intestinal absorption of intake antigenic protein (Warshaw and Walker), 495
anastomosis, special reference to, in follow-up study of endorectal pull-through operation for treatment of Hirschsprung's disease (Satomura et al.), 581
Intraoperative tests in vagotomy, value of (Gullickson) (letter to editors), 357
Intravascular coagulation, disseminated (Hardaway) (letter to editors), 682; reply (Schwartz), 684
Irradiation, single dose, effect of, on isolated perfused canine kidney (Malek et al.), 272
Ischemia and gastric mucosal barrier: note of caution (Ritchie) (editorial), 363
effect of, on hepatic parenchymal and reticuloendothelial function in baboon (Holper et al.), 423
hepatic, in baboon: reticuloendothelial function as determinant for survival following (Olcay et al.), 643
Ischemic, acutely, upper extremity: selective management (Sachatello, Ernst, and Griffen), 1002
colitis following rectal prolapse (Kawarada, Satinsky, and Matsumoto), 340
disease, below-knee amputation for, deleterious effect of immediate postoperative prosthesis in (Cohen et al.), 992
dog heart, coronary blood flow and myocardial reactive hyperemia in (Elzinga et al.), 482
nonventilated canine lung, evaluation of pulmonary function in (Fonkalsrud et al.), 527
tolerance of canine autotransplanted lung (Kondo et al.), 447
Isolated perfused rabbit thymus, lymphocyte output by (Ekwueme and Forrest), 794

J

James IV surgical traveler, perspective of: British surgery today (Kelly), 433
Juxtarenal aortic occlusion (Starrett and Stoney), 890

K

Kay-Shiley, Starr-Edwards No. 6520, and Reis-Hancock porcine xenograft mitral valves, clinical and hemodynamic comparisons of (Brown et al.), 983

Kidney/bladder ratio data and ^{131}I hippurate blood clearance, combined use of, in early detection, classification, and management of accelerated rejection of human renal transplants (Moore and Hayes), 587

cell crossmatch in retransplantation (Pierce and Lee), 101

donation, related, complications of (Spanos et al.), 741

perfused canine, effect of single dose irradiation on (Malek et al.), 272

transplants from donors with minor renal abnormalities, fate of (Spanos et al.), 252

L

Lecithin, heparin, and bile salts, dissolution of gallstones with (Cheung et al.), 500

Letters revisited, Carrel-Guthrie (Walker) (editorial), 359

Lipid, plasma, effect of complete parenteral nutrition including fat emulsion on (Koga, Ikeda, and Inokuchi), 278

Liver homografts, pig, another look at rejection in (Battersby et al.), 617

Loading, volume, of primates in endotoxin shock, cardiopulmonary effects of (Greenfield et al.), 560

Lung, canine autotransplanted, ischemic tolerance of (Kondo et al.), 447

ischemic, nonventilated, evaluation of pulmonary function in (Fonkalsrud et al.), 527

transplantation and immunosuppression, effect of, upon surfactant (Drews et al.), 80

Lymph, thoracic duct, and peripheral blood, rabbit anti–rat lymphocyte serum-induced lymphopenia in (Girardet, Friedman, and Karlson), 267

Lymphangiography, use of, in melanoma (Ariel), 654

Lymphangiomatosis, hepatic and splenic, with skeletal involvement: report of case and review of literature (Asch, Cohen, and Moore), 334

Lymphocyte globulin, chicken anti–rat: prolongation of rat cardiac allograft survival by new immunosuppressant (Morris et al.), 150

output by isolated perfused rabbit thymus (Ekwueme and Forrest), 794

rabbit anti–rat, serum-induced lymphopenia in thoracic duct lymph and peripheral blood (Girardet, Friedman, and Karlson), 267

Lymphoid cells, lymphotoxin-secreting, accumulation of, in rat heart allografts (Granger and Moore), 542

Lymphopenia in thoracic duct lymph and peripheral blood, rabbit anti–rat lymphocyte serum-induced (Girardet, Friedman, and Karlson), 267

Lymphotoxin-secreting lymphoid cells, accumulation of, in rat heart allografts (Granger and Moore), 542

M

Malignancies, spontaneous (pathologic) rupture of spleen in (Karakousis and Elias), 674

Malignant and normal human breast tissue, trace elements in (Schwartz et al.), 325

melanoma, BCG treatment for, uveitis and vitiligo associated with (Donaldson et al.), 771

Mammary tumor, mouse, virus–associated antigen, radioimmunoassay for (Lo Gerfo et al.), 16

Medical education, graduate, and credentialling, changes and trends in (Humphreys), 243

Melanoma, B_{16}, in vitro comparison of, in primary and metastatic form: immune surveillance and tumor dissemination (Goldman et al.), 50

malignant, BCG treatment for, uveitis and vitiligo associated with (Donaldson et al.), 771

use of lymphangiography in (Ariel), 654

Membrane antigen, cross-reactive streptococcal, tolerance to myocardial tissue allografts by pretreatment with (Ellis et al.), 142

oxygenator, new microporous Teflon, total cardiopulmonary bypass with (Karlson et al.), 935

Membranotomy, successful balloon, for obstruction of hepatic portion of inferior vena cava (Eguchi, Takeuchi, and Asano), 837

Mesenteric, superior, and portal veins, thrombectomy in: report of case treated with thrombectomy (Bergentz et al.), 286

Metabolism, transhepatic, after end-to-side portacaval shunt in young pig (Hickman et al.), 601

Metastases from primary methylcholanthrene-induced sarcoma, in vitro demonstration of altered antigenicity of (Faraci), 469

Metastatic and primary form, in vitro comparison of B_{16} melanoma in: immune surveillance and tumor dissemination (Goldman et al.), 50

Methylcholanthrene-induced sarcoma, primary, in vitro demonstration of altered antigenicity of metastases from (Faraci), 469

Microaggregate formation in banked blood, effect of aspirin on (Arrington and McNamara), 295

Microcrystalline collagen, control of capillary bleeding by topical application of (Vistnes et al.), 291

Microembolization, coronary artery, in calves, model for cardiogenic shock by (Satava and McGoon), 454

Microporous Teflon membrane oxygenator, new, total cardiopulmonary bypass with (Karlson et al.), 935

Mitral commissurotomy, open, experience with, in 100 consecutive patients (Mullin et al.), 974

valves, porcine xenograft, Kay-Shiley, Starr-Edwards No. 6520, and Reis-Hancock, clinical and hemodynamic comparisons of (Brown et al.), 983

Morphometrics, alveolar: effects of positive end-expiratory pressure (Daly, Hughes, and Norman), 624

Mucosa, upper gastrointestinal, in dogs, gastrin concentrations in (Watson et al.), 419

Mucosal barrier, gastric, and ischemia: note of caution (Ritchie) (editorial), 363

permeability, gastric, in man, effect of ethanol, acetylsalicylic acid, acetaminophen, and ferrous sulfate on (Gordon et al.), 405

Muscle, smooth, antagonist, topical, inhibiting wound contraction by using (Madden et al.), 8

Myocardial blood flow, regional, effects of pulmonary embolism on (Oldham et al.), 160

Myocardial—Cont'd
glycogen (Blackburn) (letter to editors), 346; reply (Hewitt), 346
reactive hyperemia and coronary blood flow in ischemic dog heart (Elzinga et al.), 482
tissue allografts, tolerance to, by pretreatment with cross-reactive streptococcal membrane antigen (Ellis et al.), 142
Myonecrosis in chronic experimental vasospasm (Alksne), 1

N

Neck, staged palliative resection of recurrent carcinoma of, using extra-anatomic carotid bypass (Hagood, Mozersky, and Fite), 671
Norepinephrine and 5-hydroxytryptamine, removal of, from pulmonary vascular space of man: influence of cardiopulmonary bypass and pulmonary arterial pressure on these processes (Gillis et al.), 608
Nutrition, complete parenteral, including fat emulsion, effect of, on plasma lipid (Koga, Ikeda, and Inokuchi), 278
wound, proteolysis of preformed protein in (Ehrlich, Tarver, Hunt), 263

O

Obstruction of hepatic portion of inferior vena cava, successful balloon membranotomy for (Eguchi, Takeuchi, and Asano), 837
pyloric, aberrant pancreas causing (Matsumoto, Kawai, and Kimura), 827
Occlusion and stenosis, internal carotid, directional Doppler studies of supraorbital artery flow in (LoGerfo and Mason), 723
juxtarenal aortic (Starrett and Stoney), 890
of popliteal artery caused by popliteal cysts (Schlenker, Johnston, and Wolkoff), 833
Open mitral commissurotomy, experience with, in 100 consecutive patients (Mullin et al.), 974
Operable carcinoma of breast, choice of treatment for (Haagensen), 685
Operating room, computer logic program in (Ravitch) (editorial), 202
Operation, endorectal pull-through, follow-up study of, for treatment of Hirschsprung's disease, with special reference to intestinal anastomosis (Satomura et al.), 581
Operative management and diagnosis of duodenal duplication cysts (Ackerman), 330
Organ allografting, aging, and surgical stress, effect of, on rat thymus histidine decarboxylase activity (Moore et al.), 733
Outlet, thoracic, penetrating vascular injuries of (Hewitt et al.), 715
syndrome, sequela of; subclavian artery aneurysm (Mathes and Salam), 506
Output, lymphocyte, by isolated perfused rabbit thymus (Ekwueme and Forrest), 794
Oxygen inhibition of pulmonary surfactant synthesis, mechanisms of (Gilder and McSherry), 72
Oxygenator, new microporous Teflon membrane, total cardiopulmonary bypass with (Karlson et al.), 935

P

Pacemaker, electrode, bipolar transvenous, technique for in situ repair (Gelfand and Blumenberg), 504
Painless removal of sutures (Bialostozky) (letter to editors), 356
Palliative, staged, resection of recurrent carcinoma of neck using extra anatomic carotid bypass (Hagood, Mozersky, and Fite), 671
Pancreas, aberrant, causing pyloric obstruction (Matsumoto, Kawai, and Kimura), 827
Pancreatitis, hemorrhagic, pulmonary hypertension in (Halmagyi et al.), 637
Parenchymal, hepatic, and reticuloendothelial function in baboon, effect of ischemia on (Holper et al.), 423
Parenteral nutrition, complete, including fat emulsion, effect of, on plasma lipid (Koga, Ikeda, and Inokuchi), 278
Patch graft, inverted Dacron (LoGerfo), 525
Pathologic, spontaneous, rupture of spleen in malignancies (Karakousis and Elias), 674
Pediatric burn unit, chickenpox epidemic in (Weintraub, Lilly, and Randolph), 490
surgeons, need for, as determined by volume of work and mode of delivery of surgical care (Ravitch and Barton), 754
Surgery—a model for evaluation of surgical manpower needs (panel discussion) (O'Neill), 185
Penetrating vascular injuries of thoracic outlet (Hewitt et al.), 715
Peptic ulcer, pathogenesis of: selective review (Skillman), 515
Peptide fraction, immunosuppressive, in serum of cancer patients (Glasgow et al.), 35
Perfused canine kidney, effect of single-dose irradiation on (Malek et al.), 272
isolated, rabbit thymus, lymphocyte output by (Ekwueme and Forrest), 794
Perfusion, ex vivo, of canine renal autografts, immunologic injury induced by (Filo et al.), 88
Peripheral blood and thoracic duct lymph, rabbit anti–rat lymphocyte serum-induced lymphopenia in (Girardet, Friedman, and Karlson), 267
Peritoneography, positive-contrast, for accurate delineation of diaphragmatic abnormalities (White, Oh, and Haller), 398
Permeability, gastric mucosal, in man, effect of ethanol, acetylsalicylic acid, acetaminophen, and ferrous sulfate on (Gordon et al.), 405
Petrov, Boris, great Russian surgeon, and Sklifosovsky Institute of Emergency Surgery (Wangensteen), 204
Phagocytosis (Gans) (letter to editors), 352; reply (Di Luzio, Olcay, and Drapanas), 353
Physician supply, residency programs, and foreign medical graduate (Leape) (editorial), 372
Phytomitogens, using to mask graft antigens in renal allograft prolongation (Toledo-Pereyra et al.), 121
Pig liver homografts, another look at rejection in (Battersby et al.), 617
young, thymectomy in: effects on level of circulating thymic hormone (Lacombe et al.), 556
transhepatic metabolism after end-to-side portacaval shunt in (Hickman et al.), 601
Plasma lipid, effect of complete parenteral nutrition including fat emulsion on (Koga, Ikeda, and Inokuchi), 278
Popliteal artery, occlusion of, caused by popliteal

Popliteal—Cont'd
cysts (Schlenker, Johnston, and Wolkoff), 833
cysts, occlusion of popliteal artery caused by (Schlenker, Johnston, and Wolkoff), 833
Porcine xenograft mitral valves, Kay-Shiley, Starr-Edwards No. 6520, and Reis-Hancock, clinical and hemodynamic comparisons of (Brown et al.), 983
Portacaval shunt, end-to-side, in young pig, transhepatic metabolism after (Hickman et al.), 601
Portal and superior mesenteric veins, thrombosis in: report of case treated with thrombectomy (Bergentz et al.), 286
hypertension, postoperative, special reference to: long-term results of hepatic portoenterostomy for biliary atresia (Miyata et al.), 234
Portoenterostomy, hepatic, for biliary atresia, long-term results of: special reference to postoperative portal hypertension (Miyata et al.), 234
Positive end-expiratory pressure, effects of, on alveolar morphometrics (Daly, Hughes, and Norman), 624
ventilation, hemodynamic response to, in hypovolemic patients (Harken et al.), 786
Preformed protein, proteolysis of, in wound nutrition (Ehrlich, Tarver, and Hunt), 263
Preservation of carotid, direct repair of carotid cavernous fistula with (Parkinson et al.), 882
Pressure, positive end-expiratory, effects of, on alveolar morphometrics (Daly, Hughes, and Norman), 624
pulmonary arterial, and cardiopulmonary bypass, influence of, on these processes: removal of 5-hydroxytryptamine and norepinephrine from pulmonary vascular space of man (Gillis et al.), 608
Primates in endotoxin shock, cardiopulmonary effects of volume loading of (Greenfield et al.), 560
Program, computer logic, in operating room (Ravitch) (editorial), 202
preliminary results of, for operative management of colon cancer (Knutson and Watson), 298
Prolapse, rectal, ischemic colitis following (Kawarada, Satinsky, and Matsumoto), 340
Prosthesis, immediate postoperative, in below-knee amputation for ischemic disease, deleterious effect of (Cohen et al.), 992
Prosthetic valve replacement, probable salmonella endocarditis treated with: case report (Yamamoto et al.), 678
Protein, intake antigenic, intestinal absorption of (Warshaw and Walker), 495
preformed, proteolysis of, in wound nutrition (Ehrlich, Tarver, and Hunt), 263
Proteolysis of preformed protein in wound nutrition (Ehrlich, Tarver, and Hunt), 263
Pull-through operation, endorectal, follow-up study of, for treatment of Hirschsprung's disease, with special reference to intestinal anastomosis (Satomura et al.), 581
Pulmonary arterial pressure and cardiopulmonary bypass, influence of, on these processes: removal of 5-hydroxytryptamine and norepinephrine from pulmonary vascular space of man (Gillis et al.), 608
Pulmonary — Cont'd
embolism, effects of, on regional myocardial blood flow (Oldham et al.), 160
function in ischemic, nonventilated canine lung, evaluation of (Fonkalsrud et al.), 527
hypertension in acute hemorrhagic pancreatitis (Halmagyi et al.), 637
chronic, pulmonary vascular impedance in (Elkins et al.), 57
surfactant synthesis, mechanisms of oxygen inhibition of (Gilder and McSherry), 72
vascular impedance in chronic pulmonary hypertension (Elkins et al.), 57
space of man, removal of 5-hydroxytryptamine and norepinephrine from: influence of cardiopulmonary bypass and pulmonary arterial pressure on these processes (Gillis et al.), 608
Pyloric obstruction, aberrant pancreas causing (Matsumoto, Kawai, and Kimura), 827
Pyloroplasty, vagotomy with, and vagotomy with antrectomy, comparison of gastric emptying before and after (Donovan et al.), 729

R

Rabbit anti–rat lymphocyte serum-induced lymphopenia in thoracic duct lymph and peripheral blood (Girardet, Friedman, and Karlson), 267
thymus, isolated perfused, lymphocyte output by (Ekwueme and Forrest), 794
Radioextraction ratio, sinusoidal shunt fraction by (Bradley et al.), 918
Radioimmunoassay for mouse mammary tumor virus–associated antigen (Lo Gerfo et al.), 16
Rat(s), effect of sepsis on acute gastric ulcerations in (Rasche and Butterfield), 764
heart allografts, accumulation of lymphotoxin-secreting lymphoid cells in (Granger and Moore), 542
and patients, normal and partially hepatectomized, effect of sera obtained from, on growth of cells in tissue culture (Demetriou, Seifter, and Levenson), 779
thymus histidine decarboxylase activity, effect of aging, organ allografting, and surgical stress on (Moore et al.), 733
Reconstruction, abdominal wall, adjuncts to, following extensive cancer surgery (Tajima and McDonald), 259
of alimentary canal after total gastrectomy, new method of (Kalemba and Lazarkiewicz), 748
Rectal prolapse, ischemic colitis following (Kawarada, Satinsky, and Matsumoto), 340
ulcer, solitary: cause of life-threatening hemorrhage (Delancy and Hitch), 830
Reis-Hancock, Kay-Shiley, and Starr-Edwards No. 6520 porcine xenograft mitral valves, clinical and hemodynamic comparisons of (Brown et al.), 983
Rejection, accelerated, of human renal transplants, combined use of ^{131}I hippurate blood clearance and bladder/kidney ratio data in early detection, classification, and management of (Moore and Hayes), 587
renal allograft, failure of anti–HL-A antibodies to correlate with (Callender et al.), 573
Related kidney donation, complications of (Spanos et al.), 741
Release, gastrin and insulin, in enteroinsular axis,

Release—Cont'd
influence of glucose on (Friesen, Bolinger, and Kyner), 804
Renal abnormalities, minor, fate of kidney transplants from donors with (Spanos et al.), 252
allograft(s), canine, passive enhancement of, with polyspecific $F(ab')_2$ fragments (Wren et al.), 112
prolongation using phytomitogens to mask graft antigens (Toledo-Pereyra et al.), 121
rejection, failure of anti–HL-A antibodies to correlate with (Callender et al.), 573
artery stenosis, deceptive patterns of (Dean et al.), 872
autografts, canine, immunologic injury induced by ex vivo perfusion of (Filo et al.), 88
transplantation, human, functional characterization of blocking antibody after (Miller et al.), 129
in 100 children, results of (DeShazo et al.), 461
transplants, human, accelerated rejection of, combined use of ^{131}I hippurate blood clearance and bladder/kidney ratio data in early detection, classification, and management of (Moore and Hayes), 587
Renovascular hypertension, post-traumatic (Sechas, Plessas, and Skalkeas), 666
Reoperation for residual defects after repair of tetralogy of Fallot (Castaneda et al.), 1010
Repair, direct, of carotid cavernous fistula, with preservation of carotid (Parkinson et al.), 882
Replacement, vena caval, current status of (Sherck, Kerstein, and Stansel), 209
Research fellowships, surgical, in United States, attitudes of British graduates on (Knight and Griffiths), 238
Resection, staged palliative, of recurrent carcinoma of neck using extra anatomic carotid bypass (Hagood, Mozersky, and Fite), 671
Residency programs, foreign medical graduate, and physician supply (Leape) (editorial), 372
training programs, surgical, should the total number be regulated? (panel discusssion) (Spencer), 188
Residents, surgical, the demand for: some preliminary observations (panel discussion) (Hughes), 176
Reticuloendothelial and hepatic parenchymal function in baboon, effect of ischemia on (Holper et al.), 423
function: determinant for survival following hepatic ischemia in baboon (Olcay et al.), 643
Retransplantation, kidney cell crossmatch in (Pierce and Lee), 101
RNA, xenogeneic "immune," immune cytolysis of human tumor cells mediated by: implications for immunotherapy (Pilch et al.), 23
Rupture of spleen, traumatic, lower abdominal tenderness following (Butsch and Butsch) (letter to editors), 524
spontaneous (pathologic), of spleen in malignancies (Karakousis and Elias), 674
Russian surgeon, great, Boris Petrov and Sklifosovsky Institute of Emergency Surgery (Wangensteen), 204

S

Salmonella endocarditis, probable, treated with prosthetic valve replacement: case report (Yamamoto et al.), 678
Sarcoma, primary, methylcholanthrene-induced, in vitro demonstration of altered antigenicity of metastases from (Faraci), 469
Scholarly journals, authorship in: reply (De Bakey) (letter to editors), 344
Sepsis, effect of, on acute gastric ulcerations in rat (Rasche and Butterfield), 764
Serum of cancer patients, immunosuppressive peptide fraction in (Glasgow et al.), 35
induced, rabbit anti–rat, lymphopenia in thoracic duct lymph and peripheral blood (Girardet, Friedman, and Karlson), 267
obtained from normal and partially hepatectomized rats and patients, effect of, on growth of cells in tissue culture (Demetriou, Seifter, and Levenson), 779
Shock, cardiogenic, by coronary artery microembolization in calves, model for (Satava and McGoon), 454
endotoxin, cardiopulmonary effects of volume loading of primates in (Greenfield et al.), 560
Shunt, portacaval, end-to-side, in young pig, transhepatic metabolism after (Hickman et al.), 601
sinusoidal, fraction by radioextraction ratio (Bradley et al.), 918
Single dose irradiation, effect of, on isolated perfused canine kidney (Malek et al.), 272
Sinusoidal shunt fraction by radioextraction ratio (Bradley et al.), 918
Skeletal involvement in hepatic and splenic lymphangiomatosis: report of case and review of literature (Asch, Cohen, and Moore), 334
Sklifosovsky Institute of Emergency Surgery, Boris Petrov, great Russian surgeon, and (Wangensteen), 204
Small-bowel allografts, preserved, role of endotoxin and bacteria in long-term survival of (Toledo-Pereyra), 474
Solitary rectal ulcer: cause of life-threatening hemorrhage (Delancy and Hitch), 830
Spleen, spontaneous (pathologic) rupture of, in malignancies (Karakousis and Elias), 674
traumatic rupture of, lower abdominal tenderness following (Butsch and Butsch) (letter to editors), 524
Splenic artery aneurysms, pathogenesis and clinical significance of (Stanley and Fry), 898
and hepatic lymphangiomatosis with skeletal involvement: report of case and review of literature (Asch, Cohen, and Moore), 334
Spontaneous (pathologic) rupture of spleen in malignancies (Karakousis and Elias), 674
Staged palliative resection of recurrent carcinoma of neck using extra anatomic carotid bypass (Hagood, Mozersky, and Fite), 671
Starr-Edwards No. 6520, Kay-Shiley, and Reis-Hancock porcine xenograft mitral valves, clinical and hemodynamic comparisons of (Brown et al.), 983
Stasis, venous, surgical therapy for (De Palma), 910
Steal syndrome, subclavian (Mozersky) (letter to editors), 355; reply (LeVeen), 355
axillo-axillary bypass with cephalic vein for correction of (Dardik and Dardik), 413
Stenosis and occlusion, internal carotid, directional

Stenosis—Cont'd
Doppler studies of supraorbital artery flow in (LoGerfo and Mason), 723
renal artery, deceptive patterns of (Dean et al.), 872
Streptococcal membrane antigen, cross-reactive, tolerance to myocardial tissue allografts by pretreatment with (Ellis et al.), 142
Subclavian artery aneurysm; sequela of thoracic outlet syndrome (Mathes and Salam), 506
steal syndrome (Mozersky) (letter to editors), 355; reply (LeVeen), 355
axillo-axillary bypass with cephalic vein for correction of (Dardik and Dardik), 413
Superior mesenteric and portal veins, thrombosis in: report of case treated with thrombectomy (Bergentz et al.), 286
Supraorbital artery flow in internal carotid stenosis and occlusion, directional Doppler studies of (LoGerfo and Mason), 723
Surfactant, effect of immunosuppression and lung transplantation upon (Drews et al.), 80
synthesis, pulmonary, mechanisms of oxygen inhibition of (Gilder and McSherry), 72
Surgeon(s)-in-training: preview (panel discussion) (Saxbe), 172
pediatric, need for, as determined by volume of work and mode of delivery of surgical care (Ravitch and Barton), 754
too many? (Welch) (editorial), 199
training of: how many, in what, and by whom? (panel discussion) (Miller), 170
Surgery, British, today: perspective of James IV surgical traveler (Kelly), 433
Emergency, Sklifosovsky Institute of, and Boris Petrov, great Russian surgeon (Wangensteen), 204
extensive cancer, adjuncts to abdominal wall reconstruction following (Tajima and McDonald), 259
Pediatric—a model for evaluation of surgical manpower needs (panel discussion) (O'Neill), 185
Vascular, beginnings of (Dale), 849
Surgical, academic, body count (Eiseman) (editorial), 367
care, mode of delivery of, and volume of work, need for pediatric surgeons as determined by (Ravitch and Barton), 754
management of trauma, experience with autotransfusion in (Reul et al.), 546
manpower needs, a model for evaluation of—Pediatric Surgery (panel discussion) (O'Neill), 185
research fellowships in United States, attitudes of British graduates on (Knight and Griffiths), 238
residency training programs, should the total number be regulated? (panel discussion) (Spencer), 188
residents, the demand for: some preliminary observations (panel discussion) (Hughes), 176
stress, aging, and organ allografting, effect of, on rat thymus histidine decarboxylase activity (Moore et al.), 733
training program of the United States, reduction in: warnings for the unwary (panel discussion) (Moore), 192
treatment, elective, of chronic duodenal ulcer: critical review (Wise and Ballinger), 811
Surveillance, immune, and tumor dissemination: in vitro comparison of B_{16} melanoma in primary and metastatic form (Goldman et al.), 50
Sutures, painless removal of (Bialostozky) (letter to editors), 356
Syndrome, celiac band, long-term evaluation of (Evans), 867
subclavian steal (Mozersky) (letter to editors), 355; reply (LeVeen), 355
axillo-axillary bypass with cephalic vein for correction of (Dardik and Dardik), 413
thoracic outlet, sequela of; subclavian artery aneurysm (Mathes and Salam), 506

T

Taboo subject, spendid statement on (Holcombe) (letter to editors), 345
Teflon membrane oxygenator, new microporous, total cardiopulmonary bypass with (Karlson et al.), 935
Teratomas in infancy and childhood: experience with 81 cases (Mahour et al.), 309
Tests, intraoperative, value of, in vagotomy (Gullickson) (letter to editors), 357
Tetralogy of Fallot, reoperation for residual defects after repair of (Castaneda et al.), 1010
Thoracic duct lymph and peripheral blood, rabbit anti–rat lymphocyte serum-induced lymphopenia in (Girardet, Friedman, and Karlson), 267
outlet, penetrating vascular injuries of (Hewitt et al.), 715
syndrome, sequela of; subclavian artery aneurysm (Mathes and Salam), 506
Thrombectomy, report of case of thrombosis in superior mesenteric and portal veins treated with (Bergentz et al.), 286
Thrombosis in superior mesenteric and portal veins: report of case treated with thrombectomy (Bergentz et al.), 286
Thymectomy in young pig: effects on level of circulating thymic hormone (Lacombe et al.), 556
Thymic hormone, circulating, effects of thymectomy in young pig on level of (Lacombe et al.), 556
Thymus histidine decarboxylase activity, rat, effect of aging, organ allografting, and surgical stress on (Moore et al.), 733
isolated perfused rabbit, lymphocyte output by (Ekwueme and Forrest), 794
Tissue allografts, myocardial, tolerance to, by pretreatment with cross-reactive streptococcal membrane antigen (Ellis et al.), 142
breast, normal and malignant human, trace elements in (Schwartz et al.), 325
culture, growth of cells in, effect of sera obtained from normal and partially hepatectomized rats and patients on (Demetriou, Seifter, and Levenson), 779
Tolerance, allograft, in absence of circulating antibodies (Nowygrod et al.), 630
Total gastrectomy, new method of reconstruction of alimentary canal after (Kalemba and Lazarkiewicz), 748
Trace elements in normal and malignant human breast tissue (Schwartz et al.), 325
Transhepatic metabolism after end-to-side portacaval shunt in young pig (Hickman et al.), 601
Transplantation, human renal, functional characterization of blocking antibody after (Miller et al.), 129

Transplantation—Cont'd
lung, and immunosuppression, effect of, upon surfactant (Drews et al.), 80
renal, in 100 children, results of (DeShazo et al.), 461
Transplants, human renal, accelerated rejection of, combined use of ^{131}I hippurate blood clearance and bladder/kidney ratio data in early detection, classification, and management of (Moore and Hayes), 587
kidney, from donors with minor renal abnormalities, fate of (Spanos et al.), 252
Transposition of great arteries, complications following contoured Dacron baffle in correction of (Reul et al.), 946
Transvenous pacemaker electrode, bipolar, technique for in situ repair (Gelfand and Blumenberg), 504
Trauma, renovascular hypertension after (Sechas, Plessas, and Skalkeas), 666
surgical management of, experience with autotransfusion in (Reul et al.), 546
Traumatic rupture of spleen, lower abdominal tenderness following (Butsch and Butsch) (letter to editors), 524
Treatment, choice of, for operable carcinoma of breast (Haagensen), 685
Tumor cells, human, immune cytolysis of, mediated by xenogeneic "immune" RNA: implications for immunotherapy (Pilch et al.), 23
dissemination, immune surveillance and: in vitro comparison of B_{16} melanoma in primary and metastatic form (Goldman et al.), 50
-specific immunity, distinction of allogeneic immunity from, in man (Parks et al.), 43

U

Ulcer, chronic duodenal, elective surgical treatment of: critical review (Wise and Ballinger), 811
peptic, pathogenesis of: selective review (Skillman), 515
solitary rectal: cause of life-threatening hemorrhage (Delancy and Hitch), 830
Ulcerations, acute gastric, in rat, effect of sepsis on (Rasche and Butterfield), 764
United States, attitudes of British graduates on surgical research fellowships in (Knight and Griffiths), 238
reduction in surgical training program of: warnings for the unwary (panel discussion) (Moore), 192
Upper extremity, acutely ischemic: selective management (Sachatello, Ernst, and Griffen), 1002
gastrointestinal mucosa in dogs, gastrin concentrations in (Watson et al.), 419
Uveitis and vitiligo associated with BCG treatment for malignant melanoma (Donaldson et al.), 771

V

Vagotomy, anatomic approach to (Griffith) (letter to editors), 350; reply (Skandalakis), 352
value of intraoperative tests in (Gullickson) (letter to editors), 357
with antrectomy and vagotomy with pyloroplasty, comparison of gastric emptying before and after (Donovan et al.), 729
pyloroplasty and vagotomy with antrectomy, comparison of gastric emptying before and after (Donovan et al.), 729
Vagus, vagaries of: reply (Skandalakis) (letter to editors), 352
Valve(s), porcine xenograft mitral, Kay-Shiley, Starr-Edwards No. 6520, and Reis-Hancock, clinical and hemodynamic comparisons of (Brown et al.), 983
replacement, prosthetic, probable salmonella endocarditis treated with: case report (Yamamoto et al.), 678
Vascular impedance, pulmonary, in chronic pulmonary hypertension (Elkins et al.), 57
injuries, penetrating, of thoracic outlet (Hewitt et al.), 715
pulmonary, space of man, removal of 5-hydroxytryptamine and norepinephrine from: influence of cardiopulmonary bypass and pulmonary arterial pressure on these processes (Gillis et al.), 608
Surgery, beginnings of (Dale), 849
Vasospasm, chronic experimental, myonecrosis in (Alksne), 1
Vein(s), cephalic, axillo-axillary bypass with, for correction of subclavian steal syndrome (Dardik and Dardik), 413
superior mesenteric and portal, thrombosis in: report of case treated with thrombectomy (Bergentz et al.), 286
Vena cava, inferior, successful balloon membranotomy for obstruction of hepatic portion of (Eguchi, Takeuchi, and Asano), 837
Vena caval replacement, current status of (Sherck, Kerstein, and Stansel), 209
Venous, autogenous, grafts, structural changes during preparation of (Abbott, Wieland, and Austen), 1031
catheter maintenance, central (Kim and Fortner) (letter to editors), 357
stasis, surgical therapy for (De Palma), 910
Ventilation, positive end-expiratory, hemodynamic response to, in hypovolemic patients (Harken et al.), 786
Virus, mouse mammary tumor-associated antigen, radioimmunoassay for (Lo Gerfo et al.), 16
Vitiligo and uveitis associated with BCG treatment for malignant melanoma (Donaldson et al.), 771
Volume loading of primates in endotoxin shock, cardiopulmonary effects of (Greenfield et al.), 560
of work and mode of delivery of surgical care, need for pediatric surgeons as determined by (Ravitch and Barton), 754

W

Wound(s), experimental, contraction of. I. Inhibiting wound contraction by using topical smooth muscle antagonist (Madden et al.), 8
nutrition, proteolysis of preformed protein in (Ehrlich, Tarver, and Hunt), 263
Writer, is the author the? Who cares? (Lavin) (letter to editors), 344; reply (DeBakey), 345

X

Xenogeneic "immune" RNA, immune cytolysis of human tumor cells mediated by: implications for immunotherapy (Pilch et al.), 23
Xenograft mitral valves, porcine, Kay-Shiley, Starr-Edwards No. 6520, and Reis-Hancock, clinical and hemodynamic comparisons of (Brown et al.), 983